# Principles and Practice
# of Movement Disorders

# Principles and Practice of Movement Disorders

## Stanley Fahn, MD

H. Houston Merritt Professor of Neurology and Director
Center for Parkinson's Disease and Other Movement Disorders
Department of Neurology
Columbia University Medical Center
The Neurological Institute
New York, New York

## Joseph Jankovic, MD

Professor of Neurology and Director
Parkinson's Disease Center and Movement Disorders Clinic
Department of Neurology
Baylor College of Medicine
Houston, Texas

With Contributions From

## Mark Hallett, MD

Chief, Human Motor Control Section
National Institute of Neurological Disorders and Stroke
National Institutes of Health
Bethesda, Maryland

## Peter Jenner, BPharm (Hons), PhD, DSc, FRPharms

Professor, Neurodegenerative Disease Research Centre
Guy's, King's, and St. Thomas' School of Biomedical Sciences
King's College
London, United Kingdom

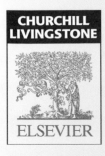

CHURCHILL
LIVINGSTONE

ELSEVIER

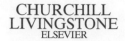

CHURCHILL
LIVINGSTONE
ELSEVIER

1600 John F. Kennedy Blvd.
Suite 1800
Philadelphia, PA 19103-2899

PRINCIPLES AND PRACTICE OF MOVEMENT DISORDERS       ISBN: 978-0-443-07941-2

---

**Notice**

Knowledge and best practice in this field are constantly changing. As new research and experience broaden our knowledge, changes in practice, treatment, and drug therapy may become necessary or appropriate. Readers are advised to check the most current information provided (i) on procedures featured or (ii) by the manufacturer of each product to be administered, to verify the recommended dose or formula, the method and duration of administration, and contraindications. It is the responsibility of the practitioners, relying on their own experience and knowledge of the patients, to make diagnoses, to determine dosages and the best treatment for each individual patient, and to take all appropriate safety precautions. To the fullest extent of the law, neither the Publisher nor the Editors assume any liability for any injury and/or damage to persons or property arising out of or related to any use of the material contained in this book.

The Publisher

---

**Library of Congress Cataloging-in-Publication Data**

Fahn, Stanley, 1933–
   Principles and practice of movement disorders/Stanley Fahn, Joseph Jankovic; with
   contributing authors, Mark Hallett, Peter Jenner.—1st ed.
     p. ; cm.
   Includes index.
   ISBN 978-0-443-07941-2
   1. Movement disorders. 2. Movement disorders—Pathophysiology. I. Jankovic,
Joseph. II. Title.
   [DNLM: 1. Movement Disorders—diagnosis. 2. Movement
Disorders—physiopathology. 3. Movement Disorders—therapy. WL 390 F157p 2007]
RC376.5.P75 2007
616.8′3—dc22

2006040304

*Publishing Director:* Susan F. Pioli
*Developmental Editor:* Joan Ryan
*Project Manager:* Mary Stermel
*Marketing Manager:* Matt Latuchie

Printed in United States of America

Last digit is the print number: 9 8 7 6 5 4 3 2 1

# DEDICATION

*We dedicate this book to our loving wives and families in acknowledgment of their understanding and unconditional support. We also hope that the book will honor the memory of our close friend and colleague David Marsden.*

# Preface

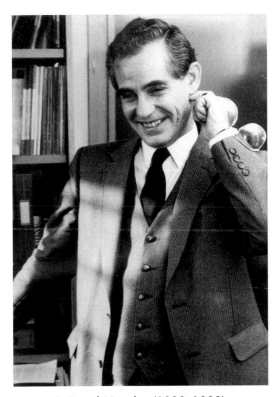

C. David Marsden (1938–1998).

The impetus for this monograph comes directly from the success of "Movement Disorders for the Clinical Practitioner," a continuing medical education course that has been held in Aspen, Colorado, each summer since 1990. Together with C. David Marsden, DSc, MB, FRCP, professor and head of the Department of Clinical Neurology at the Institute of Neurology in Queen Square, London, we originated the course. Dividing the lectures equally among us, we covered the entire field of movement disorders in four half-day sessions that included a large sampling of videos to demonstrate the variety of movement disorders that a neurologist in practice may encounter.

As the course continued to grow in popularity, we decided to produce a textbook of movement disorders, using as our starting point the annually updated course syllabus. We determined that the book would be not a collection of overlapping chapters by different authors but an integrated work in which the tasks of writing and editing were shared among the three of us as co-authors. The project began, but it came to a halt on September 29, 1998, with the untimely death of Professor Marsden.

To continue the Aspen course, we invited Mark Hallett, MD, chief of the Human Motor Control Section at the National Institute of Neurological Diseases and Stroke in Bethesda, Maryland (who had trained in the clinical physiology of movement disorders with Professor Marsden), and neuropharmacologist Peter Jenner, PhD (Professor Marsden's longtime colleague and collaborator), to join the faculty and share with us in delivering the majority of the lectures that Professor Marsden had given. In subsequent years, Drs. Hallett and Jenner continually updated the portion of the course syllabus that was originally written by Dr. Marsden and incorporated additional topics.

When we finally resumed the book project, we determined to retain the principle of an integrated work, taking on the responsibility of editing the chapters written by all four authors. We are grateful to Drs. Hallett and Jenner for their contributions to this book, and we accept full responsibility for the final version. We also thank Susan F. Pioli, publishing director in Elsevier's Health Sciences Division, for her constant guidance and encouragement, and Joan Vidal for her editorial expertise and professionalism.

We and our contributors greatly miss the intellectual and personal interaction that we enjoyed with our close friend and collaborator David Marsden for so many years. This book is dedicated to his memory, and we believe that he would be gratified that the book has finally come to fruition and that it encompasses the most important aspects of our current understanding of movement disorders.

The text is divided into three sections—overview, hypokinetic disorders, and hyperkinetic disorders—following the organization of the Aspen course. It is accompanied by an expanded collection of videos—videos from the Aspen course supplemented by new videos that illustrate the rich phenomenology and etiology of movement disorders and provide a visual guide to this most therapeutically oriented specialty of neurology. We hope that readers find the volume comprehensive, current, and enjoyable.

Stanley Fahn, MD
Joseph Jankovic, MD
July 2007

# Contents

# Overview

## Chapter 1

# Clinical Overview and Phenomenology of Movement Disorders

> To study the phenomenon of disease without books is to sail an uncharted sea, while to study books without patients is not to go to sea at all.
>
> Sir William Osler
> *Sir William Osler Aphorisms*

## FUNDAMENTALS

The quotation from William Osler is an apt introduction to this chapter, which offers a description of the various phenomenologies of movement disorders. Movement disorders can be defined as neurologic syndromes in which there is either an excess of movement or a paucity of voluntary and automatic movements, unrelated to weakness or spasticity. The former are commonly referred to as *hyperkinesias* (excessive movements), *dyskinesias* (unnatural movements), and *abnormal involuntary movements*. In this text the term *dyskinesias* is used most often, but all are interchangeable. The five major categories of dyskinesias are chorea, dystonia, myoclonus, tics, and tremor. Box 1-1 presents the complete list.

The paucity of movement group can be referred to as *hypokinesia* (decreased amplitude of movement), but *bradykinesia* (slowness of movement), and *akinesia* (loss of movement) could be reasonable alternative names. The parkinsonian syndromes are the most common cause of such paucity of movement; other hypokinetic disorders represent only a small group of patients. Basically, movement disorders can be conveniently divided into parkinsonism and all other types; each of these two groups has about an equal number of patients.

Those who are interested in keeping up to date in the field of movement disorders should refer to the journal *Movement Disorders,* a monthly publication of the Movement Disorder Society. The journal is accompanied by two DVDs per year and comes with Movement Disorders Society membership, which is open to all interested medical professionals. The reader is also referred to the World Health Organization's ICD-10NA classification of movement disorders, which has been published in *Movement Disorders* (Jankovic, 1995). The listing and codes are used for various epidemiologic studies and diagnostic codings.

## Categories of Movements

It is important to note that not all of the hyperkinesias in Box 1-1 are technically classified as abnormal involuntary movements, commonly called AIMS. A movement can be categorized into one of four classes: *automatic, voluntary, semivoluntary* (also called unvoluntary) (Lang, 1991; Tourette Syndrome Classification Study Group, 1993; Fahn, 2005), and *involuntary* (Jankovic, 1992). *Automatic* movements are learned motor behaviors that are performed without conscious effort (e.g., the act of walking or speaking and the swinging of arms during walking). *Voluntary* movements are intentional (planned or self-initiated) or externally triggered (in response to some external stimulus—e.g., turning the head toward a loud noise or withdrawing a hand from a hot plate). Intentional voluntary movements are preceded by the Bereitschaftspotential (or readiness potential), a slow negative potential that is recorded over the supplemental motor area and contralateral motor cortex and appears 1 to 1.5 seconds prior to the movement. The Bereitschaftspotential does not appear with other movements, including the externally triggered voluntary movements (Papa et al., 1991). In some cases, learned voluntary motor skills are incorporated within the repertoire of the movement disorders, such as camouflaging choreic movements or tics by immediately following them with voluntarily executed movements, so-called parakinesias. *Semivoluntary* (or *unvoluntary*) movements are induced by an inner sensory stimulus (e.g., the need to stretch a body part or the need to scratch an itch) or by an unwanted feeling or compulsion (e.g., compulsive touching or smelling). Many of the movements that occur as tics or as a response to various sensations (e.g., akathisia and the restless legs syndrome) can be considered unvoluntary because the movements are usually the result of an action to nullify an unwanted, unpleasant sensation. Unvoluntary movements usually are suppressible. *Involuntary* movements are often

Box 1-1 Movement disorders

**Hypokinesias**
Akinesia/bradykinesia (parkinsonism)
Apraxia
Blocking (holding) tics
Cataplexy and drop attacks
Catatonia, psychomotor depression, and obsessional
    slowness
Freezing
Hesitant gaits
Hypothyroid slowness
Rigidity
Stiff muscles

**Hyperkinesias**
Abdominal dyskinesias
Akathitic movements
Asynergia/ataxia/dysmetria
Athetosis
Ballism
Chorea
Dystonia
Hemifacial spasm
Hyperekplexia
Hypnogenic dyskinesias
Jumpy stumps
Moving toes and fingers
Myoclonus
Myokymia and synkinesis
Myorhythmia
Paroxysmal dyskinesias
Restless legs
Stereotypy
Tics
Tremor

nonsuppressible (e.g., most tremors and myoclonus), but some can be partially suppressible (e.g., some tremors, chorea, dystonia, stereotypies, and some tics) (Koller and Biary, 1989).

## The Origins of Abnormal Movements

Most movement disorders are associated with pathologic alterations in the basal ganglia or their connections. The basal ganglia are that group of gray matter nuclei lying deep within the cerebral hemispheres (caudate, putamen, and pallidum), the diencephalon (subthalamic nucleus), and the mesencephalon (substantia nigra) (see Chapter 3). There are some exceptions to this general rule. Pathology of the cerebellum or its pathways typically results in impairment of coordination (asynergia, ataxia), misjudgment of distance (dysmetria), and intention tremor (see Chapter 22). Myoclonus and many forms of tremors do not appear to be related primarily to basal ganglia pathology and often arise elsewhere in the central nervous system, including the cerebral cortex (cortical reflex myoclonus), brainstem (cerebellar outflow tremor, reticular reflex myoclonus, hyperekplexia, and rhythmic brainstem myoclonus such as palatal myoclonus and ocular myoclonus), and spinal cord (rhythmic segmental myoclonus and nonrhythmic propriospinal myoclonus). Moreover, many myoclonic disorders

are associated with diseases in which the cerebellum is involved, such as those that cause the Ramsay Hunt syndrome of progressive myoclonic ataxia (see Chapter 21). It is not known for certain which part of the brain is associated with tics, although the basal ganglia and the limbic structures have been implicated. Certain localizations within the basal ganglia are classically associated with specific movement disorders: substantia nigra with bradykinesia and rest tremor, subthalamic nucleus with ballism, caudate nucleus with chorea, and putamen with dystonia. A succinct overview of the anatomy, physiology, and biochemistry of the basal ganglia is presented in Chapter 3). Finally, there is a growing body of evidence supporting the notion that some movement disorders are peripherally induced (Jankovic, 1994; Marsden, 1994) (see also Chapter 24).

## Historical Perspective

The neurologic literature contains a number of seminal papers, reviews, and books that emphasized and established movement disorders as being associated with pathology of the basal ganglia (Alzheimer, 1911; Fischer, 1911; Wilson, 1912; Hunt, 1917; Vogt and Vogt, 1920; Jakob, 1923; Putnam et al., 1940; Denny-Brown, 1962; Martin, 1967).

A historical perspective of movement disorders can be gained by listing the dates when the various clinical entities were first introduced (Table 1-1).

## Epidemiology

Movement disorders are common neurologic problems, and epidemiologic studies are available for some of them (Table 1-2). There have been several studies for Parkinson disease (PD), and these have been carried out in several countries (Tanner, 1994; de Lau and Breteler, 2006). Table 1-2 lists the prevalence rates of some movement disorders. The frequency of different types of movement disorders seen in the two specialty clinics at Columbia University and Baylor College of Medicine are presented in Table 1-3. More detailed information is provided in the relevant chapters on specific diseases.

## Genetics

A large number of movement disorders are genetic in etiology; many of the diseases have now been mapped to specific regions of the genome, and some have even been localized to a specific gene (Table 1-4). For example, 13 genetic loci have so far been identified with PD or variants of classic PD. (*PARK4* is a triplication of the normal α-synuclein gene, for which mutations are listed as *PARK1*.) A detailed chapter (Harris and Fahn, 2003) and an entire book (Pulst, 2003) have been published specifically related to movement disorder genetics. Several inherited movement disorders are due to expanded repeats of the trinucleotide cytosine-adenosine-guanosine (CAG), and Friedreich ataxia is due to the expanded trinucleotide repeat of guanosine-adenosine-adenosine (GAA). Normal individuals contain an acceptable number of these trinucleotide repeats in their genes, but these triplicate repeats are unstable and, when expanded, lead to disease (Table 1-5). The gene localizations and identifications for PD are presented in Table 1-6. Neurogenetics is one of the fastest-moving research areas in neurology, so the lists in Tables 1-4 to 1-6 keep expanding rapidly.

Table 1-1 Some notable historical descriptions of movement disorders

| Year* | Source | Entity |
|---|---|---|
| | Bible | Reference to tremor in the aged |
| | | Trembling associated with fear and strong emotion |
| 1567 | Paracelsus | Mercury-induced tremor |
| 1652 | Tulpius | Spasmodic torticollis |
| 1686 | Sydenham | Sydenham chorea |
| 1817 | Parkinson | Parkinson disease |
| 1825 | Itard | Tourette syndrome |
| 1830 | Bell | Writer's cramp |
| 1837 | Couper | Manganese-induced parkinsonism |
| 1848 | Grisolle† | Primary writing tremor |
| 1871 | Hammond | Athetosis |
| 1871 | Traube | Spastic dysphonia |
| 1872 | Huntington | Huntington disease |
| 1872 | Mitchell | Jumpy stumps |
| 1874 | Kahlbaum | Catatonia |
| 1878 | Beard | Jumpers |
| 1881 | Friedreich | Myoclonus |
| 1885 | Gilles de la Tourette | Gilles de la Tourette syndrome |
| 1886 | Spencer | Palatal myoclonus |
| 1887 | Dana | Hereditary tremor |
| 1887 | Wood | Cranial dystonia |
| 1889 | Benedikt | Benedikt syndrome |
| 1891 | Unverricht | Progressive myoclonus epilepsy (Unverricht-Lundborg disease) |
| 1895 | Schultze | Myokymia |
| 1900 | Dejerine/Thomas | Olivopontocerebellar atrophy |
| 1901 | Haskovec | Akathisia |
| 1903 | Batten | Neuronal ceroid lipofuscinosis |
| 1904 | Holmes | Midbrain ("rubral") tremor |
| 1908 | Schwalbe | Familial dystonia |
| 1910 | Meige | Oromandibular dystonia |
| 1911 | Oppenheim | Dystonia musculorum deformans |
| 1911 | Lafora | Lafora disease |
| 1912 | Wilson | Wilson disease |
| 1914 | Lewy | Lewy bodies in Parkinson disease |
| 1916 | Henneberg | Cataplexy |
| 1917 | Hunt | Progressive pallidal atrophy |
| 1920 | Creutzfeldt | Creutzfeldt-Jakob disease |
| 1921 | Jakob | Creutzfeldt-Jakob disease |
| 1921 | Hunt | Dyssynergia cerebellaris myoclonica (Ramsay Hunt syndrome) |
| 1922 | Hallervorden/Spatz | Pantothenate kinase deficiency (neurodegenerative disorder with brain iron deposition) |
| 1923 | Sicard | Akathisia |
| 1924 | Fleischhacker | Striatonigral degeneration |
| 1926 | Davidenkow | Myoclonic dystonia |
| 1927 | Goldsmith | Hereditary chin quivering |
| 1927 | Orzechowski | Opsoclonus |
| 1931 | Herz | Myorhythmia |
| 1931 | Guillain/Mollaret | Palato-pharyngo-laryngo oculo-diaphragmatic myoclonus |
| 1932 | De Lisi | Hypnic jerks |
| 1933 | Spiller | Fear of falling |
| 1933 | Scherer | Striatonigral degeneration |
| 1940 | Mount/Reback | Paroxysmal nonkinesigenic dyskinesia (paroxysmal dystonic choreoathetosis) |
| 1941 | Louis-Bar | Ataxia-telangiectasia |
| 1946 | Titeca/van Bogaert | Dentatorubral-pallidoluysian degeneration |
| 1953 | Adams/Foley | Asterixis |

*Other important dates in the history of movement disorders are 1912, the coining of the term *extrapyramidal* by Wilson; 1985, the founding of the Movement Disorder Society; and 1986, the publication of the first issue of the journal *Movement Disorders*.
†Cited by Castillo et al., 1993.
MPTP, 1-methyl-4-phenyl-1,2,3,6-tetrahydropyridine.

Continued

Table 1-1  Some notable historical descriptions of movement disorders—cont'd

| Year | Source | Entity |
|------|--------|--------|
| 1953 | Symonds | Nocturnal myoclonus (periodic movements in sleep) |
| 1956 | Moersch/Woltman | Stiff-person syndrome |
| 1957 | Schonecker | Tardive dyskinesia |
| 1958 | Kirstein/Silfverskiold | Startle disease (hyperekplexia) |
| 1958 | Smith et al. | Dentatorubral-pallidoluysian degeneration |
| 1958 | Monrad-Krohn/Refsum | Myorhythmia |
| 1959 | Paulson | Acute dystonic reaction |
| 1960 | Ekbom | Restless legs |
| 1960 | Shy/Drager | Dysautonomia with parkinsonism |
| 1961 | Hirano et al. | Parkinsonism-dementia complex of Guam |
| 1961 | Andermann et al. | Facial myokymia |
| 1961 | Isaacs | Neuromyotonia, Isaacs syndrome |
| 1962 | Kinsbourne | Opsoclonus-myoclonus |
| 1963 | Lance/Adams | Posthypoxic action myoclonus |
| 1964 | Adams et al | Striatonigral degeneration |
| 1964 | Steele et al. | Progressive supranuclear palsy |
| 1964 | Levine | Neuroacanthocytosis |
| 1964 | Kinsbourne | Sandifer syndrome |
| 1964 | Lesch/Nyhan | Lesch-Nyhan syndrome |
| 1965 | Hakim/Adams | Normal pressure hydrocephalus |
| 1965 | Goldstein/Cogan | Apraxia of lid opening |
| 1966 | Suhren et al. | Hyperekplexia |
| 1966 | Rett | Rett syndrome |
| 1967 | Haerer et al. | Hereditary nonprogressive chorea |
| 1968 | Rebeiz et al. | Cortical-basal ganglionic degeneration |
| 1968 | Delay/Denniker | Neuroleptic malignant syndrome |
| 1969 | Horner/Jackson | Hypnogenic paroxysmal dyskinesias |
| 1969 | Graham/Oppenheimer | Multiple system atrophy |
| 1970 | Spiro | Minipolymyoclonus |
| 1970 | Ritchie | Jumpy stumps |
| 1971 | Spillane et al. | Painful legs and moving toes |
| 1976 | Segawa et al. | Dopa-responsive dystonia |
| 1976 | Allen/Knopp | Dopa-responsive dystonia |
| 1977 | Hallett et al. | Reticular myoclonus |
| 1978 | Satoyoshi | Satoyoshi syndrome |
| 1978 | Fahn | Tardive akathisia |
| 1979 | Hallett et al. | Cortical myoclonus |
| 1979 | Rothwell et al. | Primary writing tremor |
| 1980 | Fukuhara et al. | Myoclonus epilepsy associated with ragged red fibers (MERFF) |
| 1980 | Coleman et al. | Periodic movements in sleep |
| 1981 | Fahn/Singh | Oscillatory myoclonus |
| 1981 | Lugaresi/Cirignotta | Hypnogenic paroxysmal dystonia |
| 1982 | Burke et al. | Tardive dystonia |
| 1983 | Langston et al. | MPTP-induced parkinsonism |
| 1984 | Heilman | Orthostatic tremor |
| 1985 | Aronson | Breathy dysphonia |
| 1986 | Bressman et al. | Biotin-responsive myoclonus |
| 1986 | Schwartz et al. | Oculomasticatory myorhythmia |
| 1987 | Tominaga et al. | Tardive myoclonus |
| 1987 | Little/Jankovic | Tardive myoclonus |
| 1990 | Iliceto et al. | Abdominal dyskinesias |
| 1990 | Ikeda et al. | Cortical tremor/myoclonus |
| 1991c | Brown et al. | Propriospinal myoclonus |
| 1991 | Hymas et al. | Obsessional slowness |
| 1992 | Stacy/Jankovic | Tardive tremor |
| 1993 | Bhatia et al. | Causalgia-dystonia |
| 1993 | Atchison et al. | Primary freezing gait |
| 1993 | Achiron et al. | Primary freezing gait |

**Table 1-2** The prevalence of movement disorders

| Disorder | Rate 100,000 (per population) | Reference |
|---|---|---|
| Restless legs | 9800* | Rothdach et al. (2000) |
| Essential tremor | 415 | Haerer et al. (1982) |
| Parkinson disease | 187† | Kurland (1958) |
| Tourette syndrome | 29–1052 | Caine et al. (1988), Comings et al. (1990) |
| | 2990 | Mason et al. (1998) |
| Primary torsion dystonia | 33 | Nutt et al. (1988) |
| Hemifacial spasm | 7.4–14.5 | Auger and Whisnant (1990) |
| Blepharospasm | 13.3 | Defazio et al. (2001) |
| Hereditary ataxia | 6 | Schoenberg (1978) |
| Huntington disease | 2–12 | Harper (1992), Kokmen et al. (1994) |
| Wilson disease | 3 | Reilly et al. (1993) |
| Progressive supranuclear palsy | 2 | Golbe (1994) |
| | 2.4 | Nath et al. (2001) |
| | 6.4 | Schrag et al. (1999) |
| Multiple system atrophy | 4.4 | Schrag et al. (1999) |

*For restless legs, the rate cited is in a population 65 to 83 years of age.
†For Parkinson disease, the rate is 347 per 100,000 for ages over 40 years (Schoenberg et al., 1985).

## Quantitative Assessments

The assessment of severity of disease is a process that is carried out by all clinicians when evaluating a patient. Quantifying the severity provides the means determining the progression of the disorder and the effect of intervention by pharmacologic or surgical approaches. Many mechanical and electronic devices, including accelerometers, can quantitate specific signs, such as tremor, rigidity, and bradykinesia. These have been developed by physicians and engineers over at least 80 years (Lewy, 1923; Carmichael and Green, 1928), and newer computerized devices continue to be conceived and developed (Larsen et al., 1983; Tryon, 1984; Potvin and Tourtelotte, 1985; Cohen et al., 2003). The advantages of mechanical and electronic measurements are objectivity, consistency, uniformity among different investigators, and rapidity of database storage and analysis. However, these measurements might not be as sensitive as more subjective clinical measurements. In one study comparing objective measurements of reaction and movement times with clinical evaluations, Ward and his colleagues (1983) found the latter to be more sensitive.

The mechanical and electronic methods of measurement have other disadvantages. Instrumentation can usually measure only a single sign at a single point in time and in a single part of the body. Disorders such as parkinsonism encompass a wide range of motor abnormalities as well as behavioral features. Clinical measurements can cover a wider range of the parkinsonian spectrum of impairments and have the advantage of being carried out at the bedside or in the office or clinic at the time the patient is being examined by the physician. Equally important, clinical assessment can evaluate disability in terms of activities of daily living (ADL), and the one developed by England and Schwab (1956) and modified slightly (Fahn and Elton, 1987) has proven highly useful.

A number of clinical rating scales have been proposed (e.g., see Marsden and Schachter, 1981). Several that are now considered standards and are in wide use can be recommended:

the Unified Parkinson's Disease Rating Scale (Fahn and Elton, 1987) is the standard scale for rating severity of signs and symptoms; a videotaped demonstration of the assigned ratings has been published (Goetz et al., 1995). Other standard scales for PD and its complications are the Schwab and England Activities of Daily Living scale for parkinsonism (Schwab and England, 1969) as modified (Fahn and Elton, 1987); the Hoehn and Yahr Parkinson Disease Staging Scale (Hoehn and Yahr, 1967) as modified (Fahn and Elton, 1987); the Goetz dopa dyskinesia severity scale (Goetz et al., 1994); the Lang-Fahn dopa dyskinesia ADL scale (Parkinson Study Group, 2001); the Parkinson psychosis scale (Friedberg et al., 1998); the daily diary to record fluctuations and dyskinesias (Hauser et al., 2004); the core assessment program for intracerebral transplantation (Langston et al., 1992); the Fahn-Marsden Dystonia Rating Scale (Burke et al., 1985); the Unified Dystonia Rating Scale (Comella et al., 2003); the Fahn-Tolosa clinical rating scale for tremor (Fahn et al., 1993); the Bain tremor scale (Bain et al., 1993); and the Unified Huntington's Disease Rating Scale, which also has a published videotaped demonstration of assigned ratings (Huntington Study Group, 1996).

## DIFFERENTIAL DIAGNOSIS OF HYPOKINESIAS

For a list of hypokinesias, refer to Box 1-1.

### Akinesia/Bradykinesia

*Akinesia*, *bradykinesia*, and *hypokinesia* literally mean "absence," "slowness," and "decreased amplitude of movement," respectively. The three terms are commonly grouped together for convenience under the term *bradykinesia*. These phenomena are prominent and most important features of parkinsonism and are often considered a sine qua non for parkinsonism. Although *akinesia* means "lack of movement," the label is often used to

Table 1-3 The prevalence of movement disorders encountered in two large movement disorder clinics

| Movement Disorder | Number of Patients | Percent |
| --- | --- | --- |
| **Parkinsonism** | **7564** | **32.9** |
| Parkinson disease | 5410 | |
| Progressive supranuclear palsy | 381 | |
| Multiple system atrophy | 349 | |
| Cortical-basal ganglionic degeneration | 143 | |
| Vascular | 265 | |
| Drug-induced | 227 | |
| Hemiparkinsonism-hemiatrophy | 81 | |
| Gait disorder | 187 | |
| Other | 521 | |
| **Dystonia** | **6798** | **31.3** |
| Primary dystonia | 5247 | |
|     Focal | | (61%) |
|     Segmental | | (30%) |
|     Generalized | | (9%) |
| Secondary dystonia | 1551 | |
|     Hemidystonia | 191 | |
|     Tardive | 472 | |
|     Other | 888 | |
| **Tremor** | **3013** | **13.9** |
| Essential tremor | 2082 | |
| Cerebellar | 151 | |
| Midbrain ('rubral') | 86 | |
| Primary writing | 59 | |
| Orthostatic | 16 | |
| Other | 619 | |
| **Tics (Tourette syndrome)** | **1022** | **4.7** |
| **Chorea** | **658** | **3.1** |
| Huntington disease | 282 | |
| Hemiballism | 62 | |
| Other | 314 | |
| **Tardive syndromes** | **583** | **2.7** |
| **Myoclonus** | **547** | **2.5** |
| **Hemifacial spasm** | **359** | **1.7** |
| **Ataxia** | **316** | **1.5** |
| **Paroxysmal dyskinesias** | **169** | **0.8** |
| **Stereotypies (other than tardive dyskinesia)** | **163** | **0.7** |
| **Restless legs syndrome** | **108** | **0.5** |
| **Stiff-person syndrome** | **32** | **0.1** |
| **Psychogenic movement disorder** | **434** | **2.0** |
| Grand total | 21,766 | 100 |

Data were obtained from the combined databases of the Movement Disorder Clinics at Columbia University Medical Center (New York City) and Baylor College of Medicine (Houston) for patients encountered through 1996. Because some patients might have more than one type of movement disorder (such as a combination of essential tremor and Parkinson disease), they would be listed more than once. Therefore, the figures in the table represent the types of movement disorder phenomenology encountered in two large clinics rather than the exact number of patients.

Table 1-4 Gene localization of movement disorders

| CATEGORY Disease | Pattern of Inheritance | Chromosome Region | Name of Gene | Gene Identified | Triplet Repeat | Name of Protein | Function of Protein |
|---|---|---|---|---|---|---|---|
| **Parkinson Disease** | | | | | | | |
| (1) Familial Parkinson disease | Autosomal-dominant | 4q21–q22 | PARK1 | Yes | No | α-synuclein | Synaptic protein |
| (2) Young-onset Parkinson disease | Autosomal-recessive/dominant | 6q25.2–q27 | PARK2 | Yes | No | Parkin | Ubiquitin-protein ligase |
| (3) Susceptibility locus | Autosomal-dominant | 2p13 | PARK3 | No | N/I | N/I | N/I |
| (4) Familial Parkinson disease | Autosomal-dominant | 4q region | PARK4 | Yes | No | Duplication or triplication of α-synuclein region of chromosome | Excess amount of normal α-synuclein |
| (5) Familial Parkinson disease | Autosomal-recessive | 4p15 | PARK5 | Yes | No | Ubiquitin carboxy-terminal hydrolase L1 | Hydrolase ubiquitin |
| (6) Young-onset Parkinson disease | Autosomal-recessive | 1p35–p36 | PARK6 | Yes | No | PINK1 | Mitochondrial, anti-stress-induced degeneration |
| (7) Young-onset Parkinson disease | Autosomal-recessive | 1p36 | PARK7 | Yes | No | DJ-1 | Sumolyation pathway |
| (8) Familial Parkinson disease | Autosomal-dominant | 12p11.2–q13.1 | PARK8 | Yes | No | LRRK2, dardarin | Phosphorylates protein |
| (9) Familial Parkinson disease | Autosomal-recessive | 1p32 | PARK10 | No | No | N/I | N/I |
| (10) Familial Parkinson disease | Autosomal-dominant | 2q36–q37 | PARK11 | No | N/I | N/I | N/I |
| (11) Familial Parkinson disease | Autosomal-dominant | 1q21 | Glucocere-brosidase | Yes | No | Glucocerebrosidase | Membrane lipid |
| (12) Familial Parkinson disease | Autosomal-dominant | 2q22–q23 | Nurr1 | Yes | No | Nurr1 | DA cell development; transcription activator |
| (13) Infantile/childhood Parkinson disease | Autosomal-recessive | 11p11.5 | Tyrosine hydroxylase | Yes | No | Tyrosine hydroxylase | Converts tyrosine to levodopa |
| **See also Ataxia and Dystonia sections: #40 Ataxia SCA2 and #73 DRD** | | | | | | | |
| (14) Familial Parkinson disease | Mitochondrial | Mitochondria | N/I | No | No | N/I | Complex I |
| (15) Familial Parkinson disease | Mitochondrial gene | Mitochondria | ND4 | Yes | No | N/I | Complex I |
| (16) Familial Parkinson disease | Susceptibility gene | 17q21 | Tau | Yes | No | Tau | Fibrils |
| (17) Frontotemporal dementia | Autosomal-dominant | 17q21–q23 | FTD-17 Tau | Yes | No | Tau | N/I |
| (18) Frontotemporal dementia | Autosomal-dominant | Chromosome 3 | FTD-3 | No | No | N/I | N/I |
| (19) Pick disease | ? | 17q21–q23 | Tau | Yes | No | Tau | N/I |
| (20) PSP and CBGD | Susceptibility locus | 17q21–q23 | Tau | Yes | No | Tau | Fibrils |
| (21) MSA | ? | 3P21 | ZNF231 | Yes | No | Zinc finger protein | Nuclear protein |
| (22) Kufor-Rakeb syndrome | Autosomal-recessive | 1p36 | PARK9 | Yes | No | ATP 13 A2 | Lysosomal ATPase |

CBGD, cortical-basal ganglionic degeneration; DRD, dopa-responsive dystonia; MSA, multiple system atrophy; N/I, not yet identified; PSP, progressive supranuclear palsy.
*Note:* References are listed at the end of the table.

Continued

Table 1-4 Gene localization of movement disorders—cont'd

| CATEGORY Disease | Pattern of Inheritance | Chromosome Region | Name of Gene | Gene Identified | Triplet Repeat | Name of Protein | Function of Protein |
|---|---|---|---|---|---|---|---|
| **Parkinson Disease—cont'd** | | | | | | | |
| (23) Parkinson-MELAS syndrome | Mitochondrial gene | Mitochondria | Cytochrome b | Yes | No | Cytochrome b | Complex III |
| (24) Familial ALS | Autosomal-dominant | 21q | SOD1 | Yes | No | Cu/Zn superoxide dismutase | Convert superoxide to $H_2O_2$ |
| **Ataxia Syndromes** | | | | | | | |
| (25) Friedreich ataxia | Autosomal-recessive | 9q13-q21.1 | X25 | Yes | GAA | Frataxin | Phosphoinositide/Fe homeostasis in mitochondria |
| (26) Friedreich ataxia 2 | Autosomal-recessive | 9p23-p11 | FRDA2 | No | N/I | N/I | N/I |
| (27) Early-onset cerebellar ataxia | Autosomal-recessive | 13q11-q12 | No | No | N/I | N/I | N/I |
| (28) X-linked congenital ataxia | X-linked recessive | X | No | No | N/I | N/I | N/I |
| (29) Ataxic cerebral palsy | Autosomal-recessive | 9p12-q12 | No | No | N/I | N/I | N/I |
| (30) Posterior column ataxia with retinitis pigmentosa | Autosomal-recessive | 1q31-q32 | AXPC1 | No | No | N/I | N/I |
| (31) Adult-onset ataxia with tocopherol deficiency | Autosomal-recessive | 8q13.1-q13.3 | α-TTP | Yes | No | α-Tocopherol-transfer protein gene | Transfers α-tocopherol to mitochondria |
| (32) Ataxia-telangiectasia | Autosomal-recessive | 11q22-q23 | ATM | Yes | No | PI-3 kinase | DNA repair |
| (33) Nonprogressive congenital ataxia | Autosomal-recessive | 9q34-9qter | No | No | N/I | N/I | N/I |
| (34) Nonprogressive infantile ataxia | Autosomal-recessive | 20q11-q13 | No | No | N/I | N/I | N/I |
| (35) Early onset cerebellar ataxia with oculomotor apraxia | Autosomal-recessive | 9p13 | APTX | Yes | No | Aprataxin | N/I |
| (36) Hereditary spastic ataxia | Autosomal-dominant | 12p13 | SAX1 | No | No | N/I | N/I |
| (37) Sensory/motor neuropathy with ataxia | Autosomal-dominant | 7q22-q32 | SMNA also SCA18 | No | No | N/I | N/I |
| (38) Ataxia with saccadic intrusions | Autosomal-recessive | 1p36 | No | No | N/I | N/I | N/I |
| (39) SCA-1 | Autosomal-dominant | 6p23 | SCA1 | Yes | CAG 40-83 | Ataxin-1 | N/I |
| (40) SCA-2 | Autosomal-dominant | 12q23-24.1 | SCA2 | Yes | CAG 34-59 | Ataxin-2 | N/I |
| (41) SCA-3 (Machado-Joseph disease) | Autosomal-dominant | 14q32.1 | SCA3 | Yes | CAG 56-86 | Ataxin-3 | N/I |
| (42) SCA-4 | Autosomal-dominant | 16q22.1 | SCA4 | No | N/I | N/I | N/I |
| (43) SCA-5 | Autosomal-dominant | 11p11-q11 | SCA5 | No | N/I | N/I | N/I |
| (44) SCA-6 [CACNA1A] | Autosomal-dominant | 19p13 | CACNA1A | Yes | CAG 21-31 | — | $Ca^{2+}$ channel |
| (45) SCA-7 | Autosomal-dominant | 3q12-13 | SCA7 | Yes | CAG 38-200 | Ataxin-7 | Cone-rod homeobox protein |
| (46) SCA-8 | Autosomal-dominant | 13q21 | SCA8 | Yes | CTG 100-155 | N/I | N/I |

| | | | | | | | |
|---|---|---|---|---|---|---|---|
| (47) SCA-10 | Autosomal-dominant | 22q13 | SCA10 | No | ATTC 800–3800 | N/I | N/I |
| (48) SCA-11 | Autosomal-dominant | 15q14–21.3 | SCA11 | No | N/I | N/I | N/I |
| (49) SCA-12 | Autosomal-dominant | 5q31–q33 | PPP2R2B | Yes | CAG 66–93 | Phosphatase 2A | Phosphatase |
| (50) SCA-13 | Autosomal-dominant | 19q13.3–q13.4 | SCA13 | No | N/I | N/I | N/I |
| (51) SCA-14 | Autosomal-dominant | 19q13.4–qter | SCA14 | Yes | No | Protein Kinase C-γ | Zinc binding |
| (52) SCA-15 | Autosomal-dominant | 3p24.2–3pter | SCA15 | N/I | No | N/I | N/I |
| (53) SCA-16 | Autosomal-dominant | 8q23–24.1 | SCA16 | No | N/I | N/I | N/I |
| (54) SCA-17 [TBP] | Autosomal-dominant | 6q27 | SCA17 | Yes | CAG 45–63 | TATA-binding protein | Transcription initiation factor |
| (55) SCA-18 with muscular atrophy | Autosomal-dominant | 7q22–q32 | SCA18 | N/I | N/I | N/I | N/I |
| (56) SCA-19 | Autosomal-dominant | 1p21–q21 | SCA19 | N/I | N/I | N/I | N/I |
| (57) SCA-20 | Autosomal-dominant | 11p13–q11 | SCA20 | N/I | N/I | N/I | N/I |
| (58) SCA-21 | Autosomal-dominant | 7p21.3–p15.1 | SCA21 | N/I | N/I | N/I | N/I |
| (59) SCA-22 | Autosomal-dominant | 1p21–q23 | SCA22 | N/I | N/I | N/I | N/I |
| (60) SCA-23 | Autosomal-dominant | 20p13–p12.3 | SCA23 | N/I | N/I | N/I | N/I |
| (61) SCA-25 Ataxia with sensory neuropathy | Autosomal-dominant | 2p15–p21 | SCA25 | N/I | N/I | N/I | N/I |
| **CHOREIC SYNDROMES** | | | | | | | |
| (62) Huntington disease | Autosomal-dominant | 4p16.3 | IT15 | Yes | CAG | Huntingtin | N/I |
| (63) Huntington-like disease-1 | Autosomal-dominant | 20p | HDL1 | Yes | Octapeptide repeat | Prion protein | N/I |
| (64) Huntington-like disease-2 | Autosomal-dominant | 16q23 | HDL2 | Yes | CAG | Junctophilin-3 | Links the plasma membrane and the endoplasmic reticulum |
| (65) Huntington-like disease-3 | Autosomal-recessive | 4p15.3 | N/I | No | No | N/I | N/I |
| (66) Neuroacanthocytosis | Autosomal-recessive | 9q21–q22 | CHAC | Yes | No | Chorein | Protein sorting |
| (67) McLeod syndrome | X-linked recessive | Xp21.2–p21.1 | XK | Yes | No | XK | Unknown |
| (68) Benign hereditary chorea | Autosomal-dominant | 14q13.1–q21.1 | TITF-1 | Yes | No | N/I | N/I |
| **CHOREOATHETOSIS** | | | | | | | |
| (69) Choreoathetosis and mental retardation | X-linked recessive | Xp11 | N/I | N/I | N/I | N/I | N/I |
| (70) Lesch-Nyhan syndrome | X-linked recessive | Xq26–q27.2 | HPRT | Yes | No | Hypoxanthine-guanine-phosphoribosyl transferase | N/I |
| **Dystonia** | | | | | | | |
| (71) Oppenheim torsion dystonia | Autosomal-dominant | 9q34 | DYT1 | Yes | No, GAG deletion | Torsin A | ATP binding, chaperone |
| (72) Lubag (X-linked dystonia-parkinsonism) | X-linked recessive | Xq13.1 | DYT3 | Yes | No | Multiple transcript system | N/I |

ALS, amyotrophic lateral sclerosis; BH4, tetrahydrobiopterin; CAG, cytosine-adenosine-guanosine trinucleotide; GAA, guanosine-adenosine-adenosine; MELAS, mitochondrial myopathy, encephalopathy, lactic acidosis, and stroke-like episodes.

Continued

Table 1-4 Gene localization of movement disorders—cont'd

| CATEGORY Disease | Pattern of Inheritance | Chromosome Region | Name of Gene | Gene Identified | Triplet Repeat | Name of Protein | Function of Protein |
|---|---|---|---|---|---|---|---|
| **Dystonia—cont'd** | | | | | | | |
| (73) Dopa-responsive dystonia | Autosomal-dominant | 14q22.1-q22.2 | DYT5 | Yes | No | GTP cyclohydrolase 1 | Synthesis of BH4 |
| (74) Craniocervical dystonia | Autosomal-dominant | 8p21-q22 | DYT6 | No | N/I | N/I | N/I |
| (75) Familial torticollis | Autosomal-dominant | 18p? | DYT7 | N/I | N/I | N/I | N/I |
| (76) Myoclonus-dystonia | Autosomal-dominant | 7q21-q31 | DYT11 | Yes | No | ε-Sarcoglycan | N/I |
| (77) Myoclonus-dystonia | Autosomal-dominant | 18p11 | DYT15 | N/I | N/I | N/I | N/I |
| (78) Rapid-onset dystonia-parkinsonism | Autosomal-dominant | 19q13 | DYT12 | Yes | No | Na(+)/K(+)-ATPase alpha 3 subunit (ATP1A3) | Sodium pump |
| (79) Alternating hemiplegia of childhood | Autosomal-dominant | 1q23 | ATP1A2 | Yes | No | Na(+)/K(+)-ATPase alpha 2 subunit (ATP1A2) | Sodium pump |
| (80) Cervical-cranial-brachial | Autosomal-dominant | 1p36.13–p36.32 | DYT13 | No | N/I | N/I | N/I |
| (81) Dopa-responsive dystonia | Autosomal-dominant | 14q13 | DYT14 | No | N/I | N/I | N/I |
| (82) Aromatic amino acid decarboxylase deficiency | Autosomal-recessive | 7p11 | Aromatic amino acid decarboxylase | Yes | No | Aromatic amino acid decarboxylase | Converts dopa to dopamine |
| (83) Torticollis | Susceptibility gene | 4p16.1-p15.3 | Dopamine D5 receptor | Yes | No | Dopamine D5 receptor | Dopamine D5 receptor |
| (84) Blepharospasm | Susceptibility gene | 4p16.1-p15.3 | Dopamine D5 receptor | Yes | No | Dopamine D5 receptor | Dopamine D5 receptor |
| (85) Deafness-dystonia-optic atrophy | X-linked recessive | Xq22 | DDP | Yes | No | DDP | Intermembrane protein transport in mitochondria |
| (86) Dystonic lipidosis (Niemann-Pick Type C) | Autosomal-recessive | 18q11-q12 | NPC1 | Yes | No | — | Esterification of LDL-derived cholesterol |
| (87) Neurodegeneration with iron deposition | Autosomal-recessive | 20p12.3-p13 | PANK2 | N/I | N/I | N/I | Pantothenate kinase |
| (88) Neuroferritinopathy | Autosomal-dominant | 19q13.3 | FTL | Yes | No | Ferritin light polypeptide | Iron binding |
| (89) Striatal necrosis | Mitochondrial | Mitochondrial | Nd5 | Yes | No | — | Decrease complex 1 activity |
| **Hyperekplexia** | | | | | | | |
| (90) Hereditary hyperekplexia | Autosomal-dominant | 5q34-q35 | STHE | Yes | No | GLRA1 | Glycine receptor |
| **Myoclonus** | | | | | | | |
| (91) Unverricht-Lundborg disease | Autosomal-recessive | 21q22.3 | EPM1 | No | N/I | Cystatin B | Cysteine protease inhibitor |

| Disorder | Inheritance | Locus | Gene | | | Protein | Function |
|---|---|---|---|---|---|---|---|
| (92) Lafora body disease | Autosomal-recessive | 6q24 | EPM2A | Yes | No | Laforin | Tyrosine phosphatase |
| (93) Lafora body disease | Autosomal-recessive | 6p22 | EPM2B | Yes | No | Malin | E3 ubiquitin ligase |
| (94) Progressive myoclonus epilepsy | Mitochondrial gene | Mitochondria | tRNA (Ser (UCNJ)) | Yes | No | N/I | N/I |
| (95) Familial adult myoclonus epilepsy | Autosomal-dominant | 8q23.3–q24.1 | FAME | No | No | N/I | N/I |
| (96) Familial Creutzfeldt-Jakob disease | Autosomal-dominant | 20pter–p12 | PRNP | Yes | No | Prion protein | N/I |
| (97) Dentatorubral-pallidoluysian atrophy (DRPLA) | Autosomal-dominant | 12p12–ter | — | Yes | CAG | Atrophin-1 | N/I |
| (98) Infantile spasms | X-linked recessive | Xp–22.13 | ARX | Yes | N/I | N/I | N/I |
| Paroxysmal dyskinesias | | | | | | | |
| (99) Episodic ataxia-1/ myokymia | Autosomal-dominant | 12p13 | Kv1.1 | Yes | No | KCNA1 | K+ channel |
| (100) Episodic ataxia-2/ vestibular | Autosomal-dominant | 19p13 | CACNL1A4 | Yes | No | CACNL 1A4 | Ca$^{2+}$ channel |
| (101) Paroxysmal kinesigenic dyskinesia (PKD) | Autosomal-dominant | 16p11.2–q11.2 | — | No | N/I | N/I | N/I |
| (102) Paroxysmal kinesigenic dyskinesia (PKD) | Autosomal-dominant | 16q13–q22.1 | EKD2 | No | N/I | N/I | N/I |
| (103) Paroxysmal nonkinesigenic dyskinesia (PKND) (Mount-Reback syndrome) | Autosomal-dominant | 2q34 | FPD1 | Yes | No | Myofibrillogenesis regulator 1 (MR-1) gene | Detoxify compounds |
| (104) Paroxysmal dyskinesia and spasticity | Autosomal-dominant | 1p | CSE | No | N/I | N/I | N/I |
| (105) Paroxysmal dyskinesia and infantile convulsions and childhood exercise-induced dyskinesia | Autosomal-recessive | 16p12–q11.2 | Sodium/ glucose cotrans-porter gene (KST1) | Yes | No | N/I | Cotransport of sodium and glucose |
| (106) Familial hypnogenic seizures/dystonia | Autosomal-dominant | 20q12.2–13.3 | CHRNA4 | Yes | No | CHRNA4 | Nicotinic ACh receptor |
| (107) Familial hypnogenic seizures/dystonia | Autosomal-dominant | 15q24 | CHRNB2 | Yes | No | CHRNB2 | Nicotinic ACh receptor |
| (108) Familial hypnogenic seizures/dystonia | Autosomal-dominant | Chromosome 1 | N/I | N/I | N/I | N/I | Nicotinic ACh receptor |
| Restless Legs Syndrome | | | | | | | |
| (109) Restless legs syndrome | Susceptibility locus | 12q12–q21 | RLS1 | N/I | N/I | N/I | N/I |
| Stereotypies | | | | | | | |
| (110) Rett syndrome | X-linked dominant | Xq28 | MECP2 | Yes | No | Methyl-CpG-binding protein | Binds CpG proteins |

Continued

Table 1-4 Gene localization of movement disorders—cont'd

| CATEGORY Disease | Pattern of Inheritance | Chromosome Region | Name of Gene | Gene Identified | Triplet Repeat | Name of Protein | Function of Protein |
|---|---|---|---|---|---|---|---|
| **Tics** | | | | | | | |
| (111) Tourette syndrome | Autosomal-dominant | 11q23 | — | No | N/I | N/I | N/I |
| (112) Tourette syndrome | Susceptibility loci | 7q31; 2p11; 8q22 | — | No | N/I | N/I | N/I |
| (113) Tourette syndrome, OCD, chronic tics | Candidate gene | 18q22 | — | No | N/I | N/I | N/I |
| **Tremor** | | | | | | | |
| (114) Familial essential tremor | Autosomal-dominant | 2p22–p25 | ETM | N/I | N/I | N/I | N/I |
| (115) Familial essential tremor | Autosomal-dominant | 3q13 | FET1 | N/I | N/I | N/I | N/I |
| (116) Hereditary geniospasm | Autosomal-dominant | 9q13–q21 | | N/I | N/I | N/I | N/I |
| (117) Roussy-Lévy syndrome | Autosomal-dominant | 17p11.2 | CMT-1B | Yes | No | Peripheral myelin protein | Myelin |
| (118) Fragile X tremor-ataxia syndrome | X-linked recessive | Xq27.3 | FMR1 | Yes | CGG repeat 50–200 | FMRP | Synaptic structure development |
| **A VARIETY OF MOVEMENTS** | | | | | | | |
| *Wilson disease* | | | | | | | |
| (119) Wilson disease | Autosomal-recessive | 13q14.3 | ATB7B | Yes | No | Cu-ATPase | Copper transport |
| *Neuronal ceroid lipofuscinoses (Batten disease)* | | | | | | | |
| (120) Infantile | Autosomal-recessive | 1p32 | CLN1 | Yes | No | Palmitoyl protein thioesterase | Lysosomal proteolysis |
| (121) Late-infantile classic | Autosomal-recessive | 9q13–q21 | CLN2 | Yes | No | Pepstatin-insensitive protease | Lysosomal proteolysis |
| (122) Finnish late infantile | Autosomal-recessive | 13q22 | CLN5 | Yes | No | Unnamed membrane protein | Lysosomal proteolysis |
| (123) Variant late infantile | Autosomal-recessive | 15q21–23 | CLN6 | No | N/I | N/I | N/I |
| (124) Variant late infantile | Autosomal-recessive | N/I | CLN7 | No | N/I | N/I | N/I |
| (125) Variant late infantile | Autosomal-recessive | 1p32 | CLN1 | Yes | N/I | Palmitoyl protein thioesterase | Lysosomal proteolysis |
| (126) Juvenile | Autosomal-recessive | 16p12 | CLN3 | Yes | No | Battenin | Lysosomal proteolysis |
| (127) Variant juvenile | Autosomal-recessive | 1p32 | CLN1 | Yes | N/I | Palmitoyl protein thioesterase | Lysosomal proteolysis |

OCD, obsessive compulsive disorder; PSP, progressive supranuclear palsy.

References for the listings in this table are, in order (1) Polymeropoulos et al., 1996, 1997; Kruger et al., 1998; Ibanez et al., 2004; Zarranz et al., 2004; (2) Matsumine et al., 1997, 1998; Kitada et al., 1998; Abbas et al., 1999; Shimura et al., 2000; Farrer et al., 2001; (3) Gasser et al., 1998; Pankratz et al., 2004; (4) Singleton et al., 2003; (5) Leroy et al., 1998; (6) Bentivoglio et al., 2001; Valente et al., 2001b, 2002; Valente, Abou-Sleimen, et al., 2004; Valente, Salvi, et al., 2004b; (7) van Duijn et al., 2000; Bonifati et al., 2003; Healy et al., 2004a; (8) Funayama et al., 2002; Paisan-Ruiz et al., 2004; Zimprich et al., 2004; (9) Hicks et al., 2002; (10) Pankratz et al., 2003; (11) Aharon-Peretz et al., 2004; Goker-Alpan et al., 2004; Clark et al., 2005; (12) Le et al., 2002; Xu et al., 2002; Zheng et al., 2003; (13) Knappskog et al., 1995; Ludecke et al., 1995, 1996; (14) Swerdlow et al., 1998; (15) Simon et al., 1999; (16) Healy et al., 2004b; (17) Lynch et al., 1994; Foster et al., 1997; Hutton et al., 1998; Pastor et al., 2004; Pittman et al., 2004; Skipper et al., 2004; (18) Gydesen et al., 2002; (19) Pickering-Brown et al., 2000; (20) Baker et al., 1999; Bugiani et al., 1999; Morris et al., 1999; Delisle et al., 1999; Higgins et al., 1999a; Spillantini et al., 2000; Wszolek et al., 2001; (21) Hashida et al., 1998; (22) Hampshire et al., 2001; (23) De Coo et al., 1999;

(24) Rosen et al., 1993; (25) Pandolfo et al., 1993; (26) Christodoulou et al., 2001; (27) Mrissa et al., 2000; (28) Bertini et al., 2000; (29) McHale et al., 2000; (30) Higgins et al., 1999b; (31) Gotoda et al., 1995; (32) Ambrose et al., 1994; Savitsky et al., 1995; (33) Delague et al., 2001; (34) Tranebjaerg et al., 2003; (35) Date et al., 2001; Moreira et al., 2001; (36) Meijer et al., 2002; (37) Brkanac et al., 2002b; (38) Swartz et al., 2003; (39) Banfi et al., 1994; (40) Lopes-Cendes et al., 1994a; (41) Kawaguchi et al., 1994; (42) Lopes-Cendes et al., 1994b; Flanigan et al., 1996; Li et al., 2003; (43) Ranum et al., 1994; (44) Riess et al., 1997; Zhuchenko et al., 1997; (45) David et al., 1996, 1997; Lindblad et al., 1996; La Spada et al., 2001; (46) Koob et al., 1999; Zu et al., 1999; (48) Worth et al., 1999; (49) Fujigasaki et al., 2001a; Holmes et al., 2001b; O'Hearn et al., 2001; (50) Herman-Bert et al., 2000; Brkanac et al., 2002a; Chen et al., 2003; Yabe et al., 2003; (52) Storey et al., 2001; Knight et al., 2003; (53) Miyoshi et al., 2001; (54) Fujigasaki et al., 2001b; Nakamura et al., 2001; Toyoshima et al., 2004; (55) Brkanac et al., 2002b; (56) Verbeek et al., 2002; (57) Knight et al., 2004; (58) Vuillaume et al., 2002; (59) Chung et al., 2003; (60) Verbeek et al., 2004; (61) Stevanin et al., 2003; (62) Huntington's Disease Collaborative Research Group, 1993; (63) Xiang et al., 1998; Moore et al., 2001; (64) Holmes et al., 2001a; Margolis et al., 2001; Stevanin et al., 2004; (65) Kambouris et al., 2000; (66) Rubio et al., 1997, 1999; Rampoldi et al., 2001; Ueno et al., 2001; Dobson-Stone et al., 2002, 2004; (67) Danek et al., 2001; (68) de Vries et al., 2000; Fernandez et al., 2001; Breedveld et al., 2002; Kleiner-Fisman et al., 2003; (69) Reyniers et al., 1999; (70) Sege-Peterson et al., 1993; (71) Kramer et al., 1994; Ozelius et al., 1997; (72) Wilhelmsen et al., 1991; Müller et al., 1994; Nolte et al., 2003; Fabbrini et al., 2005; (73) Nygaard et al., 1993; Ichinose et al., 1994; Pittock et al., 2000; De Carvalho Aguiar et al., 2004; (79) Bassi et al., 2004; (80) Valente et al., 2001a; (81) Grotzsch et al., 2002; (82) Hyland et al., 1992; Chang et al., 2004; (83) Placzek et al., 2001; (84) Misbahuddin et al., 2002; (85) Jin et al., 1999; Koehler et al., 1999; Tranebjaerg et al., 2000; Rohbauer et al., 2001; Swerdlow and Wooten, 2001; Ujike et al., 2001; (86) Lossos et al., 1997; (87) Taylor et al., 1996; Zhou et al., 2001; Hayflick et al., 2003; (88) Curtis et al., 2001; Mir et al., 2005; (89) Solano et al., 2003; (90) Shiang et al., 1993; (91) Lehesjoki et al., 1993, 1998; (92) Minassian et al., 1998; Serratosa et al., 1999; Minassian et al., 2001; (93) Chan et al., 2003a, 2003b; (94) Jaksch et al., 1998; (95) Mikami et al., 1999; Plaster et al., 1999; (96) Prusiner, 1993; (97) Koide et al., 1994; Nagafuchi et al., 1994; Yamada et al., 2001; (98) Stromme et al., 2002; Turner et al., 2002; (99) Browne et al., 1994; Litt et al., 1994; (100) Vahedi et al., 1995; von Brederlow et al., 1995; (101) Tomita et al., 1999; Bennett et al., 2000; (102) Valente et al., 2000; (103) Fink et al., 1996, 1997; Fouad et al., 1996; Hofele et al., 1997; Jarman et al., 1997a; Raskind et al., 1998; Lee et al., 2004; (104) Auburger et al., 1996; (105) Szepetowski et al., 1997; Lee et al., 1998; Carelli et al., 1999; Guerrini et al., 1999; Roll et al., 2002; (106) Oldani et al., 1998; Nakken et al., 1999; (107) Phillips et al., 1998, 2001; (108) Gambardella et al., 2000; (109) Desautels et al., 2001; (110) Sirianni et al., 1998; Amir et al., 1999; Auranen et al., 2001; Ben-Zeev et al., 2002; (111) Merette et al., 2000; (112) Szepetowski et al., 1997; Lee et al., 1998; Carelli et al., 1999; Petek et al., 2001; Simonic 2001; (113) Cuker et al., 2004; (114) Higgins et al., 1997; Gulcher et al., 1997; (116) Jarman et al., 1997b; (117) Planté-Bordeneuve et al., 1999; (118) Jacquemont et al., 2003, 2004; (119) Bull et al., 1993; Tanzi et al., 1993; (120) Jarvela et al., 1991; Vesa et al., 1995; (121) Sharp et al., 1997; (122) Savukoski et al., 1998; (123) Sharp et al., 1997; (124) Mole, 1998; (125) Das et al., 1998; (126) Michalewski et al., 1998; Mole, 1998; (127) Das et al., 1998.

**Table 1-5** Size of trinucleotide repeats

| Disease | Type of Nucleotide | In Normals | In Disease |
|---|---|---|---|
| Huntington | CAG | 11–34 | 37–121 |
| HDL2 | CAG | <50 | 50–60 |
| SCA-1 | CAG | 19–36 | 42–81 |
| SCA-2 | CAG | 15–29 | 35–59 |
| SCA-3 (Machado-Joseph) | CAG | 12–40 | 66–>200 |
| SCA-6 | CAG | 4–16 | 21–28 |
| SCA-7 | CAG | | Estimated 64 |
| SCA-12 | CAG | 9–28 | 55–78 |
| SCA-17 | CAG | 29–42 | 47–55 |
| DRPLA | CAG | 7–34 | 49–83 |
| Friedreich ataxia | GAA | 7–22 | 120–1700 |

DRPLA, dentatorubral-pallidoluysian atrophy; SCA, spinocerebellar degeneration.

Data in part from Brooks BP, Fischbeck KH: Spinal and bulbar muscular atrophy: A trinucleotide-repeat expansion neurodegenerative disease. Trends Neurosci 1995;18:459–461; Riess O, Schols L, Bottger H, et al: SCA6 is caused by moderate CAG expansion in the alpha (1A)-voltage-dependent calcium channel gene. Hum Mol Genet 1997;6:1289–1293.

**Table 1-6** Genetics of Parkinson disease

| Gene | Locus | Protein | Transmission | Mean Age at Onset | Progression | Clinical Features | Lewy Bodies |
|---|---|---|---|---|---|---|---|
| PARK1 | 4q21–q22 | α-Synuclein; A53T, A30P, and E46K mutations | AD | 45 (20–85) | Rapid | Dementia, hypoventilation, myoclonus, abnormal EOM, incontinence | + |
| PARK2 | 6q25–q27 | Parkin | AR in juvenile onset, AD in older onset | Young (3–64) | Very slow | Dystonia at onset, ↑ reflexes, sleep benefit, sensitive to dopa | – in juvenile onset; + in older onset |
| PARK3 | 2p13 | ? | AD | 59 (37–89) | Slow | 40% penetrance, dementia associated with tangles and plaques | + |
| PARK4 | 4q region duplication and triplication | Excess α-synuclein | AD | 33 | Rapid | PD/ET, weight loss, dementia, dysautonomia | + |
| PARK5 | 4p14 | UCH-L1 | AD | 50 | ? | Typical PD, ↓ penetrance | ND |
| PARK6 | 1p35–p36 | PINK1 | AR | 40 (30–68) | Slow | Similar to parkin | ND |
| PARK7 | 1p36 | DJ-1 | AR | 33 (27–40) | Slow | As in parkin but with behavioral problems and focal dystonia | ND |
| PARK8 | 12p11.2–q13 | LRRK2 (dardarin) | AD | 51 | Regular | ↓ Penetrance | + and – |
| PARK9 | 1p36 | ATP13AL | AR | 12–16 | Kufor-Rakeb syndrome, a parkinsonism-plus disorder | One family in Jordan, rapid dementia | – |
| PARK10 | 1p32 | ? | AR | Typical late onset | Standard | Families in Iceland | |
| PARK11 | 2q36–q37 | ? | AD | ? | ? | Families in the United States | ND |
| SCA2 | 12q23–24.1 | Ataxin-2 | AD | Young and late onsets | | Can have a parkinsonian phenotype | |

A review of available molecular genetic testing for a variety of movement disorders has been published (Gasser et al., 2003). AD, autosomal dominant; AR, autosomal recessive; EOM, extraocular movement abnormality; ET, essential tremor; ND, not determined; PD, parkinson disease.

Modified from Bentivoglio AR, Cortelli P, Valente EM, et al: Phenotypic characterisation of autosomal recessive PARK6-linked parkinsonism in three unrelated Italian families. Mov Disord 2001;16:999–1006; Lansbury PT Jr, Brice A: Genetics of Parkinson's disease and biochemical studies of implicated gene products. Curr Opin Genet Develop 2002;12:299–306, with new additions.

Box 1-2 Cardinal features of parkinsonism

Tremor at rest
Bradykinesia/hypokinesia/akinesia
Rigidity
Flexed posture of neck, trunk, and limbs
Loss of postural reflexes
Freezing

indicate a very severe form of bradykinesia (Video 1-1). Bradykinesia is mild in early PD and becomes more severe as the disease worsens; similarly in other forms of parkinsonism. A discussion of the phenomenology of akinesia/bradykinesia requires a brief description of the clinical features of parkinsonism. A fuller discussion is presented in Chapter 4.

Parkinsonism is a neurologic syndrome manifested by any combination of six independent, non-overlapping cardinal motor features: tremor at rest, bradykinesia, rigidity, flexed posture, freezing, and loss of postural reflexes (Box 1-2). At least two of these six cardinal features should be present before the diagnosis of parkinsonism is made, one of them being tremor at rest or bradykinesia. There are many causes of parkinsonism; they can be divided into four major categories: primary, secondary, parkinsonism-plus disorders, and heredodegenerative disorders (Box 1-3). Primary parkinsonism (Parkinson disease) is a progressive disorder of unknown etiology or of a known gene defect, and the diagnosis is usually made by excluding other known causes of parkinsonism (Fahn, 1992). The complete classification of parkinsonian disorders is presented in Chapter 4. The specific diagnosis of the type of parkinsonism depends on details of the clinical history, the neurologic examination, and laboratory tests.

The primary parkinsonism disorder known as Parkinson disease (PD), also referred to as idiopathic parkinsonism, is the most common type of parkinsonism encountered by the neurologist. But drug-induced parkinsonism is probably the most common form of parkinsonism, since neuroleptic drugs (dopamine receptor–blocking agents), which cause drug-induced parkinsonism, are widely prescribed for treating psychosis (see Chapter 20). Here, some of the motor phenomenology of parkinsonism is discussed as part of the overview of the differential diagnosis of movement disorders based on phenomenology.

PD begins insidiously. Tremor is usually the first symptom recognized by the patient. However, the disorder can begin with slowness of movement, shuffling gait, painful stiffness of a shoulder, micrographia, or even depression. In the early stages, the symptoms and signs tend to remain on one side of the body (Video 1-2), but with time, the other side slowly becomes involved as well.

*Tremor* is present in the distal parts of the extremities and the lips while the involved body part is "at rest." "Pill-rolling" tremor of the fingers and flexion-extension or pronation-supination tremor of the hands are the most typical (see Video 1-2). The tremor ceases on active movement of the limb but reemerges when the limb remains in a posture against gravity. Resting tremor must be differentiated from postural and kinetic tremors, in which tremor appears only when the arm is being used. These tremors are typically caused by other disorders—namely, essential tremor and cerebellar disorders. An occasional patient with PD will have an action tremor of the hand instead of or in addition to tremor at rest (Video 1-3). In the cranial structures, the lips, chin, jaw, and tongue are the predominant sites for PD tremor (Video 1-4), whereas head (neck) tremor—although it can occur in PD—is more typical of essential tremor, cerebellar tremor, and dystonic tremor.

*Akinesia/bradykinesia/hypokinesia* is manifested cranially by masked facies (hypomimia), decreased frequency of blinking, impaired upgaze and convergence of the eyes, soft speech (hypophonia) with loss of inflection (aprosody), and drooling of saliva due to decreased spontaneous swallowing (Video 1-5). When examining cranial structures, one should look for other signs of PD or parkinson-plus syndromes. Repetitive tapping the glabella often reveals nonsuppression of blinking (Myerson sign) in patients with PD (Brodsky et al., 2004) (Video 1-6), whereas blinking is normally suppressed after two or three blinks (Brodsky et al, 2004). Eyelid opening after the eyelids have been forcefully closed is usually normal in PD but may be markedly impaired in progressive supranuclear palsy; this is been called "apraxia of eyelid opening" (Video 1-7), even though apraxia is a misnomer. The eyes looking straight ahead are typically quiet in PD, but in some parkinson-plus syndromes, square wave jerks may be seen, especially in progressive supranuclear palsy (Video 1-8). Ocular movements are usually normal in PD, except for impaired upgaze and convergence. When saccadic eye movements are impaired, and especially when downgaze is impaired, a parkinson-plus

Box 1-3 Four categories of parkinsonism

Primary
Secondary
Parkinsonism-plus syndromes
Heredodegenerative disorders

syndrome such as progressive supranuclear palsy or cortical-basal ganglionic degeneration is usually indicated (Video 1-9).

Bradykinesia can be detected in other parts of the body. In the arms it can be detected by slowness in raising or relaxing the shoulder (Video 1-10); slowness in raising the arm; loss of spontaneous movement, such as gesturing; smallness and slowness of handwriting (micrographia); difficulty with hand dexterity for shaving, brushing teeth, and putting on makeup; and reduced armswing when walking. Symptoms of bradykinesia in other parts of the body are complaints of a short-stepped, shuffling gait, with decreased armswing and difficulty rising from a chair, getting out of automobiles, and turning in bed. Bradykinesia thus encompasses a loss of automatic movements as well as slowness in initiating movement on command and reduction in amplitude of the voluntary movement. An early feature of reduction of amplitude is the decrementing of the amplitude with repetitive finger tapping or foot tapping (see Video 1-10), which also manifests impaired rhythm of the tapping. Decreased rapid successive movements both in amplitude and speed are characteristic of bradykinesia regardless of the etiology of parkinsonism (Video 1-11). Carrying out two activities simultaneously is impaired (Schwab et al., 1954), and this difficulty may represent bradykinesia as well (Fahn, 1990). With the stimulation of a sufficient sensory input, bradykinesia, hypokinesia, and akinesia can be temporarily overcome (Video 1-12).

*Rigidity* (described later in this chapter under "Rigidity") is another cardinal feature of parkinsonism. Rigidity is usually manifested in the distal limbs by a ratchety "give" in moving a joint throughout its range of motion, so-called cogwheel rigidity. Rigidity of proximal joints is easily appreciated by the examiner by swinging the shoulders (Wartenberg sign) (Video 1-13) or rotating the hips.

As the disease advances, the patient begins to assume a *flexed posture*, particularly of the neck, thorax, elbows, hips, and knees The patient begins to walk with the arms flexed at the elbows and the forearms placed in front of the body and with decreased armswing. With the knees slightly flexed, the patient tends to shuffle the feet, which stay close to the ground and are not lifted up as high as they would normally be; with time, there is loss of heel strike, which would normally occur when the foot moving forward is placed onto the ground. Eventually, the flexion can become extreme (see Video 1-14), leading to camptocormia (Azher and Jankovic, 2005) or pronounced kyphoscoliosis with truncal tilting.

*Loss of postural reflexes* occurs later in the disease. The patient has difficulty righting himself or herself after being pulled off balance. A simple test (the pull test) for the righting reflex is for the examiner to stand behind the patient and give a firm tug on the patient's shoulders toward the examiner, explaining the procedure in advance and directing that the patient should try to maintain his or her balance by taking a step backward (Hunt and Sethi, 2006). Typically, after a practice pull, a normal person can recover within two steps (Video 1-15). A mild loss of postural reflexes can be detected if the patient requires several steps to recover balance. A moderate loss is manifested by a greater degree of retropulsion. With a more severe loss, the patient would fall if not caught by the examiner (Video 1-16), who must always be prepared for such a possibility. With a marked loss of postural reflexes, a patient cannot withstand a gentle tug on the shoulders or cannot stand unassisted without falling. To avoid having the patient

fall to the ground, it is wise to have a wall behind the examiner, particularly if the patient is a large or bulky individual.

A combination of loss of postural reflexes and stooped posture can lead to *festination*, whereby the patient walks faster and faster, trying to catch up with his or her center of gravity to prevent falling (Video 1-17).

The *freezing phenomenon* affects gait more than other parts of the body and begins with either start hesitation—that is, the feet take short, sticking, shuffling steps when the patient initiates walking or when the patient turns while walking (Video 1-18). With progression, the feet become "glued to the ground" when the patient needs to walk through a crowded space (e.g., a revolving door) or is trying to move a distance in a short period of time (e.g., crossing the street at the green light or entering an elevator before the door closes). Often, patients develop destination freezing—that is, stopping before reaching the final destination. For example, the patient might stop too soon when reaching a chair in which he or she intends to sit down. With further progression, sudden transient freezing can occur when the patient is walking in an open space or when the patient perceives an obstacle in the walking path. The freezing phenomenon can also affect arms and speech and is discussed in more detail under "Freezing" later in this chapter).

In addition to these motor signs, most patients with PD have behavioral signs. *Bradyphrenia* is mental slowness, analogous to the motor slowness of bradykinesia. Bradyphrenia is manifested by slowness in thinking or in responding to questions. It occurs even at a young age in PD and is more common than dementia. The "tip-of-the-tongue" phenomenon (Matison et al., 1982), in which a patient cannot immediately come up with the correct answer but knows what it is, may be a feature of bradyphrenia. With time, the parkinsonian patient gradually becomes more passive, indecisive, dependent, and fearful. The spouse gradually makes more of the decisions and becomes the dominant voice. Eventually, the patient sits much of the day unless encouraged to exercise or do activities. Passivity and lack of motivation also express themselves by the patient's lack of desire to attend social events. The term *abulia* is used to describe such apathy, loss of mental and motor drive, and blunting of emotional, social, and motor expression. Abulia encompasses loss of spontaneous and responsive motor activity and loss of spontaneous affective expression, thought, and initiative.

*Depression* is a frequent feature in patients with PD, being obvious in around 30% of cases. The prevalence of *dementia* in PD is about 40%, but the proportion increases with age. Below the age of 60 years, the proportion of patients with dementia is about 8%; in patients older than 80 years, it is 69% (Mayeux et al., 1992). The risk of death is markedly increased when a PD patient becomes demented (Marder et al., 1991). This explains why the incidence of dementia in PD is quite high (69/1000 patient-years) (Mayeux et al., 1990) while the prevalence is relatively lower. Dementia, in fact, has been found to be the major risk factor in the higher mortality rate in patients with PD compared to the age-matched control population (Louis et al., 1996).

The age at onset of PD is usually older than 40, with a mean of 55 years (Hoehn and Yahr, 1967), but younger patients can be affected. Onset between ages 20 and 40 is called young-onset PD; onset before age 20 is called juvenile parkinsonism. Juvenile parkinsonism does not preclude a diagnosis of PD, but it raises questions of other etiologies, such as Wilson disease and the Westphal variant of Huntington disease. Also, familial and sporadic primary juvenile parkinsonism might not show the typical pathologic hallmark of Lewy bodies (Dwork et al., 1993). It is important to note when reading the literature that in Japan, onset before age 40 is called juvenile parkinsonism and that some research studies have called onset by age 50 young-onset.

PD is more common in men, with a male:female ratio of 3:2. The incidence in the United States is 20 new cases per 100,000 population per year (Schoenberg, 1987), with a prevalence of 187 cases per 100,000 population (Kurland, 1958). For the population over 40 years of age, the prevalence rate is 347 per 100,000 (Schoenberg et al., 1985). With the introduction of levodopa, the mortality rate dropped from 3-fold to 1.5-fold above normal. But after the first wave of impaired patients improved with this new and effective treatment, the mortality rate for PD gradually climbed back to the pre-levodopa rate (Clarke, 1995).

## Apraxia

Apraxia is traditionally defined as a disorder of voluntary movement that cannot be explained by weakness, spasticity, rigidity, akinesia, sensory loss, or cognitive impairment. It can exist and be tested for in the presence of a movement disorder provided that akinesia, rigidity, or dystonia is not so severe that voluntary movement cannot be executed. The classic work of Liepmann defined three categories of apraxia:

1. In *ideational apraxia*, the concept or plan of movement cannot be formulated by the patient. Some examiners test for ideational apraxia by asking the patient to perform a series of sequential movements (e.g., filling a pipe, lighting it, and smoking or putting a letter into an envelope, sealing it, and affixing a stamp). Ideational apraxia is due to parietal lesions, most often diffuse and degenerative.
2. In *ideomotor apraxia*, the concept or plan of movement is intact, but the individual motor engrams or programs are defective. Ideomotor apraxia is commonly tested for by asking patients to undertake specific motor acts in response to verbal or written commands, such as waving goodbye, saluting like a soldier, combing their hair, or using a hammer to fix a nail. Patients with ideomotor apraxia often improve their performance if asked to mimic an action performed by the examiner or when given the object or tool to use. Idiomotor apraxia usually does not interfere with normal spontaneous motor actions but requires specific testing for its demonstration. It usually, but not always, is associated with aphasia and is due mainly to lesions in the dominant hemisphere, particularly in the parietotemporal regions, the arcuate fasciculus, or the frontal lobe; such ideomotor apraxia is bilateral, provided that there is not a hemiplegia. Lesions of the corpus callosum can cause apraxia of the nondominant hand.
3. *Limb-kinetic apraxia* is the least understood type. It refers to a higher-order motor deficit in executing motor acts that cannot be explained by simple motor impairments. It has been attributed to lesions of premotor regions in the frontal lobe, such as the supplementary motor area.

The concepts of apraxia are being refined into more discrete identifiable syndromes as knowledge of the functions of the cortical systems controlling voluntary movement advances (for recent reviews, see Pramstaller and Marsden, 1996; Zadikoff and Lang, 2005). A quick, convenient method for testing for apraxia at the bedside is to ask the patients to copy a series of hand postures shown to them by the examiner.

Ideomotor and limb-kinetic apraxias are found in a number of movement disorders—for example, cortical-basal ganglionic degeneration (CBGD) (Video 1-19) and progressive supranuclear palsy (see Chapter 10). A number of other phenomena reflecting cerebral cortex dysfunction may be seen in such patients. Patients with CBGD frequently have signs of cortical myoclonus (Video 1-20) or cortical sensory deficit. The *alien limb* phenomenon, also seen in cortical-basal ganglionic degeneration, consists of involuntary, spontaneous movements of an arm or leg (Video 1-21), which curiously and spontaneously moves to adopt odd postures quite beyond the control or understanding of the patient. Intermanual conflict is another such phenomenon; one hand irresistibly and uncontrollably begins to interfere with voluntary action of the other. The abnormally behaving limb may also show forced grasping of objects, such as blankets or clothing. Such patients often exhibit other frontal lobe signs, such as a grasp reflex or utilization behavior, in which they compulsively pick up objects presented to them and begin to use them. For example, if a pen is presented with no instructions, they pick it up and write. If a pair of glasses is proffered, they place the glasses on the nose; if further pairs of glasses are then shown, the patient may end up with three or more spectacles on the nose.

## Blocking (Holding) Tics

Blocking (or holding) is a motor phenomenon that is seen occasionally in patients with tics and is characterized as a brief interference of social discourse and contact. There is no loss of consciousness, and although the patient does not speak during these episodes, he or she is fully aware of what has been spoken. These blocking tics appear in two situations: (1) as an accompanying feature of some prolonged tics, such as during a protracted dystonic tic (Video 1-22) or during tic status, and (2) as a specific tic phenomenon in the absence of an accompanying obvious motor or vocal tic. The latter occurrences have the abruptness and duration of a dystonic tic or a series of clonic tics, but they do not occur during an episode of an obvious motor tic.

Although both types can be called blocking tics, the first type can be considered "intrusions" because the interruption of activity is due to a positive motor phenomenon (i.e., severe, somewhat prolonged, motor tics) that interferes with other motor activities. An example would be a burst of tics that is severe enough to interrupt ongoing motor acts, including speech, as seen in Video 1-22.

The second type (i.e., inhibition of ongoing motor activity without an obvious "active" tic) can be considered a negative motor phenomenon (i.e., a "negative" tic). The negative type of *blocking tics* should be differentiated from absence seizures or other paroxysmal episodes of loss of awareness. There is never loss of awareness with blocking tics. Individuals with intrusions and negative blocking recognize that they have these interruptions of normal activity and are fully aware of the environment during them, even if they are unable to speak at that time.

## Cataplexy and Drop Attacks

*Drop attacks* can be defined as sudden falls with or without loss of consciousness, due either to collapse of postural muscle tone or to abnormal muscle contractions in the legs. About two thirds of cases are of unknown etiology (Meissner et al., 1986). Symptomatic drop attacks have many neurologic and non-neurologic causes. Neurologic disorders include leg weakness, sudden falls in parkinsonian syndromes including those due to freezing, transient ischemic attacks, epilepsy, myoclonus, startle reactions, paroxysmal dyskinesias, structural central nervous system lesions, and hydrocephalus. Syncope and cardiovascular disease account for non-neurologic causes. Idiopathic drop attacks usually appear between the ages of 40 and 59 years, the prevalence increasing with advancing age (Stevens and Matthews, 1973), and are a common cause of falls and fractures in the elderly (Sheldon, 1960; Nickens, 1985). A review of drop attacks has been provided by Lee and Marsden (1995).

*Cataplexy* is another cause of symptomatic drop attacks that does not fit the categories listed previously. Patients with cataplexy fall suddenly without loss of consciousness but with inability to speak during an attack. There is a precipitating trigger, usually laughter or a sudden emotional stimulus. The patient's muscle tone is flaccid and remains this way for many seconds. Cataplexy is usually just one feature of the narcolepsy syndrome; other features include sleep paralysis and hypnagogic hallucinations, in addition to the characteristic feature of uncontrollable falling asleep. A review of cataplexy has been provided by Guilleminault and Gelb (1995).

## Catatonia, Psychomotor Depression, and Obsessional Slowness

In 1874, Karl Ludwig Kahlbaum wrote the following description: "The patient remains entirely motionless, without speaking, and with a rigid, mask like facies, the eyes focused at a distance; he seems devoid of any will to move or react to any stimuli; there may be fully developed 'waxen' flexibility, as in cataleptic states, or only indications, distinct, nevertheless, of this striking phenomenon. The general impression conveyed by such patients is one of profound mental anguish" (Bush et al., 1996).

Gelenberg (1976) defined *catatonia* as a syndrome characterized by catalepsy (abnormal maintenance of posture or physical attitudes), waxy flexibility (retention of the limbs for an indefinite period of time in the positions in which they are placed), negativism, mutism, and bizarre mannerisms. Patients with catatonia can remain in one position for hours and move  exceedingly slowly in response to commands, usually requiring the examiner to push them along (Video 1-23). But when moving spontaneously, they move quickly, such as when scratching themselves. In contrast to patients with parkinsonism, there is no concomitant cogwheel rigidity, freezing, or loss of postural reflexes. Classically, catatonia is a feature of schizophrenia, but it can also occur with severe depression. Gelenberg also stated that catatonia can appear with conversion hysteria, dissociative states, and organic brain disease. However, his organic syndromes of akinetic mutism, abulia, encephalitis, and so forth should be distinguished from catatonia, and catatonia should preferably be considered a psychiatric disorder.

*Depression* is commonly associated with a general slowness of movement, as well as of thought, so-called psychomotor retardation, and catatonia can be considered an extreme case of this problem. Although depressed patients are widely recognized to manifest slowness in movement, some—particularly children—might not have the more classic symptoms of low mood, dysphoria, anorexia, insomnia, somatizations, and tearfulness. In this situation, slowness due to depression can be difficult to distinguish from the bradykinesia of parkinsonism. As in catatonia, lack of rigidity and preservation of postural reflexes may help to differentiate psychomotor slowness from parkinsonism. However, there can be loss of facial expression and decreased blinking in both catatonia and depression. Lack of Myerson sign, snout reflex, and palmomental reflexes are the rule, all of which are usually present in parkinsonism. In children with psychomotor depression and motor slowness (Video 1-24), the differential diagnosis is that of juvenile parkinsonism, including Wilson disease and the akinetic form of Huntington disease.

Some patients with obsessive-compulsive disorder (OCD) may present with extreme slowness of movement, so-called obsessional slowness. Hymas and colleagues (1991) evaluated 17 such patients out of 59 admitted to hospital with OCD. These patients had difficulty initiating goal-directed action and had many suppressive interruptions and perseverative behavior. Besides slowness, some patients had cogwheel rigidity, decreased armswing when walking, decreased spontaneous movement, hypomimia, and flexed posture. However, there was no decrementing of either amplitude or speed with repetitive movements, no tremor, and no micrographia. Also there was no freezing or loss of postural reflexes. Like other cases of OCD, this is a chronic illness. Fluorodopa positron emission tomography scans revealed no abnormality of dopa uptake, thereby clearly distinguishing this disorder from PD (Sawle et al., 1991). However, there is hypermetabolism in the orbital, frontal, premotor, and midfrontal cortex, suggesting excessive neural activity in these regions.

## Freezing

*Freezing* refers to transient periods, usually lasting several seconds, in which the motor act is halted, being stuck in place. It commonly develops in parkinsonism (see Chapter 4), both primary and atypical parkinsonism (Giladi et al., 1997). The freezing phenomenon has also been called motor blocks (Giladi et al., 1992). The terms *pure akinesia* (Narabayashi et al., 1976, 1986; Imai et al., 1986), and *gait ignition failure* (Atchison et al., 1993; Nutt et al., 1993) refer to syndromes in which freezing is the predominant clinical feature with only a few other features of parkinsonism.

In freezing, the voluntary motor activity being attempted is halted because agonists and antagonist muscles are simultaneously and isometrically contracting (Andrews, 1973), preventing normal execution of voluntary movement. The motor blockage, therefore, is not one of lack of muscle tone or flaccidity but rather is analogous to being glued to a position so that the patient exerts increased effort to overcome being "stuck." The stuck body part attempts to move to overcome the block, and muscle force (isometric) is exerted. So with freezing of gait, by far the most common form of the freezing phenomenon, as the patient attempts to move the feet, short, incomplete steps are attempted, but the feet tend to remain in the same place ("glued to the ground"). After a few seconds, the freezing clears spontaneously, and the patient is able to move at his or her normal pace again until the next

Box 1-4 Types of freezing phenomena

Start hesitation (freezing when gait is initiated)
Turning hesitation (freezing when turning)
Destination hesitation (freezing when approaching the target)
Freezing when an "obstacle" is encountered
Spontaneous sudden transient freezing
Palilalia or freezing of speech
"Apraxia" of eyelid opening or levator inhibition
Freezing of limbs

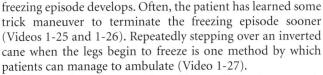

freezing episode develops. Often, the patient has learned some trick maneuver to terminate the freezing episode sooner (Videos 1-25 and 1-26). Repeatedly stepping over an inverted cane when the legs begin to freeze is one method by which patients can manage to ambulate (Video 1-27).

Although freezing most often affects walking, it can manifest in other ways (Box 1-4). Speech can be arrested, with the patient repeating a sound until it finally becomes unstuck, and speech then continues (Video 1-28). This can be considered a severe form of parkinsonian palilalia, which usually refers to a repetition of the first syllable of the word the patient is trying to verbally express. Parkinsonian palilalia differs from the palilalia seen in patients with Gilles de la Tourette syndrome, in which there is repetition of entire words or a string of words (see Video 1-22).

Freezing of the arms, such as during handwriting or teeth brushing, has also been reported (Narabayashi et al., 1976). Difficulty opening the eyes can be another example of freezing (see Video 1-7). This eyelid freezing was originally called apraxia of eyelid opening, which is a misnomer because the problem is not an apraxia. Eyelid freezing has also been called levator palpebrae inhibition (Lepore and Duvoisin, 1985) and even a form of dystonia. Although previously unrecognized as a freezing phenomenon and usually considered a form of body bradykinesia, difficulty rising from a chair may be due to freezing in some patients (see Video 1-25). Patients use many tricks to overcome freezing, but these might not always be successful. An update on the freezing phenomenon is provided in a review by Fahn (1995).

As was discussed previously, the freezing phenomenon occurs in parkinsonism, whether it be primary (PD) (Giladi et al., 1992), secondary (such as vascular parkinsonism), or parkinsonism-plus syndromes, such as progressive supranuclear palsy and multiple system atrophy. It can also appear as an idiopathic freezing gait without other features of parkinsonism, except for loss of postural reflexes and mild bradykinesia (Achiron et al., 1993; Atchison et al., 1993) (Video 1-29). In some patients, it may be an early sign of impending progressive supranuclear palsy (Riley et al., 1994) or due to nigropallidal degeneration (Katayama et al., 1998).

## Hesitant Gaits

Hesitant gaits or uncertain gaits are seen in a number of syndromes. The *cautious gait* that is seen in some elderly people is slow on a wide base with short steps and superficially may resemble that of parkinsonism except that there are no other parkinsonian features. *Fear of falling*, because of either per-

ceived instability or realistic loss of postural righting reflexes, produces an inability to walk independently without holding on to people or objects. Because this abnormal gait disappears when the person walks holding on to someone, it is often considered to be a psychiatric disorder, a phobia of open spaces (i.e., agoraphobia). But because previous falls usually play a role in patients' developing this disorder, it appears to be a true fear of falling that is distinguishable from agoraphobia, which is a separate syndrome. Fear of falling should be differentiated from other types of psychogenic gait disorders (see Chapter 26). A *cautious gait* may be superimposed on any other gait disorder.

The *senile gait disorder* (or *gait disorder of the elderly*) is a poorly understood condition that comprises a number of different syndromes (Nutt et al., 1993). In *gait ignition failure* (Atchison et al., 1993), also called primary freezing gait (Achiron et al., 1993), the problem is one of getting started. Once under way, such patients walk fairly briskly (see Video 1-29), and equilibrium is preserved. In the *frontal gait disorders*, there is also start hesitation, and walking is with slow, small, shuffling steps, similar to that in PD. However, there are few other signs of parkinsonism, and equilibrium is preserved. Such a gait can occur with frontal lobe tumors, cerebrovascular disease, and hydrocephalus, all causing frontal lobe damage. This pattern has been incorrectly called frontal ataxia or gait apraxia in the older literature.

Other hesitant gaits are those due to *severe disequilibrium*. These types of gaits have been associated with frontal cortex and deep white matter lesions (*frontal disequilibrium*) or thalamic and midbrain lesions (*subcortical disequilibrium*) (Nutt et al., 1993). Hesitant gait syndromes are covered in more depth in Chapter 11.

## Hypothyroid Slowness

Along with decreased metabolic rate, cool temperature, bradycardia, myxedema, loss of hair, hoarseness, and myotonia, severe hypothyroidism can feature motor slowness, weakness, and lethargy. These signs could be mistaken for the bradykinesia of parkinsonism, but the combination of the other signs of hypothyroidism, along with lack of rigidity and loss of postural reflexes, should aid the correct diagnosis.

## Rigidity

*Rigidity* is characterized as increased muscle tone to passive motion. It is distinguished from spasticity in that it is present equally in all directions of the passive movement, equally in flexors and extensors, and throughout the range of motion, and it does not exhibit the clasp-knife phenomenon. Rigidity can be smooth (lead-pipe) or jerky (cogwheel). Cogwheeling occurs in the same range of frequencies as action and resting tremor (Lance et al., 1963) and appears to be due to superimposition of a tremor rhythm (Denny-Brown, 1962). Cogwheel is more common than lead-pipe rigidity in parkinsonism (nigral lesion), and lead-pipe rigidity can be caused by various other central nervous system lesions (Fahn, 1987), including those involving the corpus striatum (hypoxia, vascular lesions, neuroleptic malignant syndrome [NMS], cortical-basal ganglionic degeneration) (Video 1-30), midbrain (decorticate rigidity), medulla (decerebrate rigidity), and spinal cord (tetanus).

An increase in passive muscle tone can sometimes lead to impaired motor performance or even immobility. Before there was a clear understanding of bradykinesia, rigidity was considered to be responsible for the paucity of movement in parkinsonism. But rigidity is clearly distinct from bradykinesia; the former is more easily treated by levodopa therapy or by stereotactic thalamotomy and can then be relieved, while bradykinesia with residual paucity of movement persists. When rigidity is extremely severe, such that the examiner can barely move the limbs, as in patients with neuroleptic malignant syndrome, the patient is virtually unable to move.

The extended neck that is occasionally seen in progressive supranuclear palsy (Steele-Richardson-Olszewski syndrome) may be due to rigidity (versus dystonia); the neck can be immobile in this disorder, and axial muscles are also rigid.

Rigidity is one part of neuroleptic malignant syndrome (see Chapter 20), which is an idiosyncratic adverse effect of dopamine receptor blocking agents, usually antipsychotic drugs (Smego and Durack, 1982; Kurlan et al., 1984), but it has also been reported to occur on sudden discontinuation of levodopa therapy (Friedman et al., 1985; Keyser and Rodnitzky, 1991). The clinical features of the syndrome are the abrupt onset of a combination of rigidity/dystonia, fever with other autonomic dysfunctions such as diaphoresis and dyspnea, and an altered mental state including confusion, stupor, or coma. The level of serum creatine kinase activity is usually elevated. The dopamine receptor–blocking agents may have been administered at therapeutic, not toxic, dosages. There does not seem to be any relationship to the duration of therapy. It can develop soon after the first dose or any time after prolonged treatment. This is a potentially lethal disorder unless it is treated; up to 25% of patients die (Henderson and Wooten, 1981). Neuroleptic malignant syndrome is sometimes called malignant catatonia (Boeve et al., 1994) and needs to be distinguished from malignant hyperthermia.

## Stiff Muscles

Stiff muscles are defined as being due to continuous muscle firing without muscle disease and not to rigidity or spasticity. These are reviewed in detail in Chapter 12. Briefly, there are four major categories of stiff-muscle syndromes: continuous muscle fiber activity or neuromyotonia, encephalomyelitis with rigidity, the stiff-limb syndrome, and the stiff-person syndrome (Thompson, 1994). *Neuromyotonia* is a syndrome of myotonic failure of muscle relaxation plus myokymia and fasciculations. Clinically, it manifests as continuous muscle activity causing stiffness and cramps. The best-known neuromyotonic disorder is Isaacs syndrome (Isaacs 1961).

Encephalomyelitis with rigidity, initially called spinal interneuronitis, manifests with marked rigidity and muscle irritability, with increased response to tapping the muscles, along with myoclonus (Video 1-31). It is now recognized as a severe manifestation of stiff-person syndrome and may respond to steroid therapy.

*Stiff-person syndrome* refers to a rare disorder (Spehlmann and Norcross, 1979) in which many somatic muscles are continuously contracting isometrically, resembling "chronic tetanus," in contrast to dystonic movements, which produce abnormal twisting and patterned movements and postures. The contractions of stiff-person syndrome are usually forceful and painful and most frequently involve the trunk and neck musculature (Video 1-32). The proximal limb muscles can also be involved, but rarely does the disorder first affect the distal limbs. Benzodiazepines and valproate are usually somewhat effective. Withdrawal of these agents results in an increase of painful spasms. This disorder has now been recognized to be an autoimmune disease, with circulating antibodies against the GABA-synthesizing enzyme, glutamic acid decarboxylase, and also other types of antibodies, including antibodies against insulin (Solimena et al., 1988, 1990; Blum and Jankovic, 1991). Diabetes is a common accompanying disorder. The diagnosis can now be aided by laboratory testing for these antibodies. The syndrome of interstitial neuronitis, also called encephalomyelitis with rigidity and myoclonus, is a more acute variant of the stiff-person syndrome. The so-called stiff-baby syndrome (Video 1-33) is actually due to infantile hyperekplexia, in which the muscles continue to fire repeatedly and so frequently that they appear to contract continuously.

## EVALUATION OF A DYSKINESIA

The first question to be answered in seeing a patient for the possible presence of abnormal movements is whether or not involuntary movements are actually present. One must consider whether the suspected abnormal movements might be purposeful voluntary movements, such as exaggerated gestures, mannerisms, or compulsive movements, or whether sustained contracted muscles might be "involuntary" muscle tightness to reduce pain, so-called guarding. It should be noted that as a general rule, abnormal involuntary movements are exaggerated with anxiety and diminish during sleep. They may or may not lessen with use of amobarbital or hypnosis.

Once it has been decided that abnormal movements are present, the next question is to determine the category of the involuntary movement, such as chorea, dystonia, myoclonus, tics, or tremor: in other words, to determine the nature of the involuntary movements. To do so, one evaluates features such as rhythmicity, speed, duration, pattern (e.g., repetitive, flowing, continual, paroxysmal, diurnal), induction (i.e., stimuli-induced, action-induced, exercise-induced), complexity of the movements (complex versus simple), suppressibility by volitional attention or by sensory tricks, and whether the movements are accompanied by sensations such as restlessness or the urge to make a movement that can release a built-up tension. In addition, the examiner must determine which body parts are involved. The evaluation for the type of dyskinesia is the major subject of the next section in this chapter.

The third question is to determine the etiology of the abnormal involuntary movements. Is the disorder hereditary, sporadic, or symptomatic of some known neurologic disorder? The etiology and workup for the various dyskinesias are discussed in each chapter dealing with specific types of movement disorders. As a general rule, the etiology can be ascertained on the basis of the history and judicially selected laboratory tests.

The final question is how best to treat the movement disorder. Treatments of the various movement disorders are covered in the appropriate chapters.

## DIFFERENTIAL DIAGNOSIS OF DYSKINESIAS

The differential diagnosis of movement disorders depends primarily on their clinical features. It is important to observe and describe the nature of the involuntary movements as mentioned previously. In addition, one examines for postural changes, alteration of muscle tone, loss of postural reflexes, motor impersistence, and any other neurologic abnormalities during the general neurologic examination.

A list of abnormal involuntary movements is presented alphabetically in Box 1-1 under "Hyperkinesias." A brief description of each of these is now presented, along with its major recognizable and differentiating features. Boxes 1-5 to 1-13 list the ordinary process of distinguishing one type of dyskinesia from another by the major stepwise deciphering based on a practical approach.

### Abdominal Dyskinesias

*Abdominal dyskinesias* are continuous movements of the abdominal wall or sometimes the diaphragm. The movements persist, and their sinuous, rhythmic nature has led to their being called belly dancer's dyskinesia (Iliceto et al., 1990). They may be associated with abdominal trauma in some cases, and a common result is segmental abdominal myoclonus (Kono et al., 1994) (Video 1-34). Another common cause is tardive dyskinesia (TD). *Hiccups*, which are regularly recurring diaphragmatic myoclonus, do not move the abdomen and umbilicus in a sinewy fashion but with sharp jerks and typically with noises as air is expelled by the contractions, so they should not present a diagnostic problem. Abdominal dyskinesias are discussed in Chapter 24.

### Akathitic Movements

*Akathisia* (from the Greek, meaning "unable to sit still") refers to a feeling of inner, general restlessness that is reduced or relieved by moving about. The typical akathitic patient, when seated, may caress his or her scalp, cross and uncross the legs, rock the trunk, squirm, get out of the chair often to pace back and forth (Video 1-35), and even make noises such as moaning (Video 1-36). Carrying out these motor acts brings relief from the sensations of akathisia. Akathitic movements are complex and usually stereotyped; the same type of movements are employed over and over. Other movement disorders that show complex movements are tics, compulsions, mannerisms, and the stereotypies associated with mental retardation, autism, or psychosis.

Akathisia does not necessarily affect the whole body; an isolated body part can be affected. Focal akathisia often produces a sensation of burning or pain, again relieved by moving that body part. Common sites for focal akathisia are the mouth and vagina (Ford et al., 1994). Akathisia may be expressed by vocalizations, such as continual moaning, groaning, or humming. Other movement disorders associated with moaning sounds or humming are tics, oromandibular dystonia, Huntington disease, parkinsonian disorders (Micheli et al., 1991; Friedman, 1993). and those induced by levodopa (Fahn et al., 1996). The patient can transiently suppress akathitic movements and vocalizations if he or she is asked to do so.

The most common cause of akathisia is iatrogenic. It is a frequent complication of antidopaminergic drugs, including those that block dopamine receptors (such as antipsychotic drugs and certain antiemetics) and those that deplete dopamine (such as reserpine and tetrabenazine). Akathisia can occur when drug therapy is initiated (acute akathisia), subsequently with the emergence of drug-induced parkinsonism, or after chronic treatment (tardive akathisia). Acute akathisia is eliminated on withdrawal of the medication. Tardive akathisia usually is associated with the syndrome of tardive dyskinesia (see Chapter 20). Like tardive dyskinesia, tardive akathisia is aggravated by discontinuing the neuroleptic, and it is usually relieved by increasing the dose of the offending drug, which masks the movement disorder. When associated with tardive dyskinesia, the akathitic movements can be rhythmic, such as body rocking or marching in place. In this situation, it is difficult to be certain whether such rhythmic movements are due to akathisia or to tardive dyskinesia.

The exact mechanism of akathisia is not known, but it seems that the dopamine systems are involved, possibly in the limbic system or frontal cortex. It is of interest that akathisia, both generalized and regional, can be present in patients with PD.

### Asynergia/Ataxia/Dysmetria

*Asynergia* or *dyssynergia* refers to decomposition of movement due to breakdown of normal coordinated execution of a voluntary movement. It is one of the cardinal clinical features of cerebellar disease or of lesions involving the pathways to or from the cerebellum (Video 1-37). Asynergia of a limb results in a decomposition of movement instead of a smooth, continuous movement; it is associated with a tendency to miss the target and worsens when approaching a target. Limb asynergia is also manifested by *dysdiadochokinesia*, which refers to the breakup and irregularity that occur when the limb is attempting to carry out rapid alternating movements. Because of its association with cerebellar disease, limb asynergia is frequently accompanied by *dysmetria* (the misjudging of distance), with its characteristic overshooting (hypermetria) and undershooting (hypometria) of the target, and occasionally by intention (or terminal) tremor (see under "Tremor," later in this chapter). In addition, asynergia is usually associated with hypotonia, loss of check (when a voluntary ballistic movement is unable to stop precisely on target when the limb reaches its destination), and rebound (when sudden displacement of a limb results in excessive overcorrection to return to the baseline position). Asynergia is seen only during voluntary movement and is not appreciated when the limb is at rest. *Ataxia* of gait is typified by unsteadiness with a wide base, the body swaying, and an inability to walk on tandem (heel-to-toe). Ataxia appears with active voluntary movement and not at rest.

## Athetosis

*Athetosis* has been used in two senses: to describe a class of slow, writhing, continuous, involuntary movements and to describe the syndrome of athetoid cerebral palsy. This syndrome commonly occurs as a result of injury to the basal ganglia in the prenatal or perinatal period or during infancy. Athetotic movements affect the limbs, especially distally, but can also involve axial musculature, including neck, face, and tongue. When not present in certain body parts at rest, it can often be brought out by having the patient carry out voluntary motor activity elsewhere in the body; this phenomenon is known as *overflow*. For example, speaking can induce increased athetosis in the limbs, neck, trunk, face, and tongue (Video 1-38). Athetosis often is associated with sustained contractions producing abnormal posturing. In this regard, athetosis blends with dystonia. However, the speed of these involuntary movements can sometimes be faster and blend with those of chorea, and the term *choreoathetosis* is then used. Athetosis resembles "slow" chorea in that the direction of movement changes randomly and in a flowing pattern (see Chapter 16).

*Pseudoathetosis* refers to distal athetoid movements of the fingers and toes due to loss of proprioception, which can be due to sensory deafferentation (sensory athetosis) or to central loss of proprioception (Sharp et al., 1994).

## Ballism

*Ballism* refers to very large-amplitude choreic movements of the proximal parts of the limbs, causing flinging and flailing limb movements (see Chapter 16). Ballism is most frequently unilateral, in which case it is referred to as hemiballism (Video 1-39). This is often the result of a lesion in the contralateral subthalamic nucleus or its connections or of multiple small infarcts (lacunes) in the contralateral striatum. In rare instances, ballism occurs bilaterally (*biballism*) and is due to bilateral lacunes in the basal ganglia (Sethi et al., 1987). Like chorea, ballism can sometimes occur as a result of overdosage of levodopa.

## Chorea

*Chorea* refers to involuntary, irregular, purposeless, nonrhythmic, abrupt, rapid, unsustained movements that seem to flow from one body part to another. A characteristic feature of chorea is that the movements are unpredictable in timing, direction, and distribution (i.e., random). Although some neurologists erroneously label almost all nonrhythmic, rapid involuntary movements as choreic, many are not. Nonchoreic rapid movements can be tics, myoclonus, and dystonia (see the chapters for each of these disorders); in these conditions, the movements repeat themselves in a set distribution of the body (i.e., are patterned) and do not have the changing, flowing nature of choreic movements, which travel around the body. In rapid dystonic movements, there is a recognizable repetitive recurrence to the movements in the affected body parts, unlike the random nature of chorea. The prototypical choreic movements are those seen in Huntington disease (Video 1-40), in which the brief and rapid movements are irregular and occur randomly as a function of time. In Sydenham chorea and in the withdrawal emergent syndrome

(see Chapter 20), the flowing choreic movements have a restless appearance (Video 1-41).

When choreic movements are infrequent, they appear as isolated, small-amplitude, brief movements, somewhat slower than myoclonus but sometimes difficult to distinguish from it. When chorea is more pronounced, the movements occur almost continually, presenting as involuntary movements flowing from one site on the body to another.

Choreic movements can be partially suppressed, and the patient can often camouflage some of the movements by incorporating them into semipurposeful movements, known as *parakinesia*. Chorea is usually accompanied by *motor impersistence* ("negative chorea"), the inability to maintain a sustained contraction. A common symptom of motor impersistence is the dropping of objects. Motor impersistence is detected by examining for the inability to keep the tongue protruded and by the presence of the "milkmaid" grip due to the inability to keep the fist in a sustained tight grip. For details on choreic disorders, see Chapters 15 and 16.

## Dystonia

*Dystonia* refers to twisting movements that tend to be sustained at the peak of the movement, are frequently repetitive, and often progress to prolonged abnormal postures (see Chapter 13). In contrast to chorea, dystonic movements repeatedly involve the same group of muscles—that is, they are patterned. Agonist and antagonist muscles contract simultaneously (cocontraction) to produce the sustained quality of dystonic movements. The speed of the movement varies widely from slow (athetotic dystonia) to shock-like (myoclonic dystonia). When the contractions are very brief (e.g., less than a second), they are referred to as dystonic spasms. When they are sustained for several seconds, they are called dystonic movements. When they last minutes to hours, they are known as *dystonic postures*. When present for weeks or longer, the postures can lead to permanent fixed contractures.

When dystonia first appears, the movements typically occur when the affected body part is carrying out a voluntary action (*action dystonia*) and are not present when that body part is at rest. With progression of the disorder, dystonic movements can appear at distant sites (overflow) when other parts of the body are voluntarily moving, such as occurs also in athetosis and in dopa-induced dyskinesias. With further progression, dystonic movements become present when the body is "at rest." Even at this stage, dystonic movements are usually made more severe with voluntary activity. Whereas primary dystonia often begins as action dystonia and may persist as the kinetic (clonic) form, symptomatic dystonia often begins as sustained postures (tonic form).

Different parts of the body can be affected with dystonia, and dystonia can be classified according to body distribution (Fahn et al., 1987). When a single body part is affected, the condition is referred to as focal dystonia. Common forms of focal dystonia are spasmodic torticollis (cervical dystonia), blepharospasm (upper facial dystonia), and writer's cramp (hand dystonia). Involvement of two or more contiguous regions of the body is referred to as segmental dystonia. Generalized dystonia indicates involvement of one or both legs, the trunk, and some other part of the body. Multifocal dystonia involves two or more regions, not conforming to segmental or generalized dystonia. Hemidystonia refers to

# Color Plates

Color Plate 1 Diagram of the main pathways of basal ganglia. The putamen receives excitatory input (glutamate) from the cerebral cortex and projects both via an indirect pathway to the GPe, which in turn projects to the STN and then to the GPi, and via a direct pathway to the GPi. The GPi projects rostrally to the thalamus and cortex and caudally to the brainstem, particularly to the PPN and spinal cord. Glut, glutamate; PPN, pedunculopontine nucleus. (See Fig. 3-1.) (Used with permission from J. Jankovic.)

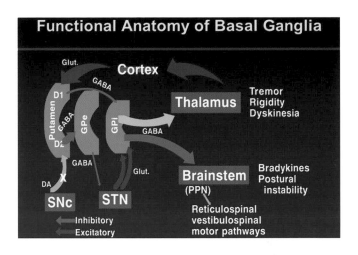

Color Plate 2 Major neural circuits of the basal ganglia. Excitatory projections are depicted as *green arrows*. Inhibitory projections are depicted as *red, orange,* or *yellow arrows*. Cerebral cortical neurons in layer 5 provide excitatory, glutamatergic projections to the striatum (corticostriatal pathway). The striatum comprises two populations of medium spiny projection neurons. Direct-pathway neurons (*red*) bear D1 receptors and provide inputs directly to the output nuclei of the basal ganglia, the internal segment of the globus pallidus (GPi), and the substantia nigra pars reticulata (SNr). Indirect-pathway neurons (*yellow*) possess D2 receptors and provide indirect projections to the output of the basal ganglia through projections to the external segment of the globus pallidus (GPe). The GPe provides inhibitory inputs to the GPi and SNr (not shown). The GPe is also interconnected with the subthalamic nucleus (STN). The STN receives inputs directly from the cortex through the hyperdirect pathway and provides excitatory inputs to the output nuclei of the basal ganglia. The GPi and SNr provide inhibitory inputs to the thalamic nuclei, the mediodorsal (MD), ventromedial (VM), and ventrolateral (VL) nuclei, which project to prefrontal, premotor, and motor cortical areas (thalamocortical pathway). Dopaminergic neurons in the ventral tegmental area (VTA) and substantia nigra pars compacta (SNc) give rise to dopamine projections to the striatum (DA [*blue arrow*]). (See Fig. 3-2.) (Reproduced with permission from Gerfen CR: Molecular effects of dopamine on striatal-projection pathways. Trends Neurosci 2000;23[suppl]:S64–S70.)

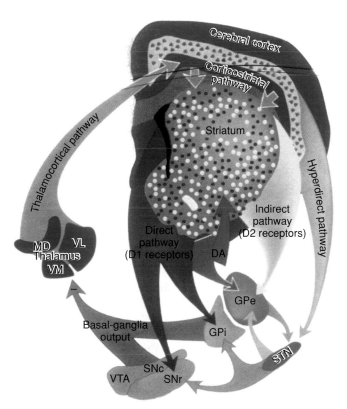

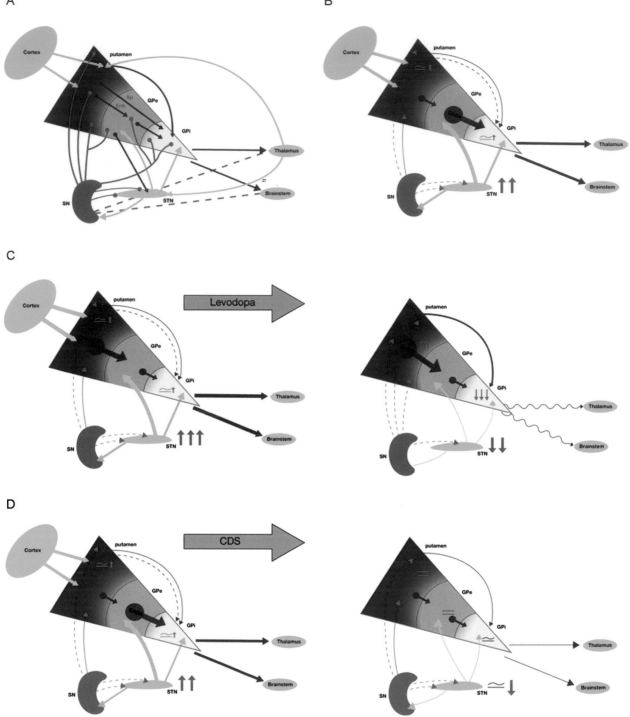

**Color Plate 3** A revisionist view of the functioning of basal ganglia and its modification in Parkinson's disease (PD) and following levodopa treatment. Diagram of the main pathways of the basal ganglia in different functional states. **A,** Normal basal ganglia, highlighting that dopaminergic innervation is not limited to the striatum and the various "internal" loops. **B,** Modification induced by dopamine depletion in early PD. Hyperactivity of the STN precedes significant dopamine putaminal depletion. Therefore, the GPe is still functionally operative and overstimulated by the STN. This leads to increased inhibition from the GPe to the GPi, which partially compensates for the augmented excitation from the STN and reduced inhibition in the "direct" pathway. **C,** Changes associated with advanced PD and the effects of levodopa. At this stage, striatal depletion has progressed and both striatopallidal projections are altered. There is increased inhibition from the GABA/enkephalin projection to the GPe, which is hypoactive and no longer compensates for STN hyperactivity. This results in overactivity of GPi output and abnormal inhibition of motor areas. In this state, levodopa does not restore the normal physiology of the basal ganglia. **D,** Putative effects of stable dopaminergic delivery (continuous dopaminergic stimulation [CDS]) in early PD. Hyperactivity of both the STN and putamino-GPe projections is normalized, restoring the homeostatic mechanisms of the basal ganglia and output activity. This has been proposed to restore the probability of developing motor complications. (See Fig. 3-3.) (Reproduced with permission from Obeso JA, Rodriguez-Oroz M, Marin C, et al: The origin of motor fluctuations in Parkinson's disease: Importance of dopaminergic innervation and basal ganglia circuits. Neurology 2004;62[suppl 1]:S17–S30.)

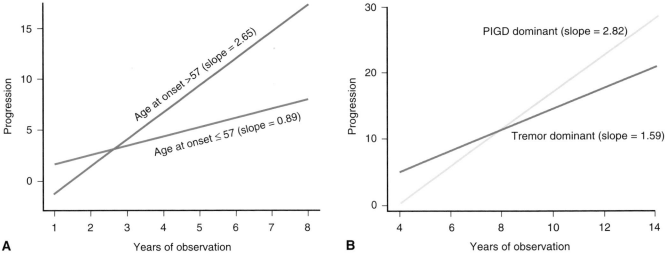

PROGRESSION (PER YEAR OF OBSERVATION) OF TOTAL UPDRS "ON" SCORE FOR AGE AT ONSET ≤ 57 (n = 158) AND AGE AT ONSET >57 (n = 133)

Age at onset >57 (slope = 2.65)

Age at onset ≤ 57 (slope = 0.89)

Progression

Years of observation

**A**

PROGRESSION (PER YEAR OF OBSERVATION) OF TOTAL UPDRS "ON" SCORES ADJUSTED FOR AGE AT INITIAL VISIT FOR PIGD DOMINANT (n = 149) AND TREMOR DOMINANT (n = 77) GROUPS

PIGD dominant (slope = 2.82)

Tremor dominant (slope = 1.59)

Progression

Years of observation

**B**

Color Plate 4 **A,** Younger patients have a slower progression of Parkinson disease symptoms than those with later age at onset. **B,** Patients with postural instability and gait difficulty at onset of their disease progress more rapidly than those with the tremor-dominant form of Parkinson disease. PIGD, postural instability and gait difficulty; UPDRS, Unified Parkinson's Disease Rating Scale. (See Fig. 4-2.) (Reprinted with permission from Jankovic J, Kapadia AS: Functional decline in Parkinson's disease. Arch Neurol 2001;58:1611–1615.)

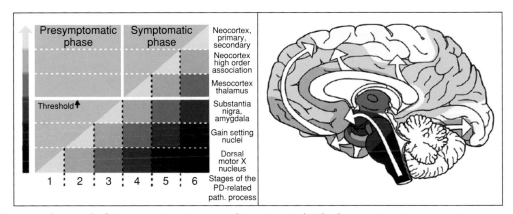

Color Plate 5 Sequential spread of Lewy neurites in nonparkinsonian individuals over time. Lewy neurites seen on histopathologic staining of α-synuclein first appear in the lower medulla oblongata and olfactory tubercle (stage 1). Succeeding stages are the appearances on these neurites more rostrally in the brainstem, with the pons (including locus coeruleus) in stage 2 and midbrain (with substantia nigra) in stage 3. Stages 4 through 6 are the more rostral spread from thalamus to mesocortex to neocortex. (See Fig. 5-1.) (From Braak H, Ghebremedhin E, Rub U, et al: Stages in the development of Parkinson's disease–related pathology. Cell Tissue Res 2004;318[1]:121–134.)

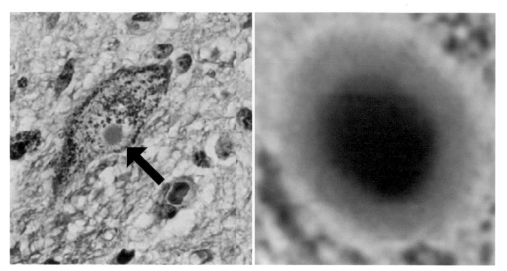

**Color Plate 6** Lewy body (H&E stain). The left-hand part of the figure is a low-power micrograph of a neuromelanin-pigmented dopaminergic neuron in the substantia nigra pars compacta from a patient with sporadic PD. The arrow points to a Lewy body inclusion with a reddish core and clear halo. The right-hand part of the figure is a high-power view of the Lewy body. (See Fig. 5-2.)

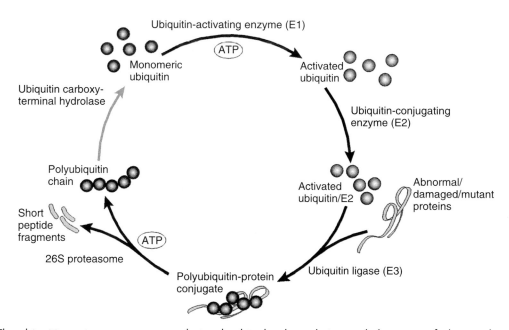

**Color Plate 7** The ubiquitin-proteasome system cycle involved in the degradation and clearance of abnormal or misfolded proteins. Ubiquitin protein is activated by the E1 enzyme, a step requiring energy from ATP. Activated ubiquitin is bound to misfolded protein by the E2 enzyme. The polyubiquitin-protein complex is processed through the proteasome, another step requiring energy from ATP. The proteasome degrades the protein into small peptide fragments. The polyubiquitin chain detached during the entry into the proteasome is split into individual ubiquitin molecules by the action of ubiquitin-carboxy-terminal hydrolase, completing the cycle. (See Fig. 5-3.) (From McNaught KS, Olanow CW, Halliwell B, et al: Failure of the ubiquitin-proteasome system in Parkinson's disease. Nat Rev Neurosci 2001;2:589–594.)

DATATOP ENDPOINTS

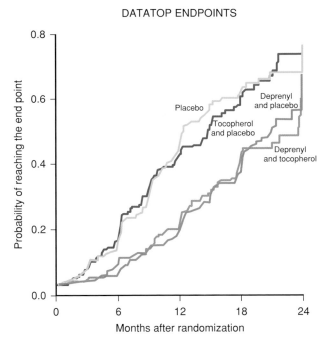

**Color Plate 8** Kaplan-Meier curves of the cumulative probability of reaching the endpoint (need for dopaminergic therapy) in the DATATOP study. Subjects receiving deprenyl (selegiline) reached endpoint statistically significantly more slowly than those not on deprenyl. (See Fig. 6-2.) (From Parkinson Study Group: Effects of tocopherol and deprenyl on the progression of disability in early Parkinson's disease. N Engl J Med 1993;328:176–183.)

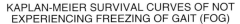

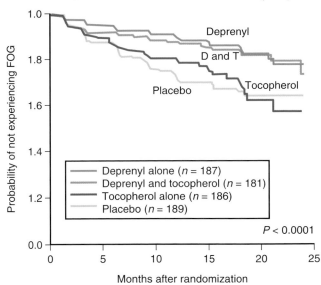

**Color Plate 9** Kaplan-Meier curves showing probability of not experiencing freezing of gait in the absence of levodopa in the DATATOP study. Subjects who had no history of freezing at the time of entry into the study were compared. Those on deprenyl (selegiline) were statistically less likely to develop freezing of gait compared to those who were not on deprenyl. (See Fig. 6-3.) (From Giladi N, McDermott MP, Fahn S, et al: Freezing of gait in PD: Prospective assessment in the DATATOP cohort. Neurology 2001;56:1712–1721.)

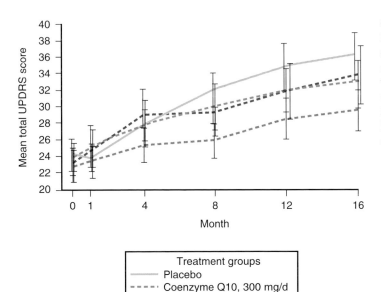

**Color Plate 10** Change in total Unified Parkinson's Disease Rating Scale (UPDRS) with different dosages of coenzyme Q10. Subjects on the highest dosage (1200 mg per day) of coenzyme Q10 had a slower rate or worsening of total UPDRS scores. (See Fig. 6-6.) (Reprinted with permission from Shults CW, Oakes D, Kieburtz K, et al: Effects of coenzyme Q10 in early Parkinson disease: Evidence of slowing of the functional decline. Arch Neurol 2002;59:1541–1550.)

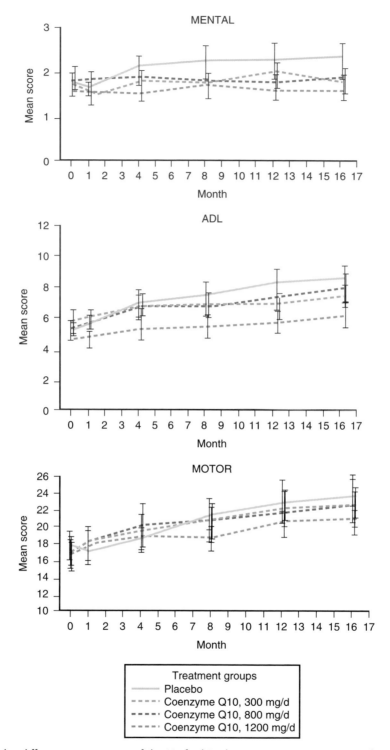

Color Plate 11 Change in the different components of the Unified Parkinson's Disease Rating Scale (UPDRS) with coenzyme Q10. The main effect of the highest dose of coenzyme Q10 on the worsening of total UPDRS was in the Activities of Daily Living (ADL) component (Part 2 of the UPDRS). This score is based on the subject's subjective estimate of how he or she is performing on a series of daily tasks. (See Fig. 6-7.) (Reprinted with permission from Shults CW, Oakes D, Kieburtz K, et al: Effects of coenzyme Q10 in early Parkinson disease: Evidence of slowing of the functional decline. Arch Neurol 2002;59:1541–1550.)

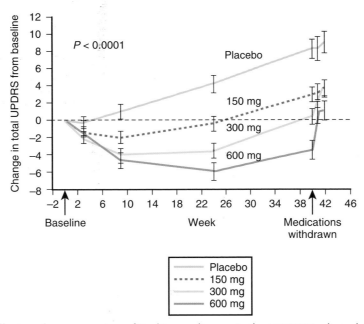

CHANGE IN UPDRS FROM BASELINE TO WEEK-42

$P < 0.0001$

Placebo

150 mg

300 mg

600 mg

Baseline

Week

Medications withdrawn

Placebo
150 mg
300 mg
600 mg

**Color Plate 12** Levodopa's effect on the progression of Parkinson disease in the ELLDOPA clinical trial. Three doses of levodopa were compared with a placebo over 40 weeks followed by a 2-week withdrawal of medications. The total UPDRS scores were dose dependent for both symptomatic benefit (the first 40 weeks) and after the medications were discontinued. Subjects on the highest dosage of levodopa (600 mg per day) had a statistically signifcant superior outcome. UPDRS, Unified Parkinson's Disease Rating Scale. (See Fig. 6-9.) (From Parkinson Study Group: Levodopa and the progression of Parkinson's disease. N Engl J Med 2004;351:2498–2508.)

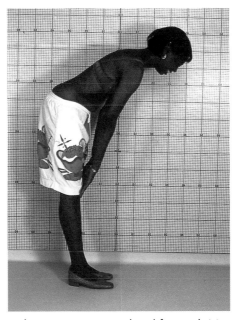

**Color Plate 13** A patient with stiff-person syndrome attempting to bend forward. Note the limitation in bending forward. (See Fig. 12-2.) (Photo courtesy of Dr. M. Dalakas.)

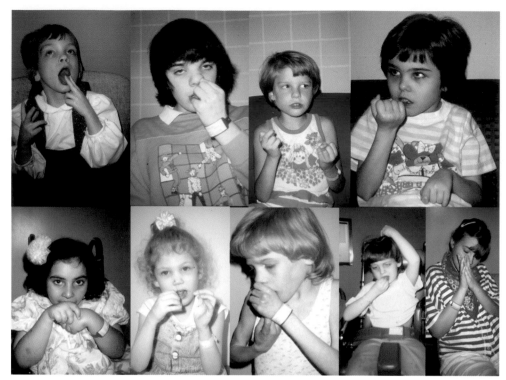

**Color Plate 14** Collage of hand and mouthing stereotypies exhibited by girls with Rett syndrome. (See Fig. 18-1.)

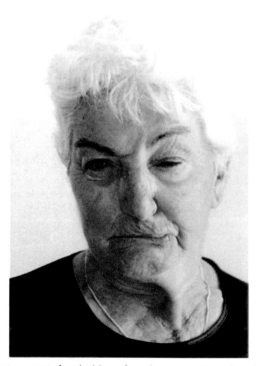

**Color Plate 15** Left-sided hemifacial spasm. Note the elevation of the left brow with the spasm due to contraction of the frontalis muscle. Elevation of the brow with closing of the eye is not easily possible voluntarily. The phenomenon was noted by Babinski and has been referred to as "the other Babinski's sign." (See Fig. 24-2.) (Reprinted with permission from Devoize JL: "The other" Babinski's sign: Paradoxical raising of the eyebrow in hemifacial spasm. J Neurol Neurosurg Psychiatry 2001;70:516.)

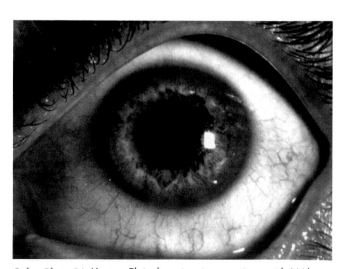

**Color Plate 16** Kayser-Fleischer ring in a patient with Wilson disease. The ring is composed of the *brownish black* pigment at the outer circumference of the iris. (See Fig. 25-2.) (From Scheinberg H, Sternlieb I: Wilson Disease. Philadelphia, Saunders, 1984, with permission.)

involvement of the arm and leg on the same side. A variety of these types of dystonias are shown in Videos 1-42 to 1-49.

One type of focal dystonia requires special mention, namely, sustained contractions of ocular muscles, resulting in tonic ocular deviation, usually upward gaze (Video 1-50). This is referred to as *oculogyric crisis*, and this sustained ocular deviation was encountered in victims of encephalitis lethargica and later in those survivors who developed postencephalitic parkinsonism. Primary torsion dystonia does *not* involve the ocular muscles; hence, oculogyria is not truly a feature of dystonia syndromes. Rather, it is more common today as a complication of dopamine receptor–blocking agents, as in drug-induced parkinsonism or other parkinsonian syndromes such as juvenile parkinsonism and the parkinsonism associated with the degenerative disease known as neuronal intranuclear inclusion disease (Kilroy et al., 1972; Funata et al., 1990), and with the biochemical deficiency of the monoamines in the metabolic disorders of aromatic amino acid decarboxylase deficiency (Hyland et al., 1992; Chang et al., 2004) and pterin deficiencies (Hyland et al., 1998). There has been a case report of oculogyric crises in a patient with dopa-responsive dystonia (Lamberti et al., 1993) and its phenocopy, tyrosine hydroxylase deficiency. *Paroxysmal tonic upgaze* has also been seen in infants and children and often eventually subsides (Ouvrier and Billson, 1988), but it may be a forerunner of developmental delay, intellectual disability, or language delay, indicating impaired corticomesencephalic control of vertical eye movements (Hayman et al., 1998).

One specific type of action dystonia should be mentioned, because is it virtually pathognomonic of a certain diagnosis. When a person with this type of dystonia is eating, the tongue is uncontrollably pushed out of the mouth, often resulting in biting the tongue and dropping food from the mouth (Video 1-51). This characteristic feeding dystonia is seen in the disorder neuroacanthocytosis.

Although classic primary torsion dystonia may appear initially only as an action dystonia, it usually progresses to manifest as continual contractions. A rarer presentation is when primary dystonia appears initially at rest and would clear when the affected body part or some other part of the body is voluntarily active; this type has been called *paradoxical dystonia* (Video 1-52). In contrast to this continual type of classic torsion dystonia, a variant of dystonia also exists in which the movements occur in attacks, which are sudden in onset and of limited duration, known as paroxysmal kinesigenic dyskinesias and paroxysmal nonkinesigenic dyskinesias (see Chapter 23). These are categorized among the paroxysmal disorders. Among the other disorders to be differentiated from dystonia are tonic tics (also called dystonic tics) (see Chapter 17), which also appear as sustained contractions.

## Hemifacial Spasm

*Hemifacial spasm*, as the name indicates, refers to unilateral facial muscle contractions. Generally, these are continual rapid, brief, repetitive spasms, but they can also be more prolonged sustained tonic spasms, mixed with periods of quiescence (Video 1-53). Often, the movements can be brought out when the patient voluntarily and forcefully contracts the facial muscles; when the patient then relaxes the face, the

involuntary movements appear. Hemifacial spasm usually affects both upper and lower parts of the face, but patients are commonly more concerned about closure of the eyelid than about the contractions of the cheek or at the corner of the mouth. The eyebrow tends to elevate with the facial contractions owing to being pulled upward by the forehead muscles. The disorder is believed to involve the facial nerve, and it is sometimes due to compression of the nerve by an aberrant blood vessel (Jannetta, 1982). Hemifacial spasm is an example of a peripherally induced movement disorder (see Chapter 24).

Hemifacial spasm can be easily distinguished from blepharospasm, since the latter involves the face bilaterally and the dystonic contractions often spread to contiguous structures, such as oromandibular and nuchal muscles. Rarely is blepharospasm due to dystonia unilaterally. In such a circumstance, it can be difficult clinically to distinguish it from hemifacial spasm. In contrast to hemifacial spasm, blepharospasm tends to pull the eyebrow down because of contraction of the procerus muscle in addition to the orbicularis oculi. Another condition that has been confused with hemifacial spasm is repetitive facial myoclonus seen with Whipple disease. In this disorder, the myoclonic jerks tend to be fairly rhythmic, the contractions usually involve the other side of the face to some extent, and the movements are not sustained. Electromyography may be of assistance, since hemifacial spasm is associated with high-frequency repetitive discharges and sometimes with evidence of facial nerve denervation and ephaptic transmission. The contractions in both hemifacial spasm and blepharospasm are intermittent, but both can be sustained.

## Hyperekplexia

Hyperekplexia ("startle disease") is an excessive startle reaction to a sudden, unexpected stimulus (Andermann and Andermann, 1986; Brown et al., 1991b; Matsumoto and Hallett, 1994). The startle response can be either a short "jump" or a more prolonged tonic spasm causing falls (Video 1-54). This condition can be familial or sporadic. It may be related to jumping disorders and other similar conditions, such as latah and myriachit, but all of these appear to be influenced by social and group behavior. In jumping disorders, after the initial jump to the unexpected stimulus, there is automatic speech or behavior, such as striking out. In some of these, there is automatic obedience to words such as "jump" or "throw" (Matsumoto and Hallett, 1994). Such automatic behaviors are not seen in hyperekplexia, which is discussed in more detail in Chapter 21. If patients have a delayed reaction to sudden noise or threat, a psychogenic problem should be considered (Hallett et al., 2006).

## Hypnogenic Dyskinesias

Most dyskinesias disappear during deep sleep, although they may emerge during light sleep. The major exception is symptomatic rhythmic *oculopalatal myoclonus*, which persists during sleep, in addition to being present while the patient is awake (Deuschl et al., 1990). There are, however, a few movement disorders that are present only when the patient is asleep. The most common hypnogenic dyskinesia is the condition known as *periodic movements in sleep* (Coleman et al.,

1980; Lugaresi et al., 1983, 1986; Hening et al., 1986), formerly referred to as *nocturnal myoclonus* (Symonds, 1953). The latter term is unacceptable because the movements are not shock-like, but in fact are rather slow. They appear as flexor contractions of one or both legs, with dorsiflexion of the big toe and the foot and flexion of the knee and hip (Video 1-55). They occur at intervals, approximately every 20 seconds and hence have been given its new, more acceptable name (Coleman et al., 1980). Periodic movements in sleep are a frequent component of restless legs syndrome (see Chapter 24). In addition to periodic movements in sleep, this syndrome also is associated with myoclonic-like and dystonic-like movements during sleep and while the patient is drowsy (Hening et al., 1986).

Another rare nocturnal dyskinesia is hypnogenic paroxysmal dystonia or other dyskinesias that occur only during sleep (Video 1-56) (see Chapter 23). Hypnogenic dystonia can be complex and with sustained contractions, similar to those occurring in torsion dystonia. As its name suggests, such movements occur as a paroxysm during sleep and last only a few minutes. They might or might not awaken the patient. Some may be frontal lobe seizures (Fish and Marsden, 1994).

## Jumpy Stumps

*Jumpy stumps* are uncontrollable and sometimes exhausting chaotic movements of the stump remaining from an amputated limb (Video 1-57). When they occur, it is after a delayed period of time following the amputation (Marion et al., 1989).

## Moving Toes and Fingers

The painful legs, moving toes syndrome (see Chapter 24) refers to a disorder in which the toes of one foot or both feet are in continual flexion-extension with some lateral motion, associated with a deep pain in the ipsilateral leg (Spillane et al., 1971). The constant movement has a sinusoidal quality (Video 1-58). The movements and pain are continuous, and both occur even during sleep, though they may be reduced, and the normal sleep pattern may be altered (Montagna et al., 1983). The leg pain is much more troublesome to the patient than are the constant movements. In some patients with this disorder, there is evidence for a lesion in the lumbar roots or in the peripheral nerves (Nathan, 1978; Montagna et al., 1983; Dressler et al., 1994). An analogous disorder, "painful arm, moving fingers," has also been described (Verhagen et al., 1985) (Video 1-59).

## Myoclonus

Myoclonic jerks are sudden, brief, shock-like involuntary movements caused by muscular contractions (positive myoclonus) or inhibitions (negative myoclonus) (see Chapter 21). The most common form of negative myoclonus is asterixis, which frequently accompanies various metabolic encephalopathies. In asterixis, the brief flapping of the outstretched limbs is due to transient inhibition of the muscles that maintain posture of those extremities (Video 1-60). Unilateral asterixis has been described with focal brain lesions of the contralateral medial frontal cortex, parietal cortex, internal capsule, and ventrolateral thalamus (Obeso et al., 1995).

Myoclonus can appear when the affected body part is at rest or when it is performing a voluntary motor act, so-called action myoclonus (Video 1-61). Myoclonic jerks are usually irregular (arrhythmic) but can be rhythmic (such as in *palatal myoclonus* (Videos 1-62 and 1-63) or in *ocular myoclonus* (Video 1-64), with a rate of approximately 2 Hz). Rhythmic ocular myoclonus due to a lesion in the dentato-olivary pathway needs to be distinguished from arrhythmic and chaotic *opsoclonus*, or dancing eyes (Video 1-65). Rhythmic myoclonus is typically due to a structural lesion of the brainstem or spinal cord (therefore also called segmental myoclonus), but not all cases of segmental myoclonus are rhythmic, and some types of cortical epilepsia partialis continua can be rhythmic. Oscillatory myoclonus is depicted as rhythmic jerks that occur in a burst and then fade (Fahn and Singh, 1981). Spinal myoclonus (Video 1-66), in addition to presenting as segmental and rhythmic, can also present as flexion axial jerks triggered by a distant stimulus that travels via a slow-conducting spinal pathway, a type that is called propriospinal myoclonus (Brown et al., 1991c).

Myoclonic jerks occurring in different body parts are often synchronized, a feature that may be specific for myoclonus. The jerks can often be triggered by sudden stimuli such as sound, light, visual threat, or movement (reflex myoclonus). Myoclonus has a relationship to seizures in that both seem to be the result of hyperexcitable neurons.

Cortical reflex myoclonus usually presents as a focal myoclonus and is triggered by active or passive muscle movements of the affected body part (see Video 1-20). It is associated with high-amplitude ("giant") somatosensory evoked potentials and with cortical spikes that are observed by computerized back averaging, time-locked to the stimulus (Obeso et al., 1985). Spread of cortical activity within the hemisphere and via the corpus callosum can produce generalized cortical myoclonus or multifocal cortical myoclonus (Brown et al., 1991a). Reticular reflex myoclonus (Hallett et al., 1977) is more often generalized or spreads along the body away from the source in the brainstem in a timed-related sequential fashion.

The fact that rhythmic myoclonus consists of contractions of agonists rather than alternating agonist-antagonists contractions and the fact that those in one body part are timerelatedly synchronized with contractions elsewhere are strong arguments for categorizing rhythmic myoclonus as a myoclonic disorder and not a type of tremor. Furthermore, rhythmic myoclonias tend to persist during sleep, whereas tremors usually disappear during sleep.

Action or intention myoclonus is often encountered after cerebral hypoxia-ischemia (Lance-Adams syndrome) and with certain degenerative disorders such as progressive myoclonus epilepsy (Unverricht-Lundborg disease) and progressive myoclonic ataxia (Ramsay Hunt syndrome). Usually, action myoclonus is more disabling than is rest myoclonus. Negative myoclonus also occurs in the Lance-Adams syndrome, and when it occurs in the thigh muscles when the patient is standing, it manifests as bouncy legs (Video 1-67). In the opsoclonus-myoclonus syndrome, originally described by Kinsbourne (1962) and subsequently called both dancing eyes, dancing feet and polymyoclonia by Dyken and Kolar (1968), the amplitude of the myoclonus is usually very tiny, resembling irregular tremors. Because of the small amplitudes of the continuous, generalized myoclonus, it is preferable to use the term *minipolymyoclonus* (see Video 1-65), a term that was originally used by Spiro (1970) to describe small-amplitude movements in childhood spinal muscular atrophy and subsequently used by Wilkins and colleagues (1985) for the type of myoclonus that is seen in primary generalized epileptic myoclonus.

## Myokymia and Synkinesis

*Myokymia* is a fine persistent quivering or rippling of muscles (sometimes called live flesh by patients). The term has evolved since first used (Schultze, 1895), when it described benign fasciculations. Although some may still refer to the benign fasciculations that frequently occur in orbicularis oculi as *myokymia*, Denny-Brown and Foley (1948) distinguished between myokymia and benign fasciculations on the basis of electromyography (EMG). In myokymia, the EMG reveals regular groups of motor unit discharges, especially doublets and triplets, occurring with a regular rhythmic discharge. Myokymia occurs most commonly in facial muscles. Most facial myokymias are due to pontine lesions, particularly multiple sclerosis (Andermann et al., 1961; Matthews, 1966), and less often to pontine glioma. When due to multiple sclerosis, facial myokymia tends to abate after weeks or months. When due to a pontine glioma, facial myokymia may persist indefinitely and can be associated with facial contracture (Video 1-68). Myokymia is also a feature of neuromyotonia (see under "Stiff Muscles," earlier in this chapter). Myokymia can persist during sleep. Continuous facial myokymia in multiple sclerosis has been found by magnetic resonance imaging to be caused by a pontine tegmental lesion involving the postnuclear, postgenu portion of the facial nerve (Jacobs et al., 1994).

Aberrant reinnervation of the facial nerve following denervation, such as from Bell palsy, is manifested by *synkinesis*, which is the occurrence of involuntary movements in one part of the face accompanying voluntary contraction of another part. For example, moving the mouth in a smile may cause the eyelid to close.

For the sake of completeness, it is important to mention fasciculations, the small-amplitude contractions of muscles innervated by a motor unit. This is seen predominantly with disease of the anterior horn cells and presents as low-amplitude intermittent twitching of muscles due to motor unit discharges, which are usually not strong enough to move a joint, although this can occur, particularly in children.

## Myorhythmia

The term *myorhythmia* has been used in different ways over time. Herz (1931, 1944) used it to refer to the somewhat rhythmic movements that are sometimes seen in patients with torsion dystonia. Today, this is simply called dystonic movements and is not distinguished from the movements that are repetitive and those that are not. Dystonic myorhythmia should not be confused with dystonic tremor, which strongly resembles other tremors but is due to dystonia. Monrad-Krohn and Refsum (1958) used the term *myorhythmia* to label what today is called palatal myoclonus or other rhythmic myoclonias. This meaning of the term *myorhythmia* has also been adopted by Masucci and colleagues (1984). The term could be used to represent a somewhat slow frequency (<3 Hz) and a prolonged, rhythmic or repetitive movement, in which the movement does not have the sharp square wave appearance of a myoclonic jerk. Therefore, it would not be applied to palatal myoclonus. Myorhythmia would also not apply to the sinusoidal cycles of most tremors (parkinsonian, essential, cerebellar) because the frequency of these tremors is faster than what is defined for myorhythmia.

The most typical disorder in which the term *myorhythmia* is applied is in Whipple disease, in which there are slow-moving, repetitive, synchronous, rhythmic contractions in ocular, facial, masticatory, and other muscles, so-called oculo-faciomasticatory myorhythmia (Schwartz et al., 1986; Hausser-Hauw et al., 1988; Tison et al., 1992). There is often also vertical supranuclear ophthalmoplegia. Ocular myorhythmia is manifested as continuous, horizontal, pendular, vergence oscillations of the eyes, usually of small amplitude, occurring about every second (Video 1-69). They may be asymmetric and may continue in sleep. They never diverge beyond the primary position. Divergence and convergence are at the same speed. They are not accompanied by pupillary miosis. The movements in the face, jaw, and skeletal muscles are about at the same frequency but may be somewhat quicker and may be more like rhythmic myoclonus (Video 1-70). The abnormal movements of facial and masticatory muscles can also persist in sleep, as is seen also with palatal myoclonus.

Sometimes the term *myorhythmia* may be applied to slow, undulating, rhythmic movements of muscles, unrelated to Whipple disease. Perhaps some of these types of movements are part of the spectrum of complex tics, while in others, they may represent psychogenic movements.

## Paroxysmal Dyskinesias

The paroxysmal dyskinesias represent various types of dyskinetic movements, particularly choreoathetosis and dystonia, that occur out of the blue and then disappear after being present for seconds, minutes, or hours (see Chapter 23). The patient can remain normal for months between attacks, or there can be many attacks per day.

*Paroxysmal kinesigenic dyskinesia* is the best described and easiest to diagnose because it is characteristically triggered by a sudden movement; the abnormal movements last seconds to a few minutes. Paroxysmal kinesigenic dyskinesia can be hereditary or symptomatic and usually is successfully treated with anticonvulsants. The abnormal movements easily habituate—that is, they fail to recur if the sudden movement is immediately repeated. These movements can be dystonic, ballistic, and choreic (Video 1-71). There may be many brief paroxysmal bursts of movements each day.

*Paroxysmal nonkinesigenic dyskinesia* is often familial; is triggered by stress, fatigue, caffeine, or alcohol; and can last minutes to hours (Video 1-72). It is more difficult to treat than is the kinesigenic variety, but it sometimes responds to clonazepam or other benzodiazepines and sometimes to acetazolamide. Paroxysmal nonkinesigenic dyskinesia can be familial or sporadic. Sporadic paroxysmal nonkinesigenic dyskinesia, experience would suggest, is more often a psychogenic movement disorder (see Chapter 26), particularly if it is a combination of both paroxysmal and continual dystonias.

*Episodic ataxias and tremors* are also part of the paroxysmal dyskinesia spectrum. They are usually familial and may include vestibular signs and symptoms. The paroxysmal dyskinesias are covered in Chapter 23.

## Restless Legs

The term *restless legs syndrome* refers to more than just the phenomenon of restless legs, in which the patient has unpleasant crawling sensations in the legs, particularly when sitting and relaxing in the evening, which then disappear on walking (Ekbom, 1960). The complete syndrome consists of several parts, in which one or more may be present in any individual. While the unpleasant dysesthesias in the legs are the most common symptom, as was mentioned previously in the discussion on hypnogenic dyskinesias, the clinical spectrum may also include periodic movements in sleep (see Video 1-55), myoclonic jerks, more sustained dystonic movements, or stereotypic movements that occur while the patient is awake, particularly in the late evening (Walters et al., 1991). Other movement disorders associated with a sensory phenomenon are akathisia (feeling of inner restlessness) and tics (feeling of relief of tension or sensory urges upon producing a tic). The restless legs syndrome is covered in Chapter 24.

## Stereotypy

*Stereotypy* refers to coordinated movements that repeat continually and identically. However, there may be long periods of minutes between movements, or the movements may be very frequent. When they occur at irregular intervals, stereotypies may not always be easily distinguished from motor tics, compulsions, gestures, and mannerisms. They can also appear as paroxysmal movements when a child is excited (Tan et al, 1997). In their classic monograph on tics, Meige and Feindel (1907) distinguished between stereotypies and motor tics by describing the latter as acts that are impelling but not impossible to resist, whereas the former, while illogical, are without an irresistible urge. Tics almost always occur intermittently and not continuously—that is, they occur paroxysmally out of a background of normal motor behavior. Although stereotypies can also be bursts of repetitive movements emerging out of a background of normal motor activity, they often repeat themselves in a uniform, repetitive fashion for long periods of time (Lees, 1985). Stereotypies typically occur in patients with tardive dyskinesia (Video 1-73) and with schizophrenia, mental retardation (especially Rett syndrome) (Video 1-74), and autism (Video 1-75), characteristics that assist in separating these from motor tics (Shapiro et al., 1988). Stereotypies apparently occur in Asperger syndrome, a form of mild autism. They have been seen in patients with Kluver-Bucy syndrome (Video 1-76) and when children are left alone and are not in contact with other people (Video 1-77).

Although motor tics are often considered to be stereotypic, when a tic bursts out, it is not necessarily a repetition of the previous tic movement. Thus, tics are usually not repetitive from one burst to the next. However, the same type of tic movement will usually recur after some period of time passes, which provides their stereotypic nature. The diversity of motor tics is one feature that sets their phenomenology apart from stereotypies. Tics are rarely continuously repetitive, and when this occurs, the term *tic status* can be applied (Fahn, 2005). As is pointed out later in the chapter, tics have many other features that aid in their diagnosis, such as their suppressibility, their accompaniment by an underlying urge or compulsion to make the movement, their variability, their

migration from one body part to another part, their abruptness, their brevity, and the repetitiveness, rather than randomness, of the particular body part affected by the movements (Fahn, 2005). Therefore, while tics have an element of stereotypy, this type of stereotypy, which can be considered paroxysmal, intermittent, or at most continual (meaning with interruptions), needs to be distinguished from continuous (uninterrupted) involuntary movements that repeat unceasingly. The latter type of continuous stereotypy is what distinguishes the disorders known as stereotypies and is the hallmark of abnormal movements in patients with classic tardive dyskinesia, which is called tardive stereotypy (Jankovic, 2005), the most common type of stereotypy seen in movement disorder clinics.

*Compulsions* are repetitive, purposeless, usually complex movements that are seen in patients with OCD. They are associated with an irresistible urge to make the movement. Patients realize that they are making the movements in response to this "need to do so." In this respect, compulsions resemble tics and not stereotypies, which are not accompanied by any urge. In fact, some patients with Gilles de la Tourette syndrome also have OCD, and in this situation, it might be impossible to distinguish between tics and compulsions (Jankovic, 2001). Like stereotypies, compulsions could be carried out in a uniform repetitive fashion for long periods of time but at the expense of all other activities because compulsions may be impossible to stop. In contrast, stereotypies can usually be stopped on command, and the patient will have normal motor behavior until they start up again, usually as soon as the patient is no longer paying attention to the command.

*Gestures* are culturally developed, expressive, voluntary movements that are calculated to indicate a particular state of mind and that may also be used as a means of adding emphasis to oratory (Lees, 1985). *Mannerisms* are sets of movements that include gestures plus more peculiar and individualistic movements that are not considered as bothersome. Mannerisms can be considered to represent a type of motor signature that individualizes a person. Sometimes, mannerisms can be bizarre, and these could be considered tics or on the borderline with tics. Because gestures and mannerisms rarely continually repeat themselves, they would not likely be confused with stereotypies, but there may be problems at times distinguishing them from tics.

From this description, stereotypies can be divided into two phenomenologically distinct groups. One type is that in which the stereotypy, although repetitive for prolonged periods, occurs intermittently, normal motor activity being the general background. It is this type that can be difficult to distinguish from tics and compulsions. The second type is that in which the repetitive movements are virtually always there, with less time spent without them. The most common of this type of continuous stereotypy is that of classic *tardive dyskinesia*. The movements that are seen in classic tardive dyskinesia are rhythmic and continuously repetitive complex chewing movements (oral-buccal-lingual dyskinesia) (see Video 1-73). Often, this tardive stereotypy will appear in the same patient together with different motor phenomena that make up the tardive dyskinesia syndromes (see Chapter 20), namely, dystonia (tardive dystonia), and akathisia (tardive akathisia). All are secondary to exposure to dopamine receptor–blocking drugs.

## Tics

*Tics* consist of abnormal movements (motor tics) or abnormal sounds (phonic tics). When both types of tics are present, the designation of *Gilles de la Tourette syndrome* or *Tourette syndrome* is commonly applied (see Chapter 17). Tics frequently vary in severity over time and can have remissions and exacerbations.

Motor and phonic tics can be simple or complex and occur abruptly for brief moments from a background of normal motor activity. Thus, they are paroxysmal in occurrence unless they are so severe as to be continual. A single simple motor tic may be impossible to distinguish from a myoclonic or choreic jerk; each of these would be an abrupt, sudden, isolated movement. Examples include a shoulder shrug, head jerk, blink, dart of the eyes, and twitch of the nose. Most of the time, such simple tics are repetitive, such as a run of eye blinking or a sequence of several simple tics in a row. In this pattern, tics can be easily distinguished from the other hyperkinesias. Even when tics are simple jerks, more complex forms of tics may also be present in the same patient, allowing one to establish the diagnosis by "the company it keeps." One type of simple tic is quite distinct, namely, ocular (Video 1-78). A single eye movement is not a feature of chorea or myoclonus but is common in tics (Frankel and Cummings, 1984).

Complex motor tics are very distinct, consisting of coordinated patterns of sequential movements that can appear in different parts of the body (Video 1-79) and are not necessarily identical from occurrence to occurrence in the same body part. Examples of complex tics include such acts as touching the nose, touching other people, head shaking with shoulder shrugging, kicking the legs, and jumping. Obscene gesturing (copropraxia) is another example.

Like akathitic movements, tics are usually preceded by an uncomfortable feeling or sensory urge that is relieved by carrying out the movement, like "scratching an itch." Thus, the movements and sounds can be considered "unvoluntary." Unless very severe, tics can be voluntarily suppressed for various periods of time. But when they are suppressed, inner tension builds up and is relieved only by an increased burst of more tics (Video 1-80).

In addition to being as rapid as myoclonic jerks, tics can be sustained contractions, resembling dystonic movements (Video 1-81). The complex sequential pattern of muscular contractions in dystonic tics makes the diagnosis obvious in most cases. Moreover, torsion dystonia is a continual hyperkinesia, whereas tics are paroxysmal bursts of varying duration.

Involuntary ocular movements can be an important feature for differentiation of tics from other dyskinesias. Whether a brief jerk of the eyes or more sustained eye deviation, ocular movements can occur as a manifestation of tics (see Video 1-78). Very few other dyskinesias involve ocular movements. The exceptions are opsoclonus (dancing eyes) (see Video 1-65), which is a form of myoclonus; ocular myoclonus (rhythmic vertical oscillations at a rate of 2 Hz) (see Video 1-64) that often accompanies palatal myoclonus; ocular myorhythmia, a slow horizontal oscillation (see Video 1-69); and oculogyric crisis (a sustained deviation of the eyes) (see Video 1-50) associated with dopamine receptor–blocking drugs or as a consequence of encephalitis lethargica or other parkinsonian disorders such as neuronal intranuclear hyaline inclusion disease and aromatic amino acid decarboxylase deficiency. See the discussion of oculogyric crises under "Dystonia" earlier in this chapter.

Phonic tics can range from simple throat-clearing sounds or grunts to complex verbalizations and the utterance of obscenities (coprolalia). Sniffing can also be a phonic tic, involving nasal passages rather than the vocal apparatus. Like motor tics, phonic tics can be divided into simple and complex tics. Throat-clearing and sniffing represent simple phonic tics, whereas verbalizations are considered complex phonic tics.

Involuntary phonations occur in only a few other neurologic disorders beside tics. These include the moaning in akathisia and in parkinsonism; the brief sounds in oromandibular dystonia and Huntington disease; and the sniffing, spitting, groaning, or singing that is occasionally encountered in Huntington disease and neuroacanthocytosis.

## Tremor

*Tremor* is an oscillatory, typically rhythmic and regular movement that affects one or more body parts, such as the limbs, neck, tongue, chin, or vocal cords. Jerky, irregular "tremor" is usually a manifestation of myoclonus. Tremor is produced by rhythmic alternating or simultaneous contractions of agonists and antagonists. The rate, location, amplitude, and constancy vary depending on the specific type of tremor and its severity. It is helpful to determine whether the tremor is present at rest (with the patient sitting or lying in repose) (Video 1-82), with posture-holding (with the arms or legs extended in front of the body) (Video 1-83), with action (such as writing or pouring water) (see Video 1-83), or with intention maneuvers (such as bringing the finger to touch the nose) (Video 1-84). Tremors can then be classified as tremor at rest, postural tremor, action tremor, or intention tremor, respectively. Some tremors may be present only during a specific task (such as writing) or with a specific posture, such as standing, as in orthostatic tremor (Video 1-85). These are called task-specific and position-specific tremors, respectively, and may overlap with task-specific and position-specific action dystonias, which may also appear as tremors (dystonic tremor) (Video 1-86). Etiologies and treatment of tremors differ according to the type of tremor phenomenology (see Chapter 19). A combination of rest tremor and a worse action and intention tremor is often a manifestation of a lesion in the midbrain (Video 1-87), commonly mislabeled as "rubral" tremor, but is more appropriately called midbrain tremor and due to involvement of both the nigrostriatal and dentato-rubro-thalamic pathways. It is important to realize that any tremor, especially wing beating and other unusual tremors, can be a manifestation of Wilson disease (Videos 1-88 and 1-89).

## THE CLINICAL APPROACH TO DIFFERENTIATE THE DYSKINESIAS

The process by which one distinguishes one type of dyskinesia from the others is by characterizing the type of abnormal movements that are present and then determining which dyskinesia definition most appropriately encompasses the overall picture and, at the same time, eliminating the dyskinesias that fail to fit. One performs this process in a hierarchic manner, first considering the immediately obvious clinical features

**Box 1-5** The clinical approaches to recognizing the various dyskinesias

**Level A: Immediate Impressions**
Rhythmic versus arrhythmic (see Box 1-6)
Sustained versus nonsustained (see Box 1-7)
Paroxysmal versus continual versus continuous (*continual* means over and over again; *continuous* means without stopping
  or unbroken) (see Box 1-8)
Sleep versus awake (see Box 1-9)

**Level B: More Prolonged Observations**
At rest versus with action (see Box 1-10)
Patterned versus nonpatterned (see Box 1-11)
Combinations of varieties of movements (see Box 1-12)

**Level C: Features Requiring Longer Observation (See Box 1-13)**
Speed: slow versus fast
Amplitude: ballistic versus not ballistic
Force: powerful (painful) versus easy to overcome
Suppressibility
Vocalizations
Self-mutilation
Complexity of movements
Sensory component

　　Level A has four equal factors, and each has its own table dividing movement disorders into those that fit these factors: rhythmicity (Box 1-6), duration of the contractions (Box 1-7), continuity of the contractions (Box 1-8), and their appearance with sleep or when awake (Box 1-9). The second level (Level B), taking a slightly longer period of observation, has three factors. The first is evaluating whether the movements occur when the affected body part is at rest, in a voluntary action, or both (Box 1-10). Box 1-10 lists those movement disorders that are present when the affected body part is at rest and disappear with action, appear only with action, or are present both at rest and continue with action. The term *action* refers to the presence of the movements when the affected body part is performing a voluntary movement. In the action category are task-specific and posture-specific dyskinesias. Box 1-11 considers whether the movements keep involving the same set of muscles recurring in a repetitive manner (patterned) rather than randomly to involve different muscle groups. Box 1-12 lists disorders in which there are commonly combinations of various dyskinesias,

　　The third level (Level C), taking still longer periods of observation, evaluates many factors: speed, amplitude, force, suppressibility, presence of vocalizations, presence of self-mutilation, complexity of the movements, and whether there are associated sensory symptoms (Box 1-13).

**Box 1-6** Differential diagnosis of rhythmic and arrhythmic hyperkinesias

| **Rhythmic** | **Arrhythmic** |
|---|---|
| Tremor | Akathitic movements |
| 　resting | Athetosis |
| 　postural | Ballism |
| 　action | Chorea |
| 　intention | Dystonia* |
| Dystonic tremor* | Hemifacial spasm |
| Dystonic myorhythmia* | Hyperekplexia |
| Myoclonus, segmental* | Arrhythmic myoclonus |
| Epilepsia partialis continua | Stereotypy* |
| Myoclonus, oscillatory | Tics |
| Moving toes/fingers | |
| Myorhythmia* | |
| Periodic movements in sleep | |
| Tardive dyskinesia (tardive stereotypy)* | |

*Any apparent incongruity of some dyskinesias appearing on both columns has been explained in the definitions of the different dyskinesias. Dystonia often, but not always, has repetitive movements, which were termed *myorhythmia* by Herz (1931, 1944) and are now labeled *dystonic tremor* and *patterned movements*. Today, the term *myorhythmia* refers to the slow, rhythmic movements that are most classically seen in Whipple disease. Segmental myoclonus is typically rhythmic, whereas other forms of myoclonus are arrhythmic. Stereotypies can occur at irregular intervals, and these are listed in the first column. In contrast, classic tardive dyskinesia movements are continuous, and these stereotypies are listed in the second column.

Box 1-7 Differential diagnosis of sustained hyperkinesias

| Sustained Contractions or Postures | Nonsustained Contractions |
| --- | --- |
| Rigidity | All others |
| Dystonia | |
| Oculogyric crisis | |
| Paroxysmal dystonia | |
| Dystonic tics | |
| Sandifer syndrome | |
| Stiff-person syndrome | |
| Neuromyotonia | |
| Congenital torticollis | |
| Orthopedic torticollis | |

(Level A) and proceeding to the next two lower levels in order, each taking longer periods of observation (see Box 1-5).

Boxes 1-5 to 1-13 are intended to assist the clinician in establishing the correct dyskinesia or syndrome. Once this has been accomplished, it is then the clinician's task to determine the correct etiology that has produced this dyskinesia. The chapters describing the details of each motor phenomenology also describe the authors' approach for evaluating patients to determine their etiologies and treatments.

## CONCLUSIONS

Working definitions and clinical characteristics of the movement disorders have been presented. Electrophysiologic recordings are adding to the definitions presented, but they must be compatible with the clinical definitions that have been in use for decades. There are nine predominant movement disorders: akinesia/bradykinesia; rhythmic tremor; the sustained contractions of dystonia (athetosis); three types of usually fast movements—myoclonus, chorea (ballism), and tics; stereotypies (compulsions); paroxysmal dyskinesias; and asynergia (ataxia). The others are less common. The pathophysiology of movement disorders is beginning to be understood. Many appear to involve the dopamine system and the basal ganglia, such as too little dopaminergic activity (parkinsonian rigidity and tremor) or too much (chorea, ballism, and tardive dyskinesia). It is hoped that much more knowledge will be gained to provide a better understanding of these disorders, but the first task of the clinician is to recognize the characteristics of the movement disorder in order to decide on the clinical syndrome that the patient presents. The next task is to unravel the etiologic diagnosis to provide information on genetics, prognosis, and treatment.

Box 1-8 Differential diagnosis of paroxysmal and nonparoxysmal hyperkinesias

| Paroxysmal | Continual* | Continuous* |
| --- | --- | --- |
| Tics | Ballism | Abdominal dyskinesias |
| PKD | Chorea | Athetosis |
| PNKD | Dystonic movements | Tremors |
| PED | Myoclonus, arrhythmic | Dystonic postures |
| Paroxysmal ataxia | Some stereotypies | Myoclonus, rhythmic |
| Paroxysmal tremor | Akathitic moaning | Tardive stereotypy[†] |
| Hypnogenic dystonia | | Myokymia |
| Stereotypies | | Tic status[†] |
| Akathitic movements | | |
| Jumpy stumps | | |
| Moving toes | | |
| Myorhythmia | | |

*Continual means over and over again; continuous means without stopping or unbroken.
[†]Tic status refers to the rare episodes in which tics become so severe that they do not stop. Stereotypy and tardive stereotypy (classic tardive dyskinesia) are distinguished in Box 1-6.
PED, paroxysmal exertional dyskinesia; PKD, paroxysmal kinesigenic dyskinesia; PNKD, paroxysmal nonkinesigenic dyskinesia.

Box 1-9 Differential diagnosis of hyperkinesias that are present while asleep or awake

| Appears during Sleep and Disappears When Awakened | Persists during Sleep | Diminishes during Sleep |
|---|---|---|
| Hypnogenic dyskinesias | Secondary palatal myoclonus | All others |
| Periodic movements in sleep | Ocular myoclonus | |
| | Oculofaciomasticatory myorhythmia | |
| | Moving toes | |
| | Myokymia | |
| | Neuromyotonia (Isaacs syndrome) | |

Box 1-10 Differential diagnosis of hyperkinesias that are present at rest or with action

| At Rest Only (Disappears with Action) | With Action Only | At Rest and Continues with Action |
|---|---|---|
| Akathitic movements | Ataxia | Abdominal dyskinesias |
| Paradoxical dystonia* | Action dystonia | Athetosis |
| Resting tremor | Action myoclonus | Ballism |
| Restless legs | Orthostatic tremor* | Chorea |
| Orthostatic tremor (only on standing) | Tremor: postural, action, intention | Dystonia* |
| | Task-specific tremor | Jumpy stumps |
| | Task-specific dystonia | Minipolymyoclonus |
| | | Moving toes/fingers |
| | | Myoclonus* |
| | | Myokymia |
| | | Pseudodystonias* |
| | | Tics |

*Paradoxical dystonia refers to dystonia that is present only at rest and disappears with action (Fahn, 1989); orthostatic tremor is tremor of the thighs and legs (spreading to the trunk) that occurs only on prolonged standing and disappears with walking or sitting; most dystonias and myoclonias that are present at rest are also present and often worse with action as well; pseudodystonias refer to neuromyotonia and other causes of stiff muscles or postures that are not due to dystonia (common causes are orthopedic deformities and pain).

Box 1-11 Patterned and nonpatterned movements

| Patterned (Same Muscle Groups) | Nonpatterned |
|---|---|
| Abdominal dyskinesias | All others |
| Dystonia | |
| Hemifacial spasm | |
| Moving toes/fingers | |
| Segmental myoclonus | |
| Myorhythmia | |
| Myokymia | |
| Tardive stereotypy | |
| Tremor | |

Box 1-12 Combinations of varieties of movements

| Movements |
|---|
| Psychogenic movement disorders |
| Tardive syndromes |
| Neuroacanthocytosis |
| Wilson disease |
| Huntington disease |
| DRPLA |
| Dystonia* |

*Patients with dystonia can have additional dyskinesias that are part of the spectrum of classic torsion dystonia (see the text discussion of dystonia). These include tremor, myoclonus, and choreic-like movements. Dystonia-plus syndromes can have features of parkinsonism or myoclonus in addition to dystonia.

Box 1-13  Clinical features requiring longer observation time

| SPEED*: | *Fastest* | *Intermediate* | *Slowest* |
|---|---|---|---|
| | Minipolymyoclonus | Chorea | Athetosis |
| | Myoclonus | Ballism | Moving toes/fingers |
| | Hyperekplexia | Jumpy stumps | Myorhythmia |
| | Hemifacial spasm | Tremors | Akathitic movements |
| | | Tardive stereotypy | |
| | | | |
| AMPLITUDE: | *Ballistic* | *Not Ballistic* | *Very Small* |
| | Ballism | Chorea and all others | Minipolymyoclonus |
| | Jumpy stumps would ballistic, but a short stump keeps the amplitude relatively small | | |
| | | | |
| FORCE: | *Powerful* | *Intermediate* | *Easy to Overcome* |
| | Stiff-person | Dystonia | All others |
| | Jumpy stumps | | |

**SUPPRESSIBILITY**
Stereotypies > tics, akathitic movements > chorea > ballism > dystonia > tremor > moving toes
Not suppressible: hemifacial spasm, myoclonus, hyperekplexia, myorhythmia, moving toes

**VOCALIZATIONS**
Vocal tics: simple or complex
Akathisia: moaning
Huntington disease
Neuroacanthocytosis
Cranial dystonia

**SELF-MUTILATION**
Lesch-Nyhan syndrome
Neuroacanthocytosis
Tourette syndrome
Psychogenic movement disorders

**COMPLEX MOVEMENTS†**
Tics
Akathitic movements
Compulsions
Stereotypies
Psychogenic movements

**SENSORY COMPONENT**
Akathisia
Moving toes, painful legs
Restless legs
Tics

**OCULAR MOVEMENTS**
Tics
Oculogyric crises
Opsoclonus
Ocular myoclonus
Ocular myorhythmia
Ocular dysmetria
Nystagmus

*Tics and dystonic movements can be of all speeds.
†Each of these can also consist of simple movements.

## References

Abbas N, Lucking CB, Ricard S, et al: A wide variety of mutations in the parkin gene are responsible for autosomal recessive parkinsonism in Europe. Hum Mol Genet 1999;8:567–574.

Achiron A, Ziv I, Goren M, et al: Primary progressive freezing gait. Mov Disord 1993;8:293–297.

Adams RD, Foley J: The neurological disorder associated with liver disease. Res Publ Assoc Nerv Ment Dis 1953;32:198–231.

Adams RD, van Bogaert L, van der Eecken H: Striato-nigral degeneration. J Neuropathol Exp Neurol 1964;23:584–608.

Aharon-Peretz J, Rosenbaum H, Gershoni-Baruch R: Mutations in the glucocerebrosidase gene and Parkinson's disease in Ashkenazi Jews. N Engl J Med 2004;351(19):1972–1977.

Allen N, Knopp W: Hereditary parkinsonism-dystonia with sustained control by L-dopa and anticholinergic medication. Adv Neurol 1976;14:201–213.

Almasy L, Bressman SB, Raymond D, et al: Idiopathic torsion dystonia linked to chromosome 8 in two Mennonite families. Ann Neurol 1997;42:670–673.

Alzheimer A: Über de Anatomische Grundlage der Huntingtonschen Chorea und der choreatisch Bewungen überhaupt. Z Gesamte Neurol Psychiatr 1911;3:566–567.

Ambrose HJ, Byrd PJ, McConville CM, et al: Physical map across chromosome 11q22–q23 containing the major locus for ataxia telangiectasia. Genomics 1994;21:612–619.

Amir RE, Vanden-Veyver IB, Wan M, et al: Rett syndrome is caused by mutations in X-linked MECP2, encoding methyl-CpG-binding protein 2. Nat Genet 1999;23:185–188.

Andermann F, Andermann E: Excessive startle syndromes: Startle disease, jumping, and startle epilepsy. Adv Neurol 1986;43:321–338.

Andermann F, Cosgrove JBR, Lloyd-Smith DL, et al: Facial myokymia in multiple sclerosis. Brain 1961;84:31–44.

Andrews CJ: Influence of dystonia on the response to long-term L-dopa therapy in Parkinson's disease. J Neurol Neurosurg Psychiatry 1973;36:630–636.

Aronson AE: Clinical Voice Disorders. New York, Thieme, 1985.

Atchison PR, Thompson PD, Frackowiak RSJ, Marsden CD: The syndrome of gait ignition failure: A report of six cases. Mov Disord 1993;8:285–292.

Auburger G, Ratzlaff T, Lunkes A, et al: A gene for autosomal dominant paroxysmal choreoathetosis spasticity (CSE) maps to the vicinity of a potassium channel gene cluster on chromosome 1p, probably within 2 cM between D1S443 and D1S197. Genomics 1996;31:90–94.

Auger RG, Whisnant JP: Hemifacial spasm in Rochester and Olmsted County, Minnesota, 1960 to 1984. Arch Neurol 1990;47:1233–1234.

Auranen M, Vanhala R, Vosman M, et al: MECP2 gene analysis in classical Rett syndrome and in patients with Rett-like features. Neurology 2001;56:611–617.

Azher SN, Jankovic J: Camptocormia: Pathogenesis, classification, and response to therapy. Neurology 2005;65(3):355–369.

Bain PG, Findley LJ, Atchison P, et al: Assessing tremor severity. J Neurol Neurosurg Psychiatry 1993;56:868–873.

Baker M, Litvan I, Houlden H, et al: Association of an extended haplotype in the tau gene with progressive supranuclear palsy. Hum Mol Genet 1999;8:711–715.

Banfi S, Servadio A, Chung MY, et al: Identification and characterization of the gene causing type 1 spinocerebellar ataxia. Nat Genet 1994;7:513–520.

Bassi MT, Bresolin N, Tonelli A, et al: A novel mutation in the ATP1A2 gene causes alternating hemiplegia of childhood. J Med Genet 2004;41(8):621–628.

Batten FE: Cerebral degeneration with symmetrical changes in the manulae in two members of a family. Trans Ophthalmol Soc UK 1903;23:386–390.

Beard GM: Remarks on jumpers or jumping Frenchmen. J Nerv Ment Dis 1878;5:526.

Bell C. Description of writers' cramp. (Attributed by Gowers [1893].)

Benedikt M: Tremblement avec paralysie croisee du moteur oculaire commun. Bull Med 1889;3:547–548. English translation published in Wolf JK: The Classical Brain Stem Syndromes, Springfield, Ill, Charles C Thomas, 1971, pp 103–109.

Bennett LB, Roach ES, Bowcock AM: A locus for paroxysmal kinesigenic dyskinesia maps to human chromosome 16. Neurology 2000;54:125–130.

Bentivoglio AR, Cortelli P, Valente EM, et al: Phenotypic characterisation of autosomal recessive PARK6-linked parkinsonism in three unrelated Italian families. Mov Disord 2001;16:999–1006.

Ben-Zeev B, Yaron Y, Schanen NC, et al: Rett syndrome: Clinical manifestations in males with MECP2 mutations. J Child Neurol 2002;17(1):20–24.

Bertini E, des Portes V, Zanni G, et al: X-linked congenital ataxia: A clinical and genetic study. Amer J Med Genet 2000;92:53–56.

Bhatia KP, Bhatt MH, Marsden CD: The causalgia-dystonia syndrome. Brain 1993;116:843–851.

Blum P, Jankovic J. Stiff-person syndrome: An autoimmune disease. Mov Disord 1991;6:12–20.

Boeve BF, Rummans TA, Philbrick KL, Callahan MJ: Electrocardiographic and echocardiographic changes associated with malignant catatonia. Mayo Clin Proc 1994;69:645–650.

Bonifati V, Rizzu P, van Baren MJ, et al: Mutations in the DJ-1 gene associated with autosomal recessive early-onset parkinsonism. Science 2003;299(5604):256–259.

Breedveld GJ, Percy AK, MacDonald ME, et al: Clinical and genetic heterogeneity in benign hereditary chorea. Neurology 2002;59(4):579–584.

Bressman S, Fahn S, Eisenberg M, et al: Biotin-responsive encephalopathy with myoclonus, ataxia, and seizures. Adv Neurol 1986;43:119–125.

Brkanac Z, Bylenok L, Fernandez M, et al: A new dominant spinocerebellar ataxia linked to chromosome 19q13.4-qter. Arch Neurol 2002a;59(8):1291–1295.

Brkanac Z, Fernandez M, Matsushita M, et al: Autosomal dominant sensory/motor neuropathy with ataxia (SMNA): Linkage to chromosome 7q22–q32. Amer J Med Genet 2002b;114(4):450–457.

Brodsky H, Vuong KD, Thomas M, Jankovic J: Glabellar and palmomental reflexes in parkinsonian disorders. Neurology 2004;63:1096–1098.

Brooks BP, Fischbeck KH: Spinal and bulbar muscular atrophy: A trinucleotide-repeat expansion neurodegenerative disease. Trends Neurosci 1995;18:459–461.

Brown P, Day BL, Rothwell JC, et al: Intrahemispheric and interhemispheric spread of cerebral cortical myoclonic activity and its relevance to epilepsy. Brain 1991a;114:2333–2351.

Brown P, Rothwell JC, Thompson PD, et al: The hyperekplexias and their relationship to the normal startle reflex. Brain 1991b;114:1903–1928.

Brown P, Thompson PD, Rothwell JC, et al: Axial myoclonus of propriospinal origin. Brain 1991c;114:197–214.

Browne DL, Gancher ST, Nutt TG, et al: Episodic ataxia/myokymia syndrome is associated with point mutations in the human potassium channel gene, KCNA1. Nat Genet 1994;8:136–140.

Bugiani O, Murrell JR, Giaccone G, et al: Frontotemporal dementia and corticobasal degeneration in a family with a P301S mutation in tau. J Neuropathol Exp Neurol 1999;58:667–677.

Bull PC, Thomas GR, Rommens JM, et al: The Wilson disease gene is a putative copper transporting P-type ATPase similar to the Menkes gene. Nat Genet 1993;5:327–337.

Burk K, Zuhlke C, Konig IR, et al: Spinocerebellar ataxia type 5: Clinical and molecular genetic features of a German kindred. Neurology 2004;62(2):327–329.

Burke RE, Fahn S, Jankovic J, et al: Tardive dystonia: Late-onset and persistent dystonia caused by antipsychotic drugs. Neurology 1982;32:1335–1346.

Burke RE, Fahn S, Marsden CD, et al: Validity and reliability of a rating scale for the primary torsion dystonias. Neurology 1985;35: 73–77.

Bush G, Fink M, Petrides G, et al: Catatonia: I. Rating scale and standardized examination. Acta Psychiatr Scand 1996;93:129–136.

Caine ED, McBride MC, Chiverton P, et al: Tourette's syndrome in Monroe County school children. Neurology 1988;38:472–475.

Carelli V, Ghelli A, Bucchi L, et al: Biochemical features of mtDNA 14484 (ND6/M64V) point mutation associated with Leber's hereditary optic neuropathy. Ann Neurol 1999;45:320–328.

Carmichael EA, Green FHK: Parkinsonian rigidity: A clinical and instrumental study of the effects of stramonium, hyoscine and other alkaloids. Quart J Med 1928;22:51.

Castillo J, Martinez F, Gonzalez-Quintela A, Noya M: Historical description of primary writer's tremor. J Neurol Neurosurg Psychiatry 1993;56:1275.

Chan EM, Bulman DE, Paterson AD, et al: Genetic mapping of a new Lafora progressive myoclonus epilepsy locus (EPM2B) on 6p22. J Med Genet. 2003a;40(9):671–675.

Chan EM, Young EJ, Ianzano L, et al: Mutations in NHLRC1 cause progressive myoclonus epilepsy. Nat Genet. 2003b;35(2):125–127.

Chang YT, Sharma R, Marsh JL, et al: Levodopa-responsive aromatic L-amino acid decarboxylase deficiency. Ann Neurol 2004;55(3): 435–438.

Chen DH, Brkanac Z, Verlinde CLMJ, et al: Missense mutations in the regulatory domain of PKC gamma: A new mechanism for dominant nonepisodic cerebellar ataxia. Amer J Hum Genet 2003; 72(4):839–849.

Christodoulou K, Deymeer F, Serdaroglu P, et al: Mapping of the second Friedreich's ataxia (FRDA2) locus to chromosome 9p23–p11: Evidence for further locus heterogeneity. Neurogenetics. 2001; 3(3):127–132.

Chung MY, Lu YC, Cheng NC, Soong BW: A novel autosomal dominant spinocerebellar ataxia (SCA22) linked to chromosome 1p21–q23. Brain 2003;126(Pt 6):1293–1299.

Clark LN, Nicolai A, Afridi S, et al: Pilot association study of the beta-glucocerebrosidase N370S allele and Parkinson's disease in subjects of Jewish ethnicity. Mov Disord 2005;20(1):100–103.

Clarke CE: Does levodopa therapy delay death in Parkinson's disease? A review of the evidence. Mov Disord 1995;10:250–256.

Cohen O, Pullman S, Jurewicz E, et al: Rest tremor in patients with essential tremor: Prevalence, clinical correlates, and electrophysiologic characteristics. Arch Neurol 2003;60(3):405–410.

Coleman RM, Pollak CP, Weitzman ED: Periodic movements in sleep (nocturnal myoclonus): relation to sleep disorders. Ann Neurol 1980;8:416–421.

Comella CL, Leurgans S, Wuu J: Rating scales for dystonia: A multicenter assessment. Mov Disord 2003;18(3):303–312.

Comings DE, Himes JA, Comings BG: An epidemiologic study of Tourette's syndrome in a single school district. J Clin Psychiatry 1990;51:463–469.

Couper J: On the effects of black oxide of manganese when inhaled into the lungs. Brit Ann Med Pharm 1837;1:41–43.

Creutzfeldt HG: Ueber eine eigenartige herdfoerimge Errnakumg des Zentralnervensystems. Z Gesamte Neurol Psychiatr 1920;57:1–19.

Cuker A, State MW, King RA, et al: Candidate locus for Gilles de la Tourette syndrome/obsessive compulsive disorder/chronic tic disorder at 18q22. Am J Med Genet Part A 2004;130A(1):37–39.

Curtis ARJ, Fey C, Morris CM, et al: Mutation in the gene encoding ferritin light polypeptide causes dominant adult-onset basal ganglia disease. Nat Genet 2001;28:345–349.

Dana CL: Hereditary tremor, a hitherto undescribed form of motor neurosis. Amer J Med Sci 1887;94:386–393.

Danek A, Rubio JP, Rampoldi L, et al: McLeod neuroacanthocytosis: Genotype and phenotype. Ann Neurol 2001;50:755–764.

Das AK, Becerra CHR, Yi W, et al: Molecular genetics of palmitoyl-protein thioesterase deficiency in the U.S. J Clin Invest 1998; 102:361–370.

Date H, Onodera O, Tanaka H, et al: Early-onset ataxia with ocular motor apraxia and hypoalbuminemia is caused by mutations in a new HIT superfamily gene. Nat Genet 2001;29:184–188.

David G, Abbas N, Coullin P, et al: The gene for autosomal dominant cerebellar ataxia type II is located in a 5-cM region in 3p12–p13: Genetic and physical mapping of the SCA7 locus. Am J Hum Genet 1996;59:1328–1336.

David G, Abbas N, Stevanin G, et al: Cloning of the SCA7 gene reveals a highly unstable CAG repeat expansion. Nat Genet 1997;17:65–70.

Davidenkow S: Auf hereditar-abiotrophischer Grundlage akut auftretende, regressierende und episodische Erkrankungen des Nervensystems und Bemerkungen uber die familiare subakute, myoklonische Dystonie. Z Gesamte Neurol Psychiatr 1926;104: 596–622.

De Carvalho Aguiar P, Sweadner KJ, Penniston JT, et al: Mutations in the Na(+)/K(+)-ATPase alpha3 gene ATP1A3 are associated with rapid-onset dystonia parkinsonism. Neuron 2004;43(2): 169–175.

De Coo IFM, Renier WO, Ruitenbeek W, et al: A 4–base pair deletion in the mitochondrial cytochrome b gene associated with parkinsonism/MELAS overlap syndrome. Ann Neurol 1999;45:130–133.

Defazio G, Livrea P, De Salvia R, et al: Prevalence of primary blepharospasm in a community of Puglia region, Southern Italy. Neurology 2001;56:1579–1581.

Dejerine J, Thomas A: L'atrophie olivo-ponto-cerebelleuse. Nouv Iconogr Salpetriere 1900;13:330–370.

Delague V, Bareil C, Bouvagnet P, et al: Nonprogressive autosomal recessive ataxia maps to chromosome 9q34– 9qter in a large consanguineous Lebanese family. Ann Neurol 2001;50:250–253.

de Lau LM, Breteler MM: Epidemiology of Parkinson's disease. Lancet Neurol 2006;5:525–535.

Delay J, Denniker P: Drug-induced extrapyramidal syndromes. In Vinken PJ, Bruyn GW (eds): Handbook of Clinical Neurology: Diseases of the Basal Ganglia, vol 6. Amsterdam, North-Holland, 1968, pp 248–266.

De Lisi L: Su di un fenomeno motorio costante del sonno normale: Le mioclonie ipniche fisiologiche. Riv Pat Nerv Ment 1932;39:481–496.

Delisle MB, Murrell JR, Richardson R, et al: A mutation at codon 279 (N279K) in exon 10 of the tau gene causes a tauopathy with dementia and supranuclear palsy. Acta Neuropathol 1999;98:62–77.

Denny-Brown D: The Basal Ganglia and their Relation to Disorders of Movement. London, Oxford University Press, 1962.

Denny-Brown D, Foley JM: Myokymia and the benign fasciculations of muscular cramps. Trans Assoc Am Physicians 1948;61:88–96.

Desautels A, Turecki G, Montplaisir J, et al: Identification of a major susceptibility locus for restless legs. Am J Hum Genet 2001;69: 1266–1270.

Deuschl G, Mischke G, Schenck E, et al: Symptomatic and essential rhythmic palatal myoclonus. Brain 1990;113:1645–1672.

De Vries BBA, Arts WFM, Breedveld GJ, et al: Benign hereditary chorea of early onset maps to chromosome 14q. Am J Hum Genet 2000;66:136–142.

Dobson-Stone C, Danek A, Rampoldi L, et al: Mutational spectrum of the CHAC gene in patients with chorea-acanthocytosis. Eur J Human Genet 2002;10(11):773–781.

Dobson-Stone C, Velayos-Baeza A, Filippone LA, et al: Chorein detection for the diagnosis of chorea-acanthocytosis. Ann Neurol 2004;56(2):299–302.

Dressler D, Thompson PD, Gledhill RF, Marsden CD: The syndrome of painful legs and moving toes. Mov Disord 1994;9:13–21.

Dwork AJ, Balmaceda C, Fazzini EA, et al: Dominantly inherited, early-onset parkinsonism: Neuropathology of a new form. Neurology 1993;43:69–74.

Dyken P, Kolar O: Dancing eyes, dancing feet: Infantile polymyoclonia. Brain 1968;91:305–320.

Ekbom KA: Restless legs syndrome. Neurology 1960;10:868–873.

England AC, Schwab RS: Postoperative evaluation of 26 selected patients with Parkinson's disease. J Am Geriat Soc 1956;4:1219–1232.

Fabbrini G, Brancati F, Vacca L, et al: A novel family with an unusual early-onset generalized dystonia. Mov Disord 2005;20(1):81–86.

Fahn S: Tardive dyskinesia and akathisia. N Engl J Med 1978; 299:202–203.

Fahn S: Clinical aspects and treatment of rigidity and dystonia. In Benecke R, Conrad B, Marsden CD (eds): Motor Disturbances, vol 1. London, Academic Press, 1987, pp 101–110.

Fahn S: Clinical variants of idiopathic torsion dystonia. J Neurol Neurosurg Psychiatry 1989;Suppl:96–100.

Fahn S: Akinesia. In Berardelli A, Benecke R, Manfredi M, Marsden CD (eds): Motor Disturbances, vol 2. London, Academic Press, 1990, pp 141–150.

Fahn S: Parkinson's disease and other basal ganglion disorders. In Asbury AK, McKhann GM, McDonald WI (eds): Diseases of the Nervous System. Clinical Neurobiology, 2nd ed. Philadelphia, W B Saunders, 1992, pp 1144–1158.

Fahn S: The freezing phenomenon in parkinsonism. In Fahn S, Hallett M, Lueders HO, Marsden CD (eds): Negative Motor Phenomena. New York, Lippincott-Raven, 1995, pp 53–63.

Fahn S: Motor and vocal tics. In Kurlan R (ed): Handbook of Tourette's Syndrome and Related Tic and Behavioral Disorders, 2nd ed. New York, Marcel Dekker, 2005, pp 1–14.

Fahn S, Brin MF, Dwork AJ, et al: Case 1, 1996: Rapidly progressive parkinsonism, incontinence, impotency, and levodopa-induced moaning in a patient with multiple myeloma. Mov Disord 1996;11:298–310.

Fahn S, Elton RL, Members of the UPDRS Development Committee: The Unified Parkinson's Disease Rating Scale. In Fahn S, Marsden CD, Calne DB, Goldstein M (eds): Recent Developments in Parkinson's Disease, vol 2. Florham Park, NJ, Macmillan Healthcare Information, 1987, pp. 153–163, 293–304.

Fahn S, Marsden CD, Calne DB: Classification and investigation of dystonia. In Marsden CD, Fahn S (eds): Movement Disorders 2. London: Butterworths, 1987, pp 332–358.

Fahn S, Singh N: An oscillating form of essential myoclonus. Neurology 1981;3(4, pt 2):80.

Fahn S, Tolosa E, Martin C: Clinical rating scale for tremor. In Jankovic J, Tolosa E (eds): Parkinson's Disease and Movement Disorders. Baltimore, Williams & Wilkins, 1993, pp 271–280.

Farrer M, Chan P, Chen R, et al: Lewy bodies and parkinsonism in families with parkin mutations. Ann Neurol 2001;50:293–300.

Fernandez M, Raskind W, Matsushita M, et al: Hereditary benign chorea: Clinical and genetic features of a distinct disease. Neurology 2001;57:106–110.

Fink JK, Hedera P, Mathay JG, Albin RL: Paroxysmal dystonic choreoathetosis linked to chromosome 2q: Clinical analysis and proposed pathophysiology. Neurology 1997;49:177–183.

Fink JK, Rainier S, Wilkowski J, et al: Paroxysmal dystonic choreoathetosis: Tight linkage to chromosome 2q. Am J Hum Genet 1996;59:140–145.

Fischer O: Zur Frage der anatomischen Grundlage der Athetose double und der posthemiplegischen Bewegungsstörung überhaupt. Z Gesamte Neurol Psychiatr 1911;7:463–486.

Fish DR, Marsden CD: Epilepsy masquerading as a movement disorder. In Marsden CD, Fahn S (eds): Movement Disorders, vol 3. Oxford, UK, Butterworth-Heinemann, 1994, pp 346–358.

Flanigan K, Gardner K, Alderson K, et al: Autosomal dominant spinocerebellar ataxia with sensory axonal neuropathy (SCA4): Clinical description and genetic localization to chromosome 16q22.1. Am J Hum Genet 1996;59:392–399.

Fleischhacker H: Afamiliare chronisch-progressive Erkrankung des mitteren Lebensalters vom Pseudosklerosetyp. Z Gesante Neurol Psychiatr 1924;91:1–22.

Ford B, Greene P, Fahn S: Oral and genital tardive pain syndromes. Neurology 1994;44:2115–2119.

Foster NL, Wilhelmsen K, Sima AAF, et al: Frontotemporal dementia and parkinsonism linked to chromosome 17: A consensus conference. Ann Neurol 1997;41:706–715.

Fouad GT, Servidei S, Durcan S, et al: A gene for familial paroxysmal dyskinesia (FPD1) maps to chromosome 2q. Am J Hum Genet 1996;59:135–139.

Frankel M, Cummings JL: Neuro-ophthalmic abnormalities in Tourette's syndrome: Functional and anatomic implications. Neurology 1984;34:359–361.

Friedberg G, Zoldan J, Weizman A, Melamed E: Parkinson psychosis rating scale: A practical instrument for grading psychosis in Parkinson's disease. Clin Neuropharmacol 1998;21: 280–284.

Friedman JH: Involuntary humming in autopsy-proven Parkinson's disease. Mov Disord 1993;8:401–402.

Friedman JH, Feinberg SS, Feldman RG: A neuroleptic malignantlike syndrome due to levodopa therapy withdrawal. JAMA 1985;254: 2792–2795.

Friedreich N: Neuropathologische Beobachtung beim paramyoklonus multiplex. Virchow's Arch Pathol Anat Physiol Klin Med 1881; 86:421–434.

Fujigasaki H, Verma IC, Camuzat A, et al: SCA12 is a rare locus for autosomal dominant cerebellar ataxia: A study of an Indian family. Ann Neurol 2001a;49:117–121.

Fujigasaki H, Martin JJ, De Deyn PP, et al: CAG repeat expansion in the TATA box-binding protein gene causes autosomal dominant cerebellar ataxia. Brain 2001b;124:1939–1947.

Fukuhara N, Tokiguchi S, Shirakawa K, Tsubaki T: Myoclonus epilepsy associated with ragged red fibers (mitochondrial abnormalities): Disease entity or a syndrome? J Neurol Sci 1980;47: 117–133.

Funata N, Maeda Y, Koike M, et al: Neuronal intranuclear hyaline inclusion disease: Report of a case and review of the literature. Clin Neuropathol 1990;9(2):89–96.

Funayama M, Hasegawa K, Kowa H, et al: A new locus for Parkinson's disease (PARK8) maps to chromosome 12p11.2–q13.1. Ann Neurol 2002;51(3):296–301.

Gambardella A, Annesi G, DeFusco M, et al: A new locus for autosomal dominant nocturnal frontal lobe epilepsy maps to chromosome 1. Neurology 2000;55:1467–1471.

Gasser T, Bressman S, Durr A, et al: Molecular diagnosis of inherited movement disorders: Movement disorders society task force on molecular diagnosis. Mov Disord 2003;18(1):3–18.

Gasser T, Mullermyhsok B, Wszolek ZK, et al: A susceptibility locus for Parkinson's disease maps to chromosome 2p13. Nat Genet 1998;18:262–265.

Gelenberg AJ: The catatonic syndrome. Lancet 1976;1:1339–1341.

Giladi N, Kao R, Fahn S: Freezing phenomenon in patients with parkinsonian syndromes. Mov Disord 1997;12:302–305.

Giladi N, McMahon D, Przedborski S, et al: Motor blocks in Parkinson's disease. Neurology 1992;42:333–339.

Gilles de la Tourette G: Etude sur une affection nerveuse caracterisee par de l'incoordination motrice accompagnee d'echolalie et de copralalie. Arch Neurol (Paris) 1885;9:19–42, 158–200.

Goetz CG, Stebbins GT, Chmura TA, et al: Teaching tape for the motor section of the Unified Parkinson's Disease Rating Scale. Mov Disord 1995;10:263–266.

Goetz CG, Stebbins GT, Shale HM, et al: Utility of an objective dyskinesia rating scale for Parkinson's disease: Interrater and intrarater reliability assessment. Mov Disord 1994;9:390–394.

Goker-Alpan O, Schiffmann R, LaMarca ME, et al: Parkinsonism among Gaucher disease carriers. J Med Genet 2004;41(12): 937–940.

Golbe LI: The epidemiology of PSP. J Neural Transm 1994; 42(suppl):263–273.

Goldsmith JB: The inheritance of "facial spasm" and the effect of a modifying factor associated with high temper. J Hered 1927; 18:185–187.

Goldstein JE, Cogan DG: Apraxia of lid-opening. Arch Ophthalmol 1965;73:155–159.

Gotoda T, Arita M, Arai H, et al: Adult-onset spinocerebellar dysfunction caused by a mutation in the gene for the α-tocopherol-transfer protein. N Engl J Med 1995;333:1313–1318.

Gowers WR: A Manual of Diseases of the Nervous System, vol 2, 2nd ed. Philadelphia, Blakiston, 1893, pp. 711 (attribution of description of writers' cramp to Charles Bell in 1830), 729 (description of musicians' cramps).

Graham JG, Oppenheimer DR: Orthostatic hypotension and nicotinic sensitivity in a case of multiple system atrophy. J Neurol Neurosurg Psychiatry 1969;32:28–34.

Grimes DA, Han F, Lang AE, et al: A novel locus for inherited myoclonus-dystonia on 18p11. Neurology 2002;59:1183–1186.

Grisolle A: Tratado de Patologia Interna. Vol. 6. De las neurosis. Madrid, Imprenta de Francisco Andres y Compania, 1848.

Grotzsch H, Pizzolato GP, Ghika J, et al: Neuropathology of a case of dopa-responsive dystonia associated with new genetic locus, DYT14. Neurology 2002;58:1839–1842.

Guerrini R, Bonanni P, Nardocci N, et al: Autosomal recessive rolandic epilepsy with paroxysmal exercise-induced dystonia and writer's cramp: Delineation of the syndrome and gene mapping to chromosome 16p12–11.2. Ann Neurol 1999;45:344–352.

Guillain G, Mollaret P: Deux cas de myoclonies synchrones et rythmées vélo-pharyngo-laryngo-oculo-diaphragmatiques: Le problème anatomique et physio-pathologique de ce syndrom. Rev Neurol 1931;2:545–566.

Guilleminault C, Gelb M: Clinical aspects and features of cataplexy. In Fahn S, Hallett MH, Lueders HO, Marsden CD (eds): Negative Motor Phenomena. New York, Lippincott-Raven, 1995, pp 65–77.

Gulcher JR, Jonsson D, Kong A, et al: Mapping of a familial essential tremor gene, FET1, to chromosome 3q13. Nat Genet 1997;17: 84–87.

Gydesen S, Brown JM, Brun A, et al: Chromosome 3 linked frontotemporal dementia (FTD-3). Neurology 2002;59(10):1585–1594.

Haerer AF, Anderson DW, Schoenberg BS: Prevalence of essential tremor: Results from the Copiah County study. Arch Neurol 1982;39:750–751.

Haerer AF, Currier RD, Jackson JF: Hereditary nonprogressive chorea of early onset. N Eng J Med 1967;276:1220–1224.

Hagerman RJ, Leavitt BR, Farzin F, et al: Fragile-X-associated tremor/ataxia syndrome (FXTAS) in females with the FMR1 premutation. Amer J Hum Genet 2004;74(5):1051–1056.

Hakim S, Adams RD: The special clinical problem of symptomatic hydrocephalus with normal cerebrospinal pressure: Observations on cerebrospinal fluid hydrodynamics. J Neurol Sci 1965;2: 307–327.

Hallervorden J, Spatz H: Eigenartige Erkrankung im extrapyramidalen System mit besonderer Beteiligung des Globus Pallidus und der Substantia nigra. Z Gesamte Neurol Psychiatr 1922;79:254–302.

Hallett M, Chadwick D, Adam J, Marsden CD: Reticular reflex myoclonus: A physiological type of human post hypoxic myoclonus. J Neurol Neurosurg Psychiatry 1977;40:253–264.

Hallett M, Chadwick D, Marsden CD: Cortical reflex myoclonus. Neurology 1979;29:1107–1125.

Hallett M, Fahn S, Jankovic J, et al (eds): Psychogenic Movement Disorders—Neurology and Neuropsychiatry, Lippincott Williams & Wilkins, Philadelphia, 2006.

Hammond WA: A Treatise on Diseases of the Nervous System. New York, Appleton, 1871.

Hampshire DJ, Roberts E, Crow Y, et al: Kufor-Rakeb syndrome, pallido-pyramidal degeneration with supranuclear upgaze paresis and dementia, maps to 1p36. J Med Genet 2001;38:680–682.

Harper PS: The epidemiology of Huntington's disease. Hum Genet 1992;89:365–376.

Harris JM, Fahn S: Genetics of movement disorders. In Rosenberg RN, Prusiner SB, DiMauro S, et al (eds): The Molecular and Genetic Basis of Neurologic and Psychiatric Disease, 3rd ed. Philadelphia, Butterworth-Heinemann, 2003, pp 351–368.

Hashida H, Goto J, Zhao ND, et al: Cloning and mapping of ZNF231, a novel brain-specific gene encoding neuronal double zinc finger protein whose expression is enhanced in a neurodegenerative disorder, multiple system atrophy (MSA). Genomics 1998;54:50–58.

Haskovec L: L'akathisie. Rev Neurol 1901;9:1107–1109.

Hauser RA, Deckers F, Lehert P: Parkinson's disease home diary: Further validation and implications for clinical trials. Mov Disord 2004;19(12):1409–1413.

Hausser-Hauw C, Roullet E, Robert R, Marteau R: Oculo-facio-skeletal myorhythmia as a cerebral complication of systemic Whipple's disease. Mov Disord 1988;3:179–184.

Hayflick SJ, Westaway SK, Levinson B, et al: Genetic, clinical and radiographic delineation of Hallervorden-Spatz syndrome. N Engl J Med 2003;348:33–40.

Hayman M, Harvey AS, Hopkins IJ, et al: Paroxysmal tonic upgaze: A reappraisal of outcome. Ann Neurol 1998;43:514–520.

Healy DG, Abou-Sleiman PM, Lees AJ, et al: Tau gene and Parkinson's disease: A case-control study and meta-analysis. J Neurol Neurosurg Psychiat 2004b;75(7):962–965.

Healy DG, Abou-Sleiman PM, Valente EM, et al: DJ-1 mutations in Parkinson's disease. J Neurol Neurosurg Psychiat 2004a;75(1): 144–145.

Heilman KM: Orthostatic tremor. Arch Neurol 1984;41:880–881.

Henderson VW, Wooten GF: Neuroleptic malignant syndrome: A pathogenetic role for dopamine receptor blockade. Neurology 1981;31:132–137.

Hening W, Walters A, Kavey N, et al: Dyskinesias while awake and periodic movements in sleep in restless legs syndrome: Treatment with opioids. Neurology 1986;36:1363–1366.

Henneberg K: Über genuine Narkolepsie. Berl Klin Wochenschr 1916;53:24.

Herman-Bert A, Stevanin G, Netter JC, et al: Mapping of spinocerebellar ataxia 13 to chromosome 19q13.3–q13.4 in a family with autosomal dominant cerebellar ataxia and mental retardation. Am J Hum Genet 2000;67:229–235.

Herz E: Die amyostatischen Unruheerscheinungen. Klinisch kinematographische Analyse ihrer Kennzeichen und Beleiterscheinungen. J Psychologie Neurol 1931;43:146–163.

Herz E: Dystonia: I. Historical review: Analysis of dystonic symptoms and physiologic mechanisms involved. Arch Neurol Psychiatry 1944;51:305–318.

Hicks AA, Petursson H, Jonsson T, et al: A susceptibility gene for late-onset idiopathic Parkinson's disease. Ann Neurol 2002;52(5): 549–555.

Higgins JJ, Adler RL, Loveless JM: Mutational analysis of the tau gene in progressive supranuclear palsy. Neurology 1999a;53: 1421–1424.

Higgins JJ, Morton DH, Loveless JM: Posterior column ataxia with retinitis pigmentosa (AXPC1) maps to chromosome 1q31–q32. Neurology 1999b;52:146–150.

Higgins JJ, Pho LT, Nee LE: A gene (ETM) for essential tremor maps to chromosome 2p22– p25. Mov Disord 1997;12:859–864.

Hirano A, Kurland LT, Krooth RS, Lessel S: Parkinsonism-dementia complex, an endemic disease on the island of Guam: I. Clinical features. Brain 1961;84:642–661.

Hoehn MM, Yahr MD: Parkinsonism: Onset, progression and mortality. Neurology 1967;17:427–442.

Hofele K, Benecke R, Auburger G: Gene locus FPD1 of the dystonic Mount-Reback type of autosomal-dominant paroxysmal choreoathetosis. Neurology 1997;49:1252–1257.

Holmes G: On certain tremors in organic cerebral lesions. Brain 1904;27:327–375.

Holmes SE, O'Hearn E, Rosenblatt A, et al: A repeat expansion in the gene encoding junctophilin-3 is associated with Huntington disease-like 2. Nat Genet 2001a;29(4):377–378.

Holmes SE, O'Hearn E, Ross CA, Margolis RL: SCA12: An unusual mutation leads to an unusual spinocerebellar ataxia. Brain Res Bull 2001b;56:397–403.

Horner FH, Jackson LC: Familial paroxysmal choreoathetosis. In Barbeau A, Brunette J-R (eds): Progress in Neuro-Genetics. Amsterdam, Excerpta Medica Foundation, 1969, pp 745–751.

Hunt AL, Sethi KD. The pull test: A history. Mov Disord. 2006; 21(7):894–899.

Hunt JR: Progressive atrophy of the globus pallidus (primary atrophy of the pallidal system): A system disease of the paralysis agitans type, characterized by atrophy of the motor cells of the corpus striatum: A contribution to the functions of the corpus striatum. Brain 1917;40:58–148.

Hunt JR: Dyssynergia cerebellaris myoclonica: Primary atrophy of the dentate system: A contribution to the pathology and symptomatology of the cerebellum. Brain 1921;44:490–538.

Huntington G: On chorea. Med Surg Reporter 1872;26:320–321.

Huntington's Disease Collaborative Research Group: A novel gene containing a trinucleotide repeat that is expanded and unstable on Huntington's disease chromosomes. Cell 1993;72:971–983.

Huntington Study Group: Unified Huntington's disease rating scale: Reliability and consistency. Mov Disord 1996;11:136–142.

Hutton M, Lendon CL, Rizzu P, et al: Association of missense and 5′-splice-site mutations in tau with the inherited dementia FTDP-17. Nature 1998;393:702–705.

Hyland K, Arnold LA, Trugman JM: Defects of biopterin metabolism and biogenic amine biosynthesis: Clinical, diagnostic, and therapeutic aspects. In Fahn S, Marsden CD, DeLong MR (eds): Dystonia, vol 3. Philadelphia, Lippincott-Raven, 1998, pp 301–308.

Hyland K, Surtees RAH, Rodeck C, Clayton PT: Aromatic L-amino acid decarboxylase deficiency: Clinical features, diagnosis, and treatment of a new inborn error of neurotransmitter amine synthesis. Neurology 1992;42:1980–1988.

Hymas N, Lees A, Bolton D, et al: The neurology of obsessional slowness. Brain 1991;114:2203–2233.

Ibanez P, Bonnet AM, Debarges B, et al: Causal relation between alpha-synuclein gene duplication and familial Parkinson's disease. Lancet 2004;364(9440):1169–1171.

Ichinose H, Ohye T, Takahashi E, et al: Hereditary progressive dystonia with marked diurnal fluctuation caused by mutations in the GTP cyclohydrolase I gene. Nat Genet 1994;8:236–242.

Ikeda A, Kakigi R, Funai N, et al: Cortical tremor: A variant of cortical reflex myoclonus. Neurology 1990;40:1561–1565.

Iliceto G, Thompson PD, Day BL, et al: Diaphragmatic flutter, the moving umbilicus syndrome, and belly dancers dyskinesia. Mov Disord 1990;5:15–22.

Imai H, Narabayashi H, Sakata E: "Pure akinesia" and the later added supranuclear ophthalmoplegia. Adv Neurol 1986;45:207–212.

Isaacs H: A syndrome of continuous muscle-fibre activity. J Neurol Neurosurg Psychiatry 1961;24:319–325.

Itard JMG: Memoire sur quelques fonctions involontaires des appareils de la locomotion de la prehension et de la voix. Arch Gen Med 1825;8:385–407.

Jacobs L, Kaba S, Pullicino P: The lesion causing continuous facial myokymia in multiple sclerosis. Arch Neurol 1994;51:1115–1119.

Jacquemont S, Hagerman RJ, Leehey M, et al: Fragile X premutation tremor/ataxia syndrome: Molecular, clinical, and neuroimaging correlates. Am J Hum Genet 2003;72:869–878.

Jacquemont S, Hagerman RJ, Leehey MA, et al: Penetrance of the fragile X-associated tremor/ataxia syndrome in a premutation carrier population. JAMA 2004;291(4):460–469.

Jakob A: Ueber eigenartigen Erkrankungen des Zentralnervensystems mit bemerkenswertem anatomischen Befund. Z Gesamte Neurol Psychiatr 1921;64;147–228.

Jakob A: Die extrapyramidalen Erkrankungen. Berlin, Springer-Verlag, 1923.

Jaksch M, Klopstock T, Kurlemann G, et al: Progressive myoclonus epilepsy and mitochondrial myopathy associated with mutations in the tRNA(Ser(UCN)) gene. Ann Neurol 1998;44:635–640.

Jankovic J: Diagnosis and classification of tics and Tourette's syndrome. Adv Neurol 1992;58:7–14.

Jankovic J: Post-traumatic movement disorders: Central and peripheral mechanisms. Neurology 1994;44:2006–2014.

Jankovic J: International classification of diseases, tenth revision. Neurological adaptation (ICD-10 NA): Extrapyramidal and movement disorders. Mov Disord 1995;10:533–540.

Jankovic J: Tourette's syndrome. N Engl J Med 2001;345:1184–1192.

Jankovic J: Tics and stereotypies. In Freund HJ, Jeannerod M, Hallett M, Leiguarda R (eds): Higher-Order Motor Disorders. Oxford, UK: Oxford University Press, 2005, pp 383–396.

Jannetta PJ: Surgical approach to hemifacial spasm: Microvascular decompression. In Marsden CD, Fahn S (eds): Movement Disorders. London, Butterworth Scientific, 1982, pp 330–333.

Jarman PR, Davis MB, Hodgson SV, et al: Paroxysmal dystonic choreoathetosis: Genetic linkage studies in a British family. Brain 1997a;120:2125–2130.

Jarman PR, Wood NW, Davis MT, et al: Hereditary geniospasm: Linkage to chromosome 9q13–q21 and evidence for genetic heterogeneity. Am J Hum Genet 1997b;61:928–933.

Jarvela I, Autti T, Lamminranta S, et al: Clinical and magnetic resonance imaging findings in Batten disease: Analysis of the major mutation (1.02-kb deletion). Ann Neurol 1997;42:799–802.

Jarvela I, Schleutker J, Haataja L, et al: Infantile form of neuronal ceroid lipofuscinosis (CLN1) maps to the short arm of chromosome 1. Genomics 1991;9:170–173.

Jin H, Kendall E, Freeman TC, et al: The human family of deafness/dystonia peptide (DDP) related mitochondrial import proteins. Genomics 1999;61:259–267.

Kahlbaum KL: Catatonia (Levi Y, Pridon T, trans). Baltimore, Johns Hopkins University Press, 1973 (originally published in 1874).

Kambouris M, Bohlega S, Al-Tahan A, Meyer BF: Localization of the gene for a novel autosomal recessive neurodegenerative Huntington-like disorder to 4p15.3. Amer J Hum Genet 2000;66:445–452.

Katayama S, Watanabe C, Khoriyama T, et al: Slowly progressive L-DOPA nonresponsive pure akinesia due to nigropallidal degeneration: A clinicopathological case study. J Neurol Sci 1998;161:169–172.

Kawaguchi Y, Okamoto T, Taniwaki M, et al: CAG expansions in a novel gene for Machado-Joseph disease at chromosome 14q32.1. Nat Genet 1994;8:221–228.

Keyser DL, Rodnitzky RL: Neuroleptic malignant syndrome in Parkinson's disease after withdrawal or alteration of dopaminergic therapy. Arch Intern Med 1991;151:794–796.

Kilroy AW, Paulsen WA, Fenichel GM: Juvenile parkinsonism treated with levodopa. Arch Neurol 1972;27:350.

Kinsbourne M: Myoclonic encephalopathy of infants. J Neurol Neurosurg Psychiatry 1962;25:271–276.

Kinsbourne M: Hiatus hernia with contortions of the neck. Lancet 1964;1:1058–1061.

Kirstein L, Silfverskiold B: A family with emotionally precipitated drop seizures. Acta Psychiatr Scand 1958;33:471–476.

Kitada T, Asakawa S, Hattori N, et al: Mutations in the parkin gene cause autosomal recessive juvenile parkinsonism. Nature 1998;392:605–608.

Klein C, Schilling K, Saunders-Pullman RJ, et al: A major locus for myoclonus-dystonia maps to chromosome 7q in eight families. Amer J Hum Genet 2000;67:1314–1319.

Kleiner-Fisman G, Rogaeva E, Halliday W, et al: Benign hereditary chorea: Clinical, genetic, and pathological findings. Ann Neurol 2003;54(2):244–247.

Knappskog PM, Flatmark T, Mallet J, et al: Recessively inherited L-DOPA-responsive dystonia caused by a point mutation (Q381K) in the tyrosine hydroxylase gene. Hum Mol Genet 1995;4:1209–1212.

Knight MA, Gardner RJM, Bahlo M, et al: Dominantly inherited ataxia and dysphonia with dentate calcification: Spinocerebellar ataxia type 20. Brain 2004;127:1172–1181.

Knight MA, Kennerson ML, Anney RJ, et al: Spinocerebellar ataxia type 15 (SCA15) maps to 3p24.2–3pter: Exclusion of the ITPR1 gene, the human orthologue of an ataxic mouse mutant. Neurobiol Disease 2003;13(2):147–157.

Koehler CM, Leuenberger D, Merchant S, et al: Human deafness dystonia syndrome is a mitochondrial disease. Proc Nat Acad Sci U S A 1999;96:2141–2146.

Koide R, Ikeuchi T, Onodera O, et al: Unstable expansion of CAG repeat in hereditary dentatorubral-pallidoluysian atrophy (DRPLA). Nat Genet 1994;6:9–13.

Kokmen E, Ozekmecki S, Beard CM, et al: Incidence and prevalence of Huntington's disease in Olmstead County, Minnesota (1950–1989). Arch Neurol 1994;51:696–698.

Koller WC, Biary NM: Volitional control of involuntary movements. Mov Disord 1989;4:153–156.

Kono I, Ueda Y, Araki K, et al: Spinal myoclonus resembling belly dance. Mov Disord 1994;9:325–329.

Koob MD, Moseley ML, Schut LJ, et al: An untranslated CTG expansion causes a novel form of spinocerebellar ataxia (SCA8). Nat Genet 1999;21:379–384.

Kramer PL, Heiman GA, Gasser T, et al: The DYTI gene on 9q34 is responsible for most cases of early limb-onset idiopathic torsion dystonia in non-Jews. Am J Hum Genet 1994;55:468–475.

Kramer PL, Mineta M, Klein C, et al: Rapid-onset dystonia-parkinsonism: Linkage to chromosome 19q13. Ann Neurol 1999; 46:176–182.

Kruger R, Kuhn W, Muller T, et al: Ala30Pro mutation in the gene encoding alpha-synuclein in Parkinson's disease. Nat Genet 1998;18:106–108.

Kurlan R, Hamill R, Shoulson I: Neuroleptic malignant syndrome. Clin Neuropharmacol 1984;7:109–120.

Kurland LT: Epidemiology: Incidence, geographic distribution and genetic considerations. In Fields WS (ed): Pathogenesis and Treatment of Parkinsonism. Springfield, Ill, Charles C Thomas, 1958, pp 5–49.

Lafora GR: Ueber das Vorkommen amyloider Koerperchen im innern der Ganglienzellen. Virchow's Arch Pathol Anat Physiol Klin Med 1911;205:295.

Lamberti P, Demari M, Iliceto G, et al: Effect of L-dopa on oculogyric crises in a case of dopa-responsive dystonia. Mov Disord 1993; 8:236–237.

Lance JW, Adams RD: The syndrome of intention or action myoclonus as a sequel to hypoxic encephalopathy. Brain 1963;86:111–136.

Lance JW, Schwab RS, Peterson EA: Action tremor and the cogwheel phenomenon in Parkinson's disease. Brain 1963;86:95–110.

Lang A: Patient perception of tics and other movement disorders. Neurology 1991;41(2):223–228.

Langston JW, Ballard P, Tetrud JW, Irwin I: Chronic parkinsonism in humans due to a product of meperidine-analog synthesis. Science 1983;219:979–980.

Langston JW, Widner H, Goetz CG, et al: Core assessment program for intracerebral transplantations (CAPIT). Mov Disord 1992; 7:2–13.

Lansbury PT Jr, Brice A: Genetics of Parkinson's disease and biochemical studies of implicated gene products. Curr Opin Genet Develop 2002;12:299–306.

Larsen TA, LeWitt PA, Calne DB: Theoretical and practical issues in assessment of deficits and therapy in parkinsonism. In Calne DB, Horowski R, McDonald RJ, Wuttke W (eds): Lisuride and Other Dopamine Agonists. New York, Raven Press, 1983, pp 363–373.

La Spada AR, Fu YH, Sopher BL, et al: Polyglutamine-expanded ataxin-7 antagonizes CRX function and induces cone-rod dystrophy in a mouse model of SCA7. Neuron 2001;31:913–927.

Le W, Xu P, Jiang H, et al: Nurr1 gene mutations in PD. Neurology 2002;58(suppl 3):A409.

Lee HY, Xu Y, Huang Y, et al: The gene for paroxysmal non-kinesigenic dyskinesia encodes an enzyme in a stress response pathway. Hum Mol Genet 2004;13(24):3161–3170.

Lee MS, Marsden CD: Drop attacks. In Fahn S, Hallett MH, Lueders HO, Marsden CD (eds): Negative Motor Phenomena. New York, Lippincott-Raven, 1995, pp 41–52.

Lee WL, Tay A, Ong HT, et al: Association of infantile convulsions with paroxysmal dyskinesias (ICCA syndrome): Confirmation of linkage to human chromosome 16p12–q12 in a Chinese family [abstract]. Hum Genet 1998;103:608–612.

Lees AJ: Tics and Related Disorders. Edinburgh, Churchill Livingstone, 1985.

Lehesjoki AE, Koskiniemi M: Clinical features and genetics of progressive myoclonus epilepsy of the Unverricht-Lundborg type. Ann Med 1998;30:474–480.

Lehesjoki AE, Koskiniemi M, Norio R, et al: Localization of the EPM1 gene for progressive myoclonus epilepsy on chromosome 21: Linkage disequilibrium allows high resolution mapping. Hum Mol Genet 1993;2:1229–1234.

Lepore FE, Duvoisin RC: "Apraxia" of eyelid opening: An involuntary levator inhibition. Neurology 1985;35:423–427.

Leroy E, Boyer R, Auburger G, et al: The ubiquitin pathway in Parkinson's disease. Nature 1998;395:451–452.

Lesch M, Nyhan WL: A familial disorder of uric acid metabolism and central nervous system function. Am J Med 1964;36:561–570.

Leube B, Rudnicki D, Ratzlaff T, et al: Idiopathic torsion dystonia: Assignment of a gene to chromosome 18p in a German family with adult onset, autosomal dominant inheritance and purely focal distribution. Hum Mol Genet 1996;5:1673–1677.

Levine IM: An hereditary neurological disease with acanthocytosis. Neurology 1964;14:272.

Lewy F: Die Lehre von Tonus und der Bewegung. Berlin, Springer, 1923.

Lewy FH: Zur pathologischen Anatomie der Paralysis agitans. Dtsch Z Nervenheilk 1914;1:50–55.

Li M, Ishikawa K, Toru S, et al: Physical map and haplotype analysis of 16q-linked autosomal dominant cerebellar ataxia (ADCA) type III in Japan. J Hum Genet 2003;48(3):111–118.

Lindblad K, Savontaus ML, Stevanin G, et al: An expanded CAG repeat sequence in spinocerebellar ataxia type 7. Genome Res 1996;6:965–971.

Litt M, Kramer P, Browne D, et al: A gene for episodic ataxia/myokymia maps to chromosome 12p13. Am J Hum Genet 1994; 55:702–709.

Little JT, Jankovic J: Tardive myoclonus. Mov Disord 1987;2:307–311.

Lopes-Cendes I, Andermann E, Attig E, et al: Confirmation of the SCA-2 locus as an alternative locus for dominantly inherited spinocerebellar ataxias and refinement of the candidate region. Am J Hum Genet 1994a;54:774–781.

Lopes-Cendes I, Andermann E, Rouleau GA: Evidence for the existence of a fourth dominantly inherited spinocerebellar ataxia locus. Genomics 1994b;21:270–274.

Lossos A, Schlesinger I, Okon E, et al: Adult-onset Niemann-pick type C disease: Clinical, biochemical, and genetic study. Arch Neurol 1997;54:1536–1541.

Louis ED, Marder K, Cote L, et al: Age at death is significantly younger in patients with Parkinson's disease who have dementia and severe extrapyramidal signs. Neurology 1996;46:A377.

Louis-Bar D: Sur un syndrome progressif comprenant des télangiectasies capillaires cutanees et conjonctivales symetriques, à disposition naevoide et des troubles cérébelleux. Confin Neurol 1941; 4:32–42.

Ludecke B, Dworniczak B, Bartholomé K: A point mutation in the tyrosine hydroxylase gene associated with Segawa's syndrome. Hum Genet 1995;95:123–125.

Ludecke B, Knappskog PM, Clayton PT, et al: Recessively inherited L-DOPA-responsive parkinsonism in infancy caused by a point mutation (L205P) in the tyrosine hydroxylase gene. Hum Mol Genet 1996;5:1023–1028.

Lugaresi E, Cirignotta F: Hypnogenic paroxysmal dystonia: Epileptic seizure or a new syndrome? Sleep 1981;4:129–138.

Lugaresi E, Cirignotta F, Coccagna G, Montagna P: Nocturnal myoclonus and restless legs syndrome. Adv Neurol 1986;43: 295–307.

Lugaresi E, Cirignotta F, Montagna P, Coccagna G: Myoclonus and related phenomena during sleep. In Chase M, Weitzman ED (eds): Sleep Disorders: Basic and Clinical Research. New York, Spectrum, 1983, pp 123–127.

Lynch T, Sano M, Marder KS, et al: Clinical characteristics of a family with chromosome 17–linked disinhibition dementia parkinsonism amyotrophy complex. Neurology 1994;44:1878–1884.

Maddox LO, Descartes M, Collins J, et al: Identification of a recombination event narrowing the Lafora disease gene region. J Med Genet 1997;34:590–591.

Marder K, Leung D, Tang M, et al: Are demented patients with Parkinson's disease accurately reflected in prevalence surveys? A survival analysis. Neurology 1991;41:1240–1244.

Margolis RL, O'Hearn E, Rosenblatt A, et al: A disorder similar to Huntington's disease is associated with a novel CAG repeat expansion. Ann Neurol 2001;50:373–380.

Marion MH, Gledhill RF, Thompson PD: Spasms of amputation stumps: A report of 2 cases. Mov Disord 1989;4:354–358.

Marsden CD: Peripheral movement disorders. In Marsden CD, Fahn S (eds): Movement Disorders, vol 3. Oxford, UK, Butterworth-Heinemann, 1994, pp 406–417.

Marsden CD, Schachter M: Assessment of extrapyramidal disorders. Br J Clin Pharmacol 1981;11:129–151.

Martin JP: The Basal Ganglia and Posture. Philadelphia, Lippincott, 1967.

Mason A, Banerjee S, Eapen V, et al: The prevalence of Tourette syndrome in a mainstream school population. Dev Med Child Neurol 1998;40:292–296.

Masucci EF, Kurtzke JF, Saini N: Myorhythmia: A widespread movement disorder: Clinicopathological correlations. Brain 1984;107:53–79.

Matison R, Mayeux R, Rosen J, Fahn S: "Tip-of-the-tongue" phenomenon in Parkinson disease. Neurology 1982;32:567–570.

Matsumine H, Saito M, Shimoda-Matsubayashi S, et al: Localization of a gene for an autosomal recessive form of juvenile parkinsonism to chromosome 6q25.2–27. Am J Hum Genet 1997;60:588–596.

Matsumine H, Yamamura Y, Kobayashi T, et al: Early onset parkinsonism with diurnal fluctuation maps to a locus for juvenile parkinsonism. Neurology 1998;50:1340–1345.

Matsumoto J, Hallett M: Startle syndromes. In Marsden CD, Fahn S (eds): Movement Disorders, vol 3. Oxford, UK, Butterworth-Heinemann, 1994, pp 418–433.

Matsuura T, Achari M, Khajavi M, et al: Mapping of the gene for a novel spinocerebellar ataxia with pure cerebellar signs and epilepsy. Ann Neurol 1999;45:407–411.

Matthews WB: Facial myokymia. J Neurol Neurosurg Psychiatry 1966;29:35–39.

Mayeux R, Chen J, Mirabello E, et al: An estimate of the incidence of dementia in patients with idiopathic Parkinson's disease. Neurology 1990;40:1513–1517.

Mayeux R, Denaro J, Hemenegildo N, et al: A population-based investigation of Parkinson's disease with and without dementia: Relationship to age and gender. Arch Neurol 1992;49:492–497.

McHale DP, Jackson AP, Campbell DA, et al: A gene for ataxic cerebral palsy maps to chromosome 9p12–q12. Eur J Human Genet 2000;8:267–272.

Meige H: Les convulsion de le face, une forme clinique de convulsion faciale bilateral et mediane. Rev Neurol 1910;21:437–443.

Meige H, Feindel E: Tics and Their Treatment (translated from the French by Wilson SAK). London, Appleton, 1907, pp 57–58.

Meijer IA, Hand CK, Grewal KK, et al: A locus for autosomal dominant hereditary spastic ataxia, SAX1, maps to chromosome 12p13. Am J Hum Genet 2002;70(3):763–769.

Meissner I, Wiebers DO, Swanson JW, O'Fallon WM: The natural history of drop attacks. Neurology 1986;36:1029–1034.

Merette C, Brassard A, Potvin A, et al: Significant linkage for Tourette syndrome in a large French Canadian family. Am J Hum Genet 2000;67:1008–1013.

Michalewski MP, Kaczmarski W, Golabek AA, et al: Evidence for phosphorylation of CLN3 protein associated with Batten disease. Biochem Biophys Res Commun 1998;253:458–462.

Micheli F, Fernandez Pardal M, Giannaula R, Fahn S: What is it? Case 3, 1991: Moaning in a man with parkinsonian signs. Mov Disord 1991;6:376–378.

Mikami M, Yasuda T, Terao A, et al: Localization of a gene for benign adult familial myoclonic epilepsy to chromosome 8q23.3–q24.1. Am J Hum Genet 1999;65:745–751.

Minassian BA, Andrade DM, Ianzano L, et al: Laforin is a cell membrane and endoplasmic reticulum-associated protein tyrosine phosphatase. Ann Neurol 2001;49:271–275.

Minassian BA, Lee JR, Herbrick JA, et al: Mutations in a gene encoding a novel protein tyrosine phosphatase cause progressive myoclonus epilepsy. Nat Genet 1998;20:171–174.

Mir P, Edwards MJ, Curtis ARJ, et al: Adult-onset generalized dystonia due to a mutation in the neuroferritinopathy gene. Mov Disord 2005;20(2):243–245.

Misbahuddin A, Placzek MR, Chaudhuri KR, et al: A polymorphism in the dopamine receptor DRD5 is associated with blepharospasm. Neurology 2002;58(1):124–126.

Mitchell SW: Injuries of Nerves and Their Consequences. New York, Lippincott, 1872.

Miyoshi Y, Yamada T, Tanimura M, et al: A novel autosomal dominant spinocerebellar ataxia (SCA16) linked to chromosome 8q22.1–24.1. Neurology 2001;57:96–100.

Moersch FP, Woltman HW: Progressive and fluctuating muscular rigidity and spasm (stiff-man syndrome): Report of a case and some observations in 13 other cases. Mayo Clin Proc 1956;31:421–427.

Mole SE: Batten disease: Four genes and still counting. Neurobiol Disease 1998;5:287–303.

Monrad-Krohn GH, Refsum S: The Clinical Examination of the Nervous System, 11th ed. New York, Paul B. Hoeber, 1958..

Montagna P, Cirignotta F, Sacquegna T, et al: "Painful legs and moving toes" associated with polyneuropathy. J Neurol Neurosurg Psychiatry 1983;46:399–403.

Moore RC, Xiang F, Monaghan J, et al: Huntington disease phenocopy is a familial prion disease. Am J Hum Genet 2001;69: 1385–1388.

Moreira MC, Barbot C, Tachi N, et al: The gene mutated in ataxia-ocular apraxia 1 encodes the new HIT/Zn-finger protein aprataxin. Nat Genet 2001;29:189–193.

Morris HR, Janssen JC, Bandmann O, et al: The tau gene A0 polymorphism in progressive supranuclear palsy and related neurodegenerative diseases. J Neurol Neurosurg Psychiat 1999;66: 665–667.

Mount LA, Reback S: Familial paroxysmal choreoathetosis. Arch Neurol Psychiat 1940;44:841–847.

Mrissa N, Belal S, BenHamida C, et al: Linkage to chromosome 13q11–12 of an autosomal recessive cerebellar ataxia in a Tunisian family. Neurology 2000;54:1408–1414.

Müller U, Haberhausen G, Wagner T, et al: DXS1O6 and DXS559 flank the X-linked dystonia-parkinsonism syndrome locus (DYT3). Genomics 1994;23:114–117.

Nagafuchi S, Yanagisawa H, Sato K, et al: Dentatorubral and pallidoluysian atrophy expansion of an unstable CAG trinucleotide on chromosome-12p. Nat Genet 1994;6:14–18.

Nakamura K, Jeong SY, Uchihara T, et al: SCA17, a novel autosomal dominant cerebellar ataxia caused by an expanded polyglutamine in TATA-binding protein. Hum Mol Genet 2001;10:1441–1448.

Nakken KO, Magnusson A, Steinlein OK: Autosomal dominant nocturnal frontal lobe epilepsy: An electroclinical study of a Norwegian family with ten affected members. Epilepsia 1999;40:88–92.

Narabayashi H, Imai H, Yokochi M, et al: Cases of pure akinesia without rigidity and tremor and with no effect by L-DOPA therapy. In Birkmayer W, Hornykiewicz O (eds): Advances in Parkinsonism. Basle, Editiones Roche, 1976, pp 335–342.

Narabayashi H, Kondo T, Yokochi F, Nagatsu T: Clinical effects of L-threo-3,4-dihydroxyphenylserine in cases of parkinsonism and pure akinesia. Adv Neurol 1986;45:593–602.

Nath U, Ben-Shlomo Y, Thomson RG, et al: The prevalence of progressive supranuclear palsy (Steele-Richardson-Olszewski syndrome) in the UK. Brain 2001;124:1438–1449.

Nathan PW: Painful legs and moving toes: Evidence on the site of the lesion. J Neurol Neurosurg Psychiatry 1978;41:934–939.

Nickens H: Intrinsic factors in falling among the elderly. Arch Int Med 1985;145:1089–1093.

Nolte D, Niemann S, Muller U: Specific sequence changes in multiple transcript system DYT3 are associated with X-linked dystonia parkinsonism. Proc Natl Acad Sci U S A 2003;100(18): 10347–10352.

Nutt JG, Marsden CD, Thompson PD: Human walking and higher-level gait disorders, particularly in the elderly. Neurology 1993;43:268–279.

Nutt JG, Muenter MD, Aronson A, et al: Epidemiology of focal and generalized dystonia in Rochester, Minnesota. Mov Disord 1988;3:188–194.

Nygaard TG, Raymond D, Chen CP, et al: Localization of a gene for myoclonus-dystonia to chromosome 7q21–q31. Ann Neurol 1999;46(5):794–798.

Nygaard TG, Wilhelmsen KC, Risch NJ, et al: Linkage mapping of dopa-responsive dystonia (DRD) to chromosome 14q. Nature Genetics 1993;5:386–391.

Obeso JA, Artieda J, Burleigh A: Clinical aspects of negative myoclonus. In Fahn S, Hallett M, Luders HO, Marsden CD (eds): Negative Motor Phenomena: Advances in Neurology, vol 67. Philadelphia, Lippincott-Raven, 1995, pp 1–7.

Obeso JA, Rothwell JC, Marsden CD: The spectrum of cortical myoclonus: From focal reflex jerks to spontaneous motor epilepsy. Brain 1985;108:193–224.

O'Hearn E, Holmes SE, Calvert PC, et al: SCA-12: Tremor with cerebellar and cortical atrophy is associated with a CAG repeat expansion. Neurology. 2001;56:287–289.

Oldani A, Zucconi M, Asselta R, et al: Autosomal dominant nocturnal frontal lobe epilepsy: A video-polysomnographic and genetic appraisal of 40 patients and delineation of the epileptic syndrome. Brain 1998;121:205–223.

Oppenheim H: Uber eine eigenartige Krampfkrankheit des kindlichen und jugendlichen Alters (Dysbasia lordotica progressiva, Dystonia musculorum deformans). Neurol Centrabl 1911;30:1090–1107.

Orzechowski K: De l'ataxie dysmetrique des yeaux: Remarque sur l'ataxie des yeux myoclonique (Opsoclonie, Opsochorie). J Psychol Neurol 1927;35:1–18.

Ouvrier RA, Billson MD: Benign paroxysmal tonic upgaze of childhood. J Child Neurol 1988;3:177–180.

Ozelius LJ, Hewett JW, Page CE, et al: The early-onset torsion dystonia gene (DYT1) encodes an ATP binding protein. Nat Genet 1997;17:40–48.

Paisan-Ruiz C, Jain S, Evans EW, et al: Cloning of the gene containing mutations that cause PARK8–linked Parkinson's disease. Neuron 2004;44(4):595–600.

Pandolfo M, Munaro M, Cocozza S, et al: A dinucleotide repeat polymorphism (d9s202) in the Friedreich's ataxia region on chromosome-9q13–q21.1. Hum Mol Genet 1993;2:822.

Pankratz N, Nichols WC, Uniacke SK, et al: Significant linkage of Parkinson disease to chromosome 2q36–37. Am J Hum Genet 2003 Apr;72(4):1053–1057.

Pankratz N, Uniacke SK, Halter CA, et al: Genes influencing Parkinson disease onset: Replication of PARK3 and identification of novel loci. Neurology 2004;62(9):1616–1618.

Papa SM, Artieda J, Obeso JA: Cortical activity preceding self-initiated and externally triggered voluntary movement. Mov Disord 1991;6:217–224.

Paracelsus TBH: Von der Bergsucht und anderen Bergkrankheiten (translated by G. Rosen as Part II: On the Miners' Sickness and Other Miners' Diseases). In Sigerist HE (ed): Four Treatises of Paracelsus. Baltimore, Johns Hopkins Press, 1941 (originally published in 1567).

Parkinson J: An Essay on the Shaking Palsy. London, Sherwood, Neely, and Jones, 1817.

Parkinson Study Group: Evaluation of dyskinesias in a pilot, randomized, placebo-controlled trial of remacemide in advanced Parkinson disease. Arch Neurol 2001;58(10):1660–1668.

Pastor P, Ezquerra M, Perez JC, et al: Novel haplotypes in 17q21 are associated with progressive supranuclear palsy. Ann Neurol 2004;56(2):249–258.

Paulson G: Phenothiazine toxicity, extrapyramidal seizures, and oculogyric crises. J Ment Sci 1959;85:798–802.

Petek E, Windpassinger C, Vincent JB, et al: Disruption of a novel gene (IMMP2L) by a breakpoint in 7q31 associated with Tourette syndrome. Amer J Hum Genet 2001;68:848–858.

Phillips HA, Favre I, Kirkpatrick M, et al: CHRNB2 is the second acetylcholine receptor subunit associated with autosomal dominant nocturnal frontal lobe epilepsy. Am J Hum Genet 2001; 8:225–231.

Phillips HA, Scheffer IE, Crossland KM, et al: Autosomal dominant nocturnal frontal-lobe epilepsy: Genetic heterogeneity and evidence for a second locus at 15q24. Am J Hum Genet 1998;63: 1108–1116.

Pickering-Brown S, Baker M, Yen SH, et al: Pick's disease is associated with mutations in the tau gene. Ann Neurol 2000;48:859–867.

Pittman AM, Myers AJ, Duckworth J, et al: The structure of the tau haplotype in controls and in progressive supranuclear palsy. Hum Mol Genet 2004;13(12):1267–1274.

Pittock SJ, Joyce C, O'Keane V, et al: Rapid-onset dystonia-parkinsonism: A clinical and genetic analysis of a new kindred. Neurology 2000;55:991–995.

Placzek MR, Misbahuddin A, Chaudhuri KR, et al: Cervical dystonia is associated with a polymorphism in the dopamine (D5) receptor gene. J Neurol Neurosurg Psychiatry 2001;71:262–264.

Plante-Bordeneuve V, Guiochon-Mantel A, Lacroix C, et al: The Roussy-Levy family: From the original description to the gene. Ann Neurol 1999;46:770–773.

Plaster NM, Uyama E, Uchino M, et al: Genetic localization of the familial adult myoclonic epilepsy (FAME) gene to chromosome 8q24. Neurology 1999;53:1180–1183.

Polymeropoulos MH, Higgins JJ, Golbe LI, et al: Mapping of a gene for Parkinson's disease to chromosome 4q21–q23. Science 1996;274:1197–1199.

Polymeropoulos MH, Lavedan C, Leroy E, et al: Mutation in the alpha-synuclein gene identified in families with Parkinson's disease. Science 1997;276:2045–2047.

Potvin AR, Tourtelotte WW: Quantitative Examination of Neurologic Functions, vols 1 and 2. Boca Raton, Fla: CRC Press, 1985.

Pramstaller PP, Marsden CD: The basal ganglia and apraxia. Brain 1996;119:319–340.

Prusiner SB: Genetic and infectious prion diseases. Arch Neurol 1993;50:1129–1153.

Pulst S-M (ed): Genetics of Movement Disorders. San Diego, Academic Press, 2003.

Putnam TJ, Frantz AM, Ransom SW (eds): The Diseases of the Basal Ganglia: Research Publications, vol 21. New York, Association for Research in Nervous and Mental Disorders, 1940.

Rampoldi L, Dobson-Stone C, Rubio JP, et al: A conserved sorting-associated protein is mutant in chorea-acanthocytosis. Nat Genet 2001;28:119–120.

Ranum LPW, Schut LJ, Lundgren JK, et al: Spinocerebellar ataxia type 5 in a family descended from the grandparents of President Lincoln maps to chromosome 11. Nat Genet 1994;8: 280–284.

Raskind WH, Bolin T, Wolff J, et al: Further localization of a gene for paroxysmal dystonic choreoathetosis to a 5-cM region on chromosome 2q34. Hum Genet 1998;102:93–97.

Rebeiz JJ, Kolodny EH, Richardson EP Jr: Corticodentatonigral degeneration with neuronal achromasia. Arch Neurol 1968;18: 20–33.

Reilly M, Daly L, Hutchinson M: An epidemiological study of Wilson's disease in the Republic of Ireland. J Neurol Neurosurg Psychiatry 1993;56:298–300.

Rett A: Ueber ein eigenartiges hirnatrophisches Syndrom bei Hyperammoniamie in Kindesalter. Wien Med Wochenschr 1966;116:723–738.

Reyniers E, Van Bogaert P, Peeters N, et al: A new neurological syndrome with mental retardation, choreoathetosis, and abnormal behavior maps to chromosome Xp11. Amer J Hum Genet 1999;65:1406–1412.

Riess O, Schols L, Bottger H, et al: SCA6 is caused by moderate CAG expansion in the alpha(1A)-voltage-dependent calcium channel gene. Hum Mol Genet 1997;6:1289–1293.

Riley DE, Fogt N, Leigh RJ: The syndrome of "pure akinesia" and its relationship to progressive supranuclear palsy. Neurology 1994; 44:1025–1029.

Ritchie RW: Neurological sequelae of amputation. Br J Hosp Med 1970;6:607–609.

Roll P, Massacrier A, Pereira S, et al: New human sodium/glucose cotransporter gene (KST1): identification, characterization, and mutation analysis in ICCA (Infantile convulsions and choreoathetosis) and BFIC (Benign familial infantile convulsions) families. Gene 2002;285(1–2):141–148.

Rosen DR, Siddique T, Patterson D, et al: Mutations in Cu/Zn superoxide dismutase gene are associated with familial amyotrophic lateral sclerosis. Nature 1993;362:59–62.

Rothbauer U, Hofmann S, Muhlenbein N, et al: Role of the deafness dystonia peptide 1 (DDP1) in import of human Tim23 into the inner membrane of mitochondria. J Biol Chem 2001;276: 37327–37334.

Rothdach AJ, Trenkwalder C, Haberstock J, et al: Prevalence and risk factors of RLS in an elderly population: The MEMO Study. Neurology 2000;54:1064–1068.

Rothwell JC, Traub MM, Marsden CD: Primary writing tremor. J Neurol Neurosurg Psychiatry 1979;42:1106–1114.

Rubio JP, Danek A, Stone C, et al: Chorea-acanthocytosis: Genetic linkage to chromosome 9q21. Am J Hum Genet 1997;61:899–908.

Rubio JP, Levy ER, Dobson-Stone C, Monaco AP: Genomic organization of the human G alpha 14 and G alpha q genes and mutation analysis in chorea-acanthocytosis (CHAC). Genomics 1999;57: 84–93.

Satoyoshi E: A syndrome of progressive muscle spasm, alopecia and diarrhea. Neurology 1978;28:458–471.

Savitsky K, Bar-Shira A, Gilad S, et al: A single ataxia telangiectasia gene with a product similar to PI-3 kinase. Science 1995; 268:1749–1753.

Savukoski M, Klockars T, Holmberg V, et al: CLN5, a novel gene encoding a putative transmembrane protein mutated in Finnish variant late infantile neuronal ceroid lipofuscinosis. Nature Genet 1998;19:286–288.

Sawle GV, Hymas NF, Lees AJ, Frackowiak RSJ: Obsessional slowness: Functional studies with positron emission tomography. Brain 1991;114:2191–2202.

Scherer HJ: Extrapyramidale Störungen bei der olivopontocerebellaren Atrophie. Ein Beitrag zum Problem des lokalen vorzeitigen Alterns. Z Gesamte Neurol Psychiatr 1933;145:406–419.

Schoenberg BS: Epidemiology of inherited ataxias. In Kark RAP, Rosenberg RN, Schut LJ (eds): The Inherited Ataxias. Adv Neurol 1978;21:15–32.

Schoenberg BS: Epidemiology of movement disorders. In Marsden CD, Fahn S (eds): Movement Disorders, vol 2. London, Butterworths, 1987, pp 17–32.

Schoenberg BS, Anderson DW, Haerer AF: Prevalence of Parkinson's disease in the biracial population of Copiah County, Mississippi. Neurology 1985;35:841–845.

Schonecker VM: Ein eigentumliches Syndrom im oralen Bereich bei Megaphenapplikation. Nervenarzt 1957;28:35–43.

Schrag A, Ben-Shlomo Y, Quinn NP: Prevalence of progressive supranuclear palsy and multiple system atrophy: A cross-sectional study. Lancet 1999;354:1771–1775.

Schultze F: Beitrage zur Muskelpathologie: I. Myokymie (Muskelwogen) besonders an den Unterextremitaten. Dtsch Z Nervenheilk 1895;6:65–70.

Schwab RS, Chafetz ME, Walker S: Control of two simultaneous voluntary motor acts in normal and in parkinsonism. Arch Neurol Psychiat 1954;72:591–598.

Schwab RS, England AC Jr: Projection technique for evaluating surgery in Parkinson's disease. In Gillingham FJ, Donaldson MC (eds): Third Symposium on Parkinson's Disease. Edinburgh, E & S Livingstone, 1969, pp 152–157.

Schwalbe W: Eine eigentumliche tonische Krampfform mit hysterischen Symptomen. Inaug Diss, Berlin, G. Schade, 1908.

Schwartz NA, Selhorst JB, Ochs AL, et al: Oculomasticatory myorhythmia: A unique movement disorder occurring in Whipple's disease. Ann Neurol 1986;20:677–683.

Segawa M, Hosaka A, Miyagawa F, et al: Hereditary progressive dystonia with marked diurnal fluctuation. Adv Neurol 1976;14:215–233.

Sege-Peterson K, Nyhan WL, Page T: Lesch-Nyhan disease and HPRT deficiency. In Rosenberg RN, Prusiner SB, DiMauro S, et al (eds): The Molecular and Genetic Basis of Neurological Disease. Stoneham, Mass, Butterworth-Heinemann, 1993, pp 241–260.

Serratosa JM, Gomez-Garre P, Gallardo ME, et al: A novel protein tyrosine phosphatase gene is mutated in progressive myoclonus epilepsy of the Lafora type (EPM2). Hum Mol Genet 1999;8:345–352.

Sethi KD, Nichols FT, Yaghmai F: Generalized chorea due to basal ganglia lacunar infarcts. Mov Disord 1987;2:61–66.

Shapiro AK, Shapiro ES, Young JG, Feinberg TE: Gilles de la Tourette Syndrome, 2nd ed. New York, Raven Press, 1988.

Sharp FR, Rando TA, Greenberg SA, et al: Pseudochoreoathetosis: Movements associated with loss of proprioception. Arch Neurol 1994;51:1103–1109.

Sharp JD, Wheeler RB, Lake BD, et al: Loci for classical and a variant late infantile neuronal ceroid lipofuscinosis map to chromosomes 11p15 and 15q21–23. Hum Mol Genet 1997;6:591–596.

Sheldon JH: On the natural history of falls in old age. Brit Med J 1960;2:1685–1690.

Shiang R, Ryan SG, Zhu YZ, et al: Mutations in the alpha 1 subunit of the inhibitory glycine receptor cause the dominant neurologic disorder, hyperekplexia. Nat Genet 1993;5:351–358.

Shimura H, Hattori N, Kubo S, et al: Familial Parkinson disease gene product, parkin, is a ubiquitin-protein ligase. Nat Genet 2000;25:302–305.

Shy GM, Drager GA: A neurological syndrome associated with orthostatic hypotension: A clinical-pathologic study. Arch Neurol 1960;2:511–527.

Sicard JA: Akathisia and taskinesia. Presse Med 1923;31:265–266.

Simon DK, Pulst SM, Sutton JP, et al: Familial multisystem degeneration with parkinsonism associated with the 11778 mitochondrial DNA mutation. Neurology 1999;53:1787–1793.

Simonic I, Nyholt DR, Gericke GS, et al: Rapid publication: Further evidence for linkage of Gilles de la Tourette syndrome (GTS) susceptibility loci on chromosomes 2p11, 8q22, and 11q23–24 in south African Afrikaners. Amer J Med Genet 2001;105: 163–167.

Singleton AB, Farrer M, Johnson J, et al: Alpha-synuclein locus triplication causes Parkinson's disease. Science 2003;302(5646):841.

Sirianni N, Naidu S, Pereira J, et al: Rett syndrome: Confirmation of X-linked dominant inheritance, and localization of the gene to Xq28. Am J Hum Genet 1998;63:1552–1558.

Skipper L, Wilkes K, Toft M, et al: Linkage disequilibrium and association of MAPT H1 in Parkinson disease. Amer J Hum Genet 2004;75(4):669–677.

Smego RA Jr, Durack DT: The neuroleptic malignant syndrome. Arch Int Med 1982;142:1183–1185.

Smith JK, Gonda VE, Malamud N: Unusual form of cerebellar ataxia: Combined dentato-rubral and pallido-Luysian degeneration. Neurology 1958;8:205–209.

Solano A, Roig M, Vives-Bauza C, et al: Bilateral striatal necrosis associated with a novel mutation in the mitochondrial ND6 gene. Ann Neurol 2003;54(4):527–530.

Solimena M, Folli F, Aparisi R, et al: Autoantibodies to GABAergic neurons and pancreatic beta cells in stiff-man syndrome. N Engl J Med 1990;322:1555–1560.

Solimena M, Folli F, Denis-Donini S, et al: Autoantibodies to glutamic acid decarboxylase in a patient with stiff-man syndrome, epilepsy, and type I diabetes mellitus. N Engl J Med 1988;318: 1012–1020.

Spehlmann R, Norcross K: Stiff-man syndrome. Clin Neuropharmacol 1979;4:109–121.

Spencer HR: Pharyngeal and laryngeal "nystagmus." Lancet 1886;2:702.

Spillane JD, Nathan PW, Kelly RE, Marsden CD: Painful legs and moving toes. Brain 94:541–556, 1971.

Spillantini MG, Yoshida H, Rizzini C, et al: A novel tau mutation (N296N) in familial dementia with swollen achromatic neurons and corticobasal inclusion bodies. Ann Neurol 2000;48:939–943.

Spiller WG: Akinesia agera. Arch Neurol Psychiatry 1933;30:842–884.

Spiro AJ: Minipolymyoclonus: A neglected sign in childhood spinal muscular atrophy. Neurology 1970;20:1124–1126.

Stacy M, Jankovic J: Tardive tremor. Mov Disord 1992;7:53–57.

Stanford PM, Halliday GM, Brooks WS, et al: Progressive supranuclear palsy pathology caused by a novel silent mutation in exon 10 of the tau gene: Expansion of the disease phenotype caused by tau gene mutations. Brain 2000;123:880–893.

Steele JC, Richardson JC, Olszewski J: Progressive supranuclear palsy: A heterogeneous degeneration involving the brainstem, basal ganglia and cerebellum with vertical gaze and pseudobulbar palsy, nuchal dystonia and dementia. Arch Neurol 1964;10:333–359.

Stevanin G, Bouslam N, Thobois S, et al: Spinocerebellar ataxia with sensory neuropathy (SCA25) maps to chromosome 2p. Ann Neurol 2004;55(1):97–104.

Stevanin G, Fujigasaki H, Lebre AS, et al: Huntington's disease-like phenotype due to trinucleotide repeat expansions in the TBP and JPH3 genes. Brain 2003;126.1599–603.

Stevens DL, Matthews WB: Cryptogenic drop attacks: An affliction of women. Br Med J 1973;1:439–442.

Storey E, Gardner RJM, Knight MA, et al: A new autosomal dominant pure cerebellar ataxia. Neurology 2001;57:1913–1915.

Stromme P, Mangelsdorf ME, Scheffer IE, Geecz J: Infantile spasms, dystonia, and other X-linked phenotypes caused by mutations in Aristaless related homeobox gene, ARX. Brain Develop 2002; 24(5):266–268.

Suhren O, Bruyn GW, Tuynman JA: Hyperekplexia: A hereditary startle syndrome. J Neurol Sci 1966;3:577–605.

Swartz BE, Li S, Bespalova I, et al: Pathogenesis of clinical signs in recessive ataxia with saccadic intrusions. Ann Neurol 2003;54(6): 824–828.

Swerdlow RH, Parks JK, Davis JN, et al: Matrilineal inheritance of complex I dysfunction in a multigenerational Parkinson's disease family. Ann Neurol 1998;44:873–881.

Swerdlow RH, Wooten GF: A novel deafness/dystonia peptide gene mutation that causes dystonia in female carriers of Mohr-Tranebjaerg syndrome. Ann Neurol 2001;50:537–540.

Sydenham T: Schedula Monitoria de Novae Febris Ingressu. London, G. Kettilby, 1686.

Symonds CP: Nocturnal myoclonus. J Neurol Neurosurg Psychiatry 1953;16:166–171.

Szepetowski P, Rochette J, Berquin P, et al: Familial infantile convulsions and paroxysmal choreoathetosis: A new neurological syndrome linked to the pericentromeric region of human chromosome 16. Am J Hum Genet 1997;61:889–898.

Tan A, Salgado M, Fahn S: The characterization and outcome of stereotypic movements in nonautistic children. Mov Disord 1997;12:47–52.

Tanner CM: Pathological clues to the cause of Parkinson's disease. In Marsden CD, Fahn S (eds): Movement Disorders, vol 3. Oxford, UK, Butterworth-Heinemann, 1994:124–146.

Tanzi RE, Petrukhin K, Chernov I, et al: The Wilson disease gene is a copper transporting ATPase with homology to the Menkes disease gene. Nat Genet 1993;5:344–350.

Taylor TD, Litt M, Kramer P, et al: Homozygosity mapping of Hallervorden-Spatz syndrome to chromosome 20p12.3–p13. Nat Genet 1996;14:479–481.

Thompson PD: Stiff people. In Marsden CD, Fahn S (eds): Movement Disorders, vol 3. Oxford, UK, Butterworth-Heinemann, 1994:373–405.

Tison F, Louvetgiendaj C, Henry P, et al: Permanent bruxism as a manifestation of the oculo-facial syndrome related to systemic Whipple's disease. Mov Disord 1992;7:82–85.

Titeca J, van Bogaert L: Heredo-degenerative hemiballismus: A contribution to the question of primary atrophy of the corpus Luysii. Brain 1946;69:251–263.

Tominaga H, Fukuzako H, Izumi K, et al: Tardive myoclonus. Lancet 1987;1:322.

Tomita H, Nagamitsu S, Wakui K, et al: Paroxysmal kinesigenic choreoathetosis locus maps to chromosome 16p11.2–q12.1. Am J Hum Genet 1999;65:1688–1697.

Tourette Syndrome Classification Study Group: Definitions and classification of tic disorders. Arch Neurol 1993;50:1013–1016.

Toyoshima Y, Yamada M, Onodera O, et al: SCA17 homozygote showing Huntington's disease-like phenotype. Ann Neurol 2004;55: 281–286.

Tranebjaerg L, Hamel BCJ, Gabreels FJM, et al: A de novo missense mutation in a critical domain of the X-linked DDP gene causes the typical deafness-dystonia-optic atrophy syndrome. Eur J Human Genet 2000;8:464–467.

Tranebjaerg L, Teslovich TM, Jones M, et al: Genome-wide homozygosity mapping localizes a gene for autosomal recessive non-progressive infantile ataxia to 20q11–q13. Hum Genet 2003; 113(3):293–295.

Traube L: Zur Lhere von den Larynxaffectionen beim Ileotyphus. Berlin:Verlag Von August Hirschwald; 1871:674–678.

Tryon WW: Principles and methods of mechanically measuring motor activity. Behavioral Assessment 1984;6:129–139.

Tulpius N: Obs med libr IV, cap LVIII, Amsterdam, 1652, according to Redard P. Le torticollis et son traitement. Paris, Carre & Naud, 1898.

Turner G, Partington M, Kerr B, et al: Variable expression of mental retardation, autism, seizures, and dystonic hand movements in two families with an identical ARX gene mutation. Amer J Med Genet 2002;112(4):405–411.

Ueno S, Maruki Y, Nakamura M, et al: The gene encoding a newly discovered protein, chorein, is mutated in chorea-acanthocytosis. Nat Genet 2001;28:121–122.

Ujike H, Tanabe Y, Takehisa Y, et al: A family with X-linked dystonia-deafness syndrome with a novel mutation of the DDP gene. Arch Neurol 2001;58:1004–1007.

Unverricht H: Die Myoclonie. Leipzig und Wien, Franz Deuticke, 1891.

Vahedi K, Joutel A, van Bogaert P, et al: A gene for hereditary paroxysmal cerebellar ataxia maps to chromosome 19p. Ann Neurol 1995;37:289–293.

Valente EM, Abou-Sleiman PM, Caputo V, et al: Hereditary early-onset Parkinson's disease caused by mutations in PINK1. Science 2004;304(5674):1158–1160.

Valente EM, Bentivoglio AR, Cassetta E, et al: DYT13, a novel primary torsion dystonia locus, maps to chromosome 1p36.13–36.32 in an Italian family with cranial-cervical or upper limb onset. Ann Neurol 2001a;49:362–366.

Valente EM, Bentivoglio AR, Dixon PH, et al: Localization of a novel locus for autosomal recessive early-onset parkinsonism, PARK6, on human chromosome 1p35–p36. Am J Hum Genet 2001b;68:895–900.

Valente EM, Brancati F, Ferraris A, et al: PARK6-linked parkinsonism occurs in several European families. Ann Neurol 2002;51(1): 14–18.

Valente EM, Salvi S, Ialongo T, et al: PINK1 mutations are associated with sporadic early-onset parkinsonism. Ann Neurol 2004;56(3): 336–341.

Valente EM, Spacey SD, Wali GM, et al: A second paroxysmal kinesigenic choreoathetosis locus (EKD2) mapping on 16q13–q22.1 indicates a family of genes which give rise to paroxysmal disorders on human chromosome 16. Brain 2000;123:2040–2045.

van Duijn CM, Dekker MC, Bonifati V, et al: Park7, a novel locus for autosomal recessive early-onset parkinsonism, on chromosome 1p36. Am J Hum Genet 2001;69:629–634.

Verbeek DS, Schelhaas JH, Ippel EF, et al: Identification of a novel SCA locus (SCA19) in a Dutch autosomal dominant cerebellar ataxia family on chromosome region 1p21–q21. Hum Genet 2002;111(4–5):388–393.

Verbeek DS, van de Warrenburg BP, Wesseling P, et al: Mapping of the SCA23 locus involved in autosomal dominant cerebellar ataxia to chromosome region 20p13–12.3. Brain 2004;127: 2551–2557.

Verhagen WIM, Horstink MWIM, Notermans SLH: Painful arm and moving fingers. J Neurol Neurosurg Psychiatry 1985;48:384–389.

Vesa J, Hellsten E, Verkruyse LA, et al: Mutations in the palmitoyl protein thioesterase gene causing infantile neuronal ceroid lipofuscinosis. Nature 1995;376:584–587.

Vogt C, Vogt O: Zur Lehre der Erkrankungen des striaren Systems. J Psychol Neurol 1920;25:627–846.

von Brederlow B, Hahn A, Koopman WJ, et al: Mapping the gene for acetazolamide responsive hereditary paryoxysmal cerebellar ataxia to chromosome 19p. Hum Mol Genet 1995;4:279–284.

Vuillaume I, Devos D, Schraen-Maschke S, et al: A new locus for spinocerebellar ataxia (SCA21) maps to chromosome 7p21.3–p15.1. Ann Neurol 2002;52(5):666–670.

Walters AS, Hening WA, Chokroverty S: Review and videotape recognition of idiopathic restless legs syndrome. Mov Disord 1991;6: 105–110.

Ward CD, Sanes JN, Dambrosia JM, Calne DB: Methods for evaluating treatment in Parkinson's disease. Adv Neurol 1983; 37:1–7.

Wilhelmsen KC, Weeks DE, Nygaard TG, et al: Genetic mapping of "lubag" (X-linked dystonia-parkinsonism) in a Filipino kindred to the pericentromeric region of the X chromosome. Ann Neurol 1991;29:124–131.

Wilkins DE, Hallett M, Erba G: Primary generalized epileptic myoclonus: A frequent manifestation of minipolymyoclonus of central origin. J Neurol Neurosurg Psychiatry 1985;48:506–516.

Wilson SAK: Progressive lenticular degeneration: A familial nervous system disease associated with cirrhosis of the liver. Brain 1912;34:295–509.

Wood HC: Nervous Diseases and Their Diagnosis. Philadelphia, Lippincott, 1887.

Worth PF, Giunti P, Gardner-Thorpe C, et al: Autosomal dominant cerebellar ataxia type III: Linkage in a large British family to a 7.6-cM region on chromosome 15q14–21.3. Am J Hum Genet 1999;65:420–426.

Wszolek ZK, Tsuboi Y, Uitti RJ, et al: Progressive supranuclear palsy as a disease phenotype caused by the S305S tau gene mutation. Brain 2001;124(8):1666–1670.

Xiang FQ, Almqvist EW, Huq M, et al: A Huntington disease-like neurodegenerative disorder maps to chromosome 20p. Am J Hum Genet 1998;63:1431–1438.

Xu PY, Liang R, Jankovic J, et al: Association of homozygous 7048G7049 variant in the intron six of Nurr1 gene with Parkinson's disease. Neurology 2002;58(6):881–884.

Yabe I, Sasaki H, Chen DH, et al: Spinocerebellar ataxia type 14 caused by a mutation in protein kinase C gamma. Arch Neurol 2003;60(12):1749–1751.

Yamada M, Wood JD, Shimohata T, et al: Widespread occurrence of intranuclear atrophin-1 accumulation in the central nervous system neurons of patients with dentatorubral-pallidoluysian atrophy. Ann Neurol 2001;49:14–23.

Yamashita I, Sasaki H, Yabe I, et al: A novel locus for dominant cerebellar ataxia (SCA14) maps to a 10.2-cM interval flanked by D19S206 and D19S605 on chromosome 19q13.4–qter. Ann Neurol 2000;48:156–163.

Zadikoff C, Lang AE: Apraxia in movement disorders. Brain. 2005;128:1480–1497.

Zarranz JJ, Alegre J, Gomez-Esteban JC, et al: The new mutation, E46K, of alpha-synuclein causes Parkinson and Lewy body dementia. Ann Neurol 2004;55(2):164–173.

Zheng KN, Heydari B, Simon DK: A common NURR1 polymorphism associated with Parkinson disease and diffuse Lewy body disease. Arch Neurol 2003;60(5):722–725.

Zhou B, Westaway SK, Levinson B, et al: A novel pantothenate kinase gene (PANK2) is defective in Hallervorden-Spatz syndrome. Nat Genet 2001;28:345–349.

Zhuchenko O, Bailey J, Bonnen P, et al: Autosomal dominant cerebellar ataxia (SCA6) associated with small polyglutamine expansions in the alpha 1A-voltage-dependent calcium channel. Nat Genet 1997;15:62–69.

Zimprich A, Biskup S, Leitner P, et al: Mutations in LRRK2 cause autosomal-dominant Parkinsonism with pleomorphic pathology. Neuron 2004;44(4):601–607.

Zimprich A, Grabowski M, Asmus F, et al: Mutations in the gene encoding epsilon-sarcoglycan cause myoclonus-dystonia syndrome. Nat Genet 2001;29:66–69.

Zu L, Figueroa KP, Grewal R, Pulst SM: Mapping of a new autosomal dominant spinocerebellar ataxia to chromosome 22. Amer J Hum Genet 1999;64:594–599.

# Chapter 2

# Motor Control
## Physiology of Voluntary and Involuntary Movements

Movement, whether voluntary or involuntary, is produced by the contraction of muscle. Muscle, in turn, is normally controlled entirely by the anterior horn cells or alpha motoneurons. Some involuntary movement disorders arise from muscle, the alpha motoneuron axon, or the alpha motoneuron itself. While this territory might be considered neuromuscular disease, the border can be fuzzy and patients may well appear in the office of the movement disorder specialist. Examples of involuntary movement arising from neuromuscular disorders that are discussed in subsequent chapters are listed in Box 2-1.

As the sole controller of muscle, the alpha motoneuron is clearly important in understanding the genesis of movement. The influences on the alpha motoneuron are many and complex, but have been extensively studied. Here, only the basics are reviewed (Hallett, 2003b). Inputs onto the alpha motoneuron can be divided into the segmental inputs and the supraspinal inputs.

## SEGMENTAL INPUTS ONTO THE ALPHA MOTONEURON

Figure 2-1 depicts the reflex connections onto the alpha motoneuron.

### Renshaw Cell

The alpha motoneuron axon has a recurrent collateral in the spinal cord that synapses onto the Renshaw cell. As at the neuromuscular junction, the neurotransmitter onto the Renshaw cell is acetylcholine. The Renshaw cell then directly inhibits the alpha motoneuron, using glycine as the neurotransmitter. This is called recurrent inhibition. It provides inhibitory feedback to the pool of alpha motoneurons to prevent excessive output.

### Ia Afferent

The Ia afferent comes from the muscle spindle and provides a sensitive measure of muscle stretch. It synapses monosynaptically with excitation onto the alpha motoneuron, using glutamate as the neurotransmitter, and is the substrate of the tendon reflex. Electrical stimulation of the Ia afferents proximal to the muscle spindle produces the H reflex.

### Ib Afferent

The Ib afferent comes from the Golgi tendon organ and responds to tension of the muscle tendon. It excites the Ib inhibitory interneuron, which in turn inhibits the alpha motoneuron in a disynaptic chain.

### Ia Afferent from an Antagonist Muscle

Ia afferents from antagonist muscles excite interneurons in the spinal cord called the Ia inhibitory interneuron. This interneuron provides direct inhibition of the alpha motoneuron disynaptically. Glycine is the neurotransmitter. This is called reciprocal inhibition.

### Flexor Reflex Afferents

Fibers, largely small myelinated and unmyelinated, carrying nociceptive information provide polysynaptic excitation onto the alpha motoneuron. These are the substrate for the flexor reflex.

### Presynaptic Inhibition

The inhibitory influences described so far are direct on the alpha motoneuron and are largely mediated by the neurotransmitter glycine. Some inhibitory influences, however, are presynaptic on excitatory synapses, such as the Ia afferent synapse. Presynaptic inhibition is commonly mediated by GABA. Some presynaptic inhibition of the Ia afferent synapse is produced by oligosynaptic input from the antagonist Ia afferent. This effect will cause a second phase of reciprocal inhibition following the disynaptic reciprocal inhibition described earlier.

All of these mechanisms can be studied in humans, although they are often limited to certain muscles. Such studies have illuminated the pathophysiology of both segmental and suprasegmental movement disorders. The reason that suprasegmental movement disorders can be evaluated with these tests is that supraspinal influences can affect segmental function.

Examples of movement disorders arising from segmental dysfunction that are discussed in subsequent chapters are listed in Table 2-1.

## SUPRASPINAL CONTROL OF THE ALPHA MOTONEURON

The main supraspinal control comes from the corticospinal tract. Approximately 30% of the corticospinal tract arises from the primary motor cortex, and other significant contributions come from the premotor cortex and sensory cortex. The fibers largely cross in the pyramid, but some remain uncrossed. Some terminate as monosynaptic projections onto alpha motoneurons, and others terminate on interneurons, including those in the dorsal horn. Other cortical neurons project to basal ganglia, to the cerebellum, and to the brainstem, and these structures can also originate spinal projections. Particularly

**Muscle**
Schwartz-Jampel syndrome

**Alpha Motor Neuron Axon**
Hemifacial spasm
Peripheral myoclonus
Fasciculation
Neuromyotonia

**Anterior Horn Cell**
Fasciculation
Spinal alpha rigidity

Table 2-1 Movement disorders arising from segmental dysfunction

| Disorder | Mechanism |
|---|---|
| Tetanus | Tetanus toxin blocks the release of GABA and glycine at spinal synapses |
| Stiff-person syndrome | Mainly a disorder of GABA and presynaptic inhibition in the spinal cord |
| Hereditary hyperekplexia | A disorder of glycine receptors with deficient inhibition at multiple synapses, including that from the Ia inhibitory interneuron |

important is the reticular formation, which originates several reticulospinal tracts with different functions (Nathan et al., 1996). The nucleus reticularis gigantocellularis mediates some long-loop reflexes and is hyperactive in a form of myoclonus. The nucleus reticularis pontis oralis mediates the startle reflex. The inhibitory dorsal reticulospinal tract may have particular relevance for spasticity (Takakusaki et al., 2001). In thinking about the cortical innervation of the reticular formation, it is possible to speak of a corticoreticulospinal tract. The rubrospinal tract, originating in the magnocellular division of the red nucleus, while important in lower primates, is virtually absent in humans.

The basal ganglia circuitry and cerebellar circuitry both can be considered subcortical loops that largely receive information from the cortex and return most of the output back to the cortex via the thalamus. Both also have smaller directly descending projections. Although both loops utilize the thalamus, the relay nuclei are separate, and the loops remain separate.

## THE BASAL GANGLIA

The basal ganglia loop anatomy is complex, with many connections, but a simplification has become popular that has some heuristic value (Bar-Gad et al., 2003; Wichmann and DeLong, 2003a, 2003b) (Fig. 2-2). In this model, there are two pathways that go from the cortex and then back to the cortex.

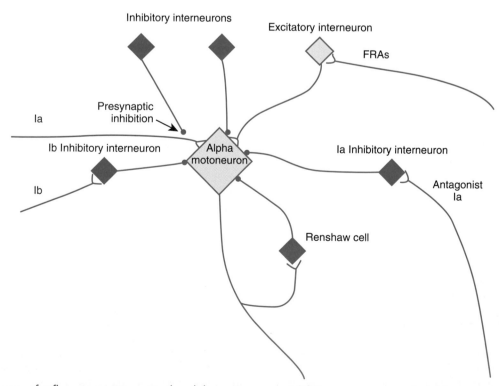

Figure 2-1 Diagram of reflex connections onto the alpha motoneuron. Inhibitory neurons are *dark blue;* excitatory neurons are *light blue.* FRAs flexor reflex afferents.

The direct pathway is the putamen, internal division of the globus pallidus (GPi), and thalamus (mainly the Vop nucleus). The indirect pathway is the putamen, external division of the globus pallidus (GPe), subthalamic nucleus (STN), GPi, and thalamus. The substantia nigra pars compacta (SNc) is the source of the important nigrostriatal dopamine pathway and appears to modulate the loop, though it is not in the loop itself. The putaminal neurons of the direct pathway have dopamine D2 receptors and are facilitated by the dopamine, while the putaminal neurons of the indirect pathway have dopamine D1 receptors and are inhibited. (Figure 2-2 also has a more complete diagram indicating more connections and some of the complexity.)

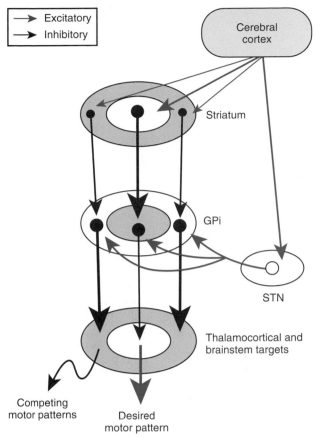

Figure 2-3 Diagrammatic view of the direct and indirect pathways of the basal ganglia showing how the direct pathway could select a desired movement and the indirect pathway could inhibit unwanted movements. (Reprinted with permission from Mink JW: The basal ganglia and involuntary movements: Impaired inhibition of competing motor patterns. Arch Neurol 2003;60:1365–1368.)

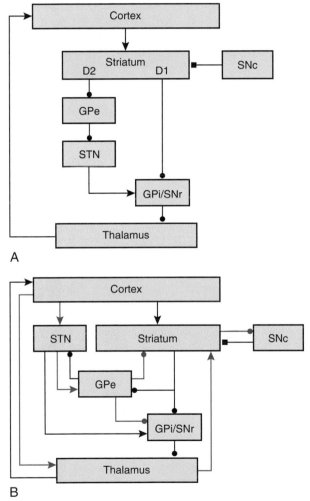

Figure 2-2 The corticobasal ganglia network. The box and arrow network of the different pathways of the basal ganglia. **A**, The early Albin-DeLong network. **B**, The up-to-date network. The early network is in *black;* later additions are in *blue.* Glutamatergic synapses are denoted by *arrows,* GABAergic synapses by *circles,* and dopaminergic synapses by *squares.* (Reprinted with permission from Bar-Gad I, Morris G, Bergman H: Information processing, dimensionality reduction and reinforcement learning in the basal ganglia. Prog Neurobiol 2003;71:439–473.)

What do the basal ganglia contribute to movement? There are likely many contributions, but the topic remains somewhat controversial.

The basal ganglia are anatomically organized to work in a center-surround mechanism. This idea of center-surround organization was one of the possible functions of the basal ganglia circuitry suggested by Alexander and Crutcher (1990). This was followed up nicely by Mink (1996), who detailed the possible anatomy (Fig. 2-3). The direct pathway has a focused inhibition in the globus pallidus, while the subthalamic nucleus has divergent excitation. The direct pathway (with two inhibitory synapses) is a net excitatory pathway, and the indirect pathway (with three inhibitory synapses) is a net inhibitory pathway. Hence, the direct pathway can be the center and the indirect pathway the surround of a center-surround mechanism.

Basal ganglia disorders are characterized by a wide variety of movement signs and symptoms. Often, they are divided into hypokinetic and hyperkinetic varieties, implying too little movement on the one hand and too much movement on the other. A full listing of these disorders is in Chapter 1. Here, the pathophysiology of Parkinson disease (PD) and dystonia are emphasized.

## PARKINSON DISEASE

PD is classically characterized by bradykinesia, rigidity, and tremor at rest. All features seem due to the degeneration of the nigrostriatal pathway, but it has not been possible to define a single underlying pathophysiologic mechanism that explains everything. Nevertheless, there are considerable data that give separate understanding to each of the three classic features (Hallett, 2003a).

### Bradykinesia

The most important functional disturbance in patients with PD is a disorder of voluntary movement prominently characterized by slowness. This phenomenon is generally called bradykinesia, although it has at least two components that can be designated bradykinesia and akinesia (Berardelli et al., 2001). Bradykinesia refers to slowness of movement that is ongoing. Akinesia refers to failure of willed movement to occur. There are two possible reasons for the absence of expected movement. One is that the movement is so slow (and small) that it cannot be seen. A second is that the time needed to initiate the movement becomes excessively long.

While self-paced movements can give information about bradykinesia, the study of reaction time movements can give information about both akinesia and bradykinesia. In the reaction time situation, a stimulus is presented to a subject, and the subject must make a movement as rapidly as possible. The time between the stimulus and the start of movement is the *reaction time*, and the time from initiation to completion of movement is the *movement time*. According to this logic, prolongation of reaction time is akinesia, and prolongation of movement time is bradykinesia. Studies of patients with PD confirm that both reaction time and movement time are prolonged. However, the extent of abnormality of one does not necessarily correlate with the extent of abnormality of the other (Evarts et al., 1981). This suggests that they may be impaired by separable physiologic mechanisms. In general, prolongation of movement time (bradykinesia) is better correlated with the clinical impression of slowness than is prolongation of reaction time (akinesia).

Some contributing features of bradykinesia are established. One is that there is a failure to energize muscles up to the level necessary to complete a movement in a standard amount of time. This has been demonstrated clearly with attempted rapid, monophasic movements at a single joint (Hallett and Khoshbin, 1980). In this circumstance, movements of different angular distances are accomplished in approximately the same time by making longer movements faster. The electromyographic (EMG) activity underlying the movement begins with a burst of activity in the agonist muscle of 50 to 100 ms, followed by a burst of activity in the antagonist muscle of 50 to 100 ms, followed variably by a third burst of activity in the agonist. This triphasic pattern has relatively fixed timing with movements of different distance, correlating with the fact of similar total time for movements of different distance. Different distances are accomplished by altering the magnitude of the EMG within the fixed-duration burst. The pattern is correct in

patients with PD, but there is insufficient EMG activity in the burst to accomplish the movement. These patients often must go through two or more cycles of the triphasic pattern to accomplish the movement. Interestingly, such activity looks virtually identical to the tremor at rest that is seen in these patients. The longer the desired movement, the more likely it is to require additional cycles. These findings were reproduced by Baroni and colleagues (1984), who also showed that levodopa normalized the pattern and reduced the number of bursts.

Berardelli and colleagues (1986) showed that PD patients could vary the size and duration of the first agonist EMG burst with movement size and added load in the normal way. However, there was a failure to match these parameters appropriately to the size of movement required. This suggests an additional problem in scaling of the actual movement to the required movement. A problem in sensory scaling of kinesthesia was demonstrated by Demirci and colleagues (1997). PD patients used kinesthetic perception to estimate the amplitude of passive angular displacements of the index finger about the metacarpophalangeal joint and to scale them as a percentage of a reference stimulus. The reference stimulus was either a standard kinesthetic stimulus preceding each test stimulus (task K) or a visual representation of the standard kinesthetic stimulus (task V). The PD patients' underestimation of the amplitudes of finger perturbations was significantly greater in task V than in task K. Thus, when kinesthesia is used to match a visual target, PD patients perceive distances to be shorter. Assuming that visual perception is normal, kinesthesia must be reduced in PD patients. This reduced kinesthesia, when combined with the well-known reduced motor output and probably reduced corollary discharges, implies that the sensorimotor apparatus is set smaller in PD patients than in normal subjects.

In a slower, multijoint movement task, PD patients show a reduced rate of rise of muscle activity that also implies deficient activation (Godaux et al., 1992). On the other hand, Jordan and colleagues (1992) showed that release of force was just as slowed as increase of force, suggesting that slowness to change and not deficient energization was the main problem. If termination of activity is an active process, then this finding really does not argue against deficient energization.

A second physiologic mechanism of bradykinesia is that there is difficulty with simultaneous and sequential movements (Benecke et al., 1987). That PD patients have more difficulty with simultaneous movements than with isolated movements was first pointed out by Schwab and colleagues (1954). Quantitative studies show that slowness in accomplishing simultaneous or sequential movements is more than would be predicted from the slowness of each individual movement. With sequential movements, there is another parameter of interest: the time between the two movements, designated the *interonset latency* by Benecke and colleagues (1987). The interonset latency is also prolonged in patients with PD. This problem, similar to the problem with simple movements, can also be interpreted as insufficient motor energy.

Akinesia would seem to be multifactorial, and a number of contributing factors are already known. As was noted earlier in the chapter, one type of akinesia is the limit of bradykinesia from the point of view of energizing muscles. If the muscle is selected but not energized, then there will be no movement. Such phenomena can be recognized on some occasions with EMG studies in which EMG activity is initiated but is insufficient to move the body part. Another type of akinesia, again as was noted previously, is prolongation of reaction time; the patient is preparing to move, but the movement has not yet occurred. Considerable attention has been paid to mechanisms of prolongation of reaction time. One factor is easily demonstrable in patients with rest tremor, who appear to have to wait to initiate the movement together with a beat of tremor in the agonist muscle of the willed movement (Hallett et al., 1977; Staude et al., 1995).

Another mechanism of prolongation of reaction time can be seen in those circumstances in which eye movement must be coordinated with limb movement (Warabi et al., 1988). In this situation, there is a visual target that moves into the periphery of the visual field. Normally, there is a coordinated movement of eyes and limb, the eyes beginning slightly earlier. In PD, some patients do not begin to move the limb until the eye movement has been completed. This might be due to a problem with simultaneous movements, as was noted previously. Alternatively, it might be that PD patients need to foveate a target before they are able to move to it.

Many studies have evaluated reaction time quantitatively with neuropsychological methods (Hallett, 1990). The goal of these studies is to determine the abnormalities in the motor processes that must occur before a movement can be initiated. To understand reaction time studies, it is useful to consider from a theoretic point of view the tasks that the brain must accomplish. The starting point is the "set" for the movement. This includes the environmental conditions, initial positions of body parts, understanding the nature of the experiment, and, in particular, some understanding of the expected movement. In some circumstances, the expected movement is described completely, without ambiguity. This is the *simple reaction time* condition. The movement can be fully planned. It then needs to be held in store until the stimulus comes to initiate the execution of the movement. In other circumstances, the set does not include a complete description of the required movement. It is intended that the description be completed at the time of the stimulus that calls for the movement initiation. This is the *choice reaction time* condition. In this circumstance, the programming of the movement occurs between the stimulus and the response. Choice reaction time is always longer than simple reaction, and the time difference is due to this movement programming.

In most studies, simple reaction time is significantly prolonged in PD patients compared with normal subjects (Hallett, 1990). On the other hand, PD patients appear to have normal choice reaction times, or the increase of choice reaction time over simple reaction time is the same in PD patients and normal subjects. Many studies in which cognitive activity was required for a decision on the correct motor response have shown that PD patients do not have apparent slowing of thinking, called bradyphrenia. Brown and colleagues (1993) extended the study of choice reaction times by considering three different choice reaction time tasks that required the same simple movement but differed in the difficulty of the decision about which movement to make. When PD patients were compared to normal subjects, the PD patients had a longer reaction time in all three conditions, but the difference was largest when the task was the easiest and smallest when the task was the most difficult. Thus, the greater the proportion of time there is in the reaction time devoted to motor program selection, the closer to normal are the PD results. Labutta and colleagues (1994) showed that PD patients have no difficulty

holding a motor program in store. Hence, the difficulty must be in executing the motor program. Execution of the movement, however, lies at the end of choice reaction time, just as it does for simple reaction time. How then can it be abnormal and choice reaction time be normal? The answer may be that in the choice reaction time situation, both the motor programming and the motor execution can proceed in parallel.

Transcranial magnetic stimulation (TMS) can be used to study the initiation of execution. With low levels of TMS, it is possible to find a level that will not produce any motor evoked potentials (MEPs) at rest but will produce an MEP when there is voluntary activation. Using such a stimulus in a reaction time situation between the stimulus to move and the response, Starr and colleagues (1988) showed that stimulation close to movement onset would produce a response even though there was still no voluntary EMG activity. A small response first appeared about 80 ms before EMG onset and grew in magnitude closer to onset. This method divides the reaction time into two periods. In the first period, the motor cortex remains unexcitable. In the second period, the cortex becomes increasingly excitable as it prepares to trigger the movement. Pascual-Leone and colleagues (1994a) found that most of the prolongation of the reaction time was due to prolongation of the later period of rising excitability. This result has been confirmed (Chen et al., 2001). The finding of prolonged initiation time in PD patients is supported by studies of motor cortex neuronal activity in reaction time movements in monkeys that had been rendered parkinsonian with 1-methyl-4-phenyl-1,2,3,6-tetrahydropyridine (Watts and Mandir, 1992). In these investigations, there was a prolonged time between initial activation of motor cortex neurons and movement onset.

Thus, an important component of akinesia is the difficulty in initiating a planned movement. This statement would not be a surprise to PD patients, who often say that they know what they want to do, but they just cannot do it. A major problem in bradykinesia is a deficiency in activation of muscles, whereas the problem in akinesia seems to be a deficiency in activation of motor cortex. The dopaminergic system apparently provides energy to many different motor tasks, and the deficiency of this system in PD leads to both bradykinesia and akinesia.

Another factor that should be kept in mind is that patients appear to have much more difficulty initiating internally triggered movements than externally triggered movements. This is clear clinically in that external clues are often helpful in movement initiation. Examples include improving walking by providing an object to step over or playing march music. This can also be demonstrated in the laboratory with a variety of paradigms (Curra et al., 1997; Majsak et al., 1998).

How does bradykinesia arise from dysfunction of the nigrostriatal pathway? According to the simple basal ganglia diagram, dopamine facilitates the direct pathway and inhibits the indirect pathway. Loss of dopamine will lead to lack of facilitation of movement in both pathways. This could certainly be represented by bradykinesia. The origin of rigidity and tremor is less understandable but also less directly linked to dopamine deficiency clinically.

## Rigidity

Tone is defined as the resistance to passive stretch. Rigidity is one form of increased tone that is seen in disorders of the basal ganglia ("extrapyramidal disorders") and is particularly prominent in PD. Increased tone can result from changes in (1) muscle properties or joint characteristics, (2) amount of background contraction of the muscle, and (3) magnitude of stretch reflexes. There is evidence for all three of these aspects contributing to rigidity. For quantitative purposes, responses can be measured to controlled stretches delivered by devices that contain torque motors. The stretch can be produced by altering the torque of the motor or by altering the position of the shaft of the motor. The perturbation can be a single step or more complex, such as a sinusoid. The mechanical response of the limb can be measured: the positional change if the motor alters force or the force change if the motor alters position. Such mechanical measurements can directly mimic and quantify the clinical impression (Hallett et al., 1994; Hallett, 1999).

Patients with PD do not relax well and often have slight contraction at rest. This is a standard clinical as well as electrophysiologic observation, and it is clear that this mechanism plays a significant part in rigidity.

There are increases in long-latency reflexes in PD patients. Generally, this is neurophysiologically distinct from the increases in the short-latency reflexes seen in spasticity, increase in tone of pyramidal type. The short-latency reflex is the monosynaptic reflex. Reflexes occurring at a longer latency than this are designated *long latency*. When a relaxed muscle is stretched, in general only a short-latency reflex is produced. When a muscle is stretched while it is active, one or more distinct long-latency reflexes are produced following the short-latency reflex and prior to the time needed to produce a voluntary response to the stretch. These reflexes are recognized as separate because of brief time gaps between them, giving rise to the appearance of distinct "humps" on a rectified EMG trace. Each component reflex, either short or long in latency, has about the same duration, approximately 20 to 40 ms. They appear to be true reflexes in that their appearance and magnitude depend primarily on the amount of background force that the muscle was exerting at the time of the stretch and the mechanical parameters of the stretch; they do not vary much with whatever the subject might want to do after experiencing the muscle stretch. By contrast, the voluntary response that occurs after a reaction time from the stretch stimulus is strongly dependent on the will of the subject.

Long-latency reflexes are best brought out with controlled stretches with a device such as a torque motor. While long-latency reflexes are normally absent at rest, they are prominent in PD patients (Rothwell et al., 1983; Tatton et al., 1984; Hallett et al., 1994; Hallett, 1999). Long-latency reflexes are also enhanced in PD with background contraction. Since some long-latency stretch reflexes appear to be mediated by a loop through the sensory and motor cortices, the enhancement of long-latency reflexes has been generally believed to indicate increased excitability of this central loop.

There is some evidence that at least one component of the increased long-latency stretch reflex in PD is a group II mediated reflex. This suggestion was first made by Berardelli and colleagues (1983) on the basis of physiologic features including insensitivity to vibration. It was subsequently supported by the observation that an enhanced late stretch reflex response could not be duplicated with a vibration stimulus (Cody et al., 1986). Some studies show a correlation between clinically measured increased tone and the magnitude of long-latency reflexes (Berardelli et al., 1983), while others do not

(Bergui et al., 1992; Meara and Cody, 1993). Long-latency reflexes contribute significantly to rigidity but are apparently not completely responsible for it.

## Tremor at Rest

The so-called tremor at rest is the classic tremor of PD and other parkinsonian states such as those produced by neuroleptics or other dopamine-blocking agents such as prochlorperazine and metoclopramide (Elble and Koller, 1990; Hallett, 1991; Elble, 1997; Hallett, 1999). It is present at rest, disappears with action, but may resume with static posture. That the tremor may also be present during postural maintenance is a significant point of confusion in regard to naming this tremor *tremor at rest*. It can involve all parts of the body and can be markedly asymmetric, but it is most typical with a flexion-extension movement at the elbow, pronation and supination of the forearm, and movements of the thumb across the fingers ("pill-rolling"). Its frequency is 3 to 7 Hz but is most commonly 4 or 5 Hz, and EMG studies show alternating activity in antagonist muscles.

The anatomic basis of the tremor at rest may well differ from the classic neuropathology of PD: that of degeneration of the nigrostriatal pathway. For example, 18F-dopa uptake in the caudate and putamen declines with bradykinesia and rigidity but is unassociated with degree of tremor (Otsuka et al., 1996). Another point in favor of this idea is that the tremor may be successfully treated with a stereotaxic lesion or deep brain stimulation of the ventral intermediate (VIM) nucleus of the thalamus, a cerebellar relay nucleus (Jankovic et al., 1995; Benabid et al., 1996).

In parkinsonian tremor at rest, there may be some mechanical-reflex component and some 8- to 12-Hz component, but the most significant component comes from a pathologic central oscillator at 3 to 5 Hz. This tremor component is unaffected by loading. Evidence for the central oscillator includes the facts that the accelerometric record and the EMG are not affected by weighting and that small mechanical perturbations do not affect it. On the other hand, it can be reset by strong peripheral stimuli such as an electrical stimulus that produces a movement of the body part five times more than the amplitude of the tremor itself (Britton et al., 1993a). Where this strong stimulus acts is not clear, but it does not have to be on the peripheral loop. Additionally, the tremor can be reset by TMS (Britton et al., 1993b; Pascual-Leone et al., 1994b), presumably indicating a role of the motor cortex in the central processes that generate the tremor. In the studies of Pascual-Leone and colleagues (1994b), using a relatively small stimulus, the tremor was reset with TMS but not with transcranial electrical stimulation. Since TMS affects the intracortical circuitry more, this seems to be further evidence for a role of the motor cortex.

While cells in the globus pallidus may have oscillatory activity, they are not as well related to the tremor as the cells in the ventral intermediate nucleus of the thalamus (Hayase et al., 1998; Hurtado et al., 1999). Lenz and colleagues have been studying the physiologic properties of cells in the ventral intermediate in relation to tremor production (Zirh et al., 1998). They have tried to determine whether the pattern of spike activity is consistent with specific hypotheses. They examined whether parkinsonian tremor might be produced by the activity of an intrinsic thalamic pacemaker or by the oscillation of an unstable long-loop reflex arc. In one study of 42 cells, they found 11 with a sensory feedback pattern, 1 with a pacemaker pattern, 21 with completely random patterns, and 9 that did not fit any pattern (Zirh et al., 1998). In another study of thalamic neuron activity, some cells with a pacemaker pattern were seen, but these did not participate in the rhythmic activity correlating with tremor (Magnin et al., 2000). These results confirm those of Lenz and colleagues, suggesting that the thalamic cells are not the pacemaker.

Wherever the pacemaker for the tremor is, it is important to note, while the tremor is synchronous within a limb, it is not synchronous between limbs (Hurtado et al., 2000). Hence, a single pacemaker does not influence the whole body.

There are other types of tremor in PD, including an action tremor that looks like essential tremor, but these have not been extensively studied.

# DYSTONIA

Dystonia is characterized by abnormal muscle spasms producing distorted motor control and undesired postures. Early on, dystonia is produced only by action, but then it can occur spontaneously. There are three general lines of work at the present time that may indicate the physiologic substrate for dystonia. Most of the data are derived from studies of focal dystonias.

## Loss of Inhibition

A principal finding in focal dystonia is that of loss of inhibition (Hallett, 2004). Loss of inhibition is likely responsible for the excessive movement that is seen in dystonia patients. Excessive movement includes abnormally long bursts of EMG activity, cocontraction of antagonist muscles, and overflow of activity into muscles not intended for the task (Cohen and Hallett, 1988). Loss of inhibition can be demonstrated in spinal and brainstem reflexes. Examples are the loss of reciprocal inhibition in the arm in patients with focal hand dystonia (Nakashima et al., 1989; Panizza et al., 1990) and abnormalities of blink reflex recovery in blepharospasm (Berardelli et al., 1985). Loss of reciprocal inhibition can be partly responsible for the presence of the cocontraction of antagonist muscles that characterizes voluntary movement in dystonia.

Loss of inhibition can also be demonstrated for motor cortical function, including short intracortical inhibition, long intracortical inhibition, and the silent period.

Short intracortical inhibition (SICI) is obtained with paired pulse methods and reflects interneuron influences in the cortex (Ziemann et al., 1996). In such studies, an initial conditioning stimulus is given, enough to activate cortical neurons but small enough that no descending influence on the spinal cord can be detected. A second test stimulus, at suprathreshold level, follows at a short interval. Intracortical influences initiated by the conditioning stimulus modulate the amplitude of the MEP produced by the test stimulus. At short intervals, less than 5 ms, there is inhibition that is likely largely a GABAergic effect, specifically GABA-A (Di Lazzaro et al., 2000). (At intervals between 8 and 30 ms, there is facilitation, called intracortical facilitation, ICF.) There is a loss of intracortical inhibition in patients with focal hand dystonia

(Ridding et al., 1995). Inhibition was less in both hemispheres of patients with focal hand dystonia; this indicates that this abnormality is more consistent as a substrate for dystonia.

The silent period (SP) is a pause in ongoing voluntary EMG activity produced by TMS. While the first part of the SP is due in part to spinal cord refractoriness, the latter part is entirely due to cortical inhibition (Fuhr et al., 1991). This type of inhibition is likely mediated by GABA-B receptors (Werhahn et al., 1999). SICI and the SP show different modulation in different circumstances and clearly reflect different aspects of cortical inhibition. The SP is shortened in focal dystonia.

Intracortical inhibition can also be assessed with paired suprathreshold TMS pulses at intervals from 50 to 200 ms (Valls-Solé et al., 1992). This is called long intracortical inhibition, or LICI, to differentiate it from SICI. LICI and SICI differ as demonstrated by the facts that with increasing test pulse strength, LICI decreases but SICI tends to increase, and that there is no correlation between the degree of SICI and LICI in different individuals (Sanger et al., 2001). The mechanisms of LICI and the SP may be similar in that both seem to depend on GABA-B receptors. Chen and colleagues (1997) investigated LICI in patients with writer's cramp and found a deficiency only in the symptomatic hand and only with background contraction. This abnormality is particularly interesting because it is restricted to the symptomatic setting and therefore might be a correlate of the development of the dystonia.

There is also neuroimaging evidence consistent with a loss of inhibition. Dopamine D2 receptors are deficient in focal dystonias (Perlmutter et al., 1997). There is also direct evidence for reduced GABA concentration in both basal ganglia and motor cortex, found by utilizing magnetic resonance spectroscopy (Levy and Hallett, 2002).

Loss of cortical inhibition in the motor cortex can give rise to dystonic-like movements in primates. Matsumura and colleagues (1991) showed that local application of bicuculline, a GABA antagonist, onto the motor cortex led to disordered movement and changed the movement pattern from reciprocal inhibition of antagonist muscles to cocontraction. In a second study, they showed that bicuculline caused cells to lose their crisp directionality, converted unidirectional cells to bidirectional cells, and increased firing rates of most cells, including making silent cells into active ones (Matsumura et al., 1992).

There is a valuable animal model for blepharospasm that supports the idea of a combination of genetics and environment and, specifically, that the background for the development of dystonia could be a loss of inhibition (Schicatano et al., 1997). In this model, rats were lesioned to cause a depletion of dopamine; this reduces inhibition. Then the orbicularis oculi muscle was weakened. This causes an increase in the blink reflex drive in order to produce an adequate blink. Together, but not separately, these two interventions produced spasms of eyelid closure, similar to blepharospasm. Shortly after the animal model was presented, several patients with blepharospasm after a Bell palsy were reported (Chuke et al., 1996; Baker et al., 1997). This could be a human analog of the animal experiments. The idea is that those patients who developed blepharospasm were in some way predisposed. A gold weight implanted into the weak lid of one patient, aiding lid closure, improved the condition, a result suggesting that when the abnormal increase in reflex drive was removed, the dystonia could be ameliorated (Chuke et al., 1996).

## Loss of Surround Inhibition

A principle for function of the motor system may be *surround inhibition*. Surround inhibition is a concept that is well accepted in sensory physiology (Angelucci et al., 2002). It is not as well known in the motor system, but it is a logical concept. To make a movement, the brain must activate the motor system. It is possible that the brain just activates the specific movement. On the other hand, it is more likely that the one specific movement is generated and, simultaneously, other possible movements are suppressed. The suppression of unwanted movements would be surround inhibition, and this should produce a more precise movement, just as surround inhibition in sensory systems produces more precise perceptions. For dystonia, a failure of "surround inhibition" may be particularly important, since overflow movement is often seen and is a principal abnormality.

There is now good evidence for surround inhibition in human movement. Sohn and colleagues (2003) have shown that with movement of one finger, there is widespread inhibition of muscles in the contralateral limb. Significant suppression of MEP amplitudes was observed when TMS was applied between 35 and 70 ms after EMG onset. Sohn and colleagues have also shown that there is some inhibition of muscles in the ipsilateral limb when those muscles are not involved in any way in the movement (Sohn and Hallett, 2004b). TMS was delivered to the left motor cortex from 3 to 1000 ms after EMG onset in the flexor digitorum superficialis muscle. MEPs from abductor digiti minimi were slightly suppressed during the movement of the index finger in the face of increased F-wave amplitude and persistence, indicating that cortical excitability is reduced.

Surround inhibition was studied similarly in patients with focal hand dystonia (Sohn and Hallett, 2004a). The MEPs were enhanced similarly in the flexor digitorum superficialis and abductor digiti minimi, indicating a failure of surround inhibition. Using another experimental paradigm, Stinear and Byblow (2004) have also found a loss of surround inhibition in the hand.

How can the abnormalities of dystonia be related to the basal ganglia? This is not completely clear, but a number of investigators have thought that there is an imbalance in the direct and indirect pathways so that the direct pathway is relatively overactive (or that the indirect pathway is relatively underactive). This should lead to excessive movement and, in particular, a loss of surround inhibition.

## Abnormal Plasticity

There is an abnormal plasticity of the motor cortex in patients with focal hand dystonia (Quartarone et al., 2006). This has been demonstrated by using the technique of paired associative stimulation (Stefan et al., 2000). In paired associative stimulation, a median nerve shock is paired with a TMS pulse to the sensorimotor cortex timed to occur immediately after the arrival of the sensory volley. This intervention increases the amplitude of the MEP produced by TMS to the motor cortex. It has been demonstrated that the process of paired associative stimulation produces motor learning similar to long-term

potentiation. In patients with dystonia, paired associative stimulation produces a larger increase in the MEP than what is seen in normal subjects. There is also an abnormality in homeostatic plasticity. Homeostatic plasticity is the phenomenon whereby plasticity remains within limits; this can be exceeded in dystonia.

Increased plasticity may arise from decreased inhibition, so the inhibitory problem may well be more fundamental. This abnormality may be an important link in demonstrating how environmental influences can trigger dystonia.

The possibility of increased plasticity in dystonia had been suspected for some time, given that repetitive activity over long periods seems to be a trigger for its development. An animal model supported this idea (Byl et al., 1996). Monkeys were trained to hold a vibrating manipulandum for long periods. After some time, they became unable to do so, and this motor control abnormality was interpreted as a possible dystonia. The sensory cortex of these animals was studied, and sensory receptive fields were found to be large. The interpretation of these results was that the synchronous sensory input caused the receptive field enlargement and that the abnormal sensory function led to abnormal motor function. The results suggested that the same thing might be happening in human focal dystonia: Repetitive activity caused sensory receptive field changes and led to the motor disorder.

## Abnormal Sensory Function

Stimulated by the findings of sensory dysfunction in the primate model, investigators began examining sensory function in patients with focal hand dystonia and found it to be abnormal. Although there is no apparent sensory loss on a clinical level, detailed testing of spatial and temporal discrimination revealed subtle impairments (Molloy et al., 2003). The abnormality is present on both hands of patients with unilateral hand dystonia and on hands of patients with cervical dystonia and blepharospasm. The identification of abnormality of sensation beyond the symptomatic body parts indicated that the sensory abnormality could not be a consequence of abnormal learning but is more likely a preexisting physiologic state.

Sensory dysfunction can also be demonstrated with somatosensory evoked potential (SEP) testing (Bara-Jimenez et al., 1998). The dipoles of the N20 from stimulation of individual fingers show disordered representation in the primary sensory cortex (Bara-Jimenez et al., 1998), and these abnormalities are present on both hands of patients with focal hand dystonia (Meunier et al., 2001). The bilateral SEP abnormality was the first indication in the literature that the sensory abnormality was more likely endophenotypic than a consequence of repetitive activity. PET studies show that the sensory cortex is more activated than normal with writing and is more activated when patients are experiencing more dystonia (Lerner et al., 2004). Voxel-based morphometry studies in patients with focal hand dystonia show an increase in gray matter in the primary sensory cortex (Garraux et al., 2004). Such observations indicate that dystonia is a sensory disorder as well as a motor disorder.

There are data from sensory function that are compatible with loss of surround inhibition. Tinazzi and colleagues (2000) studied median and ulnar nerve SEPs in patients who had dystonia involving at least one upper limb. They compared the amplitude of SEP components obtained by stimulating the median and ulnar nerves simultaneously (MU), the amplitude value being obtained from the arithmetic sum of the SEPs elicited by stimulating the same nerves separately (M + U). The ratio of MU to (M + U) indicates the interaction between afferent inputs from the two peripheral nerves. No significant difference was found between SEP amplitudes and latencies for individually stimulated median and ulnar nerves in dystonic patients and normal subjects, but recordings in dystonic patients yielded a significantly higher percentage ratio for spinal N13 brainstem P14 and cortical N20, P27, and N30 components. The authors state that "these findings suggest that the inhibitory integration of afferent inputs, mainly proprioceptive inputs, coming from adjacent body parts is abnormal in dystonia. This inefficient integration, which is probably due to altered surrounding inhibition, could give rise to an abnormal motor output and might therefore contribute to the motor impairment present in dystonia."

## DYSKINESIAS

The dyskinesias include the choreas, such as Huntington disease, hemiballismus, and dopa-induced dyskinesia. These are characterized by involuntary movements that generally appear randomly. These might arise due to a substantial failure of the indirect pathway of the basal ganglia loop. This would be a failure of the inhibitory role of the basal ganglia, and involuntary movement would result. Evidence for this in regard to Huntington disease is that the initial degeneration of the putamen is for those neurons bearing dopamine D2 receptors.

## CEREBELLUM

The anatomy of the cerebellar pathways, like the anatomy of the basal ganglia pathways, is complex, but there are simplified models that aid thinking (Schmahmann, 1994; Schmahmann and Pandya, 1997) (Fig. 2-4). The main cortico-cerebellar-cortical loop is frontal lobe, pontine nuclei, cerebellar cortex (via middle cerebellar peduncle), deep cerebellar nuclei, VL thalamus (via superior cerebellar peduncle and passing the red nucleus), and motor cortex. The input fibers to the cerebellar cortex are the mossy fibers that synapse onto granule cells, which in turn synapse onto the Purkinje cells. There is also extensive sensory input via spinocerebellar tracts, largely carried in the inferior cerebellar peduncle. A critical modulatory loop involves the inferior olivary nucleus. The inferior olive innervates both the cerebellar cortex and deep nuclei via

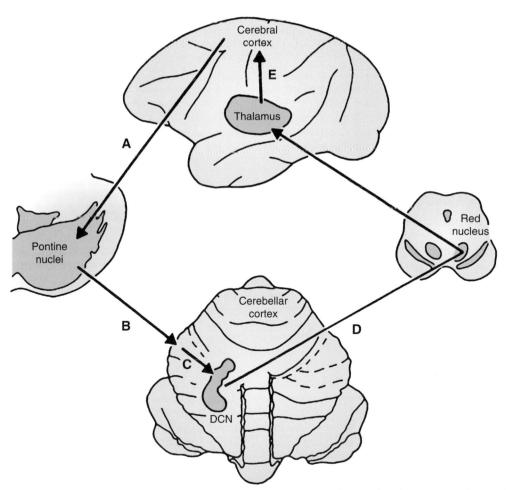

**Figure 2-4** Diagram of the cerebrocerebellar circuit. (Reprinted with permission from Schmahmann JD: The cerebellum in autism: Clinical and anatomical perspectives. In Bauman ML and Kemper TL [eds]: The Neurobiology of Autism. Baltimore, Johns Hopkins University Press, 1994, pp 195–226.)

the inferior cerebellar peduncle and the climbing fibers that synapse directly onto Purkinje cells. Feedback returns to the inferior olive by a dentate-olivary pathway that travels in the superior cerebellar peduncle, goes around the red nucleus, and descends in the central tegmental tract.

## ATAXIA

The term *ataxia*, literally meaning "without order," refers to disorganized, poorly coordinated, or clumsy movement (Massaquoi and Hallett, 2002). Since the time of Holmes, it has been applied more specifically to clumsiness that is due to lesions of the cerebellum and its immediate connecting pathways, of proprioceptive sensory pathways, or sometimes of the vestibular system. To identify the presence of ataxia, it should not be explained by any abnormality in (maximal isometric) strength, segmental reflexes, muscular tone, ability to isolate movement of individual body parts, or gross motor sequencing or spatial planning. The clumsiness is also not due to spontaneous involuntary movements. Ataxia may be associated with any voluntary movement and with many reflex movements. It commonly affects upright balance, gait, manual coordination, and speech, yielding stagger, clumsy manipulation, and slurring dysarthria, which appear drunken. Indeed, the motor coordination–impairing effects of ethanol are attributed to its specific interference with cerebellar function.

### Tonic Force Control Abnormalities: Hypotonia and Asthenia

Normal individuals have very low, barely perceptible muscle tone when they are fully relaxed. Holmes noted, however, that acutely injured soldiers with penetrating wounds to the cerebellum had further reduced resistance to passive movement. He viewed hypotonia as a fundamental abnormality that underlies many cerebellar motor deficits (Holmes, 1939). This hypotonia tended to be characteristic especially of the upper extremities and to normalize gradually over weeks to months, depending on the severity of the injury. Gilman and colleagues (1981) have shown that in primates, this change parallels the recovery of muscle spindle sensitivity, which was acutely depressed by loss of cerebellar fusimotor facilitation.

Large-scale surgical cerebellar ablation in monkeys is generally reported to produce acute weakness, especially of the extensor muscles (Gilman et al., 1981). In humans, Holmes (1939) clearly distinguished the weakness that followed acute massive damage to the cerebellar hemispheres, *asthenia*, from that associated with corticospinal tract lesions, *paresis*. The former did not affect specific muscle groups more than others and was not necessarily associated with changes in tendon reflex sensitivity. Interestingly, asthenia was noted particularly when strength was tested during movement. Static resistance to the examiner was most often normal. Indeed, weakness per se is a very inconstant complaint in cerebellar patients. Further questioning often reveals the problem to be one of easy fatigability and/or a lack of coordination or stability, not of peak strength. Holmes also drew attention to the inability of some patients to maintain steady force levels. Patients do sometimes complain of sudden losses of strength, such as a leg "giving out" or the tendency of an item to drop suddenly from the hand. Holmes attributed these episodes to hypotonia, but their nature remains unclear.

As with hypotonia, true asthenic weakness is most often seen in the context of acute cerebellar injury, especially, Holmes thought, when deep nuclei were involved. This was presumably related to the abrupt withdrawal of cerebellar facilitation from certain spinal, brainstem, and perhaps cerebral centers. Recovery usually takes place over the course of weeks to months. Although chronically ataxic patients clearly have difficulty generating force rapidly, their strength, as indicated by peak levels of isometric force that can be achieved, is most often normal. Certainly, though, coincidental weakness superimposed on cerebellar or sensory dysfunction markedly worsens the patient's disability.

Even in the presence of normal strength and muscular tone, easy fatigability (a second aspect of asthenia) is a prominent complaint of many patients with cerebellar ataxia (Holmes, 1939). The fatigue may affect an individual body part but may also be sensed more globally. Most patients report that all of the aspects of their ataxia worsen when they are fatigued. A poor night's sleep or a particularly busy previous day predisposes to a day of especially poor motor control. Patients frequently take naps during the day, which provide considerable benefit. Fatigue in cerebellar patients appears to be central and not muscular in origin. Electrophysiologic studies of fatigue in nondepressed patients with cerebellar ataxia by Samii and colleagues (1997) showed decreased postexercise facilitation of motor potentials evoked from transcranial magnetic stimulation. This is a central activation defect, similar to that seen in patients with depression and chronic fatigue syndrome. As in these disorders, patients sometimes complain of decreased concentration and mild difficulties with thinking. In this regard, the fatigue is also qualitatively similar to that seen in PD. Ultimately, the general fatigue in cerebellar disease and other movement disorders may be related to the increased mental concentration needed to compensate for degraded automatic motor control.

### Force-Rate and Movement Amplitude-Scaling Deficits: Dysmetria, Impaired Check, and Past-Pointing

Classic descriptions of cerebellar ataxia include various clinical signs such as dysmetria, dyssynergia (asynergia, decomposition of movement), dysdiadochokinesia, dysrhythmia, and kinetic (intention) and postural tremors (Holmes, 1939; Gilman et al., 1981). Characteristically, ataxic individuals have particular difficulty in properly generating, guiding, and terminating high-speed movements. Movements accelerate somewhat slowly and are relatively late in onset if executed in reaction to a cue. Movements may then either partially arrest prior to reaching their targets or gradually accelerate to excessive speed and overshoot their targets to an abnormal degree. These two types of errors are examples of dysmetria: hypometria and hypermetria, respectively. Two distinct motor control abnormalities appear to underlie dysmetria: force-rate inadequacy and step amplitude mis-scaling. The former causes brief, more consistent velocity-sensitive inaccuracies, and the latter causes more variable protracted errors.

At a fundamental level, the patient with cerebellar ataxia has difficulty changing voluntary force levels abruptly (Mai et al., 1988). Both acceleration and braking are impaired. In point-to-point movements, for example, this voluntary force-rate deficit is generally corroborated by a slowness in the buildup of agonist EMG and a prolonged agonist action with delayed onset of antagonist EMG (Hallett et al., 1991; Hallett and Massaquoi, 1993). In patients attempting rapid, single-joint movement, the first agonist burst is frequently prolonged regardless of the distance and speed of the movement, and the most striking kinematic abnormality is prolonged acceleration time. The pattern of acceleration time exceeding deceleration time is common in PD patients but uncommon in normal subjects. The duration of the first agonist burst correlates with, and is largely responsible for, the acceleration time. Altered production of appropriate acceleration for rapid voluntary movements may therefore be the primary abnormality in cerebellar dysfunction for attempted rapid voluntary movements. Hypermetria would be the expected resultant movement error unless there is compensation. Hypometria has been attributed to overcompensation, to asthenia in the acute setting, to tremor, or to failure of timely relaxation of the antagonist during movement initiation (Manto et al., 1998). Any of these mechanisms may be contributory in a given movement, and the topography of the lesion might correlate with the type of deficit (Manto et al., 1998).

For point-to-point movements of any given duration, ataxic movements exhibit greater overshoot than normal. In their study of rapid point-to-point elbow flexions, Hore and colleagues (1991) noted in normal subjects a transient overshoot of about 5% to 10% of the movement distance. Ataxic patients overshot the target by more than 20% and as much as 35% of the movement distance. On the other hand, whenever there is no observable overshoot, the movements of ataxic individuals are usually abnormally slow or are hypometric. From the point of view of Fitts's speed-accuracy trade-off, ataxic patients display decreased motor control bandwidth. Generally, therefore, in the assessment of ataxia, it is important to note both the degree of overshoot and the movement time. Appropriate abnormality of either may be consistent with ataxia. However, because there may be alternative explanations for increased movement time, slowness is a much less specific finding than overshoot. Owing to the inherent trade-off between speed and accuracy, patients often slow down intentionally to maintain error levels that are acceptable to them. Therefore, if it is important to observe maximal speed in a motor task, the examiner must explain that large errors are acceptable and may be, in fact, unavoidable. Even with this encouragement, the examiner is sometimes uncertain that the maximum achievable speed has been elicited.

In spinocerebellar atrophy type 6 (SCA 6), there is an abnormality of a voltage-sensitive calcium channel. Hyperventilation enhances the defective function of the channel and increases the behavioral dysfunction. In addition to modifying nystagmus, hypermetria in single-joint movements is exaggerated with hyperventilation (Manto, 2001). This may be a useful clinical provocative test.

Patients with cerebellar deficits also have abnormalities in termination of movement. This problem has been explicitly studied in a task in which subjects were asked to make a rapid elbow flexion on the background of tonic elbow extension needed to hold a position against a background force (Hallett et al., 1975). In this circumstance, the tonic triceps activity typically stops before the phasic biceps activity occurs (the *Hufschmidt phenomenon*). Patients with cerebellar dysfunction have a delay in terminating the triceps activity, so it overlaps the beginning of the biceps activity. This delay in stopping leads to overlap of the end of one movement with the beginning of the next.

The practical consequence of sluggishness in termination can be seen at the bedside with the sign called impaired check. If a patient's elbow that was flexed strongly against the grasp of the examiner is suddenly released, it is difficult for the patient to avoid striking himself or herself with the hand. Impaired check can also be attributed to delay in the triggering of the antagonist muscle (Terzuolo et al., 1973). The distinction between sluggish reduction and delayed changes in force is partially artificial.

In addition to transient overshoot, some patients may show movements that come to rest briefly, or nearly come to rest, at locations that are different from that of the target, most often beyond it (*past-pointing*). Unlike dynamic overshoot, which is always speed-dependent, this effective mis-scaling of the overall movement amplitude is less consistently related to the movement velocity and often improves with repetition. The sign can be elicited by using the Barany pointing test, in which the patient is asked to extend an arm forward, holding it parallel to the floor, and to note its position carefully (Gilman et al., 1981). Next, the patient closes the eyes and points the arm toward the ceiling. The arm is then rapidly brought down to a level as close to its original horizontal position as possible. The ataxic patient without demonstrable proprioceptive deficits may return at least briefly to a steady position beyond (lower than) the original, as if there is an error in the calculation of the distance moved or to have been moved. Among ataxic patients, past-pointing is less consistently observed than is dynamic overshoot, and it is not known whether past-pointing is as closely linked to movement acceleration as is dynamic overshoot. If the patient is allowed to practice and view the error a few times, he or she may become able correct the final position using a second movement while maintaining the eyes closed. It is as if a more precise proprioceptive measurement system can be employed after movement completion. Eventually, the patient may learn to produce a normally scaled movement. That the initial mis-scaling is often correctable may be related to residual cerebellar function, to a retained ability to increase dependence on proprioceptive information, or to rescaling movement at extracerebellar sites.

## Exaggerated Postural Reactions: Rebound

When the cerebellar patient is asked to maintain a steady outstretched arm position and the examiner applies a gentle downward tap, there typically follows a rapid, excessive upward displacement termed *rebound*. (Note that the term currently has a meaning slightly different from the original.) Rebound often occurs transiently in normal individuals and is usually quickly attenuated with reperturbation as the normal subject adapts to the amplitude or force of the disturbance. Owing to the excessive rate and magnitude of the response, the patient initially yields less than normal to the perturbation but overshoots in the opposite direction. Rebound may be partially due to sluggish braking, as occurs with *impaired check*. However, an excess force-rate abnormality is at least contributory.

The same phenomenon is seen as persistently excessive postural responses to platform perturbations observed by Horak and Diener in patients with injury to the anterior lobe of the cerebellum (Horak and Diener, 1994). As with rebound in the upper extremity, the excessive initial component of the platform postural response does not attenuate with repetition. Consistent with a cerebellar mechanism, attenuation of initial platform responses in normal subjects appears to be subconscious. Because of secondary, long-latency stabilizing responses, cerebellar patients were still able to avoid falling during the experiments.

## Abnormal Control of Simple Multijoint Movements: Dyssynergia

In ataxic simple multijoint movements, such as intended straight point-to-point hand movements, there is a breakdown in the normal coordination of joint rotations. This has been termed *dyssynergia* or *asynergia* and is described as a type of *movement decomposition*. This typically causes abnormal movement path deviations. As the movements of normal subjects usually display some natural deviation from perfect linearity, abnormality in path is a matter of degree of curvature and of specific pattern. Evidence is now accumulating that ataxic multijoint movements exhibit characteristic trajectory abnormalities (Massaquoi and Hallett, 1996). Thach and colleagues (1993) have attributed the pronounced ataxia that is seen in multijoint movements to a hypothetically preferential role for the cerebellum in the coordination of multijoint movement. While the neuroanatomic organization of the cerebellum makes it particularly well suited for coordinating muscle actions of different body parts, the function of the cerebellum in both single-joint and multijoint control may be fundamentally similar.

Analysis of simple, horizontal planar two-joint arm movements suggests that the deficits in acceleration and braking that are observed at single joints may account, at least in part, for the dyssynergia that is observed (Hallett and Massaquoi, 1993; Massaquoi and Hallett, 1996). It appears that the force-rate deficit may be accentuated at the joint that has the greatest torque-rate demand, which causes an imbalance in the joint accelerations, leading to hand movement curvature. This suspected mechanism is consistent with the marked worsening of dyssynergia with increases in intended acceleration. Massaquoi and Slotine (1996) have proposed a theoretical model of intermediate cerebellar function that relates the force production deficit in both single-joint and multijoint limb movements to a common failure of a long-loop feedback control system. The model accounts for the underdamped quality of ataxic motions and reproduces the characteristic curvature of cerebellar patients' hand trajectories in horizontal planar movements.

As Holmes noted, ataxia may be especially apparent in multijoint movements because the control problem is more demanding. In addition to the need for forces to launch and stop, there is a requirement for rapid compensation for the disturbing effects of multiple interaction torques between body segments, as well as the need to coordinate more muscles having different individual actions. Because of the additional degrees of force and motion freedom that are available, failure to compensate for muscular forces and body interaction torques may lead to multidirectional path errors in addition to overall dysmetria. Indeed, several groups have specifically related multijoint trajectory errors in cerebellar ataxia to deficits in interaction torque compensation (Bastian et al., 1996, 2000; Topka et al., 1998). Moreover, Sainburg and colleagues (1993) have shown deficits in interaction torque control in subjects with sensory ataxia due to peripheral neuropathy. These findings appear to point to similar mechanisms underlying both sensory and cerebellar ataxia.

Several investigators have suggested other mechanisms for asynergia that may be also or alternatively operative. Multijoint movements may be sometimes decomposed into multistep single-joint movement components as a voluntary strategy to simplify programming by minimizing interaction torques between the joints (Bastian et al., 1996). Dyssynergy may be due to the general difficulties cerebellar patients have with timing tasks (Keele and Ivry, 1990). These might yield problems with coordinating the actions of the different joints or muscles within the synergy, as was suggested by Thach and colleagues (1992). From this perspective, dysmetria and dyssynergy within simple (single intended velocity peak) single-joint and multijoint movements may have a mechanism similar to that which underlies *dysdiadochokinesia*, a disruption of compound movements involving more than one intended velocity peak (see later). On the other hand, a servo-control model, such as Massaquoi's, predicts that timing derangements within single movements occur as secondary effects of muscular activation (force) rate deficits (Massaquoi and Slotine, 1996). The latter view is supported by the prediction, based on dynamics, of a preferred direction for the inter-joint timing abnormality (i.e., lag or lead) for a given intended planar hand movement and therefore of a certain preferred trajectory pattern, rather than random path aberrations.

## Abnormalities in Timing and Coupling Movements and Other Processes: Dysrhythmia, Dysdiadochokinesia, Delayed Reaction Time, and Impaired Time Interval Assessment

Ataxia also includes the disruption of the normally smooth concatenation and coordination of compound movement subcomponents. This gives rise to a particular degradation of the rhythm of repetitively alternating single movements (*dysrhythmia*) and of the synchronization of single-joint movement components within repetitively alternating multijoint movements, yielding *dysdiadochokinesia* (*adiadochokinesia*), a second type of movement decomposition. Although clinical testing for dysrhythmia and dysdiadochokinesia typically employs rapidly alternating oppositely directed movements that maximize the sensitivity for detecting errors in the timing of movement onsets and offsets, timing difficulties may be noted in a variety of tasks that involve sequential movements. Bedside testing for dysrhythmia can be done by asking the patient to tap out a rhythm with a single-joint movement. Tests for dysdiadochokinesia include alternately slapping the palmar and dorsal surfaces of the hand on the thigh or making rapid pincer movements of the index finger tip to the opposing midthumb crease. Accurate slapping or tapping requires precise synchronization of rotations of more than one joint (the elbow and radioulnar joints in the first case, the interphalangeal and metacarpophalangeal joints in the latter). In these two tasks, ataxic patients display both an irregular underlying rhythm and inaccurately placed contacts, owing to failed multijoint coordination. Dysdiadochokinesia can therefore be seen as a combination of dysrhythmia and dyssynergia.

Thus, in multicomponent movements, considering that each subcomponent movement is subject to imprecise execution due to simple movement control deficits discussed previously, it is clear that at least some timing derangement is associated with, if not due to, abnormal acceleration, braking, or scaling. That is, it results from serial dysmetria, as well as serial dyssynergia in the multijoint case. If a patient is asked to perform even multicomponent movements very slowly, both temporal and spatial accuracy tend to improve substantially.

In addition to timing aberrations that are associated with, and in fact may result from, clumsy movement execution, there appears to be a separate timing abnormality due to failure of a cerebellum-dependent "central clock" (Keele and Ivry, 1990). Theoretically, this clock assists in the timely launching of movements with respect to preceding movements (Diener et al., 1993; Grill et al., 1997). The same system may generally help to launch movements with respect to other events, both external and internal. In all types of reaction tasks, not only does agonist EMG build up more slowly in cerebellar patients but also the EMG onset itself is significantly delayed with respect to the time of the stimulus, as if a triggering system were defective (Grill et al., 1997).

Much physiologic evidence has been accumulated to suggest that the lateral cerebellar hemispheres and dentate nucleus are preferentially involved in context-dependent triggering of movements, while the intermediate and medial regions of the cerebellum control the evolution of ongoing movement of single or multiple body parts. Supporting the existence of an internal triggering/timing system that is separate from that for movement execution control is the finding by Wing and Kristofferson that timing errors in a simple rhythmic finger-tapping task could be partitioned into implementation (executional) mistiming and internal clock mistiming, according to a two-component statistical model (Wing et al., 1984). Subsequently, Keele and Ivry (1990) found that in cerebellar patients, increased implementation errors were associated with lesions of the medial cerebellum, while clock errors occurred in those having lesions of the lateral hemispheres. Moreover, cerebellar patients with lateral hemisphere lesions also had difficulty in accurately assessing the difference in the lengths of time intervals between two pairs of tones, while those with medial cerebellar lesions did not. Also noteworthy is their observation that patients with clumsy movements due to either sensory neuropathy or deafferentation showed only executional mistiming. It is not clear, however, whether their abnormal movements appeared clinically identical to those of cerebellar ataxia.

## Abnormalities in Motion Assessment and Prediction: Impairment of Tracking and Mass Estimation

Probably closely related to their problems with assessment of time intervals and movement amplitude scaling is cerebellar patients' basic difficulty in using sensory information to assess and predict motion characteristics. This applies both to body parts, as shown by Grill and colleagues (1994) and as exhibited in past-pointing tests, and to external objects. Especially in rapid multicomponent movements, a certain amount of motion prediction ability is important for effective performance. Because of the delays in the transmission of neural signals, initiation of movement subcomponents might need to

take place well in advance of completion of the preceding subcomponent (Grill et al., 1997). Often, however, details of the plan for the second motion may depend on the progress of the first motion. For example, in throwing a ball, timing of the release must be coordinated with the movement of the arm to produce a properly directed trajectory (e.g., Becker et al., 1990). Similarly, for any control system that has nontrivial feedback delays, high-precision tracking of a moving target requires a certain amount of predictive control. This may take the form of additional open-loop (feedforward) predictive signals or the processing of higher derivatives of error information (e.g., velocity error information for position control), which inherently include some predictive information.

The cerebellum appears to be involved in both predictive feedforward and velocity feedback control. Motion prediction deficits can often be identified at the bedside by asking the patient to track, with his or her finger, the examiner's finger as it moves slowly back and forth in a smooth motion. A motion should be used that would normally be easy to predict and at a speed that would not engender overshoot in a simple point-to-point movement. Cerebellar patients will nevertheless frequently lag behind the examiner during the motion and/or overshoot at the direction reversals, presumably because they fail to assess properly the examiner's rate of acceleration and deceleration or the rhythm of the examiner's overall movement (Morrice et al., 1990). Very slow manual tracking in cerebellar patients also shows breakdown into a sequence of small movements in a staircase pattern that has been attributed to loss of velocity feedback control (Beppu et al., 1984, 1987).

Holmes (1939) and Angel (1980) have noted in hemiataxic patients a tendency to overestimate the weight of objects in the affected hand. However, Holmes found no difference between the sides in being able to discriminate accurately between two different weights placed successively in the same hand. Keele and Ivry (1990) also did not find an abnormality in the perception of static force in cerebellar patients. Thus, the cerebellar patient appears compromised in terms of absolute but not relative weight determination. The explanation favored by Holmes and Angel is that individuals tend to assess weight (or mass, as opposed to force per se) by moving an object up and down with their hands, presumably attempting to relate the applied force or, perhaps more accurately, the applied effort, to the rate of acceleration or oscillation frequency. Given patients' difficulties with the kinesthetic assessment of motion characteristics (Grill et al., 1994) and possibly an element of asthenia, it would not be surprising if patients' ability to relate movement effort to hand acceleration is compromised, thus disturbing the assessment of mass as a secondary effect.

## Sensory Information Acquisition and Analysis and Motor Control

The critical role of sensory information in successful motor control has been long recognized. On the basis of the deficits that have been noted in cerebellar patients that were described earlier and on the afferent neuroanatomic connections of the cerebellum, it is evident that the cerebellum plays an important role in processing sensory information to influence motor performance. However, the nature of this influence has been debated. Although it would appear that improved stability and accuracy of body motion are principal purposes of cerebellar function, Bower has put forward the controversial suggestion that the cerebellum is concerned primarily with fine control of the acquisition of sensory information rather than with control of movement per se (Gao et al., 1996; Bower, 1997). In particular, the cerebellum might have evolved chiefly to coordinate the positioning and movement of tactile sensory surfaces to optimize the information received.

However, the question of whether the cerebellum is primarily interested in acquiring sensory information or a motor controller is substantially moot from the point of view of modern feedback control system design, which often incorporates sophisticated afferent signal processing. The job of any motor feedback controller is to assist in minimizing the discrepancy between an intended body state (position and velocity) and the actual state as it is deduced or predicted from available information. If the output is effectively employed for continuous control, the controlled body part will be guided to so that its associated sensors register or nearly register measurements of the intended state. In a real sense, feedback-controlled motion is always planned in sensory coordinates. Whether the purpose of the motion is to acquire other sensory information or to transport the body part varies with the task. If the controller output is not applied to the motor command, the controller may be used simply for state estimation or other types of processing of its sensory input (e.g., filtering or prediction), depending on its design. For example, computation of the slide rate along the skin of a contact point is as useful for control of active tactile exploration as it is for monitoring the progress of an object slipping from a stationary hand or of a passive hand slipping from a support. Because in practice the detection of slip may be used to trigger a certain behavior when the slide approaches a critical point, even the distinction between motor control and passive sensory data acquisition is not fundamental. The state of seemingly passive sensory monitoring may in fact be readily employed within a discrete response-type motor control loop.

## Increased Movement Variability

Ataxic motor performance is frequently described as being more variable than normal (Hallett and Massaquoi, 1993; Palliyath et al., 1998). However, aside from the presence of involuntary movements, ataxic variability may arise as a consequence more of enhanced susceptibility to perturbation and of the sequential compounding of errors than of an inherent noise as might result from the presence of an unstable autonomous generator. This is suggested by the fact that when tasks are constrained sufficiently, ataxic movements become much less variable (Massaquoi and Hallett, 1996). Thus, especially for experimentally conducted single- and two-joint movements for which there is a single attempted movement speed and direction, and where head, eyes, and trunk are fixed, and in the absence of external contacts and forces (i.e., not against gravity), ataxic movements, though inaccurate, are much more consistent in their inaccuracy. Because of the loosened control over executive action in the cerebellar patient, movements and perhaps certain cognitive processes are more vulnerable to both internal and external environmental disturbances. Most natural tasks involve multijoint movements, which inherently have many degrees of movement freedom as well as ongoing efforts to guide motion. Elemental trajectory errors may therefore

interact, propagate, and become compounded; a process that effectively produces motor control noise.

## Cerebellar Tremors

Two types of action cerebellar tremor are commonly identified: kinetic and postural tremor. Lesions of the dentate, of the interpositus, and of the cerebellar outflow via the brachium conjunctivum appear to be the most frequently associated with action tremors. Both manifest alternating EMG bursting in agonist and antagonist muscles (Hallett, 1987). All types of cerebellar action tremors may be exacerbated near the point of attempted fixation if greater effort is made to maintain position precisely. Tremor frequency may differ between limbs, and the oscillations are generally not synchronous in nonadjacent body parts. However, like most tremors, cerebellar action tremors are worsened by fatigue. Cerebellar action tremors are often improved and sometimes eliminated by eye closure (Sanes et al., 1988). Propranolol has no substantial effect, and alcohol tends to worsen cerebellar action tremors.

Basic mechanisms that have been suggested to underlie cerebellar tremor have included (1) serial voluntary corrections for positioning error (serial dysmetria) (Hallett, 1987), (2) abnormality of transcortical and segmental proprioceptive feedback loops (Hore and Flament, 1986), and (3) action of central oscillators (Ito, 1984). Sufficient evidence has accumulated to indicate that each of these mechanisms is likely to be important to some component of body oscillations in ataxic patients under various circumstances. It is apparent clinically from the slowness of cerebellar voluntary reactions and in performance of rapid alternating movements that serial dysmetria is unlikely to be operative at frequencies greater than around 1 to 2 Hz at proximal joints or perhaps 3 Hz at the fingers. Thus, only the irregular, low-frequency, ataxic movements exhibited by patients' limbs as they approach a target are a manifestation of serial dysmetria. Because of the voluntary nature and gross irregularity of these movements, however, serial dysmetria is not really tremor.

Holmes (1939) also drew attention to the intermittent recoveries of posture that patients exhibit when fatigued. These movements consist of slow drifting *downward* from the intended posture followed by faster upward corrections that appeared voluntary. While these movements can be viewed as a coarse, asymmetric tremor, their nystagmoid character distinguishes them from the more regular, higher-frequency, involuntary oscillations *around* the intended posture or trajectory that would be characteristic of "true" cerebellar tremors.

The modification of cerebellar tremor by external perturbations and mechanical state (Sanes et al., 1988) indicates at least a partial dependence on peripheral factors, while the persistence of these cerebellar tremors during deafferentation indicates the presence of some central neural instability (Gilman et al., 1976). Several experimental results and models of cerebellar function include the interaction between central and peripheral feedback loops that could be consistent with these observations (Massaquoi and Slotine, 1996).

## Increased Postural Sway and Titubation

Ataxic patients exhibit increased irregular sway when standing and sometimes a more regular tremor (titubation). The characteristics of these involuntary movements vary according to the site of the cerebellar system lesion. Diener and Dichgans have performed extensive studies of postural balance in patients with cerebellar system disease (Diener et al., 1984; Diener and Dichgans, 1992). Common to all ataxic patients except those with lesions that are restricted to the hemispheres is the tendency to have abnormally large-amplitude sway when the eyes are closed. Patients with anterior lobe atrophy due to chronic alcohol intake and malnutrition and patients with Friedreich ataxia have a high "Romberg quotient," meaning that they sway considerably more with their eyes closed. In general, the eyes-closed instability is greater in Friedreich ataxia patients, who typically have significant proprioceptive loss and may fall without vision. By contrast, the anterior lobe lesion patients tend to oscillate markedly without falling when their eyes are closed. Patients with anterior lobe damage also tend to move much more in an anteroposterior direction, while those with Friedreich ataxia have an abnormal degree of lateral sway.

Patients with vestibulocerebellar lesions display increased, omnidirectional, low-frequency (~1-Hz) sway and may fall with eyes both open and closed and therefore have a normal Romberg quotient. Patients who have hemispheric lesions may exhibit slightly increased sway relative to normal subjects, but balance instability is not prominent. Those with diffuse cerebellar damage exhibit a mixture of characteristics. They may be differentiated from normal subjects but not from each other on the basis of posturography.

In addition to low-frequency (~1 Hz) sway, a characteristic 2- to 3-Hz body tremor is seen exclusively in patients with anterior lobe dysfunction when the eyes are closed. Unlike the irregular head and trunk titubation that may be seen with various other cerebellar lesions, the anterior lobe tremor consists of regular anteroposterior oscillation at the head, hip, and ankle. The hip is 180 degrees out of phase with the head, so the center of gravity moves little, and balance is maintained despite marked titubation. This tremor has been attributed to increased duration and amplitude of long-latency stretch responses. These long-latency responses are likely to be the scalable, secondary responses observed by Horak and Diener (1994) following exaggerated postural responses. Although abnormally large, these responses eventually stabilize the body after a few decaying oscillations at about 2 to 3 Hz when the eyes are open. Presumably, persistent titubation occurs especially with eyes closed because the gain of these scalable responses is increased in an effort to compensate for the loss of visual input. This is consistent with the view of titubation as a postural tremor.

## Dysarthria

When ataxia affects speech, it is manifested as a clumsy, slurring, poorly modulated dysarthria. No disruption of language usage, structure, or content is attributable to the cerebellar dysfunction. As was noted by Gilman and colleagues (1981), adjectives that are commonly used to describe cerebellar speech include scanning, slurring, staccato, explosive, hesitant, slow, altered accent, and garbled. These investigators identified 10 elemental speech abnormalities that are present to varying degrees in different cerebellar patients: (1) imprecise consonants, a feature that is basic to all dysarthrias; (2) excess and equal stress, the inappropriate allocation of emphasis and accent; (3) irregular articulatory breakdown, the elision of syllables or phonemes; (4) distorted vowels; (5) harshness;

(6) prolonged phonemes; (7) prolonged intervals; (8) monopitch; (9) monoloudness; and (10) slow rate. Cerebellar speech may also be tremulous and may trail off to a whisper. However, it should again be noted that many patients are intentionally slow and perhaps regularize their speech—that is, voluntarily generate "scanning" speech to increase its intelligibility.

Perhaps analogous to the two types of timing deficits in finger movements described by Keele and Ivry (1990), at least two levels of speech control may be abnormal in cerebellar dysarthria. First, it is evident that on simple repetition of syllables, the peak repetition rate is considerably reduced in cerebellar patients, and the sounds are not crisp. This could easily be attributed to a difficulty with rapid production and termination of force in the musculature of the vocal tract and respiration. In addition, however, there seems to be a poor regulation of the normal speech prosody or rhythm that is not simply due to decreased ability to speak quickly. Correspondingly, at least two locations for cerebellar control of speech have been suggested. Holmes described dysarthria in gunshot wound patients with damage to the cerebellar hemispheres that was more pronounced when the vermis was also damaged, suggesting important roles for both the vermis and hemispheres.

Dysarthria has been reported in cases in which lesions were apparently confined to the vermis (Kadota et al., 1994), and Chiu and colleagues (1996) have stressed the importance of the vermis and fastigial nuclei in speech integration. On the other hand, Lechtenberg and Gilman (1978) have identified a paravermal site in the left cerebellar hemisphere that is specifically related to cerebellar dysarthria. They speculate that this cerebellar region functions in association with prosody areas in the right cerebral hemisphere to help regulate the timing of speech. The left hemisphere site is probably the more important of at least two cerebellar regions involved in normal speech production.

## Gait Ataxia

A deterioration in the stability of ambulation is the chief complaint of the majority of patients afflicted with cerebellar dysfunction. This is apparently due to two factors. First, the vermis of the cerebellum appears to be preferentially or initially affected in many degenerative conditions. This is especially the case for alcoholic/nutritional degeneration but also for cases of olivopontocerebellar degeneration. Second, walking, which consists of carefully managing a series of controlled collisions with the environment, is very demanding dynamically. Unlike the vocal tract and the arms, which are mechanically stable and will come to rest on relaxation, the upright body, virtually an inverted pendulum, is unstable. Thus, the body does not automatically return to a consistent initial condition following each step. Rather, each successive step depends sensitively on the manner in which the preceding step was completed. This aspect of bipedal locomotion probably contributes significantly to the variability of foot placement in ataxic gait.

Despite the variability in ataxic locomotion, there are still consistent kinematic patterns (Palliyath et al., 1998). As in upper extremity multijoint movement tasks, lower extremity multijoint coordination is characteristically abnormal. In particular, when walking, patients show a relatively greater delay in plantarflexion at the ankle than in flexion at the knee, as well as a relatively sluggish dorsiflexion of the ankle at the onset of swing. In walking, the largest and fastest required force transients are the forceful ankle plantar flexion at the end of stance and the rapid ankle dorsiflexion that follows immediately at the onset of swing. Therefore, as is argued with respect to the shoulder in upper extremity multijoint coordination failure, each of these two lower extremity coordination abnormalities is consistent with a force-rate deficit (or perhaps force-delay) at the joint, in this case the ankle, that has the greatest force-rate demand. The situation is not completely clear, however, because a similar ankle-knee relationship may be seen in elderly subjects without ataxia. Further quantitative studies are needed. In any case, owing at least in part to the sluggishness of dorsiflexion, there is a tendency for ataxic patients to trip as their toes fail to clear the ground during swing. That no significant abnormality was noted in the height of toe lift during swing phase by Palliyath and colleagues (1998) may well be because trials in which stumbles occurred were excluded from analysis.

Ataxic gait, when under control, tends to be slower than normal and to have shortened strides. As Palliyath and colleagues (1998) argued, this is at least partially a voluntary compensation for the loss of control that occurs at higher speeds. Because walking involves controlled falling, both forward and laterally onto the next foot placement, walking with too slow a cadence demands prolonged balancing on each leg, which is difficult for the ataxic patient. Therefore, as patients slow down, they will tend to adopt a much shorter stride to maintain their cadence or a wider base to stabilize themselves laterally. Possibly because of the resulting waddle, patients sometimes report that they walk "better" when they move at a moderate speed rather than very slowly, even though they might become more prone to veer or to trip than when they waddle.

## Impaired Motor Learning

The consideration that ataxic patients should have difficulty with motor learning follows from the apparent logic that if they could learn, then why would they still be clumsy? Motor learning itself is a complex phenomenon with a number of different components (Hallett et al., 1996; Hallett and Grafman, 1997). One aspect can be defined as a change in motor performance with practice. Other aspects would include increasing the repertoire of motor behavior and maintenance of a new behavior over a period of time. Even considering only a change in motor performance, there are likely to be several different phenomena. Adaptation and skill learning can be distinguished. Adaptation is simply a change in the nature of the motor output, while skill learning is the development of a new capability.

Adaptation learning clearly involves the cerebellum. Adaptation to lateral displacement of vision as produced by prism glasses is a method for assessing learning of a visual-motor task. When prism glasses are used, there is at first a mismatch between where an object is seen and where the pointing is directed. With experience, normal human subjects adjust to this and begin to point correctly. This correct pointing can be a product of a true change in the visual-motor coordination or an intellectual decision to point in a different direction than where the object appears to be so that the correct movement is made. When the glasses are removed, typically the subject initially points in the direction opposite to that in which he or she pointed when the glasses were put on. In the naïve subject, this is an excellent measure of true change in the visual-motor task, since there is no reason for making any intellectual decision to point other than in the direction where the object appears to be. With additional experience, the subjects return to correct performance again. Patients with cerebellar damage show poor or no adaptation (Weiner et al., 1983; Martin et al., 1996). Another paradigm that can test adaptation learning is a task with a change in the visual-motor gain. An example is making movements of the elbow by matching targets on a computer screen. If the gain of the elbow with respect to the display on the computer screen is changed, then the amount of movement to match the targets will change. In the normal circumstance after a gain change, there would be an error that gradually would be reduced with continued practice. Deuschl and colleagues (1996) found that ataxic patients showed much slower learning than did the normal controls.

Eye blink conditioning is recognized as a form of motor learning and could be argued to fit the definition proposed here for adaptation learning. In nonhuman animal studies, eye blink conditioning seems to require the cerebellum, at least for the expression and timing of the response. A number of groups have studied eye blink conditioning in patients with cerebellar lesions and found them to be markedly deficient (Daum et al., 1993; Topka et al., 1993).

There have been fewer studies of motor skill learning. Topka and colleagues (1998) evaluated the ability of patients to learn a multijoint two-dimensional trajectory with the upper extremity. While the performance of the patients was clearly impaired, they improved their performance as much as the normal subjects did, as long as the task was done slowly. With rapid movements, learning did slow down abnormally in the patients. Skill learning has many components, including features such as the sequencing of the different components. Other parts of the brain play important roles in these other functions and can be responsible for the learning in the ataxic patients. Functional imaging studies, for example, show increased activation with learning in motor cortex, premotor cortex, and parietal areas (Hallett et al., 1996; Hallett and Grafman, 1997).

## Clinical Localization

Virtually any lesion of the cerebellar parenchyma can be associated with ataxia. Presumably owing to the considerable redundancy, complex interconnectedness, and plasticity of cerebellar circuits, as well as to interindividual physiologic differences, attempts at precisely localizing cerebellar function on the basis of experimental and natural lesions have yielded inconsistent results. Similarly, it is usually not possible to predict lesion sites within the cerebellum with great accuracy from the clinical examination. Thus clinicoanatomic correlations should be viewed only as predominant patterns.

The cerebellum is often considered to be functionally divided into four parts on the basis of its output nuclei. Three sagittal zones—midline, intermediate, and lateral—project to the fastigius, interpositus (globose and emboliform nuclei in combination), and dentate nuclei, respectively, while the vestibulocerebellum (flocculonodular lobe) projects to the lateral vestibular nucleus, which effectively functions as a fourth cerebellar deep nucleus. From a clinical point of view, however, partitioning into simply midline, lateral (or vermis and hemispheres), and vestibular cerebellum is usually sufficient. The vestibulocerebellum, owing to its large involvement in head, eye, and balance control, can be considered part of the midline region. At least for tasks used in bedside examination, the functions of the intermediate and lateral zones of the hemispheres are not readily distinguished. In addition, it is useful to keep in mind that tremor seldom appears to be due to lesions of the cerebellar cortex alone and that the superior/anterior portion of the vermis, in particular, is affected in relative isolation by vitamin deficiency (often secondary to chronic alcohol intoxication) and tumors (especially in children), which produce a fairly pure ataxia of upright stance and gait with minimal, if any, limb ataxia, dysarthria, or nystagmus.

In general, signs that involve only the limbs unilaterally are most often due to lesions of the ipsilateral cerebellar hemispheres. However, this is not uniformly the case. In a series of 106 patients having unilateral or predominantly unilateral hemispheric injury (most postsurgical cases) studied by Lechtenberg and Gilman (Gilman et al., 1981), predominantly right limb dysmetria was associated with right hemisphere damage in 22 of 26 (85%) cases, and left limb dysmetria was associated with left hemispheric damage in 37 of 42 (88%) cases. For dysdiadochokinesia, ipsilateral hemispheric lesions were seen in 11 of 12 (91%) right-predominant cases and 25 of 32 (78%) left-predominant cases. The mechanism of strictly contralateral hemispheric effects on limb movement is not known. The handedness of the subjects was not reported. However, assuming the usual prevalence, the findings for dysdiadochokinesia are consistent with a mild additional impairment of the nondominant hand. This is consistent with the apparent importance of cerebrocerebellar interaction with rapid alternating movements (see previous discussion). When vermal lesions affected the limbs, the deficits were usually seen bilaterally, and when there was asymmetry of deficit, the left limbs tended to be more severely affected. Overall, tremor was found less often than dysmetria or dysdiadochokinesia, but it occurred with similar rates in vermal and unilateral hemispheric disease.

Deficits involving the head, trunk, balance, and gait in isolation tend to be related preferentially to vermal lesions. However, other sites are possible. As was discussed earlier, dysarthria, deficits involving the mouth, although midline, may be due to vermal or hemispheric dysfunction.

## CORTICAL CONTROL MECHANISMS

As was noted earlier, the primary motor cortex provides the principal output to the corticospinal tract. Thus, its inputs determine the brain's contribution to movement. The main inputs come from the premotor cortices, including the lateral premotor cortex, the supplementary motor area, and the caudal parts of the cingulate motor area. These areas in turn receive their input from wide areas of brain, including the presupplementary motor area, rostral parts of the cingulate motor area, the dorsolateral prefrontal cortex, and parietal areas. Considerable attention has been given recently to the parietal-premotor connections, which are highly specific and appear to provide important links between sensory and motor function (Rizzolatti et al., 1998; Rizzolatti and Luppino, 2001) (Fig. 2-5).

## APRAXIA

The apraxias are disorders of motor control, characterized by a loss of the motor program, not explicable by more elemental motor, sensory, coordination, or language impairments (Haaland et al., 2000; Hanna-Pladdy et al., 2001; Zadikoff and Lang, 2005). Idiomotor apraxia is present when there is knowledge of the task but there are temporal and spatial errors in performance. It has long been suspected to be due to a disconnection between parietal and premotor areas. Table 2-2 lists the types of apraxias.

## WHAT IS A VOLUNTARY MOVEMENT?

While clearly much is known about the anatomy and physiology of the motor system, there is still considerable difficulty with the concept of voluntariness. Many movements are triggered by sensory stimuli, and the physiology of this mechanism is relatively clear. However, there are certainly movements that appear to be internally triggered, and humans have the sense that they have willed the movement. The self-initiation of movement and conscious awareness of movement appear to involve mesial motor structures such as the supplementary motor area and the dorsolateral prefrontal cortex (Deiber et al., 1999). As Paus (2001) pointed out, the mesial motor structures and the anterior cingulate cortex in particular are places of convergence for motor control, homeostatic drive, emotion, and cognition. Looked at critically, the sense of voluntariness is clearly a perception of consciousness (what can be called a qualia). There is very little understanding of how this comes about.

## DISORDERS OF WILLED MOVEMENT

In neurology, there are many disorders in which the issue of will arises (Hallett, 2006). There are patients who have movements that are commonly held as being involuntary. Myoclonus is such an example. The brain makes the movement, yet the patient interprets the movement as involuntary. Early in the course of Huntington disease, patients with chorea often do not recognize that there are any involuntary movements. It is not clear why this happens or why it changes later.

Although tics are generally considered involuntary, patients with tics often cannot say whether their movements are voluntary or involuntary. This might not be a relevant distinction in their minds. It is perhaps a better description to say that they can suppress their movements or they just let them happen. Tics look like voluntary movements in all respects from the point of view of EMG and kinesiology (Hallett, 2000). Interestingly, they are often not preceded by the normal brain potential, the Bereitschaftspotential; hence, the brain mechanisms for their production clearly differ from those of ordinary voluntary movement (Obeso et al., 1981; Karp et al., 1996).

The symptom of loss of voluntary movement is often called abulia or, in the extreme, akinetic mutism (Fisher, 1983). The classic lesion is in the midline frontal region affecting areas including the supplementary motor area and cingulate motor areas. The bradykinesia and akinesia of PD are related.

The alien hand phenomenon is characterized by unwanted movements that arise without any sense of their being willed.

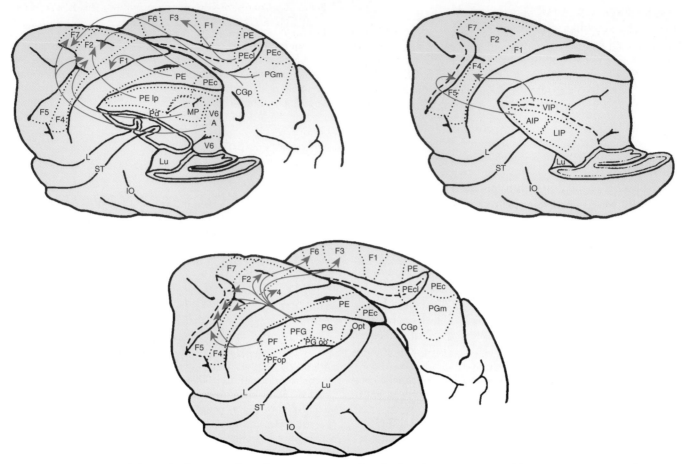

**Figure 2-5** Diagram of the multiple parietofrontal connections as identified in the primate. For abbreviations, see Rizzolatti et al., 1998. (Reprinted with permission from Rizzolatti G, Luppino G, Matelli M: The organization of the cortical motor system: New concepts. Electroencephalogr Clin Neurophysiol 1998;106:283–296.)

In addition to simple, unskilled, quasi-reflex movements (such as grasping), there can also be complex, skilled movements such as intermanual conflict or interference (Fisher, 2000). There appears to be a difficulty in self-initiating movement and excessive ease in the production of involuntary and triggered movements. In cases with discrete lesions, this seems to have its anatomic correlation in the territory of the anterior cerebral artery.

Conversion psychogenic movements are movements that the patient interprets as involuntary. Their etiology is actually obscure, since the physiology of conversion is really unknown. EEG investigation of these movements shows a normal-looking Bereitschaftpotential preceding them (Toro and Torres, 1986; Terada et al., 1995). The normal brain potential, however, indicates that there must be substantial sharing of brain voluntary movement mechanisms.

**Table 2-2** Types of apraxia

| Apraxia | Features |
|---|---|
| Limb kinetic apraxia | Loss of hand and finger dexterity; significantly affecting manipulative movements |
| Ideomotor apraxia | Deficit in pantomiming tool use and gestures with temporal and spatial errors. Knowledge of tasks is still present. |
| Ideational apraxia | Failure to carry out a series of tasks using multiple objects for an intended purpose; problem in the sequencing of actions. Tools are identifiable. |
| Conceptual apraxia | Loss of tool knowledge; inappropriate use of tools and objects; inability to solve mechanical problems. |
| (Verbal-motor) Dissociation apraxia | Failure to respond to verbal commands but use of objects is appropriate |
| Conduction apraxia | Problems with imitating but not with responding to verbal commands |

Modified from Wheaton L, Hallett M: Ideomotor apraxia: A review. J Neurol Sci 2007 (in press).

## Acknowledgments

This chapter is the work of the U.S. government and is not copyrighted. The ataxia section of the chapter is updated from a syllabus written for the 1999 meeting of the American Academy of Neurology, which itself was extensively modified and updated from a chapter by Massaquoi and Hallett (1998). The PD section is modified from an earlier chapter (Hallett, 2003a). The dystonia section is modified from earlier chapters (Hallett, 2004).

## References

Alexander GE, Crutcher MD: Functional architecture of basal ganglia circuits: Neural substrates of parallel processing. Trends Neurosci 1990;13:266–271.

Angel RW: Barognosis in a patient with hemiataxia. Ann Neurol 1980;7:73–77.

Angelucci A, Levitt JB, Lund JS: Anatomical origins of the classical receptive field and modulatory surround field of single neurons in macaque visual cortical area V1. Prog Brain Res 2002;136:373–388.

Baker RS, Sun WS, Hasan SA, et al: Maladaptive neural compensatory mechanisms in Bell's palsy-induced blepharospasm. Neurology 1997;49:223–229.

Bara-Jimenez W, Catalan MJ, Hallett M, Gerloff C: Abnormal somatosensory homunculus in dystonia of the hand. Ann Neurol 1998;44:828–831.

Bar-Gad I, Morris G, Bergman H: Information processing, dimensionality reduction and reinforcement learning in the basal ganglia. Prog Neurobiol 2003;71:439–473.

Baroni A, Benvenuti F, Fantini L, et al: Human ballistic arm abduction movements: Effects of L-dopa treatment in Parkinson's disease. Neurology 1984;34:868–876.

Bastian AJ, Martin TA, Keating JG, Thach WT: Cerebellar ataxia: Abnormal control of interaction torques across multiple joints. J Neurophysiol 1996;76:492–509.

Bastian AJ, Zackowski KM, Thach WT: Cerebellar ataxia: Torque deficiency or torque mismatch between joints? J Neurophysiol 2000;83:3019–3030.

Becker WJ, Kunesch E, Freund HJ: Coordination of a multi-joint movement in normal humans and in patients with cerebellar dysfunction. Can J Neurol Sci 1990;17:264–274.

Benabid AL, Pollak P, Gao D, et al: Chronic electrical stimulation of the ventralis intermedius nucleus of the thalamus as a treatment of movement disorders. J Neurosurg 1996;84:203–214.

Benecke R, Rothwell JC, Dick JP, et al: Simple and complex movements off and on treatment in patients with Parkinson's disease. J Neurol Neurosurg Psychiatry 1987;50:296–303.

Beppu H, Nagaoka M, Tanaka R: Analysis of cerebellar motor disorders by visually-guided elbow tracking movement: 2. Contribution of the visual cues on slow ramp pursuit. Brain 1987;110:1–18.

Beppu H, Suda M, Tanaka R: Analysis of cerebellar motor disorders by visually guided elbow tracking movement. Brain 1984;107:787–809.

Berardelli A, Dick JP, Rothwell JC, Day BL, Marsden CD: Scaling of the size of the first agonist EMG burst during rapid wrist movements in patients with Parkinson's disease. J Neurol Neurosurg Psychiatry 1986;49:1273–1279.

Berardelli A, Rothwell JC, Day BL, Marsden CD: Pathophysiology of blepharospasm and oromandibular dystonia. Brain 1985;108:593–608.

Berardelli A, Rothwell JC, Thompson PD, Hallett M: Pathophysiology of bradykinesia in Parkinson's disease. Brain 2001;124:2131–2146.

Berardelli A, Sabra AF, Hallett M: Physiological mechanisms of rigidity in Parkinson's disease. J Neurol Neurosurg Psychiatry 1983;46:45–53.

Bergui M, Lopiano L, Paglia G, et al: Stretch reflex of quadriceps femoris and its relation to rigidity in Parkinson's disease. Acta Neurol Scand 1992;86:226–229.

Bower JM: Control of sensory data acquisition. Int Rev Neurobiol 1997;41:489–513.

Britton TC, Thompson PD, Day BL, et al: Modulation of postural tremors at the wrist by supramaximal electrical median nerve shocks in essential tremor, Parkinson's disease and normal subjects mimicking tremor. J Neurol Neurosurg Psychiatry 1993a;56:1085–1089.

Britton TC, Thompson PD, Day BL, et al: Modulation of postural wrist tremors by magnetic stimulation of the motor cortex in patients with Parkinson's disease or essential tremor and in normal subjects mimicking tremor. Ann Neurol 1993b;33:473–479.

Brown VJ, Schwarz U, Bowman EM, et al: Dopamine dependent reaction time deficits in patients with Parkinson's disease are task specific. Neuropsychologia 1993;31:459–469.

Byl N, Merzenich MM, Jenkins WM: A primate genesis model of focal dystonia and repetitive strain injury: I. Learning-induced dedifferentiation of the representation of the hand in the primary somatosensory cortex in adult monkeys. Neurology 1996;47:508–520.

Chen R, Kumar S, Garg RR, Lang AE: Impairment of motor cortex activation and deactivation in Parkinson's disease. Clin Neurophysiol 2001;112:600–607.

Chen R, Wassermann E, Caños M, Hallett M: Impaired inhibition in writer's cramp during voluntary muscle activation. Neurology 1997;49:1054–1059.

Chiu MJ, Chen RC, Tseng CY: Clinical correlates of quantitative acoustic analysis in ataxic dysarthria. Eur Neurol 1996;36:310–314.

Chuke JC, Baker RS, Porter JD: Bell's palsy-associated blepharospasm relieved by aiding eyelid closure. Ann Neurol 1996;39:263–268.

Cody FW, MacDermott N, Matthews PB, Richardson HC: Observations on the genesis of the stretch reflex in Parkinson's disease. Brain 1986;109:229–249.

Cohen LG, Hallett M: Hand cramps: Clinical features and electromyographic patterns in a focal dystonia. Neurology 1988;38:1005–1012.

Curra A, Berardelli A, Agostino R, et al: Performance of sequential arm movements with and without advance knowledge of motor pathways in Parkinson's disease. Mov Disord 1997;12:646–654.

Daum I, Schugens MM, Ackermann H, et al: Classical conditioning after cerebellar lesions in humans. Behav Neurosci 1993;107:748–756.

Deiber MP, Honda M, Ibanez V, et al: Mesial motor areas in self-initiated versus externally triggered movements examined with fMRI: Effect of movement type and rate. J Neurophysiol 1999;81:3065–3077.

Demirci M, Grill S, McShane L, Hallett M: A mismatch between kinesthetic and visual perception in Parkinson's disease. Ann Neurol 1997;41:781–788.

Deuschl G, Toro C, Zeffiro T, et al: Adaptation motor learning of arm movements in patients with cerebellar diseases. J Neurol Neurosurg Psychiatry 1996;60:515–519.

Diener HC, Dichgans J: Pathophysiology of cerebellar ataxia. Mov Disord 1992;7:95–109.

Diener HC, Dichgans J, Bacher M, Gompf B: Quantification of postural sway in normals and patients with cerebellar diseases. Electroencephalogr Clin Neurophysiol 1984;57:134–142.

Diener HC, Hore J, Ivry R, Dichgans J: Cerebellar dysfunction of movement and perception. Can J Neurol Sci 1993;20(suppl 3):S62–S69.

Di Lazzaro V, Oliviero A, Meglio M, et al: Direct demonstration of the effect of lorazepam on the excitability of the human motor cortex. Clin Neurophysiol 2000;111:794–799.

Elble RJ: The pathophysiology of tremor. In Watts RL, Koller WC (eds): Movement Disorders: Neurologic Principles and Practice. New York, McGraw–Hill, 1997, pp 405–417.

Elble RJ, Koller WC: Tremor. Baltimore, Johns Hopkins University Press, 1990.

Evarts EV, Teravainen H, Calne DB: Reaction time in Parkinson's disease. Brain 1981;104:167–186.

Fisher CM: Honored guest presentation: Abulia minor vs. agitated behavior. Clin Neurosurg 1983;31:9–31.

Fisher CM: Alien hand phenomena: A review with the addition of six personal cases. Can J Neurol Sci 2000;27:192–203.

Fuhr P, Agostino R, Hallett M: Spinal motor neuron excitability during the silent period after cortical stimulation. Electroencephalogr Clin Neurophysiol 1991;81:257–262.

Gao JH, Parsons LM, Bower JM, et al: Cerebellum implicated in sensory acquisition and discrimination rather than motor control. Science 1996;272:545–547.

Garraux G, Bauer A, Hanakawa T, et al: Changes in brain anatomy in focal hand dystonia. Ann Neurol 2004;55:736–739.

Gilman S, Bloedel JR, Lechtenberg R: Disorders of the Cerebellum. Philadelphia, F A Davis, 1981.

Gilman S, Carr D, Hollenberg J: Kinematic effects of deafferentation and cerebellar ablation. Brain 1976;99:311–330.

Godaux E, Koulischer D, Jacquy J: Parkinsonian bradykinesia is due to depression in the rate of rise of muscle activity. Ann Neurol 1992;31:93–100.

Grill SE, Hallett M, Marcus C, McShane L: Disturbances of kinesthesia in patients with cerebellar disorders. Brain 1994;117:1433–1447.

Grill SE, Hallett M, McShane LM: Timing of onset of afferent responses and of use of kinesthetic information for control of movement in normal and cerebellar-impaired subjects. Exp Brain Res 1997;113:33–47.

Haaland KY, Harrington DL, Knight RT: Neural representations of skilled movement. Brain 2000;123(11):2306–2313.

Hallett M: Differential diagnosis of tremor. In Vinken PJ, Bruyn GW, Klawans HL (eds): Handbook of Clinical Neurology: Extrapyramidal Disorders, vol 5 (49). Amsterdam, Elsevier Science Publishers, 1987, pp 583–595.

Hallett M: Clinical neurophysiology of akinesia. Revue Neurologique (Paris) 1990;146:585–590.

Hallett M: Classification and treatment of tremor. JAMA 1991;266:1115–1117.

Hallett M: Electrophysiologic evaluation of movement disorders. In Aminoff MJ (ed): Electrodiagnosis in Clinical Neurology. New York, Churchill Livingstone, 1999, pp 365–380.

Hallett M: Neurophysiology of tics. In Cohen DJ, Goetz CG, Jankovic J (eds): Tourette Syndrome: Advances in Neurology, vol 85. Philadelphia, Lippincott, Williams & Wilkins, 2000, pp 237–244.

Hallett M: Parkinson revisited: Pathophysiology of motor signs. Adv Neurol 2003a;91:19–28.

Hallett M (ed): Movement Disorder, vol 1. Amsterdam, Elsevier, 2003b.

Hallett M: Dystonia: Abnormal movements result from loss of inhibition. Adv Neurol 2004;94:1–9.

Hallett M: Voluntary and involuntary movements in humans. In Hallett M, Fahn S, Jankovic J, et al (eds): Psychogenic Movement Disorders: Neurology and Neuropsychiatry. Philadelphia, Lippincott, Williams & Wilkins, 2006, pp 189–195.

Hallett M, Berardelli A, Delwaide P, et al: Central EMG and tests of motor control: Report of an IFCN Committee. Electroencephalogr Clin Neurophysiol 1994;90:404–432.

Hallett M, Berardelli A, Matheson J, et al: Physiological analysis of simple rapid movements in patients with cerebellar deficits. J Neurol Neurosurg Psychiatry 1991;53:124–133.

Hallett M, Grafman J: Executive function and motor skill learning. In Schmahmann JD (ed): The Cerebellum and Cognition: International Review of Neurobiology, vol 41. San Diego, Academic Press, 1997, pp 297–323.

Hallett M, Khoshbin S: A physiological mechanism of bradykinesia. Brain 1980;103:301–314.

Hallett M, Massaquoi S: Physiologic studies of dysmetria in patients with cerebellar deficits. Can J Neurol Sci 1993;20(suppl 3):S83–S89.

Hallett M, Pascual-Leone A, Topka H: Adaptation and skill learning: Evidence for different neural substrates. In Bloedel JR, Ebner TJ, Wise SP (eds): Acquisition of Motor Behavior in Vertebrates. Cambridge, Mass, MIT Press, 1996, pp 289–301.

Hallett M, Shahani BT, Young RR: EMG analysis of patients with cerebellar deficits. J Neurol Neurosurg Psychiatry 1975;38:1163–1169.

Hallett M, Shahani BT, Young RR: Analysis of stereotyped voluntary movements at the elbow in patients with Parkinson's disease. J Neurol Neurosurg Psychiatry 1977;40:1129–1135.

Hanna-Pladdy B, Heilman KM, Foundas AL: Cortical and subcortical contributions to ideomotor apraxia: analysis of task demands and error types. Brain 2001;124:2513–2527.

Hayase N, Miyashita N, Endo K, Narabayashi H: Neuronal activity in GP and Vim of parkinsonian patients and clinical changes of tremor through surgical interventions. Stereotact Funct Neurosurg 1998;71:20–28.

Holmes G: The cerebellum of man. Brain 1939;62:1–30.

Horak FB, Diener HC: Cerebellar control of postural scaling and central set in stance. J Neurophysiol 1994;72:479–493.

Hore J, Flament D: Evidence that a disordered servo-like mechanism contributes to tremor in movements during cerebellar dysfunction. J Neurophysiol 1986;56:123–136.

Hore J, Wild B, Diener HC: Cerebellar dysmetria at the elbow, wrist, and fingers. J Neurophysiol 1991;65:563–571.

Hurtado JM, Gray CM, Tamas LB, Sigvardt KA: Dynamics of tremor-related oscillations in the human globus pallidus: A single case study. Proc Natl Acad Sci U S A 1999;96:1674–1679.

Hurtado JM, Lachaux JP, Beckley DJ, et al: Inter- and intralimb oscillator coupling in parkinsonian tremor. Mov Disord 2000;15:683–691.

Ito M: The Cerebellum and Neural Control. New York, Raven Press, 1984.

Jankovic J, Cardoso F, Grossman RG, Hamilton WJ: Outcome after stereotactic thalamotomy for parkinsonian, essential, and other types of tremor. Neurosurgery 1995;37:680–686.

Jordan N, Sagar HJ, Cooper JA: A component analysis of the generation and release of isometric force in Parkinson's disease. J Neurol Neurosurg Psychiatry 1992;55:572–576.

Kadota O, Sakaki S, Kumon Y, et al: Large cystic cavernous angioma of the cerebellum: Case report. Neurol Med Chir (Tokyo) 1994;34:768–772.

Karp BI, Porter S, Toro C, Hallett M: Simple motor tics may be preceded by a premotor potential. J Neurol Neurosurg Psychiatry 1996;61:103–106.

Keele SW, Ivry R: Does the cerebellum provide a common computation for diverse tasks?: A timing hypothesis. Ann N Y Acad Sci 1990;608:179–207.

Labutta RJ, Miles RB, Sanes JN, Hallett M: Motor program memory storage in Parkinson's disease patients tested with a delayed response task. Mov Disord 1994;9:218–222.

Lechtenberg R, Gilman S: Speech disorders in cerebellar disease. Ann Neurol 1978;3:285–290.

Lerner A, Shill H, Hanakawa T, et al: Regional cerebral blood flow correlates of the severity of writer's cramp symptoms. Neuroimage 2004;21 904–913.

Levy LM, Hallett M: Impaired brain GABA in focal dystonia. Ann Neurol 2002;51:93–101.

Magnin M, Morel A, Jeanmonod D: Single-unit analysis of the pallidum, thalamus and subthalamic nucleus in parkinsonian patients. Neuroscience 2000;96:549–564.

Mai N, Bolsinger P, Avarello M, et al: Control of isometric finger force in patients with cerebellar disease. Brain 1988;111:973–998.

Majsak MJ, Kaminski T, Gentile AM, Flanagan JR: The reaching movements of patients with Parkinson's disease under self-determined maximal speed and visually cued conditions. Brain 1998;121:755–766.

Manto MU: Effects of hyperventilation on fast goal-directed limb movements in spinocerebellar ataxia type 6. Eur J Neurol 2001;8:401–406.

Manto MU, Setta F, Jacquy J, et al: Different types of cerebellar hypometria associated with a distinct topography of the lesion in cerebellum. J Neurol Sci 1998;158:88–95.

Martin TA, Keating JG, Goodkin HP, et al: Throwing while looking through prisms: I. Focal olivocerebellar lesions impair adaptation. Brain 1996;119:1183–1198.

Massaquoi S, Hallett M: Kinematics of initiating a two-joint arm movement in patients with cerebellar ataxia. Can J Neurol Sci 1996;23:3–14.

Massaquoi SG, Hallett M: Ataxia and other cerebellar syndromes. In Jankovic J, Tolosa E (eds): Parkinson's Disease and Movement Disorders, 3rd ed. Baltimore, Williams & Wilkins, 1998, pp 623–686.

Massaquoi SG, Hallett M: Ataxia and other cerebellar syndromes. In Jankovic J, Tolosa E (eds): Parkinson's Disease and Movement Disorders, 4th ed. Philadelphia, Lippincott, Williams & Wilkins, 2002, pp 393–408.

Massaquoi SG, Slotine JJ: The intermediate cerebellum may function as a wave-variable processor. Neurosci Lett 1996;215:60–64.

Matsumura M, Sawaguchi T, Kubota K: GABAergic inhibition of neuronal activity in the primate motor and premotor cortex during voluntary movement. J Neurophysiol 1992;68:692–702.

Matsumura M, Sawaguchi T, Oishi T, et al: Behavioral deficits induced by local injection of bicuculline and muscimol into the primate motor and premotor cortex. J Neurophysiol 1991;65: 1542–1553.

Meara RJ, Cody FW: Stretch reflexes of individual parkinsonian patients studied during changes in clinical rigidity following medication. Electroencephalogr Clin Neurophysiol 1993;89: 261–268.

Meunier S, Garnero L, Ducorps A, et al: Human brain mapping in dystonia reveals both endophenotypic traits and adaptive reorganization. Ann Neurol 2001;50:521–527.

Mink JW: The basal ganglia: Focused selection and inhibition of competing motor programs. Prog Neurobiol 1996;50:381–425.

Molloy FM, Carr TD, Zeuner KE, et al: Abnormalities of spatial discrimination in focal and generalized dystonia. Brain 2003;126: 2175–2182.

Morrice BL, Becker WJ, Hoffer JA, Lee RG: Manual tracking performance in patients with cerebellar incoordination: Effects of mechanical loading. Can J Neurol Sci 1990;17:275–285.

Nakashima K, Rothwell JC, Day BL, et al: Reciprocal inhibition in writer's and other occupational cramps and hemiparesis due to stroke. Brain 1989;112:681–697.

Nathan PW, Smith M, Deacon P: Vestibulospinal, reticulospinal and descending propriospinal nerve fibres in man. Brain 1996;119(6): 1809–1833.

Obeso JA, Rothwell JC, Marsden CD: Simple tics in Gilles de la Tourette's syndrome are not prefaced by a normal premovement potential. J Neurol Neurosurg Psychiatry 1981;44:735–738.

Otsuka M, Ichiya Y, Kuwabara Y, et al: Differences in the reduced 18F-dopa uptakes of the caudate and the putamen in Parkinson's disease: Correlations with the three main symptoms. J Neurol Sci 1996;136:169–173.

Palliyath S, Hallett M, Thomas SL, Lebiedowska MK: Gait in patients with cerebellar ataxia. Mov Disord 1998;13:958–964.

Panizza M, Lelli S, Nilsson J, Hallett M: H-reflex recovery curve and reciprocal inhibition of H-reflex in different kinds of dystonia. Neurology 1990;40:824–828.

Pascual-Leone A, Valls-Solé J, Brasil-Neto J, et al: Akinesia in Parkinson's disease: I. Shortening of simple reaction time with focal, single-pulse transcranial magnetic stimulation. Neurology 1994a;44:884–891.

Pascual-Leone A, Valls-Solé J, Toro C, et al: Resetting of essential tremor and postural tremor in Parkinson's disease with transcranial magnetic stimulation. Muscle Nerve 1994b;17:800–807.

Paus T: Primate anterior cingulate cortex: Where motor control, drive and cognition interface. Nat Rev Neurosci 2001;2:417–424.

Perlmutter JS, Stambuk MK, Markham J, et al: Decreased [18F]spiperone binding in putamen in idiopathic focal dystonia. J Neurosci 1997;17:843–850.

Quartarone A, Siebner HR, Rothwell JC: Task-specific hand dystonia: Can too much plasticity be bad for you? Trends Neurosci 2006 [Epub ahead of print (March 4)].

Ridding MC, Sheean G, Rothwell JC, et al: Changes in the balance between motor cortical excitation and inhibition in focal, task specific dystonia. J Neurol Neurosurg Psychiatry 1995;59:493–498.

Rizzolatti G, Luppino G: The cortical motor system. Neuron 2001;31:889–901.

Rizzolatti G, Luppino G, Matelli M: The organization of the cortical motor system: New concepts. Electroencephalogr Clin Neurophysiol 1998;106:283–296.

Rothwell JC, Obeso JA, Traub MM, Marsden CD: The behaviour of the long-latency stretch reflex in patients with Parkinson's disease. J Neurol Neurosurg Psychiatry 1983;46:35–44.

Sainburg RL, Poizner H, Ghez C: Loss of proprioception produces deficits in interjoint coordination. J Neurophysiol 1993;70: 2136–2147.

Samii A, Wassermann EM, Hallett M: Decreased postexercise facilitation of motor evoked potentials in patients with cerebellar degeneration. Neurology 1997;49:538–542.

Sanes JN, LeWitt PA, Mauritz KH: Visual and mechanical control of postural and kinetic tremor in cerebellar system disorders. J Neurol Neurosurg Psychiatry 1988;51:934–943.

Sanger TD, Garg RR, Chen R: Interactions between two different inhibitory systems in the human motor cortex. J Physiol 2001;530:307–317.

Schicatano EJ, Basso MA, Evinger C: Animal model explains the origins of the cranial dystonia benign essential blepharospasm. J Neurophysiol 1997;77:2842–2846.

Schmahmann JD: The cerebellum in autism: Clinical and anatomical perspectives. In Bauman ML, Kemper TL (eds): The Neurobiology of Autism. Baltimore, Johns Hopkins University Press, 1994, pp 195–226.

Schmahmann JD, Pandya DN: The cerebrocerebellar system. Int Rev Neurobiol 1997;41:31–60.

Schwab RS, Chafetz ME, Walker S: Control of two simultaneous voluntary motor acts in normals and in parkinsonism. Arch Neurol 1954;72:591–598.

Sohn YH, Hallett M: Disturbed surround inhibition in focal hand dystonia. Ann Neurol 2004a;56:595–599.

Sohn YH, Hallett M: Surround inhibition in human motor system. Exp Brain Res 2004b;158:397–404.

Sohn YH, Jung HY, Kaelin-Lang A, Hallett M: Excitability of the ipsilateral motor cortex during phasic voluntary hand movement. Exp Brain Res 2003;148:176–185.

Starr A, Caramia M, Zarola F, Rossini PM: Enhancement of motor cortical excitability in humans by non-invasive electrical stimulation appears prior to voluntary movement. Electroencephalogr Clin Neurophysiol 1988;70:26–32.

Staude G, Wolf W, Ott M, et al: Tremor as a factor in prolonged reaction times of parkinsonian patients. Mov Disord 1995;10:-153–162.

Stefan K, Kunesch E, Cohen LG, et al: Induction of plasticity in the human motor cortex by paired associative stimulation. Brain 2000;123(3):572–584.

Stinear CM, Byblow WD: Impaired modulation of intracortical inhibition in focal hand dystonia. Cereb Cortex 2004;14:555–561.

Takakusaki K, Kohyama J, Matsuyama K, Mori S: Medullary reticulospinal tract mediating the generalized motor inhibition in cats: Parallel inhibitory mechanisms acting on motoneurons and on interneuronal transmission in reflex pathways. Neuroscience 2001;103:511–527.

Tatton WG, Bedingham W, Verrier MC, Blair RD: Characteristic alterations in responses to imposed wrist displacements in parkinsonian rigidity and dystonia musculorum deformans. Can J Neurol Sci 1984;11:281–287.

Terada K, Ikeda A, Van Ness PC, et al: Presence of Bereitschaftspotential preceding psychogenic myoclonus: Clinical application of jerk-locked back averaging. J Neurol Neurosurg Psychiatry 1995;58:745–747.

Terzuolo CA, Soechting JF, Viviani P: Studies on the control of some simple motor tasks: II. On the cerebellar control of movements in relation to the formulation of intentional commands. Brain Res 1973;58:217–222.

Thach WT, Goodkin HP, Keating JG: The cerebellum and the adaptive coordination of movement. Ann Rev Neurosci 1992;15:403–442.

Thach WT, Perry JG, Kane SA, Goodkin HP: Cerebellar nuclei: Rapid alternating movement, motor somatotopy, and a mechanism for the control of muscle synergy. Rev Neurol (Paris) 1993;149:607–628.

Tinazzi M, Priori A, Bertolasi L, Fet al: Abnormal central integration of a dual somatosensory input in dystonia: Evidence for sensory overflow. Brain 2000;123:42–50.

Topka H, Konczak J, Schneider K, et al: Multijoint arm movements in cerebellar ataxia: Abnormal control of movement dynamics. Exp Brain Res 1998;119:493–503.

Topka H, Valls-Solé J, Massaquoi S, Hallett M: Deficit in classical conditioning in patients with cerebellar degeneration. Brain 1993;116:961–969.

Toro C, Torres F: Electrophysiological correlates of a paroxysmal movement disorder. Ann Neurol 1986;20:731–734.

Valls-Solé J, Pascual-Leone A, Wassermann EM, Hallett M: Human motor evoked responses to paired transcranial magnetic stimuli. Electroencephalogr Clin Neurophysiol 1992;85:355–364.

Warabi T, Yanagisawa N, Shindo R: Changes in strategy of aiming tasks in Parkinson's disease. Brain 1988;111:497–505.

Watts RL, Mandir AS: The role of motor cortex in the pathophysiology of voluntary movement deficits associated with parkinsonism. Neurol Clin 1992;10:451–69.

Weiner MJ, Hallett M, Funkenstein HH: Adaptation to lateral displacement of vision in patients with lesions of the central nervous system. Neurology 1983;33:766–772.

Werhahn KJ, Kunesch E, Noachtar S, et al: Differential effects on motorcortical inhibition induced by blockade of GABA uptake in humans. J Physiol (Lond) 1999;517:591–597.

Wichmann T, DeLong MR: Functional neuroanatomy of the basal ganglia in Parkinson's disease. Adv Neurol 2003a;91:9–18.

Wichmann T, DeLong MR: Pathophysiology of Parkinson's disease: The MPTP primate model of the human disorder. Ann N Y Acad Sci 2003b;991:199–213.

Wing AM, Keele S, Margolin DI: Motor disorder and the timing of repetitive movements. Ann N Y Acad Sci 1984;423:183–192.

Zadikoff C, Lang AE: Apraxia in movement disorders. Brain 2005;128:1480–1497.

Ziemann U, Rothwell JC, Ridding MC: Interaction between intracortical inhibition and facilitation in human motor cortex. J Physiol (Lond) 1996;496:873–881.

Zirh TA, Lenz FA, Reich SG, Dougherty PM: Patterns of bursting occurring in thalamic cells during parkinsonian tremor. Neuroscience 1998;83:107–121.

# Chapter 3

# Functional Neuroanatomy of the Basal Ganglia

The key role of basal ganglia in the initiation and integration of movement is shown by the effects of the pathologic changes that occur in illnesses such as Parkinson disease (PD) and Huntington disease. The selective loss of dopaminergic cells in the substantia nigra pars compacta in PD and the subsequent fall in caudate-putamen dopamine content led to a better understanding of the functional integration of basal ganglia circuitry (Greenfield and Bosanquet, 1953; Ehringer and Hornykiewicz, 1960; Anden et al., 1964). In addition, the discovery of toxins such as 1-methyl-4-phenyl-1,2,3,6-tetrahydropyridine (MPTP) that are capable of selectively destroying dopaminergic neurons in primates has allowed further exploration of basal ganglia function and led to the development of models of how its integration controls movement (Davis et al., 1979; Burns et al., 1983; Langston et al., 1983). On the basis of the use of experimental models of PD and other basal ganglia degenerative disorders (Langston et al., 1983; Penney and Young, 1983, 1986; Crossman, 1987, 1990; Albin et al., 1989; DeLong, 1990; Bove et al., 2005), it has been possible to predict the nature of the changes in basal ganglia circuitry that occur when there is a failure to initiate voluntary movement or when involuntary movements, such as dyskinesia, appear. However, it has been necessary to refine these models constantly as further evidence of the complex nature of basal ganglia circuitry and its associated inputs and outputs is uncovered. In this chapter, the components that make up the basal ganglia, the major inputs and outputs of the basal ganglia and the transmitters that are utilized, and the functional changes in the basal ganglia that occur in disorders of movement are discussed. In addition, the functional neuroanatomy of basal ganglia is explored in an attempt to show the deficiencies of the currently used models. Indeed, it has become clear that basal ganglia function is changed in disorders of movement in a manner that is far more complex than was originally envisaged, and new models have had to be developed to reflect the advances in knowledge of its organization.

## BASAL GANGLIA AND THEIR ORGANIZATION

Anatomically, the term *basal ganglia* refers to the deep gray masses within the telencephalon (putamen, caudate nucleus, globus pallidus, and amygdala). But physiologically and clinically, the basal ganglia include the closely connected nuclei of the subthalamic nucleus (in diencephalon), substantia nigra pars compacta (SNc) and pars reticulata (SNr) (in mesencephalon), and pedunculopontine nucleus (PPN) (in pons). The caudate and putamen are collectively called the neostriatum, often abbreviated as striatum. The globus pallidus (GP) is the paleostriatum and is divided into a lateral (external) and a medial (internal) component, abbreviated GPe and GPi,

respectively. The amygdala is the archistriatum and is more functionally associated with the limbic system than with the motor system. The nucleus accumbens is anatomically the ventral part of the striatum and is also associated with limbic function. Because the centromedian parafascicular complex of the thalamus has a major afferent input into the striatum, this complex should also be included in the physiologic basal ganglia.

The anatomic relationship of the major components of basal ganglia is shown in Figure 3-1. The major inputs to basal ganglia are the topographically arranged glutamatergic corticostriatal and thalamostriatal fibers and the dopaminergic nigrostriatal pathway innervating the caudate-putamen (Alexander and Crutcher, 1990; Parent, 1990; Flaherty and Graybiel, 1993). In addition, there is input to basal ganglia from the raphe nuclei, resulting in serotonin (5-hydroxytryptamine, 5HT) innervation, and also input from the noradrenergic locus ceruleus (Moore and Bloom, 1979; Hornykiewicz, 1982; Graybiel, 1983; Agid et al., 1987), although the terminal projection sites are poorly defined despite the presence of $\alpha$-1 and $\alpha$-2 receptors in both the striatum and substantia nigra and evidence for noradrenergic inhibition of midbrain dopaminergic neurons (Paladini and Williams, 2004). Both of these inputs, as well as the nigrostriatal pathway, degenerate in PD.

Output from basal ganglia is composed largely of GABAergic pathways projecting from the GPi and SNr to the ventrolateral (VL) and ventroanterior (VA) nuclei of the thalamus (Albin et al., 1989; Parent, 1990). The SNr also projects to a variety of brainstem nuclei, including the superior colliculus (Carpenter, 1981; Parent, 1990). However, it is the output from the striatum making up the internal organization of basal ganglia that has largely been implicated in changes that occur in disorders of movement. A classic model of striatal output is illustrated in Figure 3-2. Output from the neostriatum is organized into two major pathways: the direct and indirect pathways (Penney and Young, 1983; Alexander et al., 1986; Albin et al., 1989; DeLong, 1990; Gerfen and Wilson, 1996; Smith et al., 1998). Both originate from the cell bodies of medium spiny neurons in the striatum. The direct output pathway projects from the striatum to the GPi and SNr. This pathway utilizes GABA as a neurotransmitter and colocalizes with the neuropeptides dynorphin and substance P. The cell bodies in the striatum largely bear D1 dopamine receptors (but see later). From the GPi, there is a GABAergic output pathway to the VL/VA nuclei of the thalamus, and from there, there is a glutamatergic pathway to the premotor cortex. The indirect output pathway is again a GABAergic pathway going from the striatum to the GPe that colocalizes enkephalin as a neuropeptide modulator and largely bears D2 receptors on the cell bodies in the striatum. From the GPe, another GABAergic pathway passes to the STN, which then synapses

## Functional Anatomy of Basal Ganglia

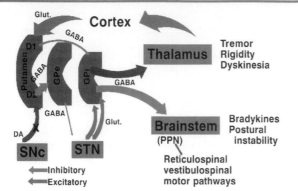

Figure 3-1 Diagram of the main pathways of basal ganglia. The putamen receives excitatory input (glutamate) from the cortex and projects both via an indirect pathway to the GPe, which in turn projects to the STN and then to the GPi, and via a direct pathway to the GPi. The GPi projects rostrally to the thalamus and cortex and caudally to the brainstem, particularly the PPN and spinal cord. Glut, glutamate; PPN, pedunculopontine nucleus. (See Color Plate 1) (Used with permission from J. Jankovic.)

with cell bodies of a glutamatergic pathway, innervating the GPi and SNr (as well as the PPN). This latter pathway may be of key importance to basal ganglia disease and is discussed again later. The alterations that occur in the indirect and direct output pathways associated with dysfunction of movement are also discussed subsequently, as are the shortcomings of the anatomic connections.

A number of key components of the basal ganglia circuitry are worthy of specific mention. In particular, the highly topographically organized corticostriatal glutamatergic input may be of special relevance to the control of motor behavior (Parent, 1990; Gerfen and Wilson, 1996). This system forms a major link of the basal ganglia with cortical input in the parallel loop process. Within the basal ganglia, there seem to be multiple, apparently segregated, circuits, defined by their source of input from different areas of the cerebral cortex and the final destination of their outputs to the frontal lobe (Parent, 1990). For example, it has been suggested that there may be at least five such segregated corticobasal gangliothalamocortical circuits, namely, motor, oculomotor, limbic, dorsolateral prefrontal, and lateral orbitofrontal (Alexander et al., 1986; Alexander and Crutcher, 1990). Each is conceived as remaining largely segregated from the others, both structurally and functionally. The different corticobasal ganglia circuits are thought to be the neural substrates for parallel processing of different functions. The extent to which activity in each of these parallel circuits remains segregated throughout the basal ganglia is debated. Anatomic evidence suggests that some degree of convergence between circuits is likely to occur at the level of the GPe and SNr (Percheron et al., 1984; Percheron and Filion, 1991; Parent and Hazrati, 1995a, 1995b). Altered dopaminergic control of the different parallel loops within basal ganglia may underlie the various manifestations of basal ganglia disease—for example, disorders of limb and axial movements, disorders of eye movement, and cognitive abnormalities (Rodriguez et al., 1998a).

Dysfunction of the glutamatergic system may also be one component of the processes responsible for the induction of dyskinesia in the treatment of PD (see later) (Chase and Oh, 2000). However, other glutamatergic components of basal ganglia also play a key role. In particular, the glutamatergic

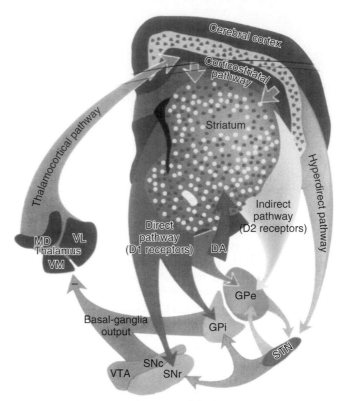

Figure 3-2 Major neural circuits of the basal ganglia. The projections from the cerebral cortex (corticostriatal and hyperdirect pathway), thalamus (thalamocortical pathway), and subthalamic nucleus (STN) are excitatory projections. The striatopallidal (both direct and indrect pathways) and the pathways to the thalamus from the pallidum and nigra reticulata are inhibitory projections. Cerebral cortical neurons in layer 5 provide excitatory, glutamatergic projections to the striatum (corticostriatal pathway). The striatum comprises two populations of medium spiny projection neurons. Direct-pathway neurons bear DI receptors and provide inputs directly to the output nuclei of the basal ganglia, the internal segment of the globus pallidus (GPi), and the substantia nigra pars reticulata (SNr). Indirect-pathway neurons possess D2 receptors and provide indirect projections to the output of the basal ganglia through projections to the external segment of the globus pallidus (GPe). The GPe is interconnected with the subthalamic nucleus (STN), which provides excitatory inputs to the output nuclei of the basal ganglia. The GPi and SNr provide inhibitory inputs to thalamic nuclei, the mediodorsal (MD), ventromedial (VM), and ventrolateral (VL) nuclei, which project to prefrontal, premotor, and motor cortical areas (thalamocortical pathway). Dopaminergic neurons in the ventral tegmental area (VTA) and substantia nigra pars compacta (SNc) give rise to dopamine projections to the striatum (labeled DA). (See Color Plate 2.) (Reproduced with permission from Gerfen CR: Molecular effects of dopamine on striatal-projection pathways. Trends Neurosci 2000;23[suppl]:S64–S70.)

pathway from the STN to the GPi and SNr may be highly important, as overactivity of the STN not only may contribute to motor deficits in PD but also has been postulated to be involved in an excitotoxic process of dopaminergic cell death in SNc (Rodriguez et al., 1998b). The key role played by STN output neurons is demonstrated by the success of both deep brain stimulation in STN and lesions of STN (Bergman et al., 1990; Pollak et al., 1997; Rodriguez-Oroz et al., 2004). A further glutamatergic input comes from the PPN to the substantia nigra and other nuclei of basal ganglia (Bevan et al., 1995; Charara et al., 1996). This pathway gets scant consideration in most schemes depicting the functional neuroanatomy of basal ganglia, despite the fact that PPN degenerates in PD (Jellinger, 1987; Heise et al., 2005). Overall, there has been little investigation of the role of the PPN pathway in the genesis of movement disorders or in the control of normal motor behavior. Relatively recently, deep brain stimulation of the PPN in PD has been shown to improve posture gait and akinesia (Jenkinson et al., 2004, 2005; Plaha and Gill, 2005; Temel and Visser-Vandewalle, 2006). Lesioning of the nigrostriatal pathway leads to overactivity of PPN neurons, and this is reversed by a lesion of the STN highlighting the intimacy of the connections between these brain regions (Breit et al., 2001).

The role of cholinergic systems in basal ganglia function is also under-researched. The presence of cholinergic interneurons in the striatum has been known for many years, and there is clearly a functional interaction between these cells and the dopaminergic input to the striatum as well as with GABAergic output and the corticostriatal glutamatergic inputs (Guyenet et al., 1975; Graybiel, 1990). The role of this system in basal ganglia is poorly described, and it is rare to find cholinergic interneurons incorporated into any current scheme of the functional neuroanatomy of the basal ganglia. Yet anticholinergic drugs can have a symptomatic effect in the treatment of PD (Jankovic and Marsden, 1998), and high doses of anticholinergics can be useful in the control of dystonia (Fahn, 1983; Burke et al., 1985). There has been little research aimed at finding novel therapeutic agents that can interact with the cholinergic system for the treatment of movement disorders. This is despite the clear data showing the presence of both muscarinic and nicotinic receptors at presynaptic and postsynaptic locations within the striatum relative to the dopaminergic input (McRae, 1998). In addition, there is a cholinergic input from the PPN to the basal ganglia (Bevan and Bolam, 1995), but once more, this is seldom considered in the control and initiation of movement and has hardly been studied in basal ganglia disease.

## DOPAMINE RECEPTORS AND BASAL GANGLIA

The key role of dopamine deficiency in PD led to the description of multiple dopamine receptor subtypes within basal ganglia (Gingrich and Caron, 1993; Seeman and Van Tol, 1994). A key component of the classic model of basal ganglia organization is that D1 dopamine receptors are selectively localized to the cell bodies of the direct output pathway, while D2 receptors are selectively found on the cell bodies of the indirect pathway (Gerfen et al., 1990; Gerfen, 2000a, 2000b). This separation of dopamine receptor function has been widely used as a basis for explaining alterations in basal ganglia output, but there may be considerably more overlap between

these receptor populations than was previously thought (Aizman et al., 2000), although this is constantly refuted. This would support the functional interaction that is known to exist between D1 and D2 receptors in the control of movement (Clark and White, 1987; Waddington, 1989). Dopamine receptors have a key functional localization within the caudate-putamen, but dopamine receptors also occur within other areas of basal ganglia, including in the substantia nigra. In SNr, dopamine receptors are located on the terminals of the glutamatergic and GABAergic inputs from the STN and from GPi, but dopamine receptors are also located on the dendrites of intrinsic dopaminergic neurons and on the cell bodies of GABA output neurons to the brainstem. These dopamine receptors appear to be functioning in the control of basal ganglia function and may have a role in the genesis of disorders of movement. Further, while the release of dopamine from dendrites serves to activate autoreceptors and postsynaptic dopamine receptors in substantia nigra, nigral dopaminergic neurons are also connected by functional electrical synapses that allow fast communication between cells (Vandecasteele et al., 2005). However, little of this important component of basal ganglia function is mentioned in describing the functional neuroanatomy of basal ganglia, and there has been little study of the role of these receptors in normal and abnormal movement.

More recently, it has been shown that the GPe, GPi, and STN also contain dopamine receptor subtypes and that these are innervated by collaterals from the nigrostriatal pathway (Hassani et al., 1997; Hedreen, 1999; Augood et al., 2000). While it is known that the nigro-GP fibers degenerate in PD, how this loss of dopaminergic input might contribute to the symptoms of PD and also how it might be involved in the normal control of basal ganglia and the onset of motor disorders are only beginning to be understood (Kreiss et al., 1996, 1997; Hauber and Fuchs, 2000; Mehta et al., 2000; Bezard, Boraud, et al., 2001; Freeman et al., 2001; Ni et al., 2001). Loss of dopaminergic input to the STN also occurs in PD, and synaptic release of dopamine has been demonstrated in this area to directly modulate the activity of STN neurons (Cragg et al., 2004). Again, these dopaminergic inputs do not feature in classic models of the functional neuroanatomy of basal ganglia (but see later).

Perhaps noteworthy, dopaminergic innervation of the thalamus may modulate its projections to the cortex, amygdala, and striatum. Previously this had not been thought to be important because of the sparse dopaminergic innervation that is found in the rodent brain arising from nigrostriatal collaterals (Freeman et al., 2001). However, in the primate, there is in addition the profuse innervation of association, limbic, and motor thalamic nuclei (Sanchez-Gonzalez et al., 2005). Dopamine receptor populations are present in the thalamus but have received scant attention. Rather than originating in SNc, dopaminergic innervation originates from the hypothalamus, the periaqueductal gray ventral mesencephalon, and the lateral parabrachial nucleus. This may represent a novel dopaminergic system, but how the thalamic dopaminergic system is affected in PD remains unknown. In contrast, the innervation arising from nigrostriatal collaterals is lost in both rats and primates following nigrostriatal destruction. This may have important consequences, since following unilateral nigrostriatal denervation in the rat, there is marked neuronal loss in the thalamus restricted to parafascicular nucleus neurons accompanied by intense hyperactivity of remaining parafascicular nucleus neurons innervating the striatum (Aymerich et al., 2006). If loss of the thalamic dopaminergic pathway occurs in PD, this may have similar important consequences in understanding the nature of the disease.

## INTERNAL ORGANIZATION OF BASAL GANGLIA NUCLEI

In looking at the anatomy of basal ganglia and at the functional neuroanatomy of these nuclei, it is invariably presumed that they are internally homogeneous, since only overall function and structure are included in concepts of basal ganglia disease. However, it is known that the striatum is made up of patches and matrix, which make up a striosomal organization. Striosomes comprise acetylcholinesterase-poor patches in the striatum within the acetylcholinesterase-rich positive-staining matrix (Graybiel et al., 1986, 1987; Jimenez-Castellanos and Graybiel, 1987a, 1987b). Within striosomes, there is a distinct anatomic localization of cell bodies, neuronal input, and receptors of importance to the genesis and treatment of movement disorders (Eblen and Graybiel, 1995).

More recently, a similar nigrosomal organization of the substantia nigra, under the influence of a variety of developmental transcription factors, has been demonstrated (Damier et al., 1999; Jankovic et al., 2005; Andersson et al., 2006), and again the internal architecture of the substantia nigra is of functional relevance to the control of movement and to basal ganglia disease. It is also highly likely that when other nuclei of basal ganglia are examined in a similar manner, their internal structure will be found to be highly defined, leading to another layer of complexity in trying to understand how basal ganglia function and the changes that occur in movement disorders. This certainly seems to be the case for the globus pallidus. Anatomic, neurochemical, and electrophysiologic studies suggest the presence of multiple neuronal populations within the rodent globus pallidus (Hoover and Marshall 1999, 2002, 2004; Billings and Marshall 2003, 2004). For example, preproenkephalin mRNA differentiates two major classes of pallidal neurons and identifies those cells that innervate the striatum from those that project to the entopeduncular nucleus or to the SNr. Some neuronal populations express D2 dopamine receptors and provide the substrate by which nigral dopaminergic innervation modulates pallidal function. The heterogeneous nature of the pallidum may relate to the associative, limbic, and sensorimotor territories within the GPe and the way they innervate target nuclei such as the STN (Karachi et al., 2005).

## DYSFUNCTION OF BASAL GANGLIA

The key role of basal ganglia in the control and initiation of voluntary movement is demonstrated by the effects of pathologic lesions of specific basal ganglia nuclei. The classic example is the degeneration of the dopaminergic cells of SNc in PD. The selective toxicity for MPTP nigral dopaminergic cells further illustrates the key role of the nigrostriatal pathway in the control of voluntary movement. The degeneration of intrinsic GABAergic striatal cells and cholinergic interneurons in Huntington disease has similarly led to an understanding of how a graded and selective degeneration of the direct and indirect output pathways results in the appearance of choreic movements

(Reiner et al., 1988). Neurons of the indirect GABA-enkephalin-containing pathway to the GPe degenerate initially, followed by the GABA-substance P–containing neurons of the direct output pathway to the GPi and SNr. Interestingly, this pattern of neuronal loss differs from the distribution of the mutant protein huntingtin, which is found in a higher proportion of direct output neurons (Fusco et al., 2003). As with PD, toxins such as quinolinic acid and 3-nitropropionic acid mimic the effects of the striatal pathology of Huntington disease (Brouillet et al., 1995; Burns et al., 1995; Palfi et al., 1996). However, in primates, the administration of 3-nitropropionic acid leads to dystonic rather than choreic movements, suggesting that the striatal lesion alone is not responsible for the motor abnormalities (Palfi et al., 1996). Similarly, pathologic lesions in the STN in hemiballism have led to an understanding of how this nucleus functions to integrate voluntary movement (Martin, 1927; Martin and Alcock, 1934; Whittier, 1947; Whittier and Mettler, 1949). Hemiballism can be produced in primate species either by lesions of STN or by manipulation of GABAergic function in STN or GPe, altering glutamatergic output from STN to GPi and SNr, or by inhibition of glutamate transmission in GPi (Carpenter et al., 1950; Hammond et al., 1979; Crossman et al., 1980, 1984; Mitchell et al., 1990).

Other disorders of movement in which no clear pathologic changes occur have proved difficult to explain. For example, dystonia has been attributed to dysfunction of the direct output pathway or to a complex alteration in the relative balance of striatal input to GPi from the direct and indirect pathways, causing a unique but abnormal spatiotemporal pattern of pallidal activity that distinguishes these changes from those that occur in PD (Eidelberg et al, 1998; Silberstein et al., 2003). However, dystonic movement can be suppressed by high-dose anticholinergic treatment, and in MPTP-treated monkeys with dyskinesia, cholinergic manipulation can turn chorea into dystonia and dystonia into chorea, suggesting a key role for cholinergic systems. It is difficult to produce dystonia in primates by lesions of the basal ganglia, although treatment with 3-nitropropionic acid to destroy both the direct and indirect pathways does induce dystonia. Yet dystonia occurs following lesions of these structures in humans (Bhatia and Marsden, 1994). Lesions that cause dystonia are found in the GP but also particularly in the putamen. Lesions of the putamen might be expected to destroy both the direct striato-GPi/SNr and the indirect striato-GPe pathway. Destruction of both output pathways should reduce thalamic output through loss of the direct pathway but increase it through loss of the indirect pathway. Indeed, degeneration of the GPe and STN can produce generalized dystonia (Wooten et al., 1993). Loss of STN excitation would reduce GPi inhibition of the thalamus. However, surprisingly, thalamic lesions also commonly result in dystonia (Lee and Marsden, 1994).

Dyskinesia resulting from levodopa treatment of PD and from repeated levodopa treatment of MPTP-treated monkeys is also poorly explained by current models of basal ganglia function (see later). A key component of the onset of dyskinesia is the loss of the nigrostriatal pathway, since the treatment of normal individuals with levodopa for long periods of time does not lead to the onset of involuntary movements (Rajput et al., 1997). Similarly, acute administration of high doses of levodopa to normal monkeys does not induce dyskinesia (Paulson, 1973; Sassin, 1975; Boyce et al., 1990). However, two recent studies have suggested that if sufficient levodopa is administered to normal primates, then dyskinesia can develop (Pearce et al., 2001; Togasaki et al., 2001). This would suggest that the nigral dopaminergic loss has a gating function for the onset of dyskinesia such that the greater the degree of denervation, the smaller is the exposure to levodopa needed to produce involuntary movements, although this is disputed (Guigoni et al., 2005). Attempts to understand the mechanisms that are involved in dyskinesia are discussed again later, but it is clear that the mechanisms that are involved in the manifestation of dyskinesia and those that are involved in priming for the appearance of dyskinesia are different. Priming appears to be a complex and persistent process that is poorly understood. A close relationship exists between dopaminergic transmission and glutamatergic function in basal ganglia. Alterations in glutamate receptors are associated with levodopa-induced motor complications, and levodopa can reverse glutamatergic activity in 6-OHDA lesioned rats (Calon et al., 2003; Picconi et al., 2004). There are two pieces of evidence that directly suggest a primary role for glutamatergic mechanisms. In patients with PD who exhibit dyskinesia, the administration of the N-methyl-D-aspartic acid antagonist amantadine can lead to a suppression of involuntary movements. Similarly, in MPTP-treated primates, established dyskinesia is suppressed by amantadine and other N-methyl-D-aspartic acid antagonists (Blanchet et al., 1998; Papa et al., 1999; Chase and Oh, 2000). Importantly, in drug-naïve MPTP-treated primates, the administration of levodopa with an N-methyl-D-aspartic acid antagonist can prevent the onset of dyskinesia, suggesting a highly important role for glutamatergic systems in the priming process. The persistence of priming for dyskinesia with levodopa bears similarities to the "neuronal memory" that underlies long-term potentiation in the hippocampus and in limbic areas. The persistent activity-dependent changes in neuronal activity that make up long-term potentiation are thought to be mediated by alterations in the sensitivity of N-methyl-D-aspartic acid–type glutamate receptors (Nicoll and Malenka, 1995). Importantly, abnormal information storage in corticostriatal synapses has recently been linked to the development of levodopa-induced dyskinesia in rats (Picconi et al., 2003; Pisani et al., 2005). Specifically, high-frequency stimulation of cortical afferents induced long-term potentiation in corticostriatal synapses of levodopa-treated rats irrespective of whether dyskinesia was observed. However, while nondyskinetic rats showed synaptic deterioration in response to subsequent low-frequency stimulation, dyskinetic rats did not. These findings provide evidence of abnormal information storage in corticostriatal synapses and strengthen arguments for the involvement of glutamatergic transmission in priming mechanisms for dyskinesia and its persistence.

Studies of the genesis of levodopa-induced dyskinesia in PD and in MPTP-treated monkeys strongly suggest that pharmacokinetic and pharmacodynamic properties of dopaminergic drugs that produce different patterns of dopamine receptor stimulation may be key to the priming process (Grondin et al., 1996; Bedard et al., 1997; Pearce et al., 1998; Maratos et al., 2001a). Thus, short-acting dopaminergic agents, including levodopa, that cause a pulsatile stimulation of dopaminergic receptors seem to set in motion a sequence of events that are more likely to promote the priming of dyskinesia than occurs with long-acting drugs that produce more continuous dopaminergic stimulation. The concept of continuous dopaminergic stimulation is now thought of as being key to the means by which the early treatment of PD should be undertaken so as to prevent dyskinesia induction until the later stages of the illness (Olanow et al., 2000). However, this concept, like many involving basal ganglia function, is also probably too simplistic. For example, the repeated administration of both apomorphine, a short-acting dopaminergic agent, and pergolide, a long-acting dopamine agonist to otherwise drug-naïve MPTP-treated primates results in less dyskinesia than is produced by levodopa (Pearce et al., 1998; Maratos et al., 2003).

## ALTERATIONS IN STRIATAL OUTPUT PATHWAYS IN PARKINSON DISEASE AND IN LEVODOPA-INDUCED DYSKINESIA

Many components of basal ganglia organization and function are not incorporated into the classic model that is used to explain dysfunction and the onset of motor abnormalities (see previous discussion). In PD, the model envisages an imbalance between the direct and indirect striatal output pathways (Grondin et al., 1996; Obeso et al., 1997, 2000; Olanow et al., 2000). The loss of dopaminergic input to the striatum removes inhibition from the D2 receptor-mediated GABA/enkephalin indirect pathway to GPe, thus increasing inhibitory GABAergic tone on the GPe-STN pathway. This pathway, which is also GABAergic, becomes underactive, and this results in increased burst firing of the glutamatergic pathways to GPi and SNr, activating GABAergic output neurons to the VL thalamus and the brainstem. Removal of excitatory dopaminergic tone on the direct D1-mediated GABA/substance P/dynorphin pathway to GPi similarly leads to decreased inhibitory tone on the GABAergic output neurons from GPi to VL thalamus. The end result of both processes is the increase of activity in GPi/SNr, and this leads to inhibition of thalamocortical pathways (as well as other output pathways) and inhibition of motor function.

The classic concept of the changes occurring in PD is supported by behavioral, electrophysiologic, biochemical, and clinical evidence. In MPTP-treated primates and in PD, there is an increase in D2 receptor protein and mRNA and in the levels of preproenkephalin mRNA in the striatum, indicative of increased activity in the striato-GPe pathway (Herrero et al., 1995; Jolkkonen et al., 1995; Nisbet, 1995). Decreased uptake of $^{14}$C-2-deoxyglucose in the STN and increased cytochrome oxidase mRNA indicate decreased GPe-STN activity and increased activity of the STN neurons, respectively (Mitchell et al., 1989; Vila et al., 1997). In the direct striato-GPi/SNr pathway, there is a decrease in mRNA for D1 receptors and for preprotachykinin and preprodynorphin mRNA. Increased activity of output neurons from GPi and SNr is shown by increases in cytochrome oxidase mRNA and glutamic acid decarboxylase (GAD) mRNA (Herrero et al., 1996; Vila et al., 1996). In MPTP-treated monkeys, levodopa treatment leads to a reduction in GAD and cytochrome oxidase mRNA in the STN, GPi, and SNr, accompanied by an improvement in motor performance (Herrero et al., 1996; Vila et al., 1996). In patients with PD and in MPTP-treated primates, lesions of the STN or GPi or stimulation of the GPi or STN can improve parkinsonian motor deficits (Aziz et al., 1991; Wichmann et al., 1994; Guridi et al., 1996; Limousin et al., 1997).

The classic model of levodopa-induced dyskinesia proposes the exact opposite of the events that occur in PD (Crossman,

1987, 1990; DeLong, 1990). It is envisaged that excessive dopaminergic stimulation of the striatal output pathways leads to decreased basal ganglia outflow to the VL thalamus. Thus, inhibition of the indirect output pathway to GPe leads to an increase in GPe-STN-induced inhibition of the glutamatergic pathway from STN-GPi/SNr. The reduced excitatory input to GPi/SNr causes a reduction in inhibitory input from GPi to VL thalamus. Similarly, excessive activation of the direct output pathway leads to an increase in striato-GPi/SNr inhibitory tone and a decrease in GABAergic output to the thalamus and brainstem. Surprisingly, there is relatively little evidence to support this sequence of events, although dyskinesia in patients with PD and MPTP-treated primates is associated with increased neuronal activity in GPe and decreased firing in GPi (Filion et al., 1991; Lozano et al., 2000).

However, since this model was developed, it has become clear that it does not fit with current knowledge of the organization of basal ganglia or with biochemical and electrophysiologic data from patients with PD and MPTP-treated primates with and without levodopa-induced dyskinesia. As was emphasized previously, current models are too simplistic and do not incorporate many features of basal ganglia circuitry and organization. In particular, the colocalization of dopamine receptors in the striatum, the presence and innervation of dopamine receptors in other basal ganglia nuclei, the omission of a role for cholinergic innervation, the omission of inputs from PPN, and the complex internal structure of the striatum and substantia nigra have been pointed out. In addition, the role of axon collaterals innervating multiple targets within basal ganglia function is only starting to be understood (Parent et al., 2000). Furthermore, the complexity of the makeup of voluntary movement and the diversity of abnormalities of movement that occur in basal ganglia disease make it clear that current models are minimalistic.

There are now major reasons why the classic models of basal ganglia organization and function that are used to explain PD and levodopa-induced dyskinesia are thought to be wrong. In PD, underactivity of GPe-STN neurons is supported by a reduced rate of neuronal firing in Gpe (Filion and Tremblay, 1991). However, in MPTP-treated primates, cytochrome oxidase mRNA in GPe is increased rather than decreased, and GAD mRNA is unchanged in comparison to normal monkeys (Herrero et al., 1996; Vila et al., 1996, 1997). So the overactivity of the STN proposed by the classic model might not be simply the result of decreased activity of the GPe-STN GABAergic pathway. Indeed, a mere reduction in GPe activity produced in monkeys by an ibotenic acid lesion did not result in parkinsonism (Soares et al., 2004). There are also clearly different territorial domains in the GPe (and GPi) associated with different behaviors and functions (Francois et al., 2004; Grabli et al., 2004; Whelan et al., 2004). So it would not be too surprising if biochemical and electrophysiologic markers of the activity of these pathways did not correlate with one another.

However, another potential explanation lies in the reciprocal connections between STN and GPe and the dense collateral networks that are formed in the target structures (Lozano et al., 2000). In addition, recurrent collaterals from the striato-GPe and GPe-STN GABAergic pathways add another level of control of basal ganglia output that was not previously envisaged. For example, there are differences between the effects of a 6-OHDA lesion of the nigrostriatal pathway on increased activity of GPe GABAergic projections to the STN/GPi and to

the striatum, the latter being more affected (Billings and Marshall, 2004). The evidence supporting the proposed decrease in activity of the direct striato-GPi pathway is based on the decrease in D1 receptor protein and mRNA and in levels of preprotachykinin and preprodynorphin mRNA, but this has not been confirmed by either electrophysiologic or metabolic investigations. Other inputs may also play an important role but are not contained in classic models of basal ganglia function. For example, thalamic lesions have been shown to reverse most of the neuronal changes that occur in the indirect output pathway following a 6-OHDA lesion of the nigrostriatal pathway in rats but without influencing parameters related to the direct pathway. This appears to involve a glutamatergic input from intralaminar thalamic nuclei (Bacci et al., 2004).

In levodopa-induced dyskinesia in MPTP-treated monkeys, the onset of involuntary movements is associated with an increase in the firing of GPe neurons and a decrease in the firing and pattern of GPi neurons, supporting the classic model of changes occurring in basal ganglia outflow (Papa et al., 1999; Filion, 2000; Boraud et al., 2001). There also appear to be differences in the response of the strio-GPi pathway in 6-OHDA-lesioned rats to levodopa, depending on whether it is administered in a continuous or intermittent manner consistent with the concept of continuous dopaminergic stimulation (Nielsen and Soghomonian, 2004). However, the responses that are measured vary between cells within these nuclei, and in dyskinetic patients with PD, there is no reduction in GPe firing associated with involuntary movements (Filion, 2000; Verhagen et al., 2000). In the striatum of MPTP-treated primates exhibiting dyskinesia, the levels of preproenkephalin mRNA are not reduced in comparison to levels in MPTP-treated animals without involuntary movements and may even be elevated further (Maneuf et al., 1994; Zeng et al., 2000). In normal monkeys treated with very high doses of levodopa to induce dyskinesia, involuntary movements are accompanied by an elevation of preproenkephalin mRNA levels that is not produced by levodopa treatment alone (Zeng et al., 2000). In GPe, levels of GAD and cytochrome oxidase mRNA are not elevated, and $^{14}$C-2-deoxyglucose utilization is not reduced in dyskinetic monkeys compared to nondyskinetic monkeys, as would be expected if striato-GPe activity was reduced and GPe-STN activity was increased (Herrero et al., 1996). In the striatum of dyskinetic monkeys, preprotachykinin and preprodynorphin mRNA levels are higher than in MPTP-treated animals without dyskinesia but are not, in general, significantly greater than are seen in normal monkeys, although marked increases in preprodynorphin mRNA have been reported (Maratos et al., 2001b; Tel et al., 2002). In the GPi of dyskinetic MPTP-treated monkeys, GAD and cytochrome oxidase mRNA are reduced in comparison to the basal parkinsonian state but remain above those seen in normal monkeys (Herrero et al., 1996; Vila et al., 1997). These findings strongly suggest that dyskinesia is not associated with a reduction in GPi activity and output to the thalamus. While all these experimental data indirectly indicate that the classic model of basal ganglia outflow in dyskinesia in PD is incorrect, it is a single clinical finding that is the final nail in the coffin. Thus, pallidotomy leading to a reduction of GPi output reduces instead of inducing dyskinesia in parkinsonian patients treated with levodopa (Marsden and Obeso, 1994). This argues against a role for GPi underactivity as the mechanism that is responsible for dyskinesia induction and focuses attention on the patterns of neuronal firing that occur in this and other parts of basal ganglia output in PD (Soares et al., 2004). Indeed, there may be a complex reshaping of the temporal structure of neuronal activity in the GP as occurs on pallidal stimulation (Bar-Gad et al., 2004). This may involve not only sensorimotor domains of basal ganglia nuclei but also limbic and associative territories (Guigoni et al., 2005). Such a conclusion makes eminent sense, considering the complexity and diversity of the movements that make up dyskinesia in patients with PD and their interaction with cognitive and limbic information processing.

## COMPENSATORY CHANGES IN PARKINSON DISEASE

The ability to maintain motor function during the early phase of nigrostriatal degeneration is commonly attributed to compensatory increases in dopamine turnover coupled with an upregulation of postsynaptic dopamine receptor function. The appearance of parkinsonian symptoms is taken to reflect the eventual breakdown of dopaminergic homeostasis. However, recent studies have challenged this view and suggest a different sequence of events based largely on findings made in primates undergoing repeated administration of low doses of MPTP to induce progressive nigral cell degeneration over a period of one month and in MPTP-treated mice with a partial lesion of the nigrostriatal pathway (Bezard et al., 2003; Meissner et al., 2003).

Following partial denervation of the striatum, dopaminergic tone is maintained with no alteration in extracellular dopamine concentration or in dopamine uptake or release (Garris et al., 1997). Only at the end of the presymptomatic phase of nigrostriatal degeneration is there an upregulation of dopamine turnover (Bezard, Dovero, et al., 2001). In contrast, postsynaptic $D_2$ receptor upregulation occurs in the middle of the presymptomatic period, suggesting that dopamine homeostasis occurs earlier than expected (Bezard, Dovero, et al., 2001). At this point, also earlier than was previously thought, changes in basal ganglia output occur as a compensatory mechanism prior to the appearance of motor symptoms. This is demonstrated by increases in PPE-A mRNA in the indirect strio-GPe output pathway in presymptomatic MPTP-treated primates together with electrophysiologic evidence for increased firing of GPi and STN neurons (Bezard, Crossman, et al., 2001; Bezard, Ravenscroft, et al., 2001). Similarly in MPTP-treated mice with a partial nigrostriatal lesion, alterations in striatal PPE-A and PPT mRNA and D3 receptor binding occur in the absence of metabolic change in output to GP and SNr, suggesting that these alterations compensate and prevent changes in neuronal firing to output neurons (Meissner et al., 2003).

Alterations in neuronal metabolic activity as judged by 2-DG studies are accepted to occur in basal ganglia in PD and in MPTP-lesioned primates, but these commence in the presymptomatic phase following MPTP treatment. Importantly, at this time, metabolic activity in the SMA is normal and declines only once motor symptoms appear. This suggests that dysfunction of basal ganglia does not necessarily lead to a loss of motor control, whereas impairment of neuronal activity in SMA does (Bezard, Crossman et al., 2001). The conclusion from this finding is that compensatory mechanisms are operating in brain regions outside of basal ganglia (Bezard, Crossman, et al., 2001). All of this information strongly suggests that compensation for abnormal

activity occurring in basal ganglia is nondopaminergic and non–basal ganglion–mediated and necessitates a reformation of the concept that is used to explain basal dysfunction in humans.

The basis of compensatory changes may also involve nigral dopaminergic projections to nonstriatal areas of basal ganglia. It has been proposed that alterations in the activity of the STN may occur prior to striatal dopamine loss reaching the threshold for the onset of motor symptoms. STN activity was proposed to be changed by loss of dopaminergic nigro-STN fibers (Obeso et al., 2004a). An increase in STN may increase GPe activity and consequently alter firing of GPi. This may also occur by a direct effect of STN on GPi. The stimulation of GPe may compensate for increasing inhibition through the strio-GPe pathway caused by increasing striatal dopamine loss. However, when dopaminergic fiber loss expands, this compensatory sequence breaks down. The concept is supported by the early overactivity of STN detected in patients with PD and by the positron emission tomography evidence for continuing decline in striatal dopaminergic function in the absence of worsening of motor symptoms in early disease, suggesting that STN may compensate for dopamine loss in the earliest stages of the illness (Kao et al., 2003; Whone et al., 2003; Sossi et al., 2004). However, this interpretation is open to criticism on the grounds that dopaminergic innervation of the STN increases burst firing through D5 receptor activation (Baufreton et al., 2003; Bezard et al., 2004). As a consequence, loss of nigro-STN input would not explain the alterations in firing observed. In addition, the various arguments that have been put forward are based on what occurs in humans and events in MPTP-treated primates, and these are different; in MPTP-treated primates, the nigro-STN pathway does not degenerate, so it would not explain the early compensatory changes that are proposed to occur in these animals (Parent et al., 1990; Jan et al., 2003). Indeed, the differences between patients with PD and toxin-treated monkeys might be too great to resolve this debate. PD is invariably unilateral and also progressive, whereas the effects of MPTP are bilateral and usually static. In PD, compensatory events may originate from the contralateral hemisphere, and there may be cross-hemispheric innervation from the substantia nigra (Obeso et al., 2004a).

If the strio-STN dopaminergic pathway is not involved, then perhaps there is a role for the strio-GPi projection. Indeed, [18]F-DOPA positron emission tomography studies in patients with early PD show increased uptake in GPi that is lost in later disease (Whone et al., 2003). This takes place in the face of increasing loss of nigrostriatal fibers but without clinical progression. So this may serve to regulate GPi output to the thalamus and provide early but transient compensation.

## UPDATING THE MODELS OF BASAL GANGLIA FUNCTION

From this discussion, it is clear that the models of basal ganglia functional neuroanatomy are too simplistic to explain the current knowledge of the circuitry and the alterations that occur in disease states and in experimental models of PD and levodopa-induced dyskinesia. A major revision has been required for some time, and Obeso and colleagues (2004b) recently proposed a new scheme that serves to explain most of the known facts (Fig. 3-3). The new model of normal basal ganglia highlights that dopaminergic innervation is not

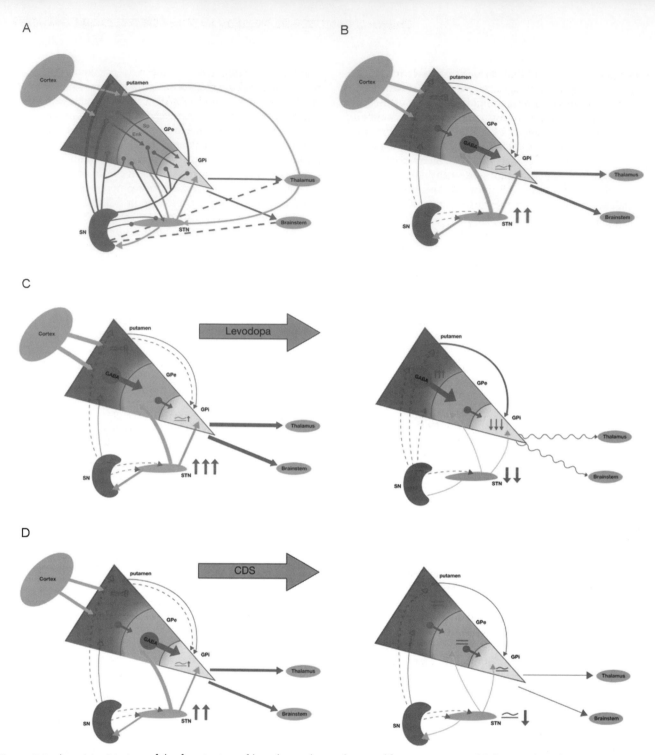

**Figure 3-3** A revisionist view of the functioning of basal ganglia and its modification in PD and following levodopa treatment. Diagram of the main pathways of the basal ganglia in different functional states. **A,** Normal basal ganglia, highlighting that dopaminergic innervation is not limited to the striatum and the various "internal" loops. **B,** Modification induced by dopamine depletion in early PD. Hyperactivity of the STN precedes significant dopamine putaminal depletion. Therefore, the GPe is still functionally operative and overstimulated by the STN. This leads to increased inhibition from the GPe to the GPi, which partially compensates for the augmented excitation from the STN and reduced inhibition in the "direct" pathway. **C,** Changes associated with advanced PD and the effects of levodopa. At this stage, striatal depletion has progressed and both striatopallidal projections are altered. There is increased inhibition from the GABA/enkephalin projection to the GPe, which is hypoactive and no longer compensates for STN hyperactivity. This results in overactivity of GPi output and abnormal inhibition of motor areas. In this state, levodopa does not restore the normal physiology of the basal ganglia. **D,** Pulative effects of stable dopaminergic delivery in early PD. Hyperactivity of both the STN and putamino-GPe projections is normalized, restoring the homeostatic mechanisms of the basal ganglia and output activity. This has been proposed to restore the probability of developing motor complications. (See Color Plate 3.) (Reproduced with permission from Obeso JA, Rodriguez-Oroz M, Marin C, et al: The origin of motor fluctuations in Parkinson's disease: Importance of dopaminergic innervation and basal ganglia circuits. Neurology 2004;62[suppl 1]:S17–S30.)

limited to the striatum and that various internal loops exist. It is proposed that following dopamine depletion in early PD, hyperactivity of the STN precedes significant dopamine depletion in the putamen, although this is controversial. Therefore, the GPe is still functionally operative and overstimulated by the STN. This leads to increased inhibition from the GPe to the GPi, which partially compensates for the augmented excitation from the STN and reduced inhibition in the direct pathway. In advanced PD and with the effects of levodopa, striatal dopamine depletion progresses, and both striatopallidal projections are altered. There is increased inhibition from the GABA/enkephalin projection to the GPe, which is hypoactive and no longer compensates for STN hyperactivity. This results in overactivity of GPi output and abnormal inhibition of motor areas.

The involvement of the corticostriatal glutamate system in the symptomatology and progression of PD is also becoming increasingly important with evidence of a breakdown of glutamatergic transmission. In PD and in experimental models of PD, the loss of the nigrostriatal input to the striatum results in a decrease in the density spines on medium spiny output neurons and the total length of remaining dendrites (Stephens et al., 2005; Day et al., 2006; Gerfen, 2006). This appears to specifically affect striopallidal neurons and to alter glutamatergic synapses in a way that must markedly affect the ability of the medium spiny neurons to function normally and to modulate basal ganglia output. This may provide a pathologic explanation for the onset of the motor symptoms of PD. Indeed, high-frequency motor cortex stimulation reverses akinesia in MPTP-treated primates with a normalization of firing in GPi and STN (Drouot et al., 2004). The incorporation of these changes into the functional neuroanatomy of the basal ganglia provides yet another facet to the wealth of alterations that contribute to the onset of movement disorders. There may be clinical implications of the alterations in glutamatergic synapses in PD. Recent clinical studies have suggested that early therapeutic intervention in PD may result in a better outcome for motor symptoms than delaying treatment. This early replacement of dopaminergic transmission makes physiologic sense and may prevent changes such as the loss of spines on medium spiny neurons that may otherwise prove irreversible and result in a loss of plasticity in basal ganglia outflow.

## CONCLUSIONS

The anatomic description of the basal ganglia is well established, and much has been done to understand the pathways that link the various nuclei making up the basal ganglia together with their specific input and output pathways and the nature of the transmitter systems that are involved. This has contributed greatly to an understanding of the basal ganglia and has helped in the development of concepts of the functional neuroanatomy of this brain region. It has also led to a realization that current views of basal ganglia function are too simplistic in many respects. Further studies examining the intricate connections within the basal ganglia and within the cortical loops are now required. As an example, the discovery of a population of tyrosine hydroxylase–positive neurons that is upregulated after destruction of the nigrostriatal pathway and coexpress GABA means that a complete reappraisal of dopaminergic function in PD is required (Mazloom and Smith,

2006). The integration of electrophysiologic, biochemical, and behavioral studies is needed to continually validate the models that have been proposed. However, a point has been reached at which the intricacy of the models and the extensiveness of the connections within basal ganglia start to make a simple description of this system almost impossible. It is therefore perhaps not too surprising that while degenerative illnesses of basal ganglia are understood at a gross pathologic level, it has not been possible to devise treatments for these disorders based on current concepts of how the basal ganglia function. Indeed, it is likely that, with the exception of PD, it may prove impossible to modulate basal ganglia disease through any single neurotransmitter system, adding a further obstacle to the future development of treatment.

## References

Agid Y, Javoy-Agid F, Ruberg M: Biochemistry of neurotransmitters in Parkinson's disease. In Marsden CD, Fahn S (eds): Movement Disorders, vol 2. London, Butterworths, 1987, pp 166–230.

Aizman O, Brismar H, Uhlen P, et al: Anatomical and physiological evidence for D1 and D2 dopamine receptor colocalization in neostriatal neurons. Nat Neurosci 2000;3:226–230.

Albin RL, Young AB, Penney JB: The functional anatomy of basal ganglia disorders. Trends Neurosci 1989;12:366–375.

Alexander GE, Crutcher MD: Functional architecture of basal ganglia circuits: Neural substrates of parallel processing. Trends Neurosci 1990;13:266–271.

Alexander GE, DeLong MR, Strick PL: Parallel organization of functionally segregated circuits linking basal ganglia and cortex. Annu Rev Neurosci 1986;9:357–381.

Anden NE, Carlsson A, Dahlstrom A, et al: Demonstration and mapping out of nigro-neostriatal dopamine neurons. Life Sci 1964;3:523–530.

Andersson E, Tryggvason U, Deng Q, et al: Identification of intrinsic determinants of midbrain dopamine neurons. Cell 2006;124: 393–405.

Augood SJ, Hollingsworth ZR, Standaert DG, et al: Localization of dopaminergic markers in the human subthalamic nucleus. J Comp Neurol 2000;421:247–255.

Aymerich MS, Barroso-Chinea P, Perez-Manso M, et al: Consequences of unilateral nigrostriatal denervation on the thalamostriatal pathway in rats. Eur J Neurosci 2006;23:2099–2108.

Aziz TZ, Peggs D, Sambrook MA, Crossman AR: Lesion of the subthalamic nucleus for the alleviation of 1-methyl-4-phenyl-1,2,3,6-tetrahydropyridine (MPTP)-induced parkinsonism in the primate. Mov Disord 1991;6:288–292.

Bacci JJ, Kachidian P, Kerkerian-Le Goff L, Salin P: Intralaminar thalamic nuclei lesions: Widespread impact on dopamine denervation-mediated cellular defects in the rat basal ganglia. J Neuropathol Exp Neurol 2004;63:20–31.

Bar-Gad I, Elias S, Vaadia E, Bergman H: Complex locking rather than complete cessation of neuronal activity in the globus pallidus of a 1-methyl-4-phenyl-1,2,3,6-tetrahydropyridine-treated primate in response to pallidal microstimulation. J Neurosci 2004;24:7410–7419.

Baufreton J, Garret M, Rivera A, de la Calle A, et al: D5 (not D1) dopamine receptors potentiate burst-firing in neurons of the subthalamic nucleus by modulating an L-type calcium conductance. J Neurosci 2003;23:816–825.

Bedard PJ, Gomez-Mancilla B, Blanchet PJ, et al: Dopamine agonists as first line therapy of parkinsonism in MPTP monkeys. In Olanow CW, Obeso JA (eds): Beyond the Decade of the Brain. Tunbridge Wells, UK, Wells, 1997, pp 101–128.

Bergman H, Wichmann T, DeLong MR: Reversal of experimental parkinsonism by lesions of the subthalamic nucleus. Science 1990;249:1436–1438.

Bevan MD, Bolam JP: Cholinergic, GABAergic, and glutamate-enriched inputs from the mesopontine tegmentum to the subthalamic nucleus in the rat. J Neurosci 1995;15:7105–7120.

Bezard E, Boraud T, Chalon S, et al: Pallidal border cells: Anatomical and electrophysiological study in the 1-methyl-4-phenyl-1,2,3,6-tetrahydropyridine-treated monkey. Neuroscience 2001;103:117–123.

Bezard E, Crossman AR, Gross CE, Brotchie JM: Structures outside the basal ganglia may compensate for dopamine loss in the presymptomatic stages of Parkinson's disease. FASEB J 2001;15:1092–1094.

Bezard E, Dovero S, Prunier C, et al: Relationship between the appearance of symptoms and the level of nigrostriatal degeneration in a progressive 1-methyl-4-phenyl-1,2,3,6-tetrahydropyridine-lesioned macaque model of Parkinson's disease. J Neurosci 2001;21:6853–6861.

Bezard E, Gross CE, Brotchie JM: Presymptomatic compensation in Parkinson's disease is not dopamine-mediated. Trends Neurosci 2003;26:215–221.

Bezard E, Gross CE, Brotchie JM: Response to Obesow et al.: Presymptomatic compensation in Parkinson's disease is not dopamine-mediated. Trends Neurosci 2004;27:127–128.

Bezard E, Ravenscroft P, Gross CE, et al: Upregulation of striatal preproenkephalin gene expression occurs before the appearance of parkinsonian signs in 1-methyl-4-phenyl-1,2,3,6-tetrahydropyridine monkeys. Neurobiol Dis 2001;8:343–350.

Bhatia KP, Marsden CD: The behavioural and motor consequences of focal lesions of the basal ganglia in man. Brain 1994;117:859–876.

Billings LM, Marshall JF: D2 antagonist-induced c-fos in an identified subpopulation of globus pallidus neurons by a direct intrapallidal action. Brain Res 2003;964:237–243.

Billings LM, Marshall JF: Glutamic acid decarboxylase 67 mRNA regulation in two globus pallidus neuron populations by dopamine and the subthalamic nucleus. J Neurosci 2004;24:3094–3103.

Blanchet PJ, Konitsiotis S, Chase TN: Amantadine reduces levodopa-induced dyskinesias in parkinsonian monkeys. Mov Disord 1998;13:798–802.

Boraud T, Bezard E, Bioulac B, Gross CE: Dopamine agonist-induced dyskinesias are correlated to both firing pattern and frequency alterations of pallidal neurones in the MPTP-treated monkey. Brain 2001;124:546–557.

Bove J, Prou D, Perier C, Przedborski S: Toxin-induced models of Parkinson's disease. NeuroRx 2005;2:484–494.

Boyce S, Rupniak NM, Steventon MJ, Iversen SD: Nigrostriatal damage is required for induction of dyskinesias by L-DOPA in squirrel monkeys. Clin Neuropharmacol 1990;13:448–458.

Breit S, Bouali-Benazzouz R, Benabid AL, Benazzouz A: Unilateral lesion of the nigrostriatal pathway induces an increase of neuronal activity of the pedunculopontine nucleus, which is reversed by the lesion of the subthalamic nucleus in the rat. Eur J Neurosci 2001;14:1833–1842.

Brouillet E, Hantraye P, Ferrante RJ, et al: Chronic mitochondrial energy impairment produces selective striatal degeneration and abnormal choreiform movements in primates. Proc Natl Acad Sci U S A 1995;92:7105–7109.

Burke RE, Fahn S, Marsden CD, et al: Validity and reliability of a rating scale for the primary torsion dystonias. Neurology 1985;35:73–77.

Burns LH, Pakzaban P, Deacon TW, et al: Selective putaminal excitotoxic lesions in non-human primates model the movement disorder of Huntington disease. Neuroscience 1995;64:1007–1017.

Burns RS, Chiueh CC, Markey SP, et al: A primate model of parkinsonism: selective destruction of dopaminergic neurons in the pars compacta of the substantia nigra by N-methyl-4-phenyl-1,2,3,6-tetrahydropyridine. Proc Natl Acad Sci U S A 1983;80:4546–4550.

Calon F, Rajput AH, Hornykiewicz O, et al: Levodopa-induced motor complications are associated with alterations of glutamate receptors in Parkinson's disease. Neurobiol Dis 2003;14:404–416.

Carpenter MB: Anatomy of the corpus striatum and brainstem integrating systems. In Brooks VB (ed): Handbook of Physiology: The Nervous System, vol 2. Washington, DC, American Physiological Society, 1981, pp 947–959.

Carpenter MB, Whittier JR, Mettler FA: Analysis of choreoid hyperkinesia in the rhesus monkey: Surgical and pharmacological analysis of hyperkinesia resulting from lesions in the subthalamic nucleus of Luys. J Comp Neurol 1950;92:293–332.

Charara A, Smith Y, Parent A: Glutamatergic inputs from the pedunculopontine nucleus to midbrain dopaminergic neurons in primates: Phaseolus vulgaris-leucoagglutinin anterograde labeling combined with postembedding glutamate and GABA immunohistochemistry. J Comp Neurol 1996;364:254–266.

Chase TN, Oh JD: Striatal dopamine- and glutamate-mediated dysregulation in experimental parkinsonism. Trends Neurosci 2000;23:S86–S91.

Clark D, White FJ: D1 dopamine receptor: The search for a function: A critical evaluation of the D1/D2 dopamine receptor classification and its functional implications. Synapse 1987;1:347–388.

Cragg SJ, Baufreton J, Xue Y, et al: Synaptic release of dopamine in the subthalamic nucleus. Eur J Neurosci 2004;20:1788–1802.

Crossman AR: Primate models of dyskinesia: The experimental approach to the study of basal ganglia-related involuntary movement disorders. Neuroscience 1987;21:1–40.

Crossman AR: A hypothesis on the pathophysiological mechanisms that underlie levodopa- or dopamine agonist-induced dyskinesia in Parkinson's disease: Implications for future strategies in treatment. Mov Disord 1990;5:100–108.

Crossman AR, Sambrook MA, Jackson A: Experimental hemiballismus in the baboon produced by injection of a gamma-aminobutyric acid antagonist into the basal ganglia. Neurosci Lett 1980;20: 369–372.

Crossman AR, Sambrook MA, Jackson A: Experimental hemichorea/hemiballismus in the monkey: Studies on the intracerebral site of action in a drug-induced dyskinesia. Brain 1984;107:579–596.

Damier P, Hirsch EC, Agid Y, Graybiel AM: The substantia nigra of the human brain: I. Nigrosomes and the nigral matrix, a compartmental organization based on calbindin D(28K) immunohistochemistry. Brain 1999;122:1421–1436.

Davis GC, Williams AC, Markey SP, et al: Chronic Parkinsonism secondary to intravenous injection of meperidine analogues. Psychiatry Res 1979;1:249–254.

Day M, Wang Z, Ding J, et al: Selective elimination of glutamatergic synapses on striatopallidal neurons in Parkinson disease models. Nat Neurosci 2006;9:251–259.

DeLong MR.: Primate models of movement disorders of basal ganglia origin. Trends Neurosci 1990;13:281–285.

Drouot X, Oshino S, Jarraya B, et al: Functional recovery in a primate model of Parkinson's disease following motor cortex stimulation. Neuron 2004;44:769–778.

Eblen F, Graybiel AM: Highly restricted origin of prefrontal cortical inputs to striosomes in the macaque monkey. J Neurosci 1995;15:5999–6013.

Ehringer H, Hornykiewicz O: Verteilung von noradrenalin und dopamin (3-Hydroxytyramin) im Gehirn des Menschen und ihr Verhalten bei Erkrank-ungen des extrapyramidalen systems. Klin Wochenschr 1960;38:1236–1239.

Eidelberg D, Moeller JR, Antonini A, et al: Functional brain networks in DYT1 dystonia. Ann Neurol 1998;44:303–312.

Fahn S: High dosage anticholinergic therapy in dystonia. Neurology 1983;33:1255–1261.

Flaherty AW, Graybiel AM: Output architecture of the primate putamen. J Neurosci 1993;13:3222–3237.

Filion M: Physiologic basis of dyskinesia. Ann Neurol 2000;47(suppl 1):S35–S40.

Filion M, Tremblay L: Abnormal spontaneous activity of globus pallidus neurons in monkeys with MPTP-induced parkinsonism. Brain Res 1991;547:142–151.

Filion M, Tremblay L, Bedard PJ: Effects of dopamine agonists on the spontaneous activity of globus pallidus neurons in monkeys with MPTP-induced parkinsonism. Brain Res 1991;547:152–161.

Francois C, Grabli D, McCairn K, et al: Behavioural disorders induced by external globus pallidus dysfunction in primates: II. Anatomical study. Brain 2004;127:2055–2070.

Freeman A, Ciliax B, Bakay R, et al: Nigrostriatal collaterals to thalamus degenerate in parkinsonian animal models. Ann Neurol 2001;50:321–329.

Fusco FR, Martorana A, De March Z, et al: Huntingtin distribution among striatal output neurons of normal rat brain. Neurosci Lett 2003;339:53–56.

Garris PA, Walker QD, Wightman RM: Dopamine release and uptake rates both decrease in the partially denervated striatum in proportion to the loss of dopamine terminals. Brain Res 1997;753:225–234.

Gerfen CR: Dopamine-mediated gene regulation in models of Parkinson's disease. Ann Neurol 2000a;47(suppl 1):S42–S50.

Gerfen CR: Molecular effects of dopamine on striatal-projection pathways. Trends Neurosci 2000b;23(suppl):S64–S70.

Gerfen CR: Indirect-pathway neurons lose their spines in Parkinson disease. Nat Neurosci 2006;9:157–158.

Gerfen CR, Engber TM, Mahan LC, et al: D1 and D2 dopamine receptor-regulated gene expression of striatonigral and striatopallidal neurons. Science 1990;250:1429–1432.

Gerfen CR, Wilson CJ: The basal ganglia. In Swanson LW (ed): Handbook of Chemical Anatomy, Integrated Systems in the CNS, Part III. New York, Elsevier, 1996, pp 371–468.

Gingrich JA, Caron MG: Recent advances in the molecular biology of dopamine receptors. Annu Rev Neurosci 1993;16:299–321.

Grabli D, McCairn K, Hirsch EC, et al: Behavioural disorders induced by external globus pallidus dysfunction in primates: I. Behavioural study. Brain 2004;127:2039–5204.

Graybiel AM: Biochemical anatomy of the striatum. In Emson PC (ed): Chemical Neuroanatomy. New York, Raven Press, 1983, pp 427–504.

Graybiel AM: Neurotransmitters and neuromodulators in the basal ganglia. Trends Neurosci 1990;13:244–254.

Graybiel AM, Baughman RW, Eckenstein F: Cholinergic neuropil of the striatum observes striosomal boundaries. Nature 1986;323:625–627.

Graybiel AM, Hirsch EC, Agid YA: Differences in tyrosine hydroxylase-like immunoreactivity characterize the mesostriatal innervation of striosomes and extrastriosomal matrix at maturity. Proc Natl Acad Sci U S A 1987;84:303–307.

Greenfield JG, Bosanquet FD: The brain-stem lesions in parkinsonism. J Neurol Neurosurg Psychiatry 1953;16:213–226.

Grondin R, Goulet M, Di Paolo T, Bedard PJ: Cabergoline, a long-acting dopamine D2-like receptor agonist, produces a sustained antiparkinsonian effect with transient dyskinesias in parkinsonian drug-naive primates. Brain Res 1996;735:298–306.

Guigoni C, Dovero S, Aubert I, et al: Levodopa-induced dyskinesia in MPTP-treated macaques is not dependent on the extent and pattern of nigrostrial lesioning. Eur J Neurosci 2005;22:283–287.

Guridi J, Herrero MT, Luquin MR, et al: Subthalamotomy in parkinsonian monkeys: Behavioural and biochemical analysis. Brain 1996;119:1717–1727.

Guyenet PG, Javory AF, Beaujouan JC, et al: Effects of dopaminergic receptor agonists and antagonists on the activity of the neo-striatal cholinergic system. Brain Res 1975;84:227–244.

Hammond C, Feger J, Bioulac B, Souteyrand JP: Experimental hemiballism in the monkey produced by unilateral kainic acid lesion in corpus Luysii. Brain Res 1979;171:577–580.

Hassani OK, Francois C, Yelnik J, Feger J: Evidence for a dopaminergic innervation of the subthalamic nucleus in the rat. Brain Res 1997;749:88–94.

Hauber W, Fuchs H: Dopamine release in the rat globus pallidus characterised by in vivo microdialysis. Behav Brain Res 2000;111:39–44.

Hedreen JC: Tyrosine hydroxylase-immunoreactive elements in the human globus pallidus and subthalamic nucleus. J Comp Neurol 1999;409:400–410.

Heise CE, Teo ZC, Wallace BA, et al: Cell survival patterns in the pedunculopontine tegmental nucleus of methyl-4-phenyl-1,2,3,6-tetrahydropyridine-treated monkeys and 6OHDA-lesioned rats: Evidence for differences to idiopathic Parkinson disease patients? Anat Embryol (Berl) 2005;210(4):287–302.

Herrero MT, Augood SJ, Hirsch EC, et al: Effects of L-DOPA on preproenkephalin and preprotachykinin gene expression in the MPTP-treated monkey striatum. Neuroscience 1995;68:1189–1198.

Herrero MT, Levy R, Ruberg M, et al: Consequence of nigrostriatal denervation and L-dopa therapy on the expression of glutamic acid decarboxylase messenger RNA in the pallidum. Neurology 1996;47:219–224.

Hoover BR, Marshall JF: Population characteristics of preproenkephalin mRNA-containing neurons in the globus pallidus of the rat. Neurosci Lett 1999;265:199–202.

Hoover BR, Marshall JF: Further characterization of preproenkephalin mRNA-containing cells in the rodent globus pallidus. Neuroscience 2002;111:111–125.

Hoover BR, Marshall JF: Molecular, chemical, and anatomical characterization of globus pallidus dopamine D2 receptor mRNA-containing neurons. Synapse 2004;52:100–113.

Hornykiewicz O: Brain neurotransmitter changes in Parkinson's disease. In Marsden CD, Fahn S (eds): Movement Disorders. London, Butterworths, 1982, pp 41–74.

Jan C, Pessiglione M, Tremblay L, et al: Quantitative analysis of dopaminergic loss in relation to functional territories in MPTP-treated monkeys. Eur J Neurosci 2003;18:2082–2086.

Jankovic J, Chen S, Le WD: The role of Nurr1 in the development of dopaminergic neurons and Parkinson's disease. Prog Neurobiol 2005;77:128–138.

Jankovic J, Marsden D: Therapeutic strategies in Parkinson's disease. In Jankovic J, Tolosa E (eds): Parkinson's Disease and Movement Disorders. Baltimore, Williams & Wilkins, 1998, pp 191–220.

Jellinger K: The pathology of parkinsonism. In Marsden CD, Fahn S (eds): Movement Disorders, vol 2. London, Butterworths, 1987, pp 124–165.

Jenkinson N, Nandi D, Aziz TZ, Stein JF: Pedunculopontine nucleus: A new target for deep brain stimulation for akinesia. Neuroreport 2005;16:1875–1876.

Jenkinson N, Nandi D, Miall RC, et al: Pedunculopontine nucleus stimulation improves akinesia in a Parkinsonian monkey. Neuroreport 2004;15:2621–2624.

Jimenez-Castellanos J, Graybiel AM: Subdivisions of the dopamine-containing A8-A9-A10 complex identified by their differential mesostriatal innervation of striosomes and extrastriosomal matrix. Neuroscience 1987a;23:223–242.

Jimenez-Castellanos J, Graybiel AM: Subdivisions of the primate substantia nigra pars compacta detected by acetylcholinesterase histochemisty. Brain Res 1987b;437:349–354.

Jolkkonen J, Jenner P, Marsden CD: L-DOPA reverses altered gene expression of substance P but not enkephalin in the caudate-putamen of common marmosets treated with MPTP. Brain Res Mol Brain Res 1995;32:297–307.

Kao C, Albea JR, Konrad PE: Asymmetry of hyperactivity between left and right subthalamic nucleus parallels severity of extremity symptoms in Parkinson's disease patients. In Abstract Viewer and Itinerary Planner, Program No. 390.314, Society for Neuroscience Online, 2003.

Karachi C, Yelnik J, Tande D, et al: The pallidosubthalamic projection: An anatomical substrate for nonmotor functions of the subthalamic nucleus in primates. Mov Disord 2005;20:172–180.

Kreiss DS, Anderson LA, Walters JR: Apomorphine and dopamine D(1) receptor agonists increase the firing rates of subthalamic nucleus neurons. Neuroscience 1996;72:863–876.

Kreiss DS, Mastropietro CW, Rawji SS, Walters JR: The response of subthalamic nucleus neurons to dopamine receptor stimulation in a rodent model of Parkinson's disease. J Neurosci 1997;17:6807–6819.

Langston JW, Ballard P, Tetrud JW, Irwin I: Chronic Parkinsonism in humans due to a product of meperidine-analog synthesis. Science 1983;219:979–980.

Lee MS, Marsden CD: Movement disorders following lesions of the thalamus or subthalamic region. Mov Disord 1994;9:493–507.

Limousin P, Greene J, Pollak P, et al: Changes in cerebral activity pattern due to subthalamic nucleus or internal pallidum stimulation in Parkinson's disease. Ann Neurol 1997;42:283–291.

Lozano AM, Lang AE, Levy R, et al: Neuronal recordings in Parkinson's disease patients with dyskinesias induced by apomorphine. Ann Neurol 2000;47(suppl 1):S141–S146.

Maneuf YP, Mitchell IJ, Crossman AR, Brotchie JM: On the role of enkephalin cotransmission in the GABAergic striatal efferents to the globus pallidus. Exp Neurol 1994;125:65–71.

Maratos EC, Jackson MJ, Pearce RKB, et al: Both short- and long-acting D-1/D-2 dopamine agonists induce less dyskinesia than L-DOPA in the MPTP-lesioned common marmoset *(Callithrix jacchus)*. Exp Neurol 2003;179(1):90–102.

Maratos EC, Jackson MJ, Pearce RK, Jenner P: Antiparkinsonian activity and dyskinesia risk of ropinirole and L-DOPA combination therapy in drug naive MPTP-lesioned common marmosets (*Callithrix jacchus*). Mov Disord 2001a;16:631–641.

Maratos EC, Jenner P, Duty S: Preproenkephalin-B gene expression in the caudate-putamen of normal monkeys exhibiting L-dopa-induced dyskinesia. Br Neurosci Assoc Abstr 2001b;16:36–11.

Marsden CD, Obeso JA: The functions of the basal ganglia and the paradox of stereotaxic surgery in Parkinson's disease. Brain 1994;117:877–897.

Martin JP: Hemichorea resulting from a local lesion of the brain (the syndrome of the body of Luys). Brain 1927;50:637–651.

Martin JP, Alcock NS: Hemichorea associated with a lesion of the corpus Luysii. Brain 1934;57:504–516.

Mazloom M, Smith Y: Synaptic microcircuitry of tyrosine hydroxylase-containing neurons and terminals in the striatum of 1 methyl-4-phenyl-1,2,3,6-tetrahydropyridine-treated monkeys. J Comp Neurol 2006;495:453–469.

McRae A: Neurotransmitters and pharmacology of the basal ganglia. In Jankovic J, Tolosa E (eds): Parkinson's Disease and Movement Disorders. Baltimore, Williams & Wilkins, 1998, pp 47–66.

Mehta A, Thermos K, Chesselet MF: Increased behavioral response to dopaminergic stimulation of the subthalamic nucleus after nigrostriatal lesions. Synapse 2000;37:298–307.

Meissner W, Dovero S, Bioulac B, et al: Compensatory regulation of striatal neuropeptide gene expression occurs before changes in metabolic activity of basal ganglia nuclei. Neurobiol Dis 2003;13:46–54.

Mitchell IJ, Clarke CE, Boyce S, et al: Neural mechanisms underlying parkinsonian symptoms based upon regional uptake of 2-deoxyglucose in monkeys exposed to 1-methyl-4-phenyl-1,2,3,6-tetrahydropyridine. Neuroscience 1989;32:213–226.

Mitchell IJ, Luquin R, Boyce S, et al: Neural mechanisms of dystonia: Evidence from a 2-deoxyglucose uptake study in a primate model of dopamine agonist-induced dystonia. Mov Disord 1990;5:49–54.

Moore RY, Bloom FE: Central catecholamine neuron systems: Anatomy and physiology of the norepinephrine and epinephrine systems. Annu Rev Neurosci 1979;2:113–168.

Ni Z, Bouali-Benazzouz R, Gao D, et al: Intrasubthalamic injection of 6-hydroxydopamine induces changes in the firing rate and pattern of subthalamic nucleus neurons in the rat. Synapse 2001;40:145–153.

Nicoll RA, Malenka RC: Contrasting properties of two forms of long-term potentiation in the hippocampus. Nature 1995;377:115–118.

Nielsen KM, Soghomonian JJ: Normalization of glutamate decarboxylase gene expression in the entopeduncular nucleus of rats with a unilateral 6-hydroxydopamine lesion correlates with increased GABAergic input following intermittent but not continuous levodopa. Neuroscience 2004;123:31–42.

Nisbet AP, Foster OJ, Kingsbury A, et al: Preproenkephalin and preprotachykinin messenger RNA expression in normal human basal ganglia and in Parkinson's disease. Neuroscience 1995;66:361–376.

Obeso JA, Rodriguez MC, DeLong MR: Basal ganglia pathophysiology: A critical review. Adv Neurol 1997;74:3–18.

Obeso JA, Rodriguez-Oroz MC, Lanciego JL, Rodriguez DM: How does Parkinson's disease begin? The role of compensatory mechanisms. Trends Neurosci 2004a;27:125–127.

Obeso JA, Rodriguez-Oroz MC, Marin C, et al: The origin of motor fluctuations in Parkinson's disease: Importance of dopaminergic innervation and basal ganglia circuits. Neurology 2004b;62: S17–S30.

Obeso JA, Rodriguez-Oroz MC, Rodriguez M, et al: Pathophysiology of the basal ganglia in Parkinson's disease. Trends Neurosci 2000;23(suppl):S8–S19.

Olanow CW, Schapira AHV, Rascol O: Continuous dopamine-receptor stimulation in early Parkinson's disease. Trends Neurosci 2000;23:S117–S126.

Paladini CA, Williams JT: Noradrenergic inhibition of midbrain dopamine neurons. J Neurosci 2004;24:4568–4575.

Palfi S, Ferrante RJ, Brouillet E, et al: Chronic 3-nitropropionic acid treatment in baboons replicates the cognitive and motor deficits of Huntington's disease. J Neurosci 1996;16:3019–3025.

Palfi S, Leventhal L, Goetz CG, et al: Delayed onset of progressive dystonia following subacute 3-nitropropionic acid treatment in Cebus apella monkeys. Mov Disord 2000;15:524–530.

Papa SM, Desimone R, Fiorani M, Oldfield EH: Internal globus pallidus discharge is nearly suppressed during levodopa-induced dyskinesias. Ann Neurol 1999;46:732–738.

Parent A: Extrinsic connections of the basal ganglia. Trends Neurosci 1990;13:254–258.

Parent A, Hazrati LN: Functional anatomy of the basal ganglia: I. The cortico-basal ganglia-thalamo-cortical loop. Brain Res Brain Res Rev 1995a;20:91–127.

Parent A, Hazrati LN: Functional anatomy of the basal ganglia: II. The place of subthalamic nucleus and external pallidum in basal ganglia circuitry. Brain Res Brain Res Rev 1995b;20:128–154.

Parent A, Lavoie B, Smith Y, Bedard P: The dopaminergic nigropallidal projection in primates: Distinct cellular origin and relative sparing in MPTP-treated monkeys. Adv Neurol 1990;53:111–116.

Parent A, Sato F, Wu Y, et al: Organization of the basal ganglia: The importance of axonal collateralization. Trends Neurosci 2000; 23(suppl):S20–S27.

Paulson GW: Dyskinesias in monkeys. In Barbeau A, Chase BA, Paulson GW (eds): Advances in Neurology, vol 1: Huntington's Chorea. New York, Raven Press, 1973, pp 647–650.

Pearce RK, Banerji T, Jenner P, Marsden CD: De novo administration of ropinirole and bromocriptine induces less dyskinesia than L-dopa in the MPTP-treated marmoset. Mov Disord 1998;13:234–241.

Pearce RK, Heikkila M, Linden IB, Jenner P: L-dopa induces dyskinesia in normal monkeys: Behavioural and pharmacokinetic observations. Psychopharmacology (Berl) 2001;156:402–409.

Penney JB Jr, Young AB: Speculations on the functional anatomy of basal ganglia disorders. Annu Rev Neurosci 1983;6:73–94.

Penney JB Jr, Young AB: Striatal inhomogeneities and basal ganglia function. Mov Disord 1986;1:3–15.

Percheron G, Filion M: Parallel processing in the basal ganglia: Up to a point. Trends Neurosci 1991;14:55–59.

Percheron G, Yelnik J, Francois C: A Golgi analysis of the primate globus pallidus: III. Spatial organization of the striato-pallidal complex. J Comp Neurol 1984;227:214–227.

Picconi B, Centonze D, Hakansson K, et al: Loss of bidirectional striatal synaptic plasticity in L-DOPA-induced dyskinesia. Nat Neurosci 2003;6:501–506.

Picconi B, Centonze D, Rossi S, et al: Therapeutic doses of L-dopa reverse hypersensitivity of corticostriatal D2-dopamine receptors and glutamatergic overactivity in experimental parkinsonism. Brain 2004;127:1661–1669.

Pisani A, Centonze D, Bernardi G, Calabresi P: Striatal synaptic plasticity: Implications for motor learning and Parkinson's disease. Mov Disord 2005;20:395–402.

Plaha P, Gill SS: Bilateral deep brain stimulation of the pedunculopontine nucleus for Parkinson's disease. Neuroreport 2005;16:1883–1887.

Pollak P, Benabid AL, Limousin P, Benazzouz A: Chronic intracerebral stimulation in Parkinson's disease. Adv Neurol 1997;74:213–220.

Rajput AH, Fenton M, Birdi S, Macaulay R: Is levodopa toxic to human substantia nigra? Mov Disord 1997;12:634–638.

Reiner A, Albin RL, Anderson KD, et al: Differential loss of striatal projection neurons in Huntington disease. Proc Natl Acad Sci U S A 1988;85:5733–5737.

Rodriguez MC, Guridi OJ, Alvarez L, et al: The subthalamic nucleus and tremor in Parkinson's disease. Mov Disord 1998a;13(suppl 3):111–118.

Rodriguez MC, Obeso JA, Olanow CW: Subthalamic nucleus-mediated excitotoxicity in Parkinson's disease: A target for neuroprotection. Ann Neurol 1998b;44(suppl 1):S175–S188.

Rodriguez-Oroz MC, Zamarbide I, Guridi J, et al: Efficacy of deep brain stimulation of the subthalamic nucleus in Parkinson's disease 4 years after surgery: Double blind and open label evaluation. J Neurol Neurosurg Psychiatry. 2004;75(10):1382–1385.

Sanchez-Gonzalez MA, Garcia-Cabezas MA, Rico B, Cavada C: The primate thalamus is a key target for brain dopamine. J Neurosci 2005;25:6076–6083.

Sassin JF: Drug-induced dyskinesia in monkeys. In Advances in Neurology. New York, Raven Press, 1975, pp 47–54.

Seeman P, Van Tol HH: Dopamine receptor pharmacology. Trends Pharmacol Sci 1994;15:264 270.

Silberstein P, Kuhn AA, Kupsch A, et al: Patterning of globus pallidus local field potentials differs between Parkinson's disease and dystonia. Brain 2003;126:2597–2608.

Smith Y, Bevan MD, Shink E, Bolam JP: Microcircuitry of the direct and indirect pathways of the basal ganglia. Neuroscience 1998;86:353–387.

Soares J, Kliem MA, Betarbet R, et al: Role of external pallidal segment in primate parkinsonism: Comparison of the effects of 1-methyl-4-phenyl-1,2,3,6-tetrahydropyridine-induced parkinsonism and lesions of the external pallidal segment. J Neurosci 2004;24:6417–6426.

Sossi V, Fuente-Fernandez R, Holden JE, et al: Changes of dopamine turnover in the progression of Parkinson's disease as measured by positron emission tomography: Their relation to disease-compensatory mechanisms. J Cereb Blood Flow Metab 2004;24:869–876.

Stephens B, Mueller AJ, Shering AF, et al: Evidence of a breakdown of corticostriatal connections in Parkinson's disease. Neuroscience 2005;132:741–754.

Tel BC, Zeng B-Y, Cannizzaro C, et al: Alterations in striatal neuropeptide mRNA produced by repeated administration of L-dopa, ropinirole or bromocriptine correlate with dyskinesia induction in MPTP-treated common marmosets. Neuroscience 2002;115(4):1047–1058.

Temel Y, Visser-Vandewalle V: Targets for deep brain stimulation in Parkinson's disease. Expert Opin Ther Targets 2006;10:355–362.

Togasaki DM, Tan L, Protell P, et al: Levodopa induces dyskinesias in normal squirrel monkeys. Ann Neurol 2001;50:254–257.

Vandecasteele M, Glowinski J, Venance L: Electrical synapses between dopaminergic neurons of the substantia nigra pars compacta. J Neurosci 2005;25:291–298

Verhagen LM, Lee JI, Chen P, et al: Apomorphine-induced dyskinesia and single-cell discharges in globus pallidus internus of parkinsonian subjects. Neurol 2000;54(suppl 3):456–457.

Vila M, Herrero MT, Levy R, et al: Consequences of nigrostriatal denervation on the gamma-aminobutyric acidic neurons of substantia nigra pars reticulata and superior colliculus in parkinsonian syndromes. Neurology 1996;46:802–809.

Vila M, Levy R, Herrero MT, et al: Consequences of nigrostriatal denervation on the functioning of the basal ganglia in human and non-human primates: An in situ hybridization study of cytochrome oxidase subunit I mRNA. J Neurosci 1997;17:765–773.

Waddington JL: Functional interactions between D-1 and D-2 dopamine receptor systems: Their role in the regulation of psychomotor behaviour, putative mechanisms, and clinical relevance. J Psychopharmacol 1989;3:54–63.

Whelan BM, Murdoch BE, Theodoros DG, et al: Redefining functional models of basal ganglia organization: Role for the posteroventral pallidum in linguistic processing? Mov Disord 2004;19:1267–1278.

Whittier JR: Ballism and the subthalamic nucleus (nucleus hypothalamicus; corpus Luysi). Arch Neurol Psychiatry 1947;58:672–692.

Whittier JR, Mettler FA: Studies on the subthalamus of the rhesus monkey: II. Hyperkinesia and other physiologic effects of subthalamic lesions, with special reference to the subthalamic nucleus of Luys. J Comp Neurol 1949;90:319–372.

Whone AL, Moore RY, Piccini PP, Brooks DJ: Plasticity of the nigropallidal pathway in Parkinson's disease. Ann Neurol 2003;53:206–213.

Wichmann T, Bergman H, DeLong MR: The primate subthalamic nucleus: III. Changes in motor behavior and neuronal activity in the internal pallidum induced by subthalamic inactivation in the MPTP model of parkinsonism. J Neurophysiol 1994;72:521–530.

Wooten GF, Lopes MB, Harris WO, et al: Pallidoluysian atrophy: Dystonia and basal ganglia functional anatomy. Neurology 1993;43:1764–1768.

Zeng BY, Pearce RK, MacKenzie GM, Jenner P: Alterations in pre-proenkephalin and adenosine-2a receptor mRNA, but not pre-protachykinin mRNA correlate with occurrence of dyskinesia in normal monkeys chronically treated with L-DOPA. Eur J Neurosci 2000;12:1096–1104.

# Hypokinetic Disorders

## Chapter 4

# Parkinsonism
## Clinical Features and Differential Diagnosis

Parkinsonism is a syndrome manifested by a combination of the following six cardinal features: tremor at rest, rigidity, bradykinesia, loss of postural reflexes, flexed posture, and freezing (motor blocks). A combination of these signs is used to clinically define definite, probable, and possible parkinsonism (Box 4-1). The most common form of parkinsonism is the idiopathic variety known as Parkinson disease (PD), first described by James Parkinson in 1817 (Parkinson, 1817). With the recognition of marked clinical-pathologic heterogeneity of parkinsonism from a single mutation and with some uncertainty whether PD should be defined clinically, pathologically, or genetically, a variety of other names have been proposed for this neurodegenerative disorder, including Parkinson complex and Parkinson Lewy disease (Langston, 2006), but it is unlikely that these names will replace the name Parkinson disease. It was not until 100 years after Parkinson's landmark paper that the loss of dopamine-containing cells in the substantia nigra (SN) was recognized (Tretiakoff et al., 1919). In 1960, Ehringer and Hornykiewicz first noted that the striatum of patients with PD was deficient in dopamine, and the following year, Birkmayer and Hornykiewicz (1961) injected levodopa in 20 patients with PD and postencephalitic parkinsonism and noted marked improvement in akinesia but not in rigidity. Later in the same decade, Cotzias and colleagues (1967 and 1969) are credited with making levodopa clinically useful in patients with PD. The recent disclosure of the diagnosis of PD in several public figures has contributed to increased awareness about the disease, which should translate into greater research funding.

Several diagnostic criteria have been developed for PD, including the U.K. Parkinson's Disease Society Brain Bank criteria used in various clinical-pathologic studies (Hughes, Ben-Shlomo, et al., 1992; Hughes, Daniel, et al., 1992) (Box 4-2). During a workshop sponsored by the National Institute of Neurological Disorders and Stroke (NINDS), a set of diagnostic criteria for PD was proposed, based on a review of the literature regarding the sensitivity and specificity of the characteristic clinical features (Gelb et al., 1999) (Box 4-3). The reliability of the different diagnostic criteria, however, has not been vigorously tested by an autopsy examination, which is commonly considered the gold standard (de Rijk et al., 1997). Two separate clinical-pathologic series concluded that only 76% of patients with a clinical diagnosis of PD actually met the pathologic criteria; the remaining 24% had evidence of other causes of parkinsonism. One of the studies was based on autopsied brains collected from 100 patients who had been clinically diagnosed with PD by the U.K. Parkinson's Disease Society Brain Bank (Hughes, Ben-Shlomo, et al., 1992; Hughes, Daniel, et al., 1992), and the other study consisted of autopsy examinations of brains from 41 patients who were followed prospectively by the same neurologist over a 22-year period (Rajput et al., 1991). In a study of 143 cases of parkinsonism that came to autopsy and had a clinical diagnosis made by neurologists, the positive predictive value of the clinical diagnosis was 98.6% for PD and 71.4% for the other parkinsonian syndromes (Hughes et al., 2002). In the DATATOP study, 800 patients were prospectively followed by trained parkinsonologists from early, untreated stages of clinically diagnosed PD for a mean of 7.6 years (Jankovic et al., 2000). An analysis of autopsy data, imaging studies, response to levodopa, and atypical clinical features indicated an 8.1% inaccuracy of initial diagnosis of PD by Parkinson experts. Although this is considerably less than the 24% diagnostic error rate reported previously, the final diagnosis was not based on pathologic confirmation in all cases. In a community-based study of 402 patients taking antiparkinsonian medications, parkinsonism was confirmed in 74% and clinically probable PD in 53%. The commonest causes of misdiagnosis were essential tremor (ET), Alzheimer disease, and vascular parkinsonism. Over one quarter of subjects did not benefit from antiparkinsonian medication (Meara et al., 1999). Parkinsonian signs, including rigidity, gait disturbance, and bradykinesia, may also occur as a consequence of normal aging, although comorbid medical conditions, such as diabetes, may significantly increase the risk of these motor signs (Arvanitakis et al., 2004).

## CLINICAL FEATURES

Nearly all studies of PD show that there is a 3:2 ratio of males to females. While there is no obvious explanation for this observed male preponderance, exposure to toxins, head trauma, neuroprotection by estrogen, mitochondrial dysfunction, or X-linked genetic factors have been suggested (Wooten et al., 2004).

There are dozens of symptoms and signs associated with PD, and the clinician must become skilled in eliciting the appropriate history and targeting the neurologic examination in a way that will bring out and document the various neurologic signs (Jankovic, 2003; Jankovic and Lang, 2004; Tolosa

**Box 4-1** Parkinsonism diagnostic criteria

1. Tremor at rest
2. Bradykinesia
3. Rigidity
4. Loss of postural reflexes
5. Flexed posture
6. Freezing (motor blocks)

*Definite*: At least two of these features must be present, one of them being 1 or 2.
*Probable*: Feature 1 or 2 alone is present.
*Possible*: At least two of features 3 to 6 must be present

et al., 2006). The manifestation of PD may vary from a barely perceptible tremor to a severe disability during the end stage of the disease. In a retrospective study of patients with PD, early nonspecific symptoms that were reported included generalized stiffness, pain or paresthesias of the limbs, constipation, sleeplessness, and reduction in volume of the voice (Przuntek, 1992). More specific complaints that were elicited on a detailed history as the disease progressed included problems with fine motor skills, decreased sense of smell, loss of appetite, and a tremor occurring with anxiety. Family members retrospectively reported decreased patient armswing on the affected side, decreased emotional expression, and personality changes, including more introversion and inflexibility. Using strict criteria for asymmetry, 46% of patients with PD had

**Box 4-2** U.K. Parkinson's Disease Society Brain Bank's clinical criteria for the diagnosis of probable Parkinson disease

*Step 1*
1. Bradykinesia
2. At least one of the following criteria:
   A. Rigidity
   B. 4- to 6-Hz rest tremor
   C. Postural instability not caused by primary visual, vestibular, cerebellar, or proprioceptive dysfunction

*Step 2*: Exclude other causes of parkinsonism
*Step 3*: At least three of the following supportive (prospective) criteria:

1. Unilateral onset
2. Rest tremor present
3. Progressive disorder
4. Persistent asymmetry affecting side of onset most
5. Excellent response (70% to 100%) to levodopa
6. Severe levodopa-induced chorea (dyskinesia)
7. Levodopa response for 5 years or more
8. Clinical course of 10 years or more

Data from Hughes AJ, Daniel SE, Kilford L, Lees AJ: Accuracy of clinical diagnosis of idiopathic Parkinson's disease: A clinico-pathological study of 100 cases. J Neurol Neurosurg Psychiatry 1992;55:181–184; and Hughes AJ, Ben-Shlomo Y, Daniel SE, Lees AJ: What features improve the accuracy of clinical diagnosis in Parkinson's disease: A clinical pathological study. Neurology 1992;42:1142–1146.

**Box 4-3** NINDS diagnostic criteria for Parkinson disease

**Group A Features: Characteristic of Parkinson's Disease**
1. Resting tremor
2. Bradykinesia
3. Rigidity
4. Asymmetric onset

**Group B Features: Suggestive of Alternative Diagnoses**
1. Features unusual early in the clinical course
   a. Prominent postural instability in the first 3 years after symptom onset
   b. Freezing phenomenon in the first 3 years
   c. Hallucinations unrelated to medications in the first 3 years
   d. Dementia preceding motor symptoms or in the first year

2. Supranuclear gaze palsy (other than restriction of upward gaze) or slowing of vertical saccades
3. Severe, symptomatic dysautonomia unrelated to medications
4. Documentation of condition known to produce parkinsonism and plausibly connected to the patient's symptoms (such as suitably located focal brain lesions or neuroleptic use within the past 6 months)

I. Criteria for DEFINITE PD
   A. All criteria for POSSIBLE PD are met and
   B. Histopathologic confirmation of the diagnosis is obtained at autopsy

II. Criteria for PROBABLE PD
   A. At least three of the four features in Group A are present
   and
   B. None of the features in Group B is present (Note: symptom duration of at least three years is necessary to meet this requirement)
   and
   C. Substantial and sustained response to levodopa or a dopamine agonist has been documented

III. Criteria for POSSIBLE PD
   A. At least two of the four features in Group A are present; at least one of these is tremor or bradykinesia
   and
   B. Either (1) none of the features in Group B is present or (2) symptoms have been present for less than three years and none of the features in Group B is present to date
   and
   C. Either (1) substantial and sustained response to levodopa or a dopamine agonist has been documented or (2) patient has not had adequate trial of levodopa or a dopamine agonist

Reprinted with permission from Gelb DJ, Oliver E, Gilman S: Diagnostic criteria for Parkinson's disease. Arch Neurol 1999;56:33–39.

characteristic asymmetric presentation that correlated with handedness (Uitti et al., 2005). In a survey of 181 treated PD patients, Bulpitt and colleagues (1985) found at least 45 different symptoms that were attributable to the disease, nine of which were reported by the patients with more than fivefold excess compared with a control population of patients randomly selected from a general practice. These common symptoms included being frozen or rooted to a spot, grimacing, jerking of the arms and legs, shaking hands, clumsy hands, salivation, poor concentration, severe apprehension, and hallucinations. Hallucinations, although usually attributed to dopaminergic therapy, may be part of PD, particularly when there is a coexistent dementia and depression (Fenelon et al., 2006; Marsh et al., 2006). However, even these frequent symptoms are relatively nonspecific and do not clearly differentiate PD patients from diseased controls. Gonera and colleagues (1997) found that 4 to 6 years prior to the onset of classic PD symptoms, patients experience a prodromal phase characterized by more frequent visits to general practitioners and specialists in comparison to normal controls. During this period, PD patients, compared to normal controls, had a higher frequency of mood disorder, fibromyalgia, and shoulder pain.

Patients who manifest predominantly axial symptoms, such as dysarthria (Ho et al., 1999), dysphagia, loss of equilibrium, and freezing of gait, are particularly disabled by their disease in comparison to those who have predominantly limb manifestations (Jankovic et al., 1990). The poor prognosis of patients in whom axial symptoms predominate is partly due to a lack of response of these symptoms to dopaminergic drugs (Kompoliti et al., 2000). Rest tremor in the hands or in the lips, however, might be not just socially embarrassing but might cause a severe handicap in people whose occupation depends on a normal appearance. Therefore, it is important that the severity of the disease be objectively assessed in the context of the individual's goals and needs.

Although a variety of neurophysiologic and computer-based methods have been proposed to quantitate the severity of the various parkinsonian symptoms and signs, most studies rely on clinical rating scales, particularly the Unified Parkinson's Disease Rating Scale (UPDRS), Hoehn-Yahr Staging Scale (Goetz et al., 2004), and Schwab-England Scale of activities of daily living (Fahn et al., 1987; Goetz et al., 1994, 1995; Bennett et al., 1997; Stebbins et al., 1999; Ramaker et al., 2002). The historical section of the UPDRS can be self-administered and reliably completed by nondemented patients (Louis et al., 1996). A short (0 to 3) Parkinson's Evaluation Scale (SPES) and Scale for Outcomes in Parkinson's Disease (SCOPA) are short, reliable scales that can be used in both research and practice (Marinus et al., 2004). Although the UPDRS has a number of limitations (Movement Disorder Society Task Force on Rating Scales for Parkinson's Disease, 2003), such as ambiguities in the written text, inadequate instructions for raters, some metric flaws, and inadequate screening questions for nonmotor symptoms, the scale is now the most frequently used instrument in numerous clinical trials. In some studies, the UPDRS is supplemented by more objective timed tests, such as the Purdue Pegboard test and movement and reaction times (Jankovic, 2003; Jankovic and Lang, 2004). When a particular aspect of parkinsonism requires more detailed study, separate scales should be employed, such as certain tremor scales or the Gait and Balance Scale (GABS) (Thomas et al., 2004). Also, it is important that in performing the UPDRS, the instructions are followed exactly. For example,

one study of 66 pull tests performed by 25 examiners showed marked variability in the technique among the examiners, and only 9% of the examinations were rated as error-free (Munhoz et al., 2004). There are also many scales, such as the Parkinson disease questionnaire-39 (PDQ-39) and the Parkinson disease quality-of-life questionnaire (PDQL) (deBoer et al., 1996), that attempt to assess the overall health-related or preference-based quality of life (Marinus et al., 2002; Siderowf et al., 2002) and the impact of the disease on the performance of activities of daily living (Lindeboom et al., 2003). The Parkinson's Disease Quality of Life Scale (PDQUALIF), developed by the Parkinson Study Group, is being used in clinical trials designed to assess the impact of PD on quality of life (Welsh et al., 2003). In addition to these quantitative measures of PD-related disability, screening tools have been developed and validated to enhance early recognition of parkinsonism. One such instrument has used nine questions that were found to reliably differentiate patients with early PD from those without parkinsonism (Hoglinger et al., 2004). The generic 15D instrument has been found to be valid for measuring health-related quality of life in PD (Haapaniemi et al., 2004). One of the most important factors contributing to quality of life is the ability to drive. Using a standardized open-route method of assigning driving abilities and safety, Wood and colleagues (2005) found that patients with PD are significantly less safe than are controls and, more important, that the driver's perception of his or her ability to drive correlated poorly with the examiner's assessment.

## BRADYKINESIA

Bradykinesia, the most characteristic clinical hallmark of PD, may be initially manifested by slowness in activities of daily living and slow movement and reaction times (Cooper et al., 1994; Touge et al., 1995; Giovannoni et al., 1999; Jankovic, Ben-Arie, et al., 1999). In addition to whole-body slowness and impairment of fine motor movement, other manifestations of bradykinesia include drooling due to failure to swallow saliva (Bagheri et al., 1999), monotonic and hypophonic dysarthria, loss of facial expression (hypomimia), and reduced armswing when walking (loss of automatic movement). Micrographia has been postulated to result from an abnormal response due to reduced motor output or weakness of agonist force coupled with distortions in visual feedback (Teulings et al., 2002). Bradyphrenia refers to slowness of thought. Bradykinesia, like other parkinsonian symptoms, is dependent on the emotional state of the patient. With a sudden surge of emotional energy, the immobile patient may catch a ball or make other fast movements. This curious phenomenon, called kinesia paradoxica, demonstrates that the motor programs are intact in PD but that patients have difficulty utilizing or accessing the programs without the help of an external trigger. Therefore, parkinsonian patients are able to make use of prior information to perform an automatic or preprogrammed movement, but they cannot use this information to initiate or select a movement.

The pathophysiology of bradykinesia is not well understood, but it is thought to result from failure of basal ganglia output to reinforce the cortical mechanisms that prepare and execute the commands to move (Jankovic, 2003). This is manifested by slowness of self-paced movements and prolongation of reaction and movement time. Evarts and colleagues (1981) first showed that both reaction (RT) and movement (MT) times are independently impaired in PD. The RT is influenced not only by the degree of motor impairment but also by the interaction between the cognitive processing and the motor response. This is particularly evident when choice RT is used and compared to simple RT. Bradykinetic patients with PD have more specific impairment in choice RT, which involves a stimulus categorization and a response selection and reflects disturbance at more complex levels of cognitive processing. Ward and colleagues (1983) found that of the various objective assessments of bradykinesia, the MT correlates best with the total clinical score, but it is not as sensitive an indicator of the overall motor deficit as is the clinical rating.

Reduced dopaminergic function has been hypothesized to disrupt normal motor cortex activity, leading to bradykinesia. In recordings from single cortical neurons in free-moving rats, a decrease in firing rate correlated with haloperidol-induced bradykinesia, demonstrating that reduced dopamine action impairs the ability to generate movement and cause bradykinesia (Parr-Brownlie and Hyland, 2005). The premovement EEG potential (Bereitschaftspotential) is reduced in PD, probably reflecting inadequate basal ganglia activation of the supplementary motor area (Dick et al., 1989). On the basis of electromyographic (EMG) recordings in the antagonistic muscles of parkinsonian patients during a brief ballistic elbow flexion, Hallett and Khoshbin (1980) concluded that the most characteristic feature of bradykinesia was the inability to energize the appropriate muscles to provide a sufficient rate of force required for the initiation and maintenance of a large, fast (ballistic) movement. Therefore, PD patients need a series of multiple agonist bursts to accomplish a larger movement. Thus, the amount of EMG activity in PD is underscaled (Berardelli et al., 2001). Secondary factors that may contribute to bradykinesia include muscle weakness, tremor, and rigidity.

Of the various parkinsonian signs, bradykinesia correlates best with a reduction in the striatal fluorodopa uptake measured by positron emission tomography (PET) scans and in turn with nigral damage (Vingerhoets et al., 1997). This is consistent with the findings that decreased density of SN neurons correlates with parkinsonism in the elderly, even without PD (Ross et al., 2004). PET scans in PD patients have demonstrated decreased $^{18}$F-fluorodeoxyglucose uptake in the striatum and accumbens-caudate complex roughly proportional to the degree of bradykinesia (Playford and Brooks, 1992). Studies performed initially in monkeys that had been made parkinsonian with the toxin 1-methyl-4-phenyl-1,2,3,6-tetrahydropyridine (MPTP) (Bergman et al., 1990) and later in patients with PD provide evidence that bradykinesia results from excessive activity in the subthalamic nucleus (STN) and the internal segment of the globus pallidus (GPi) (Dostrovsky et al., 2002). Thus, there is both functional and biochemical evidence of increased activity in the outflow nuclei, particularly the subthalamic nucleus and GPi, in patients with PD.

## TREMOR

By using the term *shaking palsy*, James Parkinson in his *An Essay on the Shaking Palsy* (1817) drew attention to tremor as a characteristic feature of PD. Indeed, some parkinsonologists regard rest tremor as the most typical sign of PD, and its absence should raise the possibility that the patient's parkinsonism is caused by a disorder other than PD. The typical rest tremor has

a frequency between 4 and 6 Hz, and the tremor is almost always most prominent in the distal part of an extremity. In the hand, the tremor has been called a pill-rolling tremor. In the head region, tremor is most common in the lips, chin, and jaw, and infrequent in the neck. Some patients with PD complain of an internal, not visible, tremor, called inner tremor.

As pointed out later, presentation with tremor as the initial symptom often confers a favorable prognosis with slower progression of the disease, and some have suggested the term *benign tremulous parkinsonism* for a subset of patients with minimal progression, frequent family history of tremor, and poor response to levodopa (Josephs et al., 2006; O'Suilleabhain, 2006). Rajput and colleagues (1991) noted that 100% of 30 patients with pathologically proven PD experienced some degree of rest tremor at some time during the course of their disease. However, in another clinical-pathologic study, only 76% of pathologically proven cases of PD had tremor (Hughes, Daniel, et al., 1992). In an expanded series of 100 pathologically proven cases of PD, tremor was present at onset in 69%; 75% had tremor during the course of the illness, and 9% lost their tremor late in the disease (Hughes et al., 1993).

Although rest tremor is a well-recognized cardinal feature of PD, many PD patients have a postural tremor that is more prominent and disabling than the classic rest tremor. Postural tremor without parkinsonian features and without any other known etiology is often diagnosed as ET, but isolated postural tremor may be the initial presentation of PD, and it may be found with higher-than-expected frequency in relatives of patients with PD (Brooks, et al., 1992b; Jankovic et al., 1995; Jankovic, 2002; Louis et al., 2003). Jankovic and colleagues (1995) and others (Louis et al., 2003) have shown that relatives of patients with tremor-dominant PD have a significantly higher risk of having action tremor than do relatives of patients with the postural instability and gait-disturbance (PIGD) form of PD, but it is not yet clear whether the isolated tremor in the relatives is ET or whether it represents and isolated manifestation of PD. The two forms of postural tremor, ET and PD, can be differentiated by a delay in the onset of tremor when arms assume an outstretched position. Most patients with PD tremor have a latency of a few seconds (up to a minute) before the tremor reemerges during postural holding—hence the term *reemergent tremor* (Jankovic, Schwartz, et al., 1999) (Video 4-1). In contrast, postural tremor of ET usually appears immediately after arms assume a horizontal posture. Since the reemergent tremor has a frequency similar to that of rest tremor and both tremors generally respond to dopaminergic drugs, reemergent tremor most likely represents a variant of the more typical rest tremor. In addition to the rest and postural tremors, a kinetic tremor, possibly related to enhanced physiologic tremor, may also impair normal reach-to-grasp movement (Wenzelburger et al., 2000). As a result of the abnormal neuronal activity at the level of the GPi, the muscle discharge in patients with PD changes from the normal high (40 Hz) to a pulsatile (10 Hz) contraction. The muscle discharge, which may be viewed as another form of PD-associated tremor, can be auscultated with a stethoscope (Brown, 1997).

## RIGIDITY AND FLEXED POSTURE

Rigidity, tested by passively flexing, extending, and rotating the body part, is manifested by increased resistance throughout the range of movement. Cogwheeling is often encountered, particularly if there is associated tremor or an underlying, not yet visible, tremor. Rigidity may occur proximally (e.g., neck, shoulders, and hips) and distally (e.g., wrists and ankles). At times, it can cause discomfort and actual pain. Painful shoulder, possibly due to rigidity but frequently misdiagnosed as arthritis, bursitis, or rotator cuff, is one of the most frequent initial manifestations of PD (Riley et al., 1989). In a prospective, longitudinal study of 6038 individuals, mean age 68.5 years, who participated in the Rotterdam study and had no dementia or parkinsonian signs at baseline, subjective complaints of stiffness, tremor, and imbalance were associated with increased risk of PD with hazard ratios of 2.11, 2.09, and 3.47, respectively (de Lau et al, 2006). During the mean 5.8 years of follow-up, 56 new cases of PD were identified.

Rigidity is often associated with postural deformity resulting in flexed neck and trunk posture and flexed elbows and knees. But rigidity is a common sign in early PD, whereas flexed posture occurs later in the disease. Some patients develop "striatal hand" deformity, characterized by ulnar deviation of hands, flexion of the metacarpophalangeal joints, and extension of the interphalangeal joints, and there may be extension of the big toe ("striatal toe") or flexion of the other toes, which can be confused with arthritis (Jankovic, 1992; Jankovic and Tintner, 2001; Ashour et al., 2005; Ashour and Jankovic, 2006) (Fig. 4-1). Striatal toe was found to be present in 13 of 62 (21%) of patients with clinically diagnosed PD (Winkler et al., 2002).

Other skeletal abnormalities include extreme neck flexion ("dropped head" or "bent spine") (Oerlemans and de Visser, 1998; Askmark et al., 2001) and truncal flexion (camptocormia) (Djaldetti et al., 1999; Umapathi et al., 2002; Azher and Jankovic, 2005). Camptocormia is characterized by

extreme flexion of the thoracolumbar spine that increases during walking and resolves in the supine position (Videos 4-2, 4-3, and 4-4). The term was coined during World War I, when young soldiers who were apparently attempting to escape the stress of battle developed this peculiar posture, perhaps promoted by a stooped posture when walking in the trenches. Askmark and colleagues (2001) found 7 patients out of 459 with parkinsonism who had a head drop attributed to neck extensor weakness. Myopathic changes on EMG were noted in all seven, and five patients who consented had abnormal muscle biopsy, with mitochondrial abnormalities in two. Isolated neck extensor myopathy was reported in other patients with anterocollis associated with parkinsonism (Lava and Factor, 2001), although its true frequency in patients with PD, multiple-system atrophy (MSA), and other parkinsonian disorders is unknown. The following etiologies have been identified in various series of patients with head drop (head ptosis), bent spine, or camptocormia: dystonia, amyotrophic lateral sclerosis, focal myopathy, inclusion body myositis, polymyositis, nemaline myopathy, facioscapulohumeral dystrophy, myasthenia gravis, encephalitis, and valproate toxicity (Umapathi et al., 2002; Gourie-Devi et al., 2003; Schabitz et al., 2003; Azher and Jankovic, 2005). Other truncal deformities include scoliosis and tilting of the trunk, referred to as the pisa syndrome (Villarejo et al., 2003). In some cases, dystonia may be the presenting symptom of PD, particularly the young-onset variety such as is seen in patients with the *parkin* mutation (Lücking et al., 2000; Jankovic and Tintner, 2001; Hedrich et al., 2002). Paroxysmal exercise-induced foot dystonia has been reported to be the presenting feature of young-onset PD (YOPD) (Bozi and Bhatia, 2003).

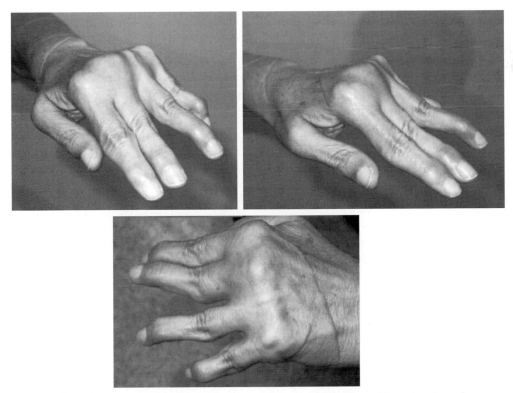

Figure 4-1 Deformities, referred to as striatal hands, seen typically in patients with parkinsonism but often wrongly attributed to arthritis. (Reprinted with permission from Ashour R, Tintner R, Jankovic J: "Striatal" hand and foot deformities in Parkinson's disease. Lancet Neurol 2005;4:423–431.)

## LOSS OF POSTURAL REFLEXES

Loss of postural reflexes usually occurs in more advanced stages of the disease and, along with freezing of gait, is the most common cause of falls that can result in hip fractures. The loss of protective reactions further contributes to fall-related injuries. Female gender, symmetric onset, postural instability, and autonomic instability appear to be the most reliable predictors of falls in PD (Williams et al., 2006). The average period from onset of symptoms to the first fall in progressive supranuclear palsy (PSP) is 16.8 months, as compared to 108 months in PD, 42 months in MSA, 54 months in dementia with Lewy bodies, and 40.8 months in vascular parkinsonism. Many patients with postural instability, particularly when associated with flexed truncal posture (camptocormia), have festination, manifested by faster and faster walking as if chasing its center of gravity to prevent falling. When combined with axial rigidity and bradykinesia, loss of postural reflexes causes the patient to collapse into the chair when attempting to sit down. The pull test (pulling the patient by the shoulders) is commonly used to determine the degree of patient's retropulsion or propulsion.

## FREEZING

One of the most disabling symptoms of PD is freezing, also referred as motor blocks, a form of akinesia (loss of movement) (Giladi et al., 1997, 2001) (Videos 4-5 and 4-6). Although it most often affects the legs when walking, it can also involve upper limbs and the eyelids (apraxia of eyelid opening or eyelid closure) (Boghen et al., 1997). Freezing consists of sudden, transient (a few seconds) inability to move. It typically causes start hesitation when initiating walking and the sudden inability to move feet (as if glued to the ground) when turning or walking through narrow passages (such as the door or the elevator), when crossing streets with heavy traffic, or when approaching a destination (target hesitation). Patients often learn a variety of tricks to overcome the freezing attacks: marching to command ("left, right, left, right"), stepping over objects (the end of a walking stick, a pavement stone, cracks in the floor, etc.), walking to music or a metronome, shifting body weight, rocking movements, and others (Dietz et al., 1990; Fahn, 1995; Marchese et al., 2001; Rubinstein et al., 2002; Suteerawattananon et al., 2004). "Off" gait freezing was found to correlate with dopa-responsive abnormal discriminatory processing as determined by abnormally increased temporal discrimination threshold (Lee et al., 2005). Freezing may be a manifestation of the "off" phenomenon in PD patients who fluctuate but may also occur during "on" time ("on freezing"), independent of bradykinesia and tremor (Bartels et al., 2003). When freezing occurs early in the course of the disease or is the predominant symptom, a diagnosis other than PD should be considered. Disorders associated with prominent freezing include PSP, MSA, and vascular (lower body) parkinsonism (FitzGerald and Jankovic, 1989; Elble et al., 1996; Winikates and Jankovic, 1999; Jankovic et al., 2001). Freezing has been thought to be related to noradrenergic deficiency as a result of degeneration of the locus coeruleus (Zarow et al., 2003), as suggested by possible response to noradrenergic agents such as L-threo-dihydroxy-phenylserine, or DOPS (Narabayashi, 1999). Neurophysiologic studies in monkeys treated with 1-methyl-4-phenyl-1,2,3,6-tetrahydropyridine found that

dopamine depletion is associated with impaired selection of proprioceptive inputs in the supplementary motor area, which could interfere with motor planning and may be related to motor freezing (Escola et al., 2002). Integrating EMG signals over real time while recording EMG activity from lower extremities before and during freezing, Nieuwboer and colleagues (2004) showed significantly abnormal timing in the tibialis anterior and gastrocnemius muscles, although reciprocity is preserved. Thus, before freezing, the tibialis anterior and gastrocnemius contract prematurely, and the duration of contraction is shortened in the tibialis anterior, but the amplitude of the EMG burst is increased (probably a compensatory strategy pulling the leg into swing), whereas the contraction is prolonged in the gastrocnemius during the actual swing phase.

## OTHER MOTOR ABNORMALITIES

Some patients exhibit the reemergence of primitive reflexes attributed to a breakdown of the frontal lobe inhibitory mechanisms that are normally present in infancy and early childhood—hence the term *release signs* (Vreeling et al., 1993; Thomas, 1994; Rao et al., 2003). The glabellar tap reflex, also known as Myerson sign, has often been associated with PD. However, its diagnostic accuracy has not been subjected to rigorous studies. The glabellar tap reflex is elicited through repeated stimuli to the glabellar region of the forehead, inducing concomitant blinking with each tap. In the normal subject, the reflex blinking habituates or the subject stops blinking with each stimulus tap after the second to fifth tap. Brodsky and colleagues (2004) examined the glabellar reflex and the palmomental reflex in 100 subjects, which included patients with PD ($n = 41$), patients with PSP ($n = 12$), patients with MSA ($n = 7$), and healthy, age-matched controls ($n = 40$). Using a standardized protocol and a "blinded" review of videotapes, they found that (1) both reflexes were present significantly more frequently in patients with PD as compared to normal controls; (2) glabellar, but not palmomental, reflex was more frequently present in patients with PSP than in controls; (3) there was no difference in the frequency of these reflexes between normal controls and patients with MSA; (4) the two reflexes occurred with similar frequency among the three parkinsonian disorders; (5) glabellar, but not palmomental, reflex correlated with parkinsonian motor deficit; and (6) the primitive reflexes correlated with mental deficit. While they are relatively sensitive signs of parkinsonian disorders, particularly PD, these primitive reflexes lack specificity, as they do not differentiate among the three most common parkinsonian disorders (Brodsky et al., 2004).

Besides the classic cardinal signs, there are many other motor abnormalities that may be equally or even more disabling. The bulbar symptoms (dysarthria, hypophonia, dysphagia, and sialorrhea) are thought to result from orofacial-laryngeal bradykinesia and rigidity (Hunker et al., 1982). PD-associated speech and voice impairment, often referred to as hypokinetic dysarthria, is characterized by low volume (hypophonia), uniform (monotonous) loudness and pitch (aprosody), imprecise consonants, hesitation, and short rushes of speech (tachyphemia). Other speech characteristics include a variable (abnormally slow or increased) speech rate, palilalia, and stuttering. A history of childhood stuttering that had remitted can subsequently recur with onset of PD, suggesting an involvement of the dopaminergic system in this speech disorder (Shahed and Jankovic, 2001). When speech therapy designed to stimulate increased vocal fold adduction with instructions to "think loud, think shout," the Lee Silverman Voice Treatment (Ramig et al., 2001), was compared with "speak loud and low," the Pitch Limiting Voice Treatment (de Swart et al., 2003), the two methods produced the same increase in loudness, but the latter method was found to prevent strained voicing. Other treatment strategies for PD-related dysarthria include the use of various verbal cues to regulate speech volume (Ho et al., 1999), but deep brain stimulation has a variable effect (Pinto et al., 2004). The low-volume voice in PD has been attributed in part to vocal fold bowing due to loss of muscle mass and control (Schulz et al., 1999), and augmentation of vocal folds with collagen injections provides improvement in voice quality and has a significantly beneficial impact on quality of life (Hill et al., 2003). Respiratory difficulties result from a variety of mechanisms, including a restrictive component due to rigid respiratory muscles and levodopa-induced respiratory dyskinesias (Rice et al., 2002).

## AUTONOMIC DYSFUNCTION

Autonomic failure is typically associated with MSA and may be the presenting feature of that disease, but it may also herald the onset of PD (Kaufmann et al., 2004). Dysautonomia, such as orthostatic hypotension, sweating dysfunction, sphincter dysfunction, and sexual impotence occur frequently in patients with PD (Senard et al., 1997; Swinn et al., 2003). In one study, 7 of 51 (14%) patients with PD had decrease of more than 20 mmHg in systolic blood pressure (Bonuccelli et al., 2003). Another community-based study of a cohort of PD patients showed that 42 of 89 (47%) met the diagnostic criteria for orthostatic hypotension (Allcock et al., 2004). Although dysautonomia is typically associated with MSA (Wenning et al., 1995), it may also be prominent in PD. Furthermore, autonomic testing might not always differentiate between PD and MSA (Riley and Chelimsky, 2003).

Orthostatic hypotension in patients with PD has been traditionally attributed to dopaminergic therapy, but recent studies have provided evidence that orthostatic hypotension in PD is due to failure of reflexive sympathetically mediated cardiovascular stimulation from sympathetic denervation, as demonstrated by markedly decreased 6-[$^{18}$F]-fluorodopamine-derived radioactivity in septal and ventricular myocardium (Goldstein et al., 2002). This sympathetic nervous system deficit involved postganglionic catecholaminergic, not cholinergic, nerves (Sharabi et al., 2003).

Sweating dysfunction, hyperhidrosis, and to a lesser extent hypohidrosis, were reported by 64% of patients with PD as compared to 12.5% of controls ($P < .005$) (Swinn et al., 2003). These symptoms did not correlate with the severity of the disease but occurred most frequently during the "off" periods and during "on with dyskinesia" periods. Urologic symptoms are frequent; one recent survey found that over one fourth of men with PD had urinary difficulty, most often causing urinary urgency (Araki and Kuno, 2000). Drooling (sialorrhea) is one of the most embarrassing symptoms of PD. While some studies have shown that PD patients actually have less saliva production (Proulx et al., 2005) than normal controls, others have suggested that the excessive drooling is due to a difficulty with swallowing (Bagheri et al., 1999). Salivary sympathetic

denervation, however, could not be demonstrated by 6-[$^{18}$F]-fluorodopamine scanning (Goldstein et al., 2002). Dysphagia (Hunter et al., 1997) along with delayed gastric emptying (Hardoff et al., 2001) and constipation (Ashraf et al., 1997; Bassotti et al., 2000; Winge et al., 2003) represent the most frequent gastrointestinal manifestations of PD. On the basis of information on the frequency of bowel movements in 6790 men in the Honolulu Heart Program, Abbott and colleagues (2001) concluded that infrequent bowel movements are associated with increased risk for future PD. Constipation in patients with PD is associated with slow colonic transit, weak abdominal strain, decreased phasic rectal contraction, and paradoxic sphincter contraction on defecation (Sakakibara et al., 2003). Dermatologic changes such as seborrhea, hair loss, and leg edema may represent evidence of peripheral involvement in PD, although some of these changes may be exacerbated by anti-PD drugs (Tabamo and DiRicco, 2002; Tan and Ondo, 2002).

Autonomic complications, coupled with motor and mental decline, contribute to a higher risk for hospitalization and nursing home placement. Examination of hospital records of 15,304 cases of parkinsonism and 30,608 age- and sex-matched controls showed that PD patients are six times more likely to be admitted to hospital with aspiration pneumonia than are nonparkinsonian controls (Gutman et al., 2004). Other comorbid medical conditions significantly more common in patients with PD include fractures of the femur, urinary tract disorders, septicemia, and fluid/electrolyte disorders. But similarly to other reports (Jansson and Jankovic, 1985; Gorell et al., 1994; Vanacore et al., 1999), this study showed that cancer might be less common in patients with PD, with the major exception being malignant melanoma with an almost twofold increased risk (Olsen et al., 2005).

Although in his original description James Parkinson focused on the motor symptoms, he also drew attention to several nonmotor features, including problems associated with sleep and gastrointestinal function (Parkinson, 1817). These nonmotor, nondopaminergic symptoms have been largely ignored, but several recent studies highlighted their frequency and their serious impact on quality of life, particularly in more advanced stages of the disease (Lang and Obeso, 2004; Chaudhuri et al., 2006).

## COGNITIVE AND NEUROBEHAVIORAL ABNORMALITIES

While most descriptions of PD focus on the motor manifestations, nonmotor manifestations and fluctuations in nonmotor symptoms have been found to be more disabling than the motor symptoms in 28% of PD patients (Witjas et al., 2002). A structured interview of 50 patients with PD found that anxiety (66%), drenching sweats (64%), slowness of thinking (58%), fatigue (56%), and akathisia (54%) were the most frequent nonmotor fluctuations. Many patients, for example, exhibit neurobehavioral disturbances, such as depression, dementia, tip-of-the-tongue phenomenon, various psychiatric symptoms, and sleep disorders (van Hilten et al., 1994; Aarsland et al., 1999; Pal et al., 1999; Tandberg et al., 1999; Olanow et al., 2000; Wetter et al., 2000; Ondo et al., 2001; Emre, 2003; Grandas and Iranzo, 2004; Adler and Thorpy, 2005). On the basis of the most frequently affected cognitive domains in PD, Marinus and colleagues (2003) proposed the SCOPA-COG (Scales for Outcomes of Parkinson's disease-cognition). Using this scale and the search of the literature, they concluded that the cognitive functions that are most frequently affected in PD include attention, active memory, executive, and visuospatial functions, whereas verbal functions, thinking, and reasoning are relatively spared. PD patients may have a limited perception of large spatial configurations (seeing the trees but not the forest) (Barrett et al., 2001). Aarsland and colleagues (2001) found in a community-based, prospective study that patients with PD have an almost sixfold increased risk of dementia. In an 8-year prospective study of 224 patients with PD, they found that 78.2% fulfilled the DSM-III criteria for dementia (Aarsland et al., 2003). The mean annual decline on Mini-Mental State Examination in patients with PD is 1 point; in patients with PD and dementia, it is 2.3 points (Aarsland et al., 2004).

Temporoparietal cortical hypometabolism is present in patients with PD and may be a useful predictor of future cognitive impairment (Hu et al., 2000). Another predictor of cognitive dysfunction appears to be reduced $^{18}$F-fluorodopa uptake in the caudate nucleus and frontal cortex (Rinne et al., 2000) as well as in the mesolimbic pathways (Ito et al., 2002). Using event-related functional magnetic resonance imaging to compare groups of cognitively impaired and unimpaired patients, Lewis and colleagues (2003) showed a significant signal intensity reduction during a working-memory paradigm in specific striatal and frontal lobe sites in PD patients with cognitive impairment. These studies indicate that cognitive impairments in early PD are related to reductions in activity of frontostriatal neural circuitry. In studies utilizing PET to study brain activation during frontal tasks, such as trial-and-error learning, Mentis and colleagues (2003) found that even in early PD when learning is still relatively preserved, PD patients had to activate four times as much neural tissue as the controls in order to achieve learning performance equal to controls. Although the sequence learning is impaired even in early PD, this learning deficit does not appear to reflect impairments in motor execution or bradykinesia and may be related to reduced attention (Ghilardi et al., 2003).

Patients with PD have nearly twice the risk for developing dementia as controls, and siblings of demented PD patients have an increased risk for Alzheimer disease (Marder et al., 1999). In addition to the Mini-Mental State Examination, other tests (e.g., the Frontal Assessment Battery) have been developed and validated to assess the cognitive and frontal lobe function (Dubois et al., 2000) in patients with dementia with or without parkinsonism. There are several reasons why patients with PD have an associated dementia. Pathologically, dementia correlates with cortical pathology, including Lewy bodies (Hughes et al., 1993; Hurtig et al., 2000), especially in the cingulate and entorhinal cortex (Kovari et al., 2003). But the significance of cortical Lewy bodies is not clear, since most patients with PD have some detectable Lewy bodies in the cerebral cortex, and patients with PD with no dementia during life have been found to have neuropathologic findings diagnostic of Lewy body dementia (Colosimo et al., 2003). In contrast to earlier studies showing relatively low frequency of dementia in PD, more recent studies suggest that the cumulative prevalence may be as high as 78%, correlating best with cortical and limbic Lewy bodies (Emre, 2004).

A community-based study showed that 7.7% of PD patients met the criteria for major depression, 5.1% met those for moderate to severe depression, and another 45.5% had mild depressive symptoms (Tandberg et al., 1996). In 139 patients with PD, Aarsland and colleagues (1999) found at least one psychiatric symptom in 61% of the patients. These included depression (38%), hallucinations (27%), and a variety of other behavioral and cognitive changes. Patients with depression may be three times more likely to later develop PD (Schuurman et al., 2002). In one study, depression was found in 15% of patients with PD, and it had more impact on the activities of daily living than on the motor subscale of UPDRS (Holroyd et al., 20005). Anhedonia is another frequent symptom of PD, which is independent from depression or motor deficits (Isella et al., 2003). Using ($^{11}$C)RTI-32 PET as a marker of both dopamine and norepinephrine transporter binding in 8 PD patients with and 12 without depression, Remy and colleagues (2005) showed significantly lower binding of this ligand in the locus coeruleus and various limbic regions in depressed and anxious patients compared to those without these psychiatric symptoms. In a group of 94 patients with primary depression, Starkstein and colleagues (2001) found that 20% of patients had parkinsonism that was reversible on treatment of the depression. Some investigators have attributed the various nonmotor symptoms associated with PD, such as depression, anxiety, lack of energy, and sexual dysfunction, to comorbid testosterone deficiency (found in 35% of PD patients) and suggested that testosterone treatment may be the appropriate therapy for these patients (Okun et al., 2002) and may also improve apathy associated with PD (Ready et al., 2004). However, in a subsequent control clinical trial, testestorone was not found to be beneficial in men with PD (Okun et al., 2006).

Several studies have shown that the occurrence of psychosis is frequently associated with other psychiatric comorbidities, especially depression, anxiety, and apathy (Marsh et al., 2004), and with dementia (Factor et al., 2003). One study concluded that the presence of hallucinations is the strongest predictor of nursing home placement and death (Aarsland et al., 2000). The prognosis of PD-associated psychosis, however, has improved with the advent of atypical neuroleptics in that the incidence of death within 2 years of nursing home placement decreased from 100% to 28%. Minor hallucinations may occur in as many as 40% of patients with PD, illusions in 25%, formed visual hallucinations in 22%, and auditory hallucinations in 10% (Fénelon et al., 2000). Risk factors for hallucinations include older age, duration of illness, depression, cognitive disorder, daytime somnolence, poor visual acuity, family history of dementia (Paleacu et al., 2005), and dopaminergic drugs (Barnes and David, 2001; Goetz et al., 2001; Holroyd et al., 2001). Hallucinations seem to correlate with daytime episodes of rapid eye movement (REM) sleep as well as daytime non-REM and nocturnal REM sleep, suggesting that hallucinations and psychosis may represent a variant of narcolepsy-like REM sleep disorder (Arnulf et al., 2000) and that dream imagery plays an important role in visual hallucinations (Manni et al., 2002). Other studies, however, have found no correlation between hallucinations and abnormal sleep patterns (Goetz et al., 2005).

Besides the cardinal motor signs, there are many behavioral and cognitive symptoms associated with PD, such as depression, sleep disorders, and fatigability, that can adversely influence the overall quality of life in patients with PD (Karlsen et al., 1999). In one study, 50% of patients with PD had significant fatigue that had a major impact on health-related quality of life (Herlofson and Larsen., 2003). PD-related fatigue contributes to poor functional capacity and physical function (Garber and Friedman, 2003; Chaudhuri and Behan, 2004). A 16-item self-report instrument designed to measure fatigue associated with PD has been developed (Brown et al., 2005). One study showed that depression, postural instability, and cognitive impairment have the greatest influence on quality of life (Schrag et al., 2000). In a prospective longitudinal study of 111 patients followed for 4 years, Karlsen and colleagues (2000) showed significantly increased distress, based on health-related quality of life, not only due to motor symptoms but also because of pain, social isolation, and emotional reactions.

Variants of bradyphrenia (slowness of thought), such as abulia (severe apathy and lack of initiative and spontaneity) as well as akinetic mutism and catatonia (immobility, mutism, refusal to eat or drink, staring, rigidity, posturing, grimacing, negativism, waxy flexibility, echophenomenon, and stereotypy), have been recognized in patients with parkinsonism. Apathy in PD appears to be related to the underlying disease process rather than being a psychological reaction to disability and is closely associated with cognitive impairment (Pluck and Brown, 2002). Whether these symptoms represent a continuum of bradykinesia-bradyphrenia or different disorders is not easy to answer with the current rudimentary knowledge of these disorders (Muqut et al., 2001).

In addition to these behavioral problems, many patients with PD develop obsessive-compulsive behavior and addictive personality, particularly exemplified by compulsive gambling (Molina et al., 2000; Alegret et al., 2001; Geschwandtner et al., 2001). Pathologic gambling has been attributed by some to the use of dopamine agonists, but this putative association has not been confirmed (Driver-Dunckley et al., 2003). Various intrusive cognitive events with associated repetitive behaviors, representing the spectrum of obsessive-compulsive disorder in PD, include the following domains: (1) checking, religious, and sexual obsessions; (2) symmetry and ordering; (3) washing and cleaning; and (4) punding. Punding is characterized by intense fascination with repetitive handling, examining, sorting, and arranging of objects (Evans et al., 2004; Voon, 2004). The behavior may be based on one's past experiences and hobbies or may be more related to obsessive-compulsive disorder features such as gambling, which in turn may be exacerbated by dopaminergic drugs (Kurlan, 2004). Pathologic gambling has been attributed most frequently to the use of dopamine agonists (Kurlan, 2004; Dodd et al., 2005), but levodopa and even subthalamic nucleus deep brain stimulation also have been reported to cause pathologic gambling. The obsessive-compulsive disorder that is associated with PD has been reported to improve with high-frequency stimulation of the subthalamic nucleus (Mallett et al., 2002). Another behavioral abnormality, possibly related to underlying obsessive-compulsive disorder, is "hedonistic homeostatic dysregulation." This behavior is seen particularly in males with early-onset PD who misuse and abuse dopaminergic drugs and develop cyclic mood disorder with hypomania or manic psychosis (Giovannoni et al., 2000; Pezzella et al., 2005). Other behavioral symptoms associated with dopamine dysregulation syndrome include compulsive dopaminergic replacement (Lawrence et al., 2003), craving, binge eating, compulsive foraging, euphoria, dysphoria, hyper sexuality, pathologic gambling, compulsive shopping, aggression, insulting gestures, paranoia, jealousy, phobias, and other behaviors (Evans and Lees, 2004).

## SLEEP DISORDERS

Sleep disorders are being increasingly recognized as a feature of PD. An instrument consisting of 15 questions for assessing sleep and nocturnal disability has been described (Chaudhuri et al., 2002). While most studies have attributed the excessive daytime drowsiness and irresistible sleep episodes (sleep attacks) to anti-PD medications (Ondo et al., 2001), some authors believe that these sleep disturbances are an integral part of PD and that increasing the nighttime sleep with antidepressants or benzodiazepines will not alleviate daytime drowsiness (Arnulf et al., 2002). In a study of 303 PD patients, 63 (21%) had symptoms of restless legs syndrome, possibly associated with low ferritin levels, but there is no evidence that restless legs syndrome leads to PD (Ondo et al., 2002). In another study, 10 of 126 (7.9%) patients with PD and 1 of 129 (0.8%) controls had symptoms of restless legs syndrome (Krishnan et al., 2003). Tan and colleagues (2002) found motor restlessness in 15.2% of their patients with PD, but the prevalence of restless legs syndrome, based on diagnostic criteria proposed by the International Restless Legs Syndrome Study Group, in the PD population was the same as that in the general or clinic population.

In one study, 38% of patients presenting with idiopathic rapid eye movement (REM) sleep behavior disorder (RBD) eventually developed parkinsonism (Schenk et al., 1996; Ferini-Strambi and Zucconi, 2000; Matheson and Saper, 2003; Postuma et al., 2006). In yet another study, 86% of patients with RBD had associated parkinsonism (PD: 47%; MSA: 26%; PSP: 2%) (Olson et al., 2000). Several other studies reported this association of RBD and parkinsonism (Plazzi et al., 1997; Comella et al., 1998; Wetter et al., 2000; Gagnon et al., 2002), and idiopathic RBD is now considered to represent a preparkinsonian state. RBD was found in 11 of 33 (33%) patients with PD, and 19 of 33 (58%) had REM sleep without atonia (Gagnon et al., 2002). In another study, RBD preceded the onset of parkinsonism in 52% of patients with PD (Olson et al., 2000). The strong male preponderance that is seen in patients with RBD is much less evident in patients who eventually develop MSA. [11 C]-dihydrotetrabenazine PET (Albin et al., 2000) and [123I]-iodobenzamide single-photon emission computed tomographic (SPECT) (Eisensehr et al., 2000) found evidence of significantly reduced dopaminergic terminals and striatal D2 receptor density, respectively, in patients with RBD, though not to the same degree as in patients with PD.

There is a growing body of evidence supporting the notion that dopamine activity is normally influenced by circadian factors (Rye and Jankovic, 2002). For example, tyrosine hydroxylase falls several hours before the person wakes, and its increase correlates with motor activity. It has been postulated that low doses of dopaminomimetic drugs stimulate D2 inhibitory autoreceptors located on cell bodies of neurons in the ventral tegmental area, resulting in sedation. This is consistent with the findings that local (ventral tegmental area) application of D2 antagonists causes sedation while administration of amphetamines initiates and maintains wakefulness. Although the cerebrospinal fluid levels of hypocretin (Sutcliffe and de Lecea, 2002) have been reported to be normal in three PD patients with excessive daytime drowsiness, further studies are needed to explore the relationship between hypocretin and sleep disorders associated with PD (Overeem et al., 2002). Since the loss of dopamine in PD generally progresses from the putamen to the caudate and eventually to the limbic areas, it has been postulated that it is loss of dopamine in these latter circuits, most characteristic of advanced disease, that is a potential factor in the expression of excessive daytime drowsiness and sleep-onset REM in PD (Rye and Jankovic, 2002).

## SENSORY ABNORMALITIES

In addition to motor and behavioral symptoms, PD patients often exhibit a variety of sensory deficits. Sensory complaints, such as paresthesias, akathisia, and oral and genital pain (Comella and Goetz, 1994; Ford et al., 1996; Djaldetti et al., 2004) are frequently not recognized as parkinsonian symptoms and result in an inappropriate and exhaustive diagnostic evaluation.

As was noted previously, olfactory function is typically impaired in PD, even in very early stages (Stern et al., 1994; Katzenschlager and Lees, 2004). One study showed that idiopathic olfactory dysfunction (hyposmia) may be associated with a 10% increased risk of developing PD (Ponsen et al., 2004). Camicioli and colleagues (2002) found that a combination of finger tapping, olfaction ability (assessed by the University of Pennsylvania Smell Identification Test, or UPSIT), and visual contrast sensitivity, or Paired Associates Learning, discriminated between PD patients and controls with 90% accuracy. To determine which signs in the very early, presymptomatic stage of the disease predict the subsequent development of PD, Montgomery and colleagues (1999) studied 80 first-degree relatives of patients with PD and 100 normal controls using a battery of tests of motor function, mood, and olfaction (Tissingh et al., 2001; Double et al., 2003). They found that 22.5% of the relatives and only 9% of the normal controls had abnormal scores. It is, of course, not known how many of the relatives with abnormal scores will develop PD; therefore, the specificity and sensitivity of the test battery in predicting PD cannot be determined. UPSIT administered to 62 twin pairs who were discordant for PD showed that smell identification was reduced in the twins affected with PD in comparison to those without symptoms (Marras et al., 2005). After a mean interval of 7.3 years, 19 of the twins were retested. Neither of two twins who developed new PD had had impaired smell identification at baseline, although their UPSIT scores declined more than those of the other 17 twins. The authors concluded that "smell identification ability may not be a sensitive indicator of future PD 7 or more years before the development of motor signs." Impaired olfaction correlates well with decreased β-CIT uptake and may precede the onset of motor symptoms of PD (Berendse et al., 2002; Siderowf et al., 2005). Reduced olfaction in PD may be related to a neuronal loss in the corticomedial amygdala (Harding et al., 2002) or to an increase of dopaminergic neurons in the olfactory bulb (dopamine inhibits olfactory transmission), as determined by increased TH-reactive neurons (Huisman et al., 2004). It is important to point out, however, that olfaction is impaired in the elderly population. Using the San Diego Odor Identification Test and self-report, Murphy and colleagues (2002) found that 24.5% of people between the ages of 53 and 97 have impaired olfaction, and the incidence is 62.5% in people over age 80. Loss of smell is characteristic of PD and Alzheimer disease but is usually not present in ET, PSP, corticobasal degeneration, vascular parkinsonism (Katzenschlager et al., 2004), or parkinsonism due to *parkin* mutation (Khan et al., 2004). Within PD, patients with the tremor-dominant form with family history were found to have less olfaction loss than were those without family history, suggesting that the familial tremor-dominant form of PD might be a different disease from sporadic PD (Ondo and Lai, 2005). Biopsy of olfactory nasal neurons does not aid in differentiating PD and Alzheimer disease from the other neurodegenerative disorders (Hawkes, 2003). Some investigators think that olfactory testing is comparable to other diagnostic tests, such as magnetic resonance imaging (MRI), SPECT, and neuropsychological testing, in differentiating PD from other parkinsonian disorders and in early detection of PD (Katzenschlager and Lees, 2004).

There are other sensory abnormalities in patients with PD. One study showed that patients with PD who experience pain have increased sensitivity to painful stimuli (Djaldetti et al., 2004). Joint position has been found to be impaired in some patients with PD (Zia et al., 2000). There is some evidence that while the visual acuity in PD is usually spared, some patients experience progressive impairment of color discrimination and contrast sensitivity (Bodis-Wollner, 2002; Diederich et al., 2002). It is not known, however, whether this visual dysfunction is due to retinal or postretinal abnormality. In their review of ophthalmologic features of PD, Biousse and colleagues (2004) noted that any of the following may contribute to the ocular and visual complaints in patients with PD: decreased blink rate, ocular surface irritation, altered tear film, visual hallucinations, blepharospasm, decreased blink rate, and decreased convergence.

Motor fluctuations related to levodopa therapy are well recognized, but what is not readily appreciated is that many patients also experience nonmotor fluctuations, such as sensory symptoms, dyspnea, facial flushing, hunger (and sweets cravings), and other symptoms (Hillen and Sage, 1996). Weight loss is another, though poorly understood, typical manifestation of PD (Jankovic et al., 1992; Ondo et al., 2000; Chen et al., 2003; Lorefalt et al., 2004). In Huntington disease, weight loss has been attributed to higher sedentary energy expenditure (Pratley et al., 2000), but the mechanism of weight loss in PD is not well understood, though it is not thought to be due to reduced energy intake (Chen et al., 2003). It is important to note that these nonmotor symptoms may be as disabling as the classic motor symptoms or even more so (Lang and Obeso, 2004).

## CLINICAL-PATHOLOGIC CORRELATIONS

The clinical heterogeneity in parkinsonian patients suggests that there is variable involvement of the dopaminergic and other neurotransmitter systems. Alternatively, the subgroups might represent different clinical-pathologic entities, thus indicating that PD is not a uniform disease but a syndrome. Highly predictive diagnostic criteria are essential to select an appropriate patient population for genetic studies and clinical trials (Gelb et al., 1999). In support of the notion that the PIGD subgroup represents a distinct disorder, separate from PD, is the finding that only 27% of patients with the PIGD form of idiopathic parkinsonism have Lewy bodies at autopsy (Rajput et al., 1993). In the London brain bank series, only 11% of the 100 pathologically proven cases of PD had tremor-dominant disease, and 23% had "akinetic/rigid" disease; the rest (64%) were diagnosed as having a "mixed pattern" (Hughes et al., 1993). In contrast to the 76% to 100% occurrence of tremor in PD, only 31% of those with atypical parkinsonism (progressive supranuclear palsy, or PSP-4; striatonigral degeneration, or SND-2; Shy-Drager syndrome, or SDS-5; and the combination of SND and olivopontocerebellar atrophy, or OPCA-2) had rest tremor (Rajput et al., 1991), and 50% of the 24 cases with non-PD parkinsonism in the London series had tremor, type not specified (Hughes, Daniel, et al., 1992).

In another clinical-pathologic study, Hirsch and colleagues (1992) have demonstrated that patients with PD and prominent tremor have degeneration of a subgroup of midbrain (A8) neurons, whereas this area is spared in PD patients without tremor. Other clinical-pathologic studies have confirmed that the tremor-dominant type of PD shows more damage to the retrorubral field A8, containing mainly calretinin-staining cells but only few tyrosine hydroxylase and dopamine transporter immunoreactive neurons (Jellinger, 1999). Also the tremor-dominant PD seems to be associated with more severe neuron loss in medial than in lateral SNzc. In contrast, A8 is rather preserved in the PIGD, rigid-akinetic PD, possibly owing to the protective role of calcium-binding protein. These findings support the hypothesis that differential damage of subpopulations of neuronal systems is responsible for the diversity of phenotypes seen in PD and other parkinsonian disorders. Detailed clinical-pathologic-biochemical studies will be required to prove or disprove this hypothesis.

Using $^{18}$F-6-fluorodopa, Vingerhoets and colleagues (1997) demonstrated that bradykinesia is the parkinsonian sign that correlates best with nigrostriatal deficiency. In contrast, patients with the tremor-dominant PD have increased metabolic activity in the pons, thalamus, and motor association cortices (Antonini et al., 1998). The presence of tremor in PD also seems to correlate with serotonergic dysfunction, as suggested by a 27% reduction in the midbrain raphe 5-HT$_{1A}$ binding demonstrated by $^{11}$C-WAY 100635 PET scans (Doder et al., 2003). By using statistical cluster analysis of 120 patients with early PD, four main subgroups were identified: (1) young-onset, (2) tremor-dominant, (3) nontremor-dominant with cognitive impairment and mild depression, and (4) rapid disease progression but no cognitive impairment (Lewis et al., 2005).

There is a growing appreciation not only for the clinical heterogeneity of PD but also for genetic heterogeneity. As a result, the notion of PD is evolving from the traditional view of a single clinical-pathologic entity to "Parkinson diseases" with different etiologies and clinical presentations. For example, the autosomal-recessive juvenile parkinsonism (AR-JP) due to mutation in the *parkin* gene on chromosome 6q25.2–27 (*PARK2*) may present with a dystonic gait or camptocormia during adolescence or early adulthood (or even in the sixth or seventh decade) and with levodopa-responsive dystonia and may be characterized by symmetric

onset, marked sleep benefit, early levodopa-induced dyskinesias, hemiparkinsonism-hemiatrophy, hyperreflexia, and "slow" orthostatic tremor. Patients with *parkin* mutation seem to have a slower disease course (Lücking et al., 2000; Rawal et al., 2003; Schrag and Schott, 2006). Furthermore, similar to YOPD, patients with *parkin* mutations show marked decrease in striatal $^{18}$F-dopa PET, but in contrast to PD, *PARK2* patients show additional reductions in caudate and midbrain as well as significantly decreased raclopride binding in striatal, thalamic, and cortical areas (Scherfler et al., 2004). *PARK2* is the most common cause of juvenile parkinsonism, but there are many other causes of levodopa-responsive juvenile parkinsonism, such as dopa-responsive dystonia, SCA2, SCA3, and even more causes of levodopa-unresponsive parkinsonism (Paviour et al., 2004).

## NATURAL HISTORY OF PARKINSON DISEASE

The rich and variable clinical expression of PD has encouraged a search for distinct patterns of neurologic deficits that may define parkinsonian subtypes and predict the future course (Jankovic, 2005). On the basis of an analysis of a cohort of 800 PD patients, two major subtypes were identified: one characterized by tremor as the dominant parkinsonian feature and the other dominated by PIGD (Zetusky et al., 1985; Jankovic et al., 1990; McDermott et al., 1995). The tremor-dominant form of PD seems to be associated with a relatively preserved mental status, earlier age at onset, and a slower progression of the disease than the PIGD subtype, which is characterized by more severe bradykinesia, dementia, and a relatively rapidly progressive course. A presentation with bradykinesia and the PIGD type of PD seems to be associated with a relatively malignant course, whereas PD patients who are young and have tremor at the onset of their disease seem to have a slower progression and a more favorable prognosis. In one study, the relative risk of death in patients with the tremor-dominant form of PD was significantly lower than in PD patients without rest tremor (1.52 versus 2.04, $P < .01$) (Elbaz et al., 2003). The American Association of Neurologists Practice Parameter on diagnosis and prognosis of new onset PD made the following conclusions: (1) Early falls, poor response to levodopa, symmetry of motor manifestations, lack of tremor, and early autonomic dysfunction are probably useful in distinguishing other parkinsonian syndromes from Parkinson disease (PD). (2) Levodopa or apomorphine challenge and olfactory testing are probably useful in distinguishing PD from other parkinsonian syndromes. (3) Predictive factors for more rapid motor progression, nursing home placement, and shorter survival time include older age at onset of PD, associated comorbidities, presentation with rigidity and bradykinesia, and decreased dopamine responsiveness (Suchowersky et al, 2006).

The more favorable course of the tremor-dominant form of PD is also supported by the finding that the reduction in F-dopa uptake, as measured by PET and expressed as $K_i$, was 12.8% over a 2-year period in PD patients with severe tremor compared with a 19.4% reduction in the mild or no tremor group ($P = .04$) (Whone et al., 2002). Furthermore, Hilker and colleagues (2005) provided evidence for a variable progression of the disease based on the clinical phenotype. Similar to other studies (Jankovic and Kapadia, 2001), they showed that patients with the tremor-dominant form of PD progressed at a slower rate than did patients with the other PD subtypes. In addition, the tremor-dominant form of PD is associated with a more frequent family history of tremor, and it is more likely to have coexistent ET (Jankovic et al., 1995). Axial impairment, probably mediated predominantly by nondopaminergic systems, is associated with incident dementia (Levy et al., 2000). While executive function was found to be impaired in both familial and sporadic PD, explicit memory recall is more impaired in the sporadic form of PD (Dujardin et al., 2001).

To determine whether age at onset is a predictor of the future course and response to levodopa, 48 patients with YOPD (onset between 20 and 40 years of age) were compared to 123 late-onset PD (LOPD) patients (onset at 60 years of age or older) (Jankovic et al., 1997). YOPD patients presented more frequently with rigidity, while LOPD presented more frequently with PIGD; there was no difference in the occurrence of tremor at onset. YOPD patients generally respond to levodopa better but are more likely to develop dyskinesias and "wearing-off" (Quinn et al., 1987; Jankovic et al., 1997; Schrag et al., 1998; Kumar et al., 2005; Schrag and Schott, 2006). Furthermore, the late-onset subtype is characterized by rapidly progressive motor and cognitive disability (Graham and Sagar, 1999; Diederich et al., 2003). Many, if not most, YOPD patients have been found to have *parkin* mutations (*PARK 2*) or other mutations in other gene loci (*PARK 6* and *PARK 7*), but their clinical characteristics and $^{18}$F-dopa uptake are similar to those in other YOPD patients without mutations (Thobois et al., 2003). PD seems to have a much greater psychosocial impact on YOPD patients in terms of loss of employment, disruption of family life, perceived stigmatization, and depression than on LOPD patients (Schrag et al., 2003).

There is growing evidence that the progression of PD is not linear and that the rate of deterioration is much more rapid in the early phase of the disease (Jankovic, 2005; Schapira and Obeso, 2006). To study the overall rate of functional decline and to assess the progression of different signs of PD, 297 patients (181 males) with clinically diagnosed PD for at least 3 years were prospectively followed (Jankovic and Kapadia, 2001) (Fig. 4-2A and 4-2B). Data from 1731 visits over a period of an average of 6.36 years (range: 3 to 17) were analyzed. The annual rate of decline in the total UPDRS scores was 1.34 units when assessed during "on" and 1.58 when assessed during "off." Patients with older age at onset had a more rapid progression of disease than did those with younger age at onset. Furthermore, the older-onset group had significantly more progression in mentation, freezing, and parts I and II UPDRS subscores. Handwriting was the only component of UPDRS that did not significantly deteriorate during the observation period. Regression analysis of 108 patients, whose symptoms were rated during their "off" state, showed a faster rate of cognitive decline as the age at onset increased. The slopes of progression in UPDRS scores, when adjusted for age at initial visit, were steeper for the PIGD group of patients than in the tremor-dominant group. These findings, based on longitudinal follow-up data, provide evidence for a variable course of progression of the different PD symptoms, thus implying different biochemical or degenerative mechanisms for the various clinical features associated with PD. These results are similar to the 1.5-point annual decline, based on longitudinal assessments using the motor function (part III) portion of the UPDRS, reported by Louis and colleagues (1999) in a community-based study of 237 patients with PD who were followed up prospectively for a mean of 3.30 years.

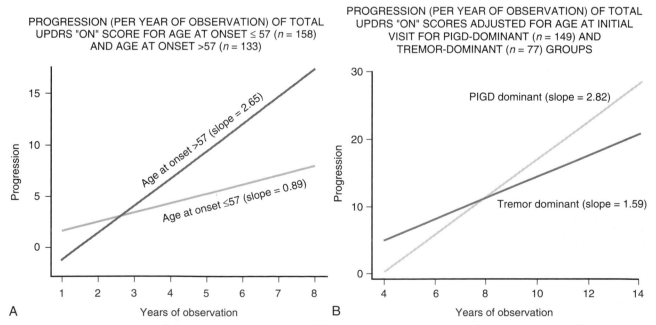

**Figure 4-2 A,** Younger patients have a slower progression of PD symptoms than those with later age at onset. **B,** Patients with postural instability and gait difficulty (PIGD) at onset of their disease progress more rapidly than those with the tremor-dominant form of PD. (See Color Plate 4.) (Reprinted with permission from Jankovic J, Kapadia AS: Functional decline in Parkinson's disease. Arch Neurol 2001;58:1611–1615.)

Another prospective study, involving 232 patients with PD, showed an annual decline in UPDRS motor score of 3.3 points (range 0–108; 3.1%) and 0.16 points in Hoehn-Yahr stage (range 0–5; 3.2%), with slower and more restricted decline in YOPD cases (Alves et al., 2005). The study by Greffard and colleagues (2006) has also suggested that the rate of progression might not be linear and that the disease might progress more rapidly initially (about 8–10 UPDRS points in the first year) and the rate of deterioration slows in more advanced stages of the disease. This is supported by the findings in moderately advanced cases of PD requiring levodopa treatment compared with patients in early stages of the disease such as those enrolled in the DATATOP study (Parkinson Study Group, 1998). In that study of early, previously untreated patients, the rate of annual decline in the total UPDRS score was 14.02 ± 12.32 (mean ± SD) in the placebo-treated group. This is nearly identical to the 1 UPDRS unit of decline per month in the ELLDOPA study (Fahn et al., 2004). In contrast, in a group of 238 patients treated with levodopa, bromocriptine, or both in whom progression was estimated on the basis of a retrospectively determined duration of the symptoms, the annual rate of decline in bradykinesia score was 3.5% during the first year but was estimated to be only 1.5% in the tenth year (Lee et al., 1994).

Interestingly, in a study of 787 older (mean age at baseline: 75.4 years) Catholic clergy without clinically diagnosed PD who were prospectively followed for up to 7 years, the average decline in UPDRS units was 0.69 per year (Wilson et al., 2002). In those subjects who had some worsening of their global UPDRS score (79% of all subjects), the risk of death was 2.93 times the rate in those without progression (21%). The risk of death was associated with worsening of gait and posture but not with rigidity or postural reflex impairment, even though the latter two signs (but not bradykinesia or tremor) also worsened. The average reported rate of decline in total UPDRS is about 8 units per year. A systematic review of 13 studies that investigated predictors of prognosis concluded that greater baseline impairment, early cognitive disturbance, older age, and lack of tremor at onset are relatively predictive of a poor prognosis (Marras et al., 2002). The aging process has been found to contribute particularly to the axial (gait and postural) impairment in PD (Levy et al., 2005).

The natural history of PD appears to be influenced not only by the age at onset and the clinical presentation but also by a number of other factors, such as stress (Tanner and Goldman, 1996), pregnancy (Shulman et al., 2000), intercurrent illness (Onofrj and Thomas, 2005), and therapy. Infection, gastrointestinal disorder, and surgery are among the most common causes of the syndrome of acute akinesia, a sudden deterioration in motor performance that usually last 4 to 26 days and represents a life-threatening complication of PD, usually requiring hospitalization (Onofrj and Thomas, 2005). Although therapeutic advances have had a positive impact on the quality of life, epidemiologic studies have not been able to demonstrate that levodopa significantly prolongs life (Clarke, 1995). Several studies, however, have concluded that PD patients have a nearly normal life expectancy (Lilienfeld et al., 1990; Clarke, 1995; Parkinson Study Group, 1998). In a prospective study of 800 patients who were followed longitudinally from the early stages of their disease for an average of 8.2 years, the overall death rate was 2.1% per year, which was similar to that of an age- and gender-matched U.S. population without PD (Parkinson Study Group, 1998). In a 10-year Sydney multicenter follow-up of 149 patients with PD initially enrolled in a double-blind study of levodopa-carbidopa versus bromocriptine, the standardized mortality ratio was 1.58, which was significantly higher than that of the Australian population ($P < .001$) (Hely et al., 1999). In a subsequent report, based on a population-based study, Morgante and colleagues (2000) showed a relative risk of death in patients with PD of 2.3 (95% confidence interval: 1.60 to 3.39). In another study of 170 elderly patients with PD, with a mean age at death of 82 years, who were followed for a median of 9.4 years, the relative risk of death compared to referent subjects was 1.60 (95% confidence interval: 1.30 to 1.8), and the mean duration of illness was 12.8 years (Fall et al., 2003). Pneumonia was the most frequent cause of death in both studies. The standardized mortality ratio was reported to be 1.52 in a community-based study of a Norwegian population (Herlofson et al., 2004). The hazard ratio for mortality was 1.64 for patients with PD compared to controls, but the mortality increased if there was associated dementia, depression, or both (Hughes et al., 2004). In a 15-year follow-up of patients who were originally enrolled in the Sydney Multicenter Study of PD comparing levodopa with low-dose bromocriptine, the standardized mortality ratio was 1.86. On the basis of 296 deaths in a cohort of patients who were originally enrolled in the DATATOP study and followed for 13 years, survival was found to be strongly related to response to levodopa (Marras et al., 2005).

Besides clinical rating, neuroimaging techniques have been used to assess progression of PD and other neurodegenerative disorders (Antonini and DeNotaris, 2004; Jankovic, 2005). Jennings and colleagues (2001) found, on the basis of sequential β-CIT [2β-carboxymethoxy-3β-(4[$^{123}$I]iodophenyl)tropane] and SPECT imaging at intervals ranging from 9 to 24 months, the annual rate of loss of striatal β-CIT uptake to be 7.1% in subjects having a diagnosis of PD for fewer than 2 years compared with a 3.7% rate in those having a diagnosis of PD for longer than 4.5 years. In another study using 6-[$^{18}$F]-fluoro-L-dopa (FDOPA) PET, Nurmi and colleagues (2001) showed a 10.3 ± 4.8% decline in the uptake in the putamen over a 5-year period. Using serial FDOPA PET in a prospective, longitudinal study of 31 patients with PD followed for more than 5 years (mean follow-up: 64.5 ± 22.6 months), Hilker and colleagues (2005) found an annual decline in striatal FDOPA ranging from 4.4% (caudate) to 6.3% (putamen), consistent with most other similar studies (Morrish et al., 1998). They concluded that "the neurodegenerative process in PD follows a negative exponential course," and in contrast to the long-latency hypothesis, they estimated that the preclinical disease period is relatively short: only about 6 years. Morrish and colleagues (1998), using a similar design, but with an interscan interval of only 18 months, came to the same conclusion. This is similar to the results of other longitudinal studies of PD progression, using imaging ligands either measuring dopamine metabolism (FDOPA PET) or targeting dopamine transporter (β-CIT SPECT), demonstrating an annualized rate of reduction in these striatal markers of about 4% to 13% in PD patients compared with a 0% to 2.5% change in healthy controls (Parkinson Study Group, 2002). In a PET follow-up brain graft study of patients with advanced PD,

Nakamura and colleagues (2001) found a 4.4% annual decline in the sham operated patients. Thus, longitudinal studies of PD progression, imaging ligands targeting dopamine metabolism ([$^{18}$F]-dopa) and dopamine transporter density (β-CIT) using PET and SPECT, respectively, have demonstrated an annualized rate of reduction in striatal [$^{18}$F]-dopa or [$^{123}$I]β-CIT uptake of about 6% to 13% in PD patients compared with a 0% to 2.5% change in healthy controls (Marek et al., 2001).

With improved methodology of β-CIT SPECT scans, the annualized rate of decline is now estimated to be 4% to 8% (Parkinson Study Group, 2002). These imaging studies are consistent with pathologic studies showing that the rate of nigral degeneration in PD patients is eightfold to tenfold higher than that of healthy age-matched controls. The several studies, including the one by Hilker and colleagues (2005), that suggest that the rate of progression of PD is not linear over time, being more rapid initially and slowing in more advanced stages of the disease, argue against the long-latency hypothesis for the presymptomatic period in PD (Jankovic, 2005). Finally, on the basis of clinical-pathologic correlation, Fearnley and Lees (1991) suggested that there is a 30% age-related nigral cell loss at disease onset, again indicating rapid decline in nigral dopaminergic cells in the early stages of the disease. Genetic studies have found that the age at onset of PD (and of Alzheimer disease) is strongly influenced by a gene on chromosome 10q (Li et al., 2002).

## DIFFERENTIAL DIAGNOSIS OF PARKINSON DISEASE

Causes of parkinsonism other than PD can be classified as secondary, multiple-system degeneration or the parkinsonism-plus syndromes and heredodegenerative disorders (Stacy and Jankovic, 1992) (Box 4-4). Features that are found to be particularly useful in differentiating PD from other parkinsonian disorders include absence or paucity of tremor, early gait abnormality (such as freezing), postural instability, pyramidal tract findings, and poor response to levodopa (Table 4-1). Although good response to levodopa is often used as an index of well-preserved postsynaptic receptors, supporting the diagnosis of PD, only 77% of pathologically proven cases had "good" or "excellent" initial levodopa response in the London series (Hughes et al., 1993). Furthermore, two patients with pathologically proven Lewy body parkinsonism but without response to levodopa have been reported (Mark et al., 1992). Therefore, while improvement with levodopa supports the diagnosis of PD, response to levodopa cannot be used to reliably differentiate PD from other parkinsonian disorders (Parati et al., 1993). Subcutaneous injection of apomorphine, a rapidly active dopamine agonist, has been used to predict response to levodopa and thus to differentiate between PD and other parkinsonian disorders (Hughes et al., 1990; D'Costa et al., 1991; Bonuccelli et al., 1993). Although PD patients are much more likely to improve with apomorphine, this test is cumbersome, and it does not reliably differentiate

---

**Box 4-4** Classification of parkinsonism

**I. Primary (Idiopathic) Parkinsonism**
- Parkinson disease
- Juvenile parkinsonism

**II. Multisystem Degenerations (Parkinsonism-Plus)**
- Progressive supranuclear palsy (PSP), Steele-Richardson-Olszewski disease (SRO)
- Multiple-system atrophy (MSA)
- Striatonigral degeneration (SND or MSA-P)
- Olivopontocerebellar atrophy (OPCA or MSA-C)
- Shy-Drager syndrome (SDS)
- Lytico-Bodig or parkinsonism-dementia-ALS complex of Guam (PDACG)
- Cortical-basal ganglionic degeneration (CBGD)
- Progressive pallidal atrophy
- Parkinsonism-dementia complex
- Pallidopyramidal disease

**III. Heredodegenerative Parkinsonism**
- Hereditary juvenile dystonia-parkinsonism
- Autosomal dominant Lewy body disease
- Huntington disease
- Wilson disease
- Hereditary ceruloplasmin deficiency
- Hallervorden-Spatz disease
- Olivopontocerebellar and spinocerebellar degenerations
- Machado-Joseph disease
- Familial amyotrophy-dementia-parkinsonism
- Disinhibition-dementia-parkinsonism-amyotrophy-complex

- Gerstmann-Strausler-Scheinker disease
- Familial progressive subcortical gliosis
- Lubag (X-linked dystonia-parkinsonism)
- Familial basal ganglia calcification
- Mitochondrial cytopathies with striatal necrosis
- Ceroid lipofuscinosis
- Familial parkinsonism with peripheral neuropathy
- Parkinsonian-pyramidal syndrome
- Neuroacanthocytosis
- Hereditary hemochromatosis

**IV. Secondary (Acquired, Symptomatic) Parkinsonism**
- Infectious: postencephalitic, AIDS, SSPE, Creuzfeldt-Jakob disease, prion diseases
- Drugs: dopamine receptor – blocking drugs (antipsychotic, antiemetic drugs), reserpine, tetrabenazine, alpha-methyl-dopa, lithium, flunarizine, cinnarizine
- Toxins: 1-methyl-4-phenyl-1,2,3,6-tetrahydropyridine, CO, Mn, Hg, $CS_2$, cyanide, methanol, ethanol
- Vascular: multi-infarct, Binswanger disease
- Trauma: pugilistic encephalopathy
- Other: parathyroid abnormalities, hypothyroidism, hepatocerebral degeneration, brain tumor, paraneoplastic, normal pressure hydrocephalus, noncommunicating hydrocephalus, syringomesencephalia, hemiatrophy-hemiparkinsonism, peripherally induced tremor and parkinsonism, and psychogenic

Reprinted with permission from Jankovic J, Lang AE: Classification of movement disorders. In Germano IM (ed): Surgical Treatment of Movement Disorders. Lebanon, NH, American Association of Neurological Surgeons, 1998, pp 3–18.

Table 4-1 Features suggestive of atypical parkinsonism

| Clinical Feature | Likely Cause of Parkinsonism |
| --- | --- |
| Poor or no response to levodopa | PSP, CBD, MSA |
| No dyskinesia despite high levodopa dose | PSP, CBD |
| Unilateral signs | HA-HP, CBD |
| No rest tremor | PSP, CBD, MSA |
| Unilateral rigidity (painful) | CBD |
| Unilateral myoclonus (cortical) | CBD |
| Asymmetric apraxia | CBD |
| Alien limb | CBD |
| Fluctuations in cognition | DLB |
| Early hallucinations, psychosis | DLB |
| Psychotic symptoms with levodopa | DLB |
| Extreme sensitivity to neuroleptics | DLB |
| Impaired downgaze | PSP |
| Deep facial folds | PSP |
| Palilalia | PSP |
| Early loss of postural reflexes and falls | PSP, MSA |
| Pure freezing | PSP |
| Stiff gait with knee-extended legs | PSP |
| Levodopa-induced facial dystonia | MSA |
| Anterocollis | MSA |
| Contractures | MSA, PSP |
| Laryngeal stridor | MSA (SND) |
| Ataxia | MSA (OPCA) |
| Dysautonomia | MSA |
| LMN and/or UMN signs | MSA |
| Excessive snoring, inspiratory sighs | MSA |

CBD, corticobasal degeneration; DLB, dementia with Lewy bodies; HA-HP, hemiatrophy-hemiparkinsonism; MSA, multiple system atrophy; OPCA, olivopontocerebellar atrophy; SND, striatonigral degeneration.

PD from the atypical parkinsonian disorders. Furthermore, response to the apomorphine test is not superior to chronic levodopa therapy in diagnosis of PD; therefore, this test adds little or nothing to the diagnostic evaluation (Clarke and Davies, 2000). The differences in response to dopaminergic drugs may be partly explained by differences in the density of postsynaptic dopamine receptors. These receptors are preserved in PD, in which the brunt of the pathology is in the SN, whereas they are usually decreased in other parkinsonian disorders in which the striatum is additionally affected.

Perhaps expression analysis of genes in brains of patients with various neurodegenerative and recognizing disease-specific patterns will in the future assist in differentiating PD from other parkinsonian disorders. For example, using microarray technology in SN samples from six patients with PD, two with PSP, one with FTDP, and five controls, Hauser and colleagues (2005) found 142 genes that were differentially expressed in PD cases and controls, 96 in the combination of PSP-FTDP, and 12 that were common to all three disorders. Further studies are needed to confirm this intriguing finding.

## LABORATORY TESTS

Although there is no blood or cerebrospinal fluid test that can diagnose PD, certain neuroimaging techniques may be helpful in differentiating PD from other parkinsonian disorders. MRI in patients with typical PD is usually normal, but a high-field-strength (1.5 T) heavily $T_2$-weighted MRI may show a wider area of lucency in the SN that is probably indicative of increased accumulation of iron (Olanow, 1992). In using this technique, prominent hypointensity in the putamen that exceeds that normally found in the globus pallidus strongly indicates the presence of atypical parkinsonism, particularly MSA. By using [18F]-fluorodopa PET scans to assess the integrity of the striatal dopaminergic terminals, characteristic reduction of the [18F]-fluorodopa uptake, particularly in the putamen, can be demonstrated in virtually all patients with PD, even in the early stages (Brooks, 1991). Using [11C]-raclopride to image dopamine D2 receptors, Brooks and colleagues (1992a) showed that in patients with untreated PD, the striatal D2 receptors are well preserved, whereas patients with atypical parkinsonism have a decrease in the density of dopamine receptors. Involvement of the postsynaptic, striatal dopamine receptor–containing neurons in the atypical parkinsonian syndromes is also suggested by decreased binding of iodobenzamide, a dopamine receptor ligand, as demonstrated by SPECT scans (Schwarz et al., 1992). In addition to reduced density of the dopamine receptors, patients with atypical parkinsonism have decreased striatal metabolism, as demonstrated by PET scans (Eidelberg et al., 1993). Besides imaging of postsynaptic D2 receptors, SPECT imaging of the striatal dopamine reuptake sites with I-123 labeled β-CIT and of presynaptic vesicles with [11C]-dihydrotetrabenazine may also be helpful in differentiating PD from atypical parkinsonism (Gilman et al., 1996; Marek et al., 1996; Booij et al., 1997). Although the imaging tests cannot yet be used to reliably differentiate PD from other parkinsonian disorders, future advances in this technology will undoubtedly improve their diagnostic potential.

Brain parenchyma sonography has been used in one study to differentiate PD from atypical parkinsonism, mostly MSA (Walter et al., 2003). The investigators found that 24 of 25 (96%) patients with PD exhibited hyperechogenicity, whereas only 2 of 23 (9%) patients with atypical parkinsonism showed a similar pattern. They concluded that brain parenchyma sonography may be highly specific in differentiating between PD and atypical parkinsonism.

## PRESYMPTOMATIC DIAGNOSIS

One of the most important challenges in PD research is to identify individuals who are at risk for PD and to diagnose the disease even before the initial appearance of symptoms. Searching for sensitive biomarkers, such as clinical, motor, physiologic, and olfactory testing, cerebrospinal fluid proteomics, genetic testing, and neuroimaging, that detect evidence of PD even before clinical symptoms first appear, has been the primary focus in many research centers around the world (Michell et al., 2004). As was noted previously, impaired olfaction is one of the earliest signs of PD, present even before the onset of motor symptoms.

Many studies provide evidence suggesting that the latency between the onset of neuronal degeneration (or onset of the disease process) and clinical symptoms might not be as long as was initially postulated (Morrish, 1996). On the basis of a study of 36 control and 20 PD brains, Fearnley and Lees (1991) suggested that the presymptomatic phase of PD from the onset of neuronal loss to the onset of symptoms might be only 5 years, thus arguing against aging as an important cause of PD. With advancing age, there is 4.7% per decade rate of loss of pigmented neurons from the SNpc, whereas in PD, there is 45% loss in the first decade. Since the rate of progression is so highly variable, it is perhaps not surprising that the estimates of the presymptomatic period vary between 40 years and 3.1 years, depending on the method used (Morrish et al., 1996). The shorter presymptomatic period has been suggested by longitudinal [18]F-dopa PET studies (Morrish et al., 1996). Although UPDRS has been used in these longitudinal studies as a measure of clinical progression, the instrument is currently being revised to include additional items, including nonmotor experiences of daily living, to capture symptoms that reflect nondopaminergic involvement in PD. Whether the progression as measured with the current or revised UPDRS correlates with nigral and extranigral pathology associated with PD awaits future clinical-pathologic validation.

One of the benefits of longitudinal imaging studies, such as the one by Hilker and colleagues (2005; see also Jankovic, 2005), is that they can be used to estimate duration of the presymptomatic period. Assuming that the threshold at which symptoms are first manifested is at 69% of the normal putaminal FDOPA uptake, Hilker and colleagues (2005) concluded that the preclinical disease period must be relatively short: only about 6 years. This is consistent with other imaging and with autopsy data (Fearnley and Lees, 1991). The 31% loss of striatal dopaminergic terminals needed before onset of symptoms, demonstrated by Hilker and colleagues (2005), is substantially lower than the 60% to 80% loss of dopaminergic neurons in the SN that is traditionally cited as being required before symptoms of PD first become evident. The difference may be explained by compensatory changes in response to presynaptic dopaminergic loss, such as enhanced synthesis of dopamine in surviving dopaminergic neurons, upregulation of striatal dopa-decarboxylase activity, and increased dopaminergic innervation of the striatum (Jankovic, 2005). Furthermore, there may be functional compensatory changes, as is suggested by the finding of increased FDOPA uptake in the globus pallidus internus, in early PD. This enhanced function of the nigropallidal dopaminergic projection maintains a more normal pattern of pallidal output in early stages of the disease, but these compensatory mechanisms eventually fail, and the disease starts to progress. Thus, because of the compensatory changes, FDOPA PET more accurately reflects dopaminergic function at the striatal terminal than a cell loss in the SN. These compensatory mechanisms may also explain why despite age-related loss of nigral neurons, there is little or no change in FDOPA uptake with normal aging (Sawle et al., 1990) and why up to 15% of patients with signs of PD, as determined by experienced parkinsonologists, have normal FDOPA or β-CIT scans without evidence of dopaminergic deficit (SWEDD) (Table 4-2) (Marek et al., 2003; Whone et al., 2003; Clarke, 2004; Fahn et al., 2004; Jankovic, 2005). These scans without evidence of dopaminergic deficit might represent patients with PD and compensatory striatal changes or with other parkinsonian disorders. They might also represent false-negative results and therefore highlight the relative lack of sensitivity of these functional neuroimaging studies as potential biomarkers for detection of PD, particularly at early stages of the disease (Michell et al., 2004). But since individuals with SWEDDs fail to develop dopaminergic deficit and fail

**Table 4-2** Scans without evidence of dopaminergic deficit (SWEDD)

| Study | Imaging | FU (mos) | SWEDDs | Reference |
|---|---|---|---|---|
| REAL-PET | FDOPA | 24 | 21/186 (11.3%) | Whone et al., 2003 |
| CALM-PD | β-CIT SPECT | 22 | 3/82 (3.6%) | Marek et al., 2003 |
| ELLDOPA | β-CIT SPECT | 9 | 21/142 (14.8%) | Marek et al., 2003 |

to show clinical worsening, it is likely that these individuals were incorrectly diagnosed. A critical review of the role of radiotracer imaging in PD concluded that "current evidence does not support the use of imaging as a diagnostic tool in clinical practice or as a surrogate endpoint in clinical trials" (Ravina et al., 2005).

In addition to the plasticity of the dopaminergic system, the presymptomatic compensation might also involve nondopaminergic mechanisms (Fig. 4-3) (Jankovic, 2005). While the emphasis in PD research has been on dopaminergic deficiency underlying motor dysfunction, there is a growing body of evidence that the caudal brainstem nuclei (e.g., dorsal motor nucleus of the glossopharyngeal and vagal nerves), anterior olfactory nucleus, and other nondopaminergic neurons might be affected long before the classic loss of dopaminergic neurons in the SN, based on accumulation of Lewy neurites detected by staining for α-synuclein (Braak et al., 2003, 2004). According to the Braak staging, during presymptomatic stage 1, the Lewy neurite pathology remains confined to the medulla oblongata and olfactory bulb. In Stage 2, it has spread to involve the pons. In stages 3 and 4, the SN and other nuclear grays of the midbrain and basal forebrain are the focus of initially subtle and then more pronounced changes, at which time the illness reaches its symptomatic phase. In end stages 5 and 6, the pathologic process encroaches on the telencephalic cortex. This staging proposal, however, has been challenged, as there is have been no cell counts to correlate with the described synuclein pathology, and there was no observed asymmetry in the pathologic findings that would correlate with the well-recognized asymmetry of clinical findings. In addition, there is controversy as to the classification of dementia with Lewy bodies; Braak viewed it as part of stage 6, but others suggest that it is a separate entity, since these patients often have behavioral and psychiatric problems before the onset of motor or other signs of PD.

To the extent that future protective therapies may prevent or even halt the neurodegenerative process, it is essential that they be implemented early in the course of the disease. Therefore, recent clinical and basic studies have focused on a search for presymptomatic biomarkers of PD (Michell et al., 2004). An identification of a disease-specific diagnostic test would be immensely helpful not only in defining the various PD subtypes and in differentiating PD from atypical parkinsonian syndromes but also, more important, in identifying populations that are at increased risk for developing PD. Such potentially vulnerable populations could then be targeted for protective therapy.

Novel imaging techniques are being developed not only to monitor the progression of the disease but also as diagnostic tools in clinically uncertain cases. Using the dopamine trans-

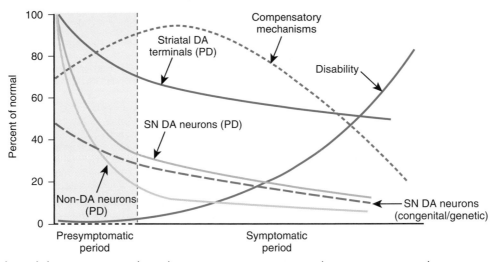

**Figure 4-3** Hypothetical dopaminergic and nondopaminergic progression and compensatory mechanisms postulated for PD and other presynaptic (congenital or genetic) parkinsonian disorders. (Reprinted with permission from Jankovic J: Progression of Parkinson's disease: Are we making progress in charting the course? Arch Neurol 2005;62:351–352.)

porter ligand, [I-123] (N)-(3-iodopropene-2-yl)-2beta-carbomethoxy-3beta-(4-chlorophenyl) tropane (IPT), and SPECT, Schwarz and colleagues (2000) showed a reduction of dopamine transporter binding in patients with early PD, suggesting that this technique has a potential in detection of preclinical disease. Comparing inversion recovery MRI and $^{18}$F-dopa PET in 10 patients with H and Y stage III and IV PD and 8 normal controls, Hu and colleagues (2001) found that discriminant function analysis of the quantified MRI nigral signal correctly classified the combined PD patient/control group, but three patients with PD were incorrectly classified as "normal," whereas with PET, 100% of PD patients and controls were correctly classified. In a study of 118 patients with clinically uncertain parkinsonian syndromes, all patients with presynaptic parkinsonism had abnormal $^{123}$I-Ioflupane SPECT (DaTSCAN, Amersham Health), whereas 94% with "nonpresynaptic" parkinsonism had a normal scan (Catafau et al., 2004).

## AUTOPSY DIAGNOSIS

In the absence of a specific biologic marker or a diagnostic test, the diagnosis of PD can be made with certainty only at autopsy. PD is pathologically defined as a neurodegenerative disorder characterized chiefly by (1) depigmentation of the SN associated with degeneration of melanin- and dopamine-containing neurons, particularly in the zona compacta of SN and in the norepinephrine-containing neurons in the locus coeruleus, and (2) the presence of Lewy bodies (eosinophilic cytoplasmic inclusions) in the SN zona compacta and other brain regions, including the locus coeruleus and some cortical areas (Zarow et al., 2003) (Box 4-5). In fact, some studies have found that, despite the universally accepted notion that SN is the site of the brunt of the pathology in PD, neuronal loss in the locus coeruleus is more severe (Zarow et al., 2003). These criteria are open to question, however, since typical cases of levodopa-responsive parkinsonism have been reported with-

out Lewy bodies and with or without neurofibrillary tangles in the SN (Rajput et al., 1991). In contrast, the pathologically typical form of Lewy body parkinsonism has been described with atypical clinical features such as poor response to levodopa (Mark et al., 1992). Both the Canadian (Rajput et al., 1991) and the London Parkinson's Disease Society Brain Bank study (Hughes, Daniel, et al., 1992) showed that 24% of patients in each series had a pathologic diagnosis other than PD. Furthermore, in patients with pathologically documented PD, other disorders may be present that can cloud the clinical picture. For example, in 100 cases of pathologically proven PD, Hughes and colleagues (1993) found 34 with coexistent pathology in the striatum and 28 outside the nigrostriatal system; vascular changes involving the striatum were found in 24 patients, Alzheimer changes in 20 (3 had striatal plaques confined to the striatum), and diffuse Lewy body disease or dementia with Lewy bodies in 4. As was noted previously, in a subsequent study, the diagnostic accuracy had improved markedly (Hughes et al., 2002). Until parkinsonian disorders can be differentiated by either disease-specific biologic or etiologic markers, neuroimaging, or other laboratory tests, the

**Box 4-5** Proposed criteria for histopathologic confirmation of Parkinson disease

1. Substantial nerve cell depletion with accompanying gliosis in SN
2. At least one Lewy body in the SN or in the LC

(Note: it may be necessary to examine up to four nonoverlapping sections in each of these areas)

3. No pathologic evidence for other diseases that produce parkinsonism

Reprinted with permission from Gelb DJ, Oliver E, Gilman S: Diagnostic criteria for Parkinson's disease. Arch Neurol 1999;56:33–39.

separation of the different parkinsonian disorders still depends largely on clinical-pathologic correlations.

## References

Aarsland D, Andersen K, Larsen JP, et al Risk of dementia in Parkinson's disease. A community–based, prospective study. Neurology 2001;56:730–736.

Aarsland D, Andersen K, Larsen JP, et al: Prevalence and characteristics of dementia in Parkinson disease: An 8-year prospective study. Arch Neurol 2003;60:387–392.

Aarsland D, Andersen K, Larsen JP, et al: The rate of cognitive decline in Parkinson disease. Arch Neurol 2004;61:1906–1911.

Aarsland D, Larsen JP, Lim NG, et al: Range of neuropsychiatric disturbances in patients with Parkinson's disease. J Neurol Neurosurg Psychiatry 1999;67:492–496.

Aarsland D, Larsen JP, Tandberg E, Laake K: Predictors of nursing home placement in Parkinson's disease: A population-based, prospective study. J Am Geriatr Soc 2000;48:1–5.

Abbott RD, Petrovich H, White LR, et al: Frequency of bowel movements and the future risk of Parkinson's disease. Neurology 2001;57:456–462.

Adler CH, Thorpy MJ: Sleep issues in Parkinson's disease. Neurology 2005; 64(suppl 3):S12–S20.

Albin RL, Koeppe RA, Chervin RD, et al: Decreased striatal dopaminergic innervation in REM sleep behavior disorder. Neurology 2000;55:1410–1412.

Alegret M, Junque C, Valldeoriola F, et al: Obsessive-compulsive symptoms in Parkinson's disease. J Neurol Neurosurg Psychiatry 2001;70:394–396.

Allcock LM, Ullyart K, Kenny RA, Burn DJ: Frequency of orthostatic hypotension in a community based cohort of patients with Parkinson's disease. J Neurol Neurosurg Psychiatry 2004;75: 1470–1471.

Alves G, Wentzel-Larsen T, Aarsland D, Larsen JP: Progression of motor impairment and disability in Parkinson disease: A population-based study. Neurology 2005;65:1436–1441.

Antonini A, DeNotaris R: PET and SPECT functional imaging in Parkinson's disease. Sleep Med 2004;5:201–206.

Antonini A, Moeller JR, Nakamura T, et al: The metabolic anatomy of tremor in Parkinson's disease. Neurology 1998;51: 803–810.

Araki I, Kuno S: Assessment of voiding dysfunction in Parkinson's disease by the international prostate symptom score. J Neurol Neurosurg Psychiatry 2000;68:429–433.

Arnulf I, Bonnet A-M, Damier P, et al: Hallucinations, REM sleep, and Parkinson's disease: A medical hypothesis. Neurology 2000; 55:281–288.

Arnulf I, Konofal E, Merino-Andreu M, et al: Parkinson's disease and sleepiness: An integral part of PD. Neurology 2002;58: 1019–1024.

Arvanitakis Z, Wilson RS, Schneider JA, et al: Diabetes mellitus and progression of rigidity and gait disturbance in older persons. Neurology 2004;63:996–1001.

Ashour R, Tintner R, Jankovic J: "Striatal" hand and foot deformities in Parkinson's disease. Lancet Neurol 2005; 4:423–431.

Ashour R, Jankovic J: Joint and skeletal deformities in Parkinson's disease, multiple system atrophy, and progressive supranuclear palsy. Mov Disord 2006;21(11):1856–1863.

Ashraf W, Pfeiffer RF, Park F, et al: Constipation in Parkinson's disease: Objective assessment and response to psyllium. Mov Disord 1997;12:946–951.

Askmark H, Edebol Eeg-Olofsson K, Johnsson A, et al: Parkinsonism and neck extensor myopathy. A new syndrome or coincidental findings. Arch Neurol 2001;58:232–237.

Azher SN, Jankovic J: Camptocormia: Pathogenesis, classification, and response to therapy. Neurology 2005;65:353–359.

Bagheri H, Damase-Michel C, Lapeyre-Mestre M, et al. A study of salivary secretion in Parkinson's disease. Clin Neuropharm 1999;22:213–215.

Barnes J, David AS: Visual hallucinations in Parkinson's disease: A review and phenomenological survey. J Neurol Neurosurg Psychiatry 2001;70:727–733.

Barrett AM, Crucian GP, Schwartz R, et al: Seeing trees but not the forest: Limited perception of large configurations in PD. Neurology 2001;56:724–729.

Bartels AL, Balash Y, Gurevich T, et al: Relationship between freezing of gait (FOG) and other features of Parkinson's: FOG is not correlated with bradykinesia J Clin Neurosci 2003;10:584–588.

Bassotti G, Maggio D, Battaglia E, et al: Manometric investigation of anorectal function in early and late stage Parkinson's disease. J Neurol Neurosurg Psychiatry 2000;68:768–770.

Bennett DA, Shannon KM, Beckett LA, et al: Metric properties of nurses' ratings of parkinsonian signs with a modified Unified Parkinson's Disease Rating Scale. Neurology 1997;49:1580–1587.

Berardelli A, Rothwell JC, Thompson PD, Hallett M: Pathophysiology of bradykinesia in Parkinson's disease. Brain 2001;124:2131–2146.

Berendse HW, Booij J, Francot CM, et al: Subclinical dopaminergic dysfunction in asymptomatic Parkinson's disease patients' relatives with a decreased sense of smell. Ann Neurol 2002;50:34–41.

Bergman H, Wichmann T, DeLong MR: Reversal of experimental parkinsonism by lesions of the subthalamic nucleus. Science 1990;249:1436–1438.

Biousse V, Skibell BC, Watts RL, et al: Ophthalmologic features of Parkinson's disease. Neurology 2004;62:177–180.

Birkmayer W, Hornykiewicz O: The effect of L-3,4-dihydroxyphenyl-alanine (DOPA) on akinesia in parkinsonism. Wien Klin Wochenschr 1961;73:787–788. Translated into English in Parkinsonism Relat Disord 1998;4:59–60.

Bodis-Wollner I: Visualizing the next steps in Parkinson disease. Arch Neurol. 2002;59:1233–1234.

Boghen D: Apraxia of lid opening: A review. Neurology 1997;48: 1481–1503.

Bonuccelli U, Lucetti C, Del Dott D, et al: Orthostatic hypotension in de novo Parkinson disease. Arch Neurol 2003;60:1400–1404.

Bonuccelli U, Piccini P, Del Dotto P, et al: Apomorphine test for dopaminergic responsiveness: A dose assessment study. Mov Disord 1993;8:158–164.

Booij J, Tissingh G, Boer GJ, et al: [123I]FP-CIT SPECT shows a pronounced decline of striatal dopamine transporter labeling in early and advanced Parkinson's disease. J Neurol Neurosurg Psychiatry 1997;62:133–140.

Bozi M, Bhatia KP: Paroxysmal exercise-induced dystonia as a presenting feature of young-onset Parkinson's disease. Mov Disord 2003;18:1545–1547.

Braak H, Del Tredici K, Rub U, et al: Staging of brain pathology related to sporadic Parkinson's disease. Neurobiol Aging 2003;24:197–211.

Braak H, Ghebremedhin E, Rub U, et al: Stages in the development of Parkinson's disease-related pathology. Cell Tissue Res 2004;318: 121–134.

Brodsky H, Dat Vuong K, Thomas M, Jankovic J: Glabellar and palmomental reflexes in parkinsonian disorders. Neurology 2004;63:1096–1098.

Brooks DJ: PET: Its clinical role in neurology. J Neurol Neurosurg Psychiatry 1991;54:1–4.

Brooks DJ, Ibanez V, Sawle GV, et al: Striatal D2 receptor status in patients with Parkinson's disease, striatonigral degeneration, and progressive supranuclear palsy, measured with 11C-Raclopride and positron emission tomography. Ann Neurol 1992a;31:184–192.

Brooks DJ, Playford ED, Ibanez V, et al: Isolated tremor and disruption of the nigrostriatal dopaminergic system: An 18F-dopa PET study. Neurology 1992b;42:1554–1560.

Brown P: Muscle sounds in Parkinson's disease. Lancet 1997;349: 533–535.

Brown RG, Dittner A, Findley L, Wessely SC: The Parkinson fatigue scale. Parkinsonism Relat Disord 2005;11:49–55.

Bulpitt CJ, Shaw K, Clifton P, et al: The symptoms of patients treated for Parkinson's disease. Clin Neuropharmacol 1985;8:175–183.

Camicioli R, Grossmann SJ, Spencer PS, et al: Discriminating mild parkinsonism: Methods for epidemiological research. Mov Disord 2001;16:33–40.

Catafau AM, Tolosa E: Impact of dopamine transporter SPECT using (123)I-Ioflupane on diagnosis and management of patients with clinically uncertain parkinsonian syndromes. Mov Disord 2004;19:1175–1182.

Chaudhuri A, Behan PO: Fatigue in neurological disorders. Lancet 2004;363:978–988.

Chaudhuri KR, Healy DG, Schapira AH, et al: Non-motor symptoms of Parkinson's disease: Diagnosis and management. Lancet Neurol 2006;5:235–245.

Chaudhuri KR, Pal S, DiMarco A, et al: The Parkinson's disease sleep scale: A new instrument for assessing sleep and nocturnal disability in Parkinson's disease. J Neurol Neurosurg Psychiatry 2002;73 (6):629–635.

Chen H, Zhang SM, Hernan MA, et al: Weight loss in Parkinson's disease. Ann Neurol 2003;53:676–679.

Clarke CE: Does levodopa therapy delay death in Parkinson's disease? A review of the evidence. Mov Disord 1995;10:250–256.

Clarke CE: A "cure" for Parkinson's disease: Can neuroprotection be proven with current trial designs? Mov Disord 2004;19:491–498.

Clarke CE, Davies P: Systematic review of acute levodopa and apomorphine challenge tests in the diagnosis of idiopathic Parkinson's disease. J Neurol Neurosurg Psychiatry 2000;69:590–594.

Colosimo C, Hughes AJ, Kilford L, Lees AJ: Lewy body cortical involvement may not always predict dementia in Parkinson's disease. J Neurol Neurosurg Psychiatry 2003;74:852–856.

Comella CL, Goetz CG: Akathisia in Parkinson's disease. Mov Disord 1994;9:545–549.

Comella CL, Nardine TM, Diederich NJ, Stebbins G: Sleep-related violence, injury, and REM sleep behavior disorder in Parkinson's disease. Neurology 1998;51:526–529.

Cooper JA, Sagar HJ, Tidswell P, et al: Slowed central processing in simple and go/no-go reaction time tasks in Parkinson's disease. Brain 1994;117:517–530.

Cotzias GC, Papavasiliou PS, Gellene R: Modification of parkinsonism—chronic treatment with L-dopa. N Engl J Med 1969;280: 337–345.

Cotzias GC, Van Woert MH, Schiffer LM: Aromatic amino acids and modification of parkinsonism. N Engl J Med 1967;276:374–379.

D'Costa DF, Abbott RJ, Pye IF, Millac PAH: The apomorphine test in parkinsonian syndromes. J Neurol Neurosurg Psychiatry 1991;54:870–872.

DeBoer AGEM, Wijker W, Speelman JD, Dehaes JCJM. Quality of life in patients with Parkinson's disease: Development of a questionnaire. J Neurol Neurosurg Psychiatry 1996;61:70–74.

de Lau LM, Koudstaal PJ, Hofman A, Breteler MM: Subjective complaints precede Parkinson disease: The Rotterdam study. Arch Neurol 2006;63:362–365.

de Rijk MC, Rocca WA, Anderson DW: A population perspective on diagnostic criteria for Parkinson's disease. Neurology 1997;48: 1277–1281.

De Swart BJ, Willemse SC, Maassen BA, Horstink MW: Improvement of voicing in patients with Parkinson's disease by speech therapy. Neurology 2003;60:498–500.

Dick JPR, Rothwell JC, Day BL, et al: The Bereitschaftpotential is abnormal in Parkinson's disease. Brain 1989;112:233–244.

Diederich NJ, Moore CG, Leurgans SE, et al: Parkinson disease with old-age onset: A comparative study with subjects with middle-age onset. Arch Neurol 2003;60:529–533.

Diederich NJ, Raman R, Leurgans S, Goetz CG: Progressive worsening of spatial and chromatic processing deficits in Parkinson disease. Arch Neurol 2002;59:1249–1252.

Dietz MA.Goetz CG, Stebbins GT: Evaluation of a modified inverted walking stick as a treatment for parkinsonian freezing episodes. Mov Disord 1990;5:243–247.

Djaldetti R, Mosberg-Galili R, Sroka H, et al: Camptocormia (bent spine) in patients with Parkinson's disease: Characterization and possible pathogenesis of an unusual phenomenon. Mov Disord 1999;14:443–447.

Djaldetti R, Shifrin A, Rogowski Z, et al: Quantitative measurement of pain sensation in patients with Parkinson disease. Neurology 2004;62:2171–2175.

Dodd ML, Klos KJ, Bower JH, et al: Pathological gambling caused by drugs used to treat Parkinson disease. Arch Neurol 2005;62: 1377–1381.

Doder M, Rabiner EA, Turjanski N, et al: Tremor in Parkinson's disease and serotonergic dysfunction: An $^{11}$C-WAY 100635 PET study. Neurology 2003;60:601–605.

Dostrovsky JO, Hutchinson WD, Lozano AM: The globus pallidus, deep brain stimulation and Parkinson's disease. Neuroscientist 2002;8:284–290.

Double KL, Rowe DB, Hayes M, et al: Identifying the pattern of olfactory deficits in Parkinson disease using the brief smell identification test. Arch Neurol 2003;60:545–549.

Driver-Dunckley E, Samanta J, Stacy M: Pathological gambling associated with dopamine agonist therapy in Parkinson's disease. Neurology 2003;61:422–423.

Dubois B, Slachevsky A, Litvan I, Pillon B: The FAB: A frontal assessment battery at bedside. Neurology 2000;55:1621–1626.

Dujardin K, Defbvre L, Grunberg C, et al: Memory and executive functionin sporadic and familial Parkinson's disease. Brain 2001;124:389–398.

Ehringer H, Hornykiewicz O: Distribution of noreadrenaline and dopamine (3 hydroxytyramine) in the human brain and their behavior in disease of the extrapyramidal system. Wien Klin Wochenschrift 1960;24:1236–1239. Translated into English in Parkinsonism Relat Disord 1998;4:53–57.

Eidelberg D, Takikawa S, Moeller JR, et al: Striatal hypometabolism distinguishes striatonigral degeneration from Parkinson's disease. Ann Neurol 1993;33:518–527.

Eisensehr I, Linke R, Noachtar S, et al: Reduced striatal dopamine transporters in idiopathic rapid eye movement sleep behaviour disorder: Comparison with Parkinson's disease and controls. Brain 2000;123:1155–1160.

Elbaz A, Bower JH, Peterson BJ, et al: Survival study of Parkinson disease in Olmsted County, Minnesota. Arch Neurol 2003;60: 91–96.

Elble RJ, Cousins R, Leffler K, Hughes L: Gait initiation by patients with lower-half parkinsonism. Brain 1996;119:1705–1716.

Emre M: What causes mental dysfunction in Parkinson's disease? Mov Disord. 2003;18(suppl 6):S63–S71.

Emre M: Dementia in Parkinson's disease: Cause and treatment. Curr Opin Neurol 2004;17:399–404.

Escola L, Michelet T, Douillard G, et al: Disruption of the proprioceptive mapping in the medial wall of parkinsonian monkeys. Ann Neurol 2002;52:581–587.

Evans AH, Katzenschlager R, Paviour D, et al: Punding in Parkinson's disease: Its relation to the dopamine dysregulation syndrome. Mov Disord 2004;19:397–405.

Evans AH, Lees AJ: Dopamine dysregulation syndrome in Parkinson's disease. Curr Opin Neurol 2004;17:393–398.

Evarts EV, Teravainen M, Calne DB: Reaction time in Parkinson's disease. Brain 1981;104:167–186.

Factor SA, Feustel PJ, Friedman JH, et al: Longitudinal outcome of Parkinson's disease patients with psychosis. Neurology 2003;60: 1756–1761.

Fahn S. The freezing phenomenon in parkinsonism. Adv Neurol 1995;67:53-63.

Fahn S, Elton RL, Members of the UPDRS Development Committee: The Unified Parkinson's Disease Rating Scale. In Fahn S, Marsden CD, Calne DB, Goldstein M (eds): Recent Developments in

Parkinson's Disease, vol 2. Florham Park, NJ, Macmillan Healthcare Information, 1987, pp 153–163, 293–304.

Fahn S, Oakes D, Shoulson I, et al: Levodopa and the progression of Parkinson's disease. N Engl J Med 2004;351:2498–2508.

Fall PA, Saleh A, Fredrickson M, et al: Survival time, mortality, and cause of death in elderly patients with Parkinson's disease: A 9-year follow-up. Mov Disord 2003;18:1312–1316.

Fearnley JM, Lees AJ: Ageing and Parkinson's disease: Substantia nigra regional selectivity. Brain 1991;114:2283–2301.

Fénelon G, Mahieux F, Huon R, Ziégler M: Hallucinations in Parkinson's disease: Prevalence, phenomenology and risk factors. Brain 2000;123:733–745.

Fénelon G, Goetz CG, Karenberg A: Hallucinations in Parkinson disease in the prelevodopa era. Neurology 2006;66:93–98.

Ferini-Strambi L, Zucconi M: REM sleep behavior disorder. Clin Neurophysiol 2000;111(suppl 2):S136–S140.

FitzGerald PM, Jankovic J: Lower body parkinsonism: Evidence for vascular etiology. Mov Disord 1989;4:249–260.

Ford B, Louis ED, Greene P, Fahn S: Oral and genital pain syndromes in Parkinson's disease. Mov Disord 1996;11:421–426.

Gagnon J, Bedard M, Fantini ML, et al: REM sleep behavior disorder and REM sleep without atonia in Parkinson's disease. Neurology 2002;59:585–589.

Garber CE, Friedman JH: Effects of fatigue on physical activity and function in patients with Parkinson's disease. Neurology 2003;60:1119–1124.

Gelb DJ, Oliver E, Gilman S: Diagnostic criteria for Parkinson's disease. Arch Neurol 1999;56:33–39.

Geschwandtner U, Aston J, Renaud S, Fuhr P: Pathologic gambling in patients with Parkinson's disease. Clin Neuropharmacol 2001;24:170–172.

Ghilardi MF, Eidelberg D, Silvestri G, Ghez C: The differential effect of PD and normal aging on early explicit sequence learning. Neurology 2003;60:1313–1319.

Giladi N, Kao R, Fahn S: Freezing phenomenon in patients with parkinsonian syndromes. Mov Disord 1997;12:302–305.

Giladi N, McDermott MP, Fahn S, et al: Freezing of gait in PD: Prospective assessment of the DATATOP cohort. Neurology 2001;56:1712–1721.

Gilman S, Frey KA, Koeppe RA, et al: Decreased striatal monoaminergic terminals in olivopontocerebellar atrophy and multiple system atrophy demonstrated with positron emission tomography. Ann Neurol 1996;40:885–892.

Giovannoni G, O'Sullivan JD, Turner K, et al: Hedonistic homeostatic dysregulation in patients with Parkinson's disease on dopamine replacement therapies. J Neurol Neurosurg Psychiatry 2000;68:423–428.

Giovannoni G, Van Schalkwyk J, Fritz VU, Lees A: Bradykinesia akinesia incoordination test (BRAIN TEST): An objective computerised assessment of upper limb motor function. J Neurol Neurosurg Psychiatry 1999;67:624–629.

Goetz CG, Leurgans S, Pappert EJ, et al: Prospective longitudinal assessment of hallucinations in Parkinson's disease. Neurology 2001;57:2078–2082.

Goetz CG, Poewe W, Rascol O, et al: Movement Disorder Society Task Force report on the Hoehn and Yahr staging scale: Status and recommendations: The Movement Disorder Society Task Force on rating scales for Parkinson's disease. Mov Disord 2004;19:1020–1028.

Goetz CG, Stebbins GT, Chmura TA, et al: Teaching tape for the motor section of the Unified Parkinson's Disease Rating Scale. Mov Disord 1995;10:263–266.

Goetz CG, Stebbins GT, Shale HM, et al: Utility of an objective dyskinesia rating scale for Parkinson's disease: inter- and intrarater reliability assessment. Mov Disord 1994;9:390–394.

Goetz CG, Wuu J, Curgian LM, Leurgans S: Hallucinations and sleep disorders in PD: Six-year prospective longitudinal study. Neurology 2005;64:81–86.

Goldstein DS, Holmes CS, Dendi R, et al: Orthostatic hypotension from sympathetic denervation in Parkinson's disease. Neurology 2002;58:1247–1255.

Gonera EG, van't Hof M, Berger HJC, et al: Symptoms and duration of the prodromal phase in Parkinson's disease. Mov Disord 1997;12:871–876.

Gorell JM, Johnson CC, Rybicki BA: Parkinson's disease and its comorbid disorders: An analysis of Michigan mortality data, 1970 to 1990. Neurology 1994;44:1865–1868.

Gourie-Devi M, Nalini A, Sandhya S: Early or late appearance of "dropped head syndrome" in amyotrophic lateral sclerosis. J Neurol Neurosurg Psychiatry 2003;74:683–686.

Graham JM, Sagar HJ: A data-driven approach to the sudy of heterogeneity in idiopathic Parkinson's disease: Identification of three distinct subtypes. Mov Disord 1999;14:10–20.

Grandas F, Iranzo A: Nocturnal problems occurring in Parkinson's disease. Neurology 2004;63(8, suppl 3):S8–S11.

Greffard S, Verny M, Bonnet AM, et al: Motor score of the Unified Parkinson Disease Rating Scale as a good predictor of Lewy body–associated neuronal loss in the substantia nigra. Arch Neurol 2006;63:584–588.

Guttman M, Slaughter PM, Theriault ME, et al: Parkinsonism in Ontario: Comorbidity associated with hospitalization in a large cohort. Mov Disord 2004;19:49–53.

Haapaniemi TH, Sotaniemi KA, Sintonen H, Taimela E: The generic 15D instrument is valid and feasible for measuring health related quality of life in Parkinson's disease. J Neurol Neurosurg Psychiatry 2004;75:976–983.

Hallett M. Khoshbin S: A physiological mechanism of bradykinesia. Brain 1980;103:30l–314.

Harding AJ, Stimson E, Henderson JM, Halliday GM: Clinical correlates of selective pathology in the amygdala of patients with Parkinson's disease. Brain 2002;125(11):2431–2445.

Hardoff R, Sula M, Tamir A, et al: Gastric emptying time and gastric motility in patients with Parkinson's disease. Mov Disord 2001;16:1041–1047.

Hauser MA, Li YJ, Xu H, et al: Expression profiling of substantia nigra in Parkinson disease, progressive supranuclear palsy, and frontotemporal dementia with parkinsonism. Arch Neurol. 2005;62:917–921.

Hawkes C: Olfaction in neurodegenerative disorder. Mov Disord 2003;18:364–372.

Hedrich K, Marder K, Harris J, et al: Evaluation of 50 probands with early-onset Parkinson's disease for parkin mutations. Neurology 2002;58:1239–1246.

Hely MA, Morris JGL, Traficante R, et al: The Sydney multicentre study of Parkinson's disease: progression and mortality at 10 years. J Neurol Neurosurg Psychiatry 1999;67:300–307.

Herlofson K, Larsen JP: The influence of fatigue on health-related quality of life in patients with Parkinson's disease. Acta Neurol Scand 2003;107:1–6.

Herlofson K, Lie SA, Arsland D, Larsen JP: Mortality and Parkinson disease: A community based study. Neurology 2004;62:937–942.

Hilker R, Schweitzer K, Coburger S, et al: Progression of Parkinson's disease is non-linear as determined by serial PET imaging of striatal [18]fluorodopa activity. Arch Neurol 2005;62:378–382.

Hill AN, Jankovic J, Vuong KD, Donovan D: Treatment of hypophonia with collagen vocal cord augmentation in patients with parkinsonism. Mov Disord 2003;18:11901192.

Hillen ME, Sage JI: Nonmotor fluctuations in patients with Parkinson's disease. Neurology 1996;47:1180–1183.

Hirsch EC, Mouatt A, Faucheux B, et al: Dopamine, tremor, and Parkinson's disease [letter]. Lancet 1992;340(8811):125–126.

Ho AK, Iansek R, Bradshaw JL: Regulation of parkinsonian speech volume: The effect of interlocutor distance. J Neurol Neurosurg Psychiatry 1999;67:199–202.

Hoglinger GU, Rissling I, Metz A, et al: Enhancing recognition of early parkinsonism in the community. Mov Disord 2004;19:505–512.

Holroyd S, Currie L, Wooten GF: Prospective study of hallucinations and delusions in Parkinson's disease. J Neurol Neurosurg Psychiatry 2001;70:734–738.

Holroyd S, Currie LJ, Wooten GF: Depression is associated with impairment of ADL, not motor function in Parkinson disease. Neurology 2005;64:2134–2135.

Hu MT, Taylor-Robinson SD, Chaudhuri KR, et al. Cortical dysfunction in non-demented Parkinson's disease patients: A combined 31P-MRS and 18FDG-PET study. Brain 2000;123:340–352.

Hu MT, White SJ, Herlihy AH, et al: A comparison of (18)F-dopa PET and inversion recovery MRI in the diagnosis of Parkinson's disease. Neurology 2001;56:1195–1200.

Hughes AJ, Ben-Shlomo Y, Daniel SE, Lees AJ: What features improve the accuracy of clinical diagnosis in Parkinson's disease: A clinical pathological study. Neurology 1992;42:1142–1146.

Hughes AJ, Daniel SE, Ben-Shlomo Y, Lees AJ: The accuracy of diagnosis of parkinsonian syndromes in a specialist movement disorder service. Brain 2002;125:861–870.

Hughes AJ, Daniel SE, Blankson S, Lees AJ: A clinicopathologic study of 100 cases of Parkinson's disease. Arch Neurol 1993;50:140–148.

Hughes AJ, Daniel SE, Kilford L, Lees AJ: Accuracy of clinical diagnosis of idiopathic Parkinson's disease: A clinico-pathological study of 100 cases. J Neurol Neurosurg Psychiatry 1992;55:181–184.

Hughes AJ, Lees AJ, Stern GM: Apomorphine test to predict dopaminergic responsiveness in parkinsonian syndromes. Lancet. 1990;336(8713):518.

Hughes TA, Ross HF, Mindham RH, Spokes EG: Mortality in Parkinson's disease and its association with dementia and depression. Acta Neurol Scand 2004;110:118–123.

Huisman E, Uylings HB, Hoogland PV: A 100% increase of dopaminergic cells in the olfactory bulb may explain hyposmia in Parkinson's disease. Mov Disord 2004;19:687–692.

Hunker CJ, Abbs JH, Barlow SM: The relationship between parkinsonian rigidity and hypokinesia in the orofacial system: A quantitative analysis. Neurology 1982;32:749–754.

Hunter PC, Crameri J, Austin S, et al: Response of parkinsonian swallowing dysfunction to dopaminergic stimulation. J Neurol Neurosurg Psychiatry 1997;63:579–583.

Hurtig HI, Trojanowski JQ, Galvin J, et al: Alpha-synuclein cortical Lewy bodies correlate with dementia in Parkinson's disease. Neurology. 2000;54(10):1916–1921.

Isella V, Iurlaro S, Piolti R, et al: Physical anhedonia in Parkinson's disease. J Neurol Neurosurg Psychiatry 2003;74:1308–1311.

Ito K, Nagano-Saito A, Kato T, et al: Striatal and extrastriatal dysfunction in Parkinson's disease with dementia: A 6-[(18)F]fluoro-L-dopa PET study. Brain 2002;125:1358–1365.

Jankovic J: Pathophysiology and clinical assessment of motor symptoms in Parkinson's disease. In Koller WC (ed): Handbook of Parkinson's Disease. New York, Marcel Dekker, 1992, pp 129–158.

Jankovic J: Essential tremor: A heterogenous disorder. Mov Disord 2002;17:638–644.

Jankovic J: Pathophysiology and clinical assessment of parkinsonian symptoms and signs. In Pahwa R, Lyons K, Koller WC (ed): Handbook of Parkinson's Disease. New York, Marcel Dekker, 2003, pp 71–107.

Jankovic J: Progression of Parkinson's disease: Are we making progress in charting the course? Arch Neurol 2005;62:351–352.

Jankovic J, Beach J, Schwartz K, Contant C: Tremor and longevity in relatives of patients with Parkinson's disease, essential tremor and control subjects. Neurology 1995;45:645–648.

Jankovic J, Ben-Arie L, Schwartz K, et al: Movement and reaction times and fine coordination tasks following pallidotomy. Mov Disord 1999;14:57–62.

Jankovic J, Kapadia AS: Functional decline in Parkinson's disease. Arch Neurol 2001;58:1611–1615.

Jankovic J, Lang AE: Classification of movement disorders. In Germano IM (ed): Surgical Treatment of Movement Disorders. Lebanon, NH, American Association of Neurological Surgeons, 1998, pp 3–18.

Jankovic J, Lang AE: Movement disorders: Diagnosis and assessment. In Bradley WG, Daroff RB, Fenichel GM, Jankovic J (eds): Neurology in Clinical Practice, 4th ed. Philadelphia, Butterworth-Heinemann, 2004, pp 293–322.

Jankovic J, Linfante I, Dawson LE, Contant, C: Young-onset versus late-onset Parkinson's disease: Clinical features and disease progression. Ann Neurol 1997;42:448.

Jankovic J, McDermott M, Carter J, et al: Variable expression of Parkinson's disease: A base-line analysis of the DATATOP cohort. Neurology 1990;41:1529–1534.

Jankovic J, Nutt JG, Sudarsky L: Classification, diagnosis and etiology of gait disorders. In Ruzicka E, Hallett M, Jankovic J (eds): Gait disorders: Advances in Neurology, vol. 87. Philadelphia, Lippincott Williams & Wilkins, 2001, pp 119–134.

Jankovic J, Rajput AH, McDermott MP, Perl DP: The evolution of diagnosis in early Parkinson disease. Arch Neurol 2000;57:369–372.

Jankovic J, Schwartz, KS, Ondo W: Re-emergent tremor of Parkinson's disease. J Neurol Neurosurg Psychiatry 1999;67:646–650.

Jankovic J, Tintner R: Dystonia and parkinsonism. Parkinsonism Relat Disord 2001;8:109–121.

Jankovic J, Wooten M, Van der Linden C, Jansson B: Weight loss in Parkinson's disease. South Med J 1992;85:351–354.

Jansson B, Jankovic J: Low cancer rates among patients with Parkinson's disease. Ann Neurol 1985;17:505–509.

Jellinger KA: Is there apoptosis in Lewy body disease? Acta Neuropathol 1999;97:413–415.

Jennings DL, Innis RB, Seibyl JP, Marek K: [123]β CIT and SPECT assessment of progression in early and later Parkinson's disease. Neurology 2006;56(Suppl 3):A74.

Josephs KA, Matsumoto JY, Ahlskog JE: Benign tremulous parkinsonism. Arch Neurol 2006;63:354–357.

Karlsen KH, Larsen JP, Tandberg E, Maeland JG: Influence of clinical and demographic variables on quality of life in patients with Parkinson's disease. J Neurol Neurosurg Psychiatry 1999;66: 431–435.

Karlsen KH, Tandberg E, Arsland D, Larsen JP: Health related quality of life in Parkinson's disease: A prospective longitudinal study. J Neurol Neurosurg Psychiatry 2000;69:584–589.

Katzenschlager R, Lees AJ: Olfaction and Parkinson's syndromes: Its role in differential diagnosis. Curr Opin Neurol 2004;17:417–423.

Katzenschlager R, Zijlmans J, Evans A, et al: Olfactory function distinguishes vascular parkinsonism from Parkinson's disease. J Neurol Neurosurg Psychiatry 2004;75:1749–1752.

Kaufmann H, Nahm K, Purohit D, Wolfe D: Autonomic failure as the initial presentation of Parkinson disease and dementia with Lewy bodies. Neurology 2004;63:1093–1095.

Khan NL, Katzenschlager R, Watt H, et al: Olfaction differentiates parkin disease from early-onset parkinsonism and Parkinson disease. Neurology 2004;62:1224–1226.

Kompoliti K, Wang QE, Goetz CG, et al: Effects of central dopaminergic stimulation by apomorphine on speech in Parkinson's disease. Neurology 2000;54:458–462.

Kovari E, Gold G, Herrmann FR, et al: Lewy body densities in the entorhinal and anterior cingulate cortex predict cognitive deficits in Parkinson's disease. Acta Neuropathol (Berl) 2003;106:83–88.

Krishnan PR, Bhatia M, Behari M: Restless legs syndrome in Parkinson's disease: A case-controlled study. Mov Disord 2003; 18:181–185.

Kumar N, Van Gerpen JA, Bower JH, Ahlskog JE: Levodopa-dyskinesia incidence by age of Parkinson's disease onset. Mov Disord 2005;20:342–344.

Kurlan R: Disabling repetitive behaviors in Parkinson's disease. Mov Disord 2004;19:433–437.

Lang AE, Obeso JA: Challenges in Parkinson's disease: Restoration of the nigrostriatal dopamine system is not enough. Lancet Neurol 2004;3:309–316.

Langston JW: The Parkinson's complex: Parkinsonism is just the tip of the iceberg. Ann Neurol 2006;59:591–596.

Lava NS, Factor SA: Focal myopathy as a cause of anterocollis in parkinsonism. Mov Disord 2001;16:754–756.

Lawrence AD, Evans AH, Lees AJ: Compulsive use of dopamine replacement therapy in Parkinson's disease: Reward systems gone awry? Lancet Neurol 2003;2:595–604.

Lee CS, Schulzer M, Mak EK, et al: Clinical observations on the rate of progression of idiopathic parkinsonism. Brain 1994;117:501–507.

Lee MS, Kim HS, Lyoo CH: "Off" gait freezing and temporal discrimination threshold in patients with Parkinson disease. Neurology 2005;64:670–674.

Levy G, Louis ED, Cote L, et al: Contribution of aging to the severity of different motor signs in Parkinson disease. Arch Neurol 2005; 62:467–472.

Levy G, Tang M–X, Cote LJ: Motor impairment in PD: Relationship to incident dementia and age. Neurology 2000;55:539–544.

Lewis SJ, Dove A, Robbins TW, et al: Cognitive impairments in early Parkinson's disease are accompanied by reductions in activity in frontostriatal neural circuitry. J Neurosci 2003;23:6351–6566.

Lewis SJ, Foltynie T, Blackwell AD, et al: Heterogeneity of Parkinson's disease in the early clinical stages using a data driven approach. J Neurol Neurosurg Psychiatry 2005;76:343–348.

Li Y-J, Scott WK, Hedges DJ, et al: Onset in neurodegenerative diseases is genetically controlled. Am J Hum Genet 2002;70:985–993.

Lilienfeld DE, Chan E, Ehland J, et al: Two decades of increasing mortality from Parkinson's disease among the US elderly. Arch Neurol 1990; 47:731–734.

Lindeboom R, Vermeulen M, Holman R, De Haan RJ: Activities of daily living instruments: Optimizing scales for neurologic assessments. Neurology 2003;60:738–742.

Lorefalt B, Ganowiak W, Palhagen S, et al: Factors of importance for weight loss in elderly patients with Parkinson's disease. Acta Neurol Scand 2004;110:180–187.

Louis ED, Levy G, Mejia-Santana H, et al: Risk of action tremor in relatives of tremor-dominant and postural instability gait disorder PD. Neurology 2003;61:931–936.

Louis ED, Lynch T, Marder K, Fahn S: Reliability of patient completion of the historical section of the Unified Parkinson's Disease Rating Scale. Mov Disord 1996;11:185–192.

Louis ED, Tang MX, Cote L, et al: Progression of parkinsonian signs in Parkinson disease. Arch Neurol 1999;56:334–337.

Lücking CB, Dürr A, Bonifati V, et al: Association beween early-onset Parkinson's disease and mutations in the parkin gene. N Engl J Med 2000;342:1560–1567.

Mallet L, Mesnage V, Houeto JL, et al: Compulsions, Parkinson's disease, and stimulation. Lancet 2002;360:1302–1304.

Manni R, Pacchetti C, Terzaghi M, et al: Hallucinations and sleep-wake cycle in PD: A 24-hour continuous polysomnographic study. Neurology 2002;59:1979–1981.

Marchese R, Diverio M, Zucchi F, et al: The role of sensory cues in the rehabilitation of parkinsonian patients: A comparison of two physical therapy protocols. Mov Disord 2001;15:879–883.

Marder K, Tang MX, Alfaro B, et al: Risk of Alzheimer's disese in relatives of Parkinson's disease patients with and without dementia. Neurology 1999;52:719–724.

Marek K, Innis R, vanDyck C, et al: [$^{123}$I]β-CIT/SPECT imaging assessment of the rate of Parkinson's disease progression. Neurology 2001;57:2089–2094.

Marek KL, Seibyl J, Parkinson Study Group: β-CIT Scans without evidence of dopaminergic deficit (SWEDD) in the ELLDOPA and CALM-CIT study: Long term imaging assessment. Neurology 2003;60(suppl 1):A293.

Marek KL, Seibyl JP, Zoghbi SS, et al:. [$^{123}$I]β–CIT/SPECT imaging demonstrates bilateral loss of dopamine transporters in hemi-Parkinson's disease. Neurology 1996;46:231–237.

Marinus J, Ramaker C, Van Hilten JJ, Stiggelbout AM: Health related quality of life in Parkinson's disease: A systematic review of disease specific instruments. J Neurol Neurosurg Psychiatry 2002;72:241–248.

Marinus J, Visser M, Stiggelbout AM, et al: A short scale for the assessment of motor impairments and disabilities in Parkinson's disease: The SPES/SCOPA. J Neurol Neurosurg Psychiatry 2004;75:388–395.

Marinus J, Visser M, Verwey NA, et al: Assessment of cognition in Parkinson's disease. Neurology 2003;61:1222–1228.

Mark MH, Sage JI, Dickson DW, et al: Levodopa-nonresponsive Lewy body parkinsonism: Clinicopathologic study of two cases. Neurology 1992;42:1323–1327.

Marras C, Goldman S, Smith A, et al: Smell identification ability in twin pairs discordant for Parkinson's disease. Mov Disord 2005;20:687–693.

Marras C, McDermott MP, Rochon PA, et al: Survival in Parkinson disease: Thirteen-year follow-up of the DATATOP cohort. Neurology 2005;64:87–93.

Marras C, Rochon P, Lang AE: Predicting motor decline and disability in Parkinson disease: A systematic review. Arch Neurol 2002;59:1724–1728.

Marsh L, McDonald WM, Cummings J, et al: Provisional diagnostic criteria for depression in Parkinson's disease: Report of an NINDS/NIMH Work Group. Mov Disord 2006;21:148–158.

Marsh L, Williams JR, Rocco M, et al: Psychiatric comorbidities in patients with Parkinson disease and psychosis. Neurology 2004;63:293–300.

Matheson JK, Saper CB: REM sleep behavior disorder: A dopaminergic deficiency disorder? Neurology. 2003;61:1328–1329.

McDermott MP, Jankovic J, Carter J, et al: Factors predictive of the need for levodopa therapy in early, untreated Parkinson's disease. Arch Neurol 1995;52:565–570.

Meara J, Bhowmick BK, Hobson P: Accuracy of diagnosis in patients with presumed Parkinson's disease. Age Ageing 1999;28:99–102.

Mentis MJ, Dhawan V, Nakamura T, et al: Enhancement of brain activation during trial-and-error sequence learning in early PD. Neurology 2003;60:612–619.

Michell AW, Lewis SJ, Foltynie T, Barker RA: Biomarkers and Parkinson's disease. Brain 2004;127:1693–1705.

Molina JA, Sainz-Artiga MJ, Fraile A, et al: Pathologic gambling in Parkinson's disease: A behavioral manifestation of pharmacologic treatment? Mov Disord 2000;15:869–872.

Montgomery EB, Baker KB, Lyons K, Koller WC: Abnormal performance on the PD test battery by asymptomatic first-degree relatives. Neurology 1999;52:757–762.

Morgante L, Salemi G, Meneghini F, et al: Parkinson disease survival: A population-based study. Arch Neurol 2000;57:507–512.

Morrish PK, Rakshi JS, Bailey DL, et al: Measuring the rate of progression and estimating the preclinical period of Parkinson's disease with [18F]dopa PET. J Neurol Neurosurg Psychiatry 1998;64:314–319.

Morrish PK, Sawle GV, Brooks DJ: An [18F]dopa-PET and clinical study of the rate of progression in Parkinson's disease. Brain 1996;119:558–591.

Movement Disorder Society Task Force on Rating Scales for Parkinson's Disease: The Unified Parkinson's Disease Rating Scale (UPDRS): Status and recommendations. Mov Disord 2003;18:738–750.

Munhoz RP, Li JY, Kurtinecz M, et al: Evaluation of the pull test technique in assessing postural instability in Parkinson's disease. Neurology 2004;62:125–127.

Murphy C, Schubert CR, Cruickshanks KJ, et al: Prevalence of olfactory impairment in older adults. JAMA 2002;288:2307–2312.

Muqit MMK, Rakshi JS, Shakir RA, Larner AJ: Catatonia or abulia? A difficult differential diagnosis. Mov Disord 2001;16:360–362.

Nakamura T, Dhawan V, Chaly T, et al: Blinded positron emission tomography study of dopamine cell implantation for Parkinson's disease. Ann Neurol 2001;50:181–187.

Narabayashi H: Evidence suggesting the role of norepinephrine deficiency in late stages of Parkinson's disease. Adv Neurol 1999; 80:501–504.

Nieuwboer A, Dom R, De Weerdt W, et al: Electromyographic profiles of gait prior to onset of freezing episodes in patients with Parkinson's disease. Brain 2004;127:1650–1660.

Nurmi E, Ruottinen HM, Bergman J, et al: Rate of progression in Parkinson's disease: A 6-year [18]fluoro-L-dopa PET study. Mov Disord 2001;16:608–615.

Oerlemans WGH, de Visser M: Dropped head syndrome and bent spine syndrome: Two separate clinical entities or different manifestations of axial myopathy. J Neurol Neurosurg Psychiatry 1998;65:258–259.

Okun MS, Fernandez HH, Rodriguez RL, et al: Testosterone therapy in men with Parkinson disease: Results of the TEST-PD Study. Arch Neurol 2006;63(5):729–735.

Okun MS, McDonald WM, DeLong MR: Refractory nonmotor symptoms in male patients with Parkinson disease due to testosterone deficiency: A common unrecognized comorbidity. Arch Neurol 2002;59:807–811.

Olanow CW: Magnetic resonance imaging in parkinsonism. Neurol Clin 1992;10:405–420.

Olanow CW, Schapira AHV, Roth T: Waking up to sleep episodes in Parkinson's disease. Mov Disord 2000;15:212–215.

Olsen JH, Frils S, Frederiksen K, et al: Atypical cancer pattern in patients with Parkinson's disease. Br J Cancer 2005;92(1):201–205.

Olson EJ, Boeve BF, Silber MH: Rapid eye movement sleep behaviour disorder: Demographic, clinical and laboratory findings in 93 cases. Brain 2000;123:331–339.

Ondo WG, Ben-Aire L, Jankovic J, et al: Weight gain following unilateral pallidotomy in Parkinson's disease. Acta Neurol Scand 2000;101:79–84.

Ondo WG, Lai D: Olfaction testing in patients with tremor-dominant Parkinson's disease: Is this a distinct condition? Mov Disord 2005;20:471–475.

Ondo WG, Vuong DK, Jankovic J: Exploring the relationship between Parkinson's disease and restless legs syndrome. Arch Neurol 2002;59:421–424.

Ondo WG, Vuong KV, Khan H, et al: Daytime sleepiness and other sleep disorders in Parkinson's disease. Neurology 2001;57: 1392–1396.

Onofrj M, Thomas A: Acute akinesia in Parkinson disease. Neurology 2005;64:1162–1169.

O'Suilleabhain PE: Parkinson disease with severe tremor but otherwise mild deterioration. Arch Neurol 2006;63:321–322.

Overeem S, van Hilten JJ, Ripley B, et al: Normal hypocretin-1 levels in Parkinson's disease patients with excessive daytime sleepiness. Neurology 2002;58:498–449.

Pal PK, Calne S, Samii A, Fleming JAE: A review of normal sleep and its disturbances in Parkinson's disease. Parkinsonism Relat Disords 1999;5:1–17.

Paleacu D, Schechtman E, Inzelberg R: Association between family history of dementia and hallucinations in Parkinson disease. Neurology 2005;64:1712–1715.

Parati EA, Fetoni V, Germiniani GC, et al: Response to L-DOPA in multiple system atrophy. Clin Neuropharmacol 1993;16:139–144.

Parkinson J: An Essay on the Shaking Palsy. London: Sherwood, Neely and Jones, 1817.

Parkinson Study Group: Mortality in DATATOP: A multicenter trial in early Parkinson's disease. Ann Neurol 1998;43:318–325.

Parkinson Study Group: Dopamine transporter brain imaging to assess the effects of pramipexole vs levodopa on Parkinson disease progression. JAMA 2002;287:1653–1661.

Parr-Brownlie LC, Hyland BI: Bradykinesia induced by dopamine D2 receptor blockade is associated with reduced motor cortex activity in the rat. J Neurosci 2005;25:5700–5709.

Paviour DC, Surtees RA, Lees AJ: Diagnostic considerations in juvenile parkinsonism. Mov Disord 2004;19:123–135.

Pezzella FR, Colosimo C, Vanacore N, et al: Prevalence and clinical features of hedonistic homeostatic dysregulation in Parkinson's disease. Mov Disord 2005;20:77–81.

Pinto S, Ozsancak C, Tripoliti E, et al: Treatments for dysarthria in Parkinson's disease. Lancet Neurol 2004;3:547–556.

Playford ED, Brooks DJ: In vivo and in vitro studies of the dopaminergic system in movement disorders. Cerebrovasc Brain Metab Rev 1992;4:144–171.

Plazzi G, Corsini R, Provini F, et al: REM sleep behavior disorders in multiple system atrophy. Neurology 1997;48:1094–1097.

Pluck GC, Brown RG: Apathy in Parkinson's disease. J Neurol Neurosurg Psychiatry 2002;73:636–642.

Ponsen MM, Stoffers D, Booij J, et al: Idiopathic hyposmia as a preclinical sign of Parkinson's disease. Ann Neurol 2004;56: 173–181.

Postuma RB, Lang AE, Massicotte-Marquez J, Montplaisir J: Potential early markers of Parkinson disease in idiopathic REM sleep behavior disorder. Neurology 2006;66:845–851.

Pratley RE, Salbe AD, Ravussin E, Caviness JN: Higher sedentary energy expenditure in patients with Huntington's disease. Ann Neurol 2000;47:64–70.

Proulx M, De Courval FP, Wiseman MA, Panisset M: Salivary production in Parkinson's disease. Mov Disord 2005;20:204–207.

Przuntek, H: Early diagnosis in Parkinson's disease. J Neural Transm Suppl 1992;38:105–114.

Quinn M, Critchley P, Marsden CD: Young onset Parkinson's disease. Mov Disord 1987;2:73–91.

Rajput AH, Pahwa R, Pahwa P: Prognostic significance of the onset mode in parkinsonism. Neurology 1993;43:829–830.

Rajput AH, Rozdilsky B, Rajput A: Accuracy of clinical diagnosis in parkinsonism: A prospective study. Can J Neurol Sci 1991;18: 275–278.

Ramaker C, Marinus J, Stiggelbout AM, Van Hilten BJ: Systematic evaluation of rating scales for impairment and disability in Parkinson's disease. Mov Disord 2002;17:867–876.

Ramig LO, Sapir S, Fox C, et al: Changes in vocal loudness following intensive voice treatment (LSVT®) in individuals with Parkinson's disease: A comparison with untreated patients and normal age-matched controls. Mov Disord 2001;16:79–83.

Rao G, Fisch L, Srinivasan S, et al: Does this patient have Parkinson disease? JAMA 2003;289:347–353.

Ravina B, Eidelberg D, Ahlskog JE, et al: The role of radiotracer imaging in Parkinson disease. Neurology 2005;64:208–215.

Rawal N, Periquet M, Lohmann E, et al: New parkin mutations and atypical phenotypes in families with autosomal recessive parkinsonism. Neurology 2003;60:1378–1381.

Ready RE, Friedman J, Grace J, Fernandez H: Testosterone deficiency and apathy in Parkinson's disease: A pilot study. J Neurol Neurosurg Psychiatry 2004;75:1323–1326.

Remy P, Doder M, Lees A, et al: Depression in Parkinson's disease: Loss of dopamine and noradrenaline innervation in the limbic system. Brain 2005;128:1314–1322.

Rice JE, Antic R, Thompson PD: Disordered respiration as a levodopa-induced dyskinesia in Parkinson's disease. Mov Disord 2002;17:524–527.

Riley D, Lang AE, Blair RDG, et al: Frozen shoulder and other disturbances in Parkinson's disease. J Neurol Neurosurg Psychiatry 1989;52:63–66.

Riley DE, Chelimsky TC: Autonomic nervous system testing may not distinguish multiple system atrophy from Parkinson's disease. J Neurol Neurosurg Psychiatry 2003;74:56–60.

Rinne JO, Portin R, Ruottinen H, et al: Cognitive impairment and the brain dopaminergic system in Parkinson disease: [18F]fluorodopa positron emission tomographic study. Arch Neurol 2000;57: 470–475.

Ross GW, Petrovitch H, Abbott RD, et al: Parkinsonian signs and substantia nigra neuron density in decendents elders without PD. Ann Neurol 2004;56:532–539.

Rubinstein TC, Giladi N, Hausdorff JM: The power of cueing to circumvent dopamine deficits: A review of physical therapy treatment of gait disturbances in Parkinson's disease. Mov Disord 2002;17:1148–1160.

Rye DB, Jankovic J: Emerging views of dopamine in modulating sleep/wake state from an unlikely source: PD. Neurology 2002;58:341–346.

Sakakibara R, Odaka T, Uchiyama T, et al: Colonic transit time and rectoanal videomanometry in Parkinson's disease. J Neurol Neurosurg Psychiatry 2003;74:268–272.

Sawle GV, Colebatch JG, Shah A, et al: Striatal function in normal aging: Implications for Parkinson's disease. Ann Neurol 1990;28:799–804.

Schabitz WR, Glatz K, Schuhan C, et al: Severe forward flexion of the trunk in Parkinson's disease: Focal myopathy of the paraspinal muscles mimicking camptocormia. Mov Disord 2003;18:408–414.

Schapira AH, Obeso J: Timing of treatment initiation in Parkinson's disease: A need for reappraisal? Ann Neurol 2006;59:559–562.

Schenk CH, Bundlie SR, Mahowald MW: Delayed emergence of a parkinsonian disorder in 38% of 29 older men initially diagnosed with idiopathic rapid eye movement sleep behavior disorder. Neurology 1996;46:388–393.

Scherfler C, Khan NL, Pavese N, et al. Striatal and cortical pre- and postsynaptic dopaminergic dysfunction in sporadic parkin-linked parkinsonism. Brain 2004;127:1332–1342.

Schrag A, Ben-Shlomo Y, Brown R, et al. Young-onset Parkinson's disease revisited: Clinical features, natural history, and mortality. Mov Disord 1998;13:885–894.

Schrag A, Hovris A, Morley D, et al: Young-versus older-onset Parkinson's disease: Impact of disease and psychosocial consequences. Mov Disord 2003;18:1250–1256.

Schrag A, Janashahi M, Quinn N: What contributes to quality of life in patients with Parkinson's disease? J Neurol Neurosurg Psychiatry 2000;69:308–312.

Schrag A, Schott JM: Epidemiological, clinical, and genetic characteristics of early-onset parkinsonism. Lancet Neurol 2006;5:355–363.

Schulz GM, Peterson T, Sapienza CM, et al: Voice and speech characteristics of persons with Parkinson's disease pre- and post-pallidotomy surgery: Preliminary findings. J Speech Lang Hear Res 1999;42:1176–1194.

Schuurman AG, Van Den Akker M, Ensinck KT, et al: Increased risk of Parkinson's disease after depression: A retrospective cohort study. Neurology 2002;58:1501–1504.

Schwarz J, Linke R, Kerner M, et al: Striatal dopamine transporter binding assessed by [1-123]IPT and single photon emission computed tomography in patients with early Parkinson's disease: Implications for a preclinical diagnosis. Arch Neurol 2000;57:205–208.

Schwarz J, Tatsch K, Arnold G, et al: 123I-iodobenzamide-SPECT predicts dopaminergic responsiveness in patients with de novo parkinsonism. Neurology 1992;42:556–561.

Senard JM, Rai S, Lapeyre-Mestre M, et al: Prevalence of orthostatic hypotension in Parkinson's disease. J Neurol Neurosurg Psychiatry 1997;63:584–589.

Shahed J, Jankovic J: Re-emergence of childhood stuttering in Parkinson's disease: A hypothesis. Mov Disord 2001;16:114–118.

Sharabi Y, Li ST, Dendi R, et al: Neurotransmitter specificity of sympathetic denervation in Parkinson's disease. Neurology 2003;60:1036–1039.

Shulman LM, Minagar A, Weiner WJ: The effect of pregnancy in Parkinson's disease. Mov Disord 2000;15:132–135.

Siderowf A, Newberg A, Chou KL, et al: [99mTc]TRODAT-1 SPECT imaging correlates with odor identification in early Parkinson disease. Neurology 2005;64:1716–1720.

Siderowf A, Ravina B, Glick HA: Preference-based quality-of-life in patients with Parkinson's disease. Neurology 2002;59:103–108.

Stacy M, Jankovic J: Differential diagnosis of Parkinson's disease and the parkinsonism plus syndromes. Neurol Clin 1992;10:341–345.

Starkstein SE, Petracca G, Chemerinski E, et al: Prevalence and correlates of parkinsonism in patients with primary depression. Neurology 2001;57:553–555.

Stebbins GT, Goetz CG, Lang AE, Cubo E: Factor analysis of the motor section of the Unified Parkinson's Disease Rating Scale during the off-state. Mov Disord 1999;14:585–589.

Stern MB, Doty RL, Dotti M, et al: Olfactory function in Parkinson's disease subtypes. Neurology 1994;44:266–268.

Suchowersky O, Reich S, Perlmutter J, et al: Practice Parameter: Diagnosis and prognosis of new onset Parkinson disease (an evidence-based review): Report of the Quality Standards Subcommittee of the American Academy of Neurology. Neurology 2006;66:968–975.

Sutcliffe JG, de Lecea L: The hypocretins: Setting the arousal threshold. Nat Rev 2002;3:339–349.

Suteerawattananon M, Morris GS, Etnyre BR, et al: Effects of visual and auditory cues on gait in individuals with Parkinson's disease. J Neurol Sci 2004;219:63–69.

Swinn L, Schrag A, Viswanathan R, et al: Sweating dysfunction in Parkinson's disease. Mov Disord 2003;18:1459–1463.

Tabamo RE, Di Rocco A: Alopecia induced by dopamine agonists. Neurology 2002;58:829–830.

Tan EK, Lum SY, Wong MC: Restless legs syndrome in Parkinson's disease. J Neurol Sci 2002;196:33–36.

Tan EK, Ondo W: Clinical characteristics of pramipexole-induced peripheral edema. Arch Neurol 2000;57:729–732.

Tandberg E, Larsen JP, Aarsland D, Cummings JL: The occurrence of depression in Parkinson's disease. Arch Neurol 1996;53:175–179.

Tandberg E, Larsen JP, Karlsen K: Excessive daytime sleepiness and sleep benefit in Parkinson's disease: A community-based study. Mov Disord 1999;14:922–927.

Tanner CM, Goldman SM: Epidemiology of Parkinson's disease. Neurol Clin 1996;14:317–336.

Teulings H-L, Contreras-Vidal JL, Stelmach GE, Adler CH: Adaptation of handwriting size under distorted visual feedback in patients with Parkinson's disease and elderly and young controls. J Neurol Neurosurg Psychiatry 2002;72:315–324.

Thobois S, Ribeiro M-J, Lohman E, et al: Young-onset Parkinson disease with and without parkin gene mutations: A Fluorodopa F 18 positron emission tomography study. Arch Neurol 2003;60:713–718.

Thomas M, Jankovic J, Suteerawattananon M, et al: Clinical gait and balance scale (GABS): Validation and utilization. J Neurol Sci 2004;217:89–99.

Thomas RJ: Blinking and the release reflexes: Are they clinically useful? J Am Geriatr Soc 1994;42:609–613.

Tissingh G, Berendse HW, Bergmans P, et al: Loss of olfaction in de novo and treated Parkinson's disease: Possible implications for early diagnosis. Mov Disord 2001;16:41–46.

Tolosa E, Wenning G, Poewe W: The diagnosis of Parkinson's disease. Lancet Neurol 2006;5:75–86.

Touge T, Werhalm KJ, Rothwell JC, et al: Movement-related cortical potentials preceding repetitive and random-choice hand movements in Parkinson's disease. Ann Neurol 1995;37:791–799.

Tretiakoff C: Contribution a l'etude de l'anatomie pathologique du locus niger de Soemmering avec quelques deductions relatives a le pathogenie des troubles du tonius musculaire et de la maladie de Parkinson [thesis]. Paris, University of Paris, 1919.

Uitti RJ, Baba Y, Whaley NR, et al: Parkinson disease: Handedness predicts asymmetry. Neurology 2005;64:1925–1930.

Umapathi T, Chaudry V, Cornblath D, et al: Head drop and camptocormia. J Neurol Neurosurg Psychiatry 2002;73:1–7.

Vanacore N, Spila-Alegiani S, Raschetti R, Meco G: Mortality cancer risk in parkinsonian patients: A population-based study. Neurology 1999;52:395–398.

van Hilten B, Hoff JI, Middelkoop HAM, et al: Sleep disruption in Parkinson's disease: Assessment by continuous activity monitoring. Arch Neurol 1994;52:922–928.

Villarejo A, Camacho A, Garcia-Ramos R, et al: Cholinergic-dopaminergic imbalance in Pisa syndrome. Clin Neuropharmacol 2003;26:119–121.

Vingerhoets FJG, Schulzer M, Calne DB, et al: Which clinical sign of Parkinson's disease best reflects the nigrostriatal lesion? Ann Neurol 1997;41:58–64.

Voon V: Repetition, repetition, and repetition: Compulsive and punding behaviors in Parkinson's disease. Mov Disord 2004;19:367–370.

Vreeling FW, Jollens J, Verhey FRJ, Houx PJ: Primitive reflexes in healthy, adult volunteers and neurological patients: Methodological issues. J Neurol 1993;240:495–504.

Walter U, Niehaus L, Probst T, et al: Brain parenchyma sonography discriminates Parkinson's disease and atypical parkinsonian syndromes. Neurology 2003;60:74–77.

Ward CD, Sanes JN, Dambrosia JM, Calne DB: Methods for evaluating treatment in Parkinson's disease. In Fahn S, Calne DB, Shoulson I (eds): Experimental Therapeutics of Movement Disorders. New York: Raven Press. 1983, pp 1–7.

Welsh M, McDermott MP, Holloway RG, et al: Development and testing of the Parkinson's disease quality of life scale. Mov Disord 2003;18:637–645.

Wenning GK, Ben-Shlomo Y, Magalhaes M, et al: Clinicopathological study of 35 cases of multiple system atrophy. J Neurol Neurosurg Psychiatry. 1995;58(2):160–166.

Wenzelburger R, Raethjen J, Löffler K, et al: Kinetic tremor in a reach-to-grasp movement in Parkinson's disease. Mov Disord 2000;15:1084–1094.

Wetter TC, Collado-Seidel V, Pollmacher T, et al: Sleep and periodic leg movement patterns in drug-free patients with Parkinson's disease and multiple system atrophy. Sleep 2000;23:361–367.

Whone AL, Brefel-Courbon C, Moore RY, et al: Tremor at diagnosis is predictive of slower disease progression in Parkinson's disease: An 18F dopa PET study. Mov Disord 2002;17(suppl 5):S140–S141.

Whone AL, Watts RL, Stoessl AJ, et al: Slower progression of Parkinson's disease with ropinirole versus levodopa: The REAL-PET study. Ann Neurol 2003;54:93–101.

Williams DR, Watt HC, Lees AJ: Predictors of falls and fractures in bradykinetic rigid syndromes: A retrospective study. J Neurol Neurosurg Psychiatry 2006;77:468–473.

Wilson RS, Schneider JA, Beckett LA, et al: Progression of gait disorder and rigidity and risk of death in older persons. Neurology 2002;58:1815–1819.

Winge K, Rasmussen D, Werdelin LM: Constipation in neurological diseases. J Neurol Neurosurg Psychiatry 2003;74:13–19.

Winikates J, Jankovic J: Clinical correlates of vascular parkinsonism. Arch Neurol 1999;56:98–102.

Winkler AS, Reuter I, Harwood G, Chaudhuri KR: The frequency and significance of "striatal toe" in parkinsonism. Parkinsonism Relat Disord 2002;9:97–101.

Witjas T, Kaphan E, Azulay JP, et al: Nonmotor fluctuations in Parkinson's disease: Frequent and disabling. Neurology 2002;59:408–413.

Wood JM, Worringham C, Kerr G, et al: Quantitative assessment of driving performance in Parkinson's disease. J Neurol Neurosurg Psychiatry 2005;76:176–180.

Wooten GF, Currie LJ, Bovbjerg VE, et al: Are men at greater risk for Parkinson's disease than women? J Neurol Neurosurg Psychiatry 2004;75:637–639.

Zarow C, Lyness SA, Mortimer JA, Chui HC: Neuronal loss is greater in the locus coeruleus than nucleus basalis and substantia nigra in Alzheimer and Parkinson diseases. Arch Neurol 2003;60(3):337–341.

Zetusky WJ, Jankovic J, Pirozzolo FJ: The heterogeneity of Parkinson's disease: Clinical and prognostic implications. Neurology 1985;35:522–526.

Zia S, Cody F, O'Boyle D: Joint position sense is impaired by Parkinson's disease. Ann Neurol 2000;47:218–228.

## Chapter 5

# Current Concepts on the Etiology and Pathogenesis of Parkinson Disease

The primary pathology of Parkinson disease (PD) that is responsible for the onset of motor symptoms is attributed to the degeneration of dopaminergic neurons in the zona compacta of the substantia nigra (Ehringer and Hornykiewicz, 1960). However, pathology in PD is much more widespread, affecting brainstem nuclei such as the locus coeruleus and raphe nuclei as well as more frontal regions, such as the substantia innominata (Jellinger, 1987). Indeed, most areas of the brain seem to be affected by pathologic damage in PD, and this results in alterations in a wide range of neurotransmitters (Agid et al., 1987). So in addition to dopamine, there are also changes in the content of noradrenaline, 5HT, acetylcholine, GABA, glutamate, and neuropeptides, among others. In fact, the pathology and biochemistry of PD illustrate that it is anything but a simple disorder and show that it affects many parts of the brain that are not directly related to the control of motor function. As a consequence, there is considerable interest in the nonmotor, nondopaminergic components of PD, as these underline the complexity of the disorder, and they reflect the symptoms of the illness that do not respond to current dopaminergic medication.

An important recent hypothesis is that PD might not originate in the substantia nigra as was previously thought; rather, pathologic change starts in the olfactory regions and areas around the dorsal motor nucleus of the vagus (Braak et al., 2003, 2004). Subsequently, it sweeps forward through the brain, affecting the locus coeruleus and raphe nuclei, and only then starts to produce the pathologic change in basal ganglia that gives rise to the motor symptoms that characterize PD and leads to its clinical diagnosis (Fig. 5-1). In due course, pathology may progress into frontal regions, thus producing the cognitive decline and dementia that occur in a proportion of patients with PD. Even more controversial is the suggestion that PD starts as a peripheral disorder as illustrated by the presence of Lewy bodies in the myenteric plexus and elsewhere (Braak et al., 2006). These concepts might explain why olfactory loss, constipation, sleep fragmentation, REM sleep behavior disorder, and depression are common parts of the history of patients who go on to develop the motor symptoms of PD (Doty et al., 1993; Leentjens et al., 2003; Chaudhuri et al., 2006; Iranzo et al., 2006; Langston, 2006; Weintraub et al., 2006). If true, such hypotheses have important consequences for an understanding of the cause of PD. However, the spectrum of pathologic change is linked by the presence of Lewy bodies, and it appears that the formation of these proteinaceous inclusions provides one of the major clues to the pathogenic mechanisms that are involved (Fig. 5-2).

In trying to understand what causes PD and the nature of the pathogenic processes, it is invariably presumed that PD is a single illness. However, as this chapter shows, nigral degeneration can arise from a variety of causes, and as a consequence, it is likely that PD should be viewed as a syndrome. This would account for the complex symptomatology and the roles that different pathogenic mechanisms may play in causing cell death. In viewing the illness in a more global sense, perhaps the best approach is to consider PD as an illness that has a genetic component but in which environmental factors also lead to the onset of neurodegeneration, and this has been adopted in the following discourse.

## GENETICS AND PARKINSON DISEASE

The suspicion that PD has a genetic component had been debated for many years. Currently, there is evidence from rare familial forms of PD, studies of twin pairs, and family cluster studies to support the concept of gene defects as an underlying cause of nigral cell degeneration. Other nonfamilial clusterings of PD cases may indicate the importance of environment (Kumar et al., 2004). Indeed, the idea that susceptibility genes may increase the risk of developing PD has also been extensively investigated, furthering the concept of an interaction between genetic and environmental factors as another cause of the illness.

The study of gene defects in familial forms of PD has probably had the greatest impact on current understanding of the pathogenic process. At least 11 gene loci have been identified in familial PD (Table 5-1), and so far, six gene products have been detected that appear to be associated with pathogenic mechanisms. The first to be described involved two mutations (A30P and A53T) in α-synuclein (*PARK1*) (Polymeropoulos et al., 1997; Kruger et al., 1998), a synaptic vesicle protein that may result in altered vesicular storage of dopamine and toxicity through the formation of reactive oxygen species (Lotharius and Brundin, 2002; Perez and Hastings, 2004). However, mutations in α-synuclein lead to alterations in its structure that make the protein prone to misfolding and aggregation (Bertoncini et al., 2005). α-Synuclein mutants form soluble protofibrils leading to fibril formation and intracellular protein aggregates, and dopamine may itself enhance the accumulation of toxic protofibrils (Conway et al., 2000; Li et al., 2001; Eriksen et al., 2003; Rochet et al., 2004). The transfection of genes for mutant α-synuclein into cell lines sensitizes them to the actions of toxins, including dopamine, while overexpression of the wild-type protein can be protective (Lee et al., 2001). The mutants stimulate oxidative stress and mitochondrial impairment, both components of the cell death process that is known to occur in nigral dopaminergic neurons in PD (see later). The toxicity of the A53T mutant was shown to involve endoplasmic reticulum stress and mitochondrial cell death pathways (Smith et al., 2005a).

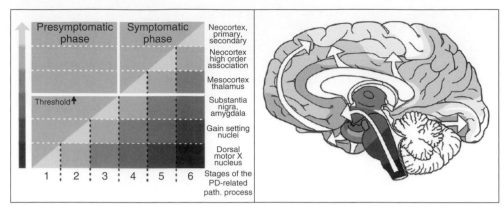

**Figure 5-1** Sequential spread of Lewy neurites in nonparkinsonian individuals over time. Lewy neurites seen on histopathologic staining of α-synuclein first appear in the lower medulla oblongata and olfactory tubercle (stage 1). Succeeding stages are the appearances on these neurites more rostrally in the brainstem, with the pons (including locus coeruleus) in stage 2 and midbrain (with substantia nigra) in stage 3. Stages 4 through 6 are the more rostral spread from thalamus to mesocortex to neocortex. (See Color Plate 5.) (From Braak H, Ghebremedhin E, Rub U, et al:. Stages in the development of Parkinson's disease–related pathology. Cell Tissue Res 2004;318[1]:121–134.)

The importance of α-synuclein to sporadic PD and related disorders was made by the discovery of the presence of the wild-type protein in Lewy bodies and Lewy neurites together with nitrated α-synuclein and other unique forms of the protein (Goedert et al., 2001; Tofaris et al., 2001; Iwatsubo, 2003; Pountney et al., 2004). Further, α-synuclein redistributes to neuromelanin lipid in the substantia nigra early in PD, potentially predisposing neurons to degeneration and to Lewy body formation (Halliday et al., 2005). This has led to the concept that α-synuclein is responsible for the pathology that occurs in substantia nigra in sporadic PD, but this is still being debated (see later). Recently, phosphorylation of α-synuclein was shown to result from its overexpression, to enhance inclusion formation and to control neurotoxicity (Yamada et al., 2004; Chen and Feany, 2005; Smith et al., 2005b). Truncation of α-synuclein at the C-terminus also occurs and may be important, since it is enriched in inclusions, its formation is enhanced by familial mutations, and it leads to inclusion formation in the substantia nigra in transgenic mice, although cell death does not occur (Li et al., 2005; Tofaris et al., 2006) In contrast, nitration of α-synuclein may inhibit fibril formation due to the formation of stable soluble oligomers (Uversky et al., 2005).

Recent discoveries have reignited the importance of α-synuclein to PD. Another α-synuclein mutant (E46K) has been discovered that causes a more fundamental change in protein function than previous mutations and stimulates protoaggregate formation that may be enhanced by dopamine itself (Golbe and Mouradian, 2004; Zarranz et al., 2004; Pandey et al., 2006). Perhaps more important has been the discovery in families with autosomal-dominant early-onset PD of a normal α-synuclein gene sequence but in which gene locus triplication occurred resulting in a doubling of α-synuclein formation that then appears pathogenic (*PARK4*) (Singleton et al., 2003; Farrer et al., 2004). Subsequently,

**Figure 5-2** Lewy body. A protein-rich Lewy body in a neuromelanin-pigmented dopaminergic neuron in the SNc in sporadic PD revealed by H&E staining. (See Color Plate 6.)

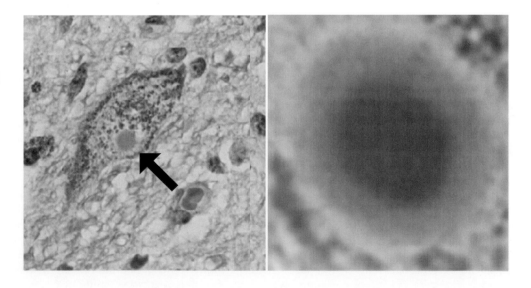

Table 5-1 Gene locations and identifications in familial Parkinson Disease

| Name and Locus | Gene | Mode of Inheritance; Pathologic and Clinical Features | Protein Function | Where Found | Pathogenic Mutations |
|---|---|---|---|---|---|
| *PARK1* 4q21.3 | α-Synuclein | Autosomal-dominant; Lewy bodies; young onset; dementia occurs | Possibly synaptic vesicle trafficking; elevated in bird song learning | Families in Germany, Italy-U.S. (Contoursi kindred), Greece, Spain | A53T and A30P, may promote aggregation; Lewy body and Alzheimer plaque component; protofibrils (toxic) accumulation |
| *PARK2* 6q25.2–q27 | Parkin | Autosomal-recessive; (also dominant?); often juvenile onset without Lewy bodies; slowly progressive | Ubiquitin E3 ligase, attaches short ubiquitin peptide chains to a range of proteins, likely to mark degradation | Ubiquitous, originally in Japan, very common in juvenile onset | Over 70 mutations identified; most likely loss of function mutations |
| *PARK3* 2p13 | Unknown | Autosomal-dominant; Lewy bodies, indistinguishable from idiopathic PD | | Four families in southern Denmark and northern Germany, probable common ancestor | |
| *PARK4* 4q | Multiple copies of wild-type α-synuclein | Autosomal-dominant; wide range of symptoms from idiopathic PD to dementia with Lewy bodies | See *PARK1* | "Spellman-Muenter" and the "Waters-Miller" families with common ancestor in the United States, European families | Duplications/triplications of chromosomal region that contains wild-type α-synuclein gene |
| *PARK5* 4p14 | Ubiquitin-C-terminal hydrolase L1 | Possibly autosomal-dominant | Removes polyubiquitin | One family in Germany | |
| *PARK6* 1p35–p36 | PINK-1 | Autosomal-recessive; juvenile onset | Mitochondrial protein; provides protection against multiple stress factors | One family in Sicily | |
| *PARK7* 1p36 | DJ-1 | Autosomal-recessive; early onset | Sumoylation pathway | Families in Holland, Italy, Uruguay | L166P, M261, and a variety of other candidates |
| *PARK8* 12p11.2–q13.1 | Dardarin (leucine-rich repeat kinase 2, LRRK2) | Autosomal-dominant; nigral degeneration, no Lewy bodies; onset at age 65; tremor, benign; responds to low doses of L-dopa. | Probably a cytoplasmic kinase | First family in Japan; eight now around the world. Gene identified in four Basque families (Spain) and one family in England | |
| *PARK9* 1p36 | Unknown | Autosomal-recessive; Kufor-Rakeb syndrome, a Parkinson-plus disorder | | One family in Jordan | |
| *PARK10* 1p32 | Unknown | Autosomal-recessive; typical late onset | | Families in Iceland | |
| *PARK11* 2q36–q37 | | Autosomal-dominant | | Families in the United States | |

Modified from Fahn S, Sulzer D: Neurodegeneration and neuroprotection in Parkinson disease. NeuroRx 2004;1:139–154.

α-synuclein gene duplication has been uncovered in individuals with inherited late-onset disease more closely resembling sporadic PD (Chartier-Harlin et al., 2004; Ibanez et al., 2004; Nishioka et al., 2006). A quantitative rather than qualitative change in α-synuclein might therefore have important implications for events occurring in sporadic PD, suggesting that even modest increases in α-synuclein can initiate nigral degeneration (Golbe and Mouradian, 2004). However, α-synuclein gene multiplication or gene dosage does not appear to be a common cause of familial disease (Gispert et al., 2005; Hofer et al., 2005).

The misfolding, overexpression, and inadequate clearance of wild-type and mutant forms of α-synuclein can all lead to aggregation along with its nitration and adduct formation. But what happens in sporadic PD remains less clear. The presence of α-synuclein in Lewy bodies and Lewy neurites is significant but does not necessarily indicate involvement in pathogenesis (Goedert, 2001; Goedert et al., 2001). There may be a change in the normal physiologic function of α-synuclein that is influenced by altered presynaptic dopaminergic transmission. Dopamine may form adducts with α-synuclein that are more prone to protofibril formation (Conway et al., 2000). However, overexpression of α-synuclein is unlikely to account for Lewy body formation (Kingsbury et al., 2004). The distribution of α-synuclein is not restricted to dopaminergic synaptic boutons (Totterdell et al., 2004), and insoluble filamentous α-synuclein and nitrated α-synuclein are found in most brain regions in A53T mutations (Kotzbauer et al., 2004). This suggests a particular sensitivity of dopaminergic cells to events initiated by α-synuclein if it is a primary cause of pathologic change; but, of course, many nondopaminergic nuclei also degenerate in PD. The clearance of α-synuclein in PD might be impaired by a failure of proteasomal function, and α-synuclein itself can impair proteasomal activity through a direct interaction (Giasson and Lee, 2003). However, wild-type α-synuclein might be removed not only by ubiquitination and proteasomal degradation, and lysosomal mechanisms might be more important (Cuervo et al., 2004; Lee et al., 2004). Interestingly, the construction of the activated 20S proteasome in substantia nigra in PD may be unusual, and this might direct α-synuclein degradation toward lysosomes (see later). Alternatively, the role of α-synuclein, its genetic variants, and its gene load may confer susceptibility to develop sporadic PD rather than direct involvement in the pathogenic process (Pals et al., 2004; Mellick et al., 2005; Mueller et al., 2005; Tan et al., 2005; Mizuta et al., 2006).

The presence of α-synuclein-containing proteinaceous inclusions is not restricted to PD and occurs in a range of other neurodegenerative disorders (Jellinger, 2003; Marti et al., 2003). This has led to the description of a group of diseases as *synucleinopathies* and suggests either a wider role for the toxic effects of α-synuclein or that it is a bystander that is swept up by pathologic processes that occur for a variety of reasons in different cell types. The direct involvement of α-synuclein in dopaminergic cell death is not clearly reflected in many of the transgenic models that have so far been generated (Maries et al., 2003). While some alterations in motor behavior have been observed together with loss of striatal presynaptic dopaminergic terminals and the presence of α-synuclein-positive inclusions, nigral cell loss has not occurred using human wild-type or mutant overexpression or knock-out mice (see Maries et al., 2003, for a review), (Chandra et al., 2004; Shults et al., 2005; Yavich et al., 2005; Martin et al., 2006). Rather, loss of motor neurons and gliosis and a range of other changes have occurred (Giasson et al., 2002).

Mice without α-synuclein are actually resistant to the toxic effects of 1-methyl-4-phenyl-1,2,3,6-tetrahydropyridine (MPTP) (Dauer et al., 2002). Mice that overexpress human α-synuclein show greater mitochondrial abnormalities in response to MPTP treatment than do wild-type mice (Song et al., 2004). This appears to be specific to the striatum and substantia nigra and is associated with the formation of α-synuclein-positive inclusions. Such findings may provide a link to the mitochondrial dysfunction that is known to occur in PD (Beal, 2004). Only in *Drosophila* or *C. elegans* overexpressing wild-type or mutant α-synuclein has dopaminergic neuronal degeneration occurred and then not in every study (Feany and Bender, 2000; Lakso et al., 2003). There is also no agreement as to whether α-synuclein expression in mice protects against toxic insult or increases susceptibility to toxin action (Robertson et al., 2004; Song et al., 2004; Thiruchelvam et al., 2004). Perhaps the problem lies in the extent of α-synuclein expression in different brain regions, since lentiviral or adenosine delivery of wild-type protein or A30P or A53T mutants into rat substantia nigra causes dopaminergic cell death and inclusion formation (Klein et al., 2002; Lo et al., 2002; Yamada et al., 2004). Importantly, however, in human α-synuclein transgenic mice, the generation of antibodies to α-synuclein promoted the degradation of aggregates, possibly by lysosomal pathways (Masliah et al., 2005). This suggests that vaccination might be effective in PD, depending on whether α-synuclein is a key player in pathogenesis and whether aggregates are pathogenic or protective.

A key discovery in familial PD has been the description of *parkin* mutations (*PARK2*) (Kitada et al., 1998). The gene encoding for parkin is large, and multiple *parkin* mutations have been uncovered (see Zhang et al., 2001; Hedrich et al., 2004; Mata et al., 2004, for reviews). Although *parkin* mutations were initially associated with autosomal-recessive juvenile parkinsonism (AR-JP), they now appear to be a major cause of inherited young-onset-disease PD as well as cases of sporadic young-onset disease and some cases of older-onset illness (Dekker et al., 2003; Oliveira et al., 2003; Periquet et al., 2003; Pramstaller et al., 2005; Wu et al., 2005). Parkin is an E3 ubiquitin ligase that is involved in the polyubiquitination of proteins prior to their degradation by the proteasome (Shimura et al., 2000). Mutations of *parkin* invariably lose ubiquitin ligase activity; as a consequence, this impairs normal physiologic handling of proteins (Shimura et al., 2000), but the mechanism that is involved may vary between pathogenic mutations (Henn et al., 2005; Sriram et al., 2005). Dopamine covalently modifies parkin so as to increase parkin insolubility and inactivate its E3 ubiquitin ligase activity (LaVoie et al., 2005). Indeed, in brains from patients with sporadic PD, parkin solubility is decreased, consistent with its functional inactivation.

A variety of substrates for parkin have been identified, including CDCrel-1, synphilin-1, O-glycosylated α-synuclein, PAEL-R and p38 (Cookson, 2003a). One suggestion is that these substrates can potentially be toxic if they are not degraded (Ko et al., 2005; Springer et al., 2005). Indeed, parkin protects monoaminergic neurons against CDCrel-1, α-synuclein, and proteasomal inhibitor toxicity (Petrucelli et al., 2002; Dong et al., 2003). In agreement, the lentiviral delivery of *parkin* prevents the degeneration of nigral dopaminergic neurons induced by A30P α-synuclein in rats (Lo et al., 2004). Parkin may also promote the degradation of mitochondrial substrates involved in apoptosis, and in *parkin* knockout *Drosophila*, altered mitochondrial morphology is observed as well as an upregulation of the JNK signaling pathway (Greene et al., 2003; Cha et al., 2005). Transfection of mutant *parkin* into cell lines increases markers of oxidative and nitrative stress, while these are induced by overexpression of wild-type protein (Hyun et al., 2002). Parkin may also act to inhibit aggresome formation in cells in response to staurosporine or dopamine toxicity, while mutant parkin lacks this action (Muqit et al., 2004). Aggresomes are linked to Lewy body formation, and its inhibition may reduce neuronal survival, suggesting the protective nature of inclusions. Overall, the data that are currently available suggest that parkin has a key role in controlling a number of important pathways leading to neuronal death.

The functional relevance of loss of parkin activity to nigral dopaminergic cell loss has been explored by inactivation of *parkin* using exon 3 knockout in mice, the most common site of mutations in humans (Goldberg et al., 2003; Itier et al., 2003). These animals show alterations in dopaminergic transmission but no damage to the nigrostriatal pathway, except for reduced dopamine transporter levels in the striatum, although such findings are disputed (Perez and Palmiter, 2005). Parkin loss induced decreased mitochondrial activity linked to complex I and IV defects, although no morphologic abnormalities were found (Palacino et al., 2004). Increased oxidative damage and decreased antioxidant capacity also occurred, and these may interact with mitochondrial dysfunction to enhance cell death. Proteomic analysis has shown alterations in energy metabolism, protein handling, and synaptic function in parkin knockout mice (Periquet et al., 2005). In *parkin*-null mice produced by deletion of exon 7, again no damage to the nigrostriatal system was observed, but the number of noradrenergic neurons in the locus coeruleus was reduced (von Coelln et al., 2004), although this too is disputed (Perez and Palmiter, 2005). *Parkin*-null *Drosophila* exhibit mitochondrial pathology and flight muscle degeneration and show alterations in markers associated with oxidative stress and inflammation (Greene et al., 2003, 2005; Pesah et al., 2004; Haywood and Staveley, 2006). Parkin may also have relevance to sporadic PD, since it is present in Lewy bodies (Shimura et al., 1999). Recently, nitrosylation of parkin was demonstrated in vitro and in vivo, leading to a loss of E3 ligase activity (Chung et al., 2004). Importantly, nitrosylated parkin was also detected in brain in PD and following MPTP toxicity. Its formation appears to be linked to nitric oxide (NO) formed from both neuronal nitric oxide synthase (NOS) and glial-derived inducible nitric oxide synthase (i-NOS). Nitrosylated parkin lacks the wild type's ability to protect against toxic insult, and this would be consistent with evidence for an involvement of NO in sporadic PD as well as the induction of nitrative stress in *parkin* mutants resulting from loss of E3 ligase activity.

The gene product of *PARK3* remains unknown, but *PARK5* encodes for UCH-L1, which plays a major role in the decomposition of polyubiquitin chains to monomeric ubiquitin, which is essential for the normal functioning of the ubiquitin-proteasome system (UPS) and hence protein degradation (Leroy et al., 1998). The mutant enzyme has 50% of the activity of the wild-type form, but the pathogenic nature of this

mutation has been disputed. Inhibition of UCH-L1 in cultures of fetal mesencephalic dopaminergic cells causes neuronal death, but there is no other evidence of toxicity (McNaught, Mytilineou, et al., 2002). However, very recently, a key function of UCH-L1 was shown to be its ability to bind to and stabilize monomeric ubiquitin in neurons (Osaka et al., 2003). It has also been suggested that reduced UCH-L1 function might jeopardize the survival of CNS neurons (Lombardino et al., 2005). In gracile axonal dystrophy mice, dysfunction of UCH-L1 leads to increased oxidation of specific proteins, suggesting a link to the oxidative stress that is known to occur during nigral degeneration in PD (Castegna et al., 2004). These mice also show inclusion formation; however, these contain β- and γ-synuclein and not α-synuclein (Wang et al., 2004). In addition, UCH-L1 may play a role in inclusion formation in PD through aggresome formation (Ardley et al., 2004). Recently, an inverse association between the polymorphic S18Y variant of UCH-L1 and PD was detected that was most apparent in younger cases (Elbaz et al., 2003; Maraganore et al., 2004). This is the only polymorphism that has so far been investigated, and it might act by preventing the dimerization of UCH-L1 necessary for normal enzyme activity. How this then leads to susceptibility to develop PD is unknown.

*PARK6* encodes for PTEN-induced kinase 1 (PINK1) in families with autosomal-recessive early-onset PD (Valente et al., 2004a). A variety of mutations have now been reported suggesting that PINK1 might be a common defect gene rivaling *parkin* (Hatano et al., 2004; Rohe et al., 2004). While PINK1 may not be associated with most common forms of PD, there might be an association with sporadic early-onset disease (Groen et al., 2004; Hatano et al., 2004; Healy et al., 2004; Rohe et al., 2004; Valente et al., 2004b; Albanese et al., 2005; Bonifati et al., 2005; Deng et al., 2005; Fung et al., 2006; Ibanez et al., 2006). PINK1 is a putative mitochondrial kinase with a proven mitochondrial localization for both the wild-type and mutated forms (Silvestri et al., 2005). PINK1 mutations confer different autophosphorylation activity that is regulated by the C-terminal of the protein. The mutation does not alter production of the full-length protein, suggesting no effect on its stability. How a mutation in PINK1 causes nigral cell degeneration is not known, but it might alter mitochondrial function. The G309D PINK1 mutation by itself had no effect on mitochondrial membrane potential in transfected cells, but in the presence of the proteasomal inhibitor MG-132, it was decreased, an effect that was not observed with the wild-type protein. Consistent with this, wild-type PINK1 overexpression protected against MG-132-induced apoptosis, but this did not occur with the E309D mutant. So overall, PINK1 appears protective, and at least the E309D mutant lacks this protective activity.

The gene product DJ-1 arising from *PARK7* was recently described in familial early-onset PD (Abou-Sleiman et al., 2003; Bonifati et al., 2003; Hague et al., 2003), although mutations appear rare (Clark et al., 2004) and may occur also in parkinsonism-dementia-amyotropic lateral sclerosis complex (Annesi et al., 2005) Wild-type DJ-1 is abundant in the brain, but the m-RNA has greater expression in subcortical tissues. In human brain, DJ-1 is markedly expressed by astrocytes, and only small amounts appear to be in neurons (Bandopadhyay et al., 2004, 2005). In rat brain, DJ-1 is ubiquitously expressed in neurons, with low expression in astrocytes, but in the mouse, there is expression in both neurons and all glial cell types (Bader et al., 2005; Bandopadhyay et al., 2005). In idiopathic PD, DJ-1 does not appear to be a major constituent of Lewy bodies, and polymorphisms are not associated with sporadic PD or DLB (Morris et al., 2003; Clark et al., 2004; Lockhart et al., 2004). It is perhaps important that oxidative damage of DJ-1 has been demonstrated in idiopathic PD (Choi et al., 2006), although many other proteins are also known to be oxidized. Perhaps surprisingly, levels of DJ-1 are increased in CSF in idiopathic PD, but this might be a response to oxidative stress (Waragai et al., 2006). DJ-1 may play a role in a variety of other neurodegenerative diseases in humans, as it is abundantly expressed in astrocytes in a wide range of disorders (Neumann et al., 2004). It is also found to be associated with neuronal tau inclusions. In mice that overexpress A30P α-synuclein, DJ-1 is present in astrocytes in the brainstem.

The function of DJ-1 is not known. It is a hydroperoxide-responsive protein that responds to oxidative stress produced by $H_2O_2$ or paraquat (Mitsumoto et al., 2001). Indeed, downregulation of DJ-1 enhances cell death due to oxidative stress and alters the expression of genes related to oxidative stress and apoptosis (Yokota et al., 2003; Martinat et al., 2004; Nishinaga et al., 2005). It might act by buffering cytosolic redox changes produced by such oxidative insults. DJ-1 forms a dimer that is necessary for its biologic activity, and the mutation might prevent this from occurring. In patients with the mutation, the level of L166P is low, and the turnover is more rapid than that of the wild-type protein, suggesting instability (Macedo et al., 2003). Both the loss of dimer formation and increased turnover might contribute to a loss of function (Cookson, 2003b; Moore et al., 2003). Wild-type DJ-1 is present in both the cytoplasm and nucleus of cells, and there is some localization to mitochondria, which is not different from that seen with mutants (Blackinton et al., 2005; Zhang et al., 2005a). However, the mitochondrial localization of DJ-1 is increased by oxidative stress. This appears to be due to a shift in the nuclear and mitochondrial distribution of the protein driven by the acidification of a key cysteine residue during oxidative stress (Canet-Aviles et al., 2004). This might be highly important, as under normal circumstances DJ-1 may function as a transcriptional coactivator and inhibit apoptosis by an interaction with a number of nuclear proteins, such as p54nrb and Daxx (Junn et al., 2005; Xu et al., 2005). There may also be interactions between DJ-1 and both parkin and α-synuclein that may be enhanced under conditions of oxidative stress (Meulener et al., 2005; Moore et al., 2005). As with other gene defects in familial PD, attempts to produce a transgenic model have been largely unsuccessful. Inactivation of DJ-1 in mice does not cause nigral cell degeneration, although dopaminergic transmission is altered (Goldberg et al., 2005). DJ-1-deficient mice are, however, more sensitive to MPTP toxicity and to oxidative stress (Kim et al., 2005). In *Drosophila*, DJ-1 is important in protecting against oxidative stress, but its deficiency does not lead to the degeneration of dopaminergic neurons (Moore et al., 2006).

*PARK8* is a common cause of autosomal-dominant PD of varying phenotype (Funayama et al., 2002). Very recently, two missense mutations in *PARK8* were associated with the production of a previously unknown protein, leucine-rich repeat kinase 2 (LRRK2, also called dardarin), in familial PD (Paisan-Ruiz et al., 2004; Zimprich et al., 2004), and more recently, other mutations have been detected (Skipper et al., 2005; Zabetian et al., 2005). Mutations in LRRK2 are important,

since they have proved to be the most common cause of familial and sporadic PD so far uncovered. The G2019S mutation, which is the most frequent form, appears to be responsible for up to 6% of autosomal-dominant cases (Di et al., 2005; Kachergus et al., 2005; Lesage et al., 2005; Mata et al., 2005; Nichols et al., 2005) and up to 8% of sporadic cases (Gilks et al., 2005; Goldwurm et al., 2005; Infante et al., 2006; Kay et al., 2006), although there are marked variations between populations (Bialecka et al., 2005; Biskup et al., 2005; Farrer et al., 2005; Funayama et al., 2005), with a particularly high prevalence in the North African Arab population (Lesage et al., 2006) and in the Ashkenazi Jewish population (Ozelius et al., 2006).

The phenotype of disease resembles classical PD (Adams et al., 2005; Khan et al., 2005; Paisan-Ruiz et al., 2005a, 2005b) but is diverse in nature and although initially associated with late onset PD, LRRK2 mutations have recently been found in early onset cases (Goldwurm et al., 2005; Hedrich et al., 2006). The pathology is pleomorphic, with patients having or not having Lewy bodies and other histopathologic features (Zimprich et al., 2004). Mutations have generally not, however, been found in other neurodegenerative diseases (Hernandez et al., 2005). LRRK2 and its mRNA are found both in the peripheral and central nervous system and are widely distributed in the brain (Paisan-Ruiz et al., 2004; Zimprich et al., 2004; Giasson et al., 2006; Simon-Sanchez et al., 2006; Taymans et al., 2006). LRRK2 is a complex cytosolic protein that belongs to the ROCO superfamily and possesses multiple functions. LRRK2 has a kinase domain that may be crucial to its pathogenic actions and that shows homology to MAP kinase kinase kinases. LRRK2 mutations show increased phosphorylation activity that suggests a gain of function rather than loss of activity (West et al., 2005; Gloeckner et al., 2006). Expression of LRRK2 mutations in cells leads to degeneration associated with inclusion formation (Greggio et al., 2006). Inactivation of the kinase domain delays cell death and prevents inclusion formation, supporting its importance in pathogenesis in PD.

The gene products of *PARK9, PARK10,* and *PARK11* remain unknown.

A recent report showed mutations in the *NR4A2* (Nurr1) gene associated with late-onset PD leading to a decrease in Nurr1 mRNA levels (Le et al., 2003). Although this has proved difficult to replicate (Levecque et al., 2004; Nichols et al., 2004), Nurr1 is essential for the differentiation and survival of dopaminergic neurons, thus making it highly relevant to nigral cell death (Saucedo-Cardenas et al., 1998; Le et al., 1999). Loss of dopaminergic neurons in Nurr1 knockout mice strongly supports a role in PD, but further study is necessary to discover its true pathogenic nature and relevance to PD in humans.

There appears to be an association of mutations in the β-glucocerebrosidase gene and PD in the Ashkenazi Jewish population (Aharon-Peretz et al., 2004, 2005; Clark et al., 2005). In a study of autopsy-proven synucleinopathies, mutations in the glucocerebrosidase gene were found in 23% of cases of dementia with Lewy bodies (Goker-Alpan et al., 2006). Large numbers of other potential candidates for susceptibility genes for sporadic PD, including those for dopamine-related events, cytochrome P450, and antioxidant enzymes have been investigated, but overall, very little has so far emerged in terms of identifying factors that fit into the known pathologic processes occurring in the substantia nigra (Riedl et al., 1998; Jenner, 1999; Olanow and Tatton, 1999).

The task is challenging, however, because of the lack of knowledge of the primary pathologic processes that occur in PD, the random nature by which potential susceptibility genes are selected, and the presence of several hundred potential gene changes in nigral tissue, the importance of which remains to be assessed (Hauser et al., 2003; Toda et al., 2003). A meta-analysis of 14 individuals' gene polymorphisms shows associations of PD with NAT-2, type B MAO, glutathione transferase-1, and a mitochondrial gene (Tan et al., 2000). However, complete genomic screens in PD have concluded that either no specific linkage was involved or multiple genetic factors may be important (DeStefano et al., 2001; Scott et al., 2001; Mellick et al., 2004). Interestingly, *PARK10* has recently been proposed as a susceptibility gene for late-onset sporadic PD (Hicks et al., 2002).

## ENVIRONMENTAL FACTORS AND PARKINSON DISEASE

There is convincing evidence for environmental factors contributing to the occurrence of PD. Epidemiologic studies have previously suggested a role for industrialization and exposure to agrochemicals as risk factors in late-onset disease and for rural environment and the drinking of well water as increasing risk in early-onset illness (Di Monte et al., 2002). Other factors that might be important include wood preservatives, heavy metals, solvents, exhaust fumes, head trauma, and general anesthesia, although most remain controversial (Seidler et al., 1996). Specific toxins that are known to cause parkinsonism in humans include MPTP, isoquinolines, β-carbolines, n-hexane, carbon monoxide, carbon disulfide, and manganese (Aaserud et al., 1988; Neafsey et al., 1989; McNaught et al., 1998; Pal et al., 1999; Pezzoli et al., 2000; Choi, 2002). In some cases, such as the involvement of manganese toxicity in parkinsonism among welders, there is considerable controversy (Jankovic, 2005; McMillan, 2005; Fored et al., 2006; Park et al., 2006) It is perhaps important that caffeine consumption, cigarette smoking, and use of aspirin and nonsteroidal anti-inflammatory drugs are routinely proposed as decreasing the risk of developing PD (Ascherio et al., 2001; Hernan et al., 2001; Chen et al., 2003; Allam et al., 2004). Recent studies have again confirmed the protective effects of cigarette smoking (Galanaud et al., 2005; Scott et al., 2005; Wirdefeldt et al., 2005) The effects of caffeine appear clear in men but not in premenopausal woman, suggesting an involvement of estrogen (Ascherio et al., 2004). In contrast, the protective effects of aspirin and NSAIDs in PD have been repeatedly questioned for their validity (Chen et al., 2005; Hernan et al., 2006; Ton et al., 2006)

Epidemiologic studies have repeatedly found a connection between the use of agrochemicals and the risk of developing PD (Seidler et al., 1996; Liou et al., 1997; Priyadarshi et al., 2000), in particular, previous long-term use of herbicides and pesticides, notably paraquat, organochlorines, and alkylated phosphates (Liu et al., 2003; Kamel and Hoppin, 2004; Ascherio et al., 2006; Brown et al., 2006; Frigerio et al., 2006). The risk from pesticides is increased in those who are poor CYP2D6 metabolizers (Elbaz et al., 2004). This has led to important experimental studies of pesticide and herbicide toxicity to nigral dopaminergic neurons.

The herbicide paraquat has a close structural resemblance to the active metabolite of MPTP, MPP[+]. This was recognized at the time of the discovery of MPTP, and intranigral injection of paraquat can selectively destroy dopaminergic neurons (Fredriksson et al., 1993). However, paraquat is a highly charged molecule, and it was thought that it did not pass the blood-brain barrier or cause nigral damage on systemic administration (Widdowson et al., 1996a, 1996b). This was despite some studies showing that systemic paraquat administration depletes striatal dopamine content and induces behavioral change (Endo et al., 1988; Fredriksson et al., 1993). Recently, however, repeated intraperitoneal injections of paraquat in mice and rats were shown to cause selective toxicity to nigral dopaminergic neurons (Brooks et al., 1999; McCormack et al., 2002; Ossowska et al., 2005a, 2005b, 2006). There was no dopamine loss in the striatum, but dopamine turnover was increased. Treatment with L-valine, L-phenylalanine, or L-dopa prevented paraquat toxicity, suggesting that it is transported into the brain by the neutral amino acid transporter (McCormack and Di Monte, 2003). Perhaps, importantly, in vitro paraquat increases α-synuclein fibril formation (an effect that is also seen with rotenone and dieldrin; see later), while paraquat toxicity to substantia nigra is associated with increased levels of α-synuclein and aggregate formation (Uversky et al., 2001; Manning-Bog et al., 2002). Indeed, paraquat induced nigral toxicity is prevented by overexpression of human wild-type or A53T α-synuclein in mice, although aggregate formation still occurs (Manning-Bog et al., 2003). Decreased toxicity is associated with increased levels of HSP70, which is known to be associated with protection against paraquat toxicity. The potential toxicity of paraquat to dopaminergic neurons might be enhanced by other agrochemicals; combined treatment with the dithiocarbamate fungicide maneb appears to have synergistic effects (Thiruchelvam et al., 2000a, 2000b, 2002). This might be due to alterations in synaptosomal dopamine content and brain levels of paraquat (Barlow et al., 2003).

Another commonly used pesticide, dieldrin, might also have potentially toxic effects on dopaminergic neurons (Sanchez-Ramos et al., 1998; Kanthasamy et al., 2005; Richardson et al., 2006). Dieldrin can deplete brain dopamine content, induce abnormal motor behaviors, and inhibit mitochondrial function. Importantly, dieldrin was toxic by apoptotic mechanisms to dopaminergic cells in culture, although it also has some toxicity to GABAergic cells (Kitazawa et al., 2001). The effects that were observed were suppressed by antioxidants, suggesting the involvement of oxidative stress. Recently, dieldrin (and other pesticides) were shown to inhibit proteasomal function, which may contribute to dopaminergic cell death (Wang et al., 2006).

The pesticide rotenone is also toxic to dopaminergic nigrostriatal neurons. Rotenone is of particular interest because it is naturally occurring, being a constituent of a range of plants, notably derris. Rotenone is highly lipophilic and a known inhibitor of complex I of the mitochondrial respiratory chain, a deficiency that also occurs in the substantia nigra in PD (see later).

Focal injection of rotenone into the nigrostriatal pathway or chronic systemic administration of rotenone to rats results in a selective inhibition of complex I and is reported to cause motor deficits and selective destruction of the nigrostriatal pathway associated with the presence of α-synuclein- and ubiquitin-positive inclusions (Betarbet et al., 2000; Alam et al., 2004; Saravanan et al., 2005). However, rotenone does not selectively accumulate in nigral cells, and more widespread basal ganglia and brain degeneration affecting 5HT, noradrenergic, and cholinergic neurons can occur, reflecting generalized impairment of mitochondrial function (Hoglinger et al., 2003b; Perier et al., 2003).

Rotenone toxicity appears to be initiated by its mitochondrial actions, since transfection of cells with a rotenone-insensitive single-subunit NADH dehydrogenase as a replacement for complex I blocks its actions (Sherer et al., 2003). Cell death is mediated by cytochrome c– and caspase-3–dependent apoptosis, but this is associated with oxidative stress and oxidative damage (Sherer et al., 2002; Ahmadi et al., 2003). NO might also play a role, since rotenone treatment induces NOS activity in both the striatum and the substantia nigra (He et al., 2003; Bashkatova et al., 2004). The effects of rotenone are prevented by a neuronal NOS inhibitor 7-NI, but its toxicity appears also dependent on the presence of microglial cells (Gao et al., 2002). In agreement, there is synergistic toxicity between rotenone and the inflammogen lipopolysaccharide (LPS) that acts to activate glial cells (Gao et al., 2003; Ling et al., 2004).

So there are three examples of commonly available agrochemicals that can have degenerative effects within the basal ganglia, and at the present time, it remains unknown how many other substances in either manufactured or natural forms might also be toxic. For example, fruit and tea from annonaceae species contain annonacin, a lipophilic complex I inhibitor that produces nigral and striatal degeneration in rats and might be responsible for atypical parkinsonism in Guadeloupe (Caparros-Lefebvre, 2004; Champy et al., 2004).

## PATHOGENIC MECHANISMS IN PARKINSON DISEASE

The pathogenic mechanisms that are involved in PD have been extensively investigated by using postmortem tissues and by the study of the actions of toxins such as 6-hydroxydopamine and MPTP (Olanow et al., 1998, 2002). Not surprisingly, the vast majority of work has centered on the events that occur in the substantia nigra, and relatively little is known about the same processes in other areas of the brain that are affected by pathologic change. These studies have uncovered important clues to the biochemical events that take place during cell death in PD and have led to a more detailed understanding of the sequence of change that occurs. However, a remarkable amount remains that is unknown, and some of the following illustrates the complexity of the current situation.

Dopaminergic neurons in the substantia nigra pars compacta (SNc) in PD will die either by necrosis or by programmed cell death (also known as apoptosis). For some years, controversy has existed over whether apoptosis is the major route for cellular degeneration in the SNc. Morphologic criteria for defining apoptosis have not been met in a number of the studies involving postmortem tissues from patients with PD, leading to its dismissal as the cell death mechanism. Equally, measures of nuclear DNA cleavage using TUNEL have been equivocal, with reports of no labeling, high levels of labeling in control tissues, or labeling being restricted to glial cells (Anglade et al., 1995; Walkinshaw and Waters, 1995; Olanow et al., 1998). The reasons for the variation between the ability of different studies to detect apoptotic cells appear

diverse. There are many methodologic issues as well as effects of postmortem delay and methods of tissue fixation (Charriaut-Mariangue, 1995; Petito and Roberts, 1995; Kingsbury et al., 1998; Tatton et al., 1998; Tatton and Rideout, 1999). But the most rigorous studies, utilizing a range of approaches to the detection of DNA cleavage, have arrived at figures of 1% or fewer of dopaminergic cells in the SNc undergoing apoptotic change, which would be consistent with the rate of progression of PD. The involvement of apoptosis in dopaminergic cell death is also strongly supported by a variety of in vitro and in vivo studies showing its involvement in the actions of toxins such as 6-OHDA and MPTP/MPP+ (Dipasquale et al., 1991; Mochizuki et al., 1994; Walkinshaw and Waters, 1995).

Biochemical markers of the cascades involved in apoptosis have caused equal controversy in postmortem studies of PD (Tatton et al., 2003). Both caspase-dependent and caspase-independent pathways have been proposed as being involved. Thus, there are reports in PD of increases in the antiapoptotic protein Bcl-2 and the proapoptotic protein Bax and caspase 3 in remaining dopaminergic neurons in the SNc, indicating the involvement of mitochondria in this process (Marshall et al., 1997; Hartmann et al., 2000; Tatton, 2000). But in addition, there are increased levels of the tumor suppressor protein p53 and nuclear translocation of glyceraldehyde-3-phosphate dehydrogenase, both of which are involved in apoptotic cascades (Ferrer et al., 2000; Tatton, 2000). But other studies have failed to show any change in a range of markers of apoptotic cell death in neurons, although these could be seen in glial cells (Jellinger, 2000). Inflammation in PD linked to glial cell activation leads to upregulation of the tumor necrosis factor (TNF) receptor superfamily and specifically to alterations in Fas and its adapter protein FADD that then activate caspase 8, leading to apoptosis, all of which have been shown to occur in postmortem nigral tissue (Mogi et al., 1996; Ferrer et al., 2000; Hartmann et al., 2001, 2002).

The complexity of the range and variety of biochemical processes involved in the initiation and control of apoptotic cell death in relation to PD has been extensively reviewed (Tatton and Chalmers-Redman, 1996; Tatton and Olanow, 1999; Jellinger, 2000; Tatton et al., 2003). Despite the controversy that exists, it appears very likely that apoptosis does play some role in pathologic change occurring in the SNc in PD. The importance might lie in the manner in which these processes converge to alter mitochondrial function by causing a lowering of mitochondrial membrane potential that leads to the opening of the permeability transition pore and the release of cytochrome c, which then initiates caspase cascades leading to apoptosis (Tatton et al., 1994, 2003; Tatton and Chalmers-Redman, 1996).

In contrast, it is clear that a range of specific biochemical events occur during the degeneration of dopaminergic neurons, including oxidative stress, mitochondrial dysfunction, excitotoxicity, and the toxic effects of NO/peroxynitrite (Jenner, 1991, 1993, 2003; Jenner, Dexter, et al., 1992; Jenner, Schapira, et al., 1992; Jenner and Olanow, 1998; Olanow et al., 2002; Halliwell, 2006; Schapira, 2006). These processes have been extensively investigated and form an intertwined series of events that occur once cell death has been initiated at any point in this cascade. For example, mitochondrial dysfunction leads to the production of reactive oxygen species, while reactive oxygen species can lead to mitochondrial dysfunction. So the wheel turns, and it becomes almost impossible to disentangle the events in terms of which is an initiator and which is secondary to some primary event. However, there are some components within the biochemical sequence of change that require further discussion as to their specific role in the pathogenesis of PD.

The evidence for oxidative stress occurring in the substantia nigra in PD is based on a series of observations showing elevations in the level of iron, alterations in levels of iron-binding proteins, increased levels of Mn-SOD, and decreased levels of reduced glutathione (GSH) (Olanow et al., 2002). This leads to oxidative damage, since there is evidence for increased lipid peroxidation, DNA damage, and increased protein oxidation. Many of these changes also occur in other neurodegenerative diseases, but the decrease in nigral GSH content was thought to be selective to PD and not to occur in other areas of the brain or in related illnesses. However, recently, decreased GSH levels were also found in the substantia nigra in multiple-system atrophy and progressive supranuclear palsy, suggesting that, like other indices of oxidative stress, it is neither selective nor specific to PD (Fitzmaurice et al., 2003). Another mystery relates to the source of the reactive oxygen species responsible for causing oxidative stress and oxidative damage in PD. There is virtually no direct evidence of increased formation of $H_2O_2$ or $O_2$ radicals, although these might originate from changes in mitochondrial function or from the release of dopamine from the vesicular monoamine transporter (Jenner, 2003). Indeed, oxidative stress and damage might be more a result of the excessive formation of NO and/or peroxynitrite (see later).

Inhibition of complex I of the mitochondrial respiratory chain in the substantia nigra in PD and the known complex I inhibitory effects of rotenone and $MPP^+$ suggest one obvious pathogenic mechanism (Schapira et al., 1990; Mann et al., 1994). The role of mitochondria in pathogenesis in PD has received considerable attention recently because of the ability of mutant proteins in familial PD to alter mitochondrial function (Beal, 2005; Poon et al., 2005; Ved et al., 2005; Kwong et al., 2006; Muqit et al., 2006). Complex I inhibition may also result in platelet and muscle in PD, although there has continued to be dispute over whether this occurs or not (Winkler-Stuck et al., 2005). Certainly, complex I inhibition will induce free radical formation, oxidative stress, and excitotoxicity, leading to apoptotic cell death, and thus would be consistent with current concepts of neuronal destruction in PD. Studies of complex I encoding have failed to find any consistent defect explaining the loss of enzyme activity. However, it has been proposed that complex I inhibition might result from clusters of mitochondrial DNA polymorphisms (Autere et al., 2004). This is supported by the construction of cybrids using platelet mitochondrial DNA from patients with PD. These show complex I deficiency associated with oxidative stress, suggesting that the decrease in activity in PD is linked to gene encoding (Cassarino et al., 1997; Veech et al., 2000). Recently, high levels of mitochondrial DNA deletions have been found in the substantia nigra, both in the aged brain and in PD, that are of functional importance (Bender et al., 2006; Kraytsberg et al., 2006). In addition, there are oxidatively damaged subunits that are functionally impaired and misassembled (Keeney et al., 2006).

The degree of complex I deficiency that causes functional defects in adenosine triphosphate (ATP) production has been debated. But in PD, there is also a deficiency in α-ketoglutarate dehydrogenase activity, a key Krebs cycle enzyme (Mizuno et al., 1994). Together, they may exert a greater effect than either defect alone. Complex I defects do not occur in all patients with PD, since the distribution of values for control individuals show a considerable overlap with those for PD. Indeed, only a proportion of patients with PD have complex I levels that are more than two standard deviations below the mean for the control group. So there is a subset of patients with PD in whom mitochondrial deficits might be a primary contributor to nigral degeneration, but in others, complex I inhibition might not be the major factor underlying neuronal destruction.

Excitotoxicity through the excessive action of glutamate has been proposed as a component of cell death mechanisms in PD (Beal, 1992; Green and Greenamyre, 1996). Excitotoxicity might occur as a result of vulnerability of dopaminergic neurons to physiologic concentrations for glutamate through weak excitotoxic mechanisms over long periods of time. However, there does not appear to be any direct evidence that this is the case. Excitotoxicity could be generated as a result of the overactivity of the subthalamic nucleus in PD, leading to increased glutamatergic transmission to the internal globus pallidus and to the zona reticulata of the substantia nigra or indeed changes in other glutamatergic pathways innervating the basal ganglia (Rodriguez et al., 1998). While subthalamic nucleus overactivity certainly occurs in PD (DeLong, 1990), there is little evidence to suggest that it contributes to the pathogenic process. Excitotoxicity could also arise as a result of alterations in mitochondrial function, but as has already been argued, this might not be a consistent event in all cases of PD. The bulk of the evidence for excitotoxicity stems from the use of experimental models of PD in which glutamate antagonists are able to protect against the toxic effects of MPTP, $MPP^+$, or 6-hydroxydopamine in mice, rats, or primates (Turski et al., 1991).

The results of such studies have been controversial; for example, Jenner (unpublished data) was unable to show any effects of either glutamate antagonists riluzole or remacemide in protecting against a partial 6-hydroxydopamine lesion of the nigrostriatal pathway in the rat. Whether these models systems are representative of the pathogenic events that occur in PD is debatable; since the evidence for excitotoxicity is low, the ineffectiveness of riluzole as a neuroprotectant in PD (Rascol et al., 2003) argues that such strategies might not be of functional significance.

In contrast to other pathogenic mechanisms occurring in PD, there appears to be increasingly strong evidence that reactive nitrogen species rather than reactive oxygen species may have a key role to play. In PD itself, there is activation of i-NOS in glial cells and evidence of peroxynitrite formation and nitrative damage to proteins in the substantia nigra and the presence of nitrated α-synuclein in Lewy bodies (Hunot et al., 1996; Good et al., 1998; Duda et al., 2000; Giasson et al., 2000). Peroxynitrite is highly reactive and is formed as a result of the interaction of NO with superoxide. It degrades to produce a number of different species, among which are the highly toxic hydroxyl radical and which explain the oxidative stress and oxidative damage occurring in substantia nigra in PD. Other evidence (Moncada and Bolanos, 2006) for the involvement of NO comes from the protection that is afforded against MPTP toxicity by selective i-NOS and neuronal NOS (n-NOS) inhibitors, although some of these findings have been disputed (Schulz et al., 1995; Hantraye et al., 1996; Mackenzie et al., 1997). Additionally, both i-NOS and n-NOS knockout mice show resistance to the toxicity of MPTP to dopaminergic cells (Przedborski et al., 1996; Liberatore et al., 1999). So at least for reactive nitrogen species, there is evidence of increased formation, evidence of their toxicity and evidence from experimental models to support the concept that NO/peroxynitrite formation might be an important mechanism in the pathogenesis of PD.

The processes leading to nigral cell death in PD are commonly attributed to events occurring solely within the dopaminergic neurons. However, oxidative stress, mitochondrial dysfunction, excitotoxicity, and NO toxicity also occur in a range of other neurodegenerative diseases and cause some concern as to their roles as a specific primary cause of pathogenesis in PD. In addition, the extent to which changes in biochemical parameters occur in human postmortem nigral tissue in PD cannot be explained solely by neuronal involvement. The increase in iron content, the decrease in GSH concentration, the decrease in complex I activity, and the decrease in proteasomal enzyme activity (see later), all occur to the same degree (30% to 40%). These are assessed in tissue homogenates in which dopaminergic neurons make up only 1% to 2% of the total number of cells, and it is hence impossible for alterations of 30% to 40% to occur solely within that neuronal population. This implies that other cells are also contributors to the pathogenic process, and the most likely type of cell would be glial cells (see later). Indeed, alterations in iron content and in GSH occur in glial cells in the substantia nigra in PD. So the nature of the cell type remains in question, as does the nature of the pathogenic process and the identification of those components that merely form part of the cell death cascade against those events that are relevant to the primary mechanism initiating neuronal loss in PD.

## A NEW WAY FORWARD?

Most of the pathogenic events that have been studied in depth in PD appear to be part of a closely integrated cascade initiated as cell death progresses. It would be comforting if these events provided a handle with which to interfere in the cell death process and thus halt or slow neurodegeneration. However, it appears unlikely that interference in any one point in this cascade will stop the inevitable descent to neuronal death. So what can be done that is directly related to events occurring in PD and that might lead to understanding primary alterations in cellular function that initiate rather than follow the cascade so far unraveled. Two possibilities seem to point in directions that have more direct relevance to pathogenesis in PD as currently understood. The first is the concept that cell death in PD is inevitably accompanied by glial cell activation and inflammatory change (for review, see Hunot and Hirsch, 2003; Teismann et al., 2003b; Herrera et al., 2005). The second is that there is a common link between familial and sporadic forms of PD in the form of alterations in the handling of mutant or damaged proteins (for review, see McNaught, Olanow, et al., 2001). Both seem to be highly relevant to events occurring in humans and also may provide model systems with which to evaluate potential neuroprotective drugs and that truly reflect the cell death process.

## GLIAL CELLS AND PARKINSON DISEASE

Pathologic change in substantia nigra in PD is accompanied by a reactive microgliosis and, to a lesser extent, astrocytosis (McGeer et al., 1988; Damier et al., 1993; Banati et al., 1998) that occurs early in the disease course (Ouchi et al., 2005). While microglia activation appears to be associated with neuronal degeneration, there is an inverse relationship between the localization of GFAP-positive astroglial cells and surviving dopaminergic neurons (Damier et al., 1993). Inflammatory change is indicated by increased levels of a range of cytokines, including IL-Iβ, IL-6, TNF-α, and IFN-γ in cerebrospinal fluid and brain tissue (Boka et al., 1994; Hunot et al., 1999; Nagatsu et al., 2000). This leads to an induction of i-NOS and COX-1 and -2 and their product prostaglandin-2 in the substantia nigra in PD (Hunot et al., 1996; Knott et al., 2000). There is also upregulation of the macrophage cell surface antigen CD23, which may activate other glial cells and cause i-NOS induction (Hunot et al., 1999). TNF-α acts on receptors on dopaminergic neurons to cause the nuclear translocation of $NF_{K\beta}$ and apoptotic cascades that are observed in the substantia nigra in PD (Hunot et al., 1997). It is also possible that peripheral mediators are involved in nigral inflammatory change, and there may be alterations in vascularization of substantia nigra in PD, allowing the entry of T-cells (Faucheux et al., 1999; Farkas et al., 2000; Barcia et al., 2005a; Kortekaas et al., 2005).

Two important aspects of the gliosis and inflammatory change that occur in PD may have relevance to the rate of disease progression. First, evidence from MPTP-exposed humans and primates shows that microglial cell activation is still present years after toxin exposure (Langston et al., 1999; Hurley et al., 2003; Barcia et al., 2004). This might suggest that once initiated, it serves to perpetuate cell death, although this has not been demonstrated, or, alternatively, that damage to the blood-brain barrier occurs as a result of toxin action, as occurs with 6-OHDA (Carvey et al., 2005), thus allowing peripheral monocytes to establish an inflammatory presence in the substantia nigra. This may involve the intracellular adhesion molecule-1 (ICAM-1) that is present in astrocytes in both patients with PD and MPTP-treated monkeys (Miklossy et al., 2006). In addition, plasma levels of TNF-α are elevated a year following MPTP treatment of primates (Barcia et al., 2005b). Second, the risk of developing PD in individuals who regularly use nonsteroidal anti-inflammatory drugs or two or more aspirin per day may be reduced (but see later).

Under normal circumstances, glial cells support neuronal function and increase survival through the production of trophic factors such as brain-derived neurotrophic factor and glial-derived neurotrophic factor. However, in vitro and in vivo activation of glial cells using the bacterial endotoxin LPS leads to a reduction in brain-derived neurotrophic factor and glial-derived neurotrophic factor secretion while increasing levels of superoxide, hydrogen peroxide, glutamate, NO, cytokines, and TNF-α (McNaught and Jenner, 2000a, 2000b; Chang et al., 2001; McNaught, Lee, et al., 2001; Gao et al., 2002). Hence, a number of potentially toxic substances are produced; and cocultured with dopaminergic neurons, activated glial cells induce neuronal death and potentiate the toxic actions of 6-OHDA and MPP+ (McNaught and Jenner, 1999; Le et al., 2001).

The acute or chronic intranigral application of LPS also leads to dopaminergic cell death as a result of both microglial and astroglial activation (Castano et al., 1998; Herrera et al., 2000). LPS might alter the permeability of the blood-brain barrier, allowing the entry of mononuclear cells that contribute to neuronal loss (Ng and Ling, 1997). It might be presumed that cytokine production is responsible for the LPS-mediated effect. However, intranigral application of proinflammatory cytokines TNF-$\alpha$, IL-1$\beta$, and IFN-$\gamma$ failed to reproduce its actions (Castano et al., 2002). Marked induction of i-NOS occurs in microglial cells that appears to produce toxicity through NO or peroxynitrite formation as levels of 3-nitrotyrosine (3-NT) immunoreactivity increase, indicating nitrative damage to proteins (Iravani et al., 2002). The role of NO is emphasized by the ability of a selective i-NOS inhibitor to partially prevent the loss of nigral dopaminergic neurons. Since NO may play a key role in pathogenesis in PD, these findings might have relevance to potential neuroprotective strategies aimed at preventing disease progression.

An illustration of the potential protective effects is shown by the ability of the glucocortioid dexamethasone to prevent glial cell activation and to protect against LPS toxicity to nigral dopaminergic neurons (Castano et al., 2002). However, methylprednisolone increases LPS toxicity to neurons, arguing against a steroid-induced approach to neuroinflammation. LPS toxicity is also inhibited by the nonsteroidal anti-inflammatory drug indomethacin and the anti-inflammatory antibiotic minocycline, although the neuroprotective effects of the latter are disputed (Shibata et al., 2003; Diguet et al., 2004; Tomas-Camardiel et al., 2004). The latter prevent glial cell activation and reduce nitrative damage. However, these drugs might not be acting through COX-linked mechanisms, since selective COX-2 inhibitors did not exert similar effects and minocycline has a range of other activities.

As in PD, toxin-based destruction of nigral dopaminergic cells using 6-OHDA, MPTP, or MPP$^+$ induces an inflammatory response that is characterized by both activated microglial and astroglial cells (Kohutnicka et al., 1998; Kurkowska-Jastrzebska et al., 1999; Sugama et al., 2003). This is accompanied by increased cytokine production, i-NOS expression, 3-NT immunoreactivity, and COX-2 levels, showing a marked similarity to events that occur in humans (Teismann et al., 2003a). In a manner similar to that of LPS-induced cell death, aspirin, salicylate, and other anti-inflammatory agents, such as dexamethasone and minocycline, reduce MPTP or MPP$^+$ toxicity with corresponding reductions in markers of inflammatory response, i-NOS, and nitrative damage (Wu et al., 2002; Sairam et al., 2003; Maharaj et al., 2004). Whether these effects are mediated through COX pathways and prostaglandin synthesis is debated. In COX-2 knockout mice, the toxicity of MPTP to dopaminergic neurons is reduced, while COX-1 knockout has no effect (Teismann et al., 2003a). The selective COX-2 inhibitor rofecoxib also reduced MPTP toxicity in mice. However, neither the nonselective COX inhibitor diclofenac nor the selective COX-2 inhibitor celecoxib had any effect on MPP$^+$ toxicity in rats (Sairam et al., 2003). Indeed, other mechanisms might be involved, since a range of anti-inflammatory agents and immunosuppressants, including thalidomide, cyclosporine A, and FK506, appear to be effective in these toxin-based models (Hunot and Hirsch, 2003). Effects of NO and/or peroxynitrite might account for the reduction

in MPTP toxicity produced by manipulation of inflammatory events, since i-NOS inhibitors and i-NOS knockout attenuate cell death (see earlier). In addition, the PPAR-$\gamma$ agonist pioglitazone reduces MPTP toxicity and nitrative damage by reducing i-NOS expression (Dehmer et al., 2004).

At this time, glial-related toxicity appears to be an important component of the cell death cascade in PD, and its inhibition might affect the progression of nigral pathology. However, manipulation of activated glial cells could be a double-edged sword, as there is also evidence that other components of their actions might be linked to neuroprotection and thus to the survival of remaining dopaminergic neurons (Sortwell et al., 2000; Diem et al., 2003).

## THE UBIQUITIN-PROTEASOME SYSTEM AND PARKINSON DISEASE

There is a current upsurge in interest in the concept that altered protein handling, in particular a failure of the ubiquitin-proteasome system (UPS), might contribute to the pathogenesis of PD (McNaught and Olanow, 2003) (Fig. 5-3). This has stemmed from the recognition of the presence of oxidized and nitrated proteins in sporadic PD and the discovery of misfolded or mutant proteins in familial disease coupled to genetic modification of important components of the UPS, such as parkin and UCHL-1 (see earlier). In addition, the presence of multiple wild-type proteins and radical damaged proteins and protein adducts in the Lewy body has given rise to the concept that these could act as storage vesicles serving to protect against potential toxicity. The key role played by the UPS in the degradation of unwanted or abnormal proteins makes it a prime target for disruption at various levels. Changes in the polyubiquitination of proteins that is necessary for their identification for degradation can alter protein handling, as can changes in the regulation of proteasomal function linked to direct or indirect damage or genetic modification.

One concept of PD would be that it is a proteasomal disorder involving impaired proteasomal function and the presence of damaged or mutant proteins that leads to a failure of proteolysis. The accumulation of proteins would lead to cross-linking, aggregation, and deposition within the cell, and this in turn would cause a failure of intracellular transport and cell death. As a result, the Lewy body can be viewed as a protective measure utilized by the cell to sequester potentially toxic proteins into a vesicular system.

There is evidence from studies of postmortem brain material in PD that supports the concept of proteasomal impairment. Measurement of the catalytic activity of the proteasome has demonstrated normal activity in most areas of the brain, but in the substantia nigra, there is an approximately 40% reduction in total activity (McNaught, Olanow, et al., 2001; Furukawa et al., 2002; Tofaris et al., 2003). This exceeds the loss that can be accounted for by changes occurring in neurons, so there must be a failure of proteasomal function in other cell types, notably glial cells. Investigation of proteasomal subunits in the substantia nigra in PD has, perhaps surprisingly, shown no change in the expression of the $\beta$-subunits of the 20S proteasomal that are responsible for catalytic activity (McNaught, Shashidharan, et al., 2002). Rather, there is a decrease in the expression of $\alpha$-subunits that

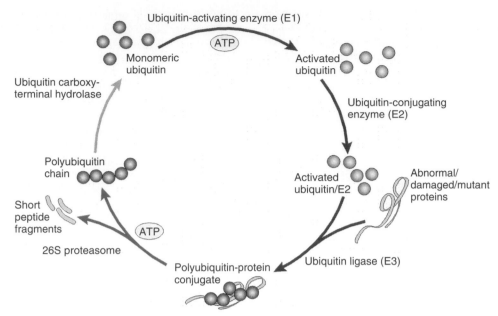

**Figure 5-3** The ubiquitin-proteasome system mediates the degradation and clearance of abnormal or misfolded proteins. (See Color Plate 7.) (From McNaught KS, Olanow CW, Halliwell B, et al: Failure of the ubiquitin-proteasome system in Parkinson's disease. Nat Rev Neurosci 2001;2:589–594.

form the structural elements of the proteasomal core. The activated 20S and 26S proteasome can be attached to one of two regulatory caps that recognize both ubiquitinated and nonubiquitinated proteins. In the 26S proteasome, PA700 is an adenosine triphosphatase (ATPase) that is responsible for the degradation of polyubiquitinated proteins. In PD, there is no loss of PA700 in the substantia nigra, but upregulation appears to occur in other brain regions (McNaught, Shashidharan, et al., 2002). This suggests that the substantia nigra does not adapt to altered protein load as occurs in other areas. In the activated 20S proteasome, the regulatory cap is PA28 responsible for the handling of nonubiquitinated proteins. Very surprisingly, neither in the normal aged substantia nigra nor in PD was the presence of PA28 detected. However, PA28 was expressed in other brain regions, suggesting that proteasomal composition might be different in the substantia nigra or that with aging, PA28 is no longer expressed.

The functional importance of proteasomal inhibition was shown by the effect of the proteasomal inhibitor lactacystin in cell cultures. In concentrations that inhibited proteasomal enzyme activity but had little effect on cell viability, it caused the cytoplasmic accumulation of a wide range of proteins (Hyun et al., 2003). In primary fetal ventral mesencephalon cultures or PC12 cells, lactacystin is selectively toxic to dopaminergic cells, and cell death is accompanied by the formation of α-synuclein- and ubiquitin-positive inclusions (McNaught et al., 2003; Biasani et al., 2004). Therefore, dopaminergic neurons appear more vulnerable to disruption of proteasomal function than occurs with other cell types. In a similar manner, the supranigral or intrastriatal infusion of proteasomal inhibitors in rats leads to the selective destruction of nigral dopaminergic cells, again accompanied by the formation of α-synuclein- and ubiquitin-positive inclusions (McNaught, Belizaire, et al., 2002; Fornai et al., 2003). This might be dependent on the presence of endogenous

dopamine, since dopamine depletion decreased both apoptotic cell death and inclusion formation. The effects of proteasomal inhibition might be more complex than was originally envisaged and might be time and concentration dependent. For example, while proteasomal inhibitors sensitize cells to oxidative damage, they have also been reported to protect against the toxicity of 6-OHDA and glutamate (Inden et al., 2005; van Leyen et al., 2005; Lev et al., 2006). However, this may be explained by acute versus chronic effects of proteasomal inhibitors in regulating prosurvival and proapoptotic transcription factors (Butts et al., 2005).

Recently, the systemic administration of the proteasomal inhibitors epoxomicin and carbobenzoxy-L-isoleucyl-gamma-t-butyl-L-glutamyl-L-alanyl-L-leucinal (PSI) to rats was shown to lead to the slow and progressive onset of motor deficits accompanied by degeneration of the nigrostriatal pathway and the presence of proteinaceous inclusions (McNaught et al., 2004). This study is the first to illustrate the selective toxicity of a proteasomal inhibitor to nigral dopaminergic cells by systemic administration. Importantly, these animals also showed pathology in the raphe nuclei, the locus coeruleus, and other areas of the brain that are known to degenerate in PD, with Lewy body pathology. This study provides strong evidence that inhibition of proteasomal function might be one mechanism by which PD can occur; however, these findings have proved difficult to reproduce in laboratories. Although several laboratories (Bove et al., 2006; Kordower et al., 2006; Manning-Bog et al., 2006) have not be able to replicate the loss of dopamine neurons after PSI administration, two others have partially reproduced the results (Schapira et al., 2006; Zeng et al., 2006), but the changes were less marked, and no definite inclusion bodies could be demonstrated. While systemic administration of proteasome inhibitor might not consistently produce nigral degeneration, local stereotactic injection of lactacystin in the median forebrain bundle has been shown to produce neurodegeneration (Zhang et al., 2005b). Since many proteasomal inhibitors are natural products, this might be an environmentally related means of disease inhibition that is particularly relevant to the risk associated with rural living and well water. This is seen in the ability of pesticides such as rotenone and dieldrin to inhibit proteasomal function, to disorganize centrosomal function and inclusion formation, and to increase susceptibility to apoptotic cell death (az-Corrales et al., 2005; Sun et al., 2005). Interestingly, actinomycetes, which produce epoxomicin and lactacystin, have been found in the brain in PD.

How proteasomal inhibition leads to inclusion formation may be key to understanding the genesis of Lewy bodies. Inclusion formation appears to start in the perinuclear region of dopaminergic cells (McNaught, Shashidharan, et al., 2002). Centrosomes then become converted into aggresomes through the transport of proteasomal elements and protein along the microtubule network to microtubule organizing centers. Lewy bodies are immunoreactive for many components of the centrosomal and proteasomal system, as are inclusions formed by the action of proteasomal inhibitors in cell systems. Recent data also suggest that inhibition of microtubule transport affects the ability of cells to form inclusions and to provide protection against the accumulation of unwanted proteins (Jenner, unpublished data). It is important to note that inclusion formation does not appear to be restricted to the sequestration of α-synuclein, and many ubiquitin-protein complexes are found in inclusions in both neurons and neurites (McNaught, Mytilineou, et al., 2002). Since some are not α-synuclein-positive, this suggests a more general defect in protein handling. The potential importance of α-synuclein-mediated toxicity remains high, but it should not be viewed as the only pathogenic component of this process.

The reasons for the failure of catalytic activity within the proteasome in PD also remain to be elucidated. It is feasible that genetic alterations in proteasomal function could occur and might account for other cases of familial PD. The regulation and encoding of the proteasome are complex, but recently, insertion of a mutant β5 subunit involving a single amino acid change and causing an increase in catalytic activity was shown to increase cell sensitivity to oxidative stress and led to the formation of inclusions containing a range of proteins and induced cell death (Li et al., 2004). Other reasons for proteasomal dysfunction might relate to damage by products of oxidative or nitrative stress. For example, incubation of cells with 4-hydroxynonenal (4-HNE), a highly reactive and toxic product of lipid peroxidation that is found in the substantia nigra in PD, decreases proteasomal enzyme activity and initiates the accumulation of oxidized and nitrated proteins, which can themselves impair proteasomal activity (Hyun et al., 2003). A 4-HNE-proteasomal adduct was also detected, suggesting that direct damage to the proteasome reduces catalytic activity, although alternatively, it might have caused protein overload. Recently, cybrids containing mtDNA from patients with PD with low complex I activity were shown to form inclusions with the fine ultrastructure of Lewy bodies and containing multiple proteins (Trimmer et al., 2004). This might form an alternative means of inclusion formation that does not involve proteasomal dysfunction, although the inclusions also contained centrosomal and proteasomal proteins. However, impaired mitochondrial function might affect adenosine triphosphatases necessary for proteasomal function and might also reduce its catalytic activity. Indeed, the complex I inhibitors rotenone and MPP$^+$ inhibit proteasomal function in concentrations that are relevant for mitochondrial inhibition (Hoglinger et al., 2003a).

Alterations in the UPS do not necessarily have to be restricted to the proteasome itself for a failure of protein handling to occur. In a recent study, the overexpression of a mutant form of ubiquitin in cell lines that prevents polyubiquitination from occurring resulted in an accumulation of ubiquitinated proteins, induced oxidative and nitrative stress, and led to a decrease in proteasomal activity (Hyun et al., 2004). While the presence of the mutant ubiquitin was itself not toxic to the cell line, it caused an increase in susceptibility to the toxic effects of 4-HNE. This suggests that impairment of the UPS at many different points is able to induce a series of events, all of which lead to a failure of proteolysis and can then impair cell viability either directly or indirectly.

A key feature of PD is the age-related nature of the illness, which is not included in many concepts of the pathogenesis of the disorder. However, proteasomal function does decline with age, and there is evidence from the rat brain and from the human spinal cord that this can affect proteolysis and protein handling (Keller et al., 2000a, 2000b). Indeed, in rats and mice, the substantia nigra is particularly vulnerable to age-related changes compared to other brain regions (Zeng et al., 2005). In addition, in young animals, the primate substantia nigra has a higher degree of proteasomal enzyme activity than is found in rodents, suggesting a greater need to clear unwanted proteins and perhaps indicating a specific vulnerability to a failure of proteolysis.

## CONCLUSIONS

The understanding of the pathogenesis of PD is progressing significantly both through the study of familial disease and from biochemical changes that have been discovered in the substantia nigra of those with the sporadic form. There are now well-substantiated biochemical changes associated with the destruction of dopaminergic neurons, but at this time, it is difficult to put these into a sequence, and they appear to form part of a general cycle of events initiated by a range of primary triggers. The concept of studying those pathogenic events that are known to occur in the substantia nigra in PD seems to form a rational way forward for understanding pathogenesis rather than investigating the actions of toxic materials that destroy dopaminergic cells through mechanisms that might be unrelated to the pathogenic process. The activation of glial cells is clearly an important event in PD, and its role in disease progression needs to be clarified. Understanding how glial cell activation can be controlled might well allow truly neuroprotective therapies to be introduced for the illness. The concept that the UPS may be a core component of pathogenesis and its failure might underlie the formation of Lewy bodies has advanced the debate about pathogenesis. If the UPS is involved, it becomes a question of proving it and then determining why this failure occurs, how it might be prevented or reversed, and how it is linked to the other biochemical changes that are known to occur in PD. In any case, the possible involvement of the UPS has focused on another aspect of cell physiology, namely, protein degradation, that could lead to a clearer understanding of why PD occurs and might help in providing a means of limiting the effects of the disease and eradicating one of its causes. However, preventing inclusion formation might not stop the progression of PD, since promotion of the formation of aggregates reduces α-synuclein toxicity (Bodner et al., 2006).

## References

Aaserud O, Gjerstad L, Nakstad P, et al: Neurological examination, computerized tomography, cerebral blood flow and neuropsychological examination in workers with long-term exposure to carbon disulfide. Toxicology 1988;49:277–282.

Abou-Sleiman PM, Healy DG, Quinn N, et al: The role of pathogenic DJ-1 mutations in Parkinson's disease. Ann Neurol 2003;54: 283–286.

Adams JR, van Netten H, Schulzer M, et al: PET in LRRK2 mutations: Comparison to sporadic Parkinson's disease and evidence for presymptomatic compensation. Brain 2005;128:2777–2785.

Agid Y, Javoy-Agid F, Ruberg M: Biochemistry of neurotransmitters in Parkinson's disease. In Marsden CD, Fahn S (eds): Movement Disorders, vol 2. London, Butterworths, 1987, pp 166–230.

Aharon-Peretz J, Badarny S, Rosenbaum H, Gershoni-Baruch R: Mutations in the glucocerebrosidase gene and Parkinson disease: Phenotype-genotype correlation. Neurology 2005;65(9): 1460–1461.

Aharon-Peretz J, Rosenbaum H, Gershoni-Baruch R: Mutations in the glucocerebrosidase gene and Parkinson's disease in Ashkenazi Jews. N Engl J Med 2004;351(19):1972–1977.

Ahmadi FA, Linseman DA, Grammatopoulos TN, et al: The pesticide rotenone induces caspase-3-mediated apoptosis in ventral mesencephalic dopaminergic neurons. J Neurochem 2003;87:914–921.

Alam M, Mayerhofer A, Schmidt WJ: The neurobehavioral changes induced by bilateral rotenone lesion in medial forebrain bundle of rats are reversed by L-DOPA. Behav Brain Res 2004;151:117–124.

Albanese A, Valente EM, Romito LM, et al: The PINK1 phenotype can be indistinguishable from idiopathic Parkinson disease. Neurology 2005;64:1958–1960.

Allam MF, Campbell MJ, Hofman A, et al: Smoking and Parkinson's disease: Systematic review of prospective studies. Mov Disord 2004;19:614–621.

Anglade P, Michel PP, Marquez J: Apoptotic degeneration of nigral dopaminergic neurons in Parkinson's disease. Abs Soc Neurosci 1995;21:1250.

Annesi G, Savettieri G, Pugliese P, et al: DJ-1 mutations and parkinsonism-dementia-amyotrophic lateral sclerosis complex. Ann Neurol 2005;58:803–807.

Ardley HC, Scott GB, Rose SA, et al: UCH-L1 aggresome formation in response to proteasome impairment indicates a role in inclusion formation in Parkinson's disease. J Neurochem 2004;90: 379–391.

Ascherio A, Chen H, Weisskopf MG, et al: Pesticide exposure and risk for Parkinson's disease. Ann Neurol 2006;60:197–203.

Ascherio A, Weisskopf MG, O'Reilly EJ, et al: Coffee consumption, gender, and Parkinson's disease mortality in the cancer prevention study II cohort: The modifying effects of estrogen. Am J Epidemiol 2004;160:977–984.

Ascherio A, Zhang SM, Hernan MA, et al: Prospective study of caffeine consumption and risk of Parkinson's disease in men and women. Ann Neurol 2001;50:56–63.

Autere J, Moilanen JS, Finnila S, et al: Mitochondrial DNA polymorphisms as risk factors for Parkinson's disease and Parkinson's disease dementia. Hum Genet 2004;115:29–35.

az-Corrales FJ, Asanuma M, Miyazaki I, et al: Rotenone induces aggregation of gamma-tubulin protein and subsequent disorganization of the centrosome: Relevance to formation of inclusion bodies and neurodegeneration. Neuroscience 2005;133:117–135.

Bader V, Ran ZX, Lubbert H, Stichel CC: Expression of DJ-1 in the adult mouse CNS. Brain Res 2005;1041:102–111.

Banati RB, Daniel SE, Blunt SB: Glial pathology but absence of apoptotic nigral neurons in long-standing Parkinson's disease. Mov Disord 1998;13:221–227.

Bandopadhyay R, Kingsbury AE, Cookson MR, et al: The expression of DJ-1 (PARK7) in normal human CNS and idiopathic Parkinson's disease. Brain 2004;127:420–430.

Bandopadhyay R, Miller DW, Kingsbury AE, et al: Development, characterisation and epitope mapping of novel monoclonal antibodies for DJ-1 (PARK7) protein. Neurosci Lett 2005;383: 225–230.

Barcia C, Bautista V, Sanchez-Bahillo A, et al: Changes in vascularization in substantia nigra pars compacta of monkeys rendered parkinsonian. J Neural Transm 2005a;112:1237–1248.

Barcia C, de Pablos V, Bautista-Hernandez V, et al: Increased plasma levels of TNF-α but not of IL1-β in MPTP-treated monkeys one year after the MPTP administration. Parkinsonism Relat Disord 2005b;11:435–439.

Barcia C, Sanchez BA, Fernandez-Villalba E, et al: Evidence of active microglia in substantia nigra pars compacta of parkinsonian monkeys 1 year after MPTP exposure. Glia 2004;46:402–409.

Barlow BK, Thiruchelvam MJ, Bennice L, et al: Increased synaptosomal dopamine content and brain concentration of paraquat produced by selective dithiocarbamates. J Neurochem 2003;85: 1075–1086.

Bashkatova V, Alam M, Vanin A, Schmidt WJ: Chronic administration of rotenone increases levels of nitric oxide and lipid peroxidation products in rat brain. Exp Neurol 2004;186:235–241.

Beal MF: Does impairment of energy metabolism result in excitotoxic neuronal death in neurodegenerative illnesses? Ann Neurol 1992;31:119–130.

Beal MF: Commentary on "Alpha-synuclein and mitochondria: A tangled skein." Exp Neurol 2004;186:109–111.

Beal MF: Mitochondria take center stage in aging and neurodegeneration. Ann Neurol 2005;58:495–505.

Bender A, Krishnan KJ, Morris CM, et al: High levels of mitochondrial DNA deletions in substantia nigra neurons in aging and Parkinson disease. Nat Genet 2006;38:515–517.

Bertoncini CW, Fernandez CO, Griesinger C, et al: Familial mutants of alpha-synuclein with increased neurotoxicity have a destabilized conformation. J Biol Chem 2005;280:30649–30652.

Betarbet R, Sherer TB, MacKenzie G, et al: Chronic systemic pesticide exposure reproduces features of Parkinson's disease. Nat Neurosci 2000;3:1301–1306.

Bialecka M, Hui S, Klodowska-Duda G, et al: Analysis of LRRK 2 G 2019 S and I 2020 T mutations in Parkinson's disease. Neurosci Lett 2005;390:1–3.

Biasini E, Fioriti L, Ceglia I, et al: Proteasome inhibition and aggregation in Parkinson's disease: A comparative study in untransfected and transfected cells. J Neurochem 2004;88: 545–553.

Biskup S, Mueller JC, Sharma M, et al: Common variants of LRRK2 are not associated with sporadic Parkinson's disease. Ann Neurol 2005;58:905–908.

Blackinton J, Ahmad R, Miller DW, et al: Effects of DJ-1 mutations and polymorphisms on protein stability and subcellular localization. Brain Res Mol Brain Res 2005;134:76–83.

Bodner RA, Outeiro TF, Altmann S, et al: Pharmacological promotion of inclusion formation: A therapeutic approach for Huntington's and Parkinson's diseases. Proc Natl Acad Sci U S A 2006;103:4246–4251.

Boka G, Anglade P, Wallach D, et al: Immunocytochemical analysis of tumor necrosis factor and its receptors in Parkinson's disease. Neurosci Lett 1994;172:151–154.

Bonifati V, Rizzu P, van Baren MJ, et al: Mutations in the DJ-1 gene associated with autosomal recessive early-onset parkinsonism. Science 2003;299:256–259.

Bonifati V, Rohe CF, Breedveld GJ, et al: Early-onset parkinsonism associated with PINK1 mutations: Frequency, genotypes, and phenotypes. Neurology 2005;65:87–95.

Bove J, Zhou C, Jackson-Lewis V, et al: Proteasome inhibition and Parkinson's disease modeling. Ann Neurol 2006;60(2):260–264.

Braak H, Del Tredici K, Rub U, et al: Staging of brain pathology related to sporadic Parkinson's disease. Neurobiol Aging 2003; 24:197–211.

Braak H, de Vos RA, Bohl J, Del TK: Gastric alpha-synuclein immunoreactive inclusions in Meissner's and Auerbach's plexuses in cases staged for Parkinson's disease-related brain pathology. Neurosci Lett 2006;396:67–72.

Braak H, Ghebremedhin E, Rub U, et al:. Stages in the development of Parkinson's disease-related pathology. Cell Tissue Res 2004; 318(1):121–134.

Brooks AI, Chadwick CA, Gelbard HA, et al: Paraquat elicited neurobehavioral syndrome caused by dopaminergic neuron loss. Brain Res 1999;823:1–10.

Brown TP, Rumsby PC, Capleton AC, et al: Pesticides and Parkinson's disease: Is there a link? Environ Health Perspect 2006;114:156–164.

Butts BD, Hudson HR, Linseman DA, et al: Proteasome inhibition elicits a biphasic effect on neuronal apoptosis via differential regulation of pro-survival and pro-apoptotic transcription factors. Mol Cell Neurosci 2005;30:279–289.

Canet-Aviles RM, Wilson MA, Miller DW, et al: The Parkinson's disease protein DJ-1 is neuroprotective due to cysteine-sulfinic acid-driven mitochondrial localization. Proc Natl Acad Sci U S A 2004;101:9103–9108.

Caparros-Lefebvre D: Atypical parkinsonism in New Caledonia: Comparison with Guadeloupe and association with Annonaceae consumption. Mov Disord 2004;19:604.

Carvey PM, Zhao CH, Hendey B, et al: 6-Hydroxydopamine-induced alterations in blood-brain barrier permeability. Eur J Neurosci 2005;22:1158–1168.

Cassarino DS, Fall CP, Swerdlow RH, et al: Elevated reactive oxygen species and antioxidant enzyme activities in animal and cellular models of Parkinson's disease. Biochim Biophys Acta 1997;1362: 77–86.

Castano A, Herrera AJ, Cano J, Machado A: Lipopolysaccharide intranigral injection induces inflammatory reaction and damage in nigrostriatal dopaminergic system. J Neurochem 1998;70: 1584–1592.

Castano A, Herrera AJ, Cano J, Machado A: The degenerative effect of a single intranigral injection of LPS on the dopaminergic system is prevented by dexamethasone, and not mimicked by rh-TNF-alpha, IL-1beta and IFN-gamma. J Neurochem 2002;81:150–157.

Castegna A, Thongboonkerd V, Klein J, et al: Proteomic analysis of brain proteins in the gracile axonal dystrophy (gad) mouse, a syndrome that emanates from dysfunctional ubiquitin carboxyl-terminal hydrolase L-1, reveals oxidation of key proteins. J Neurochem 2004;88:1540–1546.

Cha GH, Kim S, Park J, et al: Parkin negatively regulates JNK pathway in the dopaminergic neurons of Drosophila. Proc Natl Acad Sci U S A 2005;102:10345–10350.

Champy P, Hoglinger GU, Feger J, et al: Annonacin, a lipophilic inhibitor of mitochondrial complex I, induces nigral and striatal neurodegeneration in rats: Possible relevance for atypical parkinsonism in Guadeloupe. J Neurochem 2004;88:63–69.

Chandra S, Fornai F, Kwon H B, et al: Double-knockout mice for alpha- and beta-synucleins: Effect on synaptic functions. Proc Natl Acad Sci U S A 2004;101:14966–14971.

Chang RC, Chen W, Hudson P, et al: Neurons reduce glial responses to lipopolysaccharide (LPS) and prevent injury of microglial cells from over-activation by LPS. J Neurochem 2001;76:1042–1049.

Charriaut-Mariangue C: A cautionary note on the use of TUNEL stain to determine aptosis. Neuroreport 1995;7:61–64.

Chartier-Harlin MC, Kachergus J, Roumier C, et al: Alpha-synuclein locus duplication as a cause of familial Parkinson's disease. Lancet 2004;364:1167–1169.

Chaudhuri KR, Healy DG, Schapira AH: Non-motor symptoms of Parkinson's disease: Diagnosis and management. Lancet Neurol 2006;5:235–245.

Chen H, Jacobs E, Schwarzschild MA, et al: Nonsteroidal antiinflammatory drug use and the risk for Parkinson's disease. Ann Neurol 2005;58:963–967.

Chen H, Zhang SM, Hernan MA, et al: Nonsteroidal anti-inflammatory drugs and the risk of Parkinson disease. Arch Neurol 2003;60: 1059–1064.

Chen L, Feany MB: Alpha-synuclein phosphorylation controls neurotoxicity and inclusion formation in a Drosophila model of Parkinson disease. Nat Neurosci 2005;8:657–663.

Choi IS: Parkinsonism after carbon monoxide poisoning. Eur Neurol 2002;48:30–33.

Choi J, Sullards MC, Olzmann JA, et al: Oxidative damage of DJ-1 is linked to sporadic Parkinson and Alzheimer diseases. J Biol Chem 2006;281:10816–10824.

Chung KK, Thomas B, Li X, et al: S-nitrosylation of parkin regulates ubiquitination and compromises parkin's protective function. Science 2004;304:1328–1331.

Clark LN, Afridi S, Mejia-Santana H, et al: Analysis of an early-onset Parkinson's disease cohort for DJ-1 mutations. Mov Disord 2004;19:796–800.

Clark LN, Nicolai A, Afridi S, et al: Pilot association study of the beta-glucocerebrosidase N370S allele and Parkinson's disease in subjects of Jewish ethnicity. Mov Disord 2005;20(1):100–103.

Conway KA, Lee SJ, Rochet JC, et al: Acceleration of oligomerization, not fibrillization, is a shared property of both alpha-synuclein mutations linked to early-onset Parkinson's disease: Implications for pathogenesis and therapy. Proc Natl Acad Sci U S A 2000; 97:571–576.

Cookson MR: Parkin's substrates and the pathways leading to neuronal damage. Neuromolecular Med 2003a;3:1–13.

Cookson MR: Pathways to Parkinsonism. Neuron 2003b;37:7–10.

Cuervo AM, Stefanis L, Fredenburg R, et al: Impaired degradation of mutant alpha-synuclein by chaperone-mediated autophagy. Science 2004;305:1292–1295.

Damier P, Hirsch EC, Zhang P, et al: Glutathione peroxidase, glial cells and Parkinson's disease. Neuroscience 1993;52:1–6.

Dauer W, Kholodilov N, Vila M, et al: Resistance of $\alpha$-synuclein null mice to the parkinsonian neurotoxin MPTP. Proc Natl Acad Sci U S A 2002;99(22):14524–14529.

Dehmer T, Heneka MT, Sastre M, et al: Protection by pioglitazone in the MPTP model of Parkinson's disease correlates with I kappa B alpha induction and block of NF kappa B and iNOS activation. J Neurochem 2004;88:494–501.

Dekker MC, Bonifati V, van Duijn CM: Parkinson's disease: Piecing together a genetic jigsaw. Brain 2003;126:1722–1733.

DeLong MR: Primate models of movement disorders of basal ganglia origin. Trends Neurosci 1990;13:281–285.

Deng H, Le W, Guo Y, et al: Genetic and clinical identification of Parkinson's disease patients with LRRK2 G2019S mutation. Ann Neurol 2005;57:933–934.

DeStefano AL, Golbe LI, Mark MH, et al: Genome-wide scan for Parkinson's disease: The GenePD Study. Neurology 2001;57: 1124–1126.

Di FA, Rohe CF, Ferreira J, et al: A frequent LRRK2 gene mutation associated with autosomal dominant Parkinson's disease. Lancet 2005;365:412–415.

Diem R, Hobom M, Maier K, et al: Methylprednisolone increases neuronal apoptosis during autoimmune CNS inflammation by inhibition of an endogenous neuroprotective pathway. J Neurosci 2003;23:6993–7000.

Diguet E, Gross CE, Tison F, Bezard E: Rise and fall of minocycline in neuroprotection: Need to promote publication of negative results. Exp Neurol 2004;189:1–4.

Di Monte DA, Lavasani M, Manning-Bog AB: Environmental factors in Parkinson's disease. Neurotoxicology 2002;23:487–502.

Dipasquale B, Marini AM, Youle RJ: Apoptosis and DNA degradation induced by 1-methyl-4-phenylpyridinium in neurons. Biochem Biophys Res Commun 1991;181:1442–1448.

Dong Z, Ferger B, Paterna JC, et al: Dopamine-dependent neurodegeneration in rats induced by viral vector-mediated overexpression of the parkin target protein, CDCrel-1. Proc Natl Acad Sci U S A 2003;100:12438–12443.

Doty RL, Golbe LI, McKeown DA, et al: Olfactory testing differentiates between progressive supranuclear palsy and idiopathic Parkinson's disease. Neurology 1993;43:962–965.

Duda JE, Giasson BI, Chen Q, et al: Widespread nitration of pathological inclusions in neurodegenerative synucleinopathies. Am J Pathol 2000;157:1439–1445.

Ehringer H, Hornykiewicz O: Distribution of noradrenaline and dopamine (3-hydroxytyramine) in the human brain and their behavior in diseases of the extrapyramidal system. Klin Wochenschr 1960;38:1236–1239.

Elbaz A, Levecque C, Clavel J, et al: S18Y polymorphism in the UCH-L1 gene and Parkinson's disease: Evidence for an age-dependent relationship. Mov Disord 2003;18:130–137.

Elbaz A, Levecque C, Clavel J, et al: CYP2D6 polymorphism, pesticide exposure, and Parkinson's disease. Ann Neurol 2004;55:430–434.

Endo T, Hara S, Kuriiwa F, Kano S: Effects of a paraquat-containing herbicide, Gramoxon, on the central monoamines and acetylcholine in mice. Commun Psychol Psych Behav 1988;13:261–270.

Eriksen JL, Dawson TM, Dickson DW, Petrucelli L: Caught in the act: Alpha-synuclein is the culprit in Parkinson's disease. Neuron 2003;40:453–456.

Fahn S, Sulzer D: Neurodegeneration and neuroprotection in Parkinson disease. NeuroRx 2004;1:139–154.

Farkas E, De Jong GI, de Vos RA, et al: Pathological features of cerebral cortical capillaries are doubled in Alzheimer's disease and Parkinson's disease. Acta Neuropathol (Berl) 2000;100:395–402.

Farrer M, Kachergus J, Forno L, et al: Comparison of kindreds with parkinsonism and alpha-synuclein genomic multiplications. Ann Neurol 2004;55:174–179.

Farrer M, Stone J, Mata IF, et al: LRRK2 mutations in Parkinson disease. Neurology 2005;65:738–740.

Faucheux BA, Bonnet AM, Agid Y, Hirsch EC: Blood vessels change in the mesencephalon of patients with Parkinson's disease. Lancet 1999;353:981–982.

Feany MB, Bender WW: A Drosophila model of Parkinson's disease. Nature 2000;404:394–398.

Ferrer I, Blanco R, Cutillas B, Ambrosio S: Fas and Fas-L expression in Huntington's disease and Parkinson's disease. Neuropathol Appl Neurobiol 2000;26:424–433.

Fitzmaurice PS, Ang L, Guttman M, et al: Nigral glutathione deficiency is not specific for idiopathic Parkinson's disease. Mov Disord 2003;18:969–976.

Fored CM, Fryzek JP, Brandt L, et al: Parkinson's disease and other basal ganglia or movement disorders in a large nationwide cohort of Swedish welders. Occup Environ Med 2006;63:135–140.

Fornai F, Lenzi P, Gesi M, et al: Fine structure and biochemical mechanisms underlying nigrostriatal inclusions and cell death after proteasome inhibition. J Neurosci 2003;23:8955–8966.

Fredriksson A, Fredriksson M, Eriksson P: Neonatal exposure to paraquat or MPTP induces permanent changes in striatum dopamine and behavior in adult mice. Toxicol Appl Pharmacol 1993;122:258–264.

Frigerio R, Sanft KR, Grossardt BR, et al: Chemical exposures and Parkinson's disease: A population-based case-control study. Mov Disord 2006;

Funayama M, Hasegawa K, Kowa H, et al: A new locus for Parkinson's disease (PARK8) maps to chromosome 12p11.2-q13.1. Ann Neurol 2002;51:296–301.

Funayama M, Hasegawa K, Ohta E, et al: An LRRK2 mutation as a cause for the parkinsonism in the original PARK8 family. Ann Neurol 2005;57:918–921.

Fung HC, Chen CM, Hardy J, et al: Analysis of the PINK1 gene in a cohort of patients with sporadic early-onset parkinsonism in Taiwan. Neurosci Lett 2006;394:33–36.

Furukawa Y, Vigouroux S, Wong H, et al: Brain proteasomal function in sporadic Parkinson's disease and related disorders. Ann Neurol 2002;51:779–782.

Galanaud JP, Elbaz A, Clavel J, et al: Cigarette smoking and Parkinson's disease: A case-control study in a population characterized by a high prevalence of pesticide exposure. Mov Disord 2005;20:181–189.

Gao HM, Hong JS, Zhang W, Liu B: Synergistic dopaminergic neurotoxicity of the pesticide rotenone and inflammogen lipopolysaccharide: Relevance to the etiology of Parkinson's disease. J Neurosci 2003;23:1228–1236.

Gao HM, Jiang J, Wilson B, et al: Microglial activation-mediated delayed and progressive degeneration of rat nigral dopaminergic neurons: Relevance to Parkinson's disease. J Neurochem 2002; 81:1285–1297.

Giasson BI, Covy JP, Bonini NM, et al: Biochemical and pathological characterization of Lrrk2. Ann Neurol 2006;59:315–322.

Giasson BI, Duda JE, Murray IV, et al: Oxidative damage linked to neurodegeneration by selective alpha-synuclein nitration in synucleinopathy lesions. Science 2000;290:985–989.

Giasson BI, Duda JE, Quinn SM, et al: Neuronal alpha-synucleinopathy with severe movement disorder in mice expressing A53T human alpha-synuclein. Neuron 2002;34:521–533.

Giasson BI, Lee VM: Are ubiquitination pathways central to Parkinson's disease? Cell 2003;114:1–8.

Gilks WP, bou-Sleiman PM, Gandhi S, et al: A common LRRK2 mutation in idiopathic Parkinson's disease. Lancet 2005;365: 415–416.

Gispert S, Trenkwalder C, Mota-Vieira L, et al: Failure to find alpha-synuclein gene dosage changes in 190 patients with familial Parkinson disease. Arch Neurol 2005;62:96–98.

Gloeckner CJ, Kinkl N, Schumacher A, et al: The Parkinson disease causing LRRK2 mutation I2020T is associated with increased kinase activity. Hum Mol Genet 2006;15:223–232.

Goedert M: Alpha-synuclein and neurodegenerative diseases. Nat Rev Neurosci 2001;2:492–501.

Goedert M, Jakes R, Crowther RA, Spillantini MG: Parkinson's disease, dementia with Lewy bodies, and mutiple system atrophy as alpha-synucleinopathies. In Mouradian MM (ed): Parkinson's disease: Methods and Protocols. Totowa, NJ, Humana Press, 2001, pp 33–59.

Goker-Alpan O, Giasson BI, Eblan MJ, et al: Glucocerebrosidase mutations are an important risk factor for Lewy body disorders. Neurology 2006 [Epub ahead of print].

Golbe LI, Mouradian MM: Alpha-synuclein in Parkinson's disease: Light from two new angles. Ann Neurol 2004;55:153–156.

Goldberg MS, Fleming SM, Palacino JJ, et al: Parkin-deficient mice exhibit nigrostriatal deficits but not loss of dopaminergic neurons. J Biol Chem 2003;278:43628–43635.

Goldberg MS, Pisani A, Haburcak M, et al: Nigrostriatal dopaminergic deficits and hypokinesia caused by inactivation of the familial Parkinsonism-linked gene DJ-1. Neuron 2005;45:489–496.

Goldwurm S, Di FA, Simons EJ, et al: The G6055A (G2019S) mutation in LRRK2 is frequent in both early and late onset Parkinson's disease and originates from a common ancestor. J Med Genet 2005;42: e65.

Good PF, Hsu A, Werner P, et al: Protein nitration in Parkinson's disease. J Neuropathol Exp Neurol 1998;57:338–342.

Green JG, Greenamyre JT: Bioenergetics and excitotoxicity: The weak excitotoxic hypothesis. In Olanow CW, Jenner P, Youdim M (eds): Neurodegeneration and neuroprotection in Parkinson's disease. London, Academic Press, 1996, pp 125–142.

Greene JC, Whitworth AJ, Andrews LA, et al: Genetic and genomic studies of Drosophila parkin mutants implicate oxidative stress and innate immune responses in pathogenesis. Hum Mol Genet 2005;14:799–811.

Greene JC, Whitworth AJ, Kuo I, et al: Mitochondrial pathology and apoptotic muscle degeneration in Drosophila parkin mutants. Proc Natl Acad Sci U S A 2003;100:4078–4083.

Greggio E, Jain S, Kingsbury A, et al: Kinase activity is required for the toxic effects of mutant LRRK2/dardarin. Neurobiol Dis 2006;23: 329–341.

Groen JL, Kawarai T, Toulina A, et al: Genetic association study of PINK1 coding polymorphisms in Parkinson's disease. Neurosci Lett 2004;372:226–229.

Hague S, Rogaeva E, Hernandez D, et al: Early-onset Parkinson's disease caused by a compound heterozygous DJ-1 mutation. Ann Neurol 2003;54:271–274.

Halliday GM, Ophof A, Broe M, et al: Alpha-synuclein redistributes to neuromelanin lipid in the substantia nigra early in Parkinson's disease. Brain 2005;128:2654–2664.

Halliwell B: Oxidative stress and neurodegeneration: Where are we now? J Neurochem 2006;97:1634–1658.

Hantraye P, Brouillet E, Ferrante R, et al: Inhibition of neuronal nitric oxide synthase prevents MPTP-induced parkinsonism in baboons. Nat Med 1996;2:1017–1021.

Hartmann A, Hunot S, Michel PP, et al: Caspase-3: A vulnerability factor and final effector in apoptotic death of dopaminergic neurons in Parkinson's disease. Proc Natl Acad Sci U S A 2000; 97:2875–2880.

Hartmann A, Mouatt-Prigent A, Faucheux BA, et al: FADD: A link between TNF family receptors and caspases in Parkinson's disease. Neurology 2002;58:308–310.

Hartmann A, Troadec JD, Hunot S, et al: Caspase-8 is an effector in apoptotic death of dopaminergic neurons in Parkinson's disease, but pathway inhibition results in neuronal necrosis. J Neurosci 2001;21:2247–2255.

Hatano Y, Li Y, Sato K, et al: Novel PINK1 mutations in early-onset parkinsonism. Ann Neurol 2004;56:424–427.

Hauser MA, Li YJ, Takeuchi S, et al: Genomic convergence: Identifying candidate genes for Parkinson's disease by combining serial analysis of gene expression and genetic linkage. Hum Mol Genet 2003;12:671–677.

Haywood AF, Staveley BE: Mutant alpha-synuclein-induced degeneration is reduced by parkin in a fly model of Parkinson's disease. Genome 2006;49:505–510.

He Y, Imam SZ, Dong Z, et al: Role of nitric oxide in rotenone-induced nigro-striatal injury. J Neurochem 2003;86:1338–1345.

Healy DG, Abou-Sleiman PM, Ahmadi KR, et al: The gene responsible for PARK6 Parkinson's disease, PINK1, does not influence common forms of parkinsonism. Ann Neurol 2004;56:329–335.

Hedrich K, Eskelson C, Wilmot B, et al: Distribution, type, and origin of Parkin mutations: Review and case studies. Mov Disord 2004;19:1146–1157.

Hedrich K, Winkler S, Hagenah J, et al: Recurrent LRRK2 (Park8) mutations in early-onset Parkinson's disease. Mov Disord 2006;21:1506–1510.

Henn IH, Gostner JM, Lackner P, et al: Pathogenic mutations inactivate parkin by distinct mechanisms. J Neurochem 2005;92:114–122.

Hernan MA, Logroscino G, Garcia Rodriguez LA: Nonsteroidal anti-inflammatory drugs and the incidence of Parkinson disease. Neurology 2006;66:1097–1099.

Hernan MA, Zhang SM, Rueda-deCastro AM, et al: Cigarette smoking and the incidence of Parkinson's disease in two prospective studies. Ann Neurol 2001;50:780–786.

Hernandez D, Paisan RC, Crawley A, et al: The dardarin G 2019 S mutation is a common cause of Parkinson's disease but not other neurodegenerative diseases. Neurosci Lett 2005;389:137–139.

Herrera AJ, Castano A, Venero JL, et al: The single intranigral injection of LPS as a new model for studying the selective effects of inflammatory reactions on dopaminergic system. Neurobiol Dis 2000;7:429–447.

Herrera AJ, Tomas-Camardiel M, Venero JL, et al: Inflammatory process as a determinant factor for the degeneration of substantia nigra dopaminergic neurons. J Neural Transm 2005;112: 111–119.

Hicks AA, Petursson H, Jonsson T, et al: A susceptibility gene for late-onset idiopathic Parkinson's disease. Ann Neurol 2002;52: 549–555.

Hofer A, Berg D, Asmus F, et al: The role of alpha-synuclein gene multiplications in early-onset Parkinson's disease and dementia with Lewy bodies. J Neural Transm 2005;112:1249–1254.

Hoglinger GU, Carrard G, Michel PP, et al: Dysfunction of mito-chondrial complex I and the proteasome: Interactions between two biochemical deficits in a cellular model of Parkinson's disease. J Neurochem 2003a;86:1297–1307.

Hoglinger GU, Feger J, Prigent A, et al: Chronic systemic complex I inhibition induces a hypokinetic multisystem degeneration in rats. J Neurochem 2003b;84:491–502.

Hunot S, Boissiere F, Faucheux B, et al: Nitric oxide synthase and neuronal vulnerability in Parkinson's disease. Neuroscience 1996;72: 355–363.

Hunot S, Brugg B, Ricard D, Michel PP, et al: Nuclear translocation of NF-kappaB is increased in dopaminergic neurons of patients with parkinson disease. Proc Natl Acad Sci U S A 1997;94:7531–7536.

Hunot S, Dugas N, Faucheux B, et al: FcepsilonRII/CD23 is expressed in Parkinson's disease and induces, in vitro, production of nitric oxide and tumor necrosis factor-alpha in glial cells. J Neurosci 1999;19:3440–3447.

Hunot S, Hirsch EC: Neuroinflammatory processes in Parkinson's disease. Ann Neurol 2003;53(suppl 3):S49–S58.

Hurley SD, O'Banion MK, Song DD, et al: Microglial response is poorly correlated with neurodegeneration following chronic, low-dose MPTP administration in monkeys. Exp Neurol 2003; 184:659–668.

Hyun DH, Gray DA, Halliwell B, Jenner P: Interference with ubiquitination causes oxidative damage and increased protein nitration: Implications for neurodegenerative diseases. J Neurochem 2004;90:422–430.

Hyun DH, Lee M, Halliwell B, Jenner P: Proteasomal inhibition causes the formation of protein aggregates containing a wide range of proteins, including nitrated proteins. J Neurochem 2003;86:363–373.

Hyun DH, Lee M, Hattori N, et al: Effect of wild-type or mutant Parkin on oxidative damage, nitric oxide, antioxidant defenses, and the proteasome. J Biol Chem 2002;277:28572–28577.

Ibanez P, Bonnet AM, Debarges B, et al: Causal relation between alpha-synuclein gene duplication and familial Parkinson's disease. Lancet 2004;364:1169–1171.

Ibanez P, Lesage S, Lohmann E, et al: Mutational analysis of the PINK1 gene in early-onset parkinsonism in Europe and North Africa. Brain 2006;129:686–694.

Inden M, Kondo J, Kitamura Y, et al: Proteasome inhibitors protect against degeneration of nigral dopaminergic neurons in hemi-parkinsonian rats. J Pharmacol Sci 2005;97:203–211.

Infante J, Rodriguez E, Combarros O, et al: LRRK2 G2019S is a common mutation in Spanish patients with late-onset Parkinson's disease. Neurosci Lett 2006;395:224–226.

Iranzo A, Molinuevo JL, Santamaria J, et al: Rapid-eye-movement sleep behaviour disorder as an early marker for a neurodegenerative disorder: A descriptive study. Lancet Neurol 2006;5:572–577.

Iravani MM, Kashefi K, Mander P, et al: Involvement of inducible nitric oxide synthase in inflammation-induced dopaminergic neurodegeneration. Neuroscience 2002;110:49–58.

Itier JM, Ibanez P, Mena MA, et al: Parkin gene inactivation alters behaviour and dopamine neurotransmission in the mouse. Hum Mol Genet 2003;12:2277–2291.

Iwatsubo T: Aggregation of alpha-synuclein in the pathogenesis of Parkinson's disease. J Neurol 2003;250(suppl 3):11–14.

Jankovic J: Searching for a relationship between manganese and welding and Parkinson's disease. Neurology 2005;64:2021–2028.

Jellinger K: The pathology of parkinsonism. In Marsden CD, Fahn S (eds): Movement Disorders. London, Butterworths, 1987, pp 124–165.

Jellinger KA: Cell death mechanisms in Parkinson's disease. J Neural Transm 2000;107:1–29.

Jellinger KA: Neuropathological spectrum of synucleinopathies. Mov Disord 2003;18(suppl 6):S2–S12.

Jenner P: Oxidative stress as a cause of Parkinson's disease. Acta Neurol Scand Suppl 1991;136:6–15.

Jenner P: Altered mitochondrial function, iron metabolism and glutathione levels in Parkinson's disease. Acta Neurol Scand Suppl 1993;146:6–13.

Jenner P: Genetic susceptibility and the occurrence of Parkinson's disease. Parkinsonism Relat Disord 1999;5:173–177.

Jenner P: Oxidative stress in Parkinson's disease. Ann Neurol 2003;53(suppl 3):S26–S36.

Jenner P, Dexter DT, Sian J, et al: Oxidative stress as a cause of nigral cell death in Parkinson's disease and incidental Lewy body disease: The Royal Kings and Queens Parkinson's Disease Research Group. Ann Neurol 1992;32(suppl):S82–S87.

Jenner P, Olanow CW: Understanding cell death in Parkinson's disease. Ann Neurol 1998;44(suppl):S72–S84.

Jenner P, Schapira AH, Marsden CD: New insights into the cause of Parkinson's disease. Neurology 1992;42:2241–2250.

Junn E, Taniguchi H, Jeong BS, et al: Interaction of DJ-1 with Daxx inhibits apoptosis signal-regulating kinase 1 activity and cell death. Proc Natl Acad Sci U S A 2005;102:9691–9696.

Kachergus J, Mata IF, Hulihan M, et al: Identification of a novel LRRK2 mutation linked to autosomal dominant parkinsonism: Evidence of a common founder across European populations. Am J Hum Genet 2005;76:672–680.

Kamel F, Hoppin JA: Association of pesticide exposure with neurologic dysfunction and disease. Environ Health Perspect 2004;112:950–958.

Kanthasamy AG, Kitazawa M, Kanthasamy A, Anantharam V: Dieldrin-induced neurotoxicity: Relevance to Parkinson's disease pathogenesis. Neurotoxicology 2005;26:701–719.

Kay DM, Zabetian CP, Factor SA, et al: Parkinson's disease and LRRK2: Frequency of a common mutation in U.S. movement disorder clinics. Mov Disord 2006;21:519–523.

Keeney PM, Xie J, Capaldi RA, Bennett JP Jr: Parkinson's disease brain mitochondrial complex I has oxidatively damaged subunits and is functionally impaired and misassembled. J Neurosci 2006;26:5256–5264.

Keller JN, Hanni KB, Markesbery WR: Possible involvement of proteasome inhibition in aging: Implications for oxidative stress. Mech Ageing Dev 2000a;113:61–70.

Keller JN, Huang FF, Markesbery WR: Decreased levels of proteasome activity and proteasome expression in aging spinal cord. Neuroscience 2000b;98:149–156.

Khan NL, Jain S, Lynch JM, et al: Mutations in the gene LRRK2 encoding dardarin (PARK8) cause familial Parkinson's disease: Clinical, pathological, olfactory and functional imaging and genetic data. Brain 2005;128:2786–2796.

Kim RH, Smith PD, Aleyasin H, et al: Hypersensitivity of DJ-1-deficient mice to 1-methyl-4-phenyl-1,2,3,6-tetrahydropyrindine (MPTP) and oxidative stress. Proc Natl Acad Sci U S A 2005;102:5215–5220.

Kingsbury AE, Daniel SE, Sangha H, et al: Alteration in alpha-synuclein mRNA expression in Parkinson's disease. Mov Disord 2004;19:162–170.

Kingsbury AE, Mardsen CD, Foster OJ: DNA fragmentation in human substantia nigra: Apoptosis or perimortem effect? Mov Disord 1998;13:877–884.

Kitada T, Asakawa S, Hattori N, et al: Mutations in the parkin gene cause autosomal recessive juvenile parkinsonism. Nature 1998;392:605–608.

Kitazawa M, Anantharam V, Kanthasamy AG: Dieldrin-induced oxidative stress and neurochemical changes contribute to apoptopic cell death in dopaminergic cells. Free Radic Biol Med 2001;31:1473–1485.

Klein RL, King MA, Hamby ME, Meyer EM: Dopaminergic cell loss induced by human A30P alpha-synuclein gene transfer to the rat substantia nigra. Hum Gene Ther 2002;13:605–612.

Knott C, Stern G, Wilkin GP: Inflammatory regulators in Parkinson's disease: iNOS, lipocortin-1, and cyclooxygenases-1 and -2. Mol Cell Neurosci 2000;16:724–739.

Ko HS, von Coelln R, Sriram SR, et al: Accumulation of the authentic parkin substrate aminoacyl-tRNA synthetase cofactor, p38/JTV-1, leads to catecholaminergic cell death. J Neurosci 2005;25:7968–7978.

Kohutnicka M, Lewandowska E, Kurkowska-Jastrzebska I, et al: Microglial and astrocytic involvement in a murine model of Parkinson's disease induced by 1-methyl-4-phenyl-1,2,3,6-tetrahydropyridine (MPTP). Immunopharmacology 1998;39:167–180.

Kordower JH, Kanaan NM, Chu Y, et al: Failure of proteasome inhibitor administration to provide a model of Parkinson's disease in rats and monkeys. Ann Neurol 2006;60(2):264–268.

Kortekaas R, Leenders KL, van Oostrom JC, et al: Blood-brain barrier dysfunction in parkinsonian midbrain in vivo. Ann Neurol 2005;57:176–179.

Kotzbauer PT, Giasson BI, Kravitz AV, et al: Fibrillization of alpha-synuclein and tau in familial Parkinson's disease caused by the A53T alpha-synuclein mutation. Exp Neurol 2004;187:279–288.

Kraytsberg Y, Kudryavtseva E, McKee AC, et al: Mitochondrial DNA deletions are abundant and cause functional impairment in aged human substantia nigra neurons. Nat Genet 2006;38:518–520.

Kruger R, Kuhn W, Muller T, et al: Ala30Pro mutation in the gene encoding alpha-synuclein in Parkinson's disease. Nat Genet 1998;18:106–108.

Kumar A, Calne SM, Schulzer M, et al: Clustering of Parkinson disease: Shared cause or coincidence? Arch Neurol 2004;61:1057–1060.

Kurkowska-Jastrzebska I, Wronska A, Kohutnicka M, et al: The inflammatory reaction following 1-methyl-4-phenyl-1,2,3,6-tetrahydropyridine intoxication in mouse. Exp Neurol 1999;156:50–61.

Kwong JQ, Beal MF, Manfredi G: The role of mitochondria in inherited neurodegenerative diseases. J Neurochem 2006;97:1659–1675.

Lakso M, Vartiainen S, Moilanen AM, et al: Dopaminergic neuronal loss and motor deficits in Caenorhabditis elegans overexpressing human alpha-synuclein. J Neurochem 2003;86:165–172.

Langston JW: The Parkinson's complex: Parkinsonism is just the tip of the iceberg. Ann Neurol 2006;59(4):591–596.

Langston JW, Forno LS, Tetrud J, et al: Evidence of active nerve cell degeneration in the substantia nigra of humans years after 1 methyl-4-phenyl-1,2,3,6-tetrahydropyridine exposure. Ann Neurol 1999;46:598–605.

LaVoie MJ, Ostaszewski BL, Weihofen A, et al: Dopamine covalently modifies and functionally inactivates parkin. Nat Med 2005;11:1214–1221.

Le W, Conneely OM, He Y, et al: Reduced Nurr1 expression increases the vulnerability of mesencephalic dopamine neurons to MPTP-induced injury. J Neurochem 1999;73:2218–2221.

Le W, Rowe D, Xie W, et al: Microglial activation and dopaminergic cell injury: An in vitro model relevant to Parkinson's disease. J Neurosci 2001;21:8447–8455.

Le WD, Xu P, Jankovic J, et al: Mutations in NR4A2 associated with familial Parkinson disease. Nat Genet 2003;33:85–89.

Lee HJ, Khoshaghideh F, Patel S, Lee SJ: Clearance of alpha-synuclein oligomeric intermediates via the lysosomal degradation pathway. J Neurosci 2004;24:1888–1896.

Lee M, Hyun D, Halliwell B, Jenner P: Effect of the overexpression of wild-type or mutant alpha-synuclein on cell susceptibility to insult. J Neurochem 2001;76:998–1009.

Leentjens AF, Van den Akker M, Metsemakers JF, et al: Higher incidence of depression preceding the onset of Parkinson's disease: A register study. Mov Disord 2003;18:414–418.

Leroy E, Boyer R, Auburger G, et al: The ubiquitin pathway in Parkinson's disease. Nature 1998;395:451–452.

Lesage S, Dürr A, Tazir M, et al: LRRK2 G2019S as a cause of Parkinson's disease in North African Arabs. N Engl J Med 2006;354:422–423.

Lesage S, Ibanez P, Lohmann E, et al: G2019S LRRK2 mutation in French and North African families with Parkinson's disease. Ann Neurol 2005;58:784–787.

Lev N, Melamed E, Offen D: Proteasomal inhibition hypersensitizes differentiated neuroblastoma cells to oxidative damage. Neurosci Lett 2006;399:27–32.

Levecque C, Destee A, Mouroux V, et al: Assessment of Nurr1 nucleotide variations in familial Parkinson's disease. Neurosci Lett 2004;366:135–138.

Li J, Uversky VN, Fink AL: Effect of familial Parkinson's disease point mutations A30P and A53T on the structural properties, aggregation, and fibrillation of human alpha-synuclein. Biochemistry 2001;40:11604–11613.

Li W, West N, Colla E, et al: Aggregation promoting C-terminal truncation of alpha-synuclein is a normal cellular process and is enhanced by the familial Parkinson's disease-linked mutations. Proc Natl Acad Sci.U S A 2005;102:2162–2167.

Li Z, Arnaud L, Rockwell P, et al: A single amino acid substitution in a proteasome subunit triggers aggregation of ubiquitinated proteins in stressed neuronal cells. J Neurochem 2004;90:19–28.

Liberatore GT, Jackson-Lewis V, Vukosavic S, et al: Inducible nitric oxide synthase stimulates dopaminergic neurodegeneration in the MPTP model of Parkinson disease. Nat Med 1999; 5:1403–1409.

Ling Z, Chang QA, Tong CW, et al: Rotenone potentiates dopamine neuron loss in animals exposed to lipopolysaccharide prenatally. Exp Neurol 2004;190:373–383.

Liou HH, Tsai MC, Chen CJ, et al: Environmental risk factors and Parkinson's disease: A case-control study in Taiwan. Neurology 1997;48:1583–1588.

Liu B, Gao HM, Hong JS: Parkinson's disease and exposure to infectious agents and pesticides and the occurrence of brain injuries: Role of neuroinflammation. Environ Health Perspect 2003;111:1065–1073.

Lo BC, Ridet JL, Schneider BL, et al: Alpha-synucleinopathy and selective dopaminergic neuron loss in a rat lentiviral-based model of Parkinson's disease. Proc Natl Acad Sci U S A 2002;99:10813–10818.

Lo BC, Schneider BL, Bauer M, et al: Lentiviral vector delivery of parkin prevents dopaminergic degeneration in an alpha-synuclein rat model of Parkinson's disease. Proc Natl Acad Sci U S A 2004;101:17510–17515.

Lockhart PJ, Bounds R, Hulihan M, et al: Lack of mutations in DJ-1 in a cohort of Taiwanese ethnic Chinese with early-onset parkinsonism. Mov Disord 2004;19:1065–1069.

Lombardino AJ, Li XC, Hertel M, Nottebohm F: Replaceable neurons and neurodegenerative disease share depressed UCHL1 levels. Proc Natl Acad Sci U S A 2005;102:8036–8041.

Lotharius J, Brundin P: Pathogenesis of Parkinson's disease: Dopamine, vesicles and alpha-synuclein. Nat Rev Neurosci 2002; 3:932–942.

Macedo MG, Anar B, Bronner IF, et al: The DJ-1L166P mutant protein associated with early onset Parkinson's disease is unstable and forms higher-order protein complexes. Hum Mol Genet 2003; 12:2807–2816.

Mackenzie GM, Jackson MJ, Jenner P, Marsden CD: Nitric oxide synthase inhibition and MPTP-induced toxicity in the common marmoset. Synapse 1997;26:301–316.

Maharaj DS, Saravanan KS, Maharaj H, ,et al: Acetaminophen and aspirin inhibit superoxide anion generation and lipid peroxidation, and protect against 1-methyl-4-phenyl pyridinium-induced dopaminergic neurotoxicity in rats. Neurochem Int 2004;44:355–360.

Mann VM, Cooper JM, Daniel SE, et al: Complex I, iron, and ferritin in Parkinson's disease substantia nigra. Ann Neurol 1994;36:876–881.

Manning-Bog AB, McCormack AL, Li J, et al: The herbicide paraquat causes up-regulation and aggregation of alpha-synuclein in mice: Paraquat and alpha-synuclein. J Biol Chem 2002;277:1641–1644.

Manning-Bog AB, McCormack AL, Purisai MG, et al: Alpha-synuclein overexpression protects against paraquat-induced neurodegeneration. J Neurosci 2003;23:3095–3099.

Manning-Bog AB, Reaney SH, Chou VP, et al: Lack of nigrostriatal pathology in a rat model of proteasome inhibition. Ann Neurol 2006;60(2):256–260.

Maraganore DM, Lesnick TG, Elbaz A, et al: UCHL1 is a Parkinson's disease susceptibility gene. Ann Neurol 2004;55:512–521.

Maries E, Dass B, Collier TJ, et al: The role of alpha-synuclein in Parkinson's disease: Insights from animal models. Nat Rev Neurosci 2003;4:727–738.

Marshall KA, Daniel SE, Cairns N, et al: Upregulation of the anti-apoptotic protein Bcl-2 may be an early event in neurodegeneration: Studies on Parkinson's and incidental Lewy body disease. Biochem Biophys Res Commun 1997;240:84–87.

Marti MJ, Tolosa E, Campdelacreu J: Clinical overview of the synucleinopathies. Mov Disord 2003;18(suppl 6):S21–S27.

Martin LJ, Pan Y, Price AC, et al: Parkinson's disease alpha-synuclein transgenic mice develop neuronal mitochondrial degeneration and cell death. J Neurosci 2006;26:41–50.

Martinat C, Shendelman S, Jonason A, et al: Sensitivity to oxidative stress in DJ-1-deficient dopamine neurons: An ES-derived cell model of primary Parkinsonism. PLoS. Biol 2004;2:e327.

Masliah E, Rockenstein E, Adame A, et al: Effects of alpha-synuclein immunization in a mouse model of Parkinson's disease. Neuron 2005;46:857–868.

Mata IF, Lockhart PJ, Farrer MJ: Parkin genetics: One model for Parkinson's disease. Hum Mol Genet 2004;13(Spec No 1):R127–R133.

Mata IF, Taylor JP, Kachergus J, et al: LRRK2 R1441G in Spanish patients with Parkinson's disease. Neurosci Lett 2005;382:309–311.

McCormack AL, Di Monte DA: Effects of L-dopa and other amino acids against paraquat-induced nigrostriatal degeneration. J Neurochem 2003;85:82–86.

McCormack AL, Thiruchelvam M, Manning-Bog AB, et al: Environmental risk factors and Parkinson's disease: Selective degeneration of nigral dopaminergic neurons caused by the herbicide paraquat. Neurobiol Dis 2002;10:119–127.

McGeer PL, Itagaki S, Boyes BE, McGeer EG: Reactive microglia are positive for HLA-DR in the substantia nigra of Parkinson's and Alzheimer's disease brains. Neurology 1988;38:1285–1291.

McMillan G: Is electric arc welding linked to manganism or Parkinson's disease? Toxicol Rev 2005;24:237–257.

McNaught KS, Belizaire R, Isacson O, et al: Altered proteasomal function in sporadic Parkinson's disease. Exp Neurol 2003;179:38–46.

McNaught KS, Belizaire R, Jenner P, et al: Selective loss of 20S proteasome alpha-subunits in the substantia nigra pars compacta in Parkinson's disease. Neurosci Lett 2002;326:155–158.

McNaught KS, Carrupt PA, Altomare C, et al: Isoquinoline derivatives as endogenous neurotoxins in the aetiology of Parkinson's disease. Biochem Pharmacol 1998;56:921–933.

McNaught KS, Jenner P: Altered glial function causes neuronal death and increases neuronal susceptibility to 1-methyl-4-phenylpyridinium- and 6-hydroxydopamine-induced toxicity in astrocytic/ventral mesencephalic co-cultures. J Neurochem 1999;73:2469–2476.

McNaught KS, Jenner P: Dysfunction of rat forebrain astrocytes in culture alters cytokine and neurotrophic factor release. Neurosci Lett 2000a;285:61–65.

McNaught KS, Jenner P: Extracellular accumulation of nitric oxide, hydrogen peroxide, and glutamate in astrocytic cultures following glutathione depletion, complex I inhibition, and/or lipopolysaccharide-induced activation. Biochem Pharmacol 2000b;60:979–988.

McNaught KS, Lee M, Hyun DH, Jenner P: Glial cells and abnormal protein handling in the pathogenesis of Parkinson's disease. Adv Neurol 2001;86:73–82.

McNaught KS, Mytilineou C, Jnobaptiste R, et al: Impairment of the ubiquitin-proteasome system causes dopaminergic cell death and inclusion body formation in ventral mesencephalic cultures. J Neurochem 2002;81:301–306.

McNaught KS, Olanow CW: Proteolytic stress: A unifying concept for the etiopathogenesis of Parkinson's disease. Ann Neurol 2003; 53(suppl 3):S73–S84.

McNaught KS, Olanow CW, Halliwell B, et al: Failure of the ubiquitin-proteasome system in Parkinson's disease. Nat Rev Neurosci 2001;2:589–594.

McNaught KS, Perl DP, Brownell AL, Olanow CW: Systemic exposure to proteasome inhibitors causes a progressive model of Parkinson's disease. Ann Neurol 2004;56:149–162.

McNaught KS, Shashidharan P, Perl DP: Aggresome-related biogenesis of Lewy bodies. Eur J Neurosci 2002;16:2136–2148.

Mellick GD, Maraganore DM, Silburn PA: Australian data and meta-analysis lend support for alpha-synuclein (NACP-Rep1) as a risk factor for Parkinson's disease. Neurosci Lett 2005;375:112–116.

Mellick GD, Silburn PA, Prince JA, Brookes AJ: A novel screen for nuclear mitochondrial gene associations with Parkinson's disease. J Neural Transm 2004;111:191–199.

Meulener MC, Graves C., Sampathu DM, et al: DJ-1 is present in a large molecular complex in human brain tissue and interacts with alpha-synuclein. J Neurochem 2005;93:1524–1532.

Miklossy J, Doudet DD, Schwab C, et al: Role of ICAM-1 in persisting inflammation in Parkinson disease and MPTP monkeys. Exp Neurol 2006;197:275–283.

Mitsumoto A, Nakagawa Y, Takeuchi A, et al: Oxidized forms of peroxiredoxins and DJ-1 on two-dimensional gels increased in response to sublethal levels of paraquat. Free Radic Res 2001;35: 301–310.

Mizuno Y, Matuda S, Yoshino H, et al: An immunohistochemical study on alpha-ketoglutarate dehydrogenase complex in Parkinson's disease. Ann Neurol 1994;35:204–210.

Mizuta I, Satake W, Nakabayashi Y, et al: Multiple candidate gene analysis identifies alpha-synuclein as a susceptibility gene for sporadic Parkinson's disease. Hum Mol Genet 2006;15:1151–1158.

Mochizuki H, Nakamura N, Nishi K, Mizuno Y: Apoptosis is induced by 1-methyl-4-phenylpyridinium ion (MPP+) in ventral mesencephalic-striatal co-culture in rat. Neurosci Lett 1994;170: 191–194.

Mogi M, Harada M, Kondo T, et al: The soluble form of Fas molecule is elevated in parkinsonian brain tissues. Neurosci Lett 1996;220: 195–198.

Moncada S, Bolanos JP: Nitric oxide, cell bioenergetics and neurodegeneration. J Neurochem 2006;97:1676–1689.

Moore DJ, Dawson VL, Dawson TM: Genetics of Parkinson's disease: What do mutations in DJ-1 tell us? Ann Neurol 2003;54:281–282.

Moore DJ, Dawson VL, Dawson TM: Lessons from Drosophila models of DJ-1 deficiency. Sci Aging Knowledge Environ 2006; 2006(2):e2.

Moore DJ, Zhang L, Troncoso J, et al: Association of DJ-1 and parkin mediated by pathogenic DJ-1 mutations and oxidative stress. Hum Mol Genet 2005;14:71–84.

Morris CM, O'Brien KK, Gibson AM, et al: Polymorphism in the human DJ-1 gene is not associated with sporadic dementia with Lewy bodies or Parkinson's disease. Neurosci Lett 2003;352: 151–153.

Mueller JC, Fuchs J, Hofer A, et al: Multiple regions of alpha-synuclein are associated with Parkinson's disease. Ann Neurol 2005; 57:535–541.

Muqit MM, Davidson SM, Payne S, et al: Parkin is recruited into aggresomes in a stress-specific manner: Over-expression of parkin reduces aggresome formation but can be dissociated from parkin's effect on neuronal survival. Hum Mol Genet 2004;13: 117–135.

Muqit MM, Gandhi S, Wood NW: Mitochondria in Parkinson disease: Back in fashion with a little help from genetics. Arch Neurol 2006;63:649–654.

Nagatsu T, Mogi M, Ichinose H, Togari A: Changes in cytokines and neurotrophins in Parkinson's disease. J Neural Transm Suppl 2000;277–290.

Neafsey EJ, Drucker G, Raikoff K, Collins MA: Striatal dopaminergic toxicity following intranigral injection in rats of 2-methyl-norharman, a beta-carbolinium analog of N-methyl-4-phenylpyridinium ion (MPP+). Neurosci Lett 1989;105:344–349.

Neumann M, Muller V, Gorner K, et al: Pathological properties of the Parkinson's disease-associated protein DJ-1 in alpha-synucleinopathies and tauopathies: Relevance for multiple system atrophy and Pick's disease. Acta Neuropathol (Berl) 2004;107: 489–496.

Ng YK, Ling EA: Induction of major histocompatibility class II antigen on microglial cells in postnatal and adult rats following intraperitoneal injections of lipopolysaccharide. Neurosci Res 1997;28:111–118.

Nichols WC, Pankratz N, Hernandez D, et al: Genetic screening for a single common LRRK2 mutation in familial Parkinson's disease. Lancet 2005;365:410–412.

Nichols WC, Uniacke SK, Pankratz N, et al: Evaluation of the role of Nurr1 in a large sample of familial Parkinson's disease. Mov Disord 2004;19:649–655.

Nishinaga H, Takahashi-Niki K, Taira T, et al: Expression profiles of genes in DJ-1-knockdown and L 166 P DJ-1 mutant cells. Neurosci Lett 2005;390:54–59.

Nishioka K, Hayashi S, Farrer MJ, et al: Clinical heterogeneity of alpha-synuclein gene duplication in Parkinson's disease. Ann Neurol 2006;59:298–309.

Olanow CW, Jenner P, Tatton N, Tatton WG: Neurodegeneration in Parkinson's disease. In Jankovic J, Tolosa E (eds): Parkinson's Disease and Movement Disorders. Baltimore, Williams & Wilkins, 1998, pp 67–103.

Olanow CW, Tatton WG: Etiology and pathogenesis of Parkinson's disease. Annu Rev Neurosci 1999;22:123–144.

Olanow CW, Tatton WG, Jenner P: Mechanisms of cell death in Parkinson's disease. In Jankovic J, Tolosa E (eds): Parkinson's Disease and Movement Disorders. Philadelphia, Lippincott Williams & Wilkins, 2002, pp 39–59.

Oliveira SA, Scott WK, Martin ER, et al: Parkin mutations and susceptibility alleles in late-onset Parkinson's disease. Ann Neurol 2003;53:624–629.

Osaka H, Wang YL, Takada K, et al: Ubiquitin carboxy-terminal hydrolase L1 binds to and stabilizes monoubiquitin in neuron. Hum Mol Genet 2003;12:1945–1958.

Ossowska K, Smialowska M, Kuter K, et al: Degeneration of dopaminergic mesocortical neurons and activation of compensatory processes induced by a long-term paraquat administration in rats: Implications for parkinson's disease. Neuroscience 2006;141: 2155–2165.

Ossowska K, Wardas J, Kuter K, et al: Influence of paraquat on dopaminergic transporter in the rat brain. Pharmacol Rep 2005a; 57:330–335.

Ossowska K, Wardas J, Smialowska M, et al: A slowly developing dysfunction of dopaminergic nigrostriatal neurons induced by long-term paraquat administration in rats: An animal model of preclinical stages of Parkinson's disease? Eur J Neurosci 2005b; 22:1294–1304.

Ouchi Y, Yoshikawa E, Sekine Y, et al: Microglial activation and dopamine terminal loss in early Parkinson's disease. Ann Neurol 2005;57;168–175.

Ozelius LJ, Senthil G, Saunders-Pullman R, et al: LRRK2 G2019S as a cause of Parkinson's disease in Ashkenazi Jews. N Engl J Med 2006;354(4):424–425.

Paisan-Ruiz C, Jain S, Evans EW, et al: Cloning of the gene containing mutations that cause PARK8-linked Parkinson's disease. Neuron 2004;44:595–600.

Paisan-Ruiz C, Lang AE, Kawarai T, et al: LRRK2 gene in Parkinson disease: Mutation analysis and case control association study. Neurology 2005a;65:696–700.

Paisan-Ruiz C, Saenz A, Lopez de MA, et al: Familial Parkinson's disease: Clinical and genetic analysis of four Basque families. Ann Neurol 2005b;57:365–372.

Pal PK, Samii A, Calne DB: Manganese neurotoxicity: A review of clinical features, imaging and pathology. Neurotoxicology 1999; 20:227–238.

Palacino JJ, Sagi D, Goldberg MS, et al: Mitochondrial dysfunction and oxidative damage in parkin-deficient mice. J Biol Chem 2004;279:18614–18622.

Pals P, Lincoln S, Manning J, et al: α-Synuclein promoter confers susceptibility to Parkinson's disease. Ann Neurol 2004;56:591–595.

Pandey N, Schmidt RE, Galvin JE: The alpha-synuclein mutation E46K promotes aggregation in cultured cells. Exp Neurol 2006;197:515–520.

Park J, Yoo CI, Sim CS, et al: A retrospective cohort study of Parkinson's disease in Korean shipbuilders. Neurotoxicology 2006; 27:445–449.

Perez FA, Palmiter RD: Parkin-deficient mice are not a robust model of parkinsonism. Proc Natl Acad Sci U S A 2005;102:2174–2179.

Perez RG, Hastings TG: Could a loss of alpha-synuclein function put dopaminergic neurons at risk? J Neurochem 2004;89:1318–1324.

Perier C, Bove J, Vila M, Przedborski S: The rotenone model of Parkinson's disease. Trends Neurosci 2003;26:345–346.

Periquet M, Corti O, Jacquier S, Brice A: Proteomic analysis of parkin knockout mice: Alterations in energy metabolism, protein handling and synaptic function. J Neurochem 2005;95:1259–1276.

Periquet M, Latouche M, Lohmann E, et al: Parkin mutations are frequent in patients with isolated early-onset parkinsonism. Brain 2003;126:1271–1278.

Pesah Y, Pham T, Burgess H, et al: Drosophila parkin mutants have decreased mass and cell size and increased sensitivity to oxygen radical stress. Development 2004;131:2183–2194.

Petito CK, Roberts B: Effect of postmortem interval on in situ end-labeling of DNA oligonucleosomes. J Neuropathol Exp Neurol 1995;54:761–765.

Petrucelli L, O'Farrell C, Lockhart PJ, et al: Parkin protects against the toxicity associated with mutant alpha-synuclein: Proteasome dysfunction selectively affects catecholaminergic neurons. Neuron 2002;36:1007–1019.

Pezzoli G, Canesi M, Antonini A, et al: Hydrocarbon exposure and Parkinson's disease. Neurology 2000;55:667–673.

Polymeropoulos MH, Lavedan C, Leroy E, et al: Mutation in the alpha-synuclein gene identified in families with Parkinson's disease. Science 1997;276:2045–2047.

Poon HF, Frasier M, Shreve N, et al: Mitochondrial associated metabolic proteins are selectively oxidized in A30P alpha-synuclein transgenic mice: A model of familial Parkinson's disease. Neurobiol Dis 2005;18:492–498.

Pountney DL, Lowe R, Quilty M, et al: Annular alpha-synuclein species from purified multiple system atrophy inclusions. J Neurochem 2004;90:502–512.

Pramstaller PP, Schlossmacher MG, Jacques TS, et al: Lewy body Parkinson's disease in a large pedigree with 77 Parkin mutation carriers. Ann Neurol 2005;58:411–422.

Priyadarshi A, Khuder SA, Schaub EA, Shrivastava S: A meta-analysis of Parkinson's disease and exposure to pesticides. Neurotoxicology 2000;21:435–440.

Przedborski S, Jackson-Lewis V, Yokoyama R, et al: Role of neuronal nitric oxide in 1-methyl-4-phenyl-1,2,3,6-tetrahydropyridine (MPTP)-induced dopaminergic neurotoxicity. Proc Natl Acad Sci U S A 1996;93:4565–4571.

Rascol O, Olanow CW, Brooks D, et al: Effect of riluzole on Parkinson's disease progression: A double-blind placebo-controlled study. Neurology 2003;60(suppl 1):A288.

Richardson JR, Caudle WM, Wang M, et al: Developmental exposure to the pesticide dieldrin alters the dopamine system and increases neurotoxicity in an animal model of Parkinson's disease. FASEB J 2006;20:1695–1697.

Riedl AG, Watts PM, Jenner P, Marsden CD: P450 enzymes and Parkinson's disease: The story so far. Mov Disord 1998;13: 212–220.

Robertson DC, Schmidt O, Ninkina N, et al: Developmental loss and resistance to MPTP toxicity of dopaminergic neurones in substantia nigra pars compacta of gamma-synuclein, alpha-synuclein and double alpha/gamma-synuclein null mutant mice. J Neurochem 2004;89:1126–1136.

Rochet JC, Outeiro TF, Conway KA, et al: Interactions among alpha-synuclein, dopamine, and biomembranes: Some clues for understanding neurodegeneration in Parkinson's disease. J Mol Neurosci 2004;23:23–34.

Rodriguez MC, Obeso JA, Olanow CW: Subthalamic nucleus-mediated excitotoxicity in Parkinson's disease: A target for neuroprotection. Ann Neurol 1998;44:S175–S188.

Rohe CF, Montagna P, Breedveld G, et al: Homozygous PINK1 C-terminus mutation causing early-onset parkinsonism. Ann Neurol 2004;56:427–431.

Sairam K, Saravanan KS, Banerjee R, Mohanakumar KP: Non-steroidal anti-inflammatory drug sodium salicylate, but not diclofenac or celecoxib, protects against 1-methyl-4-phenyl pyridinium-induced dopaminergic neurotoxicity in rats. Brain Res 2003;966:245–252.

Sanchez-Ramos J, Facca A, Basit A, Song S: Toxicity of dieldrin for dopaminergic neurons in mesencephalic cultures. Exp Neurol 1998;150:263–271.

Saravanan KS, Sindhu KM, Mohanakumar KP: Acute intranigral infusion of rotenone in rats causes progressive biochemical lesions in the striatum similar to Parkinson's disease. Brain Res 2005;1049:147–155.

Saucedo-Cardenas O, Quintana-Hau JD, Le WD, et al: Nurr1 is essential for the induction of the dopaminergic phenotype and the survival of ventral mesencephalic late dopaminergic precursor neurons. Proc Natl Acad Sci U S A 1998;95:4013–4018.

Schapira AH: Etiology of Parkinson's disease. Neurology 2006;66: S10–S23.

Schapira AH, Cleeter MW, Muddle JR, et al: Proteasomal inhibition causes loss of nigral tyrosine hydroxylase neurons. Ann Neurol 2006;60(2):253–255.

Schapira AH, Cooper JM, Dexter D, et al: Mitochondrial complex I deficiency in Parkinson's disease. J Neurochem 1990;54:823–827.

Schulz JB, Matthews RT, Muqit MM, et al: Inhibition of neuronal nitric oxide synthase by 7-nitroindazole protects against MPTP-induced neurotoxicity in mice. J Neurochem 1995;64: 936–939.

Scott WK, Nance MA, Watts RL, et al: Complete genomic screen in Parkinson disease: Evidence for multiple genes. JAMA 2001;286: 2239–2244.

Scott WK, Zhang F, Stajich JM, et al: Family-based case-control study of cigarette smoking and Parkinson disease. Neurology 2005;64: 442–447.

Seidler A, Hellenbrand W, Robra BP, et al: Possible environmental, occupational, and other etiologic factors for Parkinson's disease: A case-control study in Germany. Neurology 1996;46:1275–1284.

Shen J: Protein kinases linked to the pathogenesis of Parkinson's disease. Neuron 2004;44:575–577.

Sherer TB, Betarbet R, Stout AK, et al: An in vitro model of Parkinson's disease: Linking mitochondrial impairment to altered alpha-synuclein metabolism and oxidative damage. J Neurosci 2002;22:7006–7015.

Sherer TB, Betarbet R, Testa CM, et al: Mechanism of toxicity in rotenone models of Parkinson's disease. J Neurosci 2003;23: 10756–10764.

Shibata H, Katsuki H, Nishiwaki M, et al: Lipopolysaccharide-induced dopaminergic cell death in rat midbrain slice cultures: Role of inducible nitric oxide synthase and protection by indomethacin. J Neurochem 2003;86:1201–1212.

Shimura H, Hattori N, Kubo S, et al: Immunohistochemical and subcellular localization of Parkin protein: Absence of protein in autosomal recessive juvenile parkinsonism patients. Ann Neurol 1999;45:668–672.

Shimura H, Hattori N, Kubo S, et al: Familial Parkinson disease gene product, parkin, is a ubiquitin-protein ligase. Nat Genet 2000;25: 302–305.

Shults CW, Rockenstein E, Crews L, et al: Neurological and neurodegenerative alterations in a transgenic mouse model expressing human alpha-synuclein under oligodendrocyte promoter: Implications for multiple system atrophy. J Neurosci 2005;25: 10689–10699.

Silvestri L, Caputo V, Bellacchio E, et al: Mitochondrial import and enzymatic activity of PINK1 mutants associated to recessive parkinsonism. Hum Mol Genet 2005;14:3477–3492.

Simon-Sanchez J, Herranz-Perez V, Olucha-Bordonau F, Perez-Tur J: LRRK2 is expressed in areas affected by Parkinson's disease in the adult mouse brain. Eur J Neurosci 2006;23:659–666.

Singleton AB, Farrer M, Johnson J, et al: Alpha-synuclein locus triplication causes Parkinson's disease. Science 2003;302:841.

Skipper L, Shen H, Chua E, et al: Analysis of LRRK2 functional domains in nondominant Parkinson disease. Neurology 2005; 65:1319–1321.

Smith WW, Jiang H, Pei Z, et al: Endoplasmic reticulum stress and mitochondrial cell death pathways mediate A53T mutant alpha-synuclein-induced toxicity. Hum Mol Genet 2005a;14:3801–3811.

Smith WW, Margolis RL, Li X, et al: Alpha-synuclein phosphorylation enhances eosinophilic cytoplasmic inclusion formation in SH-SY5Y cells. J Neurosci 2005b;25:5544–5552.

Song DD, Shults CW, Sisk A, et al: Enhanced substantia nigra mitochondrial pathology in human alpha-synuclein transgenic mice after treatment with MPTP. Exp Neurol 2004;186:158–172.

Sortwell CE, Daley BF, Pitzer MR, et al: Oligodendrocyte-type 2 astrocyte-derived trophic factors increase survival of developing dopamine neurons through the inhibition of apoptotic cell death. J Comp Neurol 2000;426:143–153.

Springer W, Hoppe T, Schmidt E, Baumeister R: A Caenorhabditis elegans Parkin mutant with altered solubility couples alpha-synuclein aggregation to proteotoxic stress. Hum Mol Genet 2005; 14:3407–3423.

Sriram SR, Li X, Ko HS, et al: Familial-associated mutations differentially disrupt the solubility, localization, binding and ubiquitination properties of parkin. Hum Mol Genet 2005;14: 2571– 2586.

Sugama S, Yang L, Cho BP, et al: Age-related microglial activation in 1-methyl-4-phenyl-1,2,3,6-tetrahydropyridine (MPTP)-induced dopaminergic neurodegeneration in C57BL/6 mice. Brain Res 2003;964:288–294.

Sun F, Anantharam V, Latchoumycandane C, et al: Dieldrin induces ubiquitin-proteasome dysfunction in alpha-synuclein overexpressing dopaminergic neuronal cells and enhances susceptibility to apoptotic cell death. J Pharmacol Exp Ther 2005;315:69–79.

Tan EK, Chandran VR, Fook-Chong S, et al: Alpha-synuclein mRNA expression in sporadic Parkinson's disease. Mov Disord 2005; 20:620–623.

Tan EK, Khajavi M, Thornby JI, et al: Variability and validity of polymorphism association studies in Parkinson's disease. Neurology 2000;55:533–538.

Tatton NA: Increased caspase 3 and Bax immunoreactivity accompany nuclear GAPDH translocation and neuronal apoptosis in Parkinson's disease. Exp Neurol 2000;166:29–43.

Tatton NA, Maclean-Fraser A, Tatton WG, et al: A fluorescent double-labeling method to detect and confirm apoptotic nuclei in Parkinson's disease. Ann Neurol 1998;44:S142–S148.

Tatton NA, Rideout HJ: Confocal microscopy as a tool to examine DNA fragmentation, chromatin condensation and other apoptotic changes in Parkinson's disease. Parkinsonism Relat Disord 1999;5:179–186.

Tatton W, Ju W, Wadia J, et al.: (-)-Deprenyl reduces neuronal apoptosis by maintaining bcl-2 synthesis and mitochondrial membrane potential. Mov Disord 1994;9(suppl 1):4.

Tatton WG, Chalmers-Redman RM: Modulation of gene expression rather than monoamine oxidase inhibition: (-)-Deprenyl-related compounds in controlling neurodegeneration. Neurology 1996;47:S171–S183.

Tatton WG, Chalmers-Redman R, Brown D, Tatton N: Apoptosis in Parkinson's disease: Signals for neuronal degradation. Ann Neurol 2003;53(suppl 3):S61–S70.

Tatton WG, Olanow CW: Apoptosis in neurodegenerative diseases: The role of mitochondria. Biochim Biophys Acta 1999;1410: 195–213.

Taymans JM, Van den Haute C, Baekelandt V: Distribution of PINK1 and LRRK2 in rat and mouse brain. J Neurochem 2006;98:951–961.

Teismann P, Tieu K, Choi DK, et al: Cyclooxygenase-2 is instrumental in Parkinson's disease neurodegeneration. Proc Natl Acad Sci U S A 2003a;100:5473–5478.

Teismann P, Tieu K, Cohen O, et al: Pathogenic role of glial cells in Parkinson's disease. Mov Disord 2003b;18:121–129.

Thiruchelvam M, Brockel BJ, Richfield EK, et al: Potentiated and environmental risk factors for Parkinson's disease? Brain Res 2000a;873:225–234.

Thiruchelvam MJ, Powers JM, Cory-Slechta DA, Richfield EK: Risk factors for dopaminergic neuron loss in human alpha-synuclein transgenic mice. Eur J Neurosci 2004;19:845–854.

Thiruchelvam M, Richfield EK, Baggs RB, et al: The nigrostriatal dopaminergic system as a preferential target of repeated exposures to combined paraquat and maneb: Implications for Parkinson's disease. J Neurosci 2000b;20:9207–9214.

Thiruchelvam M, Richfield EK, Goodman BM, et al: Developmental exposure to the pesticides paraquat and maneb and the Parkinson's disease phenotype. Neurotoxicology 2002;23: 621– 633.

Toda T, Momose Y, Murata M, et al: Toward identification of susceptibility genes for sporadic Parkinson's disease. J Neurol 2003; 250(suppl 3):III40–III43.

Tofaris GK, Garcia RP, Humby T, et al: Pathological changes in dopaminergic nerve cells of the substantia nigra and olfactory bulb in mice transgenic for truncated human alpha-synuclein (1-120): Implications for Lewy body disorders. J Neurosci 2006;26:3942–3950.

Tofaris GK, Layfield R, Spillantini MG: alpha-Synuclein metabolism and aggregation is linked to ubiquitin-independent degradation by the proteasome. FEBS Lett 2001;509:22–26.

Tofaris GK, Razzaq A, Ghetti B, et al: Ubiquitination of alpha-synuclein in Lewy bodies is a pathological event not associated with impairment of proteasome function. J Biol Chem 2003;278: 44405–44411.

Tomas-Camardiel M, Rite I, Herrera AJ, et al: Minocycline reduces the lipopolysaccharide-induced inflammatory reaction, peroxynitrite-mediated nitration of proteins, disruption of the blood-brain barrier, and damage in the nigral dopaminergic system. Neurobiol Dis 2004;16:190–201.

Ton TG, Heckbert SR, Longstreth WT Jr, et al: Nonsteroidal anti-inflammatory drugs and risk of Parkinson's disease. Mov Disord 2006; 21:964–969.

Totterdell S, Hanger D, Meredith GE: The ultrastructural distribution of alpha-synuclein-like protein in normal mouse brain. Brain Res 2004;1004:61–72.

Trimmer PA, Borland MK, Keeney PM, et al: Parkinson's disease transgenic mitochondrial cybrids generate Lewy inclusion bodies. J Neurochem 2004;88:800–812.

Turski L, Bressler K, Rettig KJ, et al: Protection of substantia nigra from MPP+ neurotoxicity by N-methyl-D-aspartate antagonists. Nature 1991;349:414–418.

Uversky VN, Li J, Fink AL: Pesticides directly accelerate the rate of alpha-synuclein fibril formation: A possible factor in Parkinson's disease. FEBS Lett 2001;500:105–108.

Uversky VN, Yamin G, Munishkina LA, et al: Effects of nitration on the structure and aggregation of alpha-synuclein. Brain Res Mol Brain Res 2005;134:84–102.

Valente EM, Abou-Sleiman PM, Caputo V, et al: Hereditary early-onset Parkinson's disease caused by mutations in PINK1. Science 2004a;304:1158–1160.

Valente EM, Salvi S, Ialongo T, et al: PINK1 mutations are associated with sporadic early-onset parkinsonism. Ann Neurol 2004b;56: 336–341.

van Leyen K, Siddiq A, Ratan RR, Lo EH: Proteasome inhibition protects HT22 neuronal cells from oxidative glutamate toxicity. J Neurochem 2005;92:824–830.

Ved R, Saha S, Westlund B, et al: Similar patterns of mitochondrial vulnerability and rescue induced by genetic modification of alpha-synuclein, parkin, and DJ-1 in Caenorhabditis elegans. J Biol Chem 2005;280:42655–42668.

Veech GA, Dennis J, Keeney PM, et al: Disrupted mitochondrial electron transport function increases expression of anti-apoptotic bcl-2 and bcl-X(L) proteins in SH-SY5Y neuroblastoma and in Parkinson disease cybrid cells through oxidative stress. J Neurosci Res 2000;61:693–700.

von Coelln R, Thomas B, Savitt JM, et al: Loss of locus coeruleus neurons and reduced startle in parkin null mice. Proc Natl Acad Sci U S A 2004;101:10744–10749.

Walkinshaw G, Waters CM: Induction of apoptosis in catecholaminergic PC12 cells by L-DOPA. Implications for the treatment of Parkinson's disease. J Clin Invest 1995;95:2458–2464.

Wang XF, Li S, Chou AP, Bronstein JM: Inhibitory effects of pesticides on proteasome activity: Implication in Parkinson's disease. Neurobiol Dis 2006;23:198–205.

Wang YL, Takeda A, Osaka H, et al: Accumulation of beta- and gamma-synucleins in the ubiquitin carboxyl-terminal hydrolase L1-deficient gad mouse. Brain Res 2004;1019:1–9.

Waragai M, Wei J, Fujita M, et al: Increased level of DJ-1 in the cerebrospinal fluids of sporadic Parkinson's disease. Biochem Biophys Res Commun 2006;345:967–972.

Weintraub D, Morales KH, Duda JE, et al: Frequency and correlates of co-morbid psychosis and depression in Parkinson's disease. Parkinsonism Relat Disord 2006;12:427–431.

West AB, Moore DJ, Biskup S, et al: Parkinson's disease-associated mutations in leucine-rich repeat kinase 2 augment kinase activity. Proc Natl Acad Sci U S A 2005;102:16842–16847.

Widdowson PS, Farnworth MJ, Simpson MG, Lock EA: Influence of age on the passage of paraquat through the blood-brain barrier in rats: A distribution and pathological examination. Hum Exp Toxicol 1996a;15:231–236.

Widdowson PS, Farnworth MJ, Upton R, Simpson MG: No changes in behaviour, nigro-striatal system neurochemistry or neuronal cell death following toxic multiple oral paraquat administration to rats. Hum Exp Toxicol 1996b;15:583–591.

Winkler-Stuck K, Kirches E, Mawrin C, et al: Re-evaluation of the dysfunction of mitochondrial respiratory chain in skeletal muscle of patients with Parkinson's disease. J Neural Transm 2005;112: 499–518.

Wirdefeldt K, Gatz M, Pawitan Y, Pedersen NL: Risk and protective factors for Parkinson's disease: A study in Swedish twins. Ann Neurol 2005;57:27–33.

Wu DC, Jackson-Lewis V, Vila M, et al: Blockade of microglial activation is neuroprotective in the 1-methyl-4-phenyl-1,2,3,6-tetrahydropyridine mouse model of Parkinson disease. J Neurosci 2002;22:1763–1771.

Wu RM, Bounds R, Lincoln S, et al: Parkin mutations and early-onset parkinsonism in a Taiwanese cohort. Arch Neurol 2005;62:82–87.

Xu J, Zhong N, Wang H, et al: The Parkinson's disease-associated DJ-1 protein is a transcriptional co-activator that protects against neuronal apoptosis. Hum Mol Genet 2005;14:1231–1241.

Yamada M, Iwatsubo T, Mizuno Y, Mochizuki H: Overexpression of alpha-synuclein in rat substantia nigra results in loss of dopaminergic neurons, phosphorylation of alpha-synuclein and activation of caspase-9: Resemblance to pathogenetic changes in Parkinson's disease. J Neurochem 2004;91:451–461.

Yavich L, Oksman M, Tanila H, et al: Locomotor activity and evoked dopamine release are reduced in mice overexpressing A30P-mutated human alpha-synuclein. Neurobiol Dis 2005;20:303–313.

Yokota T, Sugawara K, Ito K, et al: Down regulation of DJ-1 enhances cell death by oxidative stress, ER stress, and proteasome inhibition. Biochem Biophys Res Commun 2003;312:1342–1348.

Zabetian CP, Samii A, Mosley AD, et al: A clinic-based study of the LRRK2 gene in Parkinson disease yields new mutations. Neurology 2005;65:741–744.

Zarranz JJ, Alegre J, Gomez-Esteban JC, et al: The new mutation, E46K, of alpha-synuclein causes Parkinson and Lewy body dementia. Ann Neurol 2004;55:164–173.

Zeng, B-Y, Medhurst, AD, Jackson M, et al: Proteasomal activity in brain differs between species and brain regions and changes with age. Mech Ageing Dev 2005;126(6–7):760–766.

Zeng BY, Bukhatwa S, Hikima A, et al: Reproducible nigral cell loss after systemic proteasomal inhibitor administration to rats. Ann Neurol 2006;60(2):248–252.

Zhang L, Shimoji M, Thomas B, et al: Mitochondrial localization of the Parkinson's disease related protein DJ-1: Implications for pathogenesis. Hum Mol Genet 2005a;14:2063–2073.

Zhang X, Qu S, Xie W, et al: Neuroprotection by iron chelator against proteasome inhibitor-induced nigral degeneration. BBRC 2005b; 333:544–549

Zhang Y, Dawson VL, Dawson TM: Parkin: Clinical aspects and neurobiology. Clin Neurosci 2001;1:467–482.

Zimprich A, Biskup S, Leitner P, et al: Mutations in LRRK2 cause autosomal-dominant parkinsonism with pleomorphic pathology. Neuron 2004;44:601–607.

# Chapter 6

# Medical Treatment of Parkinson Disease

If treatment of Parkinson disease (PD) with levodopa, the most efficacious drug available for this disorder, were uniformly successful and free of complications, there would be no controversies or complexities, and treatment of this disease would be easy. But because of levodopa's propensity to cause motor complications (wearing off and dyskinesis), which can impair a patient's quality of life, strategies have been developed to avoid or delay these motor complications. Also, strategies have been developed to overcome these complications once they have appeared. Thus, treatment strategies have evolved to deal with the different phases of the natural history of PD as well as the presence of the motor complications.

Before discussing the phases of the disease and the treatment choices for each phase, general principles of therapy for the patient with PD are discussed.

## THERAPEUTIC PRINCIPLES

### Keep the Patient Functioning Independently as Long as Possible

There are a number of drugs that have a favorable impact on the clinical features of the disease by reducing its symptoms, but to date, none have been definitively shown to stop the progression of the disease. Since PD is a progressive disease and no medication prevents ultimate worsening, the long-term goal in treating PD is to keep the patient functioning independently for as long as possible. Clearly, if medications that provide symptomatic relief continued to be effective without producing adverse effects, this would be excellent. For example, if levodopa therapy could persistently reverse parkinsonian signs and symptoms, this therapeutic strategy would not be problematic. The difficulty is that 75% of patients have serious complications after 6 years of levodopa therapy (Table 6-1) (Fahn, 1992a), and younger patients (less than 60 years of age) are particularly prone to developing the motor complications of fluctuations and dyskinesias (Quinn et al., 1987; Kostic et al., 1991; Gershanik, 1993; Wagner et al., 1996). Some physicians therefore recommend utilizing dopamine agonists rather than levodopa in younger patients when beginning therapy, in an attempt to delay the onset of these problems (Quinn, 1994b; Fahn, 1998). Controlled clinical trials comparing dopamine agonists and levodopa as the initial therapeutic agent have proven that motor complications are less likely to occur with dopamine agonists (Parkinson Study Group, 2000; Rascol et al., 2000; Oertel et al., 2006). But each of these studies also showed that levodopa was more effective in lessening parkinsonian symptoms and signs than were the dopamine agonists as measured quantitatively by the Unified Parkinson's Disease Rating Scale (UPDRS).

## Encourage Patients to Remain Active and Mobile

PD leads to decreased motivation and increased passivity. An active exercise program, even early in the disease, can often avoid this. Furthermore, such a program encourages patients to participate in their own care, allows muscle stretching and full range of joint mobility, and enhances a better mental attitude toward fighting the disease. By being encouraged to take responsibility in fighting the devastations of the disease, the patient becomes an active participant. Physical therapy, which can be implemented in the form of a well-constructed exercise program, is useful in all stages of disease. In early stages, a physical therapy program can instruct the patient in the proper exercises, and the regimen forces the patient to exercise if he or she lacks the motivation to do so on his or her own. In advanced stages of PD, physical therapy may be even more valuable by keeping joints from becoming frozen and providing guidance in how best to remain independent in mobility. Therefore, exercise is beneficial in both the early and later stages. It has been shown that PD patients who exercise intensively and regularly have better motor performance (Reuter et al., 1999; Behrman et al., 2000). If exercise is not maintained, the benefit is lost (Lokk, 2000).

A number of basic science studies have discovered that in rodents, exercise, particularly enriched exercise, shortly after the rodents were given experimental lesions of the nigrostriatal dopamine pathway, results in significantly less damage to the dopamine pathway (Tillerson et al., 2001, 2002, 2003; Bezard et al., 2003; Cohen et al., 2003; Fisher et al., 2004; Mabandla, 2004). The mechanism appears to be to the induction of increased trophic factors, such as glial-derived neurotrophic factor (GDNF) (Smith and Zigmond et al., 2003) and brain-derived neurotrophic factor (Bezard et al., 2003).

## Individualize Therapy

The treatment of PD needs to be individualized; that is, each patient presents with a unique set of symptoms, signs, and response to medications and a host of social, occupational, and emotional problems that need to be addressed. As was mentioned previously, a major goal is to keep the patient functioning independently as long as possible. Practical guides for how to direct the treatment are to consider the patient's symptoms, the degree of functional impairment, and the expected benefits and risks of available therapeutic agents. Ask the patient what specific symptoms trouble him or her the most, and then focus on these problems. Also, keep in mind that younger patients are more likely to develop motor fluctuations and dyskinesias; older patients are more likely to develop confusion, sleep-wake alterations, and psychosis from medications.

**Table 6-1** Five major responses to more than 5 years of levodopa therapy[*]

| Response | n | Percent |
|---|---|---|
| 1. Smooth, good response | 83 | 25 |
| 2. Troublesome fluctuations | 142 | 43 |
| 3. Troublesome dyskinesias | 67 | 20 |
| 4. Toxicity at therapeutic or subtherapeutic dosages | 14 | 4 |
| 5. Total or substantial loss of efficacy | 27 | 8 |

[*]n = 330 patients. Thirty-six patients had both troublesome fluctuations and troublesome dyskinesias.

Data from Fahn S: Adverse effects of levodopa. In Olanow CW, Lieberman AN (eds): The Scientific Basis for the Treatment of Parkinson's Disease. Carnforth, UK, Parthenon Publishing Group, 1992, pp. 89–112.

## Give Priority to Any Therapies, Such as Drugs or Surgery, That Have Been Established as Protective

If any drug could slow the progression of the disease process, it would make sense to use it as soon as the disease is diagnosed. As of this writing, no proven protective or restorative effect of a drug has been demonstrated with certainty. But studies are in progress looking at various agents to determine whether they have such an effect. Drugs that have been specifically evaluated in controlled clinical trials for slowing disease progression have been selegiline and tocopherol (Parkinson Study Group, 1989b, 1993a), riluzole (Rascol et al., 2003), neuroimmunophilin (not yet published), coenzyme Q10 (Shults et al., 2002), and GDNF (Lang et al., 2006). Two anti-apoptic drugs that were studied in controlled trials were a propargyline inhibitor of glyceraldehyde 3-phosphate dehydrogenase (Waldmeier et al., 2000) and an inhibitor of the mixed lineage kinase-3 family that lies upstream of the c-Jun N-terminal kinase signal transduction pathway to apoptotic cell death (Xia et al., 2001). Both studies failed to show benefit (Waldmeier et al., 2006). Controlled trials with an antibiotic, minocycline, and an energy enhancer, creatine, using a futility design (Tilley et al., 2006), failed to show these drugs to be futile; therefore, they are potential agents for a larger clinical trial (NINDS NET-PD Investigators, 2006). A discussion of the results of these completed studies is presented later in the chapter, in the section entitled "Treatment of Early-Stage Parkinson Disease."

## THERAPEUTIC CHOICES AVAILABLE FOR PARKINSON DISEASE

Treatment of patients with PD can be divided into three major categories: physical (and mental health) therapy, medications, and surgery. Physical exercise and physiotherapy were discussed in the previous section. Speech therapy plays a similar role in patients with problems of communication. Dysarthria, palilalia, and tachyphemia are difficult to treat, but hypophonia can be overcome by training the patient to shout, known as the Lee Silverman technique (Ramig et al., 2001). Psychiatric assistance may be required to handle depression and the social and familial problems that can develop with this chronic, disabling illness. Electroconvulsive therapy may have a role in patients with severe, intractable depression; some psychiatrists have been promoting this therapy to help overcome the motor symptoms of PD, but at best electroconvulsive therapy provides only short-term benefit that might not be replicated on repeat treatments. The current practice parameters on treatment of depression, psychosis, and dementia in patients with PD have been summarized in the 2006 report by the American Academy of Neurology Quality Standards Subcommittee (Miyasaki et al, 2006) (see Chapter 8).

Neurosurgery for PD is becoming increasingly available as new techniques have been developed, particularly deep brain stimulation. This major topic is covered in Chapter 7 and is mentioned here only to be complete in understanding the choices that are available.

## MEDICATIONS AVAILABLE FOR PARKINSON DISEASE

A great many drugs have been developed for PD. Boxes 6-1, 6-2, and 6-3 classify them according to their mechanisms of action. Selection of the most suitable drugs for the individual patient and deciding when to utilize them in the course of the disease are challenges to the treating clinician. In many of the parkinsonism-plus disorders, the response to treatment is not satisfactory, but the principles for treating PD are the basis for treating these disorders as well. Because PD is a chronic progressive disease, patients require lifelong treatment. Medications and their doses will change over time as adverse effects and new symptoms are encountered. Tactical strategy is based on the severity of the disease.

Almost all drug trials evaluate the drug's short-term symptomatic benefit, but the leading unmet need is stopping or slowing progression. The Sydney Multicentre Study of Parkinson disease has reported the problems experienced by people who survive 15 years from diagnosis (Hely et al., 2005). The standardized mortality ratio was significantly elevated at 1.86. Falls occurred in 81% of patients, and 23% sustained fractures. Cognitive decline was present in 84%, and 48% fulfilled the criteria for dementia. Hallucinations and depression were experienced by 50%. Choking occurred in 50%, symptomatic postural hypotension in 35%, and urinary incontinence in 41%. No patient remained employed, and 40% of patients live in aged-care facilities. Although approximately 95% have experienced dopa-induced dyskinesia/dystonia and wearing-off, in the majority, these symptoms are not disabling. Dyskinesia and dystonia were delayed by early use of bromocriptine, but wearing-off appeared at a similar time once levodopa was added. The most disabling long-term problems of PD relate to the emergence of symptoms that are not improved by levodopa.

Because most of the major motoric symptoms of PD are related to striatal dopamine deficiency (Hornykiewicz, 1966), dopamine replacement therapy is the major medical approach to treating the disease. Box 6-1 lists these dopaminergic drugs. The most powerful drug is levodopa. It is usually administered with a peripheral decarboxylase inhibitor. In Box 6-1, both carbidopa and benserazide are listed as peripheral dopa

Box 6-1 Dopaminergic agents

Dopamine precursor: levodopa (combined with
  carbidopa in standard release, slow-release, and
  dissolvable-in-mouth formulations)
Decarboxylase inhibitor: carbidopa, benserazide
Dopamine agonists: bromocriptine, pergolide,
  pramipexole, ropinirole, apomorphine, cabergoline,
  lisuride, piribedil, rotigotine
Catechol-O-methyltransferase inhibitors: entacapone,
  tolcapone
Dopamine releaser: amantadine
Dopamine receptor blocker: domperidone
Type B MAO inhibitor: selegiline, lazabemide, rasagi-
  line, zydis selegiline
Type A & B MAO inhibitor: tranylcypromine, phenelzine
Dopamine synthesizer: zonisamide

decarboxylase inhibitors, although in the United States, only carbidopa is available. In many other countries, benserazide is also available. Carbidopa/levodopa is marketed as Sinemet or as a generic drug; the combination is available in standard (e.g., Sinemet standard) and controlled-release (e.g., Sinemet CR) formulations. The former allows a more rapid "on" and shorter half-life, and the latter allows for a delayed "on" and a slightly longer plasma half life. Benserazide/levodopa is marketed as standard Madopar and Madopar HBS (for slow release). The peripheral decarboxylase inhibitors potentiate levodopa, allowing about a fourfold reduction in dosage of levodopa to obtain the same benefit. Moreover, by preventing the formation of peripheral dopamine, which can act at the area postrema (vomiting center with a lack of a blood-brain barrier), they block the development of nausea and vomiting. If additional carbidopa is needed for patients in whom nausea persists, it can be prescribed, and patients can obtain it from their pharmacy; the additional peripheral decarboxylase inhibitor may overcome the nausea. Keep in mind that levodopa is absorbed only in the small intestine. The slow release of levodopa from the slow-release versions is such that only about two thirds to three fourths of levodopa is absorbed per tablet compared to standard Sinemet. This is because some of the levodopa in the slow-dissolving tablet has not been released before the tablet reached the large intestine. Levodopa is not absorbed rectally, so suppository administration is not useful. There is also an immediate-release formulation of carbidopa/levodopa that dissolves in the mouth on top of the tongue, which goes by the trade name Parcopa. It can be taken without water, which may be an advantage for some patients (e.g., those who have trouble swallowing or who need to be without food or water pre- and postsurgery. Eradication of *Helicobacter pylori* with omeprazole, amoxicillin, and clarithromycin in PD patients documented to be infected with the bacteria has been shown to increase absorption of levodopa, but since about 50% of the general population is infected with the bacterium, it is unlikely that this observation will translate into clinical practice (Pierantozzi et al., 2006).

The question of whether to use levodopa in a patient who has a history of malignant melanoma needs to be considered. Levodopa is an intermediary metabolite in the synthesis of skin melanin, so the concern is whether lurking melanoma cells can be activated by the use of levodopa therapy. A review of the literature does not provide evidence of a definite relationship between treatment with levodopa and the development or reemergence of malignant melanoma (Pfutzner and Przybilla, 1997; Zanetti et al., 2006). Yet it would seem prudent not to treat with levodopa if other antiparkinson agents remain effective. Once it becomes necessary to use levodopa to improve quality of life in a PD patient, the patient needs to be informed that he or she should be observed carefully for changes in or development of new pigmented lesions.

Besides being metabolized by aromatic amino acid decarboxylase (also called dopa decarboxylase), levodopa is metabolized by catechol-O-methyltransferase (COMT) to form 3-O-methyldopa. Two COMT inhibitors are currently available: tolcapone and entacapone. These agents extend the plasma half-life of levodopa without increasing its peak plasma concentration and can thereby prolong the duration of action of each dose of levodopa. The net effect with multiple dosings a day, though, is to elevate the average plasma concentration but smooth out the variations in the concentration. Tolcapone has two potential adverse effects that need to be explained to the patient. A small percentage of patients will develop elevated liver transaminases, and patients need to have baseline and follow-up liver function tests. Death has occurred in three patients who had no liver function surveillance (Watkins, 2000). Entacapone has not shown these hepatic changes. With tolcapone, a small percentage of patients will develop diarrhea that does not appear for about 6 weeks after starting the drug. The diarrhea can be explosive, so the patient might not have any warning. Entacapone appears not to have these adverse effects.

Elevated total plasma homocysteine, a risk factor for strokes, heart attacks, and dementia, has been found in PD patients using levodopa. The increase of plasma homocysteine with levodopa therapy is thought to be due to the utilization of the methyl group from methionine in the COMT reaction, converting levodopa to 3-O-methyldopa while converting methionine to homocysteine. A study evaluating the immediate effects of initiating levodopa therapy found a modest elevation of homocysteine and a modest lowering of vitamin $B_{12}$ levels (O'Suilleabhain et al., 2004). These investigators did not see a reversal with levodopa reduction, agonist treatment, or entacapone treatment. Another study reported that levodopa treatment does not affect $B_{12}$ levels but does reduce folate levels (Lamberti et al., 2005). These investigators found that the addition of COMT inhibitors could reduce the amount of homocysteine. Whether the increase in plasma homocysteine with levodopa therapy puts the patient at a greater risk for other medical problems is unknown (Postuma and Lang, 2004).

Adding entacapone to patients on levodopa who are not experiencing motor fluctuations did not improve motor performance in one study (Olanow et al., 2004) but improved the activities of daily living (ADL) score in another (Brooks and Sagar, 2003).

The next most powerful drugs, after levodopa, in treating PD symptoms are the dopamine agonists. Of those listed in Box 6-1, bromocriptine, pergolide, pramipexole, ropinirole, and apomorphine are available in the United States, and these are discussed later in the chapter. Lisuride, cabergoline, and piribedil are marketed in some countries. Lisuride is water soluble and can be infused subcutaneously; it has considerable

5-HT agonist activity. Cabergoline is the longest-acting and could be taken just once a day (Ahlskog et al., 1996; Hutton et al., 1996); it might prove to be the most important in terms of preventing or reducing the wearing-off effect. Piribedil is relatively weak but has been touted as having an antitremor effect. Rotigotine is a dopamine agonist that is currently undergoing clinical trials in a transdermally applied skin patch (Fahn and Parkinson Study Group, 2001; Parkinson Study Group, 2003; Poewe and Luessi, 2005).

Other than apomorphine, the other dopamine agonists in Box 6-1 are effective orally. Bromocriptine is the weakest clinically in comparison to the others. Pergolide, pramipexole, and ropinirole appear to be comparable in clinical practice, but some patients will respond better to one than the others. There are some differences of these agonists in their affinity for the dopamine receptor subtypes, as depicted in Tables 6-2 and 6-3. Only pergolide has agonist activity at the D1 receptor (modest). The activation of the D2 receptor is known to be important in obtaining an anti-PD response, whereas it is unknown how important D3 receptor activation is for improving the anti-PD response. Bromocriptine, pergolide, pramipexole, and ropinirole activate the dopamine D3 as well as the D2 receptor, but their ratios of affinities for these two receptors are different (see Table 6-3) (Perachon et al., 1999). All dopamine agonists are less likely to induce dyskinesias compared to levodopa (Schrag et al., 1998). The agonists can be used as adjuncts to levodopa therapy (e.g., Lieberman et al., 1998; Pinter et al., 1999) or as monotherapy (e.g., Kieburtz et al., 1997b; Brooks et al., 1998; Kulisevsky et al., 1998; Rinne, Bracco, et al., 1998; Sethi et al., 1998). Adverse effects that are more common with dopamine agonists than with levodopa are drowsiness, sleep attacks, confusion, orthostatic hypotension, nausea, and ankle/leg edema associated commonly with erythema (Parkinson Study Group, 2000; Rascol et al., 2000). Edema can spread to involve other areas of the body, including the arms and face.

Apomorphine, being water soluble, is usually employed as a rapidly acting dopaminergic to overcome "off" states—that is, to provide a rescue. It is either injected subcutaneously or applied intranasally. Because of the emesis-producing propensity of apomorphine, the patient must be pretreated with an antinauseant, such as domperidone or trimethobenzamide. Apomorphine and lisuride (also water soluble) are also being used by continuous subcutaneous infusion to provide a smooth response for patients who fluctuate between dyskinetic and "off" states. Apomorphine may be the most powerful dopamine agonist; it activates both the dopamine D1 and D2 receptors.

Having several dopamine agonists to choose from allows the opportunity to find one that is better tolerated as well as one that might have more effect. Adverse effects may be the deciding factor as to which drug a patient will do best on.

**Table 6-2** Dopamine agonists and dopamine receptors

| Agonist | D1 | D2 | D3 | D4 | D5 |
|---|---|---|---|---|---|
| Bromocriptine | − | ++ | ++ | + | + |
| Lisuride | + | ++ | ? | ? | ? |
| Pergolide | + | ++ | +++ | ? | + |
| Cabergoline | − | +++ | ? | ? | ? |
| Ropinirole | − | ++ | ++++ | + | − |
| Pramipexole | − | ++ | ++++ | ++ | ? |

**Table 6-3** Dopamine agonists and affinities for the dopamine D1, D2, and D3 receptors

| Agonist | D1 | D2 | D3 | D2/D3 Ratio |
|---|---|---|---|---|
| Bromocriptine | 0 | +++ | ++ | 10:1 |
| Pergolide | + | +++ | +++ | 1:1 |
| Ropinirole | 0 | ++ | +++ | 1:10 |
| Pramipexole | 0 | ++ | +++ | 1:10 |

Data extracted from Perachon S, Schwartz JC, Sokoloff P: Functional potencies of new antiparkinsonian drugs at recombinant human dopamine D-1, D-2 and D-3 receptors. Eur J Pharmacol 1999;366:293–300.

Unfortunately, all these drugs can induce confusion and hallucinations in elderly patients. Leg edema occurs in some patients, usually after a few years. Pramipexole and ropinirole and other dopaminergics as well, though probably with less frequency, can cause sleepiness and sleep attacks. This could be dangerous for the patient who drives an automobile, and motor vehicle accidents have occurred when patients fell asleep at the wheel (Frucht et al., 1999; Ferreira et al., 2000; Hoehn, 2000; Schapira, 2000). So when deciding to place a patient on pramipexole or ropinirole, the physician should determine the extent of the driving to be done by the patient and warn the patient about this potential hazard. Short trips—for example, 10 minutes or so—should be without risk. Should sudden falling asleep occur in any nondriving activity, the event can serve as a warning against driving; if driving is necessary, it would be best to taper or even discontinue these medications.

Amantadine has several actions. It activates release of dopamine from nerve terminals, blocks dopamine uptake into the nerve terminals, has antimuscarinic effects, and blocks glutamate receptors. Its dopaminergic actions make it a useful drug in about two thirds of patients, but it can induce livedo reticularis, ankle edema, visual hallucinations, and confusion. Its antiglutamatergic action is discussed in the text that follows.

Domperidone is a peripherally active dopamine receptor blocker and is useful in preventing gastrointestinal upset from levodopa and the dopamine agonists. Although it does not enter the CNS, it can still block the dopamine receptors in the area postrema, thereby preventing nausea and vomiting. By not penetrating the CNS, it does not block the dopamine receptors in the striatum, thus not interfering with the action of dopamine or dopamine agonists. Domperidone is not marketed in the United States, but U.S. patients can obtain it from Canada.

Monoamine oxidase (MAO) inhibitors offer mildly effective symptomatic benefit. Type B MAO inhibitors eliminate concern about the "cheese effect" that can occur with type A inhibitors and a high tyramine meal. Although there is debate about possible protective benefit with selegiline, it does have mild symptomatic effects when used alone (Parkinson Study Group, 1993a, 1996a, 1996b) and also potentiates levodopa when used in combination with it (Lees, 1995). A more thorough discussion of selegiline's possible protective effect is presented later in the chapter, in the section entitled "Selegiline and Antioxidants." Selegiline has a mild ameliorating effect for mild wearing-off from levodopa (Golbe et al., 1988). Zydis selegiline is a form of selegiline that dissolves in the mouth and is absorbed through the oral mucosa, avoiding first-pass metabolism in the liver (Waters et al., 2004). This preparation of selegiline, formulated in a freeze-dried tablet that contains a fast-dissolving selegiline (Zelapar), was approved by the Food and Drug Administration in 2006 for clinical use (Clarke and Jankovic, 2006). Like selegiline, rasagiline is an irreversible type B MAO inhibitor with mild symptomatic benefit (Rabey et al., 2000; Parkinson Study Group, 2002a, 2004a) and with a similar chemical structure; both are propargylamine compounds. Rasagiline has recently become available for use in patients with PD, both in early and advanced stages, and has a good safety record (Goetz et al., 2006).

Lazabemide is another type B MAO inhibitor but is a reversible inhibitor. It shows the same symptomatic effect in PD (Parkinson Study Group, 1993b) as do selegiline and rasagiline. It is not known whether it has a neuronal rescue effect. Lazabemide is not commercially available. In contrast to selegiline, neither lazabemide nor rasagiline is metabolized to methamphetamine. Type B MAO inhibitors should not require a tyramine-restricted diet, but the Federal Drug Administration is requiring this diet for rasagiline. Inhibitors of both type A and type B MAO would offer greater inhibition of dopamine oxidation in the brain, and thus the combination would theoretically be more capable of reducing oxidative stress as well as providing more symptomatic effect (Fahn and Chouinard, 1998). But tranylcypromine and phenelzine (both nonselective inhibitors of types A and B MAO) cannot be taken in the presence of levodopa therapy because of changes in blood pressure, the so-called cheese effect; even in the absence of levodopa, patients on these drugs need to adhere to a reduced-tyramine diet (Gardner et al., 1996).

MAO inhibitors and antioxidants are examined further later in the chapter in discussing their possible role in treating early-stage PD. First, it is necessary to review the nondopaminergic drugs that are useful in treating PD, both the motoric problems (Box 6-2) and the nonmotor problems (Box 6-3).

Nondopaminergic agents (see Box 6-2) are also useful to treat PD symptoms, particularly antimuscarinic drugs (commonly referred to as anticholinergics), which have been widely used since the 1950s, but these are much less effective than the dopaminergic agents, including amantadine. Antimuscarinic drugs have been thought to be somewhat helpful in reducing all symptoms of PD, but they have found special favor in reducing the severity of tremor. But because of sensitivity to memory impairment and hallucinations in the elderly popu-

---

**Box 6-2** Nondopaminergic agents for motor symptoms

Antimuscarinics: trihexyphenidyl, benztropine, ethopropazine, and so on.
Antihistaminics: diphenhydramine, orphenadrine
Antiglutamatergics: amantadine, dextromethorphan, riluzole
Muscle relaxants: cyclobenzaprine, diazepam, baclofen
Antioxidant vitamins: ascorbate, tocopherol
Mitochondrial enhancer: coenzyme Q10
Adenosine $A_{2A}$ receptor antagonists (in clinical trials): istradefylline
Neurotrophins: neuroimmunophilins, GDNF (neither was successful in clinical trials)

---

**Box 6-3** Nondopaminergic agents for nonmotor symptoms

**Behavioral**
Dementia: donepezil (Aricept), rivastigmine (Exelon), galantamine (Rozadyne)
Depression: selective serotonin reuptake inhibitors, tricyclics, electroconvulsive therapy
Psychosis: clozapine, quetiapine, olanzapine, donepezil, rivastigmine
Stress/anxiety: benzodiazepines: diazepam, lorazepam, alprazolam
Apathy: methylphenidate
Fatigue: modafinil

**Sleep-Related**
Daytime sleepiness: modafinil
Insomnia: quetiapine, zolpidem, benzodiazepine, mirtazapine
REM-sleep behavior disorder: clonazepam
Restless legs: opioids (e.g., propoxyphene, oxycodone)

**Autonomic**
Orthostasis: fludrocortisone, midodrine (ProAmatine)
Urinary urgency: oxybutynin (Ditropan), tolterodine (Detrol)
Impotence: sildenafil (Viagra) and related drugs

**Gastrointestinal**
Constipation: fiber, "rancho recipe," polyethylene glycol (MiraLax)
Nausea: trimethobenzamide (Tigan), domperidone
Sialorrhea: propantheline, other peripheral antimuscarinics, botulinum toxin injections

---

lation, antimuscarinic drugs should usually be avoided in patients over the age of 70 years. The antihistaminics, tricyclics, and cyclobenzaprine (Flexeril) have milder anticholinergic properties that make them useful in PD, particularly in older patients who should not take the stronger anticholinergics.

Amantadine, listed in Box 6-1 as a dopaminergic agent, is listed also in Box 6-2 because it has antiglutamatergic effects; this property might account for its usefulness in reducing choreic dyskinesias induced by levodopa (Rajput et al., 1997; Metman, Del Dotto, van den Munckhof, et al., 1998). Dextromethorphan is another antiglutamatergic agent, and it has been found effective in reducing the severity of dyskinesias by 50% (Metman, Del Dotto, Natte, et al., 1998). Another useful class of drugs is the benzodiazepines to reduce anxiety and thereby decrease parkinsonian tremor that is exacerbated by stress. Diazepam is usually well tolerated and does not exacerbate parkinsonian symptoms, whereas chlordiazepoxide can (Schwarz and Fahn, 1970). Lorazepam and alprazolam are other useful benzodiazepine agents; the latter has the added benefits of being short acting and having antidepressant effects. The muscle relaxants listed in Box 6-2 might help in treating "off" and peak-dose dystonias. Because oxidative stress appears to play a role in the pathogenesis of PD, high doses of antioxidant vitamins have been tried for patients with PD. The DATATOP study showed that tocopherol by itself has no effect, but the combination of ascorbate and tocopherol may be more effective than either of these two vitamins alone (Fahn, 1992b; Yoshikawa, 1993). Ascorbate has proven effective in blocking degeneration of nerve cells in vitro induced by levodopa

(Mena et al., 1993; Mytilineou et al., 1993; Pardo et al., 1993, 1995; Lai and Wu, 1997). Adenosine A(2A) receptors are located on GABA neurons in the striatum. Antagonizing them has a behavioral effect similar to enhancing dopaminergic transmission. Thus, these receptor antagonists are undergoing clinical trials for patients with motor fluctuations (Bara-Jimenez et al., 2003; Hauser et al., 2003) (see Chapter 9).

Many nonmotor problems are commonly present in patients with PD. These are discussed in more detail in Chapter 8, but a list of the common drugs used for these nonmotor symptoms is provided in Box 6-3, and a brief explanation of some of the drugs used is provided here. Drugs that are available to improve memory in Alzheimer disease may be tried in patients with PD who have dementia, whether from diffuse Lewy body disease or from concomitant Alzheimer disease. These drugs are the centrally active cholinesterase inhibitors donepezil, rivastigmine, and galantamine. Initial concern that they might worsen tremor and bradykinesia has not been borne out, perhaps because dopaminergic agents are also being given in these patients. These drugs have also been reported to be useful in treating levodopa-induced psychosis.

Because depression is common in patients with PD, this symptom needs to be vigorously attacked if present; otherwise, it is difficult to reduce parkinsonian symptoms. The tricyclics and selective serotonin reuptake inhibitors are useful antidepressants in PD. It is not certain whether one type of antidepressant class of compounds is superior to the other in treating the depression accompanying PD. The selective serotonin uptake inhibitors may aggravate parkinsonism if antiparkinsonian drugs are not being utilized concurrently. If insomnia is a problem for the patient, using an antidepressant at bedtime that is also a soporific, such as amitriptyline, can be doubly advantageous. Amitriptyline has considerable somnolence-inducing effect. The type B MAO inhibitor selegiline is not effective as an antidepressant, unless used in a transdermal form to achieve both types A and B inhibition. The oral inhibitors of both types A and B MAO are very effective, but they cannot be given in the presence of levodopa because of swings in blood pressure, and they must also be accompanied by a tyramine-restrictive diet at all times.

Psychosis induced by levodopa and the dopamine agonists can often be controlled by clozapine and quetiapine without worsening the parkinsonism. Both agents are dibenzodiazepine antipsychotic drugs. They are called atypical antipsychotics because they rarely cause drug-induced parkinsonism. They are relatively selective D4 receptor antagonists, although they have some D2 blocking action, particularly at high doses, because akathisia (Friedman, 1993; Safferman et al., 1993), acute dystonic reaction (Kastrup et al., 1994; Thomas et al., 1994), and tardive dyskinesia (Dave, 1994) have been associated with them. Clozapine is the most effective agent in treating levodopa-induced psychosis in patients with PD without aggravating the PD (Friedman and Lannon, 1990; Pfeiffer et al., 1990; Kahn et al., 1991; Factor and Brown, 1992; Greene et al., 1993; Pinter and Helscher, 1993; Factor et al., 1994; Diederich et al., 1995; Rabey et al., 1995; Factor and Friedman, 1997; Ruggieri et al., 1997; Friedman et al., 1999). But weekly monitoring of white blood cells is necessary with clozapine to prevent irreversible agranulocytosis that can occur rarely with clozapine; this allows a timely discontinuation of this drug when a drop of leukocytes is observed. Because of this need for weekly blood counts, quetiapine is a useful though somewhat less effective substitute for clozapine, and it is now the drug of first choice. Both clozapine and quetiapine are given at bedtime because of their soporific effect. Olanzapine is an effective antipsychotic, but the dose needs to be kept small because it can worsen PD (Jimenez-Jimenez et al., 1998). There is a window of dosing with olanzapine by which psychosis can be reduced without increasing parkinsonism.

Stress, excitement, and anxiety make parkinsonian symptoms worse, especially tremor. In fact, tremor that is otherwise well controlled can reemerge under stress. The benzodiazepines, by reducing anxiety, can partially offset this worsening of tremor. Apathy and fatigue are common in PD, and no medication as yet has been found satisfactory.

Various sleep problems are encountered in PD. Excessive drowsiness can occur after a dose of levodopa or dopamine agonist. Modafinil can sometimes help to overcome this problem. Insomnia needs to be treated; otherwise, quality of life suffers, and daytime sleepiness is enhanced. Hypnotics, such as zolpiden and benzodiazepines, can be safely used in PD. Quetiapine and clozapine often allow a good night's sleep and can be utilized even in the absence of psychosis. Acting out dreams, so-called REM-sleep behavior disorder, is not uncommon and is usually treated with clonazepam at bedtime. Restless legs syndrome and periodic movements in sleep are quite common in patients with PD. If the dopaminergic agent they are taking is ineffective, then an opioid such as propoxyphene or oxycodone can be effective. These should be administered an hour or so before the usual onset of these symptoms.

Although common in multiple-system atrophy, orthostatic hypotension is not a common feature in PD except as a complication of dopaminergic or other medications. Fludrocortisone to increase salt retention and midodrine as an alpha-1-adrenergic receptor agonist can be effective in overcoming syncope. Dyssynergia of bladder sphincters can sometimes be a problem, and relief can be obtained with peripheral antimuscarinics. Oxybutynin (Ditropan) and tolterodine (Detrol) are commonly used for this condition. Difficulty obtaining erections can occur in patients with PD, and these men have reported benefit with sildenafil and related drugs.

One of the most common complaints by patients with PD is constipation. This symptom can be a factor of both the disease and the medications used to treat PD. A high-fiber diet, including dried fruits, is often sufficient to relieve constipation. The "rancho recipe" is given in Chapter 8. If that is not effective, one can try the standard laxatives or polyethylene glycol (MiraLax). Nausea can be a complication of dopamine agonists and levodopa. Domperidone, a peripheral dopamine receptor blocker, is effective. Because domperidone is not available in the United States, trimethobenzamide (Tigan) can be tried. Sialorrhea is due to infrequent and inadequate spontaneous swallowing of saliva. Peripherally active peripheral antimuscarinics such as propantheline can be quite effective. Injecting botulinum toxin into the parotid glands may benefit some patients (Racette et al., 2003).

## TREATMENT OF EARLY-STAGE PARKINSON DISEASE

The earliest stage of PD begins when the symptoms are first noticed and the diagnosis is made. At this stage, symptoms are mild, and there is no threat to the patient's activities. The designation of "early stage" lasts until the symptoms begin to become troublesome to the patient and intervention with symptomatic medications is needed. All symptomatic drugs can induce side effects, and if a patient is not troubled by mild symptoms socially or occupationally, the introduction of these drugs can be delayed until symptoms become more pronounced. The clinician needs to discuss this choice with the patient and his or her family. Most neurologists do not use levodopa or other potent antiparkinson agents when the diagnosis is first established and the disease presents with no threat to physical, social, or occupational activities (Fahn, 1991, 1999; Fahn et al., 1996).

Because symptomatically beneficial medications are not needed and because there is no proven neuroprotective treatment, patients in the early, recently diagnosed stage of PD are excellent candidates for participating in a clinical trial in which a placebo is one of the treatment arms. A literature review of clinical trials related to neuroprotection in PD has been conducted by Fahn and Sulzer (2004) and by the Quality Standards Subcommittee of the American Academy of Neurology (Suchowersky et al., 2006). Another elective option is to use one of the drugs described in this section for which hints of neuroprotection have been demonstrated in controlled clinical trials.

One should keep in mind that the generic label *neuroprotection* can be divided into at least three different classes of action: slowing the pathogenetic cascade that leads to cell death so that the natural history of the disease is less progressive (neuroprotection), restoring injured dysfunctional neurons (neurorescue, neurorestoration), and replacing dead neurons (neuroregeneration) (Fig. 6-1). In this section the rationale and results of clinical trials for neuroprotection of PD are discussed.

## Selegiline and Antioxidants

The first controlled clinical trial for the purpose of evaluating medications as neuroprotective agents for PD was the DATATOP (Deprenyl and Tocopherol Antioxidative Therapy of Parkinsonism) study (Parkinson Study Group, 1989a, 1989b). Deprenyl (selegiline) is an irreversible noncompetitive

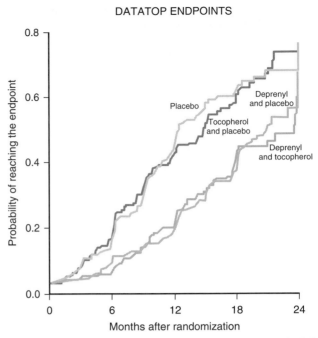

DATATOP ENDPOINTS

**Figure 6-2** Kaplan-Meier curves of the cumulative probability of reaching the endpoint (need for dopaminergic therapy) in the DATATOP study. (See Color Plate 8.) (From Parkinson Study Group: Effects of tocopherol and deprenyl on the progression of disability in early Parkinson's disease. N Engl J Med 1993;328:176–183.)

inhibitor of type B MAO with a long duration of action (type B MAO inhibition half-life of 40 days [Fowler et al., 1994]). Selegiline was tested along with the antioxidant alpha-tocopherol (vitamin E) in a $2 \times 2$ design. Patients were enrolled in the study early in the course of the illness and did not require symptomatic therapy. They were placed on selegiline (5 mg twice daily), alpha-tocopherol (1000 IU twice daily), the combination, or double placebo, with approximately 200 subjects in each of the four treatment arms. The primary endpoint was the need for dopaminergic therapy. The study showed that tocopherol had no effect in delaying parkinsonian disability, but selegiline delayed symptomatic treatment by 9 months (Fig. 6-2) (Parkinson Study Group, 1993a). It also reduced the rate of worsening of the UPDRS by half (Table 6-4). Other investigators conducted other studies testing selegiline, showing similar results (Myllyla et al., 1992; Palhagen et al., 1998).

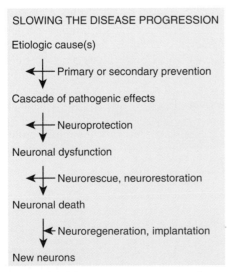

SLOWING THE DISEASE PROGRESSION

Etiologic cause(s)

◄— Primary or secondary prevention

Cascade of pathogenic effects

◄— Neuroprotection

Neuronal dysfunction

◄— Neurorescue, neurorestoration

Neuronal death

◄— Neuroregeneration, implantation

New neurons

**Figure 6-1** Neuroprotection: terminology.

**Table 6-4** Average annual rate of decline in UPDRS scores*

| Treatment | Total UPDRS |
|---|---|
| Placebo | 14.02 ± 12.32 |
| Tocopherol | 15.16 ± 16.12 |
| Selegiline | 7.00 ± 10.76 |
| Tocopherol and selegiline | 7.28 ± 11.11 |
| *P* value | <0.001 |

*Results are mean ± standard deviation.

Data from Parkinson Study Group: Effects of tocopherol and deprenyl on the progression of disability in early Parkinson's disease. N Engl J Med 1993; 328:176–183.

Because selegiline has a mild symptomatic effect that is long lasting (Parkinson Study Group, 1993a), one could explain its ability to delay progression of disability entirely on this symptomatic effect. In favor of some neuroprotective effect is that after 2 months of washout of the drug, patients had slightly milder PD than did those on placebo (Parkinson Study Group, 1993a). But because of selegiline's very long duration of action as an inhibitor of type B MAO (Parkinson Study Group, 1995), this observation could represent an insufficient washout period. Furthermore, selegiline's benefit in delaying the introduction of levodopa gradually diminishes over time (Parkinson Study Group, 1993a), the best results occurring in the first year of treatment. The odds ratio increased from 0.35 for the first 6 months to 0.38 in the second 6 months to 0.77 in the third 6 months and to 0.86 after 18 months. Follow-up of DATATOP subjects showed that placebo-treated subjects fared better than selegiline-treated subjects when the drug was reintroduced after a 2-month washout period and that the two groups were identical in developing levodopa complications (Parkinson Study Group, 1996a, 1996b). The net understanding by the year 2000 was that there is no convincing evidence that selegiline delayed the need for levodopa because of any protective effect; all results could be those of a drug with a continuing mild symptomatic benefit.

On the other hand, basic scientific research was finding that in animal models, tiny doses of selegiline have a neuronal rescue effect (Tatton, 1993). This effect is not via its MAO inhibitor mechanism of action but is believed to enhance protein synthesis of a neurotrophic agent, which is antagonized by amphetamine. Ultimately, this finding led to investigation of other agents for their rescue effect, resulting in the discovery of a propargyline drug that was tested in a clinical trial (Waldmeier et al., 2000, 2006).

When the DATATOP study was evaluated to better understand the development of freezing of gait, it was discovered that the group that was treated with selegiline had a statistically significantly decreased risk for developing freezing (Fig. 6-3) (Giladi et al., 2001b). It could not be discerned whether this benefit was because of selegiline's mild symptomatic benefit or of some unknown neuroprotection effect. Whichever it was, the authors concluded that one should consider using selegiline in patients who are likely to develop freezing of gait (absence of tremor, gait involvement as the initial symptom).

It now appears that the decreased risk of freezing of gait with selegiline is not simply from its symptomatic effect as an enhancer of dopamine. The investigators of the DATATOP study, while continuing to follow their subjects, carried out a rerandomization in a controlled trial. A total of 368 subjects who were now on both selegiline and levodopa therapy agreed to be randomized to either selegiline or placebo while remaining on levodopa. The results were dramatic. The subjects on selegiline required a lower dosage of levodopa, had a slower rate of worsening of symptoms and signs of PD (Table 6-5), and had less freezing of gait (Fig. 6-4) (Shoulson et al., 2002). These results support the view that selegiline provides some neuroprotective effect or has a symptomatic effect separate from dopamine. The possibility that this benefit is derived from an antiapoptotic effect rather than its antioxidative effect is discussed later.

A similar study was carried out by Palhagen and colleagues (2006), who followed patients for at least 7 years after they entered a controlled clinical trial that evaluated selegiline versus placebo in those with early untreated PD. Then, when any sub-

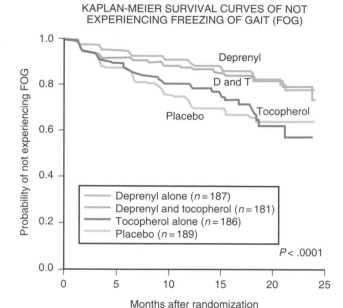

**Figure 6-3** Kaplan-Meier curves showing probability of not experiencing freezing of gait in the absence of levodopa in the DATATOP study. (See Color Plate 9.) (From Giladi N, McDermott MP, Fahn S, et al: Freezing of gait in PD: Prospective assessment in the DATATOP cohort. Neurology 2001;56:1712–1721.)

ject required symptomatic therapy, open-label levodopa was added, while maintaining the blind on selegline versus placebo. During the 7 years of follow-up from the start of the study, the selegiline-treated group had a statistically significant slower rate of worsening of clinical signs and symptoms as measured by UPDRS scores. Like the Shoulson and colleagues (2002) study mentioned earlier, this shows the added benefit that selegiline provides in slowing clinical symptoms. Whether this can be attributed to a neuroprotective effect or to a symptomatic effect that does not appear to be through dopamine is undetermined by the two studies.

**Table 6-5** Change in total UPDRS after second randomization to either selegiline or placebo while taking levodopa*

| Duration after Randomization | Placebo | Selegiline | Difference |
|---|---|---|---|
| 1 month | 0.50 ± 7.73 | −1.52 ± 7.54 | 2.02 |
| 3 months | 1.57 ± 9.41 | −0.85 ± 9.42 | 2.42 |
| 9 months | 4.18 ± 10.12 | 1.63 ± 10.61 | 2.55 |
| 15 months | 5.63 ± 10.73 | 0.46 ± 10.88 | 5.17 |
| 21 months | 7.06 ± 12.70 | 1.51 ± 10.36 | 5.55 |
| ↑Levodopa (mg/d) | 181 ± 246 | 106 ± 205 | P = .003 |

*Higher UPDRS represents more severe PD. UPDRS results, P = .0002.

Data from Shoulson I, Oakes D, Fahn S, et al: Impact of sustained deprenyl (selegiline) in levodopa-treated Parkinson's disease: A randomized placebo-controlled extension of the deprenyl and tocopherol antioxidative therapy of parkinsonism trial. Ann Neurol 2002;51:604–612.

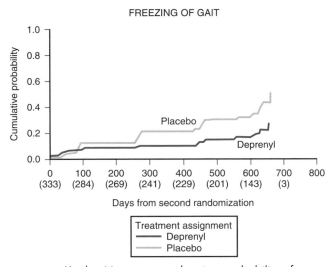

FREEZING OF GAIT

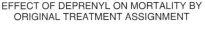

Treatment assignment
— Deprenyl
— Placebo

**Figure 6-4** Kaplan-Meier curves showing probability of experiencing freezing of gait in the presence of levodopa in the BLIND-DATE study. (From Shoulson I, Oakes D, Fahn S, et al: Impact of sustained deprenyl (selegiline) in levodopa-treated Parkinson's disease: A randomized placebo-controlled extension of the deprenyl and tocopherol antioxidative therapy of parkinsonism trial. Ann Neurol 2002;51:604–612.)

The safety of selegiline was raised, though, in an open-label clinical trial in the United Kingdom (Lees, 1995). The use of selegiline when combined with levodopa was reported to be associated with a higher mortality rate than was seen in the patients assigned to levodopa treatment alone. Analysis of this result by others found a number of flaws in the study to refute this conclusion (Olanow et al., 1996). The U.K. investigators followed up their report with a more detailed analysis of the cause of death (Ben-Shlomo et al., 1998). The excess mortality in the selegiline + levodopa group was greatest in the third and fourth years of treatment. The cause of the increase in deaths showed the excess to be from PD only and to occur particularly in patients with dementia and a history of falls. No significant differences in mortality were found for revised diagnosis, disability rating scores, autonomic or cardiovascular events, other clinical features, or drug interactions. Other studies with selegiline have failed to find any excess mortality from the combination treatment with levodopa (Myllyla et al., 1997; Aaltonen et al., 1998; Olanow et al., 1998). After being followed by the Parkinson Study Group for an average of 8.2 years, the subjects in the DATATOP study showed no difference in mortality between the groups assigned to treatment with selegiline, tocopherol, or placebo (Fig. 6-5); the death rate averaged 2.1% per year (Parkinson Study Group, 1998), much lower than that in the U.K. study.

A meta-analysis of 17 controlled clinical trials involving type B MAO inhibitors found that no significant difference in mortality existed between patients on type B MAO inhibitors and control patients (Ives et al., 2004). The analysis also found that subjects who were randomized to type B MAO inhibitors had significantly better total scores, motor scores, and ADL scores on the UPDRS at 3 months compared with patients taking placebo; they were also less likely to need additional levodopa or to develop motor fluctuations. No difference existed between

the two groups in the incidence of side effects or withdrawal of patients.

High-dose vitamin E has also been suggested to increase mortality, but analysis of the DATATOP cohort followed for up to 13 years failed to find any difference in mortality between the group on vitamin E and the group on placebo (Marras et al., 2005).

In a more recent analysis of retrospective observational data from Scotland (Donnan et al., 2000) comparing PD patients with a comparable control population, the patients with PD had a higher rate of mortality than those without PD (rate ratio [RR]: 1.76; 95% confidence interval [CI]: 1.11 to 2.81). There was significantly greater mortality in patients with PD who received levodopa monotherapy (RR: 2.45, 95% CI: 1.42 to 4.23) relative to the comparators, adjusting for previous cardiovascular drug use and diabetes. However, there was no significant difference in mortality in patients with PD who received combination therapy of selegiline with levodopa and other drugs in relation to the comparators (RR: 0.92, 95% CI: 0.37 to 2.31). Thus, from this study, selegiline did not increase the mortality rate, whether used as monotherapy or in combination with levodopa. In fact, levodopa monotherapy had the highest mortality rate.

Mortality in PD patients was also determined in a multicenter European study (Berger et al., 2000). As in the Scotland study (Donnan et al., 2000), the mortality rate was twice that of a controlled population (RR: 2.3; 95% CI: 1.8 to 3.0). The risk for death in men with PD (RR: 3.1; CI: 2.1 to 4.4) was higher than that in women with PD (RR: 1.8; CI: 1.2 to 5.1). Women with PD had a fivefold higher risk of living in a care facility than did men with PD.

The dose of selegiline should not exceed 5 mg twice daily because its specificity as a selective type B inhibitor of MAO is lost and it will also inhibit type A MAO at higher doses. Because of its long half-life, many physicians believe that a much smaller dose could be equally effective, although this

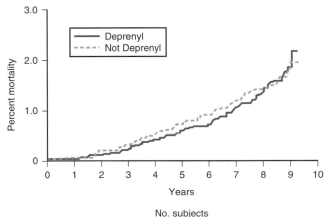

EFFECT OF DEPRENYL ON MORTALITY BY ORIGINAL TREATMENT ASSIGNMENT

**Figure 6-5** Kaplan-Meier curves showing cumulative mortality whether subjects are taking selegiline or not. (From Parkinson Study Group: Mortality in DATATOP: A multicenter trial in early Parkinson's disease. Ann Neurol 1998;43:318–325.)

has not been tested. If insomnia develops, 5 mg in the morning, avoiding later doses, usually corrects this. Male impotence is less common. When selegiline is used in the presence of levodopa, it potentiates levodopa's effect, and lower doses of levodopa can usually be achieved (Lees, 1995; Shoulson et al., 2002). Selegiline does not prevent the development of levodopa-induced complications of fluctuations and dyskinesias (Parkinson Study Group, 1996b). Selegiline decreases the risk of patients developing freezing of gait (Giladi et al., 2001b). Interestingly, type A MAO inhibitors, but not type B MAO inhibitors, have been shown to reduce stress-induced freezing behavior in rats (Maki et al., 2000).

The DATATOP study showed that selegiline inhibits MAO activity by about 20% in the central nervous system (CNS) (Parkinson Study Group, 1995). Because the original premise for the DATATOP study was that selegiline might be neuroprotective by inhibiting MAO (reducing formation of hydrogen peroxide and thereby decreasing oxidant stress), the cerebrospinal fluid analysis of homovanillic acid indicates that selegiline is a poor inhibitor of CNS MAO. This finding could explain the lack of success of selegiline as a powerful neuroprotective agent. Whether a more potent inhibitor of MAO could be more successful remains to be determined. In the meantime, it is reasonable for patients to consider an inhibitor of both types A and B as possibly augmenting inhibition of MAO in brain. Such MAO inhibitors can induce the cheese effect, so the MAO inhibitor diet, avoiding dietary tyramine, needs to be utilized. Such MAO inhibitors can be used only in the absence of levodopa because the combination will create marked blood pressure fluctuations.

Because the oxidant-stress hypothesis is widely held as a likely one in the pathogenesis of PD (Graham et al., 1978; Cohen, 1983, 1986; Fahn, 1989; Fornstedt et al., 1990; Olanow, 1990, 1992; Jenner, 1991; Fahn and Cohen, 1992; Jenner et al., 1992a, 1992b; Zigmond et al., 1992; Spencer et al., 1995; Alam et al., 1997), the use of a combination of antioxidants seems a reasonable approach.

Fahn has used tranylcypromine (Parnate), an irreversible inhibitor of both types A and B MAO, along with high doses of antioxidants (Fahn and Chouinard, 1998). As measured by cerebrospinal fluid concentration of the metabolite of dopamine, selegiline just partially inhibits dopamine oxidation, reducing hydrogen peroxide formation by only 20% (Parkinson Study Group, 1995), whereas tranylcypromine inhibits by 75% (Fahn et al., 1998). Using tranylcypromine requires the patient to be placed on an MAO inhibitor diet, which is not onerous (Gardner et al., 1996) and, if adhered to, avoids the cheese effect. In the presence of an irreversible type A MAO inhibitor, tyramine cannot be deaminated in the gut. The absorption of tyramine results in the release of norepinephrine from sympathetic nerve terminals, thereby raising blood pressure and potentially creating a hypertensive crisis (cheese effect). Some patients can develop intracerebral hemorrhage during an episode of such a crisis. The usual dose of tranylcypromine is 10 mg three times daily, but doses up to 60 mg per day can be used. Insomnia and male impotence are fairly common adverse effects that would require shifting the times of the doses from the evening hours or reducing or discontinuing the drug. A side benefit is the lifting of any existing depression. Levodopa cannot be given in the presence of an inhibitor of type A MAO because the combination produces a volatile blood pressure. Meperidine (Demerol) and the antidepressants, tricyclics, and selective serotonin uptake inhibitors are also to be avoided because of the potential for psychiatric and autonomic reactions ("serotonin syndrome") that could be fatal.

The antioxidants ascorbate (vitamin C) and tocopherol (vitamin E) are recommended solely on the basis of the oxidant stress hypothesis of the pathogenesis of PD. Although the DATATOP trial showed that tocopherol by itself is ineffective in slowing down the progression of PD, a combination of ascorbate and tocopherol potentiates the antioxidant efficacy of both (Yoshikawa, 1933; Hamilton et al., 2000). This combination of antioxidants in early PD patients has been used since 1979 and has not produced any harmful effects (Fahn, 1992b). The dosages, gradually reached in four divided doses, are 3000 mg per day of ascorbate and 3200 IU per day of D-alpha-tocopherol. Coenzyme Q10 and vitamin E need each other as antioxidants (Kagan et al., 2000). There is evidence that the natural form of tocopherol (D-alpha) achieves higher blood levels than does the synthetic racemic (D,L-alpha) tocopherol (Acuff et al., 1994).

## Riluzole

Glutamate is the major excitatory neurotransmitter in the CNS and can induce excitotoxicity. A slow excitotoxic process has been proposed by Beal (1998) to be a possible mechanism of cell death in PD. Riluzole impairs glutamatergic neurotransmission by blocking voltage-dependent sodium channel currents. In experimental animal models of PD, riluzole was found to have neuroprotective effects (Benazzouz et al., 1995; Barneoud et al., 1996; Boireau et al., 2000; Obinu et al., 2002). However, in controlled clinical trials in patients with early PD, riluzole was not found to be effective as a neuroprotective agent (Jankovic and Hunter, 2002; Rascol et al., 2003).

## Providing Trophic Factors

GDNF promotes the survival of DA neurons (Burke et al., 1998), DA neuron neurite outgrowth, and quantal size (the amount of DA released per synaptic vesicle exocytic event) (Pothos et al., 1998). When GDNF was injected into the midbrain of primates that had been rendered parkinsonian by MPTP, there was improvement of the parkinsonian features (Gash et al., 1996). Moreover, DA concentration in the substantia nigra was increased on the injected side, and the nigral DA neurons were 20% larger with an increased fiber density. In a subsequent study, primates received infusions of GDNF into a lateral ventricle (Grondin et al., 2002). This approach also showed restoration of the nigrostriatal dopaminergic system and improved the motor function in the rhesus monkeys. The functional improvements were associated with pronounced upregulation and regeneration of nigral DA neurons and their processes innervating the striatum. However, in a randomized, double-blind, placebo-controlled trial of infusing GDNF into the lateral ventricle of patients with PD, there was no clinical improvement (Nutt et al., 2003). Nausea, anorexia, and vomiting were common hours to several days after injections of GDNF. Weight loss occurred in the majority of subjects receiving 75 μg or larger doses. Paresthesias, often described as electric shocks (Lhermitte sign), were common in GDNF-treated subjects.

One subsequent open-label study in five patients with PD showed that infusing GDNF directly into the putamen improved motor performance and that there was increased FDOPA uptake in some of the patients (Gill et al., 2003). However, a subsequent larger placebo-controlled trial failed to show clinical improvement, although FDOPA uptake did increase (Lang et al., 2006).

Another approach of delivering GDNF directly into the brain was successfully achieved in primates using lentoviral vectors containing the gene for producing GDNF (Kordower et al., 2000). Lenti-GDNF was injected into the striatum and substantia nigra of rhesus monkeys that had been treated 1 week previously with MPTP. Lenti-GDNF reversed functional deficits and completely prevented nigrostriatal degeneration. Long-term gene expression (8 months) was seen in intact monkeys that were given this treatment.

A novel nonimmunosuppressive immunophilin ligand, GPI-1046 (henceforth called neuroimmunophilin), was found to have trophic activity, including regenerative sprouting from spared nigrostriatal dopaminergic neurons following MPTP toxicity in mice or 6-OHDA toxicity in rats (Steiner et al., 1997). Since then, there have been reports supporting a regenerative effect by neuroimmunophilins (Guo et al., 2001) and with a proposed mechanism of increasing glutathione in brain (Tanaka et al., 2001, 2002). On the other hand, there have been many reports that failed to find such benefits in various animal models of PD, including primates (Harper et al., 1999; Bocquet et al., 2001; Emborg et al., 2001; Eberling et al., 2002). One controlled clinical trial testing neuroimmunophilin in patients was unsuccessful, and a subsequent larger and longer one also failed to show benefit.

## Enhancing Mitochondria and Energy Function

Coenzyme Q10 is the electron acceptor for mitochondrial complexes I and II and is also a potent antioxidant. Complex I activity was found to be affected by MPTP and subsequently found to be selectively decreased postmortem in substantia nigra in patients with PD (Schapira et al., 1990). Coenzyme Q10 is reduced in the mitochondria (Shults et al., 1997) and in sera of patients with PD (Matsubara et al., 1991). Oral supplementation of coenzyme Q10 in rats resulted in increases of coenzyme Q10 in cerebral cortex mitochondria (Matthews et al., 1998). A controlled clinical pilot trial of coenzyme Q10 was undertaken in 80 patients with early PD. They were randomized into four equal arms and were assigned 300 mg per day, 600 mg per day, 1200 mg per day, or placebo and followed up to 16 months (Shults et al., 2002). There was a positive trend (P value = .09) for a linear relationship between the dosage and the mean change in the total UPDRS score. The highest-dose group (total UPDRS change of +6.69) was statistically less than the UPDRS change of +11.99 for the placebo group (Fig. 6-6). The change in UPDRS for the lower doses showed no significant difference from the placebo group. There was a slower decline in the change of all three components of the UPDRS scores in the 1200-mg-per-day group, with the greatest effect in Part II (the subjective ADL component) (Fig. 6-7). This raises the question of whether patients on 1200 mg per day of coenzyme Q10 might simply feel better rather than having an objective improvement of their motoric features of PD. After 1 month of treatment, there was improvement of the Part II UPDRS (ADL) score in the 1200-mg-per-day group of −0.66, compared to worsening in the placebo group of

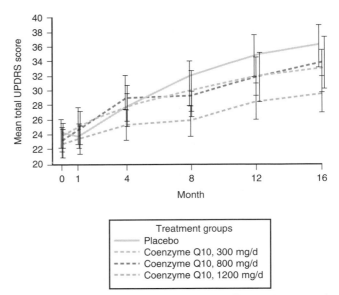

**Figure 6-6** Change in total UPDRS with different dosages of coenzyme Q10. (See Color Plate 10.) (Reprinted with permission from Shults CW, Oakes D, Kieburtz K, et al: Effects of coenzyme Q10 in early Parkinson disease: Evidence of slowing of the functional decline. Arch Neurol 2002;59:1541–1550.)

+0.52. This wash-in effect supports the concern that there might be a "feel good" response from coenzyme Q10 rather than a neuroprotective effect. Also, it should be noted that those who were treated with the 1200 mg per day failed to show a delay in the need for dopaminergic therapy. Of course, the study was not powered for a modest effect, and the study investigators urged caution in interpretation of the results until a larger study could be conducted and evaluated.

Creatine is a guanidine-derived compound that is generated in the body. The creatine/phosphocreatine system functions as an energy buffer between the cytosol and mitochondria (Beal, 2003). Creatine has been proposed to serve as a neuroprotectant in neurodegeneration and has been tested in a controlled clinical futility trial in early PD. Creatine was not found to be futile and therefore deserving of a Phase III trial (NINDS NET-PD Investigators, 2006).

## Counteracting Inflammation

Gliosis and reactive microglia are seen in the substantia nigra of patients with PD, indicating an ongoing inflammatory process. Such changes have also been seen following treatment with MPTP (Vila et al., 2001) and rotenone (Betarbet et al., 2000) neurotoxicity. Inflammation is considered to be a secondary effect but may play an important role in enhancing neurodegeneration by the production of cytokines and prostaglandins. Experimental animal models have shown that treatment with the antibiotic minocycline can reduce the level of degeneration by MPTP (Du et al., 2001; Wu et al., 2002). As a result of these reports, a controlled clinical futility trial testing minocycline was conducted, which did not show minocycline to be futile (NINDS NET-PD Investigators, 2006).

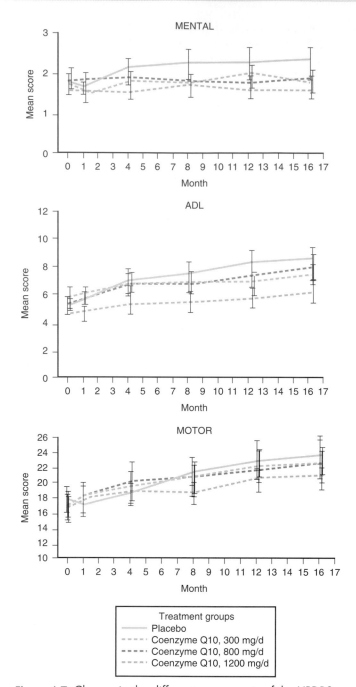

**Figure 6-7** Change in the different components of the UPDRS with coenzyme Q10. (See Color Plate 11.) (Reprinted with permission from Shults CW, Oakes D, Kieburtz K, et al: Effects of coenzyme Q10 in early Parkinson disease: Evidence of slowing of the functional decline. Arch Neurol 2002;59:1541–1550.)

## Inhibiting Apoptosis

Studies on selegiline, in an effort to explain its effectiveness in the DATATOP study, have shown it to have a neuronal rescue effect that is independent of its MAO inhibition (Tatton, 1993). This finding led to the investigation of other agents for their neuronal rescue effect, resulting in the discovery that propargylamines have an antiapoptotic action. A search for similar compounds but without inhibiting MAO resulted in the discovery of one agent that is antiapoptotic and that may act by stabilizing glyceraldehyde-3-phosphate dehydrogenase (Waldmeier et al., 2000). This drug was tested in a controlled clinical trial (Waldmeier et al., 2006) but was not found to be effective in slowing progression of PD. The propargylamine rasagiline is also antiapoptotic in laboratory and animal models. Another antiapoptotic drug, CEP1347, which inhibits mitogen linear kinases has been an effective neuroprotectant in animal models of PD. This drug was tested in a large controlled clinical trial that was ended early because of the lack of effectiveness of the drug.

## Dopamine Agonists

There are three published trials comparing a dopamine agonist and levodopa in patients with PD who were in need of symptomatic therapy. These compared ropinirole and levodopa (Rascol et al., 2000), pramipexole and levodopa (the so-called CALM-PD trial) (Parkinson Study Group, 2000), and pergolide and levodopa (Oertel et al., 2006). The clinical outcomes of these studies are discussed later in the chapter, in the section entitled "Treatment of Mild-Stage Parkinson Disease." In this section regarding neuroprotection, the results of the neuroimaging component of these trials are discussed. In the CALM-PD (pramipexole versus levodopa) trial, the 4-year imaging results show a statistically significant lesser rate of decay of dopamine transporter binding (β-CIT SPECT) (a marker of integrity of nerve terminals of the dopaminergic nigrostriatal fibers) in the striatum in the group originally assigned to pramipexole treatment (Fig. 6-8) (Parkinson Study Group, 2002b). A separate study evaluating FDOPA PET scans, a marker of dopa uptake and dopa decarboxylase activity, showed a similar statistically significant lesser rate of decay of labeling in the striatum in a controlled trial in the group assigned to ropinirole compared to the group assigned to levodopa therapy (Whone et al., 2003).

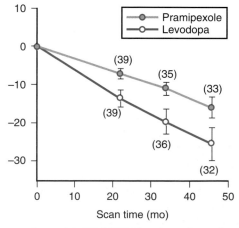

**Figure 6-8** Striatal β-CIT SPECT binding. (Data from Parkinson Study Group: Dopamine transporter brain imaging to assess the effects of pramipexole vs levodopa on Parkinson disease progression. JAMA 2002;287: 1653–1661.)

Because there was no placebo comparator in either study, interpretation is difficult. Whether dopamine agonists slow the rate of progression of PD, whether levodopa hastens it, and whether both explanations are playing a role are possibilities. Another possibility would be a pharmacodynamic effect on the dopamine transporter and dopa decarboxylase by either the agonists or levodopa. For example, if levodopa downregulated the dopamine transporter, β-CIT SPECT binding would be reduced. If levodopa downregulated dopa decarboxylase, FDOPA PET binding would be reduced. Short trials of levodopa showed no change in these imaging markers, so there is no evidence that levodopa affects either type of imaging study. Without knowing whether the agonists actually slow the rate of progression, it is not possible to recommend the starting treatment on the basis of these results alone. As is discussed later, the individual factors of patient's age, cognitive status, occupational status, and severity of symptoms all need to be taken into account in individualizing therapy to fit the patient.

## TREATMENT OF MILD-STAGE PARKINSON DISEASE

### Strategy

The mild stage of PD occurs when the signs and symptoms of the illness are beginning to interfere with daily activities or quality of life. The judgment to initiate symptomatic drug therapy is made in discussions between the patient and the treating physician. According to a survey (Parkinson Study Group, 1989a), the most common problems that clinicians consider important for the decision to initiate symptomatic agents are (1) threat to employability; (2) threat to ability to handle domestic, financial, or social affairs; (3) threat to ability to handle activities of daily living; and (4) appreciable worsening of gait or balance. According to a Norwegian quality-of-life study (Karlsen et al., 1999), the factors that produce the highest distress for PD patients compared to healthy elderly people are depressive symptoms, self-reported insomnia, and a low degree of independence, measured by the Schwab and England scale. Severity of parkinsonian motor symptoms contributed, but to a lesser extent. A sense of lack of energy was seen in half of the PD patients compared to a fifth of controls, and this could be only partially accounted for by depressive symptoms and the UPDRS motor scores.

The choice of drugs (see Boxes 6-1 and 6-2) is wide, but the degree of disability and the age (or mental acuity) of the patient are two critical factors. If the delay in initiating symptomatic treatment was so prolonged that the symptoms now threaten employment or endanger falling, one needs to begin levodopa to get a quick response. The advantages of using levodopa when the symptoms are this pronounced, in preference to a dopamine agonist or other medications, are that a therapeutic response is both rapid and virtually guaranteed, because nearly all patients with PD will respond to levodopa and relatively quickly. In contrast, only a minority of patients with severe symptoms will benefit sufficiently from a dopamine agonist given alone, and it takes more time (often months) to build up the dose to adequate levels to discover this. If levodopa is to be utilized, inhibitors of type A MAO must be discontinued. If selegiline (or another selective type B MAO inhibitor) was the MAO inhibitor that was utilized, this

drug can be continued. A type A MAO inhibitor can be used safely with dopamine agonists.

If the symptoms are not severe enough to require levodopa and the patient is younger than 60 (younger than 70 if the patient is mentally young), we prefer to employ a dopa-sparing strategy to avoid as long as possible the development of levodopa-induced dyskinesias and motor fluctuations (mainly the wearing-off effect). These complications are more likely to occur in younger patients (Quinn et al., 1987; Kostic et al., 1991; Gershanik, 1993; Wagner et al., 1996). The choices are dopamine agonists, amantadine, and anticholinergics. Tranylcypromine can be continued in the presence of any of these drugs. Dopamine agonists are the most potent antiparkinsonian agents among this group of drugs. Four-year results of the pramipexole versus levodopa trial reveal that levodopa is clinically more potent but is also much more likely to induce dyskinesias and clinical fluctuations (Holloway and Parkinson Study Group, 2004). For patients older than 70 years or those with any cognitive decline, employ levodopa as the initial therapy. Not only is there less need for a dopa-sparing strategy in these elderly patients; they are more susceptible to confusion, psychosis, or drowsiness from other antiparkinson drugs, including dopamine agonists. Levodopa provides the greatest benefit for the lowest risk of these adverse effects, compared to the other drugs.

### Rationale for Dopa-Sparing Strategy in Young Patients

As was mentioned earlier, younger patients (less than 60 years of age) are particularly prone to develop the motor complications of fluctuations and dyskinesias (Quinn et al., 1987; Kostic et al., 1991; Gershanik, 1993; Wagner et al., 1996). Some physicians therefore recommend utilizing dopamine agonists, rather than levodopa, in younger patients when beginning therapy, in an attempt to delay the onset of these problems (Quinn, 1994b; Fahn, 1998; Montastruc et al., 1999). Others prefer to start with levodopa (Weiner, 1999). A conference on this topic failed to produce a consensus (Agid et al., 1999).

### Choice of Drug When Employing a Dopa-Sparing Strategy

#### DOPAMINE AGONISTS

The dopamine agonists are the group of agents that is next most powerful in reducing the symptoms of PD after levodopa therapy. Thus, they are a good choice. Another factor is that they might slow the rate of nigrostriatal neuronal loss (Parkinson Study Group, 2002b; Whone et al., 2003) (discussed earlier, in the section entitled "Dopamine Agonists"). Finally, perhaps the main reason many patients are started with this class of drugs is that they are less likely to induce dyskinesias and motor fluctuations (Parkinson Study Group, 2000; Rascol et al., 2000).

Rinne (1989a, 1989b) first proposed that early use of the dopamine agonists will reduce the likelihood of developing complications from chronic levodopa therapy. However, the Rinne reports were on retrospective analyses, using historical rather than contemporary controls. In one double-blind study, Weiner and colleagues (1993) could not confirm Rinne's findings. However, in another controlled trial, Montastruc and colleagues (1994) reported that there were fewer motor complications in patients who started on bromocriptine to which levodopa was later added. A double-blind study comparing cabergoline and levodopa also showed that a smaller percentage of patients in the dopamine agonist group developed motor fluctuations (22% versus 34%; $P < .02$) (Rinne, Bracco, et al., 1998). Studies of dopamine agonists as primary monotherapy in early PD have shown that even with sustained treatment, drug-induced dyskinesias rarely develop but that monotherapy is successful for more than 3 years in only about 30% of all PD patients (Poewe, 1998). In addition to this benefit, the dopamine agonists are the most powerful antiparkinson medications after levodopa. Therefore, if one wants to use dopa-sparing strategies, one should choose among the dopamine agonists.

The agonists that are currently available are the ergots pergolide (Permax) and bromocriptine (Parlodel) and the nonergots pramipexole (Mirapex) and ropinirole (Requip). The longer-duration ergot cabergoline is available in some countries. Ergots rarely can induce red, inflamed skin (St. Anthony's fire), which is reversible on discontinuing the drug. They also have the potential (though rare) with long-term use to induce fibrosis: retroperitoneal, pleuropulmonary, and pericardial (Pfitzenmeyer et al., 1996; Ling et al., 1999; Shaunak et al., 1999). Pergolide has also been seen in association with fibroproliferative changes in heart valves initially reported in three patients (Pritchett et al., 2002). Since then, there have been other reports (Baseman et al., 2004; Horvath et al., 2004; Van Camp et al., 2004). The frequency of this complication is still being resolved. The reports of this complication raised new concerns and questions as to whether pergolide should be used as a drug for PD unless other dopamine agonists have been unsatisfactory in terms of benefits or adverse effects (Agarwal et al., 2004). Now echocardiograms performed on patients taking pergolide have revealed a much higher prevalence (about 33%) of restrictive valvulopathies (Van Camp et al., 2004). This indicates that all patients on pergolide need to undergo echocardiography. Fortunately, the valvulopathy is reversible in some patients if pergolide is discontinued. If this ergoline can cause this problem, then it is possible that the other ergoline agonists can do likewise. It seems prudent to utilize nonergot dopamine agonists rather than starting pergolide on other patients.

Pramipexole and ropinirole, as was mentioned earlier, appear more readily to produce drowsiness and sleep attacks in which patients fall asleep without warning, including while driving, although there have now been rare incidences of sleep attacks with all dopamine agonists and levodopa (Frucht et al., 1999; Ferreira et al., 2000; Hoehn, 2000; Schapira, 2000). The Epworth Sleepiness Scale is not predictive as to which patient may develop a sleep attack (Hobson et al., 2002). Korner and colleagues (2004) sent a questionnaire to 12,000 patients and received responses from 63%, 42% of whom reported that they had experienced sudden onset of sleep; 10% of these had not experienced sleepiness before their first sleep attack. Predicting factors were nonergoline dopamine agonists, age less than 70 years, and disease duration less than 7 years. Modafinil has successfully been used to prevent sleep attacks (Hauser et al., 2000).

Adverse effects that are more common with agonists than with levodopa are orthostatic hypotension, nausea (because nausea from levodopa is blocked by carbidopa), drowsiness, hallucinations, and leg edema. All agonists have a propensity to produce ankle and leg edema (Tan and Ondo, 2000), which is not an early problem but tends to occur after a few years of treatment. The edematous skin is often red, and some clinicians, unaware of this adverse effect, assume that there is a deep vein thrombosis. The edema and redness persist unless the drug is stopped. Diuretics are usually not effective in relieving the edema. Whether it is dangerous to continue to allow the edema to persist is not known. But continued use of the agonist can eventually result in discolored, indurated skin in the lower part of the legs where the edema was located. The tight skin prevents edema from accumulating there, so the edema is seen above the induration. Substituting one agonist for another may occasionally allow the edema to dissipate, but more often than not, once the edema has occurred, it persists in the presence of other dopamine agonists as well. The only satisfactory treatment of the edema is to discontinue the agonist and substitute levodopa, which does not cause this problem. The edema of the legs that is induced by dopamine agonists resembles that induced by amantadine.

An experimental study in MPTP-treated primates showed that treatment with dopamine agonists (ropinirole and bromocriptine in this study) was significantly less likely to cause severe dyskinesias than was treatment with levodopa (Pearce et al., 1998). The investigators titrated dosages that produced similarly increased locomotion and improved motor disability. However, the investigators also showed that an agonist will elicit comparable dyskinesia once levodopa priming has occurred; they therefore recommended early use of dopamine agonists. Controlled clinical trials comparing ropinirole (Rascol et al., 2000), pramipexole (Parkinson Study Group, 2000), and pergolide (Oertel, 2006) have shown that starting treatment with a dopamine agonist is less likely than treatment with levodopa to induce dyskinesias. On the other hand, these studies all showed that levodopa is more potent and improves UPDRS scores more than the agonists did. Moreover, the agonists are more likely to produce hallucinations and sedation than is levodopa.

Each of the dopamine agonists easily induces orthostatic hypotension, particularly when the drug is first introduced (Kujawa et al., 2000). After that period, this complication is much less common. Therefore, it is best to start with a tiny dose (bromocriptine 1.25 mg at bedtime; pergolide 0.05 mg at bedtime; pramipexole 0.125 mg at bedtime) for the first 3 days and then switch from bedtime to daytime dosing for the remainder of the first week. Ropinirole can be started at 0.25 mg three times daily for the first week. The daily dose can be increased gradually (bromocriptine 1.25 mg per day every week; pergolide 0.125 mg per day weekly; pramipexole 0.125 mg every 2 days for 10 days, then 0.125 mg per day weekly; ropinirole 0.5 mg per day twice weekly), building the dosage up on a four times a day dosing schedule until benefit or a dose around 40 mg per day (bromocriptine), 4 to 6 mg per day (pergolide and pramipexole), or 24 mg per day (ropinirole) is reached. Use the lowest dose that provides adequate benefit.

Bromocriptine appears to be the weakest of the four agonists, yet it can induce psychotoxicity just as readily as the other agonists, if not more so. The choice between the other three drugs is one of personal preference and experience and perhaps should be based on adverse effects because the benefits are similar. Some patients may benefit from all three equally; some may get adverse effects from one but not the others. By having these three drugs available, the clinician has

Table 6-6 Conversion factors for the dopamine agonists

| Agonist | Ratio |
| --- | --- |
| Pergolide | 1 |
| Pramipexole | 1 |
| Ropinirole | 5 |
| Bromocriptine | 10 |

the ability to switch from one to another should one of them not be tolerated. Switching can be done rapidly, using a ratio of 1:1:5 for pergolide:pramipexole:ropinirole, without having to build up the dose of the new drug from a much lower level. If the response is less than satisfactory and it is desired to maintain the dopa-sparing strategy for as long as possible, one can then add amantadine or an anticholinergic (see later). If none of these agents is helpful or tolerated, the patient moves into the next stage of illness, the stage in which levodopa is required. Nausea and vomiting are other potential side effects that would limit the usefulness of the dopamine agonists. These symptoms are usually avoided by increasing the dose slowly. The peripherally acting dopamine antagonist domperidone will block these gastrointestinal side effects. The usual dose is 10 to 20 mg three times daily. Even if a dopamine agonist is effective, many patients require the addition of levodopa within a year or two.

One can quickly switch from one dopamine agonist to another without having to build up the dose slowly for the new one (Canesi et al., 1999). Using a conversion factor, the new agonist can begin at full dosage at the beginning of the day while the current one is suddenly discontinued. A conversion table is provided (Table 6-6), in which pergolide is given at unity (1). Pramipexole is also 1, ropinirole is 5, and bromocriptine is 10. This means that if the dose of pergolide or pramipexole were 2 mg per day, ropinirole and bromocriptine equivalents would be 10 mg per day and 20 mg per day, respectively.

### AMANTADINE

Amantadine is a mild indirect dopaminergic, acting by augmenting dopamine release from storage sites and possibly blocking reuptake of dopamine into the presynaptic terminals. It also appears to have some anticholinergic properties as well as glutamate receptor blocking activity. In the mild stage of PD, it is effective in about two thirds of patients (Fahn and Isgreen, 1975). A major advantage is that substantial benefit, if it occurs, is seen in a couple of days. Unfortunately, its benefit in more advanced PD is often short-lived, with patients reporting a falloff effect after several months of treatment in the absence of concomitant levodopa. The mechanism appears to be a depletion of already reduced dopamine stores in the dopaminergic nerve terminals so that the effect of amantadine is exhausted. A common adverse effect is livedo reticularis (a reddish mottling of skin) around the knees; this is not dangerous, although it can be cosmetically a problem for some patients. Occasional adverse effects are ankle edema and visual hallucinosis. Sometimes when the drug is discontinued, there can be a gradual worsening of parkinsonian signs, indicating that the drug has been helpful. The usual dosage is 100 mg twice daily, but sometimes a higher dose (up to 400 mg per day) may be required.

Amantadine can be useful not only in the early phases of symptomatic therapy, thereby forestalling the introduction of levodopa or reducing the required dosage of levodopa, but also in the advanced stage of the disease as an adjunctive drug to levodopa and the dopamine agonists. It is also effective in reducing levodopa-induced dyskinesias (Rajput et al., 1997; Metman, Del Dotto, van den Munckhof, et al., 1998), probably from its antiglutamatergic activity.

Amantadine is excreted mostly unchanged in the urine, so the dose needs to be reduced in patients with renal impairment. The half-life is long, about 28 hours, so twice-daily dosing is adequate.

### ANTIMUSCARINIC DRUGS (ANTICHOLINERGICS)

The anticholinergics are less effective antiparkinson agents than are the dopamine agonists. The anticholinergics are estimated to improve parkinsonism by about 20%. Many clinicians find that if tremor is not relieved by an agonist or levodopa, then the addition of an anticholinergic drug is often effective. Sometimes, the anticholinergic can lessen tremor severity even in the absence of levodopa, so clinicians can use such an agent as monotherapy for tremor. If this is not helpful, then continuing to use the drug while a dopamine agonist or levodopa is added can be helpful. Later, if tremor is relieved by the dopaminergic agent, one can try to discontinue the anticholinergic. Commonly used anticholinergics are trihexyphenidyl (Artane) and benztropine mesylate (Cogentin), but there are many others. To minimize adverse effects, start with low doses (trihexyphenidyl 1 mg twice daily, benztropine 0.5 mg twice daily) and increase gradually to 2 mg three times daily for trihexyphenidyl and 1 mg three times daily for benztropine. As would be expected, if anticholinergics lessen parkinsonism, cholinergic agents aggravate parkinsonism (Duvoisin, 1967), including nicotine (Ebersbach et al., 1999).

Peripheral anticholinergic adverse effects include blurred vision (treated with pilocarpine eye drops, which also must be utilized if glaucoma is present), dry mouth, and urinary retention. Pyridostigmine, up to 60 mg three times daily if necessary, can sometimes be helpful in overcoming dry mouth and urinary difficulties. The predominant central side effects are forgetfulness and decreased short-term memory. Occasionally, hallucinations and psychosis can occur, particularly in the elderly. Powerful anticholinergics should be avoided in patients older than 70 years of age. If tremor persists in this age range despite the presence of levodopa or dopamine agonists, utilize drugs with a weaker anticholinergic effect, such as diphenhydramine (Benadryl), orphenadrine (Norflex), cyclobenzaprine (Flexeril), and amitriptyline (Elavil). Diphenhydramine and amitriptyline can cause drowsiness; therefore, they can also be used as a hypnotic. For tremor control, one needs to increase the dose gradually until at least 50 mg three times daily is reached for diphenhydramine and orphenadrine, 20 mg three times daily for cylclobenzaprine, and 25 mg three times daily for amitriptyline.

## Another Point of View: Utilize Levodopa as the First Drug

There are a number of neurologists who advocate starting with levodopa when symptomatic therapy is needed (Agid, 1998; Weiner, 1999; Factor, 2000), and for the sake of the reader, this point of view should be made known. The argument is that there is no proof that levodopa itself causes either neurotoxicity or the motor complications of dyskinesias and "off" states. Rather, they suggest that it is the severity of the disease that allows these complications to appear with levodopa. Therefore, they prefer to use the most effective drug first when the symptoms are mild, in order to provide the highest quality of life. However, despite the ELLDOPA trial (Parkinson Study Group, 2004b), uncertainty about neurotoxicity remains, and until a follow-up controlled clinical trial determining to answer uncertainties from that trial is conducted, the justification can be made that unless a dopamine agonist is not tolerated or effective, levodopa can be delayed until needed (Fahn, 1999).

The ELLDOPA study was a controlled clinical trial evaluating the effect of levodopa on the natural history of PD (Parkinson Study Group, 2004b). Unexpectedly, the clinical results showed that subjects treated with levodopa had less clinical progression 2 weeks after stopping the drug than did subjects treated with placebo, and this effect was dose-dependent (Fig. 6-9). But concern has been raised that perhaps the 2-week washout of levodopa was insufficient to eliminate all of its symptomatic benefit. Moreover, the ELLDOPA study showed a discordance between the neuroimaging component and the clinical results. The dopamine transporter–binding ligand imaging study was compatible with a more rapid decline of dopamine neurons. But that result has now raised the question as to whether levodopa itself interferes with this binding. Therefore, the interpretation of the ELLDOPA study remains uncertain.

Another argument is that levodopa has delayed mortality and therefore should be used early. However, the initial

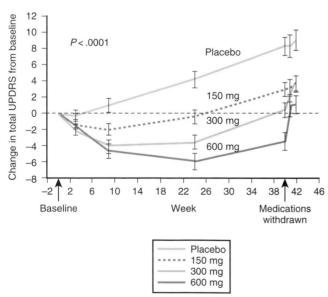

**Figure 6-9** Levodopa and the progression of Parkinson disease. Three doses of levodopa were compared with a placebo over 40 weeks, followed by a 2-week withdrawal of medications. The UPDRS scores were dose dependent for symptomatic benefit and after the medications were discontinued. (See Color Plate 12.) (From Parkinson Study Group: Levodopa and the progression of Parkinson's disease. N Engl J Med 2004;351[24]:2498–2508.)

improvement of mortality rates occurred when levodopa was first introduced and most likely was from the improvement of mobility, not from the drug itself. Improved or maintained mobility with another antiparkinson agent would probably be just as effective. Actually, mortality rates have gone back to their earlier increased level, now that levodopa has taken care of the backlog of disabled patients (Clarke, 1995). In a more recent analysis of retrospective data from Scotland (Donnan et al., 2000) comparing PD patients with their treatment assignment, levodopa monotherapy had a higher mortality rate than did selegiline monotherapy or selegiline plus levodopa.

From the DATATOP study, the 387 subjects who reached endpoint—that is, the need for symptomatic therapy—were placed on levodopa, and their UPDRS scores were reduced by approximately 33% (from approximately 43 units to 29 units) (Fig. 1 in Growdon et al., 1998).

Whether levodopa actually provides a better quality of life (Glozman et al., 1998; Martinez-Martin, 1998) for patients with mild stage PD remains to be determined, particularly as compared to dopamine agonists in patients with early PD. In one study—the levodopa versus pramipexole controlled clinical trial (Holloway and Parkinson Study Group, 2004)—health-related quality of life (HRQOL) was assessed by three different measures. All three measures resulted in similar profiles over time, characterized by initial improvement over the first 3 to 6 months and followed by a gradual decline in years 2, 3, and 4 (Noyes et al., 2006). The difference in HRQOL between the treatment arms widened in favor of pramipexole in years 3 and 4 for all HRQOL measures used. Because levodopa had a superior result in UPDRS scores, the results suggest that pramipexole and levodopa affect HRQOL via improvement on different domains of well-being: nonmotor affect for pramipexole and mobility improvement for levodopa.

Whether the motor complications that are seen with chronic levodopa therapy in patients with PD are actually caused by long-term levodopa therapy or simply reflect the progression of the disease is unknown and widely debated (de Jong et al., 1987; Quinn et al., 1987; Blin et al., 1988; Roos et al., 1990; Caraceni et al., 1991; Cedarbaum et al., 1991). Advanced disease with altered sensitivity of dopamine receptors is a critical factor, but one does not see these motor complications if the patient was never exposed to levodopa and was treated only with the other antiparkinson agents. In untreated but advanced PD, levodopa-induced dyskinesias occur shortly after levodopa is started (Onofri et al., 1998). In the parkinsonian states of postencephalitic parkinsonism and MPTP-induced parkinsonism, there is rapidly severe depletion of nigral neurons (Bernheimer et al., 1973; Davis et al., 1979; Burns et al., 1983; Langston et al., 1984). These patients may develop dyskinesias and fluctuations within weeks to months after starting levodopa (Calne et al., 1969; Sacks et al., 1970; Duvoisin et al., 1972; Sacks, 1974; Langston et al., 1983; Langston and Ballard, 1984; Ballard et al., 1985). But if patients with those diseases had been treated with dopamine agonists instead of levodopa, it is likely that those motor complications would not have occurred.

In deciding the choice of drug therapy, it is important to keep in mind the principles of therapy listed at the beginning of this chapter: individualize therapy to fit the patient and keep the goal in mind of maintaining the patient as independent as possible for as long as possible.

If one chooses to use levodopa in the mild-stage disease, there is evidence to suggest keeping the dose as low as possible to reduce the likelihood of developing motor complications (Lesser et al., 1979; Poewe et al., 1986). One strategy is to build the dosage to carbidopa/levodopa 25/100 to 50/200 mg three times daily and then add a dopamine agonist if the patient needs more symptomatic relief. (For older patients, stay with levodopa and increase that if more medication is needed; see the next section.)

## TREATMENT OF MODERATE-STAGE PARKINSON DISEASE

Moderate-stage PD is when the disability is beyond the scope of efficacy of dopamine agonists, amantadine, anticholinergics, and selegiline; treatment with levodopa is necessary to control symptoms. The rule of thumb is to utilize the lowest dosage that brings about adequate symptom reversal, not the highest dosage that the patient can tolerate, in an attempt to avoid response fluctuations and dyskinesias. Levodopa is usually given in combination with a peripheral decarboxylase inhibitor (carbidopa [Sinemet and generics] or benserazide [Madopar]) to prevent the formation of dopamine peripherally, thereby usually avoiding the otherwise common peripheral adverse effects of anorexia, nausea, and vomiting. Many patients require at least 50 to 75 mg of carbidopa a day to have adequate inhibition of peripheral dopa decarboxylase. If the dose of levodopa is less than 300 mg per day, then one should use the 25/100-mg-strength tablets and not the 10/100-mg tablets. In some patients, even 75 mg per day of carbidopa is inadequate, and nausea, anorexia, or vomiting still occurs. In such patients, one needs to use higher doses of carbidopa; carbidopa tablets (Lodosyn) are available by prescription.

Carbidopa/levodopa is marketed in both standard release (Sinemet and generics) and sustained-release (Sinemet CR and generic carbidopa/levodopa ER) tablets, which provides a longer plasma half-life and lower peak plasma levels of levodopa compared to standard Sinemet. Unfortunately, Sinemet CR has not been shown to avoid the development of response fluctuations. A 5-year study in 618 dopa-naïve patients compared Sinemet CR and standard Sinemet therapy. There was no difference between the two groups in the development of either fluctuations or dyskinesias (Block et al., 1997; Koller et al., 1999). An Italian study found that using small, divided doses during the day is more likely to lead to loss of the long-duration response (Zappia et al., 2000).

A pre-bedtime dose of Sinemet CR may allow the patient some mobility during the night. Disadvantages of Sinemet CR are the lack of a rapid response with each dose and a delayed response that can be excessive, resulting in sustained severe dyskinesias that cannot be controlled except by sedating the patient. Moreover, the response to individual doses of Sinemet CR is less predictable than the response to standard Sinemet. It is complicated to use both standard Sinemet and Sinemet CR to smooth out fluctuations, but this is often necessary. Finally, one should keep in mind that not all of the carbidopa/levodopa in Sinemet CR is absorbed, because some of the medication may have reached the large intestine before all of it was absorbed in the small intestine. A dose of Sinemet CR is equal to about two thirds to three fourths of an identical dose of standard Sinemet.

On the other hand, Sinemet CR is useful as a first-line drug in patients older than age 70 years to slow the rate of absorption and lower the peak plasma level of levodopa, making it less likely for the patient to develop peak dose drowsiness or confusion. For younger patients, in whom cognitive adverse effects are less likely to occur, standard carbidopa/levodopa is preferred in order to observe the response and better monitor the effectiveness of the drug.

Sinemet CR is available in two strengths: a carbidopa/levodopa 50/200-mg tablet, which is scored and can be broken in half, and a 25/100-mg unscored tablet. Crushing either tablet loses the slow-release property because the matrix is no longer intact. When Sinemet CR is added to a patient taking a dopamine agonist, a dose of 25/100 mg three times daily (built up gradually by 25/100 mg weekly) often suffices. When it is used alone, it often is necessary to use these dosages after meals to reduce initial nausea and vomiting; the dose can later be increased to 50/200 mg three or four times daily. If greater relief is required, a dopamine agonist should then be added.

Standard carbidopa/levodopa is available in 10/100, 25/100, and 25/250-mg tablets. Because of the desire to have at least 75 mg per day of carbidopa, one should start with the 25/100-mg tablets when the drug is introduced. An increase by 25/100 mg per day per week until three times daily dosing is achieved is often adequate. A 25/100-mg dosing three times daily is the most common plateau schedule that neurologists aim for (Fahn and Mazzoni, 2006). Not every symptom of PD responds equally well. Bradykinesia and rigidity respond best, while tremor can be more resistant. If a response is seen but with symptoms later returning or worsening, increasing to 50/200 mg three times daily is a reasonable goal before adding a dopamine agonist. If agonists are already being taken and there is still an inadequate response, the dosage of levodopa should be increased gradually, switching to the 25/250-mg tablets as necessary. A dose of 25/250 mg four times daily may be required. A reasonably high dose before concluding that levodopa is ineffective is 2000 mg of levodopa per day.

A patient's response or lack of response to levodopa is a very important piece of information to help differentiate PD from parkinsonism-plus syndromes. If the response is nil or minor, it is most likely that the disorder is not PD (Marsden and Fahn, 1982). However, a beneficial response does not ensure that a diagnosis of PD is correct. All cases of presynaptic disorders (e.g., reserpine-induced, MPTP-induced, postencephalitic parkinsonism) will respond to levodopa. Also patients in the early stages of multiple-system atrophy and progressive supranuclear palsy may improve with levodopa; later in these diseases, when dopamine receptors are lost, the response is lost. Some patients with Shy-Drager syndrome and olivopontocerebellar atrophy may continue to have intact dopamine receptors in the striatum and continue to respond to levodopa. The only effective drugs in situations in which levodopa is not effective are the anticholinergics and amantadine, even though only mildly so.

It takes a mean of $9.3 \pm 1.8$ days to achieve maximum response when beginning treatment with Sinemet CR and $6.8 \pm 3.0$ days for the parkinsonism severity to return to baseline levels after stopping chronic Sinemet CR treatment (Barbato et al., 1997). This compares to a decay time of $6.2 \pm 1.7$ days following withdrawal of the dopamine agonist ropinirole (9 to 21 mg daily). These studies support the concept that the long-duration effect of levodopa and ropinirole might be due to some slowly evolving postsynaptic pharmacodynamic change in the CNS (Barbato et al., 1997).

As PD progresses, the duration of effectiveness of a dose of levodopa becomes shorter (Contin et al., 1998a). The effective half-life of a dose of levodopa declines in relation to both worsening of symptoms and duration of disease. The half-life declines from a mean of 262 minutes in Stage I patients, to 142 minutes in Stage II, to 54 minutes in Stage III. The rate of decline becomes smaller as the disease progresses. The mean annual reduction of the effective half-life slows down as the disease worsens, dropping by 37 minutes per year in Stage I patients and by 6.5 minutes per year in Stage III and is about 17% per year of the disease. Contin and colleagues (1998a) determined this "effective" half-life by administering a standard oral fasting dose (100 mg) of levodopa (with a peripheral decarboxylase inhibitor). Motor response was measured by finger-tapping speed and walking speed. The decline in effective half-life is equivalent to the loss of the long-duration response from levodopa to only a short-duration response as the disease worsens and as first reported by Muenter and Tyce (1971).

It is important to avoid sudden withdrawal of levodopa, which is sometimes done for a surgical procedure (Stotz et al., 2004). A "neuroleptic" malignant syndrome can ensue, with fever, rigidity, and incoherence (Friedman et al., 1985; Hirschorn and Greenberg, 1988; Gordon and Frucht, 2001; Ueda et al., 2001). Tapering levodopa over 3 days appears to be safe (Parkinson Study Group, 2004b).

## TREATMENT OF ADVANCED-STAGE PARKINSON DISEASE

Advanced PD is that stage of the disease in which there is at least one of the following conditions: (1) sufficient disability to interfere with independence despite levodopa therapy, (2) sufficient loss of postural reflexes that one must be cautious when walking, (3) the presence of the freezing phenomenon to make walking difficult, (4) pronounced postural deformity, or (5) the presence of complications (fluctuations, dyskinesias, psychosis) from levodopa that have become the focus of treatment. Because it is only the last group that is somewhat amenable to therapy, the discussion will concentrate on methods to overcome these complications. In advanced PD, because of the severity of the clinical situation, all patients should be receiving levodopa therapy or at least have had a trial of this drug but have not been able to remain on it because of disabling adverse effects. The Quality Standards Subcommittee of the American Academy of Neurology conducted an evidence-based literature review of clinical trials related to treating dyskinesias and fluctuations (Pahwa et al., 2006).

### Description of Motor (and Sensory) Complications

The motor complications can be divided into two categories: fluctuations ("off" states) and dyskinesias; these are subdivided into their temporal relationship with a dose of levodopa and the clinical motor and sensory phenomena seen as features of these levodopa-related complications (Box 6-4). The "off" states usually consist of a return of parkinsonian symptoms and signs, such as bradykinesia, tremor, rigidity, immobility, and freezing (so-called off freezing). There are also other features of "off" states in many patients. Off dystonia is the presence of sustained contractions and spasms, often painful, and most common early in the morning on arising and in the feet. Because technically, off dystonia is an abnormal involuntary movement (dyskinesia), this is listed in Box 6-4 under "Dyskinesias," but it should be recognized clinically

**Box 6-4** Major fluctuations and dyskinesias as complications of levodopa

**Fluctuations ("Offs")**
Slow wearing-off
Sudden "off"
Random "off"
Yo-yo-ing
Episodic failure to respond (dose failure)
Delayed "on"
Weak response at end of day
Response varies in relationship to meals
Sudden transient freezing

**Dyskinesias**
Peak-dose chorea, ballism, and dystonia
Diphasic chorea and dystonia
"Off" dystonia
Myoclonus
Simultaneous dyskinesia and parkinsonism

**Sensory and Behavioral "Offs"**
Pain
Akathisia
Depression
Anxiety
Dysphoria
Panic

as an "off" phenomenon. Off dystonia shows an abnormal irregular firing of globus pallidus interna neurons similar to that seen in primary dystonia (Hashimoto et al., 2001). So-called sensory offs or, equivalently, behavioral offs are the sensory and behavioral phenomena that may accompany a motor (parkinsonian) "off" or be present as an "off" in the absence of any motoric parkinsonian signs. Sensory "offs" can consist of pain, akathisia, depression, anxiety, dysphoria, or panic and usually a mixture of more than one of these. Sensory "offs," like dystonic "offs," are extremely poorly tolerated. It is often the presence of one of these sensory and behavioral phenomena, more so than motoric parkinsonian or dystonic "offs," that drives the patient to take more and more levodopa, turning the patient into a "levodopa junkie." The sensory "offs" are discussed in Chapter 8.

There is usually a pattern of progressively worsening response fluctuations in patients who are on chronic levodopa therapy (Box 6-5). Response fluctuations usually begin as mild wearing-off (end-of-dose failure). Wearing-off can be defined to be present when an adequate dosage of levodopa does not last at least 4 hours. Typically, in the first couple of years of treatment, there is a long-duration response (Muenter and Tyce, 1971). As the disease progresses or as levodopa treatment continues, the long-duration response fades and the short-duration response becomes predominant, leading to the wearing-off effect.

The "offs" tend to be mild at first but, over time, often become deeper, with more severe parkinsonism; simultaneously, the duration of the "on" response becomes shorter. Eventually, many patients develop sudden "offs" in which the deep state of parkinsonism develops over minutes rather than tens of minutes, and they are less predictable in terms of timing with the dosings of

Box 6-5 Development of response fluctuations and dyskinesias

**Dyskinesias**
1. Peak-dose dyskinesias
2. Diphasic dyskinesias
3. Chorea → dystonia
4. Yo-yo-ing

**Fluctuations**
1. Mild wearing-off
2. Deeper wearing-off; shorter time "on"
3. Delayed "ons"
4. Dose failures
5. Sudden, unpredictable "offs" ("on-offs")
6. Early-morning dystonia
7. "Off" dystonia during the day

**Somatotopic Response**
For example, dyskinetic in neck, "off" in legs

**Freezing Phenomenon**
1. Freezing when "off"
2. Freezing when "on"

**Alertness**
1. Drowsy from a dose of levodopa
2. Excessive daytime sleepiness
3. Reverse sleep-wake cycle

**Myoclonus**
1. Myoclonic jerks during sleep
2. Myoclonic jerks while awake

**Behavioral and Cognitive**
1. Vivid dreams
2. Benign hallucinations
3. Malignant hallucinations
4. Delusions
5. Paranoia
6. Confusion
7. Dementia

**Sensory Offs**
1. Pain
2. Akathisia
3. Depression
4. Anxiety
5. Dysphoria
6. Panic

esias in PD can be viewed in a favorable light because the phenomenon indicates that dopamine receptors remain responsive so that motor symptoms of parkinsonism can be reduced by levodopa therapy. Also, the presence of dyskinesias does not have a significant negative effect on quality of life (Marras et al., 2004). A more detailed description and an explanation of fluctuations and dyskinesias are presented here, followed by treatment paradigms.

## Pathogenesis of Motor Complications

The major risk factor for peak-dose dyskinesia appears to be severity of the disease (Horstink et al., 1990a). On the other hand, according to some researchers, the major risk factors for fluctuations appear to be duration (Horstink et al., 1990b; Roos et al., 1990) and dosage (Poewe et al., 1986) of levodopa therapy.

### FLUCTUATIONS ("OFF" STATES)

The wearing-off phenomenon (also known as end-of-dose failure) is the gradual return of parkinsonism; it correlates with the falling concentration of levodopa in the plasma (and therefore the brain) (Muenter and Tyce, 1971; Shoulson et al., 1975; Fahn, 1982). The "on-off" phenomenon, as originally defined (Duvoisin, 1974b; Fahn, 1974), is a label for a sudden and random event in which the patient suddenly becomes parkinsonian. That is, the benefit from levodopa suddenly disappears, like turning off a light switch—hence the name. To avoid ambiguity, because the term *on-off* is sometimes used to refer to any type of fluctuation in parkinsonian patients, the phenomenon for sudden "offs" is labeled here as either *sudden off* or *on-off* in contrast to *wearing-off*. In addition to worsening of motor performance during "off" states, there is often decreased mood accompanied by anxiety and sometimes pain (Maricle et al., 1995; Ford et al., 1996; Hillen and Sage, 1996). These fluctuating mood and pain states can respond to the pharmacologic effects of levodopa.

#### On-Off Phenomenon

In "on-off," the patient can improve just as suddenly, even without taking another dose of levodopa. Pharmacologic studies have revealed plasma levels of levodopa to be in the declining phase when the "offs" appear (Fahn, 1974). It has been speculated that the "sudden off" problem is due to a sudden and transient desensitization of the dopamine receptors that would be compatible with the receptor switching from a high-affinity to a low-affinity state (Fahn, 1974). Response of a "sudden off" state to a new dose of levodopa or to a subcutaneous injection of apomorphine (Clough et al., 1984; Frankel et al., 1990) is compatible with the stimulation of a desensitized receptor; the receptor being presented with a higher concentration of dopamine (or dopamine agonist) will now respond. This result is not incompatible with the hypothesis that a desensitized receptor might be responsible for the "sudden off."

#### Wearing-Off Phenomenon

When patients have wearing-off, the clinical improvement from a dose of levodopa lasts only as long as the plasma concentration of levodopa is high (Muenter and Tyce, 1971). As the plasma level gradually falls, there is a loss of clinical response. In stable patients without clinical fluctuations, they maintain the long-duration response despite a fall in plasma levels of levodopa. Patients with wearing-off and on-off have

levodopa. Many patients who develop response fluctuations also develop abnormal involuntary movements (i.e., dyskinesias).

Levodopa-induced dyskinesias appear to be related to the degree of dopamine receptor supersensitivity. It is difficult to induce dyskinesias in normal animals or people, but with a high enough dose, this has been achieved in monkeys (Sassin et al., 1972; Pearce et al., 2001; Togasaki et al., 2001). With increasing denervation, resulting in increased receptor sensitivity, there is more likelihood of developing choreic dyskinesias at a lower dose of levodopa (Cedarbaum et al., 1991). Dystonic reactions (forceful sustained contractions) may evolve over time in patients who earlier had choreic dyskinesias. However, some patients develop peak-dose dystonia at relatively low dosages; these may be patients with multiple-system atrophy (Quinn, 1994a). In general, developing dyskin-

lost the long-duration response and have only a short-duration response. In the study by Fabbrini and colleagues (1987), discontinuation of steady intravenous infusion of levodopa was followed by a decay in the plasma concentration of levodopa, identical in all groups of patients, representing an unchanged pharmacokinetic profile. With the falling plasma concentration of levodopa, the stable patients maintain their clinical response with only a gradual decay in the response over time. However, the patients with wearing-off and "on-off" have a rapid loss of the anti-PD effect, more closely paralleling the falling plasma concentration (Fabbrini et al., 1987). If the plasma level can be maintained, the clinical response can also be maintained (Shoulson et al., 1975; Hardie et al., 1984; Mouradian et al., 1990). Providing a continuous supply of dopamine or dopamine agonist to the striatum, such as by intravenous (Nutt, 1987) or intestinal (Sage et al., 1989a, 1989b; Bredberg et al., 1993; Kurth et al., 1993b; Nyholm et al., 2005) infusion of levodopa or by subcutaneous infusion of dopamine agonist (Obeso et al., 1989b) can overcome this type of fluctuation. Thus, continuous benefit in the unstable patient (advanced PD) depends on a steady supply of levodopa in the plasma reaching the brain in a constant influx. This type of necessary bioavailability of plasma levodopa is not a factor with patients who have a smooth response to levodopa because such individuals have the same type of plasma half-life of levodopa as do those with fluctuations (Fabbrini et al., 1987). Some other factor(s) must be playing a role. It seems that central (such as small dopamine storage capacity and dopamine receptor alterations), as well as peripheral, pharmacokinetic and pharmacodynamic mechanisms are involved in the pathophysiology of these problems (Mouradian et al., 1988, 1989; Obeso et al., 1989a). The synaptic concentration of dopamine as a function of the timing of levodopa dosing was studied indirectly by evaluating D2 receptor ligand PET scans in patients who eventually developed wearing-off and those who remained stable, as nonfluctuators (de la Fuente-Fernandez et al., 2001). The former group showed higher synaptic dopamine 1 hour after a dose but lower concentrations 3 hours later than the latter group. This result suggests increased dopamine turnover—that is, decreased storage of dopamine.

### SMALL DOPAMINE-STORAGE CAPACITY
After 16 hours of infusion of levodopa intravenously and then suddenly discontinuing the infusion, patients with "on-off" and wearing-off, respectively, show the fastest return of parkinsonian symptoms, compared to those with a stable response to levodopa or those who have never been treated with levodopa (Fabbrini et al., 1987). The patients with dyskinesias have a faster decay of their dyskinesias than of their anti-PD benefit (Mouradian et al., 1989). The loss of the anti-PD effect as the plasma levodopa concentration falls in these studies strongly indicates either a small buffering capacity for levodopa storage or a short-duration receptor response in patients with fluctuations.

Supporting the concept of a small buffering capacity are studies performed in rats with different degrees of 6-hydroxy-dopamine lesions of the nigrostriatal pathway (Papa et al., 1994). The rats are then treated with twice daily injections of levodopa. Rats with over 95 percent loss of dopaminergic neurons evidenced a progressive shortening in the duration of levodopa's motor effects (equivalent to wearing-off) as well as a failure of nearly 8% of levodopa injections to elicit any response (equivalent to dose failures) after the first week of treatment. In contrast, response changes resembling those associated with wearing-off fluctuations in parkinsonian patients did not occur in the less severely lesioned rats. These results suggest that the extent of a dopamine neuron loss must exceed a relatively high threshold before intermittent levodopa treatment produces changes favoring the appearance of motor fluctuations.

Plasma concentrations of large neutral amino acids (LNAA), which compete with levodopa for transport into the brain, contribute to motor fluctuations, even when levodopa is being steadily infused (Nutt et al., 1997). These large neutral amino acids play an even bigger role when the daily dosage of levodopa is higher. On the other hand, severity of PD did not predict fluctuations during the infusions. In addition to this obvious peripheral pharmacokinetic mechanism, because fluctuations are more prominent in patients who have taken larger daily doses of levodopa, pharmacodynamic factors are also implicated.

If the wearing-off phenomenon is due, at least in part, to loss of storage sites of dopamine in the striatum, severity of parkinsonism, regardless of duration of parkinsonism, should be associated with the wearing-off effect. This would explain why fluctuations occurred early in the course of treatment in patients with MPTP-induced parkinsonism (Ballard et al., 1985); these patients had severe dopaminergic nigrostriatal pathway destruction. In contrast, those with PD develop the wearing-off problem as a function of duration of treatment (McDowell and Sweet, 1976), which could also be a reflection of duration of illness.

### LEVODOPA MAY CONTRIBUTE TO THE DEVELOPMENT OF FLUCTUATIONS
Dopamine storage capacity alone does not explain why younger patients are more prone to develop fluctuations than are older patients (Pederzoli et al., 1983). Nor would it explain why using low doses of levodopa instead of high doses would delay the development of this problem (Lesser et al., 1979; Poewe et al., 1986). Furthermore, treatment with direct-acting agonists does not eliminate the problem, although it does ameliorate it somewhat by making the depths of the "off" state less severe. These three observations would imply that levodopa itself or the peaks and valleys of supplying the brain with levodopa may also be responsible for contributing to this problem. Some investigators have found that the major risk factors for fluctuations appear to be duration (Horstink et al., 1990b; Roos et al., 1990) and dosage (Poewe et al., 1986; Fabbrini et al., 1988) of levodopa therapy.

The CALM-PD clinical trial, comparing levodopa and pramipexole, clearly showed that levodopa was statistically more likely than the dopamine agonist to induce fluctuations (and dyskinesias), after both 2 years (Parkinson Study Group, 2000) and 4 years of observation (Holloway and Parkinson Study Group, 2004). Whether the effect is inherent to levodopa, the potency of levodopa compared to the agonist, or the short duration of levodopa's half-life is uncertain. A further analysis of the CALM-PD data revealed that motor complications that occur within the first 4 years of treatment of PD do not have a significant negative effect on quality of life (Marras et al., 2004).

*Pharmacokinetic Mechanisms* Murata and Kanazawa (1993) repeatedly administered levodopa to intact rats and found that this treatment induced (1) acceleration of DOPA absorption at the gut and the blood-brain barrier, (2) reduction of dopamine retention in the striatum, and (3) loss of "supersensitive response" of dopamine receptors. These authors concluded that long-term levodopa treatment is the cause of the wearing-off effect. Murata and colleagues (1996) subsequently studied plasma pharmacokinetics in 55 parkinsonian patients. They showed that long-term levodopa therapy markedly increased the peak levodopa concentration ($C_{max}$) and the area under the time-concentration curve (AUC), whereas it decreased time to the peak concentration ($T_{max}$) and the elimination half-life ($T_{1/2}$). These results suggest that long-term levodopa therapy accelerates the absorption of levodopa. These changes were seen in patients who were stable as well as in those with the wearing-off effect, although the fluctuators had a higher $C_{max}$ and AUC and a shorter $T_{max}$ and $T_{1/2}$ than did the nonfluctuators. In a FDOPA PET study, Torstenson and colleagues (1997) showed that levodopa infusion during the scanning decreased FDOPA influx in mild PD but upregulated the influx in patients with advanced PD. These findings could help to explain the less graded clinical response to levodopa in advanced PD.

*Pharmacodynamic Mechanisms*   Direct alterations of dopamine receptors and storage sites by levodopa, dopamine, or their metabolites is another possibility. D2 receptors were studied by raclopride PET scanning in patients early in the course of treatment with levodopa and then 3 to 5 years later, when motor fluctuations had appeared (Antonini et al., 1997). Raclopride binding was elevated (supersensitive receptors) after 3 to 4 months of levodopa therapy and returned to normal (downregulated) after 3 to 5 years of treatment.

One indication that dopamine receptors play a role in the loss of the anti-PD benefit as the plasma concentration of levodopa falls is the dichotomy of the decay of dyskinesia and the return of the parkinsonism (Mouradian et al., 1989). The dyskinesia decays faster than does the loss of the anti-PD benefit. Dyskinesia half-time (time required to reduce severity score by 50%) was 25.3 minutes; the anti-PD half-time (time required to increase PD severity scores to 50% of their maximum) was 50.4 minutes. The shape of the two curves differs: The decay of dyskinesia is quadratic, and the return of PD severity is linear. This suggests that the dyskinesia effect and the anti-PD effect represent different dopamine receptors (e.g., D1 and D2 receptors, respectively).

Chase and colleagues (1993, 1998) suggest that intermittent (compared to continuous) administration of levodopa contributes to this problem. Chase proposes that there is an alteration of the striatal dopaminoceptive medium spiny neurons, with a potentiation of glutamate receptors (of the N-methyl-D-aspartate [NMDA] subtype) on these GABAergic striatal efferents, and that these cells are producing the motor complications. In 6-hydroxydopamine-lesioned rats, an animal model of PD, Chase found increased phosphorylation of striatal N-methyl-D-aspartate receptor subunits on serine and tyrosine residues. Along with this concept is the finding from his laboratory that an N-methyl-D-aspartate antagonist can reverse the shortened levodopa response time in these rats (Blanchet et al., 1997). Furthermore, the intrastriatal administration of selective inhibitors of certain serine and tyrosine kinases alleviates the motor complications (Chase et al., 2000). He believes that the same mechanism is responsible for both motor fluctuations and dyskinesias.

Although Chase incriminates intermittent administration of levodopa as the primary cause of motor complications,

another potential mechanism is that dopamine can lead to the formation of free radicals by autoxidation or by enzymatic oxidation, and these oxyradicals could be the culprits attacking dopamine receptors (Fahn and Cohen, 1992; Fahn, 1996).

Once established, motor complications are seemingly irreversible. Substituting dopamine agonists for levodopa therapy diminishes the severity of the complications but does not eliminate them. Dopamine receptors may have irreversible changes, much like the irreversible alteration that is seen with tardive syndromes after exposure to dopamine receptor–blocking agents (see Chapter 20). The healing process takes a long time without exposure to the offending agent before the process disappears, which often never happens.

## ALTERED DOPAMINE RECEPTORS

The dose-response curve to a bolus of levodopa injected intravenously was studied in patients with "on-off" and wearing-off, as well as those with a stable response to levodopa and those who had never been treated with levodopa (Mouradian et al., 1988). The antiparkinsonian response showed a linear dose-response curve in the latter two groups but an S-shaped curve for the first two groups. Thus, patients with fluctuations have a brittle response to levodopa. Because the peripheral pharmacokinetics were the same in all groups, this increased sensitivity to levodopa, despite identical antiparkinsonian threshold, strongly implies an alteration of the dopamine receptor, probably the D2 receptor, in patients with fluctuations.

Already mentioned was that the dichotomy of the decay rates for dyskinesia and anti-PD benefit when levodopa was withdrawn after a steady intravenous infusion suggested different dopamine receptors may be responsible for dyskinesias and for the anti-PD effect of levodopa (Mouradian et al., 1989). A more direct evaluation of dopamine receptors is done by using a dopaminergic agent that acts only at the postsynaptic dopamine receptors for its effect. After a steady-state optimal-dose infusion of apomorphine, a direct-acting dopamine agonist that is not dependent on storage of dopamine, the apomorphine was withdrawn, and the loss of the anti-PD effect was faster in patients who had fluctuations than in stable patients with a stable response (Bravi et al., 1994). Because apomorphine's effect is not dependent on presynaptic terminals, postsynaptic mechanisms must play a role in the loss of the long-duration response and hence the wearing-off effect.

Other studies supporting the notion that postsynaptic dopamine receptors play a role in wearing-off are those by Colosimo and colleagues (1996) and Metman and colleagues (1997a). These showed that duration of response to apomorphine is shorter in advanced, complicated parkinsonians compared to early, levodopa-naïve patients or stable patients. Also, the dose-response slope steepened, and the therapeutic window narrowed. The plasma levels of apomorphine were identical in the stable and fluctuating patients.

This conclusion was supported by another study comparing duration of response between the more and less affected sides in patients with PD to an infusion of levodopa and to subcutaneous apomorphine. Rodriguez and colleagues (1994) showed that the more affected side had a shorter response duration, increased latency, and greater response magnitude than did the less affected side. These differences were more pronounced in patients receiving chronic levodopa treatment than in untreated patients. As apomorphine is not dependent on dopamine storage capacity, these findings suggest that postsynaptic mechanisms play an important part in the origin of motor fluctuations in PD. Could these postsynaptic mechanisms develop because of inconstant and pulsating activation of receptors by dopamine related to levodopa therapy or possibly from dopamine-mediated oxyradicals or other toxins related to levodopa therapy?

### IMPLICATING THE INTERMITTENT ADMINISTRATION OF CHRONIC LEVODOPA THERAPY

Ten days of continuous, round-the-clock administration of levodopa intravenously producing a stable plasma concentration of levodopa gradually reduced fluctuations of response to levodopa in patients with the "on-off" or wearing-off effects (Mouradian et al., 1990). Because smoothing out the plasma (and brain) concentrations provided this benefit, the authors suggested that the chronic, routine method of intermittent oral treatment with levodopa may be underlying the development of motor fluctuations. Continuous intravenous treatment increased the threshold to levodopa for both the anti-PD and dyskinesia response (Table 6-7), with an increase in the therapeutic window by about 50% (computed as the difference between the dyskinesia threshold dose and the anti-PD threshold dose). The S-shape of the dose-response curve for the fluctuators remained, but with a shift of the curve to the right indicating the decreased sensitivity to levodopa. At the increased threshold dosage for dyskinesia, the anti-PD response increased 76% (despite the shift of the curve to the right) with no change in the severity of the dyskinesias. Once the continuous infusions were discontinued, the fluctuations returned. Nutt and colleagues (1993) believe that tolerance actually develops after continuous infusions; when the infusion is stopped, the duration of response is shorter after a long infusion than after a shorter one. It is well recognized that "on-off" problems, once developed, are difficult to eliminate.

A 5-year study of 618 dopa-naïve patients compared Sinemet CR and standard Sinemet therapy. There was no difference between the two groups in the development of either fluctuations or dyskinesias (Block et al., 1997; Koller et al., 1999). Whether this study adequately tested the intermittent versus continuous levodopa hypothesis for the cause of fluctuations is unlikely. But in terms of therapeutics, it showed no advantage for beginning with either preparation over the other.

### SUMMARY OF PATHOGENESIS OF FLUCTUATIONS

Chase (1998) and Metman and colleagues (2000) summarized their views on the mechanisms leading to the development of fluctuations from levodopa therapy. They believe that the fluctuations are related to altered dopaminergic mechanisms at both the presynaptic and postsynaptic levels. Wearing-off phenomena initially reflect the loss of dopamine storage capacity of the degenerating nigrostriatal system. Then, with increasing

degeneration of the nigrostriatal system, swings in plasma levodopa concentrations associated with standard dosage regimens produce nonphysiologic fluctuations in intrasynaptic dopamine. As a result of long-term discontinuous stimulation, secondary changes occur at sites downstream from the dopamine system and now appear to underlie the progressive worsening of wearing-off phenomena as well as the eventual appearance of other response complications. Chronic intermittent stimulation of normally tonically active dopaminergic receptors activates specific signaling cascades in striatal dopaminoceptive medium spiny neurons, and this evidently results in long-term potentiation of the synaptic efficacy of glutamate receptors of the N-methyl-D-aspartate subtype on these GABAergic efferents due to increased phosphorylation of the serine and tyrosine moieties in these receptors. As a consequence of their increasing sensitivity to excitation by cortical glutamatergic projections, it would, however, appear that medium spiny neuron function changes to favor the appearance of response fluctuations of the "on-off" type and peak-dose dyskinesias. The inability of standard levodopa treatment to restore striatal dopaminergic function in a more physiologic manner clearly contributes to the appearance of motor complications. Continuous dopaminergic replacement not only reverses these complications in parkinsonian patients but also prevents their development in animal models of PD.

Another explanation from both primate studies and postmortem human studies is that long-term levodopa therapy leads to glutamate receptor supersensitivity in the putamen, and this plays a role in the development of motor complications (both wearing-off and dyskinesias) following long-term levodopa therapy in PD (Calon et al., 2003).

### DYSKINESIAS

Another suggestion for a mechanism for the production of dopa-induced dyskinesias is based on postmortem chemical studies performed on primates, ranging from normal to parkinsonian to nondyskinetic dopa-treated to dyskinetic dopa-treated (Aubert et al., 2005). These investigators found that the sensitivity of the D1 receptor is linearly related to dyskinesias. This implies that dopa-induced dyskinesia results from increased dopamine D1 receptor–mediated transmission at the level of the direct pathway.

Risk factors for peak dose dyskinesias were retrospectively analyzed by using the Kaplan-Meier survival method in 100 consecutive patients treated with levodopa for 1 to 18 years. Blanchet and colleagues (1996) found that 56% of patients developed dyskinesia after a mean of 2.9 years. Dyskinetic patients were significantly younger at disease onset, but their mean latency to dyskinesia induction after levodopa initiation was not different from that of older dyskinetic individuals.

Table 6-7  Effect of continuous therapy with levodopa on its dose-response measures

| Measure | Pretreatment (mg/kg) | Posttreatment (mg/kg) | P Value |
| --- | --- | --- | --- |
| Antiparkinsonian threshold dose | 0.59 ± 0.07 | 0.9 ± 10.07 | < .0001 |
| Dyskinesia threshold dose | 0.66 ± 0.08 | 1.0 ± 0.09 | < .0001 |
| Therapeutic window | 0.061 ± 0.04 | 0.092 ± 0.04 | |

Data from Mouradian MM, Heuser IJE, Baronti F, Chase TN: Modification of central dopaminergic mechanisms by continuous levodopa therapy for advanced Parkinson's disease. Ann Neurol 1990;27:18–23.

Dyskinetic patients were on a higher daily levodopa dose than were nondyskinetic subjects when dyskinesia emerged, but the cumulative levodopa dose used prior to dyskinesia did not discriminate dyskinetic from nondyskinetic patients. A delay in initiating levodopa therapy of more than 3 years after disease onset and levodopa treatment initiation in Hoehn-Yahr stage II compared to stage I patients did not increase the probability of developing dyskinesia over time.

The levodopa dosage threshold for dyskinesia is much lower for patients with fluctuations than for patients with a stable response or for those who have never been treated before. This was determined by bolus injections of levodopa intravenously (Mouradian et al., 1989). Those who had never been treated and those with a stable response to levodopa had such a high threshold for dyskinesias that dyskinesias never appeared in some of these patients at the highest doses tested. After 16 hours of steady intravenous infusion of levodopa, followed by sudden discontinuation, the loss of dyskinesias is faster than the return of parkinsonism (Mouradian et al., 1989). These studies indicate that dyskinetic effects and antiparkinsonian effects may represent responses to different dopamine receptors. The investigators proposed that these are very likely the D1 and D2 receptors, respectively.

In a study looking at severity of PD after overnight drug withdrawal, Schuh and Bennett (1993) found that continuous intravenous levodopa shifted the dyskinesia dose-response curve to the right and reduced maximum dyskinesia activity but did not significantly alter dose response for relief of parkinsonism. These results support the hypothesis that relief of parkinsonism and production of dyskinesia by levodopa occur by separate mechanisms.

## Treatment of Motor Fluctuations Associated with Levodopa Therapy

When levodopa or other antiparkinson medication no longer provides a smooth, adequate, long-duration response, treatment requires skill; it becomes an art form utilizing approaches to control the various complications that have developed in a given patient. At this stage of treatment, the clinician is usually placed in a position analogous to that of a firefighter, being called on to "put out fires." Every time a new problem arises in a response-complicated patient, the clinician uses his or her skill to control the new developments arising from levodopa therapy. The following subsections describe various complications and the approaches that can be taken to control them.

### WEARING-OFF PHENOMENON IN THE ABSENCE OF DYSKINESIAS

There are many choices available to control wearing-off. When mild, it may be ameliorated with the addition of selegiline (Golbe et al., 1988) (introduced as 5 mg daily and increasing to 5 mg twice daily as necessary). Selegiline potentiates the action of levodopa, and its introduction can induce confusion and psychosis, particularly in the elderly, and dyskinesias. A lower dose of levodopa might be necessary. Rasagiline, another type B MAO inhibitor, also decreases the amount of daily off time, by about 1 hour per day (Parkinson Study Group, 2005), and, in a comparative study with entacapone, had the same degree of benefit (Rascol et al., 2005). Sinemet CR can also be effective in patients

with mild wearing-off (Bush et al., 1989; Hutton and Morris, 1992; Pahwa et al., 1993), and one can gradually switch from standard carbidopa/levodopa to Sinemet CR, beginning with the last dose of the day and working forward each day. Because it takes over an hour for slow-release medication to become effective, most patients will also require supplemental standard carbidopa/levodopa to obtain an adequate response. Because not all of Sinemet CR is absorbed before the tablet passes through the small intestine (absorption of carbidopa/levodopa is achieved only via the small intestine), the same dosages of Sinemet CR and standard Sinemet are not identical. Only about two thirds to three quarters of Sinemet CR is absorbed. Therefore, to achieve the equivalent of 100 mg of levodopa in standard Sinemet, a patient would require between 130 and 150 mg of levodopa in Sinemet CR.

COMT inhibitors have an advantage because if effective, they are effective immediately. They increase the amount of "on" time by about an hour per day (Kieburtz et al., 1997a; Adler et al., 1998; Rinne, Larsen, et al., 1998b). Entacapone has a shorter duration of action than tolcapone does, and its 200-mg tablet needs to be given simultaneously with carbidopa/levodopa, working with that dose only. Thus, if only one or two doses of levodopa result in wearing-off, then entacapone can be given just with those doses. Entacapone does not require any precautions for assessing liver function, whereas tolcapone does. Tolcapone can produce fulminant hepatitis; this is rare but has caused death (Assal et al., 1998; Watkins, 2000). Therefore, patients should not be given tolcapone unless the clinical fluctuations are a great problem and other medications have failed to relieve the clinical fluctuations. Patients need a baseline liver transaminase profile, which should be followed biweekly. Discontinuing tolcapone if a rise in transaminase activity is seen should be sufficient to reverse the hepatic change. Patients should also be warned that diarrhea, including explosive diarrhea, could develop in 6 to 8 weeks on tolcapone. Entacapone causes less of a problem with diarrhea, but it turns the urine a yellow-orange. Tolcapone comes in 100- and 200-mg tablets. Start with 100 mg once daily and increase it fairly rapidly to three times daily dosing. If it is not effective, switch to the 200-mg tablets. Although entacapone can reduce the amount of "off" time, it does not appear to improve quality of life (Reichmann et al., 2005).

With any of these additions to the treatment regimen, if dyskinesias develop, the dosage of carbidopa/levodopa needs to be reduced.

Another approach is to utilize standard carbidopa/levodopa alone, giving the doses closer together. But ultimately, most patients will develop progressively shorter durations of effectiveness from these doses, so patients could require as many as six or more doses per day. Then, eventually, dose failures often develop. Investigation of this problem of shorter response time with smaller, more frequent doses of levodopa has shown that response time continues to increase when suprathreshold doses of levodopa are given, although increased dyskinesias also are seen (Metman et al., 1997b).

Direct-acting dopamine agonists, which have a longer biologic half-life than does levodopa, can also be used in combination with standard Sinemet or Sinemet CR (Parkinson Study Group, 1997). As a general rule, dopamine agonists are useful to improve the severity of the "off" state but can also reduce the amount of "off" time per day. Pergolide, pramipexole, and ropinirole are more effective than bromocriptine and are preferred. These drugs in combination with levodopa can increase dyskinesias while reducing the depths of the "offs." In this situation, the levodopa dosage would need to be reduced. Because of its long half-life, cabergoline can be effective even with once-a-day dosage (Geminiani et al., 1996; Inzelberg et al., 1996).

Utilizing dopamine agonists and delaying the introduction of levodopa can delay the start of the wearing-off effect and reduce the risk of developing it (Montastruc et al., 1994; Przuntek et al., 1996; Rinne, Bracco, et al., 1998a; Parkinson Study Group, 2000; Rascol et al., 2000; Oertel et al., 2006).

Patients with a deep "off" would benefit from a rescue dose of anti-PD medication. Dissolving levodopa in carbonated water and drinking it usually provides a response in about 10 to 15 minutes. Subcutaneous injections or intranasal sprays of apomorphine provide a similar response (Dewey et al., 1998). Etilevodopa, a dispersable form of levodopa ethylester, was expected to improve these types of delayed "off" responses, but a study by the Parkinson Study Group (Blindauer et al., 2006) of 327 patients with PD who were taking levodopa and had a latency of ≥90 minutes each day before the onset of drug benefit (measured as time to "on") showed that the mean improvements were similar in the etilevodopa-carbidopa and levodopa-carbidopa groups (reductions of 0.58 and 0.79 hours, respectively).

### SUDDEN "OFFS"

The "sudden off" phenomenon is a more difficult problem to overcome. It is now clear that direct-acting dopamine agonists, slow-release levodopa, amantadine, and selegiline are ineffective. Subcutaneous injections of the dopamine agonist apomorphine are effective in turning the patient back "on" quickly (Hughes et al., 1993), as is an oral administration of dissolved Sinemet. To block nausea and vomiting by apomorphine, the peripheral dopamine receptor antagonist domperidone or trimethobenzamide needs to be taken in addition. Increasingly severe on-phase dyskinesias and postural instability mar the long-term therapeutic response of apomorphine in many patients.

Our approach is to attempt to utilize dopamine agonists as the major therapeutic agents and reduce the amount of levodopa as much as possible. If even a small amount of Sinemet added to the dopamine agonist causes too much dyskinesia, one should try to substitute plain levodopa without any carbidopa in place of Sinemet. We have not been able to eliminate sudden offs if levodopa is the major therapeutic agent.

### RANDOM "OFFS"

Often, a sudden "off" appears unrelated to the timing of the last dose of levodopa, leading to the name *random "off."* With careful plotting of these "off" periods, a pattern can often be seen, so these random "offs" might not be so random. These random "offs" are usually sudden in onset. The treatment strategy is the same as for sudden "offs."

### DOSE FAILURES (EPISODIC FAILURE TO RESPOND TO EACH DOSE) (NO "ON")

Failure of the patient to respond to each dose of levodopa is related to poor gastric emptying (Rivera-Calimlin et al., 1970; Fahn, 1977). A radionuclide gastric-emptying study showed that PD patients had prolonged gastric emptying compared with the normal control subjects and that this was increased in fluctuating patients with dose failures compared to non-fluctuators (Djaldetti et al., 1996). The problem of dose failures can be overcome by dissolving levodopa in liquid before ingesting it. For this situation, individual doses of Sinemet can be liquefied at the time it is needed. It dissolves readily in carbonated water because of the acidity of the water and the formation of bubbles that toss the Sinemet tablet around, quickly dissolving it. When a dose failure occurs, the patient can take dissolved Sinemet and will usually respond in 10 to 15 minutes. Another approach is to use apomorphine injections (Ostergaard et al., 1995).

Response failures are probably more common than is usually recognized. In a survey of his patients, Melamed and colleagues (1986) found a number of patients with this difficulty. It is not clear whether the delayed gastric emptying is due to levodopa therapy itself or whether the disorder develops because frequent dosing will statistically result in some tablets not passing through the stomach quickly enough to reach the small intestine, where absorption takes place.

### DELAYED "ON"

Melamed and colleagues (1986) reported that patients with fluctuations often also have a problem is getting an "on" with the first dose in the morning. These patients tend to have a longer delay with this dose than do nonfluctuators. The mechanism is not clear, but it might have to do with obtaining adequate plasma levels. Many patients seem to need a larger dosage of levodopa as their first dose of the day to "kick in" a response to the medication. Since the first dose is often accompanied by a higher plasma level of levodopa than later doses (Shoulson et al., 1975; Fahn, 1982), the problem might not be entirely pharmacokinetic. Rather, it is possible that the dopamine receptors are in a low-affinity state and require more dopamine agonism to activate them. To treat the delayed "on" by obtaining a higher plasma level of levodopa sooner, the patient should dissolve Sinemet before swallowing.

### WEAK RESPONSE AT END OF DAY

Most patients eventually show some diurnal variation in their responsiveness to levodopa. Often, the patient reports that she or he does best after the first morning dose, and the response is less as the day wears on. An occasional patient will report the opposite: doing better at the end of the day. The mechanism for the poorer response at the end of the day might relate to decreased plasma levels of levodopa with each subsequent dose. But increasing the dose in the afternoons usually does not help. The patient might not get any improved response and could develop drowsiness or adverse mental effects instead. Nevertheless, one should try increasing the dosage of afternoon and evening levodopa. If this fails, it is worth adding slow-release levodopa, supplemental dopamine agonist, anticholinergics, or amantadine.

### RESPONSE VARIES IN RELATION TO MEALS

Levodopa is absorbed only from the small intestine; absorption is thus dependent on passage of levodopa through the stomach to enter the small intestine. There are at least three variations of levodopa responsiveness in regard to meals. First, a full meal with delayed gastric emptying will result in a delayed and weaker response to levodopa that is ingested after or during the meal compared to taking levodopa about 20 minutes before the meal. Pharmacokinetic studies confirm that levodopa concentrations in plasma are delayed when the medication is taken in the fed state (Contin et al., 1998b). Second, patients who had normally taken levodopa with or after a meal will find that if they now take it before a meal, the response is much greater, and they might develop peak-dose dyskinesia. If either of these two variations is present, it can be corrected by accommodating the timing of dosages of levodopa according to the pathophysiology of the particular problem.

A third variation relates to high-protein meals. Competition with other amino acids in the diet can interfere with transport of levodopa across the intestinal mucosa and across the blood-brain barrier (Muenter et al., 1972; Nutt et al., 1984). Only rarely does this competition with other amino acids pose a serious problem for patients. Most accommodate to protein in their diet. In those rare individuals in whom any protein in any meal interferes with their response to levodopa, it is necessary to plan a meal strategy. Having nonprotein meals at breakfast and lunch and making up for this lack by having higher-protein meals at dinner will usually be effective. If the patient goes "off" at night when he or she can best afford to be "off," the patient can adjust to this situation.

### FREEZING

The freezing phenomenon (Fahn, 1995) is often listed as a type of fluctuation because the patient transiently has difficulty initiating movement. But this phenomenon probably should be considered distinct from the other types of fluctuations. Freezing takes many forms, and these have different names, such as start hesitation, target hesitation, turning hesitation, startle (fearfulness) hesitation, and sudden transient freezing. However, it is not clear whether any of these types has a different pathophysiologic mechanism. Of major importance is the need to distinguish between off freezing and on freezing. Off freezing is best explained as a feature of PD, and its treatment is to keep the patient from going "off." On freezing remains an enigma, and this problem tends to be aggravated by increasing the dosage of levodopa. It is not benefited by adding direct-acting dopamine agonists. Rather, it is lessened by reducing the dosage of levodopa. Both the "on" and "off" types of freezing appear to correlate with duration of illness and duration of levodopa therapy (Giladi et al., 1992). Although Narabayashi and colleagues (1986) reported benefit with L-threo-dops, supposedly a precursor of brain norepinephrine, Fahn (unpublished data) has not seen any benefit with this drug in the treatment of "on freezing." Moreover, he found no evidence that this drug increases norepinephrine in rat brain or human cerebrospinal fluid. Giladi and colleagues report some benefit with botulinum toxin injections into the legs of freezers (Giladi et al., 2001a), but the results have not been impressive on the basis of personal observations.

Interestingly, in the intravenous infusions of levodopa performed by Shoulson and colleagues (1975), a sudden stimulus, such as tilting the patient upright on a tilt table, resulted in sudden transient worsening of parkinsonism. This can be interpreted to indicate the induction of sudden transient freezing. It might be a useful model for future studies.

## Treatment of Dyskinesias Associated with Levodopa Therapy

### PEAK-DOSE DYSKINESIAS

Choreic movements can occur early in the treatment with levodopa, but the incidence of these involuntary movements increases with continuing treatment (Duvoisin, 1974a). However, the major risk factor for peak-dose dyskinesia has been considered to be severity of the disease (Horstink et al., 1990a). Chorea is more common than dystonia as the type of peak-dose dyskinesia, particularly in the early stages of levodopa therapy, but with continuing treatment, individual patients can develop more dystonia and less chorea (Fahn, 2000). Many patients probably end up having a combination of chorea and dystonia. Dystonia is a more serious problem than chorea because dystonia is usually more disabling. In fact, mild chorea is not noticed as much by the patient as by the family.

Peak-dose dyskinesia is due to too high a dose of levodopa and is representative of an overdosed state. The plasma levels of levodopa are high (Muenter et al., 1977), and there is presumably excess striatal dopamine. Reducing the individual dose can resolve this problem. The patient might need to take more frequent doses at this lower amount because reducing the amount of an individual dose also reduces the duration of benefit (Nutt et al., 1985). It was once believed that chorea appears only in the presence of supersensitive dopamine receptors, but if the dosage of levodopa were high enough, chorea could occur in normal individuals, as has been demonstrated in normal monkeys (Sassin et al., 1972).

Another method to reduce peak dose dyskinesia is to substitute higher doses of a dopamine agonist while lowering the dose of Sinemet. Dopamine agonists are less likely to cause dyskinesias and therefore can usually be used in this situation quite safely. If lowering the dose of Sinemet results in more severe "off" states, then the agonists become more important and need to be increased. Sinemet CR can help some patients by keeping the peak plasma levels of levodopa at a lower level. However, there is also the danger of increased dyskinesias at the end of the day as the blood levels become sustained from frequent dosing. Once dyskinesias appear with Sinemet CR, they last for a considerable duration of time because of the slow decay in the plasma.

In some patients, peak-dose chorea and dystonia occur at subtherapeutic doses of Sinemet, and lowering the dosage will render a patient even more parkinsonian. There is little choice but to use smaller and more frequent doses, coupled with dopamine agonists and other antiparkinsonian drugs, such as amantadine. Amantadine has been found to be a useful antidyskinetic agent (Rajput et al., 1997; Metman, Del Dotto, van den Munckhof, et al., 1998, Metman et al., 1999; Luginger et al., 2000; Snow et al., 2000), aside from its dopaminergic effect. Its antidyskinetic effect is dose dependent, and patients often require at least 400 mg per day. Start with 100 mg twice daily and increase stepwise to 200 mg twice daily as needed. Amantadine's benefit might stem from its additional action as a glutamate antagonist. Other antiglutamatergic agents that have been reported to reduce levodopa-induced dyskinesias are dextromethorphan (Metman, Del Dotto, Natte, et al., 1998), dextrorphan (Metman, Del Dotto, Blanchet, et al., 1998), and riluzole (Merims et al., 1999).

A possible approach is to use clozapine, the atypical neuroleptic that does not aggravate parkinsonism. It is increasingly being utilized as an antipsychotic in patients with dopa-induced psychosis. Clozapine can suppress dopa-induced dyskinesias while simultaneously increasing "on" time without dyskinesias (Bennett et al., 1993, 1994; Durif et al., 1997; Pierelli et al., 1998; Durif et al., 2004). Adverse effects consist of sedation, sialorrhea, and orthostatic hypotension. Clozapine also can reduce dyskinesias from apomorphine (Durif et al., 1997). Olanzapine has greater dopamine D2 receptor antagonism and usually worsens parkinsonism.

Increasing serotonin activity in the substantia nigra could induce or worsen parkinsonism, as is sometimes seen with fluoxetine treatment. A trial of fluoxetine, a selective serotonin uptake inhibitor, was shown to reduce dyskinesias induced by apomorphine treatment (Durif et al., 1995), suggesting that it be considered for levodopa-induced dyskinesias. The serotonin agonist sarizotan was developed for its possible use (Bara-Jimenez et al., 2005) as an antidyskinesia agent, but a Phase III trial was unsuccessful. Propranolol is another drug that has been reported to reduce dyskinesias (Carpentier et al., 1996). Buspirone appears to be somewhat effective in reducing the severity of dyskinesias (Bonifati et al., 1994), but because buspirone has resulted in aggravating tardive dyskinesia (LeWitt et al., 1993), it might have some dopamine receptor–blocking activity. Mirtazapine is an antidepressant with a novel pharmacologic profile (alpha-2 antagonist, $5\text{-HT}_{1A}$ agonist, and $5\text{-HT}_2$ antagonist). It was tested in a small open-label trial and found to have a modest effect in reducing dopa-induced dyskinesias (Meco et al., 2004). Although opioid antagonists have been found to reduce dopa-induced dyskinesias in parkinsonian monkeys (Henry et al., 2001), high-dose naltrexone was not effective in humans (Manson et al., 2001). Other medications such as cannabis (Carroll et al., 2004), low-dose quetiapine (Katzenschlager et al., 2004), and gabapentin (van Blercom et al., 2004) were not found to be effective.

### DIPHASIC DYSKINESIAS

Diphasic dyskinesias were first described by Muenter and colleagues (Muenter et al., 1977), who labeled them the *D-I-D phenomenon*, for "dystonia-improvement-dystonia." Although most of the affected individuals have dystonia as their pattern of dyskinesia, some have choreic movements, and others have a mixture of the two types. Diphasic dyskinesia is a situation in which the dyskinesia develops as the plasma levels of levodopa are rising or falling but not during the peak plasma level (Muenter et al., 1977; Lhermitte et al., 1978; Agid et al., 1979). Clinically, the involuntary movements predominantly involve the legs (Marsden et al., 1982; Luquin et al., 1992).

This phenomenon is difficult to explain. It is possible that there is a differential sensitivity of at least two dopamine receptors. The more sensitive one would respond to lower levels of levodopa to induce the dyskinetic state. The other receptor would be activated at higher levels and inhibit the dyskinesia. Treatment of the problem is difficult. Although Lhermitte and colleagues (1978) proposed treating this condition with higher doses of levodopa, Fahn's experience (unpublished data) is that higher dosages merely induce peak-dose dyskinesia and possibly other forms of central adverse effects. On the other hand, lowering the dosage is equally unsatisfactory because increasing parkinsonism ensues. The most effective approach is to utilize a dopamine agonist, with its longer duration of action, as the major therapeutic agent and levodopa as the supplementary drug.

### "OFF" DYSTONIA AND "OFF" PAINFUL CRAMPS

Dystonic spasms are not always a sign of levodopa overdosage. This is particularly true in many instances of painful sustained contractions. Painful dystonic cramps most often occur when the plasma level of levodopa is low, particularly in the early morning (Melamed, 1979). A survey of 383 patients with PD revealed that 16% had experienced early morning dystonia (Currie et al., 1998). But this type of dystonia can occur at any time the patient goes "off" (Ilson et al., 1984), and early-morning dystonia is a form of "off" dystonia, albeit the most common form. In this sense, "off" dystonia is a pharmacokinetic problem, and it has been correlated with low plasma levels of levodopa after an intravenous infusion was discontinued (Bravi et al., 1993). But why painful dystonic spasms should occur in addition to or instead of classic parkinsonian signs during low plasma levels of levodopa is not clear. This phenomenon might relate to some peculiarity of the dopamine receptors as well as the low plasma levels of levodopa in these patients. de Yebenes (1988) has proposed that dystonia may occur when the ratio of norepinephrine/dopamine is high. However, there are only speculations about the pathophysiology of dystonia in general, and it is difficult to be certain of the explanation of either peak-dose dystonia or of "off" dystonia such as early-morning dystonia. Preventing "offs" is the best way to control "off" dystonia. The use of pergolide is often effective when it is the major dopaminergic agent. Sinemet CR appears to be helpful for a number of patients with early-morning dystonia (Pahwa et al., 1993).

One should not forget that dystonia can also occur as a feature of PD. However, "off" dystonia does not appear to be merely a reflection of the dystonia of parkinsonism. If patients with "off" dystonia are given a drug holiday from levodopa, the painful dystonia will disappear after a few days, and the patient will be left with a baseline parkinsonian state and without painful dystonia (unpublished observations).

### COMBINATION OF FLUCTUATIONS AND DYSKINESIAS: YO-YO-ING

Many patients with advanced PD have both clinical fluctuations ("wearing-off" or "on-off") and dyskinesias (usually peak-dose and sometimes end-of-dose). Most patients are more troubled by the "off" states, in which they are fully or partially immobile, than they are by dyskinesias. In other words, they prefer having the dyskinesias rather than being unable to move freely. As a result of their discomfort with the "off" states, patients tend to overdose themselves, resulting in the alternating "offs" and dyskinesias. An extreme form of this combination is yo-yo-ing. The term comes from the repetitive ups and downs of a yo-yo and refers to a condition in which there is little time during the day of an optimally good "on" in which the patient has neither dyskinesia nor "offs." Moreover, in yo-yo-ing, the patient usually responds to a dose of levodopa almost immediately with a peak-dose dyskinesia, followed by a predictable wearing-off, with little optimum time in between these two states (Fahn, 1982).

Sudden "offs" and dose failures can further complicate the clinical situation of patients with advanced PD who have combinations of "offs" and dyskinesias (whether with good periods in between or as a yo-yo). Overcoming these highly variable clinical periods is challenging. It is a matter of attempting to smoothly activate the striatal dopamine receptors throughout the entire day. The dopamine receptors are obviously intact, but they are supersensitive to allow the dyskinesias. Hence, there appears to be a pharmacodynamic factor to account for the dyskinesias. At the same time, the short plasma half-life and the need for constant bioavailability of levodopa in the plasma account for the "off" states. Hence, the "offs" are the result of a pharmacokinetic factor. Thus, this condition should be considered a combined pharmacokinetic and pharmacodynamic problem. Treatment is virtually impossible with tablets of standard Sinemet and is even worse with Sinemet CR. The CR form has an unreliable pharmacokinetic profile. For patients who have both "offs" and dyskinesias, Sinemet CR tends to increase and prolong the dyskinesias; in some patients, the dyskinesias may be so severe that the patients have to be put to sleep to "ride them out."

Using medications with a longer biologic half-life than levodopa is a preferred method to smooth out the clinical fluctuating state. There has been partial success using direct-acting dopamine agonists as the sole or dominant form of pharmacotherapy, with carbidopa/levodopa used sparingly. In some patients, particularly those with yo-yo-ing, plain levodopa (without carbidopa) may be the preferred supplement instead of carbidopa/levodopa. The presence of carbidopa augments the potency of levodopa, so it is difficult to titrate patients for smaller dose responses in the presence of carbidopa.

Another, though more cumbersome, approach to smoothly activate the dopamine receptors without severe extremes of peaks and valleys is to place the patient on sips of small doses of liquefied Sinemet throughout the day (Metman et al., 1994). Liquefied Sinemet is not stable at room temperature unless in an acidified solution. In the absence of ascorbic acid, the concentration of levodopa in water declines significantly by 48 hours (Pappert et al., 1996a). Ascorbate prolongs stability to 72 hours. Refrigeration and freezing prevent a significant decline in concentration for the full 7 days. In place of ascorbic acid, carbonated water can be used, which is easier for many patients.

To prepare liquefied Sinemet, a simple method is to dissolve 4 tablets of 25/250-mg-strength tablets in a liter of acidified solution (dietetic soda, seltzer or other carbonated water, or ascorbic acid solution), providing a concentration of 1 mg levodopa per milliliter. Prepare it fresh daily and store the liquid in a dark environment to prevent oxidation of levodopa. It can be placed in the refrigerator. Then measure out the number of milliliters needed for a dose, which is equivalent to the milligrams of the dose. Liquefied Sinemet has been found to improve the amount of "on" time (Kurth et al., 1993a; Pappert et al., 1996b). In one double-blind trial comparing the liquid formulation versus standard tablets, no significant advantage of the liquid formulation over tablet therapy was found (Metman et al., 1994), but in another double-blind trial, there was an advantage of the liquid preparation and without increasing dyskinesias (Pappert et al., 1996b). The liquid formulation can more quickly resolve "off" states and facilitate small dose adjustments that are not possible with tablets. It seems particularly valuable for patients who have both fluctuations and dyskinesias.

A more heroic approach is to utilize the infusion of levodopa via an intraduodenal pump (Sage et al., 1989a, 1989b; Bredberg et al., 1993; Kurth et al., 1993b; Nilsson et al., 1998; Nyholm et al., 2005) or subcutaneous infusions of apomorphine (Colzi et al., 1998).

## MYOCLONUS

The lightning-like jerks of myoclonus can occur in untreated PD, but these are rarely disabling and are hardly commented on by patients. Klawans and colleagues (1975) described myoclonus as occurring as a complication of long-term levodopa therapy. They reported the movements as occurring as single unilateral or bilateral jerks in the extremities, most frequently during sleep. They found the serotonin antagonist methysergide helpful in controlling these. Such nocturnal myoclonus is infrequently encountered and is rarely disabling. Myoclonus occurs during the day as well. Its presence is usually ominous, indicating the presence of cognitive complications from levodopa, and often representing either toxicity to levodopa in PD or some other form of parkinsonism, such as diffuse Lewy body disease (Crystal et al., 1990).

## Other Motor Complications

### SIMULTANEOUS SOMATOTOPICALLY SPECIFIC DYSKINESIAS AND PARKINSONISM

Many patients have different responses to levodopa therapy in different parts of the body. For example, the head and neck regions might be more sensitive to levodopa than the legs. When the upper part of the body responds in this situation, the legs might remain parkinsonian, and the patient might not be able to walk well. In this example, on higher dosages of levodopa, the legs improve, but now the head and neck regions are dyskinetic. This problem might be due to different sensitivities of the striatal dopamine receptors on a somatotopic basis. That is, in the case described, the head and neck areas of the striatum would have more sensitive receptors than the leg area has. This problem is difficult to treat, and one can only titrate the dosage to the optimum response between the two extremes for each individual patient.

### LOSS OF EFFICACY OVER TIME

A debated point in the treatment of parkinsonism is the cause of declining efficacy from continuing treatment with levodopa in many patients (Yahr, 1976). If the postsynaptic dopamine receptors in the striatum are not lost in this disease, why should a patient get less response from medication over time? Progression of the illness with further loss of dopamine storage sites in the presynaptic terminals is the most invoked explanation. However, loss of these structures does not automatically produce a loss of response to levodopa. For example, postencephalitic parkinsonism, with its much greater loss of dopamine in the striatum (Ehringer and Hornykiewicz, 1960; Bernheimer et al., 1973), has more, not less, sensitivity to levodopa (Calne et al., 1969; Duvoisin et al., 1972). This observation is sufficient to argue against the concept that reduction in storage sites for dopamine is responsible for the declining efficacy of levodopa. Perhaps increasing PD is associated with loss of striatal dopamine receptors as well as the presynaptic dopaminergic neuron.

Even so, there may be additional factors contributing in part to the loss of efficacy that is seen with continuous treatment with levodopa. Some decline may arise in part from gradual downregulation of striatal dopamine receptors (Rinne et al., 1980). Not all patients develop this problem, but it appears to be due to the receptors being constantly exposed to high levels of dopamine. Evidence to support this concept comes from the studies of drug holidays from levodopa. After levodopa is eliminated for a short period, restoration of levodopa therapy usually provides enhanced temporary benefit (Direnfeld et al., 1980; Weiner et al., 1980). Unfortunately this enhanced sensitivity is short-lived, and the potential risks of aspiration during the drug holiday render this approach undesirable for the short-term benefit that can be obtained.

It is important to differentiate between loss of response despite a seemingly adequate dosage of medications and insufficient response due to too low a dose because of inability to tolerate adequate dosages. Secondary loss of response implies (1) a parkinsonism-plus syndrome instead of PD, (2) the development of nondopaminergic motor symptoms (flexed posture, freezing, loss of postural reflexes), (3) development of intractable bradykinesia with disease progression that had previously responded to treatment, or (4) end-stage PD. Treatment of end-stage PD requires adjusting the dosages of all medications both up and down to find the optimum level for each.

### INCREASED PARKINSONISM

A few patients on high-dosage levodopa may become more parkinsonian. This was initially reported unaccompanied by any other features of levodopa toxicity (Fahn and Barrett, 1979). This phenomenon has also been seen accompanied by confusion (Sage and Duvoisin, 1986). In both situations, improvement occurs when the dosage of levodopa is reduced. In fact, the phenomenon of increased parkinsonism without other signs of toxicity probably occurs more often than is recognized. Many physicians, unaware of this complication, are inclined to increase the dosage of antiparkinsonian medication, which does not help. Rather, a reduction of dosage should be tried first to see whether symptoms improve. This problem would appear to be related to reduced receptor sensitivity by high dosages of dopamine present in the striatum.

### INCREASED TACHYPHEMIA AND INCREASED RUNNING GAIT

A number of patients who are overdosed with levodopa will speak faster, running syllables together, so that it is difficult for the listener to understand what the patient is saying. At the same time as the speech is rapid (tachyphemia), the amplitude is lower, so the voice is softer, aggravating the situation. If the patient purposely tries to enunciate each syllable distinctly, he or she is able to do so for a few words, but then the tachyphemia takes over again. With speech therapy, sometimes using a metronome for pacing, a patient can improve the pattern of speaking, but only during the treatment session. There seems to be little carryover. Associated with tachyphemia are rapid voluntary movements in other parts of the body, displayed as such when the patient is asked to perform rapid successive movements. These are usually very fast and of small amplitude—that is, tachykinetic and hypokinetic.

This type of tachykinetic problem can also involve walking. Usually, the patient moves more rapidly but with smaller steps. Gait in this instance can be mistaken for festination, which it resembles. If postural instability is impaired, such a running gait can lead to falling. Often, lowering the dosage of levodopa will allow the patient to slow down, with a resulting clarity of speech and gait. However, parkinsonian bradykinesia can become more of a problem.

### FALLING DUE TO LOSS OF POSTURAL REFLEXES

Falling is a common feature of PD as the illness progresses and there is increasing loss of postural reflexes. Since this particular cardinal sign of PD is little benefited by levodopa therapy (Klawans, 1986), this problem persists and worsens despite pharmacotherapy (Agid et al., 1990). Because levodopa may allow the patient to be more mobile, such as allowing the patient to arise more easily from a chair and walk independently, the persistence of postural instability becomes a particular problem because it raises the hazard of increased likelihood of falling. Thus, this complication of levodopa therapy in this particular subpopulation of patients with PD is technically not a true adverse effect of the medication but a complication of the improvement in mobility in a patient who is at risk for falling, thereby increasing that risk. In this situation, the patient should use physical assistance, such as a walker. An alternative approach is to keep the patient sufficiently parkinsonian that he or she cannot arise without assistance.

### INTRACTABLE TREMOR

Persistent tremor—that is, rest tremor that has been resistant to antiparkinsonian medication—sometimes responds to clozapine (Friedman and Lannon, 1990; Jansen, 1994). If it is unresponsive to any medications, deep brain stimulation of the subthalamic nucleus should be considered.

## Treatment of Parkinson Disease during Surgery or Prolonged Conditions of Oral Unavailability

Levodopa is absorbed via the small intestine. During periods when the patient is unable to swallow or be allowed oral intake, such as during surgery, a method is needed to keep the patient's parkinsonism from being too severe. Most surgical procedures require only a short period of time for the patient to be without oral liquids or foods, and most patients can suspend taking their medications when liquids are not allowed for these periods without major difficulty. During anesthesia, parkinsonism is not a problem, so even a prolonged operation will not present a problem. It is postoperatively, if the patient is not allowed oral liquids, such as from gastric surgery, that a problem could arise. The resulting rigidity, akinesia, decreased gastrointestinal motility, and respiratory function are dangerous and could complicate the recovery process. In this situation, the three approaches are the provision of Parcopa to dissolve in the mouth, subcutaneous infusions of apomorphine with rectal domperidone (Galvez-Jimenez and Lang, 1996), and enteral administration of levodopa (Furuya et al., 1998).

## References

Aaltonen H, Kilkku O, Heinonen E, MakiIkola O: Effect of adding selegiline to levodopa in early, mild Parkinson's disease: Evidence is insufficient to show that combined treatment increases mortality. BMJ 1998;317:1586–1587.

Acuff RV, Thedford SS, Hidiroglou NN, et al: Relative bioavailability of RRR- and all-rac-alpha-tocopherol acetate in humans: Studies using deuterated compounds. Am J Clin Nutr 1994;60:397–402.

Adler CH, Singer C, O'Brien C, et al: Randomized, placebo-controlled study of tolcapone in patients with fluctuating Parkinson disease treated with levodopa-carbidopa. Arch Neurol 1998;55: 1089–1095.

Agarwal P, Fahn S, Frucht SJ: Diagnosis and management of pergolide-induced fibrosis. Mov Disord 2004;19(6):699–704.

Agid Y: Levodopa: Is toxicity a myth? Neurology 1998;50:858–863.

Agid Y, Ahlskog E, Albanese A, et al: Levodopa in the treatment of Parkinson's disease: A consensus meeting. Mov Disord 1999;14: 911–913.

Agid Y, Bonnet AM, Signoret JL, Lhermitte F: Clinical, pharmacological, and biochemical approach of "onset- and end-of-dose" dyskinesias. Adv Neurol 1979;24:401–410.

Agid Y, Graybiel AM, Ruberg M, et al: The efficacy of levodopa treatment declines in the course of Parkinson's disease: Do nondopaminergic lesions play a role? Adv Neurol 1990;53:83–100.

Ahlskog JE, Wright KF, Muenter MD, Adler CH: Adjunctive cabergoline therapy of Parkinson's disease: Comparison with placebo and assessment of dose responses and duration of effect. Clin Neuropharmacol 1996;19:202–212.

Alam ZI, Jenner A, Daniel SE, Lees AJ, et al: Oxidative DNA damage in the parkinsonian brain: An apparent selective increase in 8–hydroxyguanine levels in substantia nigra. J Neurochem 1997; 69:1196–1203.

Antonini A, Schwarz J, Oertel WH, et al: Long-term changes of striatal dopamine D-2 receptors in patients with Parkinson's disease: A study with positron emission tomography and [C-11]Raclopride. Mov Disord 1997;12:33–38.

Assal F, Spahr L, Hadengue A, et al: Tolcapone and fulminant hepatitis. Lancet 1998;352:958.

Aubert I, Guigoni C, Hakansson K, et al: Increased D-1 dopamine receptor signaling in levodopa-induced dyskinesia. Ann Neurol 2005;57(1):17–26.

Ballard PA, Tetrud JW, Langston JW: Permanent human parkinsonism due to 1-methyl-4-phenyl-1,2,3,6-tetrahydropyridine (MPTP): seven cases. Neurology 1985;35:949–956.

Bara-Jimenez W, Bibbiani F, Morris MJ, et al: Effects of serotonin 5-HT1A agonist in advanced Parkinson's disease. Mov Disord 2005;20(8):932–936.

Bara-Jimenez W, Sherzai A, Dimitrova T, et al: Adenosine A(2A) receptor antagonist treatment of Parkinson's disease. Neurology 2003;61(3):293–296.

Barbato L, Stocchi F, Monge A, et al: The long-duration action of levodopa may be due to a postsynaptic effect. Clin Neuropharmacol 1997;20:394–401.

Barneoud P, Mazadier M, Miquet JM, et al: Neuroprotective effects of riluzole on a model of Parkinson's disease in the rat. Neuroscience 1996;74:971–983.

Baseman DG, O'Suilleabhain PE, Reimold SC, et al: Pergolide use in Parkinson disease is associated with cardiac valve regurgitation. Neurology 2004;63(2):301–304.

Beal MF: Bioenergetic approaches for neuroprotection in Parkinson's disease. Ann Neurol 2003;53:S39–S47; discussion in Ann Neurol 2003;S47–S48.

Behrman AL, Cauraugh JH, Light KE: Practice as an intervention to improve speeded motor performance and motor learning in Parkinson's disease. J Neurol Sci 2000;174:127–136.

Benazzouz A, Boraud T, Dubedat P, et al: Riluzole prevents MPTP-induced parkinsonism in the rhesus monkey: A pilot study. Eur J Pharmacol 1995;284:299–307.

Bennett JP, Landow ER, Dietrich S, Schuh LA: Suppression of dyskinesias in advanced Parkinson's disease: Moderate daily clozapine doses provide long-term dyskinesia reduction. Mov Disord 1994;9:409–414.

Bennett JP, Landow ER, Schuh LA: Suppression of dyskinesias in advanced Parkinson's disease: 2. Increasing daily clozapine doses suppress dyskinesias and improve parkinsonism symptoms. Neurology 1993;43:1551–1555.

Ben-Shlomo Y, Churchyard A, Head J, et al: Investigation by Parkinson's disease Research Group of United Kingdom into excess mortality seen with combined levodopa and selegiline treatment in patients with early, mild Parkinson's disease: Further results of randomised trial and confidential inquiry. BMJ 1998;316:1191–1196.

Berger K, Breteler MMB, Helmer C, et al: Prognosis with Parkinson's disease in Europe: A collaborative study of population-based cohorts. Neurology 2000;54(suppl 5):S24–S27.

Bernheimer H, Birkmayer W, Hornykiewicz O, et al: Brain dopamine and the syndromes of Parkinson and Huntington. J Neurol Sci 1973;20:415–455.

Betarbet R, Sherer TB, MacKenzie G, et al: Chronic systemic pesticide exposure reproduces features of Parkinson's disease. Nat Neurosci 2000;3:1301–1306.

Bezard E, Dovero S, Belin D, et al: Enriched environment confers resistance to 1-methyl-4-phenyl-1,2,3,6-tetrahydropyridine and cocaine: Involvement of dopamine transporter and trophic factors. J Neurosci 2003;23(35):10999–11007.

Blanchet PJ, Allard P, Gregoire L, et al: Risk factors for peak dose dyskinesia in 100 levodopa-treated parkinsonian patients. Can J Neurol Sci 1996;23:189–193.

Blanchet PJ, Papa SM, Metman LV, et al: Modulation of levodopa-induced motor response complications by NMDA antagonists in Parkinson's disease. Neurosci Biobehav Rev 1997;21:447–453.

Blin J, Bonnet A-M, Agid Y: Does levodopa aggravate Parkinson's disease? Neurology 1988;38:1410–1416.

Blindauer K, Shoulson I, Oakes D, et al: A randomized controlled trial of etilevodopa in patients with Parkinson disease who have motor fluctuations. Arch Neurol 2006;63(2):210–216.

Block G, Liss C, Reines S, et al: Comparison of immediate-release and controlled release carbidopa/levodopa in Parkinson's disease: A multicenter 5-year study. Eur Neurol 1997;37:23–27.

Bocquet A, Lorent G, Fuks B, et al: Failure of GPI compounds to display neurotrophic activity in vitro and in vivo. Eur J Pharmacol 2001;415:173–180.

Boireau A, Dubedat P, Bordier F, et al: The protective effect of riluzole in the MPTP model of Parkinson's disease in mice is not due to a decrease in MPP(+) accumulation. Neuropharmacology 2000;39(6):1016–1020.

Bonifati V, Fabrizio E, Cipriani R, et al: Buspirone in levodopa-induced dyskinesias. Clin Neuropharmacol 1994;17:73–82.

Bravi D, Mouradian MM, Roberts JW, et al: End-of-dose dystonia in Parkinson's disease. Neurology 1993;43:2130–2131.

Bravi D, Mouradian MM, Roberts JW, et al: Wearing-off fluctuations in Parkinson's disease: Contribution of postsynaptic mechanisms. Ann Neurol 1994;36:27–31.

Bredberg E, Nilsson D, Johansson K, et al: Intraduodenal infusion of a water-based levodopa dispersion for optimisation of the therapeutic effect in severe Parkinson's disease. Eur J Clin Pharmacol 1993;45:117–122.

Brooks DJ, Abbott RJ, Lees AJ, et al: A placebo-controlled evaluation of ropinirole, a novel D-2 agonist, as sole dopaminergic therapy in Parkinson's disease. Clin Neuropharmacol 1998;21:101–107.

Brooks DJ, Sagar H: Entacapone is beneficial in both fluctuating and non-fluctuating patients with Parkinson's disease: A randomised, placebo controlled, double blind, six month study. J Neurol Neurosurg Psychiatry 2003;74(8):1071–1079.

Burke RE, Antonelli M, Sulzer D: Glial cell line-derived neurotrophic growth factor inhibits apoptotic death of postnatal substantia nigra dopamine neurons in primary culture. J Neurochem 1998; 71:517–525.

Burns RS, Chiueh CC, Markey SP, et al: A primate model of parkinsonism: Selective destruction of dopaminergic neurons in the pars compacta of the substantia nigra by N-methyl-4-phenyl-1,2,3,6-tetrahydropyridine. Proc Natl Acad Sci U S A 1983;80:4546–4550.

Bush DF, Liss CL, Morton A, Sinemet CR Multicenter Study Group: An open multicenter long-term treatment evaluation of Sinemet CR. Neurology 1989;39(suppl 2):101–104.

Calne DB, Stern GM, Laurence DR, et al: L-Dopa in postencephalitic parkinsonism. Lancet 1969;1:744–746.

Calon F, Rajput AH, Hornykiewicz O, et al: Levodopa-induced motor complications are associated with alterations of glutamate receptors in Parkinson's disease. Neurobiol Disease 2003;14(3): 404–416.

Canesi M, Antonini A, Mariani CB, et al: An overnight switch to ropinirole therapy in patients with Parkinson's disease. J Neural Transm 1999;106:925–929.

Caraceni T, Scigliano G, Musicco M: The occurrence of motor fluctuations in parkinsonian patients treated long term with levodopa: Role of early treatment and disease progression. Neurology 1991;41:380–384.

Carpentier AF, Bonnet AM, Vidailhet M, Agid Y: Improvement of levodopa-induced dyskinesia by propranolol in Parkinson's disease. Neurology 1996;46:1548–1551.

Carroll CB, Bain PG, Teare L, et al: Cannabis for dyskinesia in Parkinson disease: A randomized double-blind crossover study. Neurology 2004;63(7):1245–1250.

Cedarbaum JM, Gandy SE, McDowell FH: Early initiation of levodopa treatment does not promote the development of motor response fluctuations, dyskinesias, or dementia in Parkinson's disease. Neurology 1991;41:622–629.

Chase TN: The significance of continuous dopaminergic stimulation in the treatment of Parkinson's disease. Drugs 1998;55:1–9.

Chase TN, Mouradian MM, Engber TM: Motor response complications and the function of striatal efferent systems. Neurology 1993;43(suppl 6):S23–S27.

Chase TN, Oh JD, Blanchet PJ: Neostriatal mechanisms in Parkinson's disease. Neurology 1998;51(suppl 2):S30–S35.

Chase TN, Oh JD, Konitsiotis S: Antiparkinsonian and antidyskinetic activity of drugs targeting central glutamatergic mechanisms. J Neurol 2000;247:36–42.

Clarke A, Jankovic J: Selegiline orally disintegrating tablet in the treatment of Parkinson's disease. Therapy 2006;3:349–356.

Clarke CE: Does levodopa therapy delay death in Parkinson's disease? A review of the evidence. Mov Disord 1995;10:250–256.

Clough CG, Bergmann KJ, Yahr MD: Cholinergic and dopaminergic mechanisms in Parkinson's disease after long-term L-DOPA administration. Adv Neurol 1984;40:131–140.

Cohen AD, Tillerson JL, Smith AD, et al: Neuroprotective effects of prior limb use in 6-hydroxydopamine-treated rats: Possible role of GDNF. J Neurochem 2003;85(2):299–305.

Cohen G: The pathobiology of Parkinson's disease: Biochemical aspects of dopamine neuron senescence. J Neural Transm 1983;90(suppl 19):89–103.

Cohen G: Monoamine oxidase, hydrogen peroxide, and Parkinson's disease. Adv Neurol 1986;45:119–125.

Colosimo C, Merello M, Hughes AJ, et al: Motor response to acute dopaminergic challenge with apomorphine and levodopa in Parkinson's disease: Implications for the pathogenesis of the on-off phenomenon. J Neurol Neurosurg Psychiatry 1996;60: 634–637.

Colzi A, Turner K, Lees AJ: Continuous subcutaneous waking day apomorphine in the long term treatment of levodopa induced interdose dyskinesias in Parkinson's disease. J Neurol Neurosurg Psychiatry 1998;64:573–576.

Contin M, Riva R, Martinelli P, et al: A levodopa kinetic-dynamic study of the progression in Parkinson's disease. Neurology 1998a;51:1075–1080.

Contin M, Riva R, Martinelli P, et al: Effect of meal timing on the kinetic-dynamic profile of levodopa/carbidopa controlled release in parkinsonian patients. Eur J Clin Pharmacol 1998b;54:303–308.

Crystal HA, Dickson DW, Lizardi JE, et al: Antemortem diagnosis of diffuse Lewy body disease. Neurology 1990;40:1523–1528.

Currie LJ, Harrison MB, Trugman JM, et al: Early morning dystonia in Parkinson's disease. Neurology 1998;51:283–285.

Dave M: Clozapine-related tardive dyskinesia. Biol Psychiatry 1994;35:886–887.

Davis GC, Williams AC, Markey SP, et al: Chronic parkinsonism secondary to intravenous injection of meperidine analogues. Psychiatry Research 1979;1:249–254.

de Jong GJ, Meerwaldt JD, Schmitz PIM: Factors that influence the occurrence of response variations in Parkinson's disease. Ann Neurol 1987;22:4–7.

de la Fuente-Fernandez R, Lu JQ, Sossi V, et al: Biochemical variations in the synaptic level of dopamine precede motor fluctuations in Parkinson's disease: PET evidence of increased dopamine turnover. Ann Neurol 2001;49:298–303.

Dewey RB, Maraganore DM, Ahlskog JE, Matsumoto JY: A double-blind, placebo-controlled study of intranasal apomorphine spray as a rescue agent for off-states in Parkinson's disease. Mov Disord 1998;13:782–787.

de Yebenes JG, Vazquez A, Martinez A, et al: Biochemical findings in symptomatic dystonias. Adv Neurol 1988;50:167–175.

Diederich N, Keipes M, Grass M, Metz H: Use of clozapine for psychiatric complications of Parkinson's disease. Rev Neurol 1995;151:251–257.

Direnfeld LK, Feldman RG, Alexander MP, Kelly-Hayes M: Is L-dopa drug holiday useful? Neurology 1980;30:785–788.

Djaldetti R, Baron J, Ziv I, Melamed E: Gastric emptying in Parkinson's disease: Patients with and without response fluctuations. Neurology 1996;46:1051–1054.

Donnan PT, Steinke DT, Stubbings C, et al: Selegiline and mortality in subjects with Parkinson's disease: A longitudinal community study. Neurology 2000;55:1785–1789.

Du Y, Ma Z, Lin S, Dodel RC, et al: Minocycline prevents nigrostriatal dopaminergic neurodegeneration in the MPTP model of Parkinson's disease. Proc Natl Acad Sci U S A 98:14669–14674.

Durif F, Debilly B, Galitzky M, et al: Clozapine improves dyskinesias in Parkinson disease: A double-blind, placebo-controlled study. Neurology 2004;62(3):381–388.

Durif F, Vidailhet M, Assal F, et al: Low-dose clozapine improves dyskinesias in Parkinson's disease. Neurology 1997;48:658–662.

Durif F, Vidailhet M, Bonnet AM, et al: Levodopa-induced dyskinesias are improved by fluoxetine. Neurology 1995;45:1855–1858.

Duvoisin RC: Cholinergic-anticholinergic antagonism in parkinsonism. Arch Neurol 1967;17:124–136.

Duvoisin RC: Hyperkinetic reactions with L-DOPA. In Yahr MD (ed): Current Concepts in the Treatment of Parkinsonism. New York, Raven Press, 1974a, pp 203–210.

Duvoisin RC: Variations in the "on-off" phenomenon. Adv Neurol 1974b;5:339–340.

Duvoisin RC, Antunes JL, Yahr MD: Response of patients with postencephalitic parkinsonism to levodopa. J Neurol Neurosurg Psychiatry 1972;35:487–495.

Eberling JL, Pivirotto P, Bringas J, et al: The immunophilin ligand GPI-1046 does not have neuroregenerative effects in MPTP-treated monkeys. Exp Neurol 2002;178:236–242.

Ebersbach G, Stock M, Muller J, et al: Worsening of motor performance in patients with Parkinson's disease following transdermal nicotine administration. Mov Disord 1999;14:1011–1013.

Ehringer H, Hornykiewicz O: Verteilung von Noradrenalin und Dopamin (3–Hydroxytryramin) im Gehirn des Menschen und ihr Verhalten bei Erkrankungen des extrapyramidalen Systems. Klin Wschr 1960;38:1238–1239.

Emborg ME, Shin P, Roitberg B, et al: Systemic administration of the immunophilin ligand GPI 1046 in MPTP-treated monkeys. Exp Neurol 2001;168:171–182.

Fabbrini G, Juncos J, Mouradian MM, et al: Levodopa pharmacokinetic mechanisms and motor fluctuations in Parkinson's disease. Ann Neurol 1987;21:370–376.

Fabbrini G, Mouradian MM, Juncos JL, et al: Motor fluctuations in Parkinson's disease: Central pathophysiological mechansims, Part I. Ann Neurol 1988;24:366–371.

Factor SA: The initial treatment of Parkinson's disease. Mov Disord 2000;15:360–361.

Factor SA, Brown D: Clozapine prevents recurrence of psychosis in Parkinson's disease. Mov Disord 1992;7:125–131.

Factor SA, Brown D, Molho ES, Podskalny GD: Clozapine: A 2-year open trial in Parkinson's disease patients with psychosis. Neurology 1994;44:544–546.

Factor SA, Friedman JH: The emerging role of clozapine in the treatment of movement disorders. Mov Disord 1997;12:483–496.

Fahn S: "On-off" phenomenon with levodopa therapy in parkinsonism: Clinical and pharmacologic correlations and the effect of intramuscular pyridoxine. Neurology 1974;24:431–441.

Fahn S: Episodic failure of absorption of levodopa: A factor in the control of clinical fluctuations in the treatment of parkinsonism. Neurology 1977;27:390.

Fahn S: Fluctuations of disability in Parkinson's disease: Pathophysiological aspects. In Marsden CD, Fahn S (eds): Movement Disorders. London, Butterworth Scientific, 1982, pp 123–145.

Fahn S: The endogenous toxin hypothesis of the etiology of Parkinson's disease and a pilot trial of high dosage antioxidants in an attempt to slow the progression of the illness. Ann N Y Acad Sci 1989;570:186–196.

Fahn S: Consensus? How to proceed in treatment today: Conclusions. In Rinne UK, Nagatsu T, Horowski R (eds): International Workshop Berlin Parkinson's Disease. Bussum, The Netherlands: Medicom Europe, 1991, pp 368–371.

Fahn S: Adverse effects of levodopa. In Olanow CW, Lieberman AN (eds): The Scientific Basis for the Treatment of Parkinson's Disease. Carnforth, UK, Parthenon Publishing Group, 1992a, pp 89–112.

Fahn S: A pilot trial of high-dose alpha-tocopherol and ascorbate in early Parkinson's disease. Ann Neurol 1992b;32:S128–S132.

Fahn S: The freezing phenomenon in parkinsonism. Adv Neurol 1995;67:53–63.

Fahn S: Is levodopa toxic? Neurology 1996;47 (suppl 3):S184–S195.

Fahn S: Parkinsonism. In Rakel RE (ed): Conn's Current Therapy. Philadelphia: W B Saunders, 1998, pp 944–953.

Fahn S: Parkinson disease, the effect of levodopa, and the ELLDOPA trial. Arch Neurol 1999;56:529–535.

Fahn S: The spectrum of levodopa-induced dyskinesias. Ann Neurol 2000;47(suppl 1):S2–S11.

Fahn S, Barrett RB: Increase of parkinsonian symptoms as a manifestation of levodopa toxicity. Adv Neurol 1979;24:451–459.

Fahn S, Chouinard S: Experience with tranylcypromine in early Parkinson's disease. J Neural Transm 1998;105(suppl 52):49–61.

Fahn S, Cohen G: The oxidant stress hypothesis in Parkinson's disease: Evidence supporting it. Ann Neurol 1992;32:804–812.

Fahn S, Isgreen WP: Long-term evaluation of amantadine and levodopa combination in parkinsonism by double-blind crossover analyses. Neurology 1975;25:695–700.

Fahn S, Mazzoni P: Survey of levodopa treatment patterns by clinical practitioners. Mov Disord 2006;21(suppl 13):S109–S110.

Fahn S, Parkinson Study Group: Rotigotine transdermal system (SPM-962) is safe and effective as monotherapy in early Parkinson's disease (PD). Parkinsonism Relat Disord 2001;7(suppl):S55.

Fahn S, Rudolph A, Parkinson Study Group: Neurologists' treatment patterns for Parkinson's disease (PD). Mov Disord 1996;11:595.

Fahn S, Sulzer D: Neurodegeneration and neuroprotection in Parkinson disease. NeuroRx 2004;1:139–154.

Fahn S, Togasaki D, Chouinard S: MAO-A and -B inhibition with tranylcypromine in early Parkinson's disease: Clinical and CSF effects. Mov Disord 1998;13:148.

Ferreira JJ, Galitzky M, Montastruc JL, Rascol O: Sleep attacks and Parkinson's disease treatment. Lancet 2000;355:1333–1334.

Fisher BE, Petzinger GM, Nixon K, et al: Exercise-induced behavioral recovery and neuroplasticity in the 1-methyl-4-phenyl-1,2,3,6-tetrahydropyridine-lesioned mouse basal ganglia. J Neurosci Res 2004;77(3):378–390.

Ford B, Louis ED, Greene P, Fahn S: Oral and genital pain syndromes in Parkinson's disease. Mov Disord 1996;11:421–426.

Fornstedt B, Pileblad E, Carlsson A: In vivo autoxidation of dopamine in guinea pig striatum increases with age. J Neurochem 1990;55:655–659.

Fowler JS, Volkow ND, Logan J: Slow recovery of human brain MAO B after L-deprenyl (selegiline) withdrawal. Synapse 1994;18:86–93.

Frankel JP, Lees AJ, Kempster PA, Stern GM: Subcutaneous apomorphine in the treatment of Parkinson's disease. J Neurol Neurosurg Psychiatry 1990;53:96–101.

Friedman JH: Akathisia with clozapine. Biol Psychiatry 1993;33:852–853.

Friedman JH, Feinberg SS, Feldman RG: A neuroleptic malignantlike syndrome due to levodopa therapy withdrawal. JAMA 1985;254:2792–2795.

Friedman JH, Lannon MC: Clozapine in idiopathic Parkinson's disease. Neurology 1990;40:1151–1152.

Friedman J, Lannon M, Comella C, et al: Low-dose clozapine for the treatment of drug-induced psychosis in Parkinson's disease. N Engl J Med 1999;340:757–763.

Frucht S, Rogers JD, Greene PE, et al: Falling asleep at the wheel: Motor vehicle mishaps in persons taking pramipexole and ropinirole. Neurology 1999;52:1908–1910.

Furuya R, Hirai A, Andoh T, et al: Successful perioperative management of a patient with Parkinson's disease by enteral levodopa administration under propofol anesthesia. Anesthesiology 1998;89:261–263.

Galvez-Jimenez N, Lang AE: Perioperative problems in Parkinson's disease and their management: Apomorphine with rectal domperidone. Can J Neurol Sci 1996;23:198–203.

Gardner DM, Tailor SA, Walker SE, Shulman KI: The making of a user friendly MAOI diet. J Clin Psychiatry 1996;57(3):99–104.

Gash DM, Zhang Z, Ovadia A, et al: Functional recovery in parkinsonian monkeys treated with GDNF. Nature 1996;21:252–255.

Geminiani G, Fetoni V, Genitrini S, et al: Cabergoline in Parkinson's disease complicated by motor fluctuations. Mov Disord 1996;11:495–500.

Gershanik OS: Early-onset parkinsonism. In Jankovic J, Tolosa E (eds): Parkinson's Disease and Movement Disorders, 2nd ed. Baltimore, Williams & Wilkins, 1993, pp 235–252.

Giladi N, Gurevich T, Shabtai H, et al: The effect of botulinum toxin injections to the calf muscles on freezing of gait in parkinsonism: A pilot study. J Neurol 2001a;248:572–576.

Giladi N, McDermott MP, Fahn S, et al: Freezing of gait in PD: Prospective assessment in the DATATOP cohort. Neurology 2001b;56:1712–1721.

Giladi N, McMahon D, Przedborski S, et al: Motor blocks in Parkinson's disease. Neurology 1992;42:333–339.

Gill SS, Patel NK, Hotton GR, et al: Direct brain infusion of glial cell line-derived neurotrophic factor in Parkinson disease. Nat Med 2003;9(5):589–595.

Glozman JM, Bicheva KG, Fedorova NV: Scale of quality of life of caregivers (SQLC). J Neurol 1998;245:S39–S41.

Goetz CG, Schwid SR, Eberly SW, et al: Safety of rasagiline in elderly patients with Parkinson disease. Neurology 2006;66(9):1427–1429.

Golbe LI, Lieberman AN, Muenter MD, et al: Deprenyl in the treatment of symptom fluctuations in advanced Parkinson's disease. Clin Neuropharmacol 1988;11:45–55.

Gordon PH, Frucht SJ: Neuroleptic malignant syndrome in advanced Parkinson's disease. Mov Disord 2001;16:960–962.

Graham DG, Tiffamy SM, Bell WR, Gutknecht WF: Autooxidation versus covalent binding of quinone as the mechanism of toxicity of dopamine, 6-hydroxydopamine and related compounds toward C1300 neuroblastoma cells in vitro. Mol Pharmacol 1978;14:644–653.

Greene P, Cote L, Fahn S: Treatment of drug-induced psychosis in Parkinson's disease with clozapine. Adv Neurol 1993;60:703–706.

Grondin R, Zhang Z, Yi A, et al: Chronic, controlled GDNF infusion promotes structural and functional recovery in advanced parkinsonian monkeys. Brain 2002;125:2191–2201.

Growdon JH, Kieburtz K, McDermott MP, et al: Levodopa improves motor function without impairing cognition in mild non-demented Parkinson's disease patients. Neurology 1998;50:1327–1331.

Guo X, Dawson VL, Dawson TM: Neuroimmunophilin ligands exert neuroregeneration and neuroprotection in midbrain dopaminergic neurons. Eur J Neurosci 2001;13:1683–1693.

Hamilton ITJ, Gilmore WS, Benzie IFF, et al: Interactions between vitamins C and E in human subjects. Br J Nutr 2000;84:261–267.

Hardie RJ, Lees AJ, Stern GM: On-off fluctuations in Parkinson's disease. Brain 1984;107:487–506.

Harper S, Bilsland J, Young L, et al: Analysis of the neurotrophic effects of GPI-1046 on neuron survival and regeneration in culture and in vivo. Neuroscience 1999;88:257–267.

Hashimoto T, Tada T, Nakazato F, et al: Abnormal activity in the globus pallidus in off-period dystonia. Ann Neurol 2001;49:242–245.

Hauser RA, Hubble JP, Truong DD: Randomized trial of the adenosine A(2A) receptor antagonist istradefylline in advanced PD. Neurology 2003;61(3):297–303.

Hauser RA, Wahba MN, Zesiewicz TA, Anderson WM: Modafinil treatment of pramipexole-associated somnolence. Mov Disord 2000;15:1269–1271.

Hely MA, Morris JGL, Reid WGJ, Trafficante R: Sydney multicenter study of Parkinson's disease: Non-L-dopa-responsive problems dominate at 15 years. Mov Disord 2005;20(2):190–199.

Henry B, Fox SH, Crossman AR, Brotchie JM: Mu- and delta-opioid receptor antagonists reduce levodopa-induced dyskinesia in the MPTP-lesioned primate model of Parkinson's disease. Exp Neurol 2001;171:139–146.

Hillen ME, Sage JI: Nonmotor fluctuations in patients with Parkinson's disease. Neurology 1996;47:1180–1183.

Hirschorn KA, Greenberg HS: Successful treatment of levodopa-induced myoclonus and levodopa withdrawal-induced neuroleptic malignant syndrome: A case report. Clin Neuropharmacol 1988;2:278–281.

Hobson DE, Lang AE, Martin WR, et al: Excessive daytime sleepiness and sudden-onset sleep in Parkinson disease: A survey by the Canadian Movement Disorders Group. JAMA 2002;287(4):455–463.

Hoehn MM: Falling asleep at the wheel: Motor vehicle mishaps in people taking pramipexole and ropinirole. Neurology 2000;54:275.

Holloway RG, Parkinson Study Group: Pramipexole vs levodopa as initial treatment for Parkinson disease: A 4-year randomized controlled trial. Arch Neurol 2004;61(7):1044–1053.

Hornykiewicz O: Dopamine (3-hydroxytyramine) and brain function. Pharmacol Rev 1966;18:925–964.

Horstink MWIM, Zijlmans JCM, Pasman JW, et al: Severity of Parkinson's disease is a risk factor for peak-dose dyskinesia. J Neurol Neurosurg Psychiatry 1990a;53:224–226.

Horstink MWIM, Zijlmans JCM, Pasman JW, et al: Which risk factors predict the levodopa response in fluctuating Parkinson's disease. Ann Neurol 1990b;27:537–543.

Horvath J, Fross RD, Kleiner-Fisman G, et al: Severe multivalvular heart disease: A new complication of the ergot derivative dopamine agonists. Mov Disord 2004;19(6):656–662.

Hughes AJ, Bishop S, Kleedorfer B, et al: Subcutaneous apomorphine in Parkinson's disease: response to chronic administration for up to five years. Mov Disord 1993;8:165–170.

Hutton JT, Koller WC, Ahlskog JE, et al: Multicenter, placebo-controlled trial of cabergoline taken once daily in the treatment of Parkinson's disease. Neurology 1996;46:1062–1065.

Hutton JT, Morris JL: Long-acting carbidopa-levodopa in the management of moderate and advanced Parkinson's disease. Neurology 1992;42(suppl 1):51–56.

Ilson J, Fahn S, Cote L: Painful dystonic spasms in Parkinson's disease. Adv Neurol 1984;40:395–398.

Inzelberg R, Nisipeanu P, Rabey JM, et al: Double-blind comparison of cabergoline and bromocriptine in Parkinson's disease patients with motor fluctuations. Neurology 1996;47:785–788.

Ives NJ, Stowe RL, Marro J, et al: Monoamine oxidase type B inhibitors in early Parkinson's disease: Meta-analysis of 17 randomised trials involving 3525 patients. BMJ 2004;329(7466):593B–596B.

Jankovic J, Hunter C: A double-blind, placebo-controlled and longitudinal study of riluzole in early Parkinson's disease. Parkinsonism Relat Disord 2002;8:271–276.

Jansen ENH: Clozapine in the treatment of tremor in Parkinson's disease. Acta Neurol Scand 1994;89:262–265.

Jenner P: Oxidative stress as a cause of Parkinson's disease. Acta Neurol Scand 1991;84:6–15.

Jenner P, Dexter DT, Sian J, et al: Oxidative stress as a cause of nigral cell death in parkinson's disease and incidental Lewy body disease. Ann Neurol 1992a;32:S82–S87.

Jenner P, Schapira AHV, Marsden CD: New insights into the cause of Parkinson's disease. Neurology 1992b;42:2241–2250.

Jimenez-Jimenez FJ, Tallon-Barranco A, Orti-Pareja M, et al: Olanzapine can worsen parkinsonism. Neurology 1998;50:1183–1184.

Kagan VE, Fabisiak JP, Quinn PJ: Coenzyme Q and vitamin E need each other as antioxidants. Protoplasma 2000;214:11–18.

Kahn N, Freeman A, Juncos JL, et al: Clozapine is beneficial for psychosis in Parkinson's disease. Neurology 1991;41:1699–1700.

Karlsen KH, Larsen JP, Tandberg E, Maeland JG: Influence of clinical and demographic variables on quality of life in patients with Parkinson's disease. J Neurol Neurosurg Psychiat 1999;66:431–435.

Kastrup O, Gastpar M, Schwarz M: Acute dystonia due to clozapine. J Neurol Neurosurg Psychiatry 1994;57:119.

Katzenschlager R, Manson AJ, Evans A, et al: Low dose quetiapine for drug induced dyskinesias in Parkinson's disease: A double blind cross over study. J Neurol Neurosurg Psychiat 2004;75(2):295–297.

Kieburtz K, Shoulson I, Fahn S, et al: Entacapone improves motor fluctuations in levodopa-treated Parkinson's disease patients. Ann Neurol 1997a;42:747–755.

Kieburtz K, Shoulson I, McDermott M, et al: Safety and efficacy of pramipexole in early Parkinson disease: A randomized dose-ranging study. JAMA 1997b;278:125–130.

Klawans HL: Individual manifestations of Parkinson's disease after ten or more years of levodopa. Mov Disord 1986;1:187–192.

Klawans HL, Goetz C, Bergen D: Levodopa-induced myoclonus. Arch Neurol 1975;32:331–334.

Koller WC, Hutton JT, Tolosa E, Capilldeo R: Immediate-release and controlled-release carbidopa/levodopa in PD: A 5-year randomized multicenter study. Neurology 1999;53:1012–1019.

Kordower JH, Emborg ME, Bloch J, et al: Neurodegeneration prevented by lentiviral vector delivery of GDNF in primate models of Parkinson's disease. Science 2000;290:767–773.

Korner Y, Meindorfner C, Moller JC, et al: Predictors of sudden onset of sleep in Parkinson's disease. Mov Disord 2004;19(11):1298–1305.

Kostic V, Przedborski S, Flaster E, Sternic N: Early development of levodopa-induced dyskinesias and response fluctuations in young-onset Parkinson's disease. Neurology 1991;41:202–205.

Kujawa K, Leurgans S, Raman R, et al: Acute orthostatic hypotension when starting dopamine agonists in Parkinson's disease. Arch Neurol 2000;57:1461–1463.

Kulisevsky J, Lopez-Villegas D, Garcia-Sanchez C, et al:. A six-month study of pergolide and levodopa in de novo Parkinson's disease patients. Clin Neuropharmacol 1998;21:358–362.

Kurth MC, Tetrud JW, Irwin I, et al: Oral levodopa/carbidopa solution versus tablets in Parkinson's patients with severe fluctuations: A pilot study. Neurology 1993a;43:1036–1039.

Kurth MC, Tetrud JW, Tanner CM, et al: Double-blind, placebo-controlled, crossover study of duodenal infusion of levodopa carbidopa in Parkinson's disease patients with on-off fluctuations. Neurology 1993b;43:1698–1703.

Lai CT, Yu PH: Dopamine and L-beta-3,4-dihydroxyphenylalanine hydrochloride (L-DOPA)-induced cytotoxicity towards catecholaminergic neuroblastoma SH-SY5Y cells: Effects of oxidative stress and antioxidative factors. Biochem Pharmacol 1997;53:363–372.

Lamberti P, Zoccolella S, Iliceto G, et al: Effects of levodopa and COMT inhibitors on plasma homocysteine in Parkinson's disease patients. Mov Disord 2005;20(1):69–72.

Lang AE, Gill S, Patel NK, et al: Randomized controlled trial of intraputamenal glial cell line–derived neurotrophic factor infusion in Parkinson disease. Ann Neurol 2006;59(3):459–466.

Langston JW, Ballard PA: Parkinsonism induced by 1-methyl-4-phenyl-1,2,5,6-tetrahydropyridine: Implications for treatment and the pathophysiology of Parkinson's disease. Can J Neurosci 1984;11:160–165.

Langston JW, Ballard P, Tetrud JW, Irwin I: Chronic parkinsonism in humans due to a product of meperidine-analog synthesis. Science 1983;219:979–980.

Langston JW, Forno LS, Rebert CS, Irwin I: 1-Methyl-4-phenyl-1,2,5,6-tetrahydropyridine causes selective damage to the zona compacta of the substantia nigra in the squirrel monkey. Brain Res 1984;292:390–394.

Lees AJ: Comparison of therapeutic effects and mortality data of levodopa and levodopa combined with selegiline in patients with early, mild Parkinson's disease. BMJ 1995;311:1602–1607.

Lesser RP, Fahn S, Snider SR, et al: Analysis of the clinical problems in parkinsonism and the complications of long-term levodopa therapy. Neurology 1979;29:1253–1260.

LeWitt PA, Walters A, Hening W, McHale D: Persistent movement disorders induced by buspirone. Mov Disord 1993;8:331–334.

Lhermitte F, Agid Y, Signoret JL: Onset and end-of-dose levodopa-induced dyskinesias. Arch Neurol 1978;35:261–262.

Lieberman A, Olanow CW, Sethi K, et al: A multicenter trial of ropinirole as adjunct treatment for Parkinson's disease. Neurology 1998;51:1057–1062.

Ling LH, Ahlskog JE, Munger TM, et al: Constrictive pericarditis and pleuropulmonary disease linked to ergot dopamine agonist therapy (cabergoline) for Parkinson's disease. Mayo Clin Proc 1999;74:371–375.

Lokk J: The effects of mountain exercise in Parkinsonian persons: A preliminary study. Arch Gerontol Geriatr 2000;31:19–25.

Luginger E, Wenning GK, Bosch S, Poewe W: Beneficial effects of amantadine on L-dopa-induced dyskinesias in Parkinson's disease. Mov Disord 2000;15:873–878.

Luquin MR, Scipioni O, Vaamonde J, et al: Levodopa-induced dyskinesias in Parkinson's disease: Clinical and pharmacological classification. Mov Disord 1992;7:117–124.

Mabandla M, Kellaway L, Gibson AS, Russell VA: Voluntary running provides neuroprotection in rats after 6-hydroxydopamine injection into the medial forebrain bundle. Metab Brain Dis 2004;19(1–2):43–50.

Maki Y, Inoue T, Izumi T, et al: Monoamine oxidase inhibitors reduce conditioned fear stress-induced freezing behavior in rats. Eur J Pharmacol 2000;406:411–418.

Manson AJ, Katzenschlager R, Hobart J, Lees AJ: High dose naltrexone for dyskinesias induced by levodopa. J Neurol Neurosurg Psychiatry 2001;70:554–556.

Maricle RA, Nutt JG, Valentine RJ, Carter JH: Dose-response relationship of levodopa with mood and anxiety in fluctuating Parkinson's disease: A double-blind, placebo-controlled study. Neurology 1995;45:1757–1760.

Marras C, Lang A, Krahn M, et al: Quality of life in early Parkinson's disease: Impact of dyskinesias and motor fluctuations. Mov Disord 2004;19(1):22–28.

Marras C, McDermott MP, Rochon PA, et al: Survival in Parkinson disease: Thirteen-year follow-up of the DATATOP cohort. Neurology 2005;64(1):87–93.

Marsden CD, Fahn S: Problems in Parkinson's disease. In Marsden CD, Fahn S (eds): Movement Disorders. London, Butterworth Scientific, 1982, pp 1–7.

Marsden CD, Parkes JD, Quinn N: Fluctuations of disability in Parkinson's disease: Clinical aspects. In Marsden CD, Fahn S (eds): Movement Disorders. London, Butterworth Scientific, 1982, pp 96–122.

Martinez-Martin P: An introduction to the concept of "quality of life in Parkinson's disease." J Neurol 1998;245:S2–S6.

Matsubara T, Azuma T, Yoshida S, Yamagami T: Serum coenzyme Q10 level in Parkinson syndrome. In Folkers K, Littarru GP, Yamagami T (eds): Biomedical and Clinical Aspects of Coenzyme Q10. New York, Elsevier Science, 1991, pp 159–166.

Matthews RT, Yang L, Browne S, et al: Coenzyme Q10 administration increases brain mitochondrial concentrations and exerts neuroprotective effects. Proc Natl Acad Sci U S A 1998;95:8892–8897.

McDowell FH, Sweet RD: The "on-off" phenomenon. In Birkmayer W, Hornykiewicz O (eds): Advances in Parkinsonism. Basle, Editiones Roche, 1976, pp 603–612.

Meco G, Fabrizio E, DiRezze S, et al: Mirtazapine in L-dopa-induced dyskinesias. Clin Neuropharmacol 2003;26(4):179–181.

Melamed E: Early-morning dystonia: A late side effect of long-term levodopa therapy in Parkinson's disease. Arch Neurol 1979;36:308–310.

Melamed E, Bitton V, Zelig O: Episodic unresponsiveness to single doses of L-dopa in parkinsonian fluctuators. Neurology 1986;36:100–103.

Mena MA, Pardo B, Paino CL, de Yebenes JG: Levodopa toxicity in foetal rat midbrain neurones in culture: Modulation by ascorbic acid. Neuroreport 1993;4:438–440.

Merims D, Ziv I, Djaldetti R, Melamed E: Riluzole for levodopa-induced dyskinesias in advanced Parkinson's disease. Lancet 1999;353:1764–1765.

Metman LV, Del Dotto P, Blanchet PJ, et al: Blockade of glutamatergic transmission as treatment for dyskinesias and motor fluctuations in Parkinson's disdisdisease. Amino Acids 1998;14:75–82.

Metman LV, Del Dotto P, LePoole K, et al: Amantadine for levodopa-induced dyskinesias: A 1-year follow up study. Arch Neurol 1999;56:1383–1386.

Metman LV, Del Dotto P, Natte R, et al: Dextromethorphan improves levodopa-induced dyskinesias in Parkinson's disease. Neurology 1998;51:203–206.

Metman LV, Del Dotto P, van den Munckhof P, et al: Amantadine as treatment for dyskinesias and motor fluctuations in Parkinson's disease. Neurology 1998;50:1323–1326.

Metman LV, Hoff J, Mouradian MM, Chase TN: Fluctuations in plasma levodopa and motor responses with liquid and tablet levodopa/carbidopa. Mov Disord 1994;9:463–465.

Metman LV, Konitsiotis S, Chase TN: Pathophysiology of motor response complications in Parkinson's disease: Hypotheses on the why, where, and what. Mov Disord 2000;15:3–8.

Metman LV, Locatelli ER, Bravi D, et al: Apomorphine responses in Parkinson's disease and the pathogenesis of motor complications. Neurology 1997a;48:369–372.

Metman LV, van den Munckhof P, Klaassen AA, et al: Effects of suprathreshold levodopa doses on dyskinesias in advanced Parkinson's disease. Neurology 1997b;49:711–713.

Miyasaki JM, Shannon K, Voon V, et al: Quality Standards Subcommittee of the American Academy of Neurology. Practice Parameter: Evaluation and treatment of depression, psychosis, and dementia in Parkinson disease (an evidence-based review): Report of the Quality Standards Subcommittee of the American Academy of Neurology. Neurology 2006;66:996–1002.

Montastruc JL, Rascol O, Senard JM, Rascol A: A randomised controlled study comparing bromocriptine to which levodopa was later added, with levodopa alone in previously untreated patients with Parkinson's disease: A five year follow up. J Neurol Neurosurg Psychiatry 1994;57:1034–1038.

Montastruc JL, Rascol O, Senard JM: Treatment of Parkinson's disease should begin with a dopamine agonist. Mov Disord 1999;14:725–730.

Mouradian MM, Heuser IJE, Baronti F, Chase TN: Modification of central dopaminergic mechanisms by continuous levodopa therapy for advanced Parkinson's disease. Ann Neurol 1990;27:18–23.

Mouradian MM, Heuser IJE, Baronti F, et al: Pathogenesis of dyskinesias in Parkinson's disease. Ann Neurol 1989;25:523–526.

Mouradian MM, Juncos JL, Fabbrini G, et al: Motor fluctuations in Parkinson's disease: Central pathophysiological mechansims, Part II. Ann Neurol 1988;24:372–378.

Muenter MD, Sharpless NS, Tyce GM: Plasma 3-O-methyldopa in L-dopa therapy of Parkinson's disease. Mayo Clin Proc 1972;47:389–395.

Muenter MD, Sharpless NS, Tyce GM, Darley FL: Patterns of dystonia ('I-D-I' and 'D-I-D') in response to L-dopa therapy of Parkinson's disease. Mayo Clin Proc 1977;52:163–174.

Muenter MD, Tyce GM: L-dopa therapy of Parkinson's disease: Plasma L-dopa concentration, therapeutic response, and side effects. Mayo Clin Proc 1971;46:231–239.

Murata M, Kanazawa I: Repeated L-DOPA administration reduces the ability of dopamine storage and abolishes the supersensitivity of dopamine receptors in the striatum of intact rat. Neurosci Res 1993;16:15–23.

Murata M, Mizusawa H, Yamanouchi H, Kanazawa I: Chronic levodopa therapy enhances dopa absorption: Contribution to wearing-off. J Neural Transm 1996;103:1177–1185.

Myllyla VV, Sotaniemi KA, Hakulinen P, et al: Selegiline as the primary treatment of Parkinson's disease: A long-term double-blind study. Acta Neurol Scand 1997;95:211–218.

Myllyla VV, Sotaniemi KA, Vuorinen JA, Heinonen EH: Selegiline as initial treatment in de novo parkinsonian patients. Neurology 1992;42:339–343.

Mytilineou C, Han SK, Cohen G: Toxic and protective effects of l-DOPA on mesencephalic cell cultures. J Neurochem 1993;61:1470–1478.

Narabayashi H, Kondo T, Yokochi F, Nagatsu T: Clinical effects of L-threo-3,4-dihydroxyphenylserine in cases of parkinsonism and pure akinesia. Adv Neurol 1986;45:593–602.

Nilsson D, Hansson LE, Johansson K, et al: Long-term intraduodenal infusion of a water based levodopa-carbidopa dispersion in very advanced Parkinson's disease. Acta Neurol Scand 1998;97:175–183.

NINDS NET-PD Investigators: A randomized, double-blind, futility clinical trial of creatine and minocycline in early Parkinson disease. Neurology 2006;66(5):664–671.

Noyes K, Dick AW, Holloway RG, Parkinson Study Group: Pramipexole versus levodopa in patients with early Parkinson's disease: Effect on generic and disease-specific quality of life. Value Health 2006;9(1):28–38.

Nutt JG: On-off phenomenon: Relation to levodopa pharmacokinetics and pharmacodynamics. Ann Neurol 1987;22:535–540.

Nutt JG, Burchiel KJ, Comella CL, et al: Randomized, double-blind trial of glial cell line-derived neurotrophic factor (GDNF) in PD. Neurology 2003;60:69–73.

Nutt JG, Carter JH, Lea ES, Woodward WR: Motor fluctuations during continuous levodopa infusions in patients with Parkinson's disease. Mov Disord 1997;12:285–292.

Nutt JG, Carter JH, Woodward W, et al: Does tolerance develop to levodopa? Comparison of 2-H and 21-H levodopa infusions. Mov Disord 1993;8:139–143.

Nutt JG, Woodward WR, Anderson JL: The effect of carbidopa on the pharmacokinetics of intravenously administered levodopa: The mechanism of action in the treatment of parkinsonism. Ann Neurol 1985;18:527–543.

Nutt JG, Woodward WR, Hammerstad JP, et al: The "on-off" phenomenon in Parkinson's disease. N Engl J Med 1984;310:483–488.

Nyholm D, Remahl AIMN, Dizdar N, et al: Duodenal levodopa infusion monotherapy vs oral polypharmacy in advanced Parkinson disease. Neurology 2005;64(2):216–223.

Obeso JA, Grandas F, Vaamonde J, et al: Motor complications associated with chronic levodopa therapy in Parkinson's disease. Neurology 1989a;39 (Suppl 2):11–19.

Obeso JA, Vaamonde J, Grandas F, et al: Overcoming pharmacokinetic problems in the treatment of Parkinson's disease. Mov Disord 1989b;4(suppl 1):S70–S85.

Obinu MC, Reibaud M, Blanchard V, et al: Neuroprotective effect of riluzole in a primate model of Parkinson's disease: behavioral and histological evidence. Mov Disord 2002;17:13–19.

Oertel WH, Wolters E, Sampaio C, et al: Pergolide versus levodopa monotherapy in early Parkinson's disease patients: The PELMOPET study. Mov Disord 2006;21(3):343–353.

Olanow CW: Oxidation reactions in Parkinson's disease. Neurology 1990;40(suppl 3):32–37.

Olanow CW: An introduction to the free radical hypothesis in Parkinson's disease. Ann Neurol 1992;32:S2–S9.

Olanow CW, Fahn S, Langston JW, Godbold J: Selegiline and mortality in Parkinson's disease. Ann Neurol 1996;40:841–845.

Olanow CW, Kieburtz K, Stern M, et al: Double-blind, placebo-controlled study of entacapone in levodopa-treated patients with stable Parkinson disease. Arch Neurol 2004;61(10):1563–1568.

Olanow CW, Myllyla VV, Sotaniemi KA, et al: Effect of selegiline on mortality in patients with Parkinson's disease: A meta-analysis. Neurology 1998;51:825–830.

Onofri M, Paci C, Thomas A: Sudden appearance of invalidating dyskinesia-dystonia and off fluctuations after the introduction of levodopa in two dopaminomimetic drug naive patients with stage IV Parkinson's disease. J Neurol Neurosurg Psychiatry 1998;65:605–606.

Ostergaard L, Werdelin L, Odin P, et al: Pen injected apomorphine against off phenomena in late Parkinson's disease: A double blind, placebo controlled study. J Neurol Neurosurg Psychiatry 1995;58:681–687.

O'Suilleabhain PE, Bottiglieri T, Dewey RB, et al: Modest increase in plasma homocysteine follows levodopa initiation in Parkinson's disease. Mov Disord 2004;19(12):1403–1408.

Pahwa R, Busenbark K, Huber SJ, et al: Clinical experience with controlled-release carbidopa/levodopa in Parkinson's disease. Neurology 1993;43:677–681.

Pahwa R, Factor SA, Lyons KE, et al: Practice Parameter: Treatment of Parkinson disease with motor fluctuations and dyskinesia (an evidence-based review): Report of the Quality Standards Subcommittee of the American Academy of Neurology. Neurology 2006;66(7):983–995.

Palhagen S, Heinonen EH, Hagglund J, et al: Selegiline delays the onset of disability in de novo parkinsonian patients. Neurology 1998;51:520–525.

Palhagen S, Heinonen E, Hagglund J, et al: Selegiline slows the progression of the symptoms of Parkinson disease. Neurology 2006;66(8):1200–1206.

Papa SM, Engber TM, Kask AM, Chase TN: Motor fluctuations in levodopa treated parkinsonian rats: Relation to lesion extent and treatment duration. Brain Res 1994;662:69–74.

Pappert EJ, Buhrfiend C, Lipton JW, et al: Levodopa stability in solution: Time course, environmental effects, and practical recommendations for clinical use. Mov Disord 1996a;11:24–26.

Pappert EJ, Goetz CG, Niederman F, et al: Liquid levodopa/carbidopa produces significant improvement in motor function without dyskinesia exacerbation. Neurology 1996b;47:1493–1495.

Pardo B, Mena MA, Casarejos MJ, et al: Toxic effects of L-DOPA on mesencephalic cell cultures: Protection with antioxidants. Brain Res 1995;682:133–143.

Pardo B, Mena MA, Fahn S, De Yebenes JG: Ascorbic acid protects against levodopa-induced neurotoxicity on a catecholamine-rich human neuroblastoma cell line. Mov Disord 1993;8:278–284.

Parkinson Study Group: DATATOP: A multicenter controlled clinical trial in early Parkinson's disease. Arch Neurol 1989a;46:1052–1060.

Parkinson Study Group: Effect of deprenyl on the progression of disability in early Parkinson's disease. N Engl J Med 1989b;321:1364–1371.

Parkinson Study Group: Effects of tocopherol and deprenyl on the progression of disability in early Parkinson's disease. N Engl J Med 1993a;328:176–183.

Parkinson Study Group: A controlled trial of lazabemide (RO19-6327) in untreated Parkinson's disease. Ann Neurol 1993b;33:350–356.

Parkinson Study Group: Cerebrospinal fluid homovanillic acid in the DATATOP study on Parkinson's disease. Arch Neurol 1995;52:237–245.

Parkinson Study Group: Impact of deprenyl and tocopherol treatment on Parkinson's disease in DATATOP patients requiring levodopa. Ann Neurol 1996a;39:37–45.

Parkinson Study Group: Impact of deprenyl and tocopherol treatment on Parkinson's disease in DATATOP subjects not requiring levodopa. Ann Neurol 1996b;39:29–36.

Parkinson Study Group: Safety and efficacy of pramipexole in early Parkinson disease: A randomized dose-ranging study. JAMA 1997;278:125–130.

Parkinson Study Group: Mortality in DATATOP: A multicenter trial in early Parkinson's disease. Ann Neurol 1998;43:318–325.

Parkinson Study Group: Pramipexole vs levodopa as initial treatment for Parkinson disease: A randomized controlled trial. JAMA 2000;284:1931–1938.

Parkinson Study Group: A controlled trial of rasagiline in early Parkinson disease—the TEMPO study. Arch Neurol 2002a;59(12):1937–1943.

Parkinson Study Group: Dopamine transporter brain imaging to assess the effects of pramipexole vs levodopa on Parkinson disease progression. JAMA 2002b;287:1653–1661.

Parkinson Study Group: A controlled trial of rotigotine monotherapy in early Parkinson's disease. Arch Neurol 2003;60(12):1721–1728.

Parkinson Study Group: A controlled, randomized, delayed-start study of rasagiline in early Parkinson disease. Arch Neurol 2004a;61(4):561–566.

Parkinson Study Group: Levodopa and the progression of Parkinson's disease. N Engl J Med 2004b;351(24):2498–2508.

Parkinson Study Group: A randomized placebo-controlled trial of rasagiline in levodopa-treated patients with Parkinson disease and motor fluctuations: The PRESTO study. Arch Neurol 2005;62(2):241–248.

Pearce RKB, Banerji T, Jenner P, Marsden CD: De novo administration of ropinirole and bromocriptine induces less dyskinesia than L-dopa in the MPTP-treated marmoset. Mov Disord 1998;13:234–241.

Pearce RKB, Heikkila M, Linden IB, Jenner P: L-dopa induces dyskinesia in normal monkeys: Behavioural and pharmacokinetic observations. Psychopharmacology 2001;156:402–409.

Pederzoli M, Girotti F, Scigliano G, et al: L-Dopa long-term treatment in Parkinson's disease: Age-related side effects. Neurology 1983;33:1518–1522.

Perachon S, Schwartz JC, Sokoloff P: Functional potencies of new antiparkinsonian drugs at recombinant human dopamine D-1, D-2 and D-3 receptors. Eur J Pharmacol 1999;366:293–300.

Pfeiffer RF, Kang J, Graber B, et al: Clozapine for psychosis in Parkinson's disease. Mov Disord 1990;5:239–242.

Pfitzenmeyer P, Foucher P, Dennewald G, et al: Pleuropulmonary changes induced by ergoline drugs. Eur Resp J 1996;9:1013–1019.

Pfutzner W, Przybilla B: Malignant melanoma and levodopa: Is there a relationship? Two new cases and a review of the literature. J Am Acad Dermatol 1997;37:332–336.

Pierantozzi M, Pietroiusti A, Brusa L, et al: *Helicobacter pylori* eradication and L-dopa absorption in patients with PD and motor fluctuations. Neurology 2006;66:1824–1829.

Pierelli F, Adipietro A, Soldati G, et al: Low dosage clozapine effects on L-dopa induced dyskinesias in parkinsonian patients. Acta Neurol Scand 1998;97:295–299.

Pinter MM, Helscher RJ: Therapeutic effect of clozapine in psychotic decompensation in idiopathic Parkinson's disease. J Neural Transm Parkinsons 1993;5:135–146.

Pinter MM, Pogarell O, Oertel WH: Efficacy, safety, and tolerance of the non-ergoline dopamine agonist pramipexole in the treatment of advanced Parkinson's disease: A double blind, placebo controlled, randomised, multicentre study. J Neurol Neurosurg Psychiatry 1999;66:436–441.

Poewe W: Adjuncts to levodopa therapy: Dopamine agonists. Neurology 1998;50(suppl 6):S23–S26.

Poewe WH, Lees AJ, Stern GM: Low-dose L-dopa therapy in Parkinson's disease: A 6-year follow-up study. Neurology 1986;36:1528–1530.

Poewe W, Luessi F: Clinical studies with transdermal rotigotine in early Parkinson's disease. Neurology 2005;65(2 Suppl 1):S11–S14.

Postuma RB, Lang AE: Homocysteine and levodopa—should Parkinson disease patients receive preventative therapy? Neurology 2004;63(5):886–891.

Pothos E, Davila V, Sulzer D: Presynaptic recording of quanta from midbrain dopamine neurons and modulation of the quantal size. J Neurosci 1998;18:4106–4118.

Pritchett AM, Morrison JF, Edwards WD, et al: Valvular heart disease in patients taking pergolide. Mayo Clin Proc. 2002;77(12):1280–1286.

Przuntek H, Welzel D, Gerlach M, et al: Early institution of bromocriptine in Parkinson's disease inhibits the emergence of levodopa-associated motor side effects: Long-term results of the PRADO study. J Neural Transm 1996;103:699–715.

Quinn N: Multiple system atrophy. In Marsden CD, Fahn S (eds): Movement Disorders, vol 3. Oxford, UK, Butterworth-Heinemann, 1994a, pp 262–281.

Quinn NP: A case against early levodopa treatment of Parkinson's disease. Clin Neuropharmacol 1994b;17:S43–S49.

Quinn N, Critchley P, Marsden CD: Young onset Parkinson's disease. Mov Disord 1987;2:73–91.

Rabey JM, Sagi I, Huberman M, et al: Rasagiline mesylate, a new MAO-B inhibitor for the treatment of Parkinson's disease: A double-blind study as adjunctive therapy to levodopa. Clin Neuropharmacol 2000;23:324–330.

Rabey JM, Treves TA, Neufeld MY, et al: Low-dose clozapine in the treatment of levodopa-induced mental disturbances in Parkinson's disease. Neurology 1995;45:432–434.

Racette BA, Good L, Sagitto S, Perlmutter JS: Botulinum toxin B reduces sialorrhea in parkinsonism. Mov Disord 2003;18(9):1059–1061.

Rajput A, Wallukait M, Rajput AH: Eighteen month prospective study of amantadine (Amd) for dopa (LD) induced dyskinesias (DK) in idiopathic Parkinson's disease. Can J Neurol Sci 1997;24:S23.

Ramig LO, Sapir S, Countryman S, et al: Intensive voice treatment (LSVT (R)) for patients with Parkinson's disease: A 2 year follow up. J Neurol Neurosurg Psychiatry 2001;71:493–498.

Rascol O, Brooks DJ, Korczyn AD, et al: A five-year study of the incidence of dyskinesia in patients with early Parkinson's disease who were treated with ropinirole or levodopa. N Engl J Med 2000;342:1484–1491.

Rascol O, Brooks DJ, Melamed E, et al: Rasagiline as an adjunct to levodopa in patients with Parkinson's disease and motor fluctuations (LARGO, Lasting effect in Adjunct therapy with Rasagiline Given Once daily, study): A randomised, double-blind, parallel-group trial. Lancet 2005;365(9463):947–954.

Rascol O, Olanow CW, Brooks D, et al: Effect of riluzole on Parkinson's disease progression: A double-blind placebo-controlled study. Neurology 2003;60(suppl 1):A288.

Reichmann H, Boas J, MacMahon D, et al: Efficacy of combining levodopa with entacapone on quality of life and activities of daily living in patients experiencing wearing-off type fluctuations. Acta Neurol Scand 2005;111(1):21–28.

Reuter I, Engelhardt M, Stecker K, Baas H: Therapeutic value of exercise training in Parkinson's disease. Med Sci Sports Exerc 1999;31:1544–1549.

Rinne UK: Early dopamine agonist therapy in Parkinson's disease. Mov Disord 1989a;4(suppl 1):S86–S94.

Rinne UK: Lisuride, a dopamine agonist in the treatment of early Parkinson's disease. Neurology 1989b;39:336–339.

Rinne UK, Bracco F, Chouza C, et al: Early treatment of Parkinson's disease with cabergoline delays the onset of motor complications: Results of a double-blind levodopa controlled trial. Drugs 1998; 55:23–30.

Rinne UK, Koskinen V, Lonnberg P: Neurotransmitter receptors in the parkinsonian brain. In Rinne UK, Klingler M, Stamm G (eds): Parkinson's Disease: Current Progress, Problems and Management. Amsterdam, Elsevier/North-Holland Biomedical Press, 1980, pp 93–107.

Rinne UK, Larsen JP, Siden A, et al: Entacapone enhances the response to levodopa in parkinsonian patients with motor fluctuations. Neurology 1998;51:1309–1314.

Rivera-Calimlin L, Dujovne CA, Morgan JP, et al: L-Dopa treatment failure: Explanation and correction. BMJ 1970;4:93–94.

Rodriguez M, Lera G, Vaamonde J, et al: Motor response to apomorphine and levodopa in asymmetric Parkinson's disease. J Neurol Neurosurg Psychiatry 1994;57:562–566.

Roos RAC, Vredevoogd CB, Vandervelde EA: Response fluctuations in Parkinson's disease. Neurology 1990;40:1344–1346.

Ruggieri S, Depandis MF, Bonamartini A, et al: Low dose of clozapine in the treatment of dopaminergic psychosis in Parkinson's disease. Clin Neuropharmacol 1997;20:204–209.

Sacks OW: Awakenings. Garden City, NY, Doubleday,1974.

Sacks OW, Kohl M, Schwartz W, Messeloff C: Side-effects of L-dopa in postencephalic parkinsonism. Lancet 1970;1:1006.

Safferman AZ, Lieberman JA, Pollack S, Kane JM: Akathisia and clozapine treatment. J Clin Psychopharmacol 1993;13:286–287.

Sage JI, Duvoisin RC: Sudden onset of confusion with severe exacerbation of parkinsonism during levodopa therapy. Mov Disord 1986;1:267–270.

Sage JI, McHale DM, Sonsalla P, et al: Continuous levodopa infusions to treat complex dystonia in Parkinson's disease. Neurology 1989a;39:888–891.

Sage JI, Trooskin S, Sonsalla PK, Heikkila RE: Experience with continuous enteral levodopa infusions in the treatment of 9 patients with advanced Parkinson's disease. Neurology 1989b;39(suppl 2): 60–63.

Sassin JF, Taub S, Weitzman ED: Hyperkinesia and changes in behavior produced in normal monkeys by L-dopa. Neurology 1972; 22:1122–1125.

Schapira AHV: Sleep attacks (sleep epiodes) with pergolide. Lancet 2000;355:1332–1333.

Schapira AH, Mann VM, Cooper JM, et al: Anatomic and disease specificity of NADH CoQ1 reductase (complex I) deficiency in Parkinson's disease. J Neurochem 1990;55:2142–2145.

Schrag AE, Brooks DJ, Brunt E, et al: The safety of ropinirole, a selective nonergoline dopamine agonist, in patients with Parkinson's disease. Clin Neuropharmacol 1998;21:169–175.

Schuh LA, Bennett JP: Suppression of dyskinesias in advanced Parkinson's disease: 1. Continuous intravenous levodopa shifts dose response for production of dyskinesias but not for relief of parkinsonism in patients with advanced Parkinson's disease. Neurology 1993:43:1545–1550.

Schwarz GA, Fahn S: Newer medical treatment in parkinsonism. Med Clin North Am 1970;54:773–785.

Sethi KD, O'Brien CF, Hammerstad JP, et al: Ropinirole for the treatment of early Parkinson disease: A 12–month experience. Arch Neurol 1998;55:1211–1216.

Shaunak S, Wilkins A, Pilling JB, Dick DJ: Pericardial, retroperitoneal, and pleural fibrosis induced by pergolide. J Neurol Neurosurg Psychiatry 1999;66:79–81.

Shoulson I, Glaubiger GA, Chase TN: "On-off" response: Clinical and biochemical correlations during oral and intravenous levodopa administration. Neurology 1975;25:1144–1148.

Shoulson I, Oakes D, Fahn S, et al: Impact of sustained deprenyl (selegiline) in levodopa-treated Parkinson's disease: A randomized placebo-controlled extension of the deprenyl and tocopherol antioxidative therapy of parkinsonism trial. Ann Neurol 2002;51:604–612.

Shults CW, Haas RH, Passov D, Beal MF: Coenzyme Q(10) levels correlate with the activities of complexes I and II/III in mitochondria from parkinsonian and nonparkinsonian subjects. Ann Neurol 1997;42:261–264.

Shults CW, Oakes D, Kieburtz K, et al: Effects of coenzyme Q(10) in early Parkinson disease: Evidence of slowing of the functional decline. Arch Neurol 2002;59:1541–1550.

Smith AD, Zigmond MJ: Can the brain be protected through exercise? Lessons from an animal model of parkinsonism. Exp Neurol 2003;184(1):31–39.

Snow BJ, Macdonald L, Mcauley D, Wallis W: The effect of amantadine on levodopa-induced dyskinesias in Parkinson's disease: A double-blind, placebo-controlled study. Clin Neuropharmacol 2000;23:82–85.

Spencer JPE, Jenner P, Halliwell B: Superoxide-dependent depletion of reduced glutathione by L-DOPA and dopamine: Relevance to Parkinson's disease. Neuroreport 1995;6:1480–1484.

Steiner JP, Hamilton GS, Ross DT, et al: Neurotrophic immunophilin ligands stimulate structural and functional recovery in neurodegenerative animal models. Proc Natl Acad Sci U S A 1997;94: 2019–2024.

Stotz M, Thummler D, Schurch M, et al: Fulminant neuroleptic malignant syndrome after perioperative withdrawal of antiparkinsonian medication. Br J Anaesth 2004;93(6):868–871.

Suchowersky O, Gronseth G, Perlmutter J, et al: Practice Parameter: Neuroprotective strategies and alternative therapies for Parkinson disease (an evidence-based review): Report of the Quality Standards Subcommittee of the American Academy of Neurology. Neurology 2006;66(7):976–982.

Tan EK, Ondo W: Clinical characteristics of pramipexole-induced peripheral edcma. Arch Neurol 2000;57:729–732.

Tanaka K, Fujita N, Yoshioka M, Ogawa N: Immunosuppressive and non-immunosuppressive immunophilin ligands improve H(2)O(2)-induced cell damage by increasing glutathione levels in NG108–15 cells. Brain Res 2001;889:225–228.

Tanaka K, Yoshioka M, Miyazaki I, et al: GPI1046 prevents dopaminergic dysfunction by activating glutathione system in the mouse striatum. Neurosci Lett 2002;321:45–48.

Tatton WG: Selegiline can mediate neuronal rescue rather than neuronal protection. Mov Disord 1993;8:S20–S30.

Thomas P, Lalaux N, Vaiva G, Goudemand M: Dose-dependent stuttering and dystonia in a patient taking clozapine. Am J Psychiatry 1994;151:1096.

Tillerson JL, Caudle WM, Reveron ME, Miller GW: Exercise induces behavioral recovery and attenuates neurochemical deficits in rodent models of Parkinson's disease. Neuroscience 2003;119(3):899–911.

Tillerson JL, Cohen AD, Caudle WM, et al: Forced nonuse in unilateral parkinsonian rats exacerbates injury. J Neurosci 2002;22(15): 6790–6799.

Tillerson JL, Cohen AD, Philhower J, et al: Forced limb-use effects on the behavioral and neurochemical effects of 6-hydroxydopamine. J Neurosci 2001 Jun 15;21(12):4427–4435.

Tilley BC, Palesch YY, Kieburtz K, et al: Optimizing the ongoing search for new treatments for Parkinson disease: Using futility designs. Neurology 2006;66(5):628–633.

Togasaki DM, Tan L, Protell P, et al: Levodopa induces dyskinesias in normal squirrel monkeys. Ann Neurol 2001;50:254–257.

Torstenson R, Hartvig P, Langstrom B, et al: Differential effects of levodopa on dopaminergic function in early and advanced Parkinson's disease. Ann Neurol 1997;41:334–340.

Ueda M, Hamamoto M, Nagayama H, et al: Biochemical alterations during medication withdrawal in Parkinson's disease with and without neuroleptic malignant-like syndrome. J Neurol Neurosurg Psychiatry 2001;71:111–113.

van Blercom N, Lasa A, Verger K, et al: Effects of gabapentin on the motor response to levodopa: A double-blind, placebo-controlled, crossover study in patients with complicated Parkinson disease. Clin Neuropharmacol 2004;27(3):124–128.

Van Camp G, Flamez A, Cosyns B, et al: Treatment of Parkinson's disease with pergolide and relation to restrictive valvular heart disease. Lancet 2004;363(9416):1179–1183.

Vila M, Jackson-Lewis V, Guegan C, et al: The role of glial cells in Parkinson's disease. Curr Opin Neurol 2001;14:483–489.

Wagner ML, Fedak MN, Sage JI, Mark MH. Complications of disease and therapy: A comparison of younger and older patients with Parkinson's disease. Ann Clin Lab Sci 1996;26:389–395.

Waldmeier P, Bozyczko-Coyne D, Williams M, Vaught JL: Recent clinical features in Parkinson's disease with apoptosis inhibitors underline the need for a paradigm shift in drug discovery for neurodegenerative diseases. Biochem Pharmacol 2006;72(10): 1197–1206.

Waldmeier PC, Spooren WPJM, Hengerer B: CGP 3466 protects dopaminergic neurons in lesion models of Parkinson's disease. Naunyn Schmiedebergs Arch Pharmacol 2000;362:526–537.

Waters CH, Sethi KD, Hauser RA, et al: Zydis selegiline reduces off time in Parkinson's disease patients with motor fluctuations: A 3-month, randomized, placebo-controlled study. Mov Disord 2004;19(4):426–432.

Watkins P: COMT inhibitors and liver toxicity. Neurology 2000;55 (suppl 4):S51–S52.

Weiner WJ: The initial treatment of Parkinson's disease should begin with levodopa. Mov Disord 1999;14:716–724.

Weiner WJ, Factor SA, Sanchez-Ramos JR, et al: Early combination therapy (bromocriptine and levodopa) does not prevent motor fluctuations in Parkinson's disease. Neurology 1993;43:21–27.

Weiner WJ, Koller WC, Perlik S, et al: Drug holiday and management of Parkinson disease. Neurology 1980;30:1257–1261.

Whone AL, Watts RL, Stoessl AJ, et al: Slower progression of Parkinson's disease with ropinirole versus levodopa: the REAL-PET study. Ann Neurol 2003;54(1):93–101.

Wu D, Jackson-Lewis V, Vila M, et al: Blockade of microglial activation is neuroprotective in the 1-methyl-4-phenyl-1,2,3,6-tetrahydropyridine mouse model of Parkinson disease. J Neurosci 2002; 22:1763–1771.

Xia XG, Harding T, Weller M, et al: Gene transfer of the JNK interacting protein-1 protects dopaminergic neurons in the MPTP model of Parkinson's disease. Proc Nat Acad Sci U S A 2001;98: 10433–10438.

Yahr MD: Evaluation of long-term therapy in Parkinson's disease: Mortality and therapeutic efficacy. In Birkmayer W, Hornykiewicz O (eds): Advances in Parkinsonism. Basle, Editiones Roche, 1976, pp 444–455.

Yoshikawa T: Free radicals and their scavengers in Parkinson's disease. Eur Neurol 1993;33:60–68.

Zanetti R, Loria D, Rosso S: Melanoma, Parkinson's disease and levodopa: Causal or spurious link? A review of the literature. Melanoma Res 2006;16(3):201–206.

Zappia M, Oliveri RL, Bosco D, et al: The long-duration response to L-dopa in the treatment of early PD. Neurology 2000;54:1910–1915.

Zigmond MJ, Hastings TG, Abercrombie ED: Neurochemical responses to 6-hydroxydopamine and L-dopa therapy: Implications for Parkinson's disease. Ann N Y Acad Sci 1992;648: 71–86.

# Chapter 7

# Surgical Treatment of Parkinson Disease and Other Movement Disorders

A variety of surgical treatments for Parkinson disease (PD), including ablation or deafferentation of motor and premotor cortex, cervical cordotomy, and mesencephalic pedunculotomy, were performed in the first five decades of the 20th century (Meyers, 1968). These procedures generally yielded relief of the movement disorder at the expense of concomitant weakness and other complications. Surgery at the level of the basal ganglia for PD was pioneered by Meyers in 1939 (Meyers, 1968). These open procedures included removal of the head of the caudate and section of the anterior limb of the internal capsule and pallidofugal pathways. After Spiegel and Wycis introduced the principles of stereotactic surgery in clinical practice in 1947, this method was applied for lesioning the pallidum and ansa lenticularis in an attempt to treat the symptoms of PD and other movement disorders (Mundinger and Reichert, 1963; Hassler et al., 1979; Grossman and Hamilton, 1991). Stereotactic thalamotomy for parkinsonian symptoms was introduced by Hassler and Riechert in 1951 (Hassler et al., 1979). Thalamotomies gradually replaced pallidotomies in the late 1950s and early 1960s (Fig. 7-1) because thalamotomies were thought to produce more sustained control of tremor. The introduction of levodopa in late 1960s resulted in marked reduction in the number of functional stereotactic procedures, and only a few specialized centers continued to perform such operations.

The renewed interest in surgical treatment of movement disorders has been stimulated in part by improved understanding of the functional anatomy underlying motor control, as well as refinement of methods and techniques in neurosurgery, neurophysiology, and neuroimaging (Krauss et al., 1998; Gross et al., 1999a; Lang, 2000b; Mazziotta, 2000; Jankovic, 2001; Krauss, Jankovic, et al., 2001; Walter and Vitek, 2004). Furthermore, important strides have been made in assessments of the outcomes of surgery and in providing useful guidelines for inclusion-exclusion criteria (Defer et al., 1999; Tan and Jankovic, 2000). As a result of increased awareness about surgical options for patients with PD, the attitudes of clinicians toward referring patients for surgery have been changing, and in one survey, 99.4% of neurologists were aware of surgery for PD (Mathew et al., 1999). Although this review focuses primarily on surgical treatment of PD, there is growing interest in the application of surgical intervention in the treatment of a variety of movement disorders (Pollak, 1999; Krauss, Simpson, et al., 2001). While the interest in surgical treatment of movement disorders is growing, there is a remarkable paucity of well-designed, randomized trials (Stowe et al., 2003).

## FUNCTIONAL ANATOMY OF THE BASAL GANGLIA

Before discussing the indications for and the results of surgery for PD, it is helpful to review the current concepts about the functional anatomy of the basal ganglia (Figs. 7-2 and 7-3). This is reviewed in detail in Chapter 3. Here the essence is reiterated to help foster an understanding of the surgical targets useful in treating PD. The basal ganglia include the striatum, globus pallidus, substantia nigra, subthalamic nucleus (STN), and thalamus (Parent and Cicchetti, 1998; Hamani et al., 2004). The caudate and putamen are contiguous and comprise the striatum, and the putamen and globus pallidus are referred to as the lenticular nucleus. The cortical input from the prefrontal supplementary motor area, amygdala, and hippocampus is excitatory, mediated by glutamate. Neurons in the substantia nigra pars compacta provide major dopaminergic input to the striatum. The interaction between the afferent and efferent pathways is mediated by striatal interneurons that utilize acetylcholine as the main neurotransmitter. The substantia nigra is a melanin-containing (pigmented) nucleus in the ventral midbrain, and it consists of dopaminergic neurons. The striatal output system is mediated by the inhibitory neurotransmitter γ-amino-butyric acid (GABA). However, the basal ganglia appear to be more complex than is indicated by the current models (Parent and Cichetti, 1998). For example, it is now well recognized that the STN provides powerful excitatory projection not only to the globus pallidus interna (GPi) but also to the striatum and globus pallidus externum (GPe) and, in turn, receives input from the cerebral cortex, substantia nigra pars compacta, and various brainstem and thalamic nuclei. Although most reports emphasize the pallidal-thalamic projection, major output from the GPi is to the brainstem nuclei, such as the pedunculopontine nucleus (Jenkinson et al., 2004; Mena-Segovia et al., 2004). These complex interactions must be taken into account to explain the mechanisms of the various surgical interventions in the treatment of PD.

The reemergence of surgical treatment of PD, particularly pallidotomy and STN/GPi deep brain stimulation (DBS) (see later), has been fueled in part by improved understanding of basal ganglia circuitry, including the recognition that the STN and the GPi are overactive in experimental and human parkinsonism (Bergman et al., 1990; Limousin et al., 1995). Microelectrode-guided single-cell recordings in patients with PD showed that the average firing rate in the GPi was $91 \pm 52$ Hz and that in the GPe was $60 \pm 21$ Hz (Magnin et al., 2000). In addition, rhythmic, low-threshold calcium spike bursts are often recorded in the pallidum and medial thalamus; some but not all are synchronous (in phase) with the typical rest tremor. It has been postulated that the low-threshold calcium spike bursts contribute to rigidity and dystonia by activating the supplementary motor area. Apomorphine, a dopamine agonist, has been found to suppress the abnormal hyperactivity of the GPi and STN and to enhance the activity of the GPe on the basis of cellular recordings during surgery (Lozano et al., 2000). However, marked or complete suppression of GPi activity is

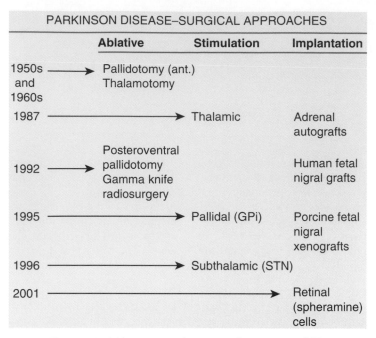

PARKINSON DISEASE–SURGICAL APPROACHES

| | Ablative | Stimulation | Implantation |
|---|---|---|---|
| 1950s and 1960s | Pallidotomy (ant.) Thalamotomy | | |
| 1987 | | Thalamic | Adrenal autografts |
| 1992 | Posteroventral pallidotomy Gamma knife radiosurgery | | Human fetal nigral grafts |
| 1995 | | Pallidal (GPi) | Porcine fetal nigral xenografts |
| 1996 | | Subthalamic (STN) | |
| 2001 | | | Retinal (spheramine) cells |

**Figure 7-1** Milestones in the surgical treatment of PD.

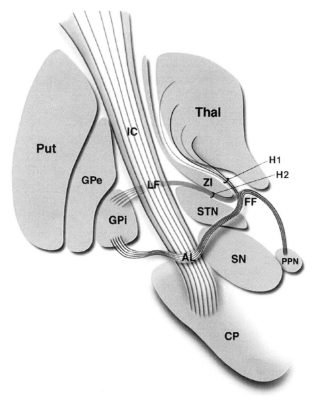

**Figure 7-2** Representation of the major anatomic structures and fiber tracts associated with the STN. AL, ansa lenticularis; CP, cerebral peduncle; FF, fields of Forel; GPe, globus pallidus externus; GPi, globus pallidus internus; H1, H1 field of Forel (thalamic fasciculus); IC, internal capsule; LF, lenticular fasciculus (H2); PPN, pedunculopontine nucleus; Put, putamen; SN, substantia nigra; STN, subthalamic nucleus; Thal, thalamus; ZI, zona incerta. (Reprinted with permission from Hamani C, Saint-Cyr JA, Fraser J, et al: The subthalamic nucleus in the context of movement disorders. Brain 2004;127:4–20.)

associated with an emergence of dyskinesias. Indeed, levodopa- or dopamine-induced dyskinesias are associated with decreased firing frequency of the GPi neurons and a modification in the firing pattern (Boraud et al., 2001). This suggests that dopaminergic drugs and pallidotomy improve parkinsonian symptoms through a similar mechanism. Single-cell recording of the STN in patients with PD showed characteristic somatotopic organization, with neurons responding to sensorimotor stimuli localized chiefly in the dorsolateral region, and were of the irregular or tonic type (Rodriguez-Oroz et al., 2001). These two groups of neurons represent 60.5% and 24% of all STN neurons, respectively; only 15.5% of the STN neurons are oscillatory. Oscillatory activity in the basal ganglia is attracting more and more attention on the basis of various surgery-related neurophysiologic studies (Dostrovsky and Bergman, 2004). Microinjection of 10 to 23 μL of lidocaine into the STN of three patients with PD produced "striking improvements in bradykinesia, limb tremor and rigidity" in all (Levy et al., 2001). Furthermore, microinjections of 5 to 10 μL of muscimol, a GABA$_A$ receptor agonist, in the region of the STN that showed oscillatory activity resulted in suppression of contralateral tremor in two patients. Simultaneous microelectrode recordings showed suppression of neuronal activity in the near vicinity (up to 1.3 mm) of the injection. In a study designed to explore the effects of GPi on the STN, Sterio and colleagues (2002) showed that GPi stimulation markedly reduced the firing rate of dorsal STN cells in the ventral STN (and substantia nigra pars reticulata). In addition to providing support for STN segregation, this suggests that there is a feedforward GPi-STN interaction that needs to be incorporated in revised models of functional anatomy of the basal ganglia. The oscillatory nature of human basal ganglia activity in relationship to movement has been recently reviewed (Brown et al., 2003). Some studies have also drawn attention to the role of the pedunculopontine nucleus in gait and locomotion. Although this has been reported to provide improvement in gait in monkeys, targeting this brainstem nucleus for therapeutic purposes in patients with

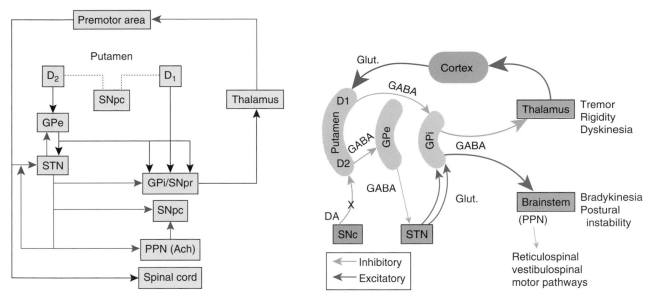

**Figure 7-3** Functional anatomy of basal ganglia circuitry relevant to PD. Ach, acetylcholine; D1, D2, dopamine receptors; GABA, γ-amino-butyric acid; Glut, glutamate; GPe, globus pallidus externus; GPi, globus pallidus internus; PPN, pedunculopontine nucleus; STN, subthalamic nucleus; SN, substantia nigra pars compacta (pc) and pars reticularis (pr).

PD or other movement disorders associated with gait difficulty will be technically challenging (Jenkinson et al., 2004).

The basal ganglia models in dystonia are even less clear; some studies have found that the GPi neuronal activity is increased in dystonia (Sanghera et al., 2003), whereas other studies have failed to find any decrease in basal ganglia output (Hutchison et al., 2003). Neurophysiologic studies performed during STN DBS have found that the STN receives direct input from the supplementary motor area and is thus involved in movement preparation, as demonstrated by recorded activity in the nucleus before voluntary movement (Paradiso et al., 2003).

Posteroventral pallidotomy (PVP) as well as GPi and STN DBS (see later) improve motor performance in patients with PD, presumably by interrupting inhibitory pallidal projections to the ventrolateral thalamus. This is supported by measurements by positron emission tomography (PET) of regional cerebral blood flow showing increased activity of supplementary motor area and premotor cortex (but not in primary motor cortex) after pallidotomy (Grafton et al., 1995;

Eidelberg et al., 1996). One possible explanation for the apparent improvement of parkinsonian features after STN or GPi ablation or simulation is that the reduced excitability of the GPe in PD prevents the normal "brake" on STN firing and leads to overactivation of the STN and GPi. Despite clear understanding of the mechanisms, surgical approaches are increasingly used in the treatment of patients with PD who fail to obtain satisfactory relief from pharmacologic therapy (Krauss and Jankovic, 1996; Hallett et al., 1999) (Table 7-1).

## TECHNIQUES OF STEREOTACTIC SURGERY

Stereotactic surgery is based on a Cartesian coordinate system, which implies that any point in space may be determined by three right-angled planes defined as the *x*, *y*, and *z* axes (Krauss and Jankovic, 1996). Functional stereotactic surgery relies on the acquisition of data from various imaging modalities and its transfer to the Cartesian coordinates referenced to an apparatus, the stereotactic frame, which is rigidly fixed to the patient's head (Hassler et al., 1979; Grossman and Hamilton, 1991). By using computed tomography, magnetic resonance imaging (MRI), or positive-contrast ventriculography, the target coordinates for functional stereotactic surgery are determined by extrapolation referring to the coordinates of the anterior and posterior commissure. The data for the spatial relation of the target to the anterior and posterior commissure are derived from stereotactic atlases. For example, the STN target, used chiefly for STN DBS, is 10 to 12 mm lateral and 2 to 3 mm posterior to the midcommissural point and 2 to 4 mm below the AC-PC line. Some surgeons have also advocated the use of the red nucleus as an internal marker for targeting the optimal region of STN stimulation (Andrade-Souza et al., 2005).

To improve the accuracy despite normal anatomic variability, physiologic verification of the target by microelectrode recordings of spontaneous neuronal activity or by electric

**Table 7-1** Results of surgical treatment for Parkinson disease

| Indication | Thalamotomy VIM DBS | Pallidotomy GPi DBS | STN DBS | Brain Grafts* |
|---|---|---|---|---|
| Bradykinesia | 0 | + | ++ | + |
| Tremor | +++ | ++ | +++ | + |
| Rigidity | + | ++ | ++ | + |
| PIGD | – | + | 0 | – |
| Freezing | 0 | + | + | 0 |
| Dyskinesia | ++ | +++ | +++ (↓L-Dopa) | † |

*Based on a double-blind study (Columbia and University of Colorado).

†Some patient experience dyskinesia even without levodopa.

–, deterioration; 0, no improvement; +, mild improvement; ++, moderate improvement; +++, marked improvement.

stimulation has been considered critical by some (Tasker, 1993; Obeso et al., 1998; Starr et al., 1998; Vitek et al., 2004), but other investigators believe that stereotactic surgery can be performed safely and effectively without microelectrode recording, using MRI-directed targeting (Dewey et al., 2000; Patel et al., 2003b; Hamid et al., 2005).

Different types of stereotactic devices are available. Functional stereotactic operations are generally performed under local anesthesia to allow examination of the patient during the physiologic investigations and during application of the lesions. In some cases, generalized anesthesia may be used safely (Maltete et al., 2004). The choice of the target and the techniques for calculation of the target as well as for physiologic localization differ (Mundinger and Reichert, 1963; Hassler et al., 1979; Grossman and Hamilton, 1991; Tasker, 1993; Tasker and Kiss, 1995). Usually, the target is chosen contralateral to the side that is more severely affected. The stereotactic frame is fixed to the skull with screws. The patient then undergoes stereotactic computed tomography scanning. While the coordinates of the target are calculated, the patient is brought back to the operating room. A small area of the head in the frontal region is shaved. A precoronal parasagittal burrhole is made via a linear incision under local anesthesia. The arch of the stereotactic device is fixed to the frame and the electrode for recording, or stimulation is directed to the precalculated target via a cannula. The tip of the microelectrode that is used for recording has a diameter of 0.01 mm, whereas the tip of the electrode that is used to produce the lesion has a diameter of 1.1 mm. After physiologic localization of the target, one to three lesions are made along the trajectory, heating the tip of the electrode to 75°C for 60 seconds. The symptomatic improvement, particularly the cessation of tremor or levodopa-induced dyskinesia, reduced rigidity, and improved performance of rapid succession movements, is usually noted immediately after placing the lesion. It is advisable to operate when the patient is "off" (before taking his or her morning dose of medication), since the effect of the surgery can be assessed more readily. The duration of the procedure varies between 2 to 3 hours for a standard thalamotomy and 4 to 5 hours for a pallidotomy. The hospital stay varies between 2 and 5 days.

## THALAMOTOMY

Prior to the advent of levodopa therapy for PD, thalamotomy offered the most effective means of controlling disabling and embarrassing tremor. Stereotactic thalamotomy has been refined substantially since its introduction in 1947 as a result of improvements in neuroimaging and electrophysiologic and surgical techniques. The application of the procedure has broadened to disorders other than tremor, particularly dystonia, hemiballism, and severe levodopa-induced dyskinesias (Cardoso et al., 1995; Jankovic, 1998; Krauss and Grossman, 1998; Starr et al., 1998; Jankovic, Lai, Krauss, et al., 1999). The outcome of 60 patients with medically intractable tremor who underwent a total of 62 stereotactic thalamotomies at Baylor College of Medicine was analyzed (Jankovic et al., 1995). The ventral intermediate (VIM) nucleus of the thalamus was the target in all patients. The patients were followed for as long as 13 years (mean: 53.4 months) after their surgery. At the most recent follow-up visit, 36 of 42 (86%) patients with PD, 5 of 6

(83%) with essential tremor (ET), 4 of 6 (67%) with cerebellar outflow tremor, and 3 of 6 (50%) with posttraumatic tremor had complete cessation of or moderate to marked improvement in their contralateral tremor. Patients who were taking levodopa ($n = 35$ patients) were able to reduce their daily dose by approximately 156 mg. Immediate postoperative complications, such as contralateral weakness (34%), dysarthria (29%), and confusion (23%), occurred in 58% of the 60 patients; these complications usually resolved rapidly during the postoperative period. These results are consistent with other reports, confirming the beneficial effects of thalamotomy on tremor and rigidity but no effect on bradykinesia in patients with PD (Zirh et al., 1999). Thalamotomy was also considered to be modestly effective in reducing the amplitude of kinetic tremor associated with multiple sclerosis (Alusi et al., 2001; Matsumoto et al., 2001). Furthermore, thalamotomy may improve levodopa-induced dyskinesia. Improved localization of the cluster of thalamic neurons with the largest amount of tremor discharges, correlated with electromyographic activity, should produce even better results. The likelihood of marked or complete tremor relief is high when the thalamic lesion is made within 2 mm of this site (Lenz et al., 1995). High-frequency stimulation (to be discussed later) rather than lesioning of the thalamic nuclei may be more effective and safer in the treatment of tremor (Schuurman et al., 2000). Since bilateral thalamotomy can cause hypophonia, dysarthria, and dysphagia, DBS is emerging as a useful alternative in those patients who require bilateral procedures. Thalamotomy has the advantage over DBS in that there is no need for hardware; and for patients with disabling bilateral tremor, unilateral thalamotomy in combination with contralateral DBS may offer the optimal tremor control with the fewest adverse side effects. Finally, microinjections of muscimol into the region of VIM thalamus that contains the tremor-synchronous cells consistently reduced tremor, suggesting that GABA agonists might be useful in the treatment of tremor (Pahapill et al., 1999).

## ABLATIVE LESIONS OF THE PALLIDUM AND SUBTHALAMIC NUCLEUS

Although a common procedure in the 1950s and 1960s, anterior pallidotomy was later abandoned because of inconsistent results, particularly concerning tremor, and because of improved results with posterior pallidotomy and later with DBS (Okun and Vitek, 2004). While some investigators had noted improvement of bradykinesia, this observation was not described by others (Hassler et al., 1979). Most surgeons at that time targeted the anterior dorsal portion of the GPi. More favorable results, with improvement of rigidity, bradykinesia, and tremor, were reported by the group of Leksell, who had chosen a different target, namely, the posterior and ventral aspect of the GPi. After Laitinen had reevaluated Leksell's approach in the early 1990s (Laitinen et al., 1992), pallidotomy was quickly reintroduced in North America and Europe (Sterio et al., 1994; Dogali et al., 1995; Lozano et al., 1995). Lesioning of the most ventral segment of the GPi provides the most antidyskinetic effect (Kishore et al., 2000).

The tentative target in the posteroventral GPi is located most commonly between 20 to 21 mm lateral to the midline,

4 to 5 mm below the intercommissural line, and 2 to 3 mm anterior to the midcommissural point. The accurate localization of the target within the pallidum is essential not only for optimal therapeutic results but also to avoid lesioning of adjacent structures. Single-cell microelectrode recording helps in delineating the borders of the GPi (Alterman et al., 1999). Different neuronal signals are identified along the pathway through the putamen, GPe, and GPi (Grafton et al., 1995). Cells with bursting discharges and low-frequency activity interrupted by pauses are characteristic for the GPe, while irregular, high-frequency discharges at a frequency of 60 to 130 Hz mark the GPi. GPi neurons may change their firing rates on movements of various joints of the limbs. It is particularly important to identify the ventral border of the GPi and the adjacent optic tract, which might be located at a distance of only 2 to 3 mm from the derived target. Stimulation via the microelectrode, which may elicit visual phenomena, is also helpful in recognizing the optic tract. The mapping might require several trajectories before the final localization for the lesion is determined. Then the radiofrequency lesioning electrode is advanced, and "macrostimulation" is applied to identify whether and at what threshold the electric current spreads to the adjacent internal capsule. If no unwanted responses are encountered, the final lesion is then made.

Because of the importance of proper localization, several reports have raised concerns about the role of gamma knife (GK) in the treatment of various movement disorders (Friedman et al., 1996; Okun et al., 2001). Okun and colleagues (2001) described eight patients who, over a period of 6 months, were treated with GK surgery for PD and developed serious complications; one died as a result of aspiration pneumonia secondary to dysphagia. Other complications included hemiplegia, hemianopsia, limb weakness, speech and voice impairment, sensory deficit, and uncontrollable laughter. The authors concluded that these complications were related in all cases to missing the intended target and a resultant involvement of adjacent structures. Some problems may also relate to delayed effects of radiation necrosis, which might not have been fully appreciated in earlier reports on GK. Since their report represents only a small subset of patients treated with GK in their institution, the overall frequency of GK-related complications is not known. Nevertheless, this study sounds a loud alarm by drawing attention to the possibility that this procedure, often promoted as safer than the surgical treatment requiring penetration of the skull and brain parenchyma with a lesioning or stimulating electrode, can be associated with serious complications. This study must be interpreted cautiously, however, as this is not a controlled study in which patients are randomized to receive GK, ablative procedure, or DBS. Nevertheless, the report by Okun and colleagues (2001) is important because it highlights two major limitations of GK in the treatment of movement disorders: It does not allow microelectrode recordings to verify the location of the target, and it is associated with an unacceptably high rate of immediate and delayed complications. GK thalamotomy has been reported to improve essential tremor and action tremor associated with multiple sclerosis (Niranjan et al., 2000) and with other movement disorders (Friedman et al., 1999).

Lesioning of the posteroventral portion of the GPi (Laitinen et al., 1992; Dogali et al., 1995; Iacono et al., 1995; Lozano et al., 1995; Baron et al., 1996; Lai et al., 1996; Olanow, 1996; Kishore et al., 1997; Lang et al., 1997; Uitti

et al., 1997; Kumar et al., 1998b; Materman et al., 1998; Starr et al., 1998; Bronstein et al., 1999; Dalvi et al., 1999; Gross et al., 1999b; Hallett et al., 1999; Lang et al., 1999; Samii et al., 1999; Schrag et al., 1999; Lai et al., 2000; Counihan et al., 2001) and the STN (Bergman et al., 1990; Guridi et al., 1993; Limousin et al., 1995; Obeso et al., 1998; Alverez et al., 2001; Barlas et al., 2001; Guridi and Obeso, 2001) has an advantage over thalamotomy because this procedure improves not only tremor but also bradykinesia and rigidity. Although some investigators (Subramanian et al., 1995) have suggested that PVP is as effective as thalamotomy in controlling parkinsonian tremor, others (Dogali et al., 1995) feel that pallidotomy provides only partial relief of tremor. The latter authors suggest, however, that thalamotomy has a higher complication rate, particularly with respect to dysarthria and impairment of balance. In one series, only 6 of 60 (10%) patients had persistent dysarthria, and none had persistent loss of balance (Jankovic et al., 1995). However, because the two procedures have never been compared in a controlled fashion, it is difficult to comment on possible differences in efficacy and complication rates.

When a lesion is precisely localized to the GPi by neuroimaging (Krauss et al., 1997; Desaloms et al., 1998; Kondziolka et al., 1999) or by microelectrode recording techniques (Lang et al., 1997), the benefits can be quite dramatic. Subsequent follow-up of 39 patients who were followed for 6 months, 27 who were followed for 1 year, and 11 who were followed for 2 years provided additional evidence of long-term efficacy of this procedure (Lang et al., 1997). There was a 28% reduction in the "off" motor score in 6 months and an 82% improvement in contralateral "on" dyskinesias. The motor improvement was generally sustained during the 2-year follow-up, although the improvement in ipsilateral and axial symptoms gradually waned. In another study of 15 PD patients who were followed postoperatively for 1 year, the total Unified Parkinson's Disease Rating Scale (UPDRS) score improved by 30% at 3 months, and the score remained improved at 1 year ($P < .001$) (Baron et al., 1996). In addition, there was a marked improvement in contralateral rigidity, tremor, and bradykinesia as well as improvement in gait, balance, and freezing. Although contralateral dyskinesia and tremor remain improved, all other symptoms of PD usually worsen 3 years after the surgery (Pal et al., 2000).

The most robust beneficial effect of pallidotomy is improvement in levodopa-induced dyskinesia (Jankovic, Lai, Ben-Arie, et al., 1999; Jankovic, Lai, Krauss, et al., 1999; Fine et al., 2000; Lai et al., 2000; Lang, 2000a; Counihan et al., 2001). At Baylor College of Medicine, 101 consecutive patients who underwent PVP procedures and who returned for at least one postoperative evaluation after 3 months were evaluated (Lai et al., 2000). All had standardized clinical evaluations within 1 week before surgery and every 3 to 6 months after surgery. Data were collected during "on" and practically defined "off" periods for the UPDRS, Hoehn and Yahr stage, Schwab and England Activities of Daily Living (ADL) scale, and movement and reaction time. In addition, the severity and anatomic distribution of dyskinesia, neuropsychological status, average percentage of "on" time with and without dyskinesia, and clinical global impression were assessed during a longitudinal follow-up. Eighty-nine patients (46 men and 43 women) underwent unilateral PVP, and 12 patients (6 men and 6 women) had staged bilateral PVP. At 3 months after unilateral or staged bilateral PVP, 84 of the 101 patients reported marked or moderate improvement in their parkinsonian symptoms. Postoperative UPDRS mean total motor score improved in the "off" state by 35.5%, and the mean ADL score improved by 33.7% ($P < .001$). Rigidity, bradykinesia, and tremor scores also markedly improved after PVP, particularly on the contralateral side. Levodopa-induced dyskinesia was markedly reduced, while daily "on" time increased by 34.5% ($P < .001$). Seven patients had transient perioperative complications, including confusion, expressive aphasia, pneumonia, and visual changes. Improvements in parkinsonian symptoms were maintained in both "off" and "on" states in 67 patients at 12 months after PVP and in 46 patients who were followed for a mean period of 26.3 months. Patients who underwent staged bilateral PVP benefited further from the second procedure. Five of 12 patients experienced some adverse event. On the basis of this large series of patients with extended follow-up, the authors concluded that PVP is an effective and relatively safe treatment for medically resistant PD, especially for dopa-induced dyskinesia, tremor, rigidity, and bradykinesia. Motor fluctuations also improved. Benefits were most noticeable on the side contralateral to the PVP. Sustained (>1 year) improvement in motor function after bilateral pallidotomy has also been demonstrated by others (Counihan et al., 2001). Clinical improvement has been sustained for longer than 2 years. In a "blinded" review of videotapes, Ondo and colleagues (1998b) showed a significant improvement in "off" UPDRS scores in patients undergoing pallidotomy. Unilateral pallidotomy was found to be an effective treatment in a randomized, single-blind, multicenter trial (de Bie et al., 1999). In comparison to a control group that did not receive surgery, the pallidotomy patients improved their UPDRS 3 "off" motor score from 47 to 32.5, whereas the score in the control group increased from 52.5 to 56.5 ($P < .0001$). Furthermore, "on" UPDRS scores improved by 50%, chiefly as a result of marked improvement in dyskinesias. Most important, there was a significant improvement in the quality of life in patients who were treated surgically in comparison to those who were treated medically. In a follow-up study, the investigators showed that the benefits persist for at least 1 year and that patients with 1000 levodopa equivalent units or lower were most likely to improve (de Bie et al., 2001). An improvement in the quality of life, using various measures, has been demonstrated by other pallidotomy series (Martinez-Martin et al., 2000). This improvement may persist for up to 5.5 years (Baron et al., 2000; Fine et al., 2000). The longest follow-up, over 10 years, after pallidotomy showed that while the patients clearly benefited from the procedure, the levodopa dosage had to be increased as a result of the disease progression, and most patients gradually became troubled by various mental and medical complications associated with the disease and aging (Hariz and Bergenheim, 2001). In a randomized trial of pallidotomy versus medical therapy, Vitek and colleagues (2003) found pallidotomy more effective as suggested by a 32% reduction in total UPDRS compared to 5% at 6 months.

Pallidotomy improves not only levodopa-induced dyskinesias but also PD-related bradykinesia. This is best demonstrated by the finding of improved movement time and reaction time during the practically defined "off" state following pallidotomy (Jankovic, Ben-Arie, et al., 1999). Unilateral pallidotomy was also associated with improved simple and choice reaction times during the optimal "on" period (Hayashi et al., 2003). Kimber and colleagues (1999) suggested that the improvement in bradykinesia after pallidotomy may be explained by "greater efficacy of external cues in facilitating movement after withdrawal of the abnormal pallidal discharge." Pfann and colleagues (1998) also showed that "off" bradykinesia improves after pallidotomy but could not demonstrate any improvement in "on" bradykinesia. A remarkable improvement in freezing contralateral to the lesion in several patients as well as objective evidence of benefits in gait and balance has been seen (Robert-Warrior et al., 2000; Jankovic et al., 2001). Improvements in gait (Baron et al., 1996; Siegel and Verhagen Metman, 2000) and postural stability (Melnick et al., 1999) were also reported in other pallidotomy series (Bakker et al., 2004).

Pallidotomy requires a multidisciplinary approach involving skilled neurologists, neurosurgeons, neuroradiologists, physiologists, physiatrists, and nurses to obtain optimal results (Bronstein et al., 1999). Even when performed by a team of experienced clinicians, pallidotomy can be associated with potentially serious complications. The reported complications include transient confusion, hemiparesis, expressive aphasia, pneumonia, and visual changes, such as homonymous hemianopia, facial paresis, and hemiparesis (Laitinen et al., 1992; Shannon et al., 1998). Cognitive function and various neuropsychological measures have been studied extensively in patients following surgery for PD, and these domains have been found to be generally preserved, particularly after unilateral pallidotomy (Masterman et al., 1998; Perrine et al., 1998; Rettig et al., 1998; York et al., 1999; Lombardi et al., 2000; Rettig et al., 2000; Saint-Cyr and Trépanier, 2000; Green et al., 2002), although subtle changes in verbal fluency and possibly executive functions have been noted after left pallidotomy (Schmand et al., 2000) and after bilateral pallidotomy (Scott et al., 1998). Staged bilateral pallidotomy, although beneficial in most patients, results in increased risk of complications, particularly worsening of speech and other bulbar functions (Intemann et al., 2001). Bilateral simultaneous pallidotomy may be associated with even more frequent and severe complications, such as depression, obsessive-compulsive disorder, abulia, pseudobulbar palsy, apraxia of eyelid opening, and visual field deficits (Ghika et al., 1999). In a systematic review of morbidity and mortality associated with unilateral pallidotomy, de Bie and colleagues (2002) found that the risk of permanent adverse effects was 13.8%, and symptomatic infarction or hemorrhage occurred in 3.9%; mortality was 1.2%. Several investigators have used implanted DBS electrodes to produce lesions in the thalamus for treating tremor and in the pallidum for treating levodopa-induced dyskinesias (Raoul et al., 2003). Although pallidotomy is used primarily to improve parkinsonian symptoms and levodopa-induced dyskinesias, bilateral pallidal lesions in otherwise normal individuals result in inadequate anticipatory and compensatory postural reflexes, bradykinesia, and other signs of motor impairment (Haaxma et al., 1995). This apparent paradox is difficult to explain with the current models of basal ganglia circuitry, but it suggests that nigrostriatal dopaminergic deficiency causing activation of the GPi is a necessary prerequisite for the beneficial effects of pallidotomy.

The mechanism by which pallidotomy improves levodopa-induced dyskinesia is not known, but single-cell recordings in the GPi of parkinsonian monkeys show a marked reduction in firing rates only when dyskinesias were present (Papa et al., 1999).

The average firing rate decreased from 46 Hz during the "off" state to 26 Hz during the "on" state and to 7.6 Hz during dyskinesia. It has been hypothesized that either overactive GPi (in a parkinsonian state) or low GPi activity (during dyskinesias) results in an abnormal ("noisy") input to the thalamocortical circuit. Pallidotomy tends to eliminate the "noise" and "normalize" the output.

Since pallidotomy has such a robust effect on levodopa-induced dyskinesia, including dystonia, the procedure has been applied in the treatment of primary and secondary dystonia (Jankovic, 1998; Ondo, Desaloms, et al., 2001; Yoshor et al., 2001). In a series of patients with generalized dystonia, about 50% improvement on various dystonia rating scales was observed following pallidotomy (Ondo et al., 1998a). Some patients, particularly those with primary generalized dystonia, however, had a marked improvement, and as a result of the surgery, their dystonia-related disability changed from a dependent state to completely independent functioning. Since the greatest effect of GPi ablation or DBS is on levodopa-induced dyskinesias, these procedures have also been tried in the treatment of other hyperkinesias, such as generalized dystonia (Jankovic, 1998; Coubes et al., 2000; Ondo, Desaloms, et al., 2001; Albright, 2003; Coubes et al., 2004; Vidailhet et al., 2005), cervical dystonia (Krauss et al., 1999; Parkin et al., 2001; Krauss et al., 2002), chorea and ballism (Thompson et al., 2000; Hashimoro et al., 2001; Krauss and Mundinger, 2001), and tics associated with Tourette syndrome (Cosgrove and Rauch, 2001).

High-frequency stimulation of the subthalamic nucleus (STN) has become an accepted treatment option for patients with moderately advanced PD (see later), but subthalamotomy has not been studied extensively. Because of its key role in the pathogenesis of PD, the STN has become a primary target for surgical treatment of PD. Although hemichorea/hemiballism is a well-recognized complication of a lesion in the STN, such hyperkinesias are very rare when the STN is lesioned (or stimulated) in the setting of PD (Barlas et al., 2001; Guridi and Obeso, 2001). This suggests that as a result of reduced activity of the "direct" GABAergic pathway from the striatum to the GPi, the parkinsonian state increases the threshold for such hyperkinesias. In PD, STN lesion reduces excitation of the GPi and simultaneously further reduces the hypoactivity of the Gpe, compensating for the GPi hypoactivity, self-stabilizing the basal ganglia output, and reducing the risk of hemichorea/hemiballism. Alvarez and colleagues (2005) reported their experience in 11 patients after unilateral dorsal subthalamotomy. They found a significant reduction in UPDRS score, which was maintained in four patients for 24 months. Despite the location of the lesion, the procedure was not complicated by hemiballism. In another study, unilateral dorsal subthalamotomy, particularly when combined with lesions in the H2 field of Forel and the zona incerta, resulted in a marked improvement in contralateral tremor, rigidity, and bradykinesia (Patel et al., 2003a). In one patient, a lesion confined to the STN produced "dyskinesia" that required H2/zona incerta DBS. In a series of 12 patients who underwent unilateral subthalamotomy, Su and colleagues (2003) showed a 30% to 38% improvement in UPDRS II and UPDRS III and an 85% improvement in dyskinesia, with a 42% reduction in levodopa dosage. The benefits persisted for about 18 months. Complications included three (25%) cases of hemiballism; two of these patients recovered spontaneously,

and one died of aspiration pneumonia. In a long-term (>3 years) follow-up of 18 patients with PD, bilateral subthalamotomy was associated with a significant improvement of ADL, reduction of levodopa-related dyskinesia by 50%, and lowering of levodopa dose by 47%, but the response was quite variable (Alvarez et al., 2005). One potential advantage of subthalamotomy compared to pallidotomy is that the latter may adversely affect subsequent response to levodopa, DBS, or other restorative therapies, since these depend on the normal function of the outflow nuclei. Subthalamotomy, however, also seems to reduce the metabolic activity of the ipsilateral GPi, midbrain, pons, and thalamus (Su et al., 2001).

## DEEP BRAIN STIMULATION

Ablative procedures, such as thalamotomy and pallidotomy, are gradually being replaced by DBS, a high-frequency stimulation of the VIM nucleus of the thalamus, GPi, STN, or other subcortical nuclei, depending on the desired effects (Benabid et al., 1991; Caparros-Lefebvre et al., 1993; Limousin et al., 1995; Benabid et al., 1996; Koller et al., 1997; Krack et al., 1998a, 1998b; Limousin et al., 1998; Ondo et al., 1998c; Pollak et al., 1998; Starr et al., 1998; Tasker, 1998; Volkmann et al., 1998; Koller et al., 1999; Limousin et al., 1999; Deep-Brain Stimulation for Parkinson's Disease Study Group, 2001; Krauss, Jankovic, et al., 2001; Lopiano et al., 2001; Volkmann et al., 2001; Kumar, 2002; Okun and Foote, 2005) (Box 7-1). Chronic high-frequency stimulation of the thalamic VIM nucleus as a treatment for parkinsonian and other tremors has been introduced in clinical practice by Benabid and colleagues (Benabid et al., 1991). It has long been known that high-frequency (>100 Hz) stimulation employed during thalamotomies at the site of the planned lesion temporarily suppresses tremor (Mundinger and Reichert, 1963; Meyers, 1968; Hassler et al., 1979). This observation led to the application of chronic thalamic stimulation in the treatment of movement disorders in the 1960s, and this procedure was later adopted for the treatment of chronic pain. Hypothalamic DBS is currently used for the treatment of various pain disorders, including migraines and cluster headaches (Leone et al., 2003).

DBS involves the implantation of the following hardware: (1) a DBS lead with four electrodes that are surgically

Box 7-1 Advantages and disadvantages of deep brain stimulation

**Advantages**
Immediate symptomatic and functional improvement
Stimulation is adjustable and can be customized
Lower risk of lesion-related complications
Lower risk with bilateral procedure

**Disadvantages**
Long-term outcome unclear
Replacement of batteries
Implantation of a foreign body (hardware)
Cost to the patient and the neurologist
Limited coverage by Medicare and other insurance carriers

inserted into the desired target and fixed at the skull with a ring and cap, (2) an extension wire that passes from the scalp area under the skin to the chest, and (3) an implantable pulse generator, a pacemaker-like device (unilateral Soletra or bilateral Kinetra, Medtronic Activa, ITREL model), which can deliver pulses with adjustable parameters (frequency, amplitude, width, modes, and polarities) (Kumar, 2002; Vesper et al., 2002). The implantable pulse generator is placed under the skin in the upper chest area near the collarbone. The patient can activate or deactivate the DBS system by placing a magnet or Access Review Device, a small mouse-like computer, over the chest area overlying the implantable pulse generator. To measure the efficacy of DBS, several quality-of-life instruments have been developed and are currently being evaluated (Kuehler et al., 2003; Diamond and Jankovic, 2005). The cost associated with STN DBS has been estimated to be about $60,000 per patient over 5 years (McIntosh et al., 2003).

The mechanism of benefits of DBS produced by the electrical stimulation is not known, but the following explanations have been offered: (1) disruption of the network ("jamming" of feedback loop from the periphery), (2) depolarization block, (3) functional ablation by desynchronizing a tremorogenic pacemaker, (4) preferential activation of large axons that inhibit GPi neurons, and (5) stimulation-evoked release of GABA (Dostrovsky et al., 2002; Garcia et al., 2005). In support of the fourth hypothesis is the observation in one patient in whom stimulation inhibited GPi firing recorded with another microelectrode 600 to 1000 μm away (Wu et al., 2001). The effects of stimulation appear to be restricted to an area of 2 to 3 mm from the macroelectrode (at 2 mA, 2 V, and impedance of 1000 ohms). This would be similar to a bipolar stimulation with two adjacent contacts 1.5 mm apart. More recent studies suggest that the observed 15- to 30-Hz oscillations of the STN might reflect synchronization with cortical beta oscillation via the corticosubthalamic pathway and might relate to mechanisms of bradykinesia, since stimulation at the 15-Hz rate worsens bradykinesia and dopaminergic drugs promote faster oscillations (about 70 Hz) and improve bradykinesia, similar to the high-frequency stimulation associated with DBS (Farmer, 2002; Levy et al., 2002). Studying the effects of STN DBS in MPTP monkeys, Hashimoto and colleagues (2003) showed that the activation of the STN efferent fibers results in a change in firing pattern of pallidal neurons, and they postulated that this could underlie the beneficial effects of chronic STN DBS. In contrast to the popular notion that DBS inhibits the target nucleus, DBS has been shown actually to activate the cerebellothalamocortical pathway (Molnar et al., 2004). Indeed, recent studies have suggested that stimulation-induced, time-locked modulation of pathologic network activity represents the most likely mechanism of the effects of DBS (McIntyre et al., 2004). DBS could have a dual effect, switching off a pathologically disrupted activity but also imposing a new discharge (in the upper γ-band frequency) that results in beneficial effects (Garcia et al., 2005). The frequency of stimulation might markedly influence the effects. For example, low-frequency (0.1 to 30 Hz) stimulation of STN has been shown to depolarize glutamatergic and GABAergic synaptic terminals, evoking excitatory and inhibitory postsynaptic potentials. Animal studies have shown that STN DBS (130 Hz for 1 hour) increases extracellular dopamine in the ipsilateral denervated striatum (Meissner et al., 2003). Although this has not yet been confirmed in patients, indirect

evidence from [¹¹C]raclopride PET studies has not indicated that STN DBS induces dopamine release (Hilker et al., 2003). In untreated parkinsonian animals and patients, the neuronal activity in STN and GPi is dominated by low-frequency (11 to 30 Hz) oscillation that is increased with levodopa to >70 Hz. The therapeutic effects of high-frequency DBS might be mediated through the same mechanism (Brown et al., 2004).

The placement of the electrode can be verified radiographically. Although computed tomography scan, rather than MRI, has been recommended by Medtronic, several studies have concluded that MRI can be safely performed in patients with implanted neurostimulation systems (Tronnier et al., 1999; Jech et al., 2001). Using PET, Ceballos-Baumann and colleagues (2001) found that VIM DBS in patients with ET was associated with increased regional cerebral blood flow in the ipsilateral motor cortex and a decrease in regional cerebral blood flow in the retroinsular (parietoinsular vestibular) cortex. They suggested that the latter affects function of the vestibular-thalamic-cortical projections and might therefore explain the frequent occurrence of disequilibrium in patients treated for tremor with VIM DBS, a reversible complication of this therapy. The authors also postulated that the increased synaptic activity in the motor cortex overrides the abnormal tremor-related rhythmic neuronal bursting. In another study (Ceballos-Baumann et al., 2001), the authors suggested that the beneficial effects of VIM DBS are due to nonphysiologic activation of thalamofrontal projections or frequency-dependent neuroinhibition. This has also been confirmed by Perlmutter and colleagues (2002). In another study involving functional MRI during DBS of STN (three patients) and thalamus (one patient), Jech and colleagues (2001) showed an increase in blood oxygenation level–dependent signal in the subcortical regions ipsilateral to the stimulated nucleus. The authors concluded that this effect cannot be simply explained by a mechanism of depolarization blockade; rather, it is caused by "overstimulation" of the target nucleus, resulting in the suppression of its spontaneous activity. The study also demonstrated that functional MRI during DBS is safe. However, diathermy treatment, which involved pulse-modulated radiofrequency to the maxilla in a 70-year-old patient with PD implanted with ITREL model 7424 in the STN, resulted in permanent diencephalic and brainstem lesions and a vegetative state (Nutt et al., 2001a). This tragic complication probably resulted from induction of radiofrequency current and heating of the electrodes, leading to edema surrounding the DBS electrode.

Thalamic stimulation appears to be particularly effective in the treatment of parkinsonian tremor and ET (Koller et al., 1997; Ondo et al., 1998c; Pollak et al., 1998; Koller et al., 1999; Pahwa et al., 1999; Koller et al., 2001; Rehncrona et al., 2003) (Videos 7-1 and 7-2). In the North American Multi-Center Trial, 25 ET and 24 PD patients were followed for 1 year after implantation (Koller et al., 1997). Combined blinded tremor ratings (0 to 4) in ET patients randomized to "on" were 0.9 compared to 2.7 for those randomized to "off" stimulation. All subjective functional measures improved, and 9 of 29 patients (31%) had complete tremor cessation. In PD patients, "on" randomized scores were 0.6 compared to 3.2 for those who were randomized to "off." Fifty-eight percent (14 of 24) of patients had complete tremor cessation. Subjective functional measures (UPDRS part II), however, were not significantly improved. Complications were manageable and included paresthesia, headache, disequilibrium, dystonia, and device failure. Results were similar at 1 month and 1 year after implantation. Although some loss of efficacy and device-related complications have been encountered after 2 years of follow-up, the authors concluded that unilateral DBS of the thalamus has long-term efficacy in patients with ET (Koller et al., 2001). In a multicenter European study in which 37 patients with ET were followed for a mean of 6.5 years, unilateral or bilateral VIM DBS offered long-term benefits and safety (Sydow et al., 2003). The experience at Baylor is similar to that reported in other centers. In a blinded and open-label trial of unilateral thalamic DBS in 33 patients (14 ET and 19 PD) with severe tremor refractory to conventional therapy, ET and PD patients demonstrated an 83% and 82% reduction ($P < .0001$), respectively, in observed contralateral arm tremor (Ondo et al., 1998c). All measures of tremor, including writing samples, pouring tests, subjective functional surveys, and disability scores, significantly improved. Bilateral thalamic DBS was more effective than unilateral DBS in controlling bilateral appendicular and midline tremors of ET and PD, and thalamic DBS did not seem to improve meaningfully any parkinsonian symptoms other than tremor (Ondo, Almaguer, et al., 2001). Although unilateral VIM DBS can markedly improve midline tremor, this improvement was significantly enhanced by bilateral procedure (Putzke et al., 2005). VIM DBS produced modest improvement, rather than tremor augmentation as was previously suggested, in ipsilateral tremor in patients with ET (Ondo, Vuong, et al., 2001). A review of long-term efficacy of VIM DBS in 39 patients (20 PD, 19 ET) showed that the benefits might be maintained for at least 6 months (Rehncrona et al., 2003). In one study, three of eight patients with PD no longer required DBS after 3 to 5 years because the tremor markedly improved (Kumar et al., 2003). In addition to reducing the amplitude, VIM DBS increased the frequency of ET by 0.5 to 2 Hz at low inertial loads, made the tremor more irregular, and reduced the tremor-electromyography coherence (Vaillancourt et al., 2003).

To compare thalamic DBS with thalamotomy, Schuurman and colleagues (2000) conducted a prospective, randomized study of 68 patients with PD, 13 with ET, and 10 with multiple sclerosis. They found that the functional status improved more in the DBS group than in the thalamotomy group, and tremor was suppressed completely or almost completely in 30 of 33 (90.9%) in the DBS group and in 27 of 34 (79.4%) in the thalamotomy group. Although one patient in the DBS group died after an intracerebral hemorrhage, DBS was associated with significantly fewer complications than was thalamotomy. In one study of VIM DBS, dysarthria worsened when both stimulators were turned on in three of six patients (Pahwa et al., 1999). DBS also has been found to be effective in rare patients with disabling task-specific tremors (Racette et al., 2001). In addition to improving distal tremor associated with PD and ET, VIM DBS can effectively control ET-related head tremor, which usually does not respond to conventional therapy (Koller et al., 1999). Other midline tremors, such as voice, tongue, and face tremor, also may improve with unilateral VIM DBS, although additional benefit can be achieved with contralateral surgery (Obwegeser et al., 2000; Putzke et al., 2005). Furthermore, unilateral thalamic DBS for ET has been found to be cognitively safe and to improve anxiety and quality of life in terms of activities of daily living and psychological

well-being (Tröster et al., 1999). In addition, VIM DBS appears to improve postural stability (Pinter et al., 1999).

VIM DBS has been found to be useful not only in the treatment of troublesome tremor associated with ET and PD but also in the treatment of cerebellar outflow tremor associated with multiple sclerosis (Montgomery et al., 1999; Matsumoto et al., 2001; Wishart et al., 2003) (Video 7-3). Thalamic DBS may also be effective in the treatment of levodopa-induced dyskinesia, possibly owing to involvement of the center median and parafascicularis complex (Caparros-Lefebvre et al., 1999). Thalamic DBS, however, does not seem to provide any benefit in PD-related gait difficulty (Defebvre et al., 1996). Bilateral ventralis oralis anterior thalamic DBS has also been reported to be effective in a patient with severe postanoxic generalized dystonia and bilateral necrosis of the basal ganglia (Ghika et al., 2002). Medically intractable myoclonus was reported to improve 80% with VIM DBS in one case of myoclonus-dystonia syndrome (Trottenberg et al., 2001a), and GPi DBS has been found to be effective in relieving myoclonus-dystonia syndrome (Magarinos-Ascone et al., 2005).

Several studies have demonstrated that DBS of the GPi and STN improves not only parkinsonian tremor but also other PD-related symptoms and prolongs the "on" time (Pahwa et al., 1997; Limousin et al., 1998; Pollak et al., 1998; Moro et al., 1999; Deep-Brain Stimulation for Parkinson's Disease Study Group, 2001; Lanotte et al., 2002; Alvarez et al., 2005) (Videos 7-4 and 7-5). Elderly patients (>70 years old) seem to benefit as much as younger patients with respect to a reduction in dyskinesias and motor fluctuations, but during the "off" times, older patients have more difficulties with ADL and axial symptoms, particularly if they had some gait problems before surgery (Russmann et al., 2004b). Depending on the location of the stimulating electrode, pallidal stimulation has a variable effect on parkinsonian features versus levodopa-induced dyskinesias. In one study, stimulation of the dorsal GPi improved parkinsonian features, but stimulation of the posteroventral GPi improved levodopa-induced dyskinesia and worsened gait and akinesia (Bejjani et al., 1997). In another study, stimulation of the most ventral part of the GPi improved rigidity and eliminated levodopa-induced dyskinesia but produced marked bradykinesia, whereas stimulation of the most dorsal contacts improved bradykinesia and induced dyskinesia (Krack et al., 1998a). Best results could be obtained by stimulating the intermediate contacts. Similar results were reported by Durif and colleagues (1999), who found that ventral GPi stimulation was more effective than dorsal stimulation for alleviating rigidity and levodopa-induced dyskinesia. But in contrast to Krack and colleagues (1998a) whose target was posterolateral to the location of the target used by Durif and colleagues (1999), the latter group found that ventral stimulation also improved bradykinesia. They concluded that "chronic stimulation in the anteromedial GPi shows that this is a safe and effective treatment for advanced PD." GPi DBS has been found not only to improve "off" state UPDRS and movement onset time and spatial errors but also to enhance motor activation responses as measured by concurrent PET recordings of regional cerebral blood flow in the sensorimotor cortex, supplementary motor area, and anterior cingulated gyrus (Fukuda et al., 2001a). Normalization of an abnormal pattern of cerebral blood flow and an increase in cerebral blood flow in the supplementary motor area and anterior cingulated cortex has also been found with STN DBS, and this correlated with improvement in bradykinesia (Strafella et al., 2003). This effect was more robust with bilateral than unilateral stimulation. Hershey and colleagues (2003), however, found that STN DBS increased blood flow in the midbrain, globus pallidus, and thalamus but decreased blood flow in cortical areas. They concluded that "STN stimulation appears to drive, rather than inhibit, STN output neurons." This is consistent with the model that increased STN output driven by STN DBS leads to excitation of pallidal neurons, which increases inhibitory output to the thalamus, resulting in thalamocortical inhibition. This is supported by the observed decrease in overactivity of SMA and other areas of overactivity presumably recruited to compensate for abnormal motor initiation as measured by resting rCBF (Grafton et al., 2006). However, it is not fully understood how rCBF reflects "normalization" of the abnormal pattern of neuronal firing.

The localization of STN has been facilitated by the neurophysiologic characterization of the STN (Hutchison et al., 1998). The mean firing rate was found to be 37 Hz. The firing pattern was irregular and movement sensitive. In addition, tremor cells were identified in the STN and ventral pallidum. Macroelectrode STN stimulation completely suppressed contralateral tremor (Ashby et al., 1999). In a 1-year follow-up of 24 PD patients treated with bilateral STN stimulation, the UPDRS, parts II and III, improved by 60%, and the mean dose of dopaminergic drugs was reduced by half (Limousin et al., 1998). Krack and colleagues (1998b) found a 71% reduction in the UPDRS score in patients treated with STN DBS. Using subjective evaluation of contralateral wrist rigidity, Rizzone and colleagues (2001) studied the effects of various STN stimulation parameters in patients with PD during a drug-free state. They found that stimulus rates higher than 90 Hz and a pulse width larger than 60 μs rarely produce additional benefits and are associated with narrowing of the therapeutic window. On the basis of longitudinal experience in a large number of patients, a monopolar stimulation with 2 V, pulse width 60 μs, and frequency of 100 to 130 Hz is usually found to provide maximal benefit (Ushe et al., 2004). There is a characteristic pattern of emergence of tremor within minutes of discontinuation of the DBS, followed by slow and steady worsening of axial signs over 3 to 4 hours, with 90% of the worsening of the UPDRS score occurring within 2 hours after DBS is turned off (Temperli et al., 2003). When the STN DBS is turned on, a similar but faster rate of improvement is observed. In an analysis of the effects of 25 electrodes used in STN DBS, placement in the dorsolateral STN border was associated with the best clinical results and least energy consumption (Herzog et al., 2004).

In a multicenter, prospective, double-blind, crossover study in 134 patients with advanced PD treated with DBS of STN or GPi, the UPDRS motor scores improved by 49% ($P < .001$) and 37% ($P < .001$), respectively, in comparison to the nonstimulated state (Deep-Brain Stimulation for Parkinson's Disease Study Group, 2001). Furthermore, 6 months following implantation as compared to baseline, the percent time "on" without dyskinesias increased from 27% to 74% ($P < .001$) and from 28% to 64% ($P < .001$) with STN and GPi DBS, respectively. While the levodopa dosage remained unchanged in the GPi group, the daily levodopa dose equivalents were reduced by 37% in the STN DBS group ($P < .001$) (Fig. 7-4). Adverse events included intracranial hemorrhage in seven patients and infection necessitating removal of the leads in two. Although

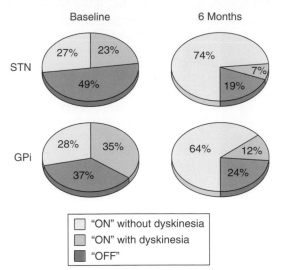

MEAN PERCENTAGE OF TIME DURING WAKING HOURS

**Figure 7-4** Results of a multicenter study of DBS in PD. (Reprinted with permission from Deep-Brain Stimulation for Parkinson's Disease Study Group: Deep-brain stimulation of the subthalamic nucleus or the pars interna of the globus pallidus in Parkinson's disease. N Engl J Med 2001;345: 956–963.)

this was the largest and best-designed study, it was criticized because of methodologic flaws (e.g., absence of true blindness), short follow-up, and underreporting of adverse effects (Obeso et al., 2002). In a blinded assessment at 1 year after implantation of STN DBS in 30 patients, the motor UPDRS decreased by only 30%, but duration of daily wearing off decreased by 69% and levodopa requirements decreased by 30% (Ford et al., 2004). In a double-blind study of 7 patients treated with STN DBS, Kumar and colleagues (1998a) found 58% improvement in the UPDRS motor score in a medication-off state when the stimulator was turned on. Furthermore, there was an 83% improvement in levodopa-induced dyskinesias, and the total drug dosage decreased by 40%. In another study involving 23 patients with PD treated with bilateral STN DBS, Houeto and colleagues (2000) showed that the procedure decreased levodopa-induced motor fluctuations, dyskinesias, and daily dose of levodopa by 61% to 78%. Similarly, Fraix and colleagues (2000) showed in 24 patients with PD treated with bilateral STN DBS that the observed improvement in levodopa-induced dyskinesia was associated with a reduction in levodopa dosage. In another study, the combination of reduced levodopa and STN stimulation reduced the duration of diphasic and peak-dose dyskinesias by 52% and reduced "off" period dystonia by 90% and "off" period pain by 66% (Krack et al., 1999). In another, much smaller, study involving only 15 patients with PD treated with bilateral STN DBS, the overall levodopa daily dose was reduced by 80.4%, and levodopa was withdrawn in 8 (53%) patients (Molinuevo et al., 2000). In a long-term follow-up, they showed that 10 of 26 (38%) patients were maintained on STN DBS monotherapy after 1.5 years of treatment (Valldeoriola et al., 2002). Similarly, Vingerhoets and colleagues (2002) found that 21 ± 8 months after implantation of bilateral STN DBS under stereotactic guidance, microelectrode recording, and clinical control in 20 patients, the UPDRS III "off medication" score decreased by 45% and was similar to the UPDRS III "on medication" score. Furthermore, medication was reduced by 79%, and 10 (50%) were able to withdraw their medications completely. In a subsequent study of two groups of six STN DBS-treated patients, the investigators showed that patients who were able to discontinue their medication and were subsequently challenged with levodopa had much less severe levodopa-induced dyskinesia than did those who had continued on levodopa, thus supporting "dopaminergic stimulation and striatal desensitization as major determinants of levodopa-induced dyskinesia in PD" (Russmann et al., 2004a). In a 2-year follow-up of 20 patients with STN DBS, the 50.9% UPDRS motor score reduction observed at 6 months was maintained during the follow-up period (Herzog et al., 2003). In a 5-year prospective study of the first 49 patients, mean age 55 years, treated with bilateral STN DBS, assessed during "on" and "off" states at 1, 3, and 5 years, the Grenoble group found a 54% improvement in "off" motor function compared to baseline and a 49% improvement in ADL (Fig. 7-5) (Krack et al., 2003). Speech was apparently the only motor function that did not improve. Except for improved dyskinesia and a lower daily levodopa dose, there was no additional improvement in "on" motor function beyond 1 year, and the axial symptoms continued to deteriorate after the first year. Of the initial 49 patients, 7 did not complete the study, 3 died, 4 were lost to follow-up, 3 developed dementia after 3 years, 1 committed suicide, and 1 had a large cerebral hemorrhage. This and other studies provide evidence for the conclusion that STN DBS is no better than levodopa, but it ameliorates levodopa-related motor complications and dyskinesias and "off" period dystonia. In a double-blind, crossover evaluation of STN DBS in ten patients during practically defined "off" (medications stopped overnight), the mean motor UPDRS score improved from 43 to 26 ($P < .04$), and various timed tests (walking and tapping) also improved significantly ($P < .04$) (Rodriguez-Oroz et al.,

2004). Open-label, 4-year follow-up also showed significant improvement in dyskinesia and levodopa reduction by half. In a 5-year follow-up of 11 patients treated with bilateral pallidal DBS, dyskinesias remained well controlled, but the initial benefit in off motor symptoms and fluctuations as well as ADL gradually declined, and the benefits were restored in 4 patients after replacement of the pallidal electrodes into STN (Volkmann et al., 2004). Reduction of dopaminergic drugs as a result of STN DBS may unmask restless legs syndrome (Kedia et al., 2004).

Besides reducing the need for levodopa, bilateral STN DBS also reduces the need for other medications, including apomorphine (Varma et al., 2003). Moro and colleagues (2002) showed that while the duration and latency of levodopa response are well maintained in patients with chronic STN DBS, the magnitude of the short-duration response tends to decrease with time. Since improvements in dyskinesia usually require a reduction in levodopa dosage, unilateral STN DBS is impractical because the side of the body contralateral to the unstimulated side would clearly worsen. Furthermore, bilateral implantation during a single procedure is less inconvenient to the patient than a staged procedure, the neurophysiologic mapping may be facilitated by anatomic symmetry, and implantation of both stimulators can be performed under a single general anesthetic.

Bilateral STN DBS appears to be more effective than unilateral STN DBS in improving parkinsonism, but unilateral STN DBS may be appropriate for patients with asymmetric parkinsonian symptoms, including a high-amplitude tremor (Kumar, Lozano, et al., 1999; Linazasoro et al., 2003; Sturman et al., 2004; Stover et al., 2005). Bilateral STN DBS greatly improves functioning and reduces levodopa-induced dyskinesias, probably by allowing a reduction in total levodopa dosage. STN DBS, however, may also somehow reverse the levodopa sensitization, since levodopa-induced dyskinesias seem to be markedly reduced after continuous bilateral STN stimulation even when the DBS is turned off (Bejjani, Gervais, et al., 2000). This may be due to the marked reduction in daily levodopa dose permitted by chronic STN DBS. Nutt and colleagues (2001b) suggested that the improvement in motor fluctuations produced by STN and GPi DBS is due to improvement in "off" disability rather than any effects on pharmacodynamics or pharmacokinetics of levodopa. Younger patients with levodopa-responsive PD are considered the best candidates for bilateral STN DBS (Charles et al., 2002; Welter et al., 2002). In a 2-year follow-up of patients with bilateral STN DBS, preoperative response to levodopa was found as the only predictor of a favorable outcome (Kleiner-Fisman et al., 2003). In patients with prior pallidotomy, bilateral (not unilateral) STN DBS may be beneficial (Su and Tseng, 2001; Kleiner-Fisman et al., 2004). The mean firing frequency of STN on the side ipsilateral to the pallidotomy is lower than on the contralateral, intact side (Mogilner et al., 2002). In a randomized trial involving 34 patients with advanced PD the "off" UPDRS score improved significantly more following bilateral STN DBS as compared to unilateral pallidotomy; "on" UPDRS motor and dyskinesia scores also improved more in the DBS group than in the pallidotomy group (Esselink et al., 2004). STN stimulation, while usually well tolerated, may produce ballistic and choreic dyskinesia when the voltage is increased above a given threshold (Moro et al., 1999) (Video 7-6).

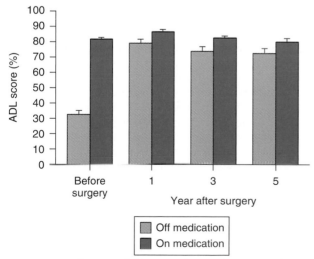

**BILATERAL STN DBS 5-YEAR FOLLOW-UP**

Off medication
On medication

**Figure 7-5** A five-year follow-up after implantation of STN DBS. (Reprinted with permission from Krack P, Batir A, Van Blercom N, et al: Five-year follow-up of bilateral stimulation of the subthalamic nucleus in advanced Parkinson's disease. N Engl J Med 2003;349:1925–1934.)

Neither memory nor executive functions seem to be affected in patients with bilateral STN or GPi DBS (Ardouin et al., 1999). Except for a mild deficit in lexical fluency, STN or GPi DBS does not appear to adversely affect cognitive performance (Pillon et al., 2000). Impaired performance in verbal fluency associated with STN DBS has been correlated with decreased regional cerebral blood flow in the left frontotemporal areas as measured by PET (Schroeder et al., 2003). While cognitive function is usually unchanged with STN DBS (Tröster et al., 1997; Gerschlager et al., 1999; Vingerhoets et al., 1999; Pillon et al., 2000; Daniele et al., 2003), even after 3 years (Funkiewiez et al., 2004), mild impairment in working memory and response inhibition performance (Hershey et al., 2004) and in frontal executive function has been found in some patients, particularly older patients (Saint-Cyr et al., 2000). This is based on a study of ten patients who were reevaluated 9 to 12 months after the implant. The investigators found significant declines in working memory, speed of mental processing, bimanual motor speed and coordination, set switching, phonemic fluency, and verbal and nonverbal memory. It is not clear, however, how these patients were selected, raising concerns about selection bias and other methodologic flaws. In another study, bilateral STN DBS was associated with moderate improvement in tasks of prefrontal function and obsessive-compulsive behavior (Mallet et al., 2002) but moderate deterioration in verbal memory and prefrontal and visuospatial function (Alegret et al., 2001). While some patients have experienced euphoria, mania, infectious laughter, and hilarity with STN DBS (Krack et al., 2001; Kulisevsky et al., 2002), others have experienced depression and other mood changes, aggressive behavior (posteromedial hypothalamus), pseudobulbar crying (Okun, Raju, et al., 2004), and other psychiatric problems (Bejjani et al., 2002; Berney et al., 2002; Mayberg and Lozano, 2002), and some have noted improvement in psychiatric symptoms, particularly obsessive-compulsive disorder (Mallet et al., 2002). Hypophonia and dysarthria were reported to be the most frequent long-term effects of STN DBS (Romito et al., 2002). Dysarthria, observed as a side effect more with left than right STN DBS (Santens et al., 2003), may develop despite improved oral control of jaw, lips, and tongue movements (Pinto et al., 2003). Several studies have now demonstrated a significant weight gain in patients with STN DBS; 32.1% show about 15% increase in body weight and a mean BMI increase of 24.7 kg/m² in 1 year (Barichella et al., 2003). While over half of patients initially considered to be DBS failures eventually had good results, 34% had persistently poor outcomes despite optimal management (Okun et al, 2005). In one study of 100 patients who were implanted with a total of 191 STN DBS devices, there were 7 (3.7%) device infections, 1 cerebral infarct, 1 intracerebral hematoma, 1 subdural hematoma, 2 (1%) skin erosions, 3 (1.6%) periprocedural seizures, and 6 (3.1%) brain electrode revisions (Goodman et al., 2006). There were 13 (6.8%) patients with postoperative confusion and 16 (8.4%) with battery failures, but there were no surgical deaths or permanent new neurologic deficits. Over a 10-year period, a total of 319 patients underwent DBS implantation at Baylor College of Medicine in Houston, Texas, 182 of whom suffered from medically refractory PD; the other patients had essential tremor (113), dystonia (18), and other hyperkinetic movement disorders (6) (Kenney et al., 2006). Intraoperative adverse effects were rare: vasovagal response in 8 patients (2.5%), syncope in 4 (1.3%), severe cough in 3 (0.9%), transient ischemic attack in 1 (0.3%), arrhythmia in 1 (0.3%),

and confusion in 1 (0.3%). Perioperative adverse effects included headache in 48 patients (15.0%), confusion in 16 (5.0%), and hallucinations in 9 (2.8%). The most serious intraoperative/perioperative adverse effects occurred in 4 patients (1.3%) with an isolated seizure, 2 patients (0.6%) with intracerebral hemorrhage, 2 patients (0.6%) with intraventricular hemorrhage, and 1 patient (0.3%) with a large subdural hematoma. Long-term complications of DBS surgery included dysarthria (4.0%), worsening gait (3.7%), cognitive decline (4.0%), and infection (4.4%). Revisions were completed in 25 patients (7.8%) for several reasons: loss of effect, lack of efficacy, infection, lead fracture, and lead migration. Hardware-related complications included 12 lead fractures and 10 lead migrations. Gender, age, and site of implantation did not predict a propensity to adverse effects.

Although bilateral STN DBS is clearly effective in improving the cardinal as well as other parkinsonian symptoms, the procedure does not necessarily improve all the symptoms, and as a result of progression of cognitive, speech, and other deficits frequently associated with PD, the quality of life might not substantially improve in patients who exhibit these additional features (Hariz et al., 2000; Diamond and Jankovic, 2005). Furthermore, pre-existing personality disorders and psychiatric disorders might not necessarily improve with STN DBS and might actually worsen and further compromise the patient's quality of life (Houeto et al., 2002), but in carefully selected patients, these behavioral problems and even apathy might improve with the procedure (Czernecki et al., 2005). Using the PD Quality of Life Questionnaire in 60 patients, Lagrange and colleagues (2002) showed improvements 1 year after bilateral STN DBS in all dimensions, including motor (+48%), systemic (+34%), emotional (+29%), and social (+63%). Other studies have demonstrated significant improvements in health-related quality of life in patients with advanced PD treated with bilateral STN DBS (Just and Ostergaard, 2002; Lagrange et al., 2002; Martinez-Martin et al., 2002). In another study, Lezcano and colleagues (2004a) applied the UPDRS, PDQ-39, and the scale of quality of life for caregivers (SQLC) in 11 PD patients 2 years after they had undergone bilateral STN DBS and found 62% improvement in PDQ-39 ($P < .001$) and 68% in SQLC ($P = .002$). A cost-effectiveness analysis suggests that DBS could be cost-effective in treating PD quality of life, which improved 18% or more compared with best medical treatment (Tomaszewski and Holloway, 2001).

The abnormal motor cortical overactivity associated with PD is reduced with STN DBS (Payoux et al., 2004). Frontal cortex function, as measured by contingent negative variation, has been improved by bilateral STN DBS (Gerschlager et al., 1999). Metabolic changes in the ipsilateral premotor cortex and cerebellum bilaterally, measured by [18F]fluorodeoxyglucose and PET, correlated with clinical improvement related to GPi DBS (Fukuda et al., 2001b). Other regional cerebral blood flow studies showed that when the STN DBS is on, the ipsilateral rostral supplementary motor area and premotor cortex are activated during contralateral movement, but there was a reduction in regional cerebral blood flow in primary motor cortex during rest (Ceballos-Baumann et al., 1999).

Although there are many reports concluding that GPi DBS is less effective than STN stimulation, there are only few studies that have objectively compared these two approaches (Okun and Foote, 2005). Before addressing this controversy, it is important to point out that GPi is a much larger target than STN (500 mm$^3$ versus 200 mm$^3$) and therefore requires larger density of stimulation. On the other hand, stimulation of the STN, because it is a smaller target, may lead to spreading of current from the intended sensorimotor area to potentially unwanted areas of the nucleus, such as the associative and limbic regions. This might account for a slightly higher frequency of cognitive and behavioral adverse effects with STN DBS (Anderson et al., 2005). Several studies have demonstrated greater antidyskinetic effects of GPi versus STN stimulation, and some studies have suggested that GPi DBS might be especially indicated in patients with a low threshold for dyskinesia (Minguez-Castellanos et al., 2005); GPi is considered the desirable target for treatment of dystonia and other hyperkinetic movement disorders. The relative safety and efficacy of STN versus GPi DBS have been compared in a few studies (Burchiel et al., 1999; Anderson et al., 2005). Although Burchiel and colleagues (1999) found no difference between the two targets, their initial study had insufficient power to detect a difference between the two groups. In their subsequent study involving 23 patients with PD complicated by marked levodopa-related motor fluctuations and dyskinesias, the investigators concluded that there were no significant differences in the overall benefits, although levodopa was decreased more in the STN group and dyskinesia improved more in the GPi group (Anderson et al., 2005). Krause and colleagues (2001) reported results in 6 patients with PD treated with GPi DBS and 12 patients with STN DBS. They found that while GPi DBS was associated with a lower frequency of levodopa-related complications, there was no improvement in bradykinesia or tremor. STN DBS, on the other hand, improved all parkinsonian symptoms and was associated with a reduced daily dose of levodopa. The authors concluded that STN was "the target of choice" for patients with severe PD who have side effects from levodopa. In a retrospective analysis of 16 patients undergoing STN DBS versus 11 treated with GPi DBS, Volkmann and colleagues (2001) showed that STN stimulation was associated with a 65% reduction in medication and required less electric power but more intensive postoperative monitoring and was associated with a higher frequency of adverse effects related to levodopa withdrawal as compared to GPi DBS. When STN and GPi DBS were compared, no difference between stimulation of the two targets on improvement of rigidity, strength, speed of movement execution, or movement initiation was found (Brown et al., 1999). For most effective results, the upper STN (sensorimotor part) and the subthalamic area containing the zona incerta, fields of Forel, and STN projections should be stimulated (Hamel et al., 2003). However, further controlled, randomized studies are needed to answer the question of which of the two methods is more effective and which patients should be considered the best candidates for either of the two procedures. Recently, the U.S. Department of Veterans Affairs initiated and sponsored a study designed to compare STN and GPi DBS in patients with PD as part of the Parkinson's Disease Research, Education, and Clinic Center (PADRECC) initiative.

DBS of the STN has been found to be effective in controlling not only parkinsonian tremor (Sturman et al., 2004) but also bradykinesia, gait difficulty, freezing (Limousin et al., 1995; Allert et al., 2001; Faist et al., 2001; Stolze et al., 2001; Bakker et al., 2004), and handwriting (Siebner et al., 1999). In addition to improving limb signs and the cardinal signs of PD,

bilateral STN DBS has also been found to improve axial parkinsonian symptoms, particularly rising from a chair and gait (Bastian et al., 2003; Bakker et al., 2004), as well as speech, neck rigidity, abnormal posture, off dystonia, balance and postural instability (Maurer et al., 2003; Colnat-Coulbois et al., 2005; Nilsson et al., 2005), and sensory symptoms (Bejjani, Damier, et al., 2000; Loher et al., 2002; Rocchi et al., 2002; Krystkowiak et al., 2003). Even sexual functioning has been shown to improve after STN DBS (Castelli et al., 2004). Using static posturography, Rocchi and colleagues (2002) found an improvement in postural sway with bilateral STN DBS but worsening with levodopa. Bilateral STN DBS has been reported to improve PD-related dysarthria in some studies (Gentil et al., 1999; Pollak, 1999). Other studies, however, have found that dysarthria, cognitive impairment, and postural instability fail to improve with STN DBS even in the same PD patient in whom the procedure improved the usual levodopa-responsive symptoms (Jarraya et al., 2003). STN or GPi DBS has been shown to improve gait velocity by increasing stride length with normalization of the gait pattern (Pahwa et al., 1997; Damier et al., 2001 Allert et al., 2001; Faist et al., 2001; Bastian et al., 2003). In one study, the "off" period cadence increased from $117 \pm 18.9$ steps per minute to $126 \pm 9.4$ steps per minute ($P < .05$) after GPi DBS (Vollmann et al., 1998). In contrast, bilateral STN DBS increased stride length but not cadence (Allert et al., 2001; Faist et al., 2001). Other studies reported significant improvements in essentially all components of gait (Krystkowiak et al., 2003; Bakker et al., 2004). Future targets should include the pedunculopontine nucleus in an attempt to improve freezing, gait, and balance.

The possibility that chronic DBS interferes with STN's excitatory output suggests a potential role of this treatment as a neuroprotective strategy (Piallat et al., 1996; Henderson and Dunnett, 1998; Krack et al., 1998b). This notion is supported by the observation that ablation of STN attenuates the loss of DA neurons in rats exposed to the mitochondrial toxin 3-nitropropionic acid (3-NP) or the catecholamine toxin 6-hydroxydopamine (6-OHDA) (Nakao et al., 1999). Furthermore, some investigators have argued that performing the procedure early in the course of the disease might prevent motor disability and adverse reactions to levodopa (Mesnage et al., 2002).

Effects of ablative surgery versus DBS on various parkinsonian features have not been adequately compared. In one prospective study, 13 patients with PD were randomized to pallidal stimulation versus pallidal ablation (Merello et al., 1999). Although the primary endpoint effects at 3 months on UPDRS and ADL were "comparable," pallidal DBS had more beneficial effects on hand-tapping speed, whereas pallidotomy had a more robust effect on levodopa-induced dyskinesias. However, additional blinded comparison studies of STN versus GPi DBS are needed before any definite conclusions about the relative effects of the two targets can be made. DBS electrodes are increasingly being used to make ablative lesions in the target areas (Raoul et al., 2003). GPe DBS might also provide benefits to patients with PD and with less delay than GPi DBS, although in one study it was associated with slightly higher frequency of dyskinesia (20% versus 9%) (Vitek et al., 2004).

As with any procedure, appropriate selection of patients as candidates for DBS surgery is critical to ensure optimal outcome (Box 7-2). Screening tools for surgical candidates have been developed and validated (Okun, Fernandez, et al., 2004).

**Box 7-2** Selection of patients for deep brain stimulation surgery

PD > 5 years (to allow for atypical features to emerge
and assess response to dopaminergic therapy)
Dopaminergic responsiveness (>3% reduction in motor
UPDRS)
Troublesome dyskinesias despite optimal medical therapy
Disabling medication-resistant tremor
Normal MRI
Exclude atypical and secondary parkinsonism
Exclude dementia and depression
Good medical health
Realistic expectations

Patients with atypical parkinsonism, such as multiple-system atrophy, are poor candidates for surgery, and STN DBS may aggravate speech, swallowing, and gait problems (Tarsy et al., 2003; Lezcano et al., 2004b). Besides GPi and STN, other targets that are being explored for DBS treatment of PD include zona incerta (Merello et al., 2006; Plaha et al., 2006) and PPN (Jenkinson et al., 2006; Stefani et al., 2007). Six patients with unsatisfactory pharmacologic control of axial signs such as gait and postural stability underwent bilateral implantation of DBS electrodes in the STN and pedunculopontine nucleus (PPN) (Stefani et al., 2007). Clinical effects were evaluated 2 to 6 months after surgery in the "off" and "on" medication state, with both STN and PPN stimulation on or off or with only one target being stimulated. Bilateral PPN-DBS at 25 Hz in "off medication" produced an immediate 45% amelioration of the motor UPDRS subscale score, followed by a decline, to give a final improvement of 32% in the score after 3 to 6 months. In contrast, bilateral STN-DBS at 130–185 Hz led to about 54% improvement. PPN-DBS was most effecitve on gait and postural items. In the "on" medication state, the association of STN and PPN-DBS provided a significant further improvement when compared to the specific benefit mediated by the activation of either single target. Moreover, the combined DBS of both targets promoted a substantial amelioration in the performance of daily living activities, The authors viewed these findings as indicating that in patients with advanced PD, PPN-DBS associated with standard STN-DBS may be useful in improving gait and in optimizing the dopamine-mediated "on" state, particularly in those whose response to STN only DBS has deteriorated over time, and may also prove useful in disorders such as progressive supranuclear palsy. Patients with significant freezing of gait (FOG) were not evaluated in this study.

## DEEP BRAIN STIMULATION FOR HYPERKINETIC AND OTHER DISORDERS

GPi DBS also has been reported to be effective in patients with primary generalized dystonia (Krauss et al., 1999; Kumar, Dagher et al., 1999; Coubes et al., 2000; Tronnier et al., 2000; Brin et al., 2001; Krack and Vercueil, 2001; Muta et al., 2001; Vercueil et al., 2001; Albright, 2003; Sanghera et al., 2003; Coubes et al., 2004; Krause et al., 2004; Diamond et al., 2005; Vidailhet et al., 2005; Jankovic, 2006; Kupsch et al., 2006; Jankovic, 2007), segmental dystonia (Wohrle et al., 2003), cervical dystonia (Bereznai et al., 2002; Krauss et al., 2002),

blepharospasm-oromandibular (cranial) dystonia (Capelle et al., 2003), tardive dyskinesia (Eltahawy, Feinstein, et al., 2004; Lenders et al., 2005), and tardive dystonia (Trottenberg et al., 2001b, 2005). Vercueil and colleagues (2001) described ten patients with bilateral GPi DBS; five had a major improvement, two had a moderate improvement, and one had a minor improvement after 14 months. They concluded that GPi DBS is much more effective than thalamic DBS for the treatment of dystonia. In a 2-year follow-up of 31 patients with primary generalized dystonia, Coubes and colleagues (2004) noted a mean improvement in the clinical and functional Burke-Fahn-Marsden Dystonia Rating Scale of 79% and 65%, respectively. There was no difference in response between DYT1-positive and DYT1-negative patients, but the magnitude of improvement was greater in children than in adults. In a presentation during the seventh International Congress of Parkinson's Disease and Movement Disorders in Miami in November 2002, Coubes provided data on 68 patients with generalized dystonia, 78% with primary dystonia, 19 of whom were DYT1-positive, and 29% with secondary dystonia, treated with GPi DBS. The MRI-guided, single-tract, bilateral implantation showed an overall 80% improvement, and this was most robust in primary, DYT1 dystonias and in the pantothenate kinase–associated neurodegeneration cases. Primary dystonia clearly responds better than secondary dystonia to either pallidotomy or GPi DBS, although patients with pantothenate kinase–associated neurodegeneration also experience marked improvement in their dystonia (Coubes, 2000; Eltahawy, Saint-Cyr, et al., 2004; Castelnau et al., 2005). Essentially all patients achieved steady state in 6 weeks. The improvement was particularly noticeable in the rapid ("ballistic") dystonic movements, pain, and bradykinesia, but there was no effect on the slow dystonia or associated bradykinesia. Except for implantable pulse generator infection in three patients and lead fracture and other lead problems in two patients, there were no other complications. The stimulating parameters were as follows: pulse rate was 450 μs, frequency was 130 Hz, and amplitude was 0.8 to 1.6 V.

In a prospective, multicenter study of 22 patients with generalized dystonia, 7 of whom had *DYT1* mutation, the Burke-Fahn-Marsden Dystonia Scale score improved after bilateral GPi DBS from a mean of $46.3 \pm 21.3$ to $21.0 \pm 14.1$ at 12 months ($P < .001$) (Vidailhet et al., 2005). A "blinded" review of the videos at 3 months showed improvement with stimulation from a mean of $34.63 \pm 12.3$ to $24.6 \pm 17.7$. The improvement in mean dystonia motor scores was 51%, and one third of the patients improved more than 75% compared to preoperative scores. In addition, there was a significant improvement in health-related quality of life as measured by the SF-36, but there was no change in cognition or mood. Although the sample was rather small, the authors were not able to find any predictors of response such as *DYT1* gene status, anatomic distribution of the dystonia, or location of the electrodes. Patients with a phasic form of dystonia improved more than those with tonic contractions and posturing. The maximum benefit was not achieved in some patients until 3 to 6 months after surgery. In six patients treated for their dystonia with bilateral GPi DBS, the contralateral prefrontal overactivity was reduced (Detante et al., 2004). In a 3-year follow-up, motor improvement observed at 1 year (51%) was maintained at 3 years (58%) and the authors concluded that "bilateral pallidal stimulation provides sustained motor benefit after 3 years" (Vidailhet et al., 2007).

It is of interest that an ablative lesion or high-frequency stimulation of the GPi can both produce and improve dystonia, suggesting that it is the pattern of discharge in the basal ganglia rather than the actual location or frequency of discharge that is pathophysiologically relevant to dystonia (Münchau et al., 2000). In one patient, a 49-year-old woman with severe generalized dystonia, bilateral GPi DBS produced an immediate improvement in dystonia, which was associated with a reduction in PET activation in certain cortical motor areas that are usually overactive in dystonia (Kumar, Dagher, et al., 1999). Bilateral GPi DBS has been found effective not only in distal or generalized dystonia but also in patients with cervical dystonia (Krauss et al., 1999; Kulisevsky et al., 2000; Parkin et al., 2001). In a report of two patients with cervical dystonia, bilateral GPi DBS produced more improvement in pain than in motor symptoms (Kulisevsky et al., 2000). Parkin and colleagues (2001) reported progressive improvement in pain and posture in three patients with cervical dystonia. Muta and colleagues (2001) described a 61-year-old woman with cranial dystonia manifested chiefly by blepharospasm, facial grimacing, cervical dystonia, and spasmodic dysphonia. She had previously failed to improve with bilateral thalamotomy but had marked improvement in all aspects of her dystonia with bilateral GPi DBS, including complete resolution of blepharospasm and oromandibular dystonia.

The expanding use of DBS in the treatment of various disorders could provide insights into the pathophysiology of other disorders (Benabid et al., 2000). For example, STN DBS has been found to be useful in the treatment of severe proximal tremor (Kitagawa et al., 2000) as well as rest and postural tremor in PD (Sturman et al., 2004). The observation that stimulation of the substantia nigra precipitates acute depression that resolves immediately when the DBS is turned off suggests that the nigrothalamic pathway may play an important role in depression (Bejjani et al., 1999). Besides left substantia nigra stimulation (Bejjani et al., 1999), stimulation superior and lateral to the right STN also produced mood changes (dysphoria) (Stefurak et al., 2003). Stimulation of white matter adjacent to the subgenual cingulated region (Brodmann area 25), which is metabolically overactive in treatment-resistant depression, has been found to be effective in treating depression in four of six patients (Mayberg et al., 2005). Globus pallidus has been increasingly used as the target in patients with disabling tics (Diederich et al., 2005). In a 16-year-old boy with disabling, medically intractable TS, bilateral GPi DBS resulted in 63% improvement in Yale Global Tic Severity Scale, 85% improvement in Tic Symptom Self Report, and 51% improvement in SF-36, a quality of life measure (Shahed et al., 2007). Furthermore, the patient was able to return to school. Although these observations must be confirmed by a controlled trial before DBS can be recommended even to severely affected patients, they suggest that stimulation of certain targets involved in the limbic striatopallidalthalamocortical system may be beneficial in the treatment of various aspects of TS.

Other emerging applications of DBS include treatment of obsessive-compulsive disorder (Gabriels et al., 2003; Nuttin et al., 2003) as well as various pain disorders, including migraines and cluster headaches (Leone et al., 2003). Normalization of bladder symptoms associated with PD-related detrusor hyperreflexia was demonstrated in a study of 16 patients with bilateral STN DBS (Seif et al., 2004).

Chronic stimulation appears to be well tolerated, and the risk of local gliosis is minimal (Caparros-Lefebvre et al., 1994; Haberler et al., 2000; Henderson et al., 2002), although more extensive damage has been rarely reported (Henderson et al., 2001). Electron microscopy examination of tissue adherent to the explanted electrode revealed foreign body multinucleate giant cell-type (some larger than 100 μm) reaction, possibly representing a response to the polyurethane component of the DBS electrode (Moss et al., 2004). Very few studies have addressed the rate and type of complications associated with DBS. During a mean follow-up period of 33 months and the cumulative follow-up of 217 patient-years of 84 consecutive cases, Oh and colleagues (2002) found that 20 patients (25.3%) had 26 hardware-related complications involving 23 (18.5%) of the electrodes. These included 4 lead fractures, 4 lead migrations, 3 short or open circuits, 12 erosions and/or infections, 2 foreign body reactions, and 1 cerebrospinal fluid leak. In addition, the hardware-related complication rate per electrode-year was 8.4%. Because of the ability to customize the stimulation parameters and the relatively low risk of complications, DBS is now considered the preferred surgical treatment for disabling PD-related tremor, ET, levodopa-related complications, generalized dystonia, and other movement disorders (Tasker, 1998). To improve the safety and efficacy of DBS, it is important to continue advancing the current understanding of the mechanisms underlying DBS and to build on and improve DBS technology (e.g., develop directional electrodes, prolong battery life, allow remote and "smart" programming).

On the basis of the observation that vagus nerve stimulation has a nonspecific "calming" effect in treated epileptics and that it suppresses harmaline-induced tremor in rats (Handforth and Krahl, 2001), a multicenter trial was conducted to study the effects of vagus nerve stimulation in patients with essential and parkinsonian tremor, but no meaningful benefit was demonstrated (Handforth et al., 2003). Encouraged by the initial reports of prefrontal rapid-rate, repetitive transcranial magnetic stimulation in PD and despite lack of effect in more recent studies (Ghabra et al., 1999), some investigators have tried extradural motor cortex simulation using a quadripolar electrostimulator and reported bilateral benefits in PD motor signs and in dyskinesias (Canavero and Paolotti, 2000). The results of these preliminary studies, however, must be confirmed by a larger study before this procedure can be considered as a potential treatment in PD.

## BRAIN GRAFTING

Neurotransplantation using fetal nigral tissue as a treatment for PD was introduced after laboratory studies demonstrated that grafts of fetal dopaminergic neurons can survive for long periods in the host striatum, that they are capable of forming synapses with striatal neurons, and that they actually produce dopamine (Freed et al., 1992; Freeman et al., 1995; Collier and Kordower, 1998; Hauser et al., 1999; Lindvall, 1999). Ventral mesencephalic grafts into parkinsonian animal models have been found to improve not only parkinsonian features but also levodopa-induced dyskinesias (Lee et al., 2000). Initial results of clinical trials have been inconsistent, and only moderate improvement has been observed. The variable results have been thought to be due to differences in surgical methods, the age and the amount of donor tissue, the methods of storage, the site of implantation, and the distribution of the tissue within the target region (Hauser et al., 1995). Controlled trials designed to determine the efficacy of fetal nigral transplantation are currently under way, but ethical concerns about the justification of sham operations, employed in these trials, have generated a lively controversy. Fetal tissue is generally obtained from elective abortions at postgestational ages ranging between 6 and 9 weeks. The tissue must be screened for infections and is implanted stereotactically in the striatum. Commonly, the putamen is chosen as the target site, sometimes in combination with the caudate. The donor tissue may be delivered via several needle tracts, either unilaterally or bilaterally. Tissue of up to eight fetal donors is grafted per patient. Whether cyclosporine or other immunosuppressants are needed has not yet been determined.

Although the initial results were encouraging, recent controlled studies have failed to show any meaningful benefit from neuronal grafting, and in one study, more than half of the implanted patients experienced "off" dyskinesias (Freed et al., 1992; Sawle et al., 1992; Spencer et al., 1992; Peschanski et al., 1994; Freeman et al., 1995; Wenning et al., 1997; Lindvall, 1998; Hauser et al., 1999; Lindvall, 1999; Freed, Greene, et al., 2001; Olanow, 2002; Mendez et al., 2005). Improvement is commonly noted between 1 and 3 months postoperatively. In single patients, functional improvement has been demonstrated up to 46 months postoperatively (Freed et al., 1992). Several patients were able to markedly reduce or even discontinue their dopaminergic drugs. Additional improvements have been noted after sequential bilateral transplantation (Hagell et al., 1999). [$^{18}$F]fluorodopa PET scans have demonstrated increased uptake following fetal transplants (Sawle et al., 1992; Freeman et al., 1995; Hauser et al., 1999), but this method has been challenged (Martin and Perlmutter, 1994). In one report, a patient received a unilateral fetal implant in 1989, with "gradual, major clinical improvement" over 3 years. Levodopa was withdrawn at 32 months, and immunosuppression was stopped at 64 months (Piccini et al., 1999). In the grafted putamen, the [11C]-raclopride positron emission tomography had normalized by 3 years with minor increases thereafter, while the untreated side showed gradual decline. While the untreated side showed increased raclopride (D2) binding (indicative of upregulation of receptors), the grafted side showed normal levels of binding. Following administration of amphetamine, which promotes dopamine release, the untreated side showed no decrease in raclopride binding, while the grafted side had a decrease in binding (due to competition from dopamine) equivalent to nondiseased controls.

Besides the in vivo evidence of graft survival, neuropathologic studies also provide evidence of graft survival and striatal reinnervation as long as 18 months after transplantation of fetal mesencephalic tissue (Kordower et al., 1995; Collier and Kordower, 1998). Survival of the human grafts can be prolonged by administering the lazaroid tirilazad mesylate, a lipid peroxidation inhibitor, into the graft tissue (Brundin et al., 2000) or possibly by immunosuppression, although postmortem studies performed 3 to 4 years after implants found that the grafts are only mildly immunogenic to the host brain (Mendez et al., 2005). Serious neurologic complications of neurotransplantation have occurred in 1% to 2% of cases and may include intracerebral hemorrhage (Hauser et al., 1995). There is also a potential risk of transmission of infectious vectors.

Freed, Greene, and colleagues (2001) reported the results of the first double-blind placebo-controlled trial of fetal graft transplantation for advanced PD. Forty patients, stratified by age into younger than 60 years and older than 60 years, with about a 7-year history of PD symptoms, were randomized to receive either four embryonic mesencephalons delivered via four needle passes to the left and right putamen or a sham operation (four drill holes to the forehead without dural penetration). After 1 year, the "sham" patients were given the option to be implanted and were then followed in an open-label manner; a total of 33 patients received an implant. Overall, there was no difference between the implanted and sham patients with respect to the primary outcome variable, a global rating by the patients (from –3, PD markedly worse, to +3, PD markedly improved). There was, however, a significant improvement in bradykinesia and rigidity, but only in the younger (<60 years old) patients. There was no improvement in freezing or motor fluctuations, and gait actually deteriorated. Although there were more adverse events in the implanted group, these were not considered directly related to the surgery. There was a marked placebo effect, sometimes lasting the whole year. Of the 20 implanted patients, 17 had evidence of fiber outgrowth from the transplanted tissue, as indicated by $^{18}$F-fluorodopa PET scans, but there was no correlation between the PET results and the UPDRS, except in the younger patient group. In a 1-year follow-up, a blinded PET study showed that patient age did not affect viability of the implant, but only in the younger group was there significant correlation between $^{18}$F-fluorodopa putaminal uptake and an improved UPDRS score for bradykinesia, though not tremor or rigidity (Nakamura et al., 2001). Most important, 5 of 33 patients who eventually received the implant experienced dyskinesias even during "off" periods, which correlates with increased F-dopa uptake on PET scans (Ma et al., 2002). GPi DBS improved these dyskinesias in three of the five patients (Freed, Breeze, et al., 2001). "Off" period dyskinesias were also reported in all 14 PD patients at a mean of 40 months following fetal transplants performed in Europe (Hagell et al., 2002). In the second, National Institutes of Health–funded, controlled trial of fetal transplants, 34 patients were randomized to receive bilateral grafting into the posterior putamen of four or one fetal tissue per side or sham surgery (partial burr hole without penetration of the dura) (Olanow et al., 2003). All patients underwent immunosuppression for 6 months after surgery and were followed for 24 months. Thirty-one patients completed the trial; two died during the trial, and three died afterward, from causes unrelated to the procedure. There was no significant overall treatment effect, but the patients with milder PD did show significant improvement ($P = .006$). Postmortem examination was performed on all patients, and in all transplanted patients, the TH staining indicated striatal innervation, particularly in those who received four tissues. PET results indicated a significant dose-dependent increase versus baseline in fluorodopa uptake, with no change in placebo patients and an approximate one third increase in patients receiving four tissues. Despite these histochemical and imaging improvements, no significant differences were seen in clinical measures. Increase (worsening) from baseline in the UPDRS motor score while off medication was 9.4 for placebo, 3.5 for one tissue, and –0.72 for four tissues ($P = .096$ for four versus placebo). Although treated patients improved for approximately 9 months, they then worsened. There was no difference between implanted and sham patients in "on" time without dyskinesias, total "off" time, ADL scores, or levodopa dose required. No placebo patients, but 13 of 23 (56%) treated patients, developed off-medication dyskinesias. The authors concluded that "Fetal nigral transplantation currently cannot be recommended as a therapy for PD based on these results." Limitations of both of the National Institutes of Health–sponsored studies have been reviewed (Winkler et al., 2005). Subsequent analysis suggested that patients with milder disease, particularly if immunosuppressed for more than 6 months, could be shown to have more robust benefit. Both studies demonstrate a marked placebo effect and the need for controlled trials in assessing surgical interventions (McRae et al., 2004).

Observations that cell division can occur in an adult brain have led to speculations that stem cell technology could be applied to neurodegenerative diseases, including PD (Barker, 2002; Bjorklund et al., 2002). One of the most exciting areas of current research is the potential use of cultured, well-characterized stem cells or adult bone marrow cells, with the ability to generate neurons and glia, for therapeutic applications in PD. This interest has been fueled by the encouraging findings from clinical trials utilizing fetal grafts into brains of PD patients (see later). It has become possible to generate central nervous system cells that express neuronal and glial properties by manipulating the tissue cultures with various cytokines and growth factors. When these progenitor cells are injected into an intact striatum, they acquire the characteristics of striatal cells (but when injected into a lesioned brain, they differentiate into glia). In one experiment, neuronal progenitor cells from a neonatal anterior subventricular zone were implanted in an adult rat with unilateral nigrostriatal denervation by 6-OHDA and were found to differentiate into neuronal phenotype as long as 5 months postimplantation (Zigova et al., 1998). In another study, embryonic stem cells derived from somatic cells via nuclear transfer differentiated into dopaminergic and serotonergic neurons in vitro and germ cells in vivo, demonstrating the full pluripotency of cloned cells and their potential usefulness in the treatment of PD (Wakayma et al., 2001). Rietze and colleagues (2001) found that a population of neuronal stem cells located in both ependymal and subventricular zones acts as a functional stem cell in vivo and has a potential to differentiate not only neuronal but also non-neuronal cells. Transplanting low-dose undifferentiated mouse embryonic stem cells into the rat striatum results in a proliferation and full differentiation into dopaminergic neurons associated with restoration of behavior and cerebral function (Bjorklund et al., 2002; Winkler et al., 2005). These studies suggest the possibility that in PD, the progenitor or stem cells can be eventually used to replace lost or degenerated cells. However, this enthusiasm must be tempered by the two negative studies of fetal transplants (see later) and the findings from animal studies that show that fetal transplants produce more robust motor and behavioral effects than transplanted embryonic stem cells. Other major limitations of stem cells are the lack of effect on nondopaminergic symptoms of PD and the potential for unregulated release of dopamine and growth.

Many questions regarding fetal tissue grafting remain open, and the procedure should be viewed as experimental (Winkler et al., 2005). Ethical concerns on the use of fetal tissue have been raised. Selection criteria for neurotransplantation differ among investigators. It has not yet been determined which patients are the ideal candidates for these procedures.

Because of logistical and ethical problems associated with harvesting human fetal mesencephalon, the use of other donor tissues has been explored. The implantation of autologous adrenal medulla into patient's striatum has been found to be helpful in about one third of patients, but the limited benefits and the potential risks of complications have resulted in the cessation of these procedures (Jankovic et al., 1989). Porcine (pig) fetal mesencephalic transplants, however, are currently being investigated as a potential therapeutic intervention (Galpern et al., 1996; Deacon et al., 1997). In 12 patients with advanced PD who received embryonic porcine ventral mesencephalic tissue, Schumacher and colleagues (2000) found 19% improvement in total UPDRS 12 months after the surgery. There were no changes in the $^{18}$F-dopa PET scans. Preliminary results from a double-blind, randomized, controlled, multicenter trial of fetal porcine implants in ten patients with PD have not produce encouraging results (Hauser et al., 2001). In addition to human embryonic tissue, other donor sources are currently being investigated, including retinal pigment epithelial cells (Spheramine) (Watts et al., 2003; Bakay et al., 2004). These cells, located in the inner layer of neural retina, produce dopamine. When attached to cross-linked gelatin microcarriers (Spheramine) and implanted stereotactically into the striatum, the cells have improved parkinsonian symptoms in rodents, nonhuman primates, and parkinsonian patients. A pilot open-label study of six patients showed 48% improvement in the UPDRS motor score 12 months after implantation (Bakay et al., 2004). A randomized controlled trial is currently being conducted in selected centers in North America and Europe.

The use of immortalized neural progenitor cells in repair and as a source of trophic factors is currently being investigated (Martinez-Serrano and Björklund, 1997). Other approaches include transplantation of polymer-coated xenografts, transfected mesencephalic neural cell lines, genetically engineered dopamine-producing fibroblasts, viral vectors modifying host cells by intrusion of the tyrosinehydroxylase gene, and others (Hauser et al., 1995). Alternative approaches also include the intraventricular or intraparenchymal infusion of neurotrophic factors such as the glial cell–derived neurotrophic factor (Gash et al., 1996). A multicenter study of this approach, however, was discontinued because of lack of efficacy.

## References

Albright AL: Neurosurgical treatment of spasticity and other pediatric movement disorders. J Child Neurol 2003;18(suppl 1): S67–S78.

Alegret M, Junque C, Valldeoriola F, et al: Effects of bilateral subthalamic stimulation on cognitive function in Parkinson disease. Arch Neurol 2001;58:1223–1227.

Allert N, Volkmann J, Dotse S, et al: Effects of bilateral pallidal or subthalamic stimulation on gait in advanced Parkinson's disease. Mov Disord 2001;16:1076–1085.

Alterman RL, Sterio D, Beric A, Kelly PJ: Microelectrode recording during posteroventral pallidotomy: Impact on target selection and complications. Neurosurgery 1999;44:315–323.

Alusi SH, Aziz TZ, Glickman S, et al: Stereotactic lesional surgery for the treatment of tremor in multiple sclerosis. A prospective case-controlled study. Brain 2001;124:1576–1589.

Alvarez L, Macias R, Lopez G, et al: Bilateral subthalamotomy in Parkinson's disease: Initial and long-term response. Brain 2005; 128:570–583.

Anderson VC, Burchiel KJ, Hogarth P, et al: Pallidal vs subthalamic nucleus deep brain stimulation in Parkinson disease. Arch Neurol 2005;62:554–560.

Andrade-Souza YM, Schwalb JM, Hamani C, et al: Comparison of three methods of targeting the subthalamic nucleus for chronic stimulation in Parkinson's disease. Neurosurgery 2005;56(2 suppl): 360–368.

Ardouin C, Pillon B, Peiffer E, et al: Bilateral subthalamic or pallidal stimulation for Parkinson's disease affects neither memory nor executive functions: A consecutive series of 62 patients. Ann Neurol 1999;46:217–223.

Ashby P, Kim YJ, Kumar R, et al: Neurophysiological effects of stimulation through electrodes in the human subthalamic nucleus. Brain 1999;122:1919–1931.

Bakay RA, Raiser CD, Stover NP, et al: Implantation of Spheramine in advanced Parkinson's disease (PD). Front Biosci 2004;9:592–602.

Bakker M, Esselink RA, Munneke M, et al: Effects of stereotactic neurosurgery on postural instability and gait in Parkinson's disease. Mov Disord 2004;19:1092–1099.

Barichella M, Marczewska AM, Mariani C, et al: Body weight gain rate in patients with Parkinson's disease and deep brain stimulation. Mov Disord 2003;18:1337–1340.

Barker RA: Repairing the brain in Parkinson's disease: Where next? Mov Disord 2002;17:233–241.

Barlas O, Hanagasi HA, Imer M, et al: Do unilateral ablative lesions of the subthalamic nucleus in parkinsonian patients lead to hemiballism? Mov Disord 2001;16:306–310.

Baron MS, Vitek JL, Bakay RAE, et al: Treatment of advanced Parkinson's disease by posterior GPi pallidotomy: 1 year results of a pilot study. Ann Neurol 1996;40:355–366.

Baron MS, Vitek JL, Bakay RAE, et al: Treatment of advanced Parkinson's disease by unilateral posterior GPi pallidotomy: 4-year results of a pilot study. Mov Disord 2000;15:230–237.

Bastian AJ, Kelly VE, Revilla FJ, et al: Different effects of unilateral versus bilateral subthalamic nucleus stimulation on walking and reaching in Parkinson's disease. Mov Disord 2003;18:1000–1007.

Bejjani B, Damier P, Arnulf I, et al: Pallidal stimulation for Parkinson's disease: Two targets? Neurology 1997;49:1564–1569.

Bejjani BP, Arnulf I, Demeret S, et al: Levodopa-induced dyskinesias in Parkinson's disease: Is sensitization reversible? Ann Neurol 2000;47:655–658.

Bejjani BP, Damier P, Arunlf I, et al: Transient acute depression induced by high-frequency deep-brain simulation. N Engl J Med 1999;340:1476–1502.

Bejjani BP, Gervais D, Arnulf I, et al: Axial parkinsonian symptoms can be improved: The role of levodopa and bilateral subthalamic stimulation. J Neurol Neurosurg Psychiatry 2000;68:595–600.

Bejjani BP, Houeto JL, Hariz M, et al: Aggressive behavior induced by intraoperative stimulation in the triangle of Sano. Neurology 2002;59:1425–1427.

Benabid AL, Koudsie A, Pollak P, et al: Future prospects of brain stimulation. Neurol Res 2000;22:237–246.

Benabid AL, Pollak P, Gao D, et al: Chronic electrical stimulation of the ventralis intermedius nucleus of the thalamus as a treatment of movement disorders. J Neurosurg 1996;84:203–214.

Benabid AL, Pollak P, Gervason C, et al: Long-term suppression of tremor by chronic stimulation of the ventral intermediate thalamic nucleus. Lancet 1991;1:403–406.

Bereznai B, Steude U, Seelos K, Botzel K: Chronic high-frequency globus pallidus internus stimulation in different types of dystonia: A clinical, video, and MRI report of six patients presenting with segmental, cervical, and generalized dystonia. Mov Disord 2002;17:138–144.

Bergman H, Wichmann T, DeLong MR: Reversal of experimental parkinsonism by lesions of the subthalamic nucleus. Science 1990;249:1436–1438.

Berney A, Vingerhoets F, Perrin A, et al: Effect on mood of subthalamic DBS for Parkinson's disease A consecutive series of 24 patients. Neurology 2002;59:1427–1429.

Bjorklund LM, Sanchez-Pernaute R, Chung S, et al: Embryonic stem cells develop into functional dopaminergic neurons after transplantation in a Parkinson rat model. Proc Natl Acad Sci U S A 2002;99:2344–2349.

Boraud T, Bezard E, Bioulac B, Gross CE: Dopamine agonist-induced dyskinesias are correlated to both firing pattern and frequency alterations of pallidal neurons in the MPTP-treated monkey. Brain 2001;124:546–557.

Brin MF, Germano I, Danisi F, et al: Deep brain stimulation in the treatment of dystonia. In Krauss JK, Jankovic J, Grossman RG (eds): Surgery for Parkinson's Disease and Movement Disorders. Philadelphia, Lippincott Williams & Wilkins, 2001, pp 307–315.

Bronstein JM, DeSalles A, DeLong MR, et al: Stereotactic pallidotomy in the treatment of Parkinson's disease. Arch Neurol 1999;56: 1064–1069.

Brown P, Mazzone P, Oliviero A, et al: Effects of stimulation of the subthalamic area on oscillatory pallidal activity in Parkinson's disease. Exp Neurol 2004;188:480–490.

Brown RG, Limousin Dowsey P, Brown P, et al: Impact of deep brain stimulation on upper limb akinesia in Parkinson's disease. Ann Neurol 1999;45:473–488.

Brundin P, Pogarell O, Hagell P, et al: Bilateral caudate and putamen grafts of embryonic mesencephalic tissue treated with lazaroids in Parkinson's disease. Brain 2000;123:1380–1390.

Burchiel KJ, Anderson VC, Favre J, Hamerstad JP: Comparison of pallidal and subthalamic nucleus deep brain stimulation for advanced Parkinson's disease: Results of a randomized, blinded pilot study. Neurosurgery 1999;45:1375–1384.

Canavero S, Paolotti R: Extradural motor cortex stimulation for advanced Parkinson's disease: A case report. Mov Disord 2000;15: 169–171.

Caparros-Lefebvre D, Blond S, Feltin M-P, et al: Improvement of levodopa induced dyskinesias by thalamic deep brain stimulation is related to slight variation in electrode placement: Possible involvement of the centre median and parafascicularis complex. J Neurol Neurosurg Psychiatry 1999;67:308–314.

Caparros-Lefebvre D, Blond S, Vermersch P, et al: Chronic thalamic stimulation improves tremor and levodopa induced dyskinesias in Parkinson's disease. J Neurol Neurosurg Psychiatry 1993;56: 268–273.

Caparros-Lefebvre D, Ruchoux MM, Blond S, et al: Long-term thalamic stimulation in Parkinson's disease: Postmortem anatomoclinical study. Neurology 1994;44:1856–1860.

Capelle HH, Weigel R, Krauss JK: Bilateral pallidal stimulation for blepharospasm-oromandibular dystonia (Meige syndrome). Neurology 2003;60:2017–2018.

Cardoso F, Jankovic J, Grossman RG, Hamilton WJ: Outcome after stereotactic thalamotomy for dystonia and hemiballismus. Neurosurgery 1995;36:501–508.

Castelli L, Perozzo P, Genesia ML, et al: Sexual well being in parkinsonian patients after deep brain stimulation of the subthalamic nucleus. J Neurol Neurosurg Psychiatry 2004;75: 1260–1264.

Castelnau P, Cif L, Valente EM, et al: Pallidal stimulation improves pantothenate kinase-associated neurodegeneration. Ann Neurol 2005;57:738–741.

Ceballos-Baumann A, Boecker H, Bartenstein P, et al: A positron emission tomographic study of subthalamic nucleus stimulation in Parkinson disease: Enhanced movement-related activity of motor-association cortex and decreased motor cortex resting activity. Arch Neurol 1999;56:997–1003.

Ceballos-Baumann AO, Boecker H, Fogel W, et al: Thalamic stimulation for essential tremor activates and deactivates vestibular cortex. Neurology 2001;56:1347–1354.

Charles PD, Van Blercom N, Krack P, et al: Predictors of effective bilateral subthalamic nucleus stimulation for PD. Neurology 2002;59:932–934.

Collier TJ, Kordower JH: Neural transplantation for the treatment of Parkinson's disease: Present-day optimism and future challenges.

In Jankovic J, Tolosa E (eds): Parkinson's Disease and Movement Disorders, 3rd ed. Baltimore, Williams & Wilkins, 1998: 1065–1083.

Colnat-Coulbois S, Gauchard GC, Maillard L, et al: Bilateral subthalamic nucleus stimulation improves balance control in Parkinson's disease. J Neurol Neurosurg Psychiatry 2005;76:780–787.

Comella CL, Leurgans S, Wuu J, et al: Rating scales for dystonia: A multicenter assessment. Mov Disord 2003;18:303–312.

Cosgrove GR, Rauch SL: Surgical treatment of Tourette syndrome and tics. In Krauss JK, Jankovic J, Grossman RG (eds): Surgery for Parkinson's Disease and Movement Disorders. Philadelphia, Lippincott Williams & Wilkins, 2001, pp 404–409.

Coubes P, Cif L, El Fertit H, et al: Electrical stimulation of the globus pallidus internus in patients with primary generalized dystonia: Long-term results. J Neurosurg 2004;101:189–194.

Coubes P, Roubertie A, Vayssiere N, et al: Treatment of DYT1-generalised dystonia by stimulation of the internal globus pallidus. Lancet 2000; 355:2220–2221.

Counihan TJ, Shinobu LA, Eskandar EN, et al: Outcomes following staged bilateral pallidotomy in advanced Parkinson's disease. Neurology 2001;56:799–802.

Czernecki V, Pillon B, Houeto JL, et al: Does bilateral stimulation of the subthalamic nucleus aggravate apathy in Parkinson's disease? J Neurol Neurosurg Psychiatry 2005;76:775–779.

Dalvi A, Winfield L, Yu Q, et al: Stereotactic posteroventral pallidotomy: Clinical methods and results at 1-year follow up. Mov Disord 1999;14:256–261.

Damier P, Houeto J-L, Bejjani B-P, et al: The role of the pallidum in Parkinson's disease gait: Lesions from pallidal stimulation. In Ruzicka E, Jankovic J, Hallett M (eds): Gait Disorders. Philadelphia, Lippincott Williams & Wilkins, 2001, pp 283–288.

Daniele A, Albanese A, Contarino MF, et al: Cognitive and behavioural effects of chronic stimulation of the subthalamic nucleus in patients with Parkinson's disease. J Neurol Neurosurg Psychiatry 2003;74:175–182.

Deacon T, Schumacher J, Dinsmore J, et al: Histological evidence of fetal pig neuronal survival after transplantation into a patient with Parkinson's disease. Nat Med 1997;3:350–353.

De Bie RMA, de Haan RJ, Nijssen PCG, et al: Unilateral pallidotomy in Parkinson's disease: A randomised, single-blind, multicentre trial. Lancet 1999;354:1665–1669.

De Bie RMA, de Haan RJ, Schuurman PR, et al: Morbidity and mortality following pallidotomy in Parkinson's disease: A systematic review. Neurology 2002;58:1008–1012.

De Bie RM, Schuurman PR, Bosch DA, et al: Outcome of unilateral pallidotomy in advanced Parkinson's disease: Cohort study of 32 patients. J Neurol Neurosurg Psychiatry 2001;71: 375–382.

Deep-Brain Stimulation for Parkinson's Disease Study Group: Deep-brain stimulation of the subthalamic nucleus or the pars interna of the globus pallidus in Parkinson's disease. N Engl J Med 2001;345:956–963.

Defebvre L, Blatt JL, Blond S, et al: Effect of thalamic stimulation on gait in Parkinson disease. Arch Neurol 1996;53:898–903.

Defer G-L, Widner H, Marié R-M, et al: Core assessment program for surgical interventional therapy in Parkinson's disease (CAPSIT-PD). Mov Disord 1999;14:572–584.

Desaloms JM, Krauss JK, Lai EC, et al: Posteroventral medial pallidotomy for Parkinson's disease: Preoperative magnetic resonance imaging features and clinical outcome. J Neurosurg 1998;89:194–199.

Detante O, Vercueil L, Thobois S, et al: Globus pallidus internus stimulation in primary generalized dystonia: A H215O PET study. Brain 2004;127:1899–1908.

Dewey RB, Giller CA, Broline SK, et al: Clinical outcome of unilateral streotactic pallidotomy without microelectrode recording for intractable Parkinson's disease. Parkinsonism Relat Disord 2000; 6:7–16.

Diamond A, Jankovic J: The effect of deep brain stimulation on quality of life in movement disorders. J Neurol Neurosurg Psychiatry 2005;76:1188–1193.

Diamond A, Shahed J, Azher S, et al: Globus pallidus deep brain stimulation in dystonia. Mov Disord 2006;21:692–695.

Diederich NJ, Kalteis K, Stamenkovic M, et al: Efficient internal pallidal stimulation in Gilles de la Tourette syndrome: A case report. Mov Disord 2005;20:1496–1499.

Dogali M, Fazzini E, Kolodny E, et al: Stereotactic ventral pallidotomy for Parkinson's disease. Neurology 1995;45:753–761.

Dostrovsky J, Bergman H: Oscillatory activity in the basal ganglia: Relationship to normal physiology and pathophysiology. Brain 2004;127:721–722.

Dostrovsky JO, Hutchison WD, Lozano AM: The globus pallidus, deep brain stimulation, and Parkinson's disease. Neuroscientist 2002;8:284–290.

Eidelberg D, Moeller JR, Ishikawa T, et al: Regional metabolic correlates of surgical outcome following unilateral pallidotomy for Parkinson's disease. Ann Neurol 1996;39:450–459.

Eltahawy HA, Feinstein A, Khan F, et al: Bilateral globus pallidus internus deep brain stimulation in tardive dyskinesia: A case report. Mov Disord 2004;19:969–972.

Eltahawy HA, Saint-Cyr J, Giladi N, et al: Primary dystonia is more responsive than secondary dystonia to pallidal interventions: Outcome after pallidotomy or pallidal deep brain stimulation. Neurosurgery 2004;54:613–619.

Esselink RA, de Bie RM, de Haan RJ, et al: Unilateral pallidotomy versus bilateral subthalamic nucleus stimulation in PD: A randomized trial. Neurology 2004;62:201–207.

Faist M, Xie J, Kurz D, et al: Effect of bilateral subthalamic nucleus stimulation on gait in Parkinson's disease. Brain 2001;124: 1590–1600.

Fine J, Duff J, Chen R, et al: Long-term follow-up of unilateral pallidotomy in advanced Parkinson's disease. N Engl J Med 2000; 342:1708–1714.

Ford B, Winfield L, Pullman SL, et al: Subthalamic nucleus stimulation in advanced Parkinson's disease: Blinded assessments at one year follow up. J Neurol Neurosurg Psychiatry 2004;75:1255–1259.

Fraix V, Pollak P, Van Blercom N, et al: Effect of subthalamic nucleus stimulation on levodopa-induced dyskinesia in Parkinson's disease. Neurology 2000;55:1921–1923.

Freed CR, Breeze RE, Fahn S: Transplantation of embryonic dopamine neurons for severe Parkinson's disease [letter to the editor]. N Engl J Med 2001;345:146–147.

Freed CR, Breeze RE, Rosenberg NL, et al: Survival of implanted fetal dopamine cells and neurologic improvement 12 to 46 months after transplantation for Parkinson's disease. N Engl J Med 1992;327:1549–1555.

Freed CR, Greene PE, Breeze RE, et al: Transplantation of embryonic dopamine neurons for severe Parkinson's disease. N Engl J Med 2001;344:710–719.

Freeman TB, Olanow CW, Hauser RA, et al: Bilateral fetal nigral transplantation into the postcommissural putamen in Parkinson's disease. Ann Neurol 1995;38:379–388.

Friedman DP, Goldman HW, Flanders AE, et al: Stereotactic radiosurgical pallidotomy and thalamotomy with the gamma knife: MR imaging findings with clinical correlation: Preliminary experience. Radiology 1999;212:143–150.

Friedman JH, Epstein M, Sanes JN, et al: Gamma knife pallidotomy in advanced Parkinson's disease. Ann Neurol 1999;39:535–538.

Fukuda M, Mentis M, Ghilardi M, et al: Functional correlates of pallidal stimulation for Parkinson's disease. Ann Neurol 2001a;49: 155–164.

Fukuda M, Mentis MJ, Ma Y, et al: Networks mediating the clinical effects of pallidal brain stimulation for Parkinson's disease: A PET study of resting-state glucose metabolism. Brain 2001b;124: 1601–1609.

Funkiewiez A, Ardouin C, Caputo E, et al: Long term effects of bilateral subthalamic nucleus stimulation on cognitive function, mood, and behaviour in Parkinson's disease. J Neurol Neurosurg Psychiatry 2004;75:834–839.

Gabriels L, Cosyns P, Nuttin B, et al: Deep brain stimulation for treatment-refractory obsessive-compulsive disorder: Psychopathological and neuropsychological outcome in three cases. Acta Psychiatr Scand 2003;107:275–282.

Galpern WR, Burns LH, Deacon TW, et al: Xenotransplantation of porcine fetal ventral mesencephalon in a rat model of Parkinson's disease: Functional recovery and graft morphology. Exp Neurol 1996;140:1–13.

Garcia L, D'Alessandro G, Bioulac B, Hammond C: High-frequency stimulation in Parkinson's disease: More or less? Trends Neurosci 2005;28:209–216.

Gash DM, Zhang Z, Ovadia A, et al: Functional recovery in parkinsonian monkeys treated with GDNF. Nature 1996;380:252–255.

Gentil M, Garcia-Ruiz P, Pollak P, Benabid A-L: Effect of stimulation of the STN on oral control of patients with parkinsonism. J Neurol Neurosurg Psychiatry 1999;67:329–333.

Gerschlager W, Alesch F, Cunnington R: Bilateral subthalamic nucleus stimulation improves frontal cortex function in Parkinson's disease: An electrophysiologic study of the contingent negative variation. Brain 1999;122:2365–2373.

Ghabra MB, Hallett M, Wassermann EM: Simultaneous repetitive transcranial magnetic stimulation does not speed fine movement in PD. Neurology 1999;52:768–770.

Ghika J, Gjika-Schmid F, Fankhauser H, et al: Bilateral contemporaneous posteroventral pallidotomy for the treatment of Parkinson's disease: Neuropsychological and neurological side effects. J Neurosurg 1999;91:313–321.

Ghika J, Villemure JG, Miklossy J, et al: Postanoxic generalized dystonia improved by bilateral Voa thalamic deep brain stimulation. Neurology 2002;58:311–313.

Goodman RR, Kim B, McClelland S III, et al: Operative techniques and morbidity with subthalamic nucleus deep brain stimulation in 100 consecutive patients with advanced Parkinson's disease. J Neurol Neurosurg Psychiatry 2006;77:12–17.

Grafton ST, Turner RS, Desmurget M, et al: Normalizing motor-related brain activity: Subthalamic nucleus stimulation in Parkinson disease. Neurology 2006;66:1192–1199.

Grafton ST, Waters C, Sutton J, et al: Pallidotomy increases activity of motor association cortex in Parkinson's disease: A positron emission tomographic study. Ann Neurol 1995;37:776–783.

Green J, McDonald WM, Vitek JL, et al: Neuropsychological and psychiatric sequelae of pallidotomy for PD: Clinical trial findings. Neurology 2002;58:858–865.

Gross CE, Boraus T, Guehl D, et al: From experimentation to the surgical treatment of Parkinson's disease: Prelude or suite in basal ganglia research? Prog Neurobiol 1999a;59:509–532.

Gross RE, Lombardi WJ, Lang AE, et al: Relationship of lesion location to clinical outcome following microelectrode-guided pallidotomy for Parkinson's disease. Brain 1999b;122:405–416.

Grossman RG, Hamilton WJ: Movement disorders. In Grossman RG, Hamilton WJ (eds): Principles of Neurosurgery. New York, Raven Press, 1991, pp 305–317.

Guridi J, Luquin MR, Herrero MT, Obeso JA: The subthalamic nucleus: A possible target for stereotaxic surgery in Parkinson's disease. Mov Disord 1993;8:421–429.

Guridi J, Obeso JA: The subthalamic nucleus, hemiballismus and Parkinson's disease: Reappraisal of a neurosurgical dogma. Brain 2001;124:5–19.

Haaxma R, van Boxtel A, Brouwer WH, et al: Motor functioning in a patient with bilateral lesions of the globus pallidus. Mov Disord 1995;10:761–777.

Haberler C, Alesch F, Mazal PR, et al: No tissue damage by chronic deep brain stimulation in Parkinson's disease. Ann Neurol 2000;48:372–376.

Hagell P, Piccini P, Bjorklund A, et al: Dyskinesias following neural transplantation in Parkinson's disease. Nat Neurosci 2002;5:627–628.

Hagell P, Schrag A, Picini P, et al: Sequential bilateral transplantation in Parkinson's disease. Effects of the second graft. Brain 1999;122:1121–1132.

Hallett M, Litvan I, Task Force on Surgery for Parkinson's Disease: Evaluation of surgery for Parkinson's disease: A report of the Therapeutics and Technology Assessment Subcommittee of the American Academy of Neurology. Neurology 1999;53:1910–1921.

Hamani C, Saint-Cyr JA, Fraser J, et al: The subthalamic nucleus in the context of movement disorders. Brain 2004;127:4–20.

Hamel W, Fietzek U, Morsnowski A, et al: Deep brain stimulation of the subthalamic nucleus in Parkinson's disease: Evaluation of active electrode contacts. J Neurol Neurosurg Psychiatry 2003;74:1036–1046.

Hamid NA, Mitchell RD, Mocroft P, et al: Targeting the subthalamic nucleus for deep brain stimulation: Technical approach and fusion of pre- and postoperative MR images to define accuracy of lead placement. J Neurol Neurosurg Psychiatry 2005;76:409–414.

Handforth A, Krahl SE: Suppression of harmaline-induced tremor in rats by vagus nerve stimulation. Mov Disord 2001;16:84–88.

Handforth A, Ondo WG, Tatter S, et al: Vagus nerve stimulation for essential tremor: A pilot efficacy and safety trial. Neurology 2003;61:1401–1405.

Hariz MI, Bergenheim AT: A 10-year follow-up review of patients who underwent Leksell's posteroventral pallidotomy for Parkinson disease. J Neurosurg 2001;94:552–558.

Hariz MI, Johansson F, Shamsgovara P, et al: Bilateral subthalamic nucleus stimulation in a parkinsonian patient with preoperative deficits in speech and cognition: Persistent improvement in mobility but increased dependency: A case study. Mov Disord 2000;15:136–139.

Hashimoto T, Elder CM, Okun MS, et al: Stimulation of the subthalamic nucleus changes the firing pattern of pallidal neurons. J Neurosci 2003;23:1916–1923.

Hashimoro T, Morita H, Tada T, et al: Neuronal activity in the globus pallidus in chorea caused by striatal lacunar infarction. Ann Neurol 2001;50:528–531.

Hassler R, Mundinger F, Riechert T: Stereotaxis in Parkinson syndrome. New York, Springer, 1979.

Hauser RA, Freeman TB, Olanow CW: Surgical therapies for Parkinson's disease. In Kurlan R (ed): Treatment of Movement Disorders. Philadelphia, Lippincott, 1995, pp 57–93.

Hauser RA, Freeman TB, Snow BJ, et al: Long term evaluation of bilateral fetal nigral transplantation in Parkinson disease. Arch Neurol 1999;56:179–187.

Hauser RA, Watts RL, Freeman TB, et al: A double-blind, randomized, controlled, multicenter clinical trial of the safety and efficacy of transplanted fetal porcine ventral mesencephalic cell versus imitation surgery in patients with Parkinson's disease. Mov Disord 2001;16:983–984.

Hayashi R, Hashimoto T, Tada T, Ikeda S: Effects of unilateral pallidotomy on voluntary movement, and simple and choice reaction times in Parkinson's disease. Mov Disord 2003;18:515–523.

Henderson JM, Dunnett SB: Targeting the subthalamic nucleus in the treatment of Parkinson's disease. Brain Res Bull 1998;46:467–474.

Henderson JM, O'Sullivan DJ, Pell M, et al: Lesion of thalamic centromedian-parafascicular complex after chronic deep brain stimulation. Neurology 2001;56:1576–1579.

Henderson JM, Pell M, O'Sullivan DJ, et al: Postmortem analysis of bilateral subthalamic electrode implants in Parkinson's disease. Mov Disord 2002;17:133–137.

Hershey T, Revilla FJ, Wernle AR, et al: Cortical and subcortical blood flow effects of subthalamic nucleus stimulation in PD. Neurology 2003;61:816–821.

Hershey T, Revilla FJ, Wernle A, et al: Stimulation of STN impairs aspects of cognitive control in PD. Neurology 2004;62:1110–1114.

Herzog J, Fietzek U, Hamel W, et al: Most effective stimulation site in subthalamic deep brain stimulation for Parkinson's disease. Mov Disord 2004;19:1050–1054.

Herzog J, Volkmann J, Krack P, et al: Two-year follow-up of subthalamic deep brain stimulation in Parkinson's disease. Mov Disord 2003;18:1332–1337.

Hilker R, Voges J, Ghaemi M, et al: Deep brain stimulation of the subthalamic nucleus does not increase the striatal dopamine concentration in parkinsonian humans. Mov Disord 2003;18:41–48.

Houeto JL, Damier P, Bejjani PB, et al: Subthalamic stimulation in Parkinson disease: A multidisciplinary approach. Arch Neurol 2000;57:461–465.

Houeto JL, Mesnage V, Mallett L, et al: Behavioral disorders, Parkinson's disease and subthalamic stimulation. J Neurol Neurosurg Psychiatry 2002;72:701–707.

Hutchison WD, Allan RJ, Opitz H, et al: Neurophysiologic identification of the subthalamic nucleus in surgery for Parkinson's disease. Ann Neurol 1998;44:622–628.

Hutchison WD, Lang AE, Dostrovsky JO, Lozano AM: Pallidal neuronal activity: Implications for models of dystonia. Ann Neurol 2003;53:480–488.

Iacono RP, Shima F, Lonser RR, et al: The results, indications, and physiology of posteroventral pallidotomy for patients with Parkinson's disease. Neurosurgery 1995;36:1118–1127.

Intemann PM, Masterman D, Subramanian I, et al: Staged bilateral pallidotomy for treatment of Parkinson disease. J Neurosurg 2001;94:437–444.

Jankovic J: Re-emergence of surgery for dystonia. J Neurol Neurosurg Psychiatry 1998;65:434.

Jankovic J: Surgery for Parkinson's disease and other movement disorders: Benefits and limitations of ablation, stimulation, restoration, and radiation. Arch Neurol 2001;58:1970–1972.

Jankovic J: Treatment of dystonia. Lancet Neurology 2006;5:864–872.

Jankovic J: Dystonic disorders. In Jankovic J, Tolosa E (eds): Parkinson's Disease and Movement Disorders, 5th ed. Philadelphia, Lippincott Williams & Wilkins, 2007, pp 321–347.

Jankovic J, Ben-Arie L, Schwartz K, et al: Movement and reaction times and fine coordination tasks following pallidotomy. Mov Disord 1999;14:57–62.

Jankovic J, Cardoso F, Grossman RG, Hamilton WJ: Outcome after stereotactic thalamotomy for parkinsonian, essential and other types of tremor. Neurosurgery 1995;45:1743–1746.

Jankovic J, Grossman R, Goodman C, et al: Clinical, biochemical and neuropathologic findings following transplantation of adrenal medulla to the caudate nucleus for treatment of Parkinson's disease. Neurology 1989;39:1227–1234.

Jankovic J, Lai E, Ben-Arie L, et al: Levodopa-induced dyskinesias treated by pallidotomy. J Neurol Sci 1999;167:62–67.

Jankovic J, Lai E, Krauss JK, Grossman RG: Surgical treatment of levodopa-induced dyskinesias. In Stern G (ed): Parkinson's Disease: Advances in Neurology, vol 80. Philadelphia, Lippincott Williams & Wilkins, 1999:603–610.

Jankovic J, Lai EC, Ondo WG, et al: Effects of pallidotomy on gait and balance. In Ruzicka E, Hallett M, Jankovic J (eds): Gait disorders. Advances in Neurology, vol 87. Philadelphia, Lippincott Williams & Wilkins, 2001, pp 271–282.

Jarraya B, Bonnet AM, Duyckaerts C, et al: Parkinson's disease, subthalamic stimulation, and selection of candidates: A pathological study. Mov Disord 2003;18:1517–1520.

Jech R, Urgošik D, Tintěra J, et al: Functional magnetic resonance imaging during deep brain stimulation: A pilot study in four patients with Parkinson's disease. Mov Disord 2001;16:1126–1132.

Jenkinson N, Nandi D, Miall RC, et al: Pedunculopontine nucleus stimulation improves akinesia in a Parkinsonian monkey. Neuroreport 2004;15:2621–2624.

Jenkinson N, Nandi D, Oram R, et al: Pedunculopontine nucleus electric stimulation alleviates akinesia independently of dopaminergic mechanisms. Neuroreport 2006;17:639–641.

Just H, Ostergaard K: Health-related quality of life in patients with advanced Parkinson's disease treated with deep brain stimulation of the subthalamic nuclei. Mov Disord 2002;17:539–545.

Kedia S, Moro E, Tagliati M, et al: Emergence of restless legs syndrome during subthalamic stimulation for Parkinson disease. Neurology 2004;63:2410–2412.

Kenney CJ, Vuong K, Hunter C, et al: Long term safety of deep brain stimulation for the treatment of Parkinson's disease. Neurology 2006;66:A49–A50.

Kimber TE, Tsai CS, Semmler J, et al: Voluntary movement after pallidotomy in severe Parkinson's disease. Brain 1999;122:895–906.

Kishore A, Panikar D, Balakrishnan S, et al: Evidence of functional somatotopy in GPi from results of pallidotomy. Brain 2000; 123:2491–2500.

Kishore A, Turnbull IM, Snow BJ, et al: Efficacy, stability and predictors of outcome of pallidotomy for Parkinson's disease: Six-month follow-up with additional 1-year observations. Brain 1997;120:729–737.

Kitagawa M, Murata J, Kikuchi S, et al: Deep brain stimulation of subthalamic area for severe proximal tremor. Neurology 2000; 55:114–116.

Kleiner-Fisman G, Fisman DN, Sime E, et al: Long-term follow up of bilateral deep brain stimulation of the subthalamic nucleus in patients with advanced Parkinson disease. J Neurosurg 2003;99:489–495.

Kleiner-Fisman G, Fisman DN, Zamir O, et al: Subthalamic nucleus deep brain stimulation for Parkinson's disease after successful pallidotomy: Clinical and electrophysiological observations. Mov Disord 2004;19:1209–1214.

Koller W, Pahwa R, Busenbark K, et al: High-frequency unilateral thalamic stimulation in the treatment of essential and parkinsonian tremor. Ann Neurol 1997;42:292–299.

Koller WC, Lyons KE, Wilkinson SB, et al: Long-term safety and efficacy of unilateral deep brain stimulation of the thalamus in essential tremor. Mov Disord 2001;16:464–468.

Koller WC, Lyons KE, Wilkinson SB, Pahwa R: Efficacy of unilateral deep brain stimulation of the VIM nucleus of the thalamus for essential head tremor. Mov Disord 1999;14:847–850.

Kondziolka D, Bonarotti E, Baser S, et al: Outcomes after stereotactically guided pallidotomy for advanced Parkinson's disease. J Neurosurg 1999;90:197–202.

Kordower JH, Freeman TB, Snow BJ, et al: Neuropathological evidence of graft survival and striatal reinnervation after the transplantation of fetal mesencephalic tissue in a patient with Parkinson's disease. N Engl J Med 1995;332:1118–1124.

Krack P, Batir A, Van Blercom N, et al: Five-year follow-up of bilateral stimulation of the subthalamic nucleus in advanced Parkinson's disease. N Engl J Med 2003;349:1925–1934.

Krack P, Kumar R, Ardouin C, et al: Mirthful laughter induced by subthalamic nucleus stimulation. Mov Disord 2001;16:867–875.

Krack P, Pollak P, Limousin P, et al: Opposite motor effects of pallidal stimulation in Parkinson's disease. Ann Neurol 1998a;43:180–192.

Krack P, Pollak P, Limousin P, et al: Subthalamic nucleus or internal pallidal stimulation in young onset Parkinson's disease. Brain 1998b;121:451–457.

Krack P, Pollak P, Limousin P, et al: From off-period dystonia to peak-dose chorea: The clinical spectrum of varying subthalamic nucleus activity. Brain 1999;122:1133–1146.

Krack P, Vercueil L: Review of the functional surgical treatment of dystonia. Europ J Neurol 2001;8:389–399.

Krause M, Fogel W, Heck A, et al: Deep brain stimulation for the treatment of Parkinson's disease: Subthalamic nucleus versus globus pallidus internus. J Neurol Neurosurg Psychiatry 2001;70:464–476.

Krause M, Fogel W, Kloss M, et al: Pallidal stimulation for dystonia. Neurosurgery 2004;55:1361–1370.

Krauss J, Grossman RG, Jankovic J (eds): Pallidal Surgery for the Treatment of Parkinson's Disease and Movement Disorders. Philadelphia, Lippincott-Raven, 1998, pp 1–324.

Krauss JK, Desaloms M, Lai EC, et al: Microelectrode-guided posteroventral pallidotomy for treatment of Parkinson's disease:

Postoperative magnetic resonance imaging analysis. J Neurosurg 1997;87:358–367.

Krauss JK, Grossman RG: Surgery for hyperkinetic movement disorders. In Jankovic J, Tolosa E (eds): Parkinson's Disease and Movement Disorders, 3rd ed. Baltimore, Williams & Wilkins, 1998, pp 1017–1047.

Krauss JK, Jankovic J: Surgical treatment of Parkinson's disease. Am Fam Physician 1996;54:1621–1629.

Krauss JK, Jankovic J, Grossman RG (eds): Surgery for Parkinson's Disease and Movement Disorders. Philadelphia, Lippincott Williams & Wilkins, 2001, pp 1–449.

Krauss JK, Loher TJ, Pohle T, et al: Pallidal deep brain stimulation in patients with cervical dystonia and severe cervical dyskinesias with cervical myelopathy. J Neurol Neurosurg Psychiatry 2002; 72:249–256.

Krauss JK, Mundinger F: Surgical treatment of hemiballism and hemichorea. In Krauss JK, Jankovic J, Grossman RG (eds): Surgery for Parkinson's Disease and Movement Disorders. Philadelphia, Lippincott Williams & Wilkins, 2001, pp 397–403.

Krauss JK, Pohle T, Weber S, et al: Bilateral stimulation of globus pallidus internus for treatment of cervical dystonia. Lancet 1999; 354:837–838.

Krauss JK, Simpson RK, Ondo WG, et al: Concepts and methods in chronic thalamic stimulation for treatment of tremor: Technique and application. Neurosurgery 2001;48:535–541.

Krystkowiak P, Blatt J-L, Bourriez J-L, et al: Effects of subthalamic nucleus stimulation and levodopa treatment on gait abnormalities in Parkinson disease. Arch Neurol 2003;60:80–84.

Kuehler A, Henrich G, Schroeder U, et al: A novel quality of life instrument for deep brain stimulation in movement disorders. J Neurol Neurosurg Psychiatry 2003;74:1023–1030.

Kulisevsky J, Berthier ML, Gironell A, et al: Mania following deep brain stimulation for Parkinson's disease. Neurology 2002;59:1421–1424.

Kulisevsky J, Lleo A, Gironell A, et al: Bilateral pallidal stimulation for cervical dystonia: Dissociated pain and motor improvement. Neurology 2000;55:1754–1755.

Kumar R: Methods for programming and patient management with deep brain stimulation of the globus pallidus for the treatment of advanced Parkinson's disease and dystonia. Mov Disord 2002; 17(suppl 3):S198–S207.

Kumar R, Dagher A, Hutchison WD, et al: Globus pallidus deep brain stimulation for generalized dystonia: Clinical and PET investigation. Neurology 1999;53:871–874.

Kumar R, Lozano AM, Kim YJ, et al: Double-blind evaluation of subthalamic nucleus deep brain stimulation in advanced Parkinson's disease. Neurology 1998a;51:850–855.

Kumar R, Lozano AM, Montgomery E, Lang AE: Pallidotomy and deep brain stimulation of the pallidum and subthalamic nucleus in advanced Parkinson's disease. Mov Disord 1998b;13(suppl 1): 73–82.

Kumar R, Lozano AM, Sime E, et al: Comparative effects of unilateral and bilateral subthalamic nucleus deep brain stimulation. Neurology 1999;53:561–566.

Kumar R, Lozano AM, Sime E, Lang AE: Long-term follow-up of thalamic deep brain stimulation for essential and parkinsonian tremor. Neurology 2003;61:1601–1604.

Kupsch A, Benecke R, Muller J, et al: Pallidal deep-brain stimulation in primary generalized or segmental dystonia. N Engl J Med 2006;355:1978–1990.

Lagrange E, Krack P, Moro E, et al: Bilateral subthalamic nucleus stimulation improves health-related quality of life in PD. Neurology 2002;59:1976–1978.

Lai EC, Jankovic J, Krauss JK, et al: Long-term efficacy of posteroventral pallidotomy in the treament of Parkinson's disease. Neurology 2000;55:1218–1222.

Lai EC, Jankovic J, Schwartz K, et al: Treatment of advanced Parkinson's disease with microelectrode-guided pallidotomy. Ann Neurol 1996;40:534–535.

Laitinen LV, Bergenheim AT, Hariz MI: Leksell's posteroventral pallidotomy in the treatment of Parkinson's disease. J Neurosurg 1992; 76:53–61.

Lang AE: Surgery for levodopa-induced dyskinesias. Ann Neurol 2000a;47(suppl 1):S193–S202.

Lang AE: Surgery for Parkinson disease: A critical evaluation of the state of art. Arch Neurol 2000b;57:1118–1125.

Lang AE, Duff J, Saint-Cyr JA, et al: Posteroventral medial pallidotomy in Parkinson's disease. J Neurol 1999;246(suppl 2):II/28–II/41.

Lang AE, Lozano A, Montgomery E, et al: Posteroventral medial pallidotomy in advanced Parkinson's disease. N Engl J Med 1997; 337:1036–1042.

Lanotte MM, Rizzone M, Bergamasco B, et al: Deep brain stimulation of the subthalamic nucleus: Anatomical, neurophysiological, and outcome correlations with the effects of stimulation. J Neurol Neurosurg Psychiatry 2002;72:53–58.

Lee CS, Cenci A, Schulzer M, Björklund A: Embryonic ventral mesencephalic grafts improve levodopa-induced dyskinesia in a rat model of Parkinson's disease. Brain 2000;123:1365–1379.

Lenders MW, Buschman HP, Vergouwen MD, et al: Long term results of unilateral posteroventral pallidotomy for antipsychotic drug induced tardive dyskinesia. J Neurol Neurosurg Psychiatry 2005;76:1039.

Lenz FA, Normand SL, Kwan HC, et al: Statistical prediction of the optimal site for thalamotomy in parkinsonian tremor. Mov Disord 1995;10:318–328.

Leone M, Franzini A, Broggi G, Bussone G: Hypothalamic deep brain stimulation for intractable chronic cluster headache: A 3-year follow-up. Neurol Sci 2003;24(suppl 2):S143–S145.

Levy R, Ashby P, Hutchison WD, et al: Dependence of subthalamic nucleus oscillations on movement and dopamine in Parkinson's disease. Brain 2002;125:1196–1209.

Levy R, Lang AE, Dostrovsky JO, et al: Lidocaine and muscimol microinjections in subthalamic nucleus reverse parkinsonian symptoms. Brain 2001;124:2105–2188.

Lezcano E, Gomez-Esteban JC, Zarranz JJ, et al: Improvement in quality of life in patients with advanced Parkinson's disease following bilateral deep-brain stimulation in subthalamic nucleus. Eur J Neurol 2004a;11:451–454.

Lezcano E, Gomez-Esteban JC, Zarranz JJ, et al: Parkinson's disease-like presentation of multiple system atrophy with poor response to STN stimulation: A clinicopathological case report. Mov Disord 2004b;19:973–977.

Limousin P, Krack P, Pollak P, et al: Electrical stimulation of the subthalamic nucleus in advanced Parkinson's disease. N Engl J Med 1998;339:1105–1111.

Limousin P, Pollak P, Benazzouz A, et al: Effect on parkinsonian signs and symptoms of bilateral subthalamic nucleus stimulation. Lancet 1995;345:91–95.

Limousin P, Speelman JD, Gielen F, et al: Multicenter European study of thalamic stimulation in parkinsonian and essential tremor. J Neurol Neurosurg Psychiatry 1999;66:289–296.

Linazasoro G, Van Blercom N, Lasa A: Unilateral subthalamic deep brain stimulation in advanced Parkinson's disease. Mov Disord 2003;18:713–716.

Lindvall O: Update on fetal transplantation: The Swedish experience. Mov Disord 1998;13:84–87.

Lindvall O: Cerebral implantation in movement disorders: State of the art. Mov Disord 1999;14:201–205.

Loher TJ, Burgunder JM, Weber S, et al: Effect of chronic pallidal deep brain stimulation on off period dystonia and sensory symptoms in advanced Parkinson's disease. J Neurol Neurosurg Psychiatry 2002;73:395–399.

Lombardi WJ, Gross RE, Trepanier LL, et al: Relationship of lesion location to cognitive outcome following microelectrode-guided pallidotomy for Parkinson's disease: Support for the existence of cognitive circuits in the human pallidum. Brain 2000;123: 746–758.

Lopiano L, Rizzone M, Bergamasco B, et al: Deep brain stimulation of the subthalamic nucleus: Clinical effectiveness and safety. Neurology 2001;56:552–554.

Lozano AM, Lang AE, Galvez-Jimenez N, et al: Effect of GPi pallidotomy on motor function in Parkinson's disease. Lancet 1995;346:1383–1387.

Lozano AM, Lang AE, Levy R, et al: Neuronal recordings in Parkinson's disease patients with dyskinesias induced by apomorphine. Ann Neurol 2000;47(suppl 1):S141–S146.

Ma Y, Feigin A, Dhawan V, et al: Dyskinesia after fetal cell transplantation for parkinsonism: A PET study. Ann Neurol 2002;52:628–634.

Magarinos-Ascone CM, Regidor I, Martinez-Castrillo JC, et al: Pallidal stimulation relieves myoclonus-dystonia syndrome. J Neurol Neurosurg Psychiatry 2005;76:989–991.

Magnin M, Morel A, Jeanmonod D: Single-unit analysis of the pallidum, thalamus and subthalamic nucleus in parkinsonian patients. Neuroscience 2000;96:549–564.

Mallet L, Mesnage V, Houeto JL, et al: Compulsions, Parkinson's disease, and stimulation. Lancet 2002;360:1302–1304.

Maltete D, Navarro S, Welter ML, et al: Subthalamic stimulation in Parkinson disease: With or without anesthesia? Arch Neurol 2004;61:390–392.

Martin WR, Perlmutter JS: Assessment of fetal tissue transplantation in Parkinson's disease: Does PET play a role? Neurology 1994;44:1777–1780.

Martinez-Martin P, Valldeoriola F, Molinuevo JL, et al: Pallidotomy and quality of life in patients with Parkinson's disease: An early study. Mov Disord 2000;15:65–70.

Martinez-Martin P, Valldeoriola F, Tolosa E, et al: Bilateral subthalamic nucleus stimulation and quality of life in advanced Parkinson's disease. Mov Disord 2002;17:372–377.

Martinez-Serrano A, Björklund A: Immortalized neuronal progenitor cells for CNS gene transfer and repair. Trends Neurosci 1997;20:530–538.

Masterman D, DeSalles A, Baloh RW, et al: Motor, cognitive, and behavioral performance following unilateral ventroposterior pallidotomy for Parkinson disease. Arch Neurol 1998;55:1201–1208.

Mathew SJ, Yudofsky SC, McCullough LB, et al: Attitudes toward neurosurgical procedures for Parkinson's disease and obsessive-compulsive disorder. J Neuropsychiatry Clin Neurosci 1999;11:259–267.

Matsumoto J, Morrow D, Kaufman K, et al: Surgical therapy for tremor in multiple sclerosis: An evaluation of outcome measures. Neurology 2001;57(10):1876–1882.

Maurer C, Mergner T, Xie J, et al: Effect of chronic bilateral subthalamic nucleus (STN) stimulation on postural control in Parkinson's disease. Brain 2003;126:1146–1163.

Mayberg HS, Lozano AM: Penfield revisited? Understanding and modifying behavior by deep brain stimulation for PD. Neurology 2002;59:1298–1299.

Mayberg HS, Lozano AM, Voon V, et al: Deep brain stimulation for treatment-resistant depression. Neuron 2005;45:651–660.

Mazziotta JC: Imaging: Window on the brain. Arch Neurol 2000;57:1413–1421.

McIntosh E, Gray A, Aziz T: Estimating the costs of surgical innovations: The case for subthalamic nucleus stimulation in the treatment of advanced Parkinson's disease. Mov Disord 2003;18:993–999.

McIntyre CC, Savasta M, Kerkerian-Le Goff L, Vitek JL: Uncovering the mechanism(s) of action of deep brain stimulation: Activation, inhibition, or both. Clin Neurophysiol 2004;115:1239–1248.

McRae C, Cherin E, Yamazaki TG, et al: Effects of perceived treatment on quality of life and medical outcomes in a double-blind placebo surgery trial. Arch Gen Psychiatry 2004;61:412–420.

Meissner W, Harnack D, Reese R, et al: High-frequency stimulation of the subthalamic nucleus enhances striatal dopamine release and metabolism in rats. J Neurochem 2003;85:601–609.

Melnick ME, Dowling GA, Aminoff MJ, et al: Effect of pallidotomy on postural control and motor function in Parkinson disease. Arch Neurol 1999;56:1361–1365.

Mena-Segovia J, Bolam JP, Magill PJ: Pedunculopontine nucleus and basal ganglia: Distant relatives or part of the same family? Trends Neurosci 2004:127:585–588.

Mendez I, Sanchez-Pernaute R, Cooper O, et al: Cell type analysis of functional fetal dopamine cell suspension transplants in the striatum and substantia nigra of patients with Parkinson's disease. Brain 2005;128:1498–1510.

Merello M, Nouzeilles MI, Kuzis G, et al: Unilateral radiofrequency lesion versus electrostimulation of posteroventral pallidum: A prospective randomized comparison. Mov Disord 1999;14:50–56.

Merello M, Tenca E, Cerquetti D: Neuronal activity of the zona incerta in Parkinson's disease patients. Mov Disord 2006;21:937–943.

Mesnage V, Houeto JL, Welter ML, et al: Parkinson's disease: Neurosurgery at an earlier stage? J Neurol Neurosurg Psychiatry 2002;73:778–779.

Meyers R: The surgery of the hyperkinetic disorders. In Vinken PJ, Bruyn GW (eds): Handbook of Clinical Neurology, vol 6. Amsterdam, North Holland, 1968, pp 844–878.

Minguez-Castellanos A, Escamilla-Sevilla F, Katati MJ, et al: Different patterns of medication change after subthalamic or pallidal stimulation for Parkinson's disease: Target related effect or selection bias? J Neurol Neurosurg Psychiatry 2005;76:34–39.

Mogilner AY, Sterio D, Rezai AR, et al: Subthalamic nucleus stimulation in patients with a prior pallidotomy. J Neurosurg 2002;96:660–665.

Molinuevo JL, Valldeoriola F, Tolosa E, et al: Levodopa withdrawal after bilateral subthalamic nucleus stimulation in advanced Parkinson disease. Arch Neurol 2000;57:983–988.

Molnar GF, Sailer A, Gunraj CA, et al: Thalamic deep brain stimulation activates the cerebellothalamocortical pathway. Neurology 2004;63:907–909.

Montgomery EB, Baker KB, Kinkel RP, Barnett G: Chronic thalamic stimulation for the tremor of multiple sclerosis. Neurology 1999;53:625–628.

Moro E, Esselink RJ, Benabid AL, Pollak P: Response to levodopa in parkinsonian patients with bilateral subthalamic nucleus stimulation. Brain 2002;125(11):2408–2417.

Moro E, Scerrati M, Romito LMA, et al: Chronic subthalamic nucleus stimulation reduced medication requirements in Parkinson's disease. Neurology 1999;53:85–90.

Moss J, Ryder T, Aziz TZ, et al: Electron microscopy of tissue adherent to explanted electrodes in dystonia and Parkinson's disease. Brain 2004;127:2755–2763.

Münchau A, Mathen D, Cox T, et al: Unilateral lesions of the globus pallidus: Report of four patients presenting with focal or segmental dystonia. J Neurol Neurosurg Psychiatry 2000;69:494–498.

Mundinger F, Riechert T: Die stereotaktischen Hirnoperationen zur Behandlung extrapyramidaler Bewegungsstörungen (Parkinsonismus und Hyperkinesen) und ihre Resultate. Fortschr Neurol Psych 1963;31:1–66, 69–120.

Muta D, Goto S, Nishikawa S, et al: Bilateral pallidal stimulation for idiopathic segmental axial dystonia advanced from Meige syndrome refractory to bilateral thalamotomy. Mov Disord 2001;16:774–778.

Nakamura T, Dhawan V, Chaly T, et al: Blinded positron emission tomography study of dopamine cell implantation for Parkinson's disease. Ann Neurol 2001;50:181–187.

Nakao N, Nakai E, Nakai K, et al: Ablation of the subthalamic nucleus supports the survival of nigral dopaminergic neurons after nigrostriatal lesions induced by the mitochondrial toxin 3-nitropropionic acid. Ann Neurol 1999;45:640–651.

Nilsson MH, Tornqvist AL, Rehncrona S: Deep-brain stimulation in the subthalamic nuclei improves balance performance in patients with Parkinson's disease, when tested without antiparkinsonian medication. Acta Neurol Scand 2005;111:301–308.

Niranjan A, Kondziolka D, Baser S, et al: Functional outcomes after gamma knife thalamotomy for essential tremor and MS-related tremor. Neurology 2000;55:443–446.

Nutt JG, Anderson VC, Peacock JH, et al: DBS and diathermy interaction induces severe CNS damage. Neurology 2001a;1384–1386.

Nutt JG, Rufener SL, Carter JH, et al: Interactions between deep brain stimulation and levodopa in Parkinson's disease. Neurology 2001b;57:1835–1842.

Nuttin BJ, Gabriels L, van Kuyck K, Cosyns P: Electrical stimulation of the anterior limbs of the internal capsules in patients with severe obsessive-compulsive disorder: Anecdotal reports. Neurosurg Clin N Am 2003;14:267–274.

Obeso JA, Guridi J, Alvarez L, et al: Ablative surgery for Parkinson's disease. In Jankovic J, Tolosa E (eds): Parkinson's Disease and Movement Disorders, 3rd ed. Baltimore, Williams & Wilkins, 1998, pp 1049–1064.

Obeso JA, Olanow CW, Lang A: Deep-brain stimulation in Parkinson's disease. N Engl J Med 2002;346:452–453.

Obwegeser AA, Uiti RJ, Turk MF, et al: Thalamic stimulation for the treatment of midline tremors in essential tremor patients. Neurology 2000;54:2342–2344.

Oh MY, Abosch A, Kim SH, et al: Long-term hardware-related complications of deep brain stimulation. Neurosurgery 2002;50:1268–1276.

Okun MS, Fernandez HH, Pedraza O, et al: Development and initial validation of a screening tool for Parkinson disease surgical candidates. Neurology 2004;63:161–163.

Okun MS, Foote KD: Subthalamic nucleus vs globus pallidus interna deep brain stimulation, the rematch: Will pallidal deep brain stimulation make a triumphant return? Arch Neurol 2005;62:533–536.

Okun MS, Raju DV, Walter BL, et al: Pseudobulbar crying induced by stimulation in the region of the subthalamic nucleus. J Neurol Neurosurg Psychiatry 2004;75:921–923.

Okun MS, Stover NP, Subramanian T, et al: Complications of gamma knife surgery for Parkinson disease. Arch Neurol 2001;58:1995–2002.

Okun MS, Tagliati M, Pourfar M, et al: Management of referred deep brain stimulation failures: A retrospective analysis from 2 movement disorders centers. Arch Neurol 2005;62:1250–1255.

Okun MS, Vitek JL: Lesion therapy for Parkinson's disease and other movement disorders: Update and controversies. Mov Disord 2004;19:375–389.

Olanow CW: GPi pallidotomy: Have we made a dent in Parkinson's disease? Ann Neurol 1996;40:341–343.

Olanow CW: Transplantation for Parkinson's disease: Pros, cons, and where do we go from here. Mov Disord 2002;17(suppl 5):S15.

Olanow CW, Goetz CG, Kordower JH, et al: A double-blind controlled trial of bilateral fetal nigral transplantation in Parkinson's disease. Ann Neurol 2003;54:403–414.

Ondo W, Almaguer M, Jankovic J, Simpson RK: Thalamic deep brain stimulation: Comparison between unilateral and bilateral placement. Arch Neurol 2001;58:218–222.

Ondo WG, Desaloms JM, Jankovic J, Grossman RG: Pallidotomy and thalamotomy for dystonia. In Krauss JK, Jankovic J, Grossman RG (eds): Surgery for Parkinson's Disease and Movement Disorders. Philadelphia, Lippincott Williams & Wilkins, 2001, pp 299–306.

Ondo WG, Desaloms M, Jankovic J, Grossman R: Surgical pallidotomy for the treatment of generalized dystonia. Mov Disord 1998a;13:693–698.

Ondo W, Jankovic J, Lai E, et al: Assessment of motor function following stereotactic pallidotomy. Neurology 1998b;50:266–270.

Ondo W, Jankovic J, Schwartz K, et al: Unilateral thalamic deep brain stimulation for refractory essential tremor and Parkinson's disease tremor. Neurology 1998c;51:1063–1069.

Ondo W, Vuong K, Almaguer M, et al: Thalamic deep brain stimulation: Effects on the nontarget limbs and rebound phenomenon. Mov Disord 2001;16:1137–1142.

Pahapill PA, Levy R, Dostrovsky J, et al: Tremor arrest with thalamic microinjections of muscimol in patients with essential tremor. Ann Neurol 1999;46:249–252.

Pahwa R, Lyons KL, Wilkinson SB, et al: Bilateral thalamic stimulation for the treatment of essential tremor. Neurology 1999;53:1447–1450.

Pahwa R, Wilkinson S, Smith D, et al: High frequency stimulation of the globus pallidus for the treatment of Parkinson's disease. Neurology 1997;49:249–253.

Pal PK, Samii A, Kishore A, et al: Long term outcome of unilateral pallidotomy: Follow up of 15 patients for 3 years. J Neurol Neurosurg Psychiatry 2000;69:337–344.

Papa SM, Desimone R, Fiorani M, Oldfield EH: Internal globus pallidus discharge is nearly suppressed during levodopa-induced dyskinesias. Ann Neurol 1999;46:732–738.

Paradiso G, Saint-Cyr JA, Lozano AM, et al: Involvement of the human subthalamic nucleus in movement preparation. Neurology 2003;61:1538–1545.

Parent A, Cicchetti F: The current model of basal ganglia organization under scrutiny. Mov Disord 1998;13:199–202.

Parkin S, Aziz T, Gregory R, Bain P: Bilateral internal globus pallidus stimulation for the treatment of spasmodic torticollis. Mov Disord 2001;16:489–493.

Patel NK, Heywood P, O'Sullivan K, et al: Unilateral subthalamotomy in the treatment of Parkinson's disease. Brain 2003a;126:1136–1145.

Patel NK, Plaha P, O'Sullivan K, et al: MRI directed bilateral stimulation of the subthalamic nucleus in patients with Parkinson's disease. J Neurol Neurosurg Psychiatry 2003b;74:1631–1637.

Payoux P, Remy P, Damier P, et al: Subthalamic nucleus stimulation reduces abnormal motor cortical overactivity in Parkinson disease. Arch Neurol 2004;61:1307–1313.

Perlmutter JS, Mink JW, Bastian AJ, et al: Blood flow responses to deep brain stimulation of thalamus. Neurology 2002;58:1388–1394.

Perrine K, Dogali M, Fazzini E, et al: Cognitive functioning after pallidotomy for refractory Parkinson's disease. J Neurol Neurosurg Psychiatry 1998;65:150–154.

Peschanski M, Defer G, N'Guyen JP, et al: Bilateral motor improvement and alteration of L-dopa effect in two patients with Parkinson's disease following intrastriatal transplantation of foetal ventral mesencephalon. Brain 1994;117:487–500.

Pfann KD, Penn RD, Shannon KM, Corcos DM: Pallidotomy and bradykinesia: Implications for basal ganglia function. Neurology 1998;51:796–803.

Piallat B, Benazzouz A, Benabid AL: Subthalamic nucleus lesion in rats prevents dopaminergic nigral neuron degeneration after striatal 6-OHDA injection: Behavioral and immunohistochemical studies. Eur J Neurosci 1996;8:1408–1414.

Piccini P, Brooks DJ, Bjorklund A, et al: Dopamine release for nigral transplants visualized in vivo in a Parkinson's patient. Nat Neurosci 1999;2:1137–1140.

Pillon B, Ardouin C, Damier P, et al: Neuropsychological changes between "off" and "on" STN or GPi stimulation in Parkinson's disease. Neurology 2000;55:411–418.

Pinter MM, Murg M, Alesch F, et al: Does deep brain stimulation of the nucleus ventralis intermedius affect postural control and locomotion in Parkinson's disease? Mov Disord 1999;14:958–963.

Pinto S, Gentil M, Fraix V, et al: Bilateral subthalamic stimulation effects on oral force control in Parkinson's disease. J Neurol 2003;250:179–187.

Plaha P, Ben-Shlomo Y, Patel NK, Gill SS: Stimulation of the caudal zona incerta is superior to stimulation of the subthalamic nucleus in improving contralateral parkinsonism. Brain 2006;129(pt 7):1732–1747.

Pollak P: Neurosurgical treatment of dyskinesias: Pathophysiological consideration. Mov Disord 1999;14:33–39.

Pollak P, Benabid AL, Krack P, et al: Deep brain stimulation. In Jankovic J, Tolosa E (eds): Parkinson's Disease and Movement Disorders, 3rd ed. Baltimore, Williams & Wilkins, 1998, pp 1085–1102.

Putzke JD, Uitti RJ, Obwegeser AA, et al: Bilateral thalamic deep brain stimulation: Midline tremor control. J Neurol Neurosurg Psychiatry 2005;76:684–690.

Racette BA, Dowling J, Randle J, Mink JW: Thalamic stimulation for primary writing tremor. J Neurol 2001;248:380–382.

Raoul S, Faighel M, Rivier I, et al: Staged lesions through implanted deep brain stimulating electrodes: A new neurosurgical procedure for treating tremor or dyskinesias. Mov Disord 2003;18: 933–938.

Rehncrona S, Johnels B, Widner H, et al: Long-term efficacy of thalamic deep brain stimulation for tremor: Double-blind assessments. Mov Disord 2003;18:163–170.

Rettig GM, Lai EC, Krauss JK, et al: Neuropsychological evaluation of patients with Parkinson's disease before and after pallidal surgery. In Krauss JK, Grossman RG, Jankovic J (eds): Pallidal Surgery for the Treatment of Parkinson's Disease and Movement Disorders. Philadelphia, Lippincott-Raven, 1998, pp 211–231.

Rettig GM, York MK, Lai EC, et al: Neuropsychological outcome following unilateral pallidotomy for the treatment of Parkinson's disease. J Neurol Neurosurg Psychiatry 2000;69:326–336.

Rietze RL, Valcanis H, Brooker GF, et al: Purification of a pluripotent neural stem cell from the adult mouse brain. Nature 2001;412: 736–739.

Rizzone M, Lanotte M, Bergamasco B, et al: Deep brain stimulation of the subthalamic nucleus in Parkinson's disease: Effects of variation in stimulation parameters. J Neurol Neurosurg Psychiatry 2001;71:215–219.

Robert-Warrior D, Overby A, Jankovic J, et al: Postural control in Parkinson's disease after unilateral posteroventral pallidotomy. Brain 2000;123:2141–2149.

Rocchi L, Chiari L, Horak FB: Effects of deep brain stimulation and levodopa on postural sway in Parkinson's disease. J Neurol Neurosurg Psychiatry 2002;73:267–274.

Rodriguez-Oroz MC, Rodriguez M, Guridi J, et al: The subthalamic nucleus in Parkinson's disease: Somatotopic organization and physiological characteristics. Brain 2001;124:1777–1790.

Rodriguez-Oroz MC, Zamarbide I, Guridi J, et al: Efficacy of deep brain stimulation of the subthalamic nucleus in Parkinson's disease 4 years after surgery: Double blind and open label evaluation. J Neurol Neurosurg Psychiatry 2004;75:1382–1385.

Romito LM, Scerrati M, Contarino MF, et al: Long-term follow up of subthalamic nucleus stimulation in Parkinson's disease. Neurology 2002;58:1546–1550.

Russmann H, Ghika J, Combrement P, et al: L-Dopa-induced dyskinesia improvement after STN-DBS depends upon medication reduction. Neurology 2004a;63:153–155.

Russmann H, Ghika J, Villemure JG, et al: Subthalamic nucleus deep brain stimulation in Parkinson disease patients over age 70 years. Neurology 2004b;63:1952–1954.

Saint-Cyr JA, Trépanier LL: Neuropsychological assessment of patients for movement disorder surgery. Mov Disord 2000;15: 771–783.

Saint-Cyr JA, Trépanier LL, Kumar R, et al: Neuropsychological consequences of chronic bilateral stimulation of the subthalamic nucleus in Parkinson's disease. Brain 2000;123:2091–2108.

Samii A, Turnbull IM, Kishore A, et al: Reassessment of unilateral pallidotomy in Parkinson's disease: A 2-year follow-up study. Brain 1999;122:417–425.

Sanghera M, Grossman RG, Kalhorn CG, et al: Basal ganglia neuronal discharge in primary and secondary dystonia in patients undergoing pallidotomy. Neurosurgery 2003;52:1358–1373.

Santens P, De Letter M, Van Borsel J, et al: Lateralized effects of subthalamic nucleus stimulation on different aspects of speech in Parkinson's disease. Brain Lang 2003;87:253–258.

Sawle GV, Bloomfield PM, Bjorklund A, et al: Transplantation of fetal dopamine neurons in Parkinson's disease: PET [18F]6-L-Fluorodopa studies in two patients with putaminal implants. Ann Neurol 1992;31:166–173.

Schmand B, de Bie RMA, Koning-Haanstra M, et al: Unilateral pallidotomy in PD: A controlled study of cognitive and behavioral effects. Neurology 2000;54:1058–1064.

Schrag A, Samuel M, Caputo E, et al: Unilateral pallidotomy for Parkinson's disease: Results after more than 1 year. J Neurol Neurosurg Psychiatry 1999;67:511–517.

Schroeder U, Kuehler A, Lange KW, et al: Subthalamic nucleus stimulation affects a frontotemporal network: A PET study. Ann Neurol 2003;54:445–450.

Schumacher JM, Ellias SA, Palmer EP, et al: Transplantation of embryonic porcine mesencephalic tissue in patients with PD. Neurology 2000;54:1042–1050.

Schuurman PR, Bosch A, Bossuyt PMM, et al: A comparison of continuous thalamic stimulation and thalamotomy for suppression of severe tremor. N Engl J Med 2000;342:461–468.

Scott R, Gregory R, Nines N, et al: Neuropsychological, neurological and functional outcome following pallidotomy for Parkinson's disease: A consecutive series of eight simultaneous bilateral and twelve unilateral procedures. Brain 1998;121:659–675.

Seif C, Herzog J, Van Der Horst C, et al: Effect of subthalamic deep brain stimulation on the function of the urinary bladder. Ann Neurol 2004;55:118–120.

Shahed J, Poysky J, Kenney C, et al: GPi deep brain stimulation for Tourette syndrome improves tics and psychiatric co-morbidities. Neurology 2007;68:159–160.

Shannon KM, Penn RD, Kroin JS, et al: Stereotactic pallidotomy for the treatment of Parkinson's disease: Efficacy and adverse effects at 6 months in 26 patients. Neurology 1998;50:434–438.

Siebner HR, Ceballos-Baumann A, Standhardt H, et al: Changes in handwriting resulting from bilateral high-frequency stimulation of the subthalamic nucleus in Parkinson's disease. Mov Disord 1999;14:964–971.

Siegel KL, Verhagen Metman L: Effects of bilateral posteroventral pallidotomy on gait of subjects with Parkinson disease. Arch Neurol 2000;57:198–204.

Spencer DD, Robbins RJ, Naftolin F, et al: Unilateral transplantation of human fetal mesencephalic tissue into the caudate nucleus of patients with Parkinson's disease. N Engl J Med 1992;327:1541–1548.

Starr PA, Vitek JL, Bakay RAE: Ablative surgery and deep brain stimulation for Parkinson's disease. Neurosurgery 1998;43:989–1015.

Stefani A, Lozano AM, Peppe A, et al: Bilateral deep brain stimulation of the pedunculopontine and subthalamic nuclei in severe Parkinson's disease. Brain 2007 (in press).

Stefurak T, Mikulis D, Mayberg H, et al: Deep brain stimulation for Parkinson's disease dissociates mood and motor circuits: A functional MRI case study. Mov Disord 2003;18:1508–1516.

Sterio D, Beric A, Dogali M, et al: Neurophysiological properties of pallidal neurons in Parkinson's disease. Ann Neurol 1994;35: 586–591.

Sterio D, Rezai A, Mogilner A, et al: Neurophysiological modulation of the subthalamic nucleus by pallidal stimulation in Parkinson's disease. J Neurol Neurosug Psychiatry 2002;72:325–328.

Stolze H, Klebe S, Poepping M, et al: Effects of bilateral subthalamic nucleus on parkinsonian gait. Neurology 2001;57:144–146.

Stover NP, Okun MS, Evatt ML, et al: Stimulation of the subthalamic nucleus in a patient with Parkinson disease and essential tremor. Arch Neurol 2005;62:141–143.

Stowe RL, Wheatley K, Clarke CE, et al: Surgery for Parkinson's disease: Lack of reliable clinical trial evidence. J Neurol Neurosurg Psychiatry 2003;74:519–521.

Strafella AP, Dagher A, Sadikot AF: Cerebral blood flow changes induced by subthalamic stimulation in Parkinson's disease. Neurology 2003;60:1039–1042.

Sturman MM, Vaillancourt DE, Metman LV, et al: Effects of subthalamic nucleus stimulation and medication on resting and postural tremor in Parkinson's disease. Brain 2004;127:2131–2143.

Su PC, Ma Y, Fukuda M, et al: Metabolic changes following subthalamotomy for advanced Parkinson's disease. Ann Neurol 2001;50: 514–520.

Su PC, Tseng H-M: Gait freezing and falling related to subthalamic stimulation in patients with previous pallidotomy. Mov Disord 2001;16:376–377.

Su PC, Tseng H-M, Liu HM, et al: Treatment of advanced Parkinson's disease by subthalamotomy: One-year results. Mov Disord 2003;18:531–538.

Subramanian T, Vitek J, Watts RL, et al: Microelectrode-guided stereotactic selective thalamotomy improves tremor but not bradykinesia in a young Parkinson's disease (PD) patient. Neurology 1995;45(suppl 4):A376.

Sydow O, Thobois S, Alesch F, et al: Multicentre European study of thalamic stimulation in essential tremor: A six year follow up. J Neurol Neurosurg Psychiatry 2003;74:1387–1391.

Tan EK, Jankovic J: Movement disorder surgery: Patient selection and evaluation of surgical results. In Lozano AM (ed): Movement Disorder Surgery: Progress and Challenges, Progress in Neurological Surgery. Basel, Karger, 2000, pp 78–90.

Tarsy D, Apetauerova D, Ryan P, Norregaard T: Adverse effects of subthalamic nucleus DBS in a patient with multiple system atrophy. Neurology 2003;61:247–249.

Tasker DR: Deep brain stimulation is preferable to thalamotomy for tremor suppression. Surg Neurol 1998;49:145–154.

Tasker RR: Movement disorders. In Apuzzo MLJ (ed): Brain Surgery: Complication Avoidance and Management. New York, Churchill Livingstone, 1993, pp 1509–1524.

Tasker RR, Kiss ZHT: The role of the thalamus in functional neurosurgery. Neurosurg Clin North Amer 1995;6:73–104.

Temperli P, Ghika J, Villemure JG, et al: How do parkinsonian signs return after discontinuation of subthalamic DBS? Neurology 2003;60:78–81.

Thompson TP, Kondziolka D, Albright AL: Thalamic stimulation for choreiform movement disorders in children: Report of two cases. J Neurosurg 2000;92:718–721.

Tronnier VM, Fogel W: Pallidal stimulation for generalized dystonia: Report of three cases. J Neurosurg 2000;92:453–456.

Tronnier VM, Staubert A, Hähnel S, et al: Magnetic resonance imaging with implanted neurostimulators: An in vitro and in vivo study. Neurosurgery 1999;44:118–126.

Tröster AI, Fields JA, Pahwa R, et al: Neuropsychological and quality of life outcome after thalamic stimulation for essential tremor. Neurology 1999;53:1774–1780.

Tröster AI, Fields JA, Wilkinson SB, et al: Unilateral pallidal stimulation for Parkinson's disease: Neurobehavioral functioning before and 3 months after electrode implantation. Neurology 1997;49:1078–1083.

Trottenberg T, Meissner W, Kabus C, et al: Neurostimulation of the ventral intermediate thalamic nucleus in inherited myoclonus-dystonia syndrome. Mov Disord 2001a;16:769–771.

Trottenberg T, Paul G, Meissner W, et al: Pallidal and thalamic neurostimulation in severe tardive dystonia. J Neurol Neurosurg Psychiatry 2001b;70:557–559.

Trottenberg T, Volkmann J, Deuschl G, et al: Treatment of severe tardive dystonia with pallidal deep brain stimulation. Neurology 2005;64:344–346.

Uitti RJ, Wharen RE, Turk MF, et al: Unilateral pallidotomy for Parkinson's disease: Comparison of outcome in younger versus elderly patients. Neurology 1997;49:1072–1077.

Ushe M, Mink JW, Revilla FJ, et al: Effect of stimulation frequency on tremor suppression in essential tremor. Mov Disord 2004;19:1163–1168.

Vaillancourt DE, Sturman MM, Verhagen Metman L, et al: Deep brain stimulation of the VIM thalamic nucleus modifies several features of essential tremor. Neurology 2003;61:919–925.

Valldeoriola F, Pilleri M, Tolosa E, et al: Bilateral subthalamic stimulation monotherapy in advanced Parkinson's disease: Long-term follow-up of patients. Mov Disord 2002;17:125–132.

Varma TRK, Fox SH, Eldridge PR, et al: Deep brain stimulation of the subthalamic nucleus: Effectiveness in advanced Parkinson's disease patients previously reliant on apomorphine. J Neurol Neurosurg Psychiatry 2003;74:170–174.

Vercueil L, Pollak P, Fraix V, et al: Deep brain stimulation in the treatment of severe dystonia. J Neurol 2001;248:695–700.

Vesper J, Chabardes S, Fraix V, et al: Dual channel deep brain stimulation system (Kinetra) for Parkinson's disease and essential tremor: A prospective multicentre open label clinical study. J Neurol Neurosurg Psychiatry 2002;73:275–280.

Vidailhet M, Vercueil L, Houeto JL, et al: Bilateral deep-brain stimulation of the globus pallidus in primary generalized dystonia. N Engl J Med 2005;352:459–467.

Vidailhet M, Vercueil L, Houeto JL, et al: Bilateral, pallidal, deep-brain stimulation in primary generalised dystonia: A prospective 3 year follow-up study. Lancet Neurol 2007;6:223–229.

Vingerhoets FJ, Villemure JG, Temperli P, et al: Subthalamic DBS replaces levodopa in Parkinson's disease: Two-year follow-up. Neurology 2002;58:396–401.

Vingerhoets G, Van der Linden C, Lannoo E, et al: Cognitive outcome after unilateral pallidal stimulation in Parkinson's disease. J Neurol Neurosurg Psychiatry 1999;66:297–304.

Vitek JL, Bakay RA, Freeman A, et al: Randomized trial of pallidotomy versus medical therapy for Parkinson's disease. Ann Neurol 2003;53:558–569.

Vitek JL, Hashimoto T, Peoples J, et al: Acute stimulation in the external segment of the globus pallidus improves parkinsonian motor signs. Mov Disord 2004;19:907–915.

Volkmann J, Albert N, Voges J, et al: Safety and efficacy of pallidal or subthalamic nucleus stimulation in advanced PD. Neurology 2001;56:548–551.

Volkmann J, Allert N, Voges J, et al: Long-term results of bilateral pallidal stimulation in Parkinson's disease. Ann Neurol 2004;55:871–875.

Walter BL, Vitek JL: Surgical treatment for Parkinson's disease. Lancet Neurol 2004;3:719–728.

Watts RL, Raiser CD, Stover NP, et al: Stereotaxic intrastriatal implantation of human retinal pigment epithelial (hRPE) cells attached to gelatin microcarriers: A potential new cell therapy for Parkinson's disease. J Neural Transm Suppl 2003;65:215–227.

Welter ML, Houeto JL, Tezenas du Montcel S, et al: Clinical predictive factors of subthalamic stimulation in Parkinson's disease. Brain 2002;125:575–583.

Wenning GK, Odin P, Morrish P, et al: Short- and long-term survival and function of unilateral instrastriatal dopaminergic grafts in Parkinson's disease. Ann Neurol 1997;42:95–107.

Winkler C, Kirik D, Bjorklund A: Cell transplantation in Parkinson's disease: How can we make it work? Trends Neurosci 2005;28:86–92.

Wishart HA, Roberts DW, Roth RM, et al: Chronic deep brain stimulation for the treatment of tremor in multiple sclerosis: Review and case reports. J Neurol Neurosurg Psychiatry 2003;74: 1392–1397.

Wohrle JC, Weigel R, Grips E, et al: Risperidone-responsive segmental dystonia and pallidal deep brain stimulation. Neurology 2003;61:546–548.

Wu YR, Levy R, Ashby P, et al: Does stimulation of the GPi control dyskinesia by activating inhibitory axons? Mov Disord 2001;16: 208–216.

York MK, Levin HS, Grossman RG, Hamilton WJ: Neuropsychological outcome following unilateral pallidotomy. Brain 1999;122: 2209–2220.

Yoshor D, Hamilton WJ, Ondo W, et al: Comparison of thalamotomy and pallidotomy for the treatment of dystonia. Neurosurgery 2001;48:818–824.

Zigova T, Pencea V, Betarbet R, et al: Neuronal progenitor cells of the neonatal subventricular zone differentiate and disperse following transplantation into the adult rat striatum. Cell Transplantation 1998;7:137–156.

Zirh A, Reich SG, Dougherty PM, Lenz FA: Stereotactic thalamotomy in the treatment of essential tremor of the upper extremity: Reassessment including a blinded measure of outcome. J Neurol Neurosurg Psychiatry 1999;66:772–775.

# Chapter 8

# Nonmotor Problems in Parkinson Disease

While the motor symptoms of Parkinson disease (PD) dominate the clinical picture—and even define the parkinsonian syndrome—many patients with PD have other complaints that have been classified as *nonmotor* (Chaudhuri et al., 2006a), and a scale has been developed to quantify them (Chaudhuri et al., 2006b). These include fatigue, depression, anxiety, sleep disturbances, constipation, bladder and other autonomic disturbances (sexual, gastrointestinal), and sensory complaints. Sensory symptoms, including pain, may occur. Orthostatic hypotension can lead to syncope. Behavioral and mental alterations include changes in mood, slowness in thinking (bradyphrenia), and a declining cognitive capacity, and these are frequent causes for concern. In one survey of nondemented PD patients, nonmotor disturbances were found to occur in the majority of patients (Table 8-1). There is even the suggestion that presentation of nonmotor symptoms commonly seen in PD patients but without any of the cardinal signs of PD may be considered part of the same disease spectrum (Langston, 2006).

Helping patients with PD to cope with these difficulties is just as important as manipulating therapy to provide control of their motor symptoms. In addition, antiparkinsonian drugs commonly induce unwanted nonmotor effects and aggravate such complaints. And so-called sensory "offs" are often underappreciated but are usually a greater source of discomfort than are motor "offs." This chapter covers nonmotor problems inherent to the disease and also those induced by medications to treat the disease.

## SENSORY SYMPTOMS

Many textbooks do not list pain and the other sensory complaints in Box 8-1 as a part of PD, and they are often not considered symptoms of the disease, but they can be (Snider et al., 1976; Koller, 1984; Goetz et al., 1986; Quinn et al., 1986; Ford et al., 1996). A constant, boring pain in the initially affected limb may be the first complaint. Aching in the shoulder and arm is often attributed to bursitis or a frozen shoulder, and pain in the hip and leg is often attributed to arthritis. That such pain is due to the PD is indicated by its relief with antiparkinsonian medication. Once adequate dosing is achieved, whether or not mobility is restored, such pain commonly abates. Of course, patients with PD may also have coincidental joint disease, so if the pain persists, patients require appropriate investigation.

Another initial complaint, particularly in younger patients, may be painful dystonic foot cramps, especially on walking. Rarely, similar painful cramp may occur in the hands. An extended big toe or curling of small toes may be seen with the cramping.

When patients with PD develop fluctuations and dyskinesias, pain may become a major feature. "Off" period dystonia often is painful. This may manifest as early morning painful cramps, particularly affecting the feet (Melamed, 1979). Similar painful dystonic cramps may emerge during "off" periods during the day and can be very distressing (Ilson et al., 1984). Some patients may experience more generalized excruciating pain during "off" periods, often a deep-seated aching but sometimes with a more superficial burning quality. Again, such pains disappear when the patient is switched "on" by appropriate medication to regain mobility. "Off" period pain may be an indication for the use of rapidly acting water-soluble preparations of levodopa or apomorphine rescue injections.

Other specific sensory symptoms, such as burning, numbness, and paresthesia, are less common in PD. However, some patients may describe rather nonspecific paresthesia in the affected limbs, but objective sensory signs are not evident (Snider et al., 1976; Koller, 1984). A rare patient may have sensory complaints from levodopa therapy, unaccompanied by dystonia. Electroconvulsive therapy can be effective in alleviating the problem. If parkinsonian pain occurs during an "off" or due to parkinsonism, one should increase medications to avoid "offs." (Sensory "offs" are considered later in this chapter.) If pain occurs during peak dose dystonia, one needs to lower the dose. If pain is secondary to levodopa or dopamine agonists, one needs to reduce or eliminate the causal agent. Occasionally, the ergot dopamine agonists bromocriptine and pergolide cause a burning pain with inflammatory skin on parts of the body, known as St. Anthony's fire. If this occurs, the agonist needs to be discontinued.

A more common sensory symptom is *akathisia*, or a sense of inner restlessness. This sometimes is focused on the legs, with uncomfortable paresthesias and the need to move them to gain relief, in which case it may be termed a true restless legs syndrome (Lang, 1987). More often, there is a sense of generalized inner restless discomfort, demanding walking for relief, when akathisia is the more appropriate description (Lang and Johnson, 1987). Akathisia may be a presenting feature of PD. The symptoms of both restless legs and akathisia may respond to dopamine replacement therapy. Akathisia may also occur during the "off" period (Lang, 1994).

Akathisia probably occurs more often in PD than is commonly recognized. It can be a sensory complaint of the disease itself and also an adverse effect from levodopa. Lang and Johnson (1987) asked patients with PD specifically for complaints of restlessness and found that 86% did have this subjective complaint. Most patients with PD who complained of an inner feeling of restlessness did not overtly manifest any signs such as moving about. From Lang and Johnson's study, it was not clear whether akathisia represented an adverse effect from levodopa or was a feature of the disease. In most of their patients, it appeared only after the introduction of antiparkinsonian drugs, but a small number had this symptom early in

**Table 8-1** Frequency of nonmotor symptoms in Parkinson disease

| Symptom | Frequency |
| --- | --- |
| Depression | 36% |
| Anxiety | 33% |
| Fatigue | 40% |
| Sleep disturbances | 47% |
| Sensory symptoms | 63% |
| No nonmotor symptom | 12% |

Data from Shulman LM, Taback RL, Bean J, Weiner WJ: Comorbidity of the nonmotor symptoms of Parkinson's disease. Mov Disord 2001;16:507–510.

the course of PD, prior to receiving any medication. It is likely that levodopa and other antiparkinsonian agents may also contribute to this complaint, for it has occurred in patients with primary torsion dystonia after starting these drugs.

*Restless legs syndrome* is encountered fairly often in patients with PD. This problem is covered in a later section, "Difficulties at Night and Daytime Sleepiness."

## BLADDER AND SEXUAL PROBLEMS

The autonomic dysfunctions in patients with PD can be segregated into urogenital problems and those that affect other functions, such as blood pressure, the gastrointestinal tract, and skin (Box 8-2). This section discusses the first group of problems.

Urinary frequency and urgency, with nocturia, are common complaints in PD (Fitzmaurice et al., 1985). Of course, PD patients are usually of an age at which prostatic problems in the male and stress incontinence in the female occur anyway. But PD itself affects bladder control, owing to detrusor hyperreflexia. As a result, premature uninhibited bladder contractions cause frequency and urgency, which can be particularly troublesome at night and during "off" periods. Araki and Kuno (2000) assessed voiding dysfunction in 203 consecutive PD patients and found that 27% had symptomatic voiding dysfunction. Its severity correlated with the severity of PD and not with disease duration, age, or gender.

Prostatic outflow obstruction can add to the problem in the male. Incontinence not explained by immobility when taken by the urge to micturate or by retention with overflow is not, however, a part of PD. True neurogenic incontinence in someone with parkinsonism suggests a diagnosis of multiple-system atrophy (MSA) (Stocchi et al., 1997). In this case, sphincter electromyography studies usually reveal signs of

**Box 8-1** Sensory symptoms in Parkinson disease

Pain
Paresthesias
Numbness
Burning
Akathisia
Restless legs syndrome

**Box 8-2** Autonomic dysfunction in Parkinson disease

Bladder problems
Sexual dysfunction
Hypotension
Gastrointestinal
Seborrhea
Sweating

denervation due to involvement of Onuf's nucleus in the sacral spinal cord, which does not occur in PD.

The diagnosis of significant prostate enlargement in PD is difficult, and prostatectomy by the unwary often leads to disaster. Prostatectomy should be considered only in those with proven outflow obstruction. A simple screening test in patients with PD is noninvasive ultrasonic estimation of post-micturition residual volume and simple mechanical measurement of urinary flow rate. If there is significant residual volume after urination (>100 mL) or if flow rate is reduced, there may be bladder outlet obstruction and further investigation by more extensive urodynamic studies, and other urologic testing is required. If there is no significant residual volume or reduction of flow rate, urinary frequency and urgency may be helped by a peripheral antimuscarinic drug such as oxybutynin (Ditropan), 5 to 10 mg at night or 5 mg three times daily. Fluid intake should be reduced at night. A tricyclic antidepressant with anticholinergic properties, such as amitriptyline, may help sleep not only through its sedative actions but also by reducing bladder irritability. Intranasal DDAVP (desmopressin) at night also may reduce nocturia.

Impotence in the male patient with PD causes distress to both partners (as do immobility and other problems in the female). PD itself does not normally cause impotence, although this is a common early complaint in MSA. Loss of libido and failure to gain or sustain erections may have some other cause in this age group, be it psychological, vascular, hormonal, or neurogenic, and appropriate investigation is warranted. Some antidepressant drugs, monoamine oxidase inhibitors, and antihypertensive medications can impair sexual performance. Failure of erection can be overcome by a variety of intrapenile or oral medications such as sildenafil (Viagra) (Zesiewicz et al., 2000). Sildenafil can be efficacious in the treatment of erectile dysfunction in both PD and MSA; however, it can unmask or exacerbate hypotension in MSA (Hussain et al., 2001). Parkinsonian symptoms are not affected, but a side benefit of reduced dyskinesias has been reported (Swope, 2000). Hypersexuality, particularly in the male, is a rare and unacceptable side effect of dopamine replacement therapy in PD, both levodopa and dopamine agonists, and usually requires reduction of antiparkinsonian medication.

## OTHER AUTONOMIC SYMPTOMS

Lewy body degeneration affects the autonomic nervous system in PD. Both sympathetic ganglion neurons and parasympathetic myenteric and cardiac plexi can be involved (Qualman et al., 1984; Kupsky et al., 1987; Wakabayashi et al., 1988). In addition, central autonomic nuclei, such as those of the hypothalamus and dorsal motor nucleus of the vagus, can show Lewy body degeneration (Eadie, 1963).

Control of blood pressure may be compromised by sympathetic failure with impaired vasoconstriction and inadequate intravascular volume. Faintness on standing (presyncope) and frank loss of consciousness on standing (postural syncope) can occur owing to postural hypotension. Orthostatic hypotension can also cause posturally induced fatigue and weakness, blurring of vision, and "coat-hanger" neck and shoulder aching. Hypotension also may occur postprandially due to gastrointestinal vasodilatation. Levodopa and dopamine agonist drugs may aggravate postural hypotension. Prominent early symptoms of postural hypotension are, of course, one of the hallmarks of MSA, so such complaints may raise concern over the diagnosis of PD. The severity of postural hypotension in PD rarely is as severe as that seen in MSA. Nevertheless, treatment might be required. A selective peripheral dopamine antagonist such as domperidone sometimes helps, as does increasing fluid and salt intake, with head uptilt at night, which reduces nocturnal polyuria. Intranasal DDAVP (desmopressin) (5 to 40 μg) at night also reduces nocturnal polyuria but can cause hyponatremia. However, a small dose of fludrocortisone (0.1 to 0.5 mg) (to promote salt retention) or midodrine (ProAmatine) (a selective α-agonist) (2.5 to 5 mg three times daily) might be required to maintain adequate blood pressure.

Gastrointestinal problems cause significant disability in PD (Edwards et al., 1991, 1992). Dysphagia is due mainly to poor masticatory and oropharyngeal muscular control, making it difficult to chew and propel the bolus of food into the pharynx and esophagus (Bushman et al., 1989; Edwards et al., 1994). Soft food is easier to eat, and antiparkinsonian medication improves swallowing.

Parasympathetic failure may contribute to gastrointestinal problems in PD, causing delay in esophageal and gastric motility. A sense of bloating, indigestion, and gastric reflux are common in PD (Edwards et al., 1992). Many factors contribute to delayed gastric emptying, including immobility, parasympathetic failure, constipation, and antiparkinsonian drugs (both anticholinergic and dopamine agonists). Levodopa is absorbed in the upper small bowel, so gastric stasis may slow or prevent levodopa assimilation, leading to "delayed-ons" and "no-ons" (dose failures) after single oral doses (either there is an excessive interval before the drug works, or it does not work at all).

Constipation is another frequent complaint in PD (Edwards et al., 1992, 1994) and is multifactorial. Again, immobility, drugs, reduced fluid and food intake, and parasympathetic involvement prolonging colonic transit time may all contribute. In addition, malfunction of the striated muscles of the pelvic floor due to the PD itself can make evacuation of the bowels difficult (Mathers et al., 1988, 1989). Constipation may exacerbate gastric stasis. Anticholinergic drugs should be stopped, and physical exercise should be increased. The role of levodopa in causing or treating constipation is uncertain. This drug usually does not relieve the problem, and some patients believe that it worsens the problem. Constipation is ameliorated by adequate fluid intake, fruit, vegetables, fiber, and lactulose (10 to 20 g per day) or other mild laxatives. The following "rancho recipe" provided by Dr. Cheryl Waters has been found useful for many patients: Mix together one cup each of bran, applesauce, and prune juice; take two tablespoons every morning; the mixture can be refrigerated for one week, then should be discarded.

Polyethylene glycol powder (marketed as MiraLax) can be effective to overcome constipation; the usual dose is 17 g per day dissolved in a glass of water at bedtime. Refractory constipation may be helped by apomorphine injections to assist defecation (Edwards et al., 1993; Merello and Leiguarda, 1994).

For patients who have abdominal bloating due to suppression of peristalsis when they are "off," keeping them "on" with levodopa or other dopaminergics is beneficial.

Excessive sebum (seborrhea) probably is due more to facial immobility that to overproduction. The greasy skin contributes to seborrheic dermatitis and dandruff. Medicated soaps and shampoos help. Blepharitis also is common, due in part to reduced blinking. Artificial teardrops can help.

Excessive sweating can be a problem, particularly in the form of sudden drenching sweats (sweating crises). Sage and Mark (1995) showed that drenching sweats is an "off" phenomenon. They found treatment with dopamine agonists to be effective. In their study, Swinn and colleagues (2003) found that sweating occurred predominantly in "off" periods and also in "on" periods with dyskinesias. Sweating can cause physical, social, and emotional impairment.

Excessive salivation (sialorrhea) is due more to failure to swallow saliva frequently than to overproduction (Bateson et al., 1973). Drooling of saliva can be helped by chewing gum or by using peripherally acting anticholinergic drugs. If these are unsuccessful, intraparotid injections of botulinum toxin B can sometimes be effective in reducing salivary secretions and drooling (Racette et al., 2003; Lipp et al., 2004; Ondo et al., 2004).

## RESPIRATORY DISTRESS

Respiratory distress such as dyspnea can occur as a symptom of PD in some patients, including during the "off" period in some (Ilson et al., 1983). It can also occur as a complication of dystonia, usually peak-dose dystonia (Braun et al., 1983), and with some dopamine agonists, particularly pergolide. Removing the offending drug is required. "Off" period dyspnea is difficult to treat, other than attempting to keep the patient "on." Despite the sensation of dyspnea, oxygen saturation is not affected because the patient will have a voluntary sigh or transient deep breathing when feeling short of breath. Some forms of parkinsonism-plus syndromes may have an accompanying apnea that is life-threatening, such as postencephalitic parkinsonism (Strieder et al., 1967; Efthimiou et al., 1987), frontotemporal dementia (Lynch et al., 1994), MSA (Chester et al., 1988; Salazar-Grueso et al., 1988), Joseph disease (SCA-3) (Kitamura et al., 1989), and other familial parkinsonian syndromes (Perry et al., 1990).

## DIFFICULTIES AT NIGHT AND DAYTIME SLEEPINESS

PD patients often have troubled nights for many reasons (Factor et al., 1990; Askenasy, 1993; Van Hilten et al., 1994; Bliwise et al., 1995). The major problem is difficulty with sleep maintenance (so-called sleep fragmentation) (Box 8-3). Frequent awakenings may be caused by tremor reappearing in the lighter stages of sleep, difficulty in turning in bed due to nocturnal akinesia as the effects of daytime administration of dopaminergic drugs wear off at night, and nocturia. In addition,

**Box 8-3** Sleep problems in Parkinson disease

Sleep fragmentation
REM sleep behavior disorder
Excessive daytime sleepiness
Altered sleep-wake cycle
Drug-induced sleep attacks

periodic leg movements in sleep (sometimes associated with restless legs), fragmentary nocturnal myoclonus, sleep apnea, REM sleep behavioral disorders (intense dream-like motor and behavioral problems), and parasomnias (nocturnal hallucinations and nocturnal wandering with disruptive behavior) may all disrupt sleep in PD. Reversal of sleep rhythm with sundowning also is common in PD (Bliwise et al., 1995). Many of these conditions probably occur more frequently in those with PD than in other aged populations. As a result, PD patients and their caregivers face disrupted nights, which lead to poor quality of life (QoL) and worse parkinsonism the next day. In fact, along with depression, poor sleep is a major factor in a PD patient's assessment of having a poor quality of life (Karlsen et al., 1999b). A good night's sleep reduces the severity of daytime parkinsonism, and many patients comment on sleep benefit, describing better mobility the morning after a restful night. Indeed, patients with marked sleep benefit might not require antiparkinsonian medication for some hours after they awaken, and some PD patients find that a daytime nap "charges the batteries." These may be the young-onset PD patients with mutations in the *parkin* gene, for they typically show sleep benefit (Elibol et al., 2000).

The reasons for the various causes of disturbed sleep also are multiple. Nocturnal tremor, akinesia, and nocturia are often due to the PD itself. Depression, which is common in PD, can cause insomnia. Drugs given to treat PD symptoms can interfere with sleep. PD pathology can also contribute to REM sleep behavioral disorders and parasomnias, especially in patients with incipient or frank dementia. The animal model of REM sleep without atonia indicates that lesions to the perilocus coeruleus disrupt the excitatory connection to the nucleus reticularis magnocellularis in the descending medullary reticular formation and disable the hyperpolarization of the alpha spinal motoneurons (Ferini-Strambi and Zucconi, 2000). The development of RBD may be an early marker for the later onset of PD (Postuma et al., 2006).

The treatment of sleep disorders in PD is important. Attention to sleep hygiene by avoiding alcohol, caffeine, nicotine, and excessive fluid intake at night is helpful. Deprenyl (selegiline), which is metabolized to methamphetamine, should not be given at night. Treatment of depression might be required. A sedative antidepressant, such as amitriptyline (10 to 25 mg at night), can be very useful, not only to induce and maintain sleep but also to reduce urinary frequency. A dose of a long-acting levodopa preparation last thing at night may improve nocturnal akinesia (Laihnen et al., 1987; Lees, 1987). However, levodopa given at night may provoke excessive dreaming and disrupted sleep in some patients (Nausieda et al., 1982). A benzodiazepine, especially clonazepam, may lessen REM sleep behavior disorders. Propoxyphene is useful for periodic leg movements of sleep and restless legs (Hening et al., 1986). A small bedtime dose of clozapine (Rabey et al.,

1995) or quetiapine may be very effective in improving sleep. For patients who have no problem falling asleep but awaken in 2 to 3 hours, the short-acting hypnotic zolpidem is useful when taken after the awakening. It helps the patient get back to sleep quickly and still be refreshed in the morning.

Excessive daytime sleepiness (EDS) occurs in about 15% of patients with PD and is associated with more severe PD and patients with cognitive decline (Tandberg et al., 1999). EDS is determined by short sleep latency and sleep-onset REM periods. When studied with tests determining these two criteria, PD patients with EDS were found to correlate not with variables related to disease severity or to total sleep time or sleep stage percentages but rather with variables related to primary impairments of waking arousal and REM-sleep expression (Rye et al., 2000). Dopamine agonists are more likely than levodopa to be associated with EDS (Ondo et al., 2001). The antisoporific agent modafinil can sometimes be beneficial in overcoming EDS in patients with PD (Happe et al., 2001).

Some patients who sleep a lot during the daytime may have their problem related to drowsiness following a dosage of levodopa. This phenomenon is usually seen in patients with developing or more pronounced dementia. With postlevodopa drowsiness, patients can sleep during much of the daytime and are then awake at night. This altered sleep-wake cycle can make life unbearable for the caregiver who requires adequate sleep at night. If a patient becomes drowsy after each dose of medication, this is a sign of overdosage. Reducing the dosage can correct this problem. Sometimes, substituting Sinemet CR for standard Sinemet will help because this provides for a slower rise in plasma and brain levels of levodopa.

If the patient's sleep problem has advanced to that of an altered sleep-wake cycle, it is important to get the patient onto a sleep-wake schedule that fits with that of the rest of the household. To correct the problem, it might be necessary to use a combination of approaches. Efforts must be made to stimulate the patient physically and mentally during the daytime and force the patient to remain awake; otherwise, he or she will not be able to sleep at night. At night, the patient should then be drowsy enough that he or she will be able to sleep. If this fails, it might be necessary to use stimulants in the morning and sedatives at night to reverse the altered state. This should be done in addition to prodding the patient to remain awake during the day. Drugs such as methylphenidate and amphetamine are usually well tolerated by patients with PD. A 10-mg dose of either of these two drugs, repeated once if necessary, may be helpful. To encourage sleep at night, a hypnotic might be necessary in addition to using daytime stimulants. It should be noted that strong sedatives, such as barbiturates, are poorly tolerated by patients with PD. Milder hypnotics, such as benzodiazepines, are usually taken without difficulty. Short-acting benzodiazepines would be preferable, but if the patient awakens too early, a longer-acting one might need to be used.

Falling asleep while driving and without warning is a serious problem that has been encountered with dopaminergic agents; it seems more likely to occur with pramipexole and ropinirole but is not limited to these drugs (Frucht et al., 1999; Ferreira et al., 2000; Hoehn, 2000; Schapira, 2000). The decision about which dopamine agonist to place a patient on is discussed in Chapter 6. Once sleep attacks have occurred, the patient should not drive, except on short trips, or the medication should be changed. Fortunately, modafinil has been reported to be helpful in preventing sleep attacks (Hauser et al., 2000). A review of the literature (Homann et al., 2002) reported that sleep attacks have been reported with all dopaminergic medications, including levodopa, the greatest number being associated with pramipexole and ropinirole. Unfortunately, not all reports refer strictly to sudden attacks without warning; some reports refer to falling asleep from drowsiness, so the interpretation is open to uncertainty.

## FATIGUE

Although fatigue can be a symptom of sleepiness or depression, it is also a symptom that may be unassociated with these other states. In patients with PD, fatigue is often a complaint during the earliest phase of the disease, before motor symptoms, such as stiffness and slowness, become prominent. As these other features of PD develop, with their important contribution to disability, they are more of a complaint than is fatigue. But when patients are specifically asked, fatigue remains a common feature in PD. In a community study of elderly people in Norway, 44% of PD patients and 18% of healthy controls reported fatigue (Karlsen et al., 1999a). Treating depression and daytime sleepiness would be helpful, but when fatigue is an independent symptom, no treatment has been found to be satisfactory. Despite the claimed benefit of amantadine in treating fatigue in multiple sclerosis, neither this drug nor the monoamine oxidase inhibitor selegiline has been found particularly beneficial in treating fatigue in PD.

## DEPRESSION AND ANXIETY

In patients with PD it is common to find a change in personality (Box 8-4), and such change may precede motor symptoms but usually develops and worsens over the course of PD. Executives with decision-making tasks might find such duties so difficult that they might not be able to continue in their work. Passivity, dependency, and lack of motivation are often more troublesome for the spouse than for the patient. Abulia is a severe form of apathy, both mental and motor apathy, with not only a loss of initiative and drive but also a general restriction of activities, including the reticence to speak. Abulia is a recognized clinical syndrome due to caudate and prefrontal dysfunction, so it might well feature in the overall symptomatology of PD. In its milder form (i.e., apathy), the loss of initiative, both mental and motor, is often noted by the spouse or close relatives, who perceive a change in personality. Spouses particularly complain about the patient's lack of desire to socialize with friends and communicate freely. Such alterations in activity may be due to depression, but not infrequently there is no change in mood. The personality alterations do not respond to dopamine replacement therapy in the way the motor problems of PD do, nor to antidepressants, unless depression is present and is itself the cause of the apathy.

Depression is common in PD, with at least one third of patients exhibiting significant depressive symptoms in cross-sectional surveys (Brown et al., 1988; Dooneief et al., 1992). Anguenot and colleagues (2002) reported a higher number of one half of PD patients having depression.

However, it often is difficult to distinguish true depression from the apathy (abulia) associated with PD, especially in the presence of the characteristic expressionless face, bowed posture, and slowed movement, which resemble the psychomotor retardation of a primary depressive illness. The critical factor is whether the patient has a true disturbance of mood (dysphoria), with low spirits, loss of interest, bleak outlook, typical depressive sleep disturbance, paranoid ruminations, and sometimes suicidal thoughts.

The reasons for depression in PD are debated. On the one hand, depressive symptoms are not surprising in vulnerable individuals who are faced with the disabilities and handicaps imposed by PD, with reduced activities and independence and the prospects of a chronic incurable condition. Such reactive depression certainly contributes to the problem. But one study suggests that depression in PD is more strongly influenced by the patients' perceptions of handicap than by actual disability (Schrag et al., 2001). However, there also is the probability that the pathology of PD in itself might predispose to depression, especially that involving serotonergic and noradrenergic systems, which have been implicated in the neurochemical basis of primary depressive illnesses. The substantia nigra itself is implicated by the report that deep brain stimulation of this structure in a patient with PD induced acute severe depression (Bejjani et al., 1999).

The recognition and treatment of depression in PD are important because depression has a major impact on the overall disability imposed by the illness. In fact, depression carries a hazard ration of 2.66 for increased mortality in PD (Hughes et al., 2004). Most antidepressant drugs can be used safely in PD. However, nonselective monoamine oxidase inhibitors are contraindicated in patients who are taking levodopa because of potential pressor reactions. There also have been concerns over the use of selective serotonin reuptake inhibitors, which in a few cases have been reported to interact with levodopa to induce the serotonin syndrome (confusion, myoclonus, rigidity, and restlessness) and to worsen PD symptoms. Despite these worries, many depressed patients with PD have been treated safely and successfully with selective serotonin reuptake inhibitors, for example, fluoxetine or paroxetine (20 to 40 mg daily). By enhancing serotonergic "tone" and thereby potentially inhibiting dopaminergic neurons in the substantia nigra, there is the potential, especially in the absence of dopaminergic drug treatment, that selective serotonin reuptake inhibitors may increase parkinsonian symptoms, but such events are rare (Jansen Steur, 1993; Jimenez-Jimenez et al., 1994; Richard et al., 1999; Ceravolo et al., 2000; Tesei et al., 2000). The traditional tricyclic antidepressants also can be employed, although their sedative and anticholinergic

---

Box 8-4 Personality and behavior in Parkinson disease

Depression
Fearfulness
Anxiety
Loss of assertive drive
Passivity
Dependency
Inability to make decisions
Loss of motivation, apathy
Abulia

properties may be detrimental in the aged. If a severely depressed patient with PD fails to respond to antidepressant drug treatment, electroconvulsive therapy can be used (Douyon et al., 1989). Indeed, electroconvulsive therapy in itself can temporarily improve mobility in PD. Tranyl-cypromine, a noncompetitive inhibitor of types A and B monoamine oxidase is an effective antidepressant (Fahn and Chouinard, 1998) but cannot be given in the presence of levodopa because of the likelihood of hypertension.

Anxiety and panic can be major difficulties in PD (Stein et al., 1990). Many patients, even early in the illness, complain of loss of confidence. In particular, they fear social occasions and public display at work, and they tend to withdraw from outside life. In part, this is due to anxiety over their friends and acquaintances perceiving that they have PD and to their loss of mobility and their nonverbal emotional responses to social interactions. However, some also develop a generalized and disturbing anxiety state, which might require psychotherapy and anxiolytic drug treatment. Those in the more advanced stages of the illness may experience profound anxiety and even terror during "off" periods (Nissenbaum et al., 1987).

Often, anxiety can be relieved by effective antiparkinsonian drug therapy, but if uncontrolled and pervasive, it might require an antidepressant, and if dysphoria is present, a benzodiazepine (e.g., lorazepam 0.5 to 2 mg three times daily) or buspirone. However, all these drugs can increase confusion in those who are cognitively impaired.

Many patients have sensory or behavioral "off" periods, either accompanying or instead of a motor "off." The behavioral symptoms can consist of depression, anxiety, dysphoria, and panic; the sensory symptoms consist of pain mainly. These sensory or behavioral "offs" are most distressing to the patient. Whereas motoric "offs" represent insufficient dopaminergic "tone" in the neostriatum, the behavioral and sensory "offs" probably represent an insufficient dopaminergic "tone" in the limbic dopaminergic areas of the brain, such as the nucleus accumbens, amygdala, and cingulate cortex.

## COGNITIVE PROBLEMS

Discussed here are cognitive defects (Box 8-5) in patients with PD who are not demented or confused (symptoms that are discussed later). If these defects are specifically looked for, about two thirds of patients with early PD will show abnormalities of cognitive function on formal neuropsychological testing (Lees and Smith, 1983; Levin et al., 1989; Brown and Marsden, 1990; Cooper et al., 1991). In particular, such patients are weak in performance of tests that are sensitive to frontal lobe dysfunction (executive function), such as verbal fluency, the Wisconsin card sorting test, the Tower of London test and its variants, and tests of working memory. Poor performance on tests such as these suggests abnormalities of

frontal lobe executive functions, which may be due to defective input from nonmotor basal ganglia regions (via thalamus) into prefrontal cerebral cortical areas. Thus, some patients with early PD may exhibit a frontostriatal cognitive syndrome, which is sometimes rather inaccurately described as a subcortical dementia, in the absence of any major defects in language, episodic memory, or visuospatial functions. The pathologic substrate of such a frontostriatal cognitive syndrome in PD is debatable. Contributing factors may include dopamine deficiency in the nonmotor regions of the striatum, especially the caudate nucleus, which receives from and projects to prefrontal cerebral cortex; loss of dopamine projections from the midbrain ventral tegmental area to the frontal lobes; loss of cortical cholinergic projections from the substantia innominata; loss of cortical noradrenergic projections from the locus coeruleus; and cortical Lewy body degeneration.

The clinical question is to what extent such neuropsychological defects intrude into everyday life in patients with PD. In this context, two clinical features of PD deserve further comment: bradyphrenia and abulia.

Bradyphrenia, or slowness of thought, probably is a real component of PD in many patients. For example, patients might comment on a slowing of mental processing and memory retrieval, and examination of neuropsychological test performance might show delay in deciding on choices, although the final decisions are correct. Finding the right word or the answer to a question may be slow. The "tip of the tongue" phenomenon refers to the patient's knowing the word he or she wants but not being able to come up with it and say it at that moment, a problem that is often encountered in PD (Matison et al., 1982). Some patients with PD spontaneously volunteer the observation that they have less ability to deal with mental problems, particularly multiple tasks at the same time. However, the extent to which depression might contribute to such problems is controversial. The general concept of bradyphrenia could be considered in the wider issue of abulia.

The overall impression of cognitive dysfunction in nondemented patients with PD may be summarized as follows: (1) Many, but not all, patients with early PD exhibit subtle frontostriatal cognitive impairments, but to begin with, these do not necessarily intrude into everyday life. (2) However, a substantial number of patients with early PD do complain of some cognitive change, in particular a slowing of thought, a difficulty or delay in memory retrieval, and problems in handling multiple tasks. (3) Such cognitive impairments may be due to depression when there is a change in mood, but often there is no dysphoria.

Unfortunately, these selective cognitive impairments do not seem to respond to dopamine replacement therapy in the way the motor problems of PD do. Nor do they respond to antidepressants unless depression is present and is itself the cause of the slowness of thinking. It is important to assess and treat any concurrent depression. It also is important to review current drug therapy. Anticholinergics, amantadine, dopamine agonists, and even levodopa in excess might well impair cognitive function, especially in the elderly PD patient.

Whether these cognitive difficulties are the precursor to frank dementia is uncertain, but obviously, they raise concern. In practice, it is likely that a minority of patients with such complaints in the early stages of PD will progress to frank dementia.

Box 8-5 Cognition and dementia in Parkinson disease

Bradyphrenia
"Tip of the tongue" phenomenon
Confusion
Dementia

## DEMENTIA AND CONFUSION

Unfortunately, a sizable proportion of patients with PD eventually develop a multifocal, pervasive dementia. This typically occurs in elderly patients. Cross-sectional studies suggest that in those with PD aged over 65 years, some 20% will be demented, compared to some 10% of non-PD individuals in this age group (Brown and Marsden, 1984). Prospective longitudinal studies suggest that up to 40% of those with PD will dement as they age (Mayeux et al., 1990; Biggins et al., 1992; Hughes et al., 2000). Aarsland and colleagues (2001) found the incidence rate for dementia to be 95.3 per 1000 person-years, which is a sixfold greater risk than that in non-PD individuals. Following patients over an 8-year period, Aarsland and colleagues (2003) found the prevalence of dementia to affect more than 75% of patients with PD, with hallucinations before baseline and akinetic-dominant or mixed tremor/akinetic PD being high risk factors. Another study also found dementia to more likely occur in the PIGD (postural instability gait disorder) category of patient than in the type presenting with tremor (Burn et al., 2006). Other correlations for developing dementia are older age, greater severity and longer duration of PD, and male gender. However, viewed from the opposite perspective, most patients with PD, particularly the young, do not have dementia. Aarsland and colleagues (2004) followed the Mini-Mental State Examination and reported that the mean annual decline for PD patients was 1 point. However, a marked variation was found. In patients with PD and dementia, the mean annual decline was 2.3, which was similar to the decline observed in patients with Alzheimer disease.

Concurrent Alzheimer disease, probably coincidental, obviously accounts for some of the dementia in PD (Boller et al., 1980). However, in recent years, it has become apparent that widespread Lewy body degeneration is another common cause of dementia (Byrne et al., 1989), some say second in frequency to Alzheimer disease. In those with prior PD, this may follow the progression and spread of Lewy neurite distribution observed by Braak and colleagues (2003). *PD dementia* is now the term applied to those whose PD symptoms began at least 1 year prior to the onset of dementia. It is called dementia with Lewy bodies (DLB) (McKeith et al., 1996) when the dementia precedes or occurs within 1 year after onset of parkinsonian motor features. Dementia with Lewy bodies may coexist with the pathologic changes of Alzheimer disease, particularly with amyloid plaques rather than neurofibrillary tangles. One hypothesis is that the two pathologies, Lewy body degeneration in cerebral cortex and the cholinergic substantia innominata and Alzheimer disease change, coexist by chance, but summate to cause dementia. Another hypothesis is that the one predisposes to the other, and it is intriguing that $\alpha$-synuclein is a component of both plaques (the nonamyloid component) and Lewy bodies. Whatever the pathogenic mechanism, this combination (which some have called the Lewy body variant of Alzheimer disease) is a common cause of dementia in PD. Pure dementia with Lewy bodies probably is less common. But it has been shown pathologically that cortical Lewy bodies can be associated with cognitive impairment independent of Alzheimer disease–type pathology (Mattila et al., 2000).

Thus, there are at least three common substrates for dementia in PD: Alzheimer disease, Alzheimer disease with Lewy bodies, and diffuse Lewy body disease (also called dementia with Lewy bodies). A fourth possibility is dementia with just the standard pathology of PD; whether such dementia in patients with PD occurs without the spread of Lewy bodies into the cortex is uncertain. In addition, all the other causes of dementia may occur in patients with PD, including cerebrovascular disease; rarer degenerations, such as frontotemporal dementia and Pick disease; cerebral tumors and other intracranial mass lesions; hydrocephalus; and metabolic, endocrine, and vitamin abnormalities. In one pathologic study, the Lewy body score was significantly associated with the rate of cognitive decline (Aarsland et al., 2005).

Accordingly, the first step in assessment of a patient with PD who is dementing is to undertake the usual investigations for known causes, especially those that are treatable. Depression causing a pseudo-dementia also must be carefully assessed.

Having excluded such symptomatic causes of dementia, the clinical picture may give important clues as to the underlying degenerative condition causing the dementia. Prominent early memory difficulties with language, praxis, and visuospatial problems pointing to temporoparietal problems suggest Alzheimer disease. A variable, fluctuating cause with prominent hallucinations (especially visual), confusion, and an unusual susceptibility to neuroleptics could indicate dementia with Lewy bodies (McKeith et al., 1996, 1999), that is, diffuse Lewy body disease. Prominent behavioral, speech, and memory difficulties could point to frontotemporal dementia or Pick disease.

FDG PET scans were correlated with the dementia score on the Unified Parkinson's Disease Rating Scale. A correlation was found with left limbic structures such as the cingulate gyrus, parahippocampal gyrus, and medial frontal gyrus (Wu et al., 2000).

Whatever the pathologic substrate of dementia in PD, the combination poses formidable management problems. These are similar to those that are discussed in the section entitled "Psychosis: Hallucinations and Paranoia." The difficulty is to maintain mobility with adequate doses of antiparkinsonian medication without exacerbating the mental and behavioral problems. Behavioral disturbances, including verbal and physical aggression, wandering, agitation, inappropriate sexual behavior, uncooperativeness, and urinary incontinence, cause major difficulties. General structured care in a familiar environment is essential. Judicious use of day care facilities and home assistants might be necessary. Drug therapy should be simplified, removing selegiline, anticholinergic agents, amantadine, and dopamine agonists. Depression might require specific treatment, preferably avoiding antidepressants with marked anticholinergic properties. Nocturnal sedation might require quetiapine, which provides both sedation and antihallucinatory effects. Clozapine does the same but requires weekly evaluation for neutropenia. Other bedtime hypnotics, such as benzodiazepines and zolpidem, can be effective. Donepezil (Aricept), which provides modest benefit in Alzheimer disease, has been found also to provide modest benefit in cognition in those with PD who are demented without aggravating the motoric symptoms of PD (Aarsland et al., 2002). Rivastigmine and other centrally active cholinesterase inhibitors were found to provide some improvement in apathy, anxiety, delusions, and hallucinations in patients with DLB (McKeith et al., 2000) and can improve dementia (Giladi et al., 2003). In a large, multicenter controlled clinical trial, rivastigmine was associated with moderate improvements in dementia associated with PD (Emre et al., 2004). An evidence-based review of treatment of PD dementia and psychosis was conducted by the American Academy of Neurology (Miyasaki et al., 2006).

Dementia, with or without a frank confusional state, is the commonest cause of final nursing home placement in those with PD and shortens life expectancy (Goetz and Stebbins, 1993).

## PSYCHOSIS: HALLUCINATIONS AND PARANOIA

The term *punding* (Box 8-6) has been used to describe an abnormal motor behavior in which there is an intense fascination with repetitive handling and examining of mechanical objects, such as picking at oneself; taking apart watches and radios; or sorting and arranging of common objects, such as lining up pebbles, rocks, or other small objects. Punding has been reported with levodopa (Fernandez and Friedman, 1999) but might be more common with dopamine agonists. A common form is repetitive cleaning/rearranging/ordering behaviors, which can be disabling. These have associated features of hypomania, occur during motor "on" periods, and often occur nocturnally (Kurlan, 2004). The repetitive behavior responds poorly to serotonin reuptake inhibitors but may benefit from atypical antipsychotics (Kurlan, 2004). Punding, a term that was first used in amphetamine abusers, is considered a dopamine dysregulation disorder (Evans et al., 2004). This behavior would appear to be a form of compulsive disorder. In this category is compulsive gambling, which is now being recognized in some patients with PD (Driver-Dunckley et al., 2003), possibly related to dopaminergic stimulation in the mesolimbic system (Gschwandtner et al., 2001). Treatment of PD with a dopamine agonist increases the lifetime risk of a PD patient to have pathologic gambling from 3.4% to 7.2% (Voon et al., 2006).

Hallucinations occur in a significant proportion of those with PD, especially in the aged. In a community study in Norway, 10% of PD patients had hallucinations with insight retained, and another 6% had more severe hallucinations or delusions (Aarsland et al., 1999). Psychotic features appear to be due to a complex interaction between the progressive and widespread pathology of the illness (diffuse cortical Lewy body degeneration; concurrent Alzheimer plaques and tangles; and cortical cholinergic, noradrenergic, and serotonergic denervation), the unwanted effects of drugs (anticholinergics, levodopa, and dopamine agonists), and intercurrent illness (such as infections or metabolic disturbances).

Isolated visual hallucinations are fairly common (Naimark et al., 1996; Sanchez-Ramos et al, 1996). Auditory hallucinations are very uncommon (Inzelberg et al., 1998). Visual hallucinations often take the form of familiar humans or animals, which the patients know are false (pseudo-hallucinations). Even milder forms of hallucinations, which do not disturb the patient because the visual images are friendly and not frightening (benign hallucinations), can worsen to a more malignant type of hallucination (Goetz et al., 2006). Such hallucinations may progress to a delusional paranoid state (often concerning infidelity) or a frank confusional state with impairment of attentiveness and disorientation.

When such symptoms occur, although antiparkinsonian drug therapy is the most likely cause, it is wise first to search for some intercurrent illness, such as a stroke or intracranial mass lesion, a chest or urinary infection, disturbance of electrolytes, renal or hepatic dysfunction, anemia, or endocrine dysfunction. Psychosis due to antiparkinsonian medications can usually be counteracted by atypical antipsychotics, drugs that usually do not aggravate parkinsonism at a dosage that has a therapeutic benefit in treating the psychosis. Start with quetiapine (Seroquel) because this drug does not cause agranulocytosis and does not require blood count monitoring (Fernandez et al., 1999; Juncos et al., 2004). A dose of 25 to 50 mg at night can often control confusion and psychosis without worsening the parkinsonism. Because of the potential for drowsiness, it is best initially to use a small dose of such drugs at night, thereafter gradually increasing the dose to that required to control the confusion without worsening the parkinsonism. The benefit of aiding sleep at night is an advantage, but try to avoid a dose that might extend the drowsiness to daytime. If quetiapine is ineffective or produces too much daytime drowsiness or other adverse effects, including worsening of parkinsonism, clozapine (Clozaril) should be tried next, starting with 12.5 mg at night to avoid daytime drowsiness and increasing the dose until benefit or adverse effects are encountered. It is probably more effective than quetiapine, but its use requires regular monitoring of blood counts to prevent the 1% to 2% risk of agranulocytosis (Scholz and Dichgans, 1985; Friedman and Lannon, 1990; Pfeiffer et al., 1990; Wolters et al., 1990; Kahn et al., 1991; Factor and Brown, 1992; Greene et al., 1993; Pinter and Helscher, 1993; Factor et al., 1994; Diederich et al., 1995; Rabey et al., 1995; Factor and Friedman, 1997; Ruggieri et al., 1997; Friedman et al., 1999; Pollak et al., 2004). In one open-label comparative trial, quetiapine and clozapine appeared equally effective; interestingly, both also reduced the severity of dyskinesias as well as controlling psychosis (Morgante et al., 2004).

Other so-called atypical antipsychotics appear to be so designated for marketing purposes. Olanzapine can be effective but easily increases parkinsonism and so needs to be used in small doses to avoid a worsening of parkinsonism (Wolters et al., 1996; Friedman, 1998; Jimenez-Jimenez et al., 1998; Goetz et al., 2000); therefore, it is relegated to third choice. Risperidone more closely resembles a typical rather than an atypical antipsychotic and worsens PD. Aripiprazole has also worsened parkinsonism (Fernandez et al., 2004). A more thorough discussion of atypical antipsychotics is found in Chapter 20. Molindone, pimozide, or another relatively weak antipsychotic might also be considered.

The muscarinic agents that are used in the treatment of dementia are an alternative to atypical antipsychotics. Surprisingly, they have been reported to have the same efficacy on psychosis as do clozapine and quetiapine (Van Laar et al., 2001; Bergman and Lerner 2002; Reading et al., 2002).

If psychosis continues without adequate benefit from the antipsychotics, selegiline, anticholinergics, and amantadine should be withdrawn. The need for anxiolytics and antidepressants should be reconsidered. If the symptoms persist,

Box 8-6 Psychiatric symptoms in Parkinson disease

Compulsive, repetitive behavior (punding)
Hallucinations
Psychosis

dopamine agonists should be reduced or stopped. If necessary, the dose of levodopa should be tapered. However, more often than not, as drugs are reduced to improve the mental state, mobility deteriorates. A brittle balance is reached at which the patient either is mobile but confused, paranoid, or hallucinating or is mentally clear but immobile. More dopamine replacement therapy is required to maintain mobility, but this causes a recurrence of the confusion, and it is very difficult to achieve a compromise. In this situation, a limited drug holiday, withdrawing dopaminergic drugs for 1 to 2 days each week, might help to dispel psychotoxicity, allowing a reasonable dose of medication to maintain mobility on other days. Sustained withdrawal of levodopa provokes unacceptable parkinsonism and, sometimes, particularly if the levodopa is withdrawn suddenly, a "neuroleptic" malignant syndrome (Friedman et al., 1985; Hirschorn and Greenberg, 1988). When it comes to balancing drug-induced psychosis and parkinsonism, keep in mind that an intact mental function is more important than an intact motor function.

The serotonin 5-HT$_3$-receptor antagonist ondansetron blocks nausea and vomiting due to anticancer drugs. It has been reported to reduce hallucinations, paranoia, and confusion in PD (Zoldan et al., 1995). Fifteen out of the 16 patients treated with 12 to 25 mg per day for up to 8 weeks showed moderate to marked improvement of visual hallucinations and paranoid delusions. There was no worsening of the parkinsonism. However, this was not replicated by Eichhorn and colleagues (1996), who failed to find benefit in most patients and found waning of benefit in the few for whom the drug was initially beneficial.

## QUALITY OF LIFE

Measuring quality of life in 124 patients with PD, Schrag and colleagues (2000) showed that it significantly deteriorated with increasing disease severity, as measured by the PDQ-39, the EQ-5D, and the physical summary of the SF 36. The greatest impairment was seen in the areas related to physical and social functioning, whereas reports of pain and poor emotional adjustment had similar prevalence in patients with PD and the general population. The impairment of QoL was seen in all age groups and was similar for men and women, but the differences between patients with PD and the general population were most marked in the younger patient groups.

From the QoL survey of patients with PD conducted in Norway by Karlsen and her colleagues (1999b), the three most important factors impacting QoL were depression, sleep disorders, and a sense of low degree of independence. The first two were addressed in this chapter, and their prominence in QoL indicates the importance of the nonmotor symptoms of PD. Independence would be affected by gait and balance disorders predominantly. Sexuality is part of quality of life, and patients with PD are more dissatisfied with their sexual functioning and relationship than are controls (Jacobs et al., 2000).

## References

Aarsland D, Andersen K, Larsen JP, et al: Risk of dementia in Parkinson's disease: A community-based, prospective study. Neurology 2001;56:730–736.

Aarsland D, Andersen K, Larsen JP, et al: Prevalence and characteristics of dementia in Parkinson disease: An 8-year prospective study. Arch Neurol 2003;60(3):387–392.

Aarsland D, Andersen K, Larsen JP, et al: The rate of cognitive decline in Parkinson disease. Arch Neurol 2004;61(12):1906–1911.

Aarsland D, Laake K, Larsen JP, Janvin C: Donepezil for cognitive impairment in Parkinson's disease: A randomised controlled study. J Neurol Neurosurg Psychiatry 2002;72(6):708–712.

Aarsland D, Larsen JP, Cummings JL, Laake K: Prevalence and clinical correlates of psychotic symptoms in Parkinson disease: A community-based study. Arch Neurol 1999;56:595–601.

Aarsland D, Perry R, Brown A, et al: Neuropathology of dementia in Parkinson's disease: A prospective, community-based study. Ann Neurol 2005;58(5):773–776.

Anguenot A, Loll PY, Neau JP, et al: Depression and Parkinson's disease: A study of 135 parkinsonian patients. Can J Neurol Sci 2002;29(2):139–146.

Araki I, Kuno S: Assessment of voiding dysfunction in Parkinson's disease by the international prostate symptom score. J Neurol Neurosurg Psychiat 2000;68:429–433.

Askenasy JJM: Sleep in Parkinson's disease. Acta Neurol Scand 1993;87(suppl 3):167–170.

Bateson MC, Gibberd FB, Wilson RSE: Salivary symptoms in Parkinson's disease. Arch Neurol 1973;29:274–275.

Bejjani BP, Damier P, Arnulf I, et al: Transient acute depression induced by high-frequency deep-brain stimulation. N Engl J Med 1999;340:1476–1480.

Bergman J, Lerner V: Successful use of donepezil for the treatment of psychotic symptoms in patients with Parkinson's disease. Clin Neuropharmacol 2002;25(2):107–110.

Biggins CA, Boyd JL, Harrop FM, et al: A controlled, longitudinal study of dementia in Parkinson's disease. J Neurol Neurosurg Psychiatry 1992;55:566–571.

Bliwise DL, Watts RL, Watts N, et al: Disruptive nocturnal behavior in Parkinson's disease and Alzheimer's disease. J Geriatr Psychiatry Neurol 1995;8:107–110.

Boller F, Mizutani T, Roessmann U, Gambetti P: Parkinson disease, dementia, and Alzheimer disease: Clinicopathological correlations. Ann Neurol 1980;7:329–335.

Braak H, Del Tredici K, Rub U, et al: Staging of brain pathology related to sporadic Parkinson's disease. Neurobiol Aging 2003;24(2):197–211.

Braun AR, Tanner CM, Goetz CG, Klawans HL: Respiratory distress due to pharyngeal dystonia: A side effect of chronic dopamine agonism. Neurology 1983;33(suppl 2):220.

Brown RG, MacCarthy B, Gotham AM, et al: Depression and disability in Parkinson's disease: A follow-up of 132 cases. Psychol Med 1988;18:49–55.

Brown RG, Marsden CD: How common is dementia in Parkinson's disease? Lancet 1984;2:1262–1265.

Brown RG, Marsden CD: Cognitive function in Parkinson's disease: From description to theory. Trends Neurosci 1990;13:21–29.

Burn DJ, Rowan EN, Allan LM, et al: Motor subtype and cognitive decline in Parkinson's disease, Parkinson's disease with dementia, and dementia with Lewy bodies. J Neurol Neurosurg Psychiatry 2006;77(5):585–589.

Bushman M, Dobmeyer SM, Leeker L, Perlmutter JS: Swallowing abnormalities and their response to treatment in Parkinson's disease. Neurology 1989;39:1309–1314.

Byrne EJ, Lennox G, Lowe J, Godwin-Austen RB: Diffuse Lewy body disease: Clinical features in 15 cases. J Neurol Neurosurg Psychiatry 1989;52:709–717.

Ceravolo R, Nuti A, Piccinni A, et al: Paroxetine in Parkinson's disease: Effects on motor and depressive symptoms. Neurology 2000;55:1216–1218.

Chaudhuri KR, Healy DG, Schapira AH: Non-motor symptoms of Parkinson's disease: Diagnosis and management. Lancet Neurol 2006a;5:235–245.

Chaudhuri KR, Martinez-Martin P, Schapira AH, et al: International multicenter pilot study of the first comprehensive self-completed nonmotor symptoms questionnaire for Parkinson's disease: The NMSQuest study. Mov Disord 2006;21(7):916–923.

Chester CS, Gottfried SB, Cameron DI, Strohl KP: Pathophysiological findings in a patient with Shy-Drager and alveolar hypoventilation syndromes. Chest 1988;94:212–214.

Cooper JA, Sagar HJ, Jordan N, et al: Cognitive impairment in early, untreated Parkinson's disease and its relationship to motor disability. Brain 1991;114:2095–2122.

Diederich N, Keipes M, Grass M, Metz H: Use of clozapine for psychiatric complications of Parkinson's disease. Rev Neurol 1995;151:251–257.

Dooneief G, Chen J, Mirabello E, et al: An estimate of the incidence of depression in idiopathic Parkinson's disease. Arch Neurol 1992;49:305–307.

Douyon R, Serby M, Klutchko B, Rotrosen J: ECT and Parkinson's disease revisited: A "naturalistic" study [see comments]. Am J Psychiatry 1989;146:1451–1455.

Driver-Dunckley E, Samanta J, Stacy M: Pathological gambling associated with dopamine agonist therapy in Parkinson's disease. Neurology 2003;61(3):422–423.

Eadie MJ: The pathology of certain medullary nuclei in parkinsonism. Aust Ann Med 1963;86:781–792.

Edwards LL, Pfeiffer RF, Quigley EMM, et al: Gastrointestinal symptoms in Parkinson's disease. Mov Disord 1991;6:151–156.

Edwards LL, Quigley EM, Harned RK, et al: Defecatory function in Parkinson's disease: Response to apomorphine. Ann Neurol 1993;33:490–493.

Edwards LL, Quigley EM, Harned RK, et al: Characterization of swallowing and defecation in Parkinson's disease. Am J Gastroenterol 1994;89:15–25.

Edwards LL, Quigley EM, Pfeiffer RF: Gastrointestinal dysfunction in Parkinson's disease: Frequency and pathophysiology. Neurology 1992;42:726–732.

Efthimiou J, Ellis SJ, Hardie RJ, Stern GM: Sleep apnea in idiopathic and postencephalitic parkinsonism. Adv Neurol 1987;45: 275–276.

Eichhorn TE, Brunt E, Oertel WH: Ondansetron treatment of L-dopa-induced psychosis. Neurology 1996;47:1608–1609.

Elibol B, Hattori N, Atac FB, Saka E, Mizuno Y. Distinguishing clinical features in patients with parkin mutations. Neurology 2000;54 (suppl 3):A444.

Emre M, Aarsland D, Albanese A, et al: Rivastigmine for dementia associated with Parkinson's disease. N Engl J Med 2004;351(24):2509–2518.

Evans AH, Katzenschlager R, Paviour D, et al: Punding in Parkinson's disease: Its relation to the dopamine dysregulation syndrome. Mov Disord 2004;19(4):397–405.

Factor SA, Brown D: Clozapine prevents recurrence of psychosis in Parkinson's disease. Mov Disord 1992;7:125–131.

Factor SA, Brown D, Molho ES, Podskalny GD: Clozapine: A 2-year open trial in Parkinson's disease patients with psychosis. Neurology 1994;44:544–546.

Factor SA, Friedman JH: The emerging role of clozapine in the treatment of movement disorders. Mov Disord 1997;12:483–496.

Factor SA, McAlarney T, Sanchez-Ramos JR, Weiner WJ: Sleep disorders and sleep effect in Parkinson's disease. Mov Disord 1990;4:280–285.

Fahn S, Chouinard S: Experience with tranylcypromine in early Parkinson's disease. J Neural Transmission 1998[suppl]52:49–61.

Ferini-Strambi L, Zucconi M: REM sleep behavior disorder. Clin Neurophysiol 2000;111:S136–S140.

Fernandez HH, Friedman JH: Punding on l-dopa. Mov Disord 1999;14:836–838.

Fernandez HH, Friedman JH, Jacques C, Rosenfeld M: Quetiapine for the treatment of drug-induced psychosis in Parkinson's disease. Mov Disord 1999;14:484–487.

Fernandez HH, Trieschmann ME, Friedman JH: Aripiprazole for drug-induced psychosis in Parkinson disease: Preliminary experience. Clin Neuropharmacol 2004;27(1):4–5.

Ferreira JJ, Galitzky M, Montastruc JL, Rascol O: Sleep attacks and Parkinson's disease treatment. Lancet 2000;355:1333–1334.

Fitzmaurice H, Fowler CJ, Rickards D, et al: Micturition disturbance in Parkinson's disease. Br J Urol 1985;57:652–656.

Ford B, Louis ED, Greene P, Fahn S: Oral and genital pain syndromes in Parkinson's disease. Mov Disord 1996;11:421–426.

Friedman J: Olanzapine in the treatment of dopaminomimetic psychosis in patients with Parkinson's disease. Neurology 1998;50:1195–1196.

Friedman JH, Lannon MC: Clozapine in idiopathic Parkinson's disease. Neurology 1990;40:1151–1152.

Friedman J, Lannon M, Comella C, et al: Low-dose clozapine for the treatment of drug-induced psychosis in Parkinson's disease. N Engl J Med 1999;340:757–763.

Friedman JH, Feinberg SS, Feldman RG: A neuroleptic malignantlike syndrome due to levodopa therapy withdrawal. JAMA 1985;254:2792–2795.

Frucht S, Rogers JD, Greene PE, et al: Falling asleep at the wheel: Motor vehicle mishaps in persons taking pramipexole and ropinirole. Neurology 1999;52:1908–1910.

Giladi N, Shabtai H, Gurevich T, et al: Rivastigmine (Exelon) for dementia in patients with Parkinson's disease. Acta Neurol Scand 2003;108(5):368–373.

Goetz CG, Blasucci LM, Leurgans S, Pappert EJ: Olanzapine and clozapine: Comparative effects on motor function in hallucinating PD patients. Neurology 2000;55:789–794.

Goetz CG, Fan W, Leurgans S, et al: The malignant course of "benign hallucinations" in Parkinson disease. Arch Neurol 2006;63(5):713–716.

Goetz CG, Stebbins GT: Risk factors for nursing home placement in advanced Parkinson's disease. Neurology 1993;43:2227–2229.

Goetz CG, Tanner CM, Levy M, et al: Pain in Parkinson's disease. Mov Disord 1986;1:45–49.

Greene P, Cote L, Fahn S: Treatment of drug-induced psychosis in Parkinson's disease with clozapine. Adv Neurol 1993;60:703–706.

Gschwandtner U, Aston J, Renaud S, Fuhr P: Pathologic gambling in patients with Parkinson's disease. Clin Neuropharmacol 2001;24:170–172.

Happe S, Pirker W, Sauter C, et al: Successful treatment of excessive daytime sleepiness in Parkinson's disease with modafinil. J Neurol 2001;248:632–634.

Hauser RA, Wahba MN, Zesiewicz TA, Anderson WM: Modafinil treatment of pramipexole-associated somnolence. Mov Disord 2000;15:1269–1271.

Hening W, Walters A, Kavey N, et al: Dyskinesias while awake and periodic movements in sleep in restless legs syndrome: Treatment with opioids. Neurology 1986;36:1363–1366.

Hirschorn KA, Greenberg HS: Successful treatment of levodopa-induced myoclonus and levodopa withdrawal–induced neuroleptic malignant syndrome: A case report. Clin Neuropharmacol 1988;2:278–281.

Hoehn MM: Falling asleep at the wheel: Motor vehicle mishaps in people taking pramipexole and ropinirole. Neurology 2000;54:275.

Homann CN, Wenzel K, Suppan K, et al: Sleep attacks in patients taking dopamine agonists: Review. Br Med J 2002;324(7352):1483–1487.

Hughes TA, Ross HF, Mindham RHS, Spokes EGS: Mortality in Parkinson's disease and its association with dementia and depression. Acta Neurol Scand 2004;110(2):118–123.

Hughes TA, Ross HF, Musa S, et al: A 10-year study of the incidence of and factors predicting dementia in Parkinson's disease. Neurology 2000;54:1596–1602.

Hussain IF, Brady CM, Swinn MJ, et al: Treatment of erectile dysfunction with sildenafil citrate (Viagra) in parkinsonism due to

Parkinson's disease or multiple system atrophy with observations. J Neurol Neurosurg Psychiat 2001;71:371–374.

Ilson J, Braun N, Fahn S: Respiratory fluctuations in Parkinson's disease. Neurology 1983;33(suppl 2):113.

Ilson J, Fahn S, Cote L: Painful dystonic spasms in Parkinson's disease. Adv Neurol 1984;40:395–398.

Inzelberg R, Kipervasser S, Korczyn AD: Auditory hallucinations in Parkinson's disease. J Neurol Neurosurg Psychiatry 1998;64: 533–535.

Jacobs H, Vieregge A, Vieregge P: Sexuality in young patients with Parkinson's disease: A population based comparison with healthy controls. J Neurol Neurosurg Psychiat 2000;69:550–552.

Jansen Steur ENH: Increase of Parkinson disability after fluoxetine medication. Neurology 1993;43:211–213.

Jimenez-Jimenez FJ, Tallon-Barranco A, Orti-Pareja M, et al: Olanzapine can worsen parkinsonism. Neurology 1998;50:1183–1184.

Jimenez-Jimenez FJ, Tejeiro J, Martinez-Junquero G, et al: Parkinsonism exacerbated by paroxetine. Neurology 1994;44:2406.

Juncos JL, Roberts VJ, Evatt ML, et al: Quetiapine improves psychotic symptoms and cognition in Parkinson's disease. Mov Disord 2004;19(1):29–35.

Kahn N, Freeman A, Juncos JL, et al: Clozapine is beneficial for psychosis in Parkinson's disease. Neurology 1991;41:1699–1700.

Karlsen K, Larsen JP, Tandberg E, Jorgensen K: Fatigue in patients with Parkinson's disease. Mov Disord 1999a;14:237–241.

Karlsen KH, Larsen JP, Tandberg E, Maeland JG: Influence of clinical and demographic variables on quality of life in patients with Parkinson's disease. J Neurol Neurosurg Psychiat 1999b;66:431–435.

Kitamura J, Kubuki Y, Tsuruta K, et al: A new family with Joseph disease in Japan: Homovanillic acid, magnetic resonance, and sleep apnea studies. Arch Neurol 1989;46:425–428.

Koller WC: Sensory symptoms in Parkinson's disease. Neurology 1984;34:957–959.

Kupsky WJ, Grimes MM, Sweeting J, et al: Parkinson's disease and megacolon: Concentric hyaline inclusions (Lewy bodies) in enteric ganglion cells. Neurology 1987;37:1253–1255.

Kurlan R: Disabling repetitive behaviors in Parkinson's disease. Mov Disord 2004;19(4):433–437.

Laihnen A, Alihanka J, Raitasuo, et al: Sleep movements and associated autonomic nervous activities in patients with Parkinson's disease. Acta Neurol Scand 1987;76:64–68.

Lang AE: Restless legs syndrome and Parkinson's disease: Insights into pathophysiology. Clin Neuropharmacol 1987;10:476–478.

Lang AE: Withdrawal akathisia: Case reports and a proposed classification of chronic akathisia. Mov Disord 1994;9:188–192.

Lang AE, Johnson K: Akathisia in idiopathic Parkinson's disease. Neurology 1987;37:477–481.

Langston JW: The Parkinson's complex: Parkinsonism is just the tip of the iceberg. Ann Neurol 2006;59(4):591–596.

Lees AJ: A sustained-release formulation of L-dopa (Madopar HBS) in the treatment of nocturnal and early-morning disabilities in Parkinson's disease. Eur Neurol 1987;27(suppl 1):126–134.

Lees AJ, Smith E: Cognitive defects in the early stages of Parkinson's disease. Brain 1983;106:257–270.

Levin BE, Llabre MM, Weiner WJ: Cognitive impairment associated with early Parkinson's disease. Neurology 1989;39:557–561.

Lipp A, Trottenberg T, Schink T, et al: A randomized trial of botulinum toxin A for treatment of drooling. Neurology 2003;61 (9):1279–1281.

Lynch T, Sano M, Marder KS, et al: Clinical characteristics of a family with chromosome 17-linked disinhibition dementia parkinsonism amyotrophy complex. Neurology 1994;44:1878–1884.

Mathers SE, Kempster PA, Law PJ, et al: Anal sphincter dysfunction in Parkinson's disease. Arch Neurol 1989;46:1061–1064.

Mathers SE, Kempster PA, Swash M, Lees AJ: Constipation and paradoxical puborectalis contraction in anismus and Parkinson's disease: A dystonic phenomenon. J Neurol Neurosurg Psychiatry 1988;51:1503–1507.

Matison R, Mayeux R, Rosen J, Fahn S: "Tip-of-the-tongue" phenomenon in Parkinson disease. Neurology 1982;32:567–570.

Mattila PM, Rinne JO, Helenius H, et al: Alpha-synuclein-immunoreactive cortical Lewy bodies are associated with cognitive impairment in Parkinson's disease. Acta Neuropathol 2000; 100:285–290.

Mayeux R, Chen J, Mirabello E, et al: An estimate of the incidence of dementia in idiopathic Parkinson's disease. Neurology 1990;40: 1513–1517.

McKeith I, DelSer T, Spano P, et al: Efficacy of rivastigmine in dementia with Lewy bodies: A randomised, double-blind, placebo-controlled international study. Lancet 2000;356:2031–2036.

McKeith IG, Galasko D, Kosaka K, et al: Consensus guidelines for the clinical and pathological diagnosis of dementia with Lewy bodies: Report of the consortium on DLB International Workshop. Neurology 1996;47:1113–1124.

McKeith IG, Perry EK, Perry RH: Report of the second dementia with Lewy body international workshop: Diagnosis and treatment. Neurology 1999;53:902–905.

Melamed E: Early-morning dystonia: A late side effect of long-term levodopa therapy in Parkinson's disease. Arch Neurol 1979;36: 308–310.

Merello M, Leiguarda R: Adynamic bowel syndrome in Parkinson's disease with dramatic response to apomorphine. Clin Neuropharmacol 1994;17:574–577.

Miyasaki JM, Shannon K, Voon V, et al: Practice Parameter: Evaluation and treatment of depression, psychosis, and dementia in Parkinson disease (an evidence-based review): Report of the Quality Standards Subcommittee of the American Academy of Neurology. Neurology 2006;66(7):996 1002.

Morgante L, Epifanio A, Spina E, et al: Quetiapine and clozapine in parkinsonian patients with dopaminergic psychosis. Clin Neuropharmacol 2004;27(4):153–156.

Naimark D, Jackson E, Rockwell E, Jeste DV: Psychotic symptoms in Parkinson's disease patients with dementia. J Am Geriatr Soc 1996;44:296–299.

Nausieda PA, Weiner WJ, Kaplan LR, et al: Sleep disruption in the course of chronic levodopa therapy: An early feature of the levodopa psychosis. Clin Neuropharmacol 1982;5:183–194.

Nissenbaum H, Quinn NP, Brown RG, et al: Mood swings associated with the "on-off" phenomenon in Parkinson's disease. Psychol Med 1987;17:899–904.

Ondo WG, Hunter C, Moore W: A double-blind placebo-controlled trial of botulinum toxin B for sialorrhea in Parkinson's disease. Neurology 2004;62(1):37–40.

Ondo WG, Vuong KD, Khan H, et al: Daytime sleepiness and other sleep disorders in Parkinson's disease. Neurology 2001;57:1392–1396.

Perry TL, Wright JM, Berry K, et al: Dominantly inherited apathy, central hypoventilation, and Parkinson's syndrome: Clinical, biochemical, and neuropathologic studies of 2 new cases. Neurology 1990;40:1882–1887.

Pfeiffer RF, Kang J, Graber B, et al: Clozapine for psychosis in Parkinson's disease. Mov Disord 1990;5:239–242.

Pinter MM, Helscher RJ: Therapeutic effect of clozapine in psychotic decompensation in idiopathic Parkinson's disease. J Neural Transm Park Dis Dement Sect 1993;5:135–146.

Pollak P, Tison F, Rascol O, et al: Clozapine in drug induced psychosis in Parkinson's disease: A randomised, placebo controlled study with open follow up. J Neurol Neurosurg Psychiatry 2004;75(5): 689–695.

Postuma RB, Lang AE, Massicotte-Marquez J, Montplaisir J: Potential early markers of Parkinson disease in idiopathic REM sleep behavior disorder. Neurology 2006;66(6):845–851.

Qualman SJ, Haupt HM, Yang P, Hamilton SJ: Esophageal Lewy bodies associated with ganglion cell loss in achalasia: Similarity to Parkinson's disease. Gastroenterology 1984;87:848–856.

Quinn NP, Koller WC, Lang AE, Marsden CD: Painful Parkinson's disease. Lancet 1986;1:1366–1369.

Rabey JM, Treves TA, Neufeld MY, et al: Low-dose clozapine in the treatment of levodopa-induced mental disturbances in Parkinson's disease. Neurology 1995;45:432–434.

Racette BA, Good L, Sagitto S, Perlmutter JS: Botulinum toxin B reduces sialorrhea in parkinsonism. Mov Disord 2003;18(9):1059–1061.

Reading PJ, Luce AK, McKeith IG: Rivastigmine in the treatment of parkinsonian hallucinosis. Neurology 2002;58:A380.

Richard IH, Maughn A, Kurlan R: Do serotonin reuptake inhibitor antidepressants worsen Parkinson's disease? A retrospective case series. Mov Disord 1999;14:155–157.

Ruggieri S, Depandis MF, Bonamartini A: Low dose of clozapine in the treatment of dopaminergic psychosis in Parkinson's disease. Clin Neuropharmacol 1997;20:204–209.

Rye DB, Bliwise DL, Dihenia B, Gurecki P: Daytime sleepiness in Parkinson's disease. J Sleep Res 2000;9:63–69.

Sage JI, Mark MH: Drenching sweats as an off phenomenon in Parkinson's disease: Treatment and relation to plasma levodopa profile. Ann Neurol 1995;37:120–122.

Salazar-Grueso EF, Rosenberg RS, Roos RP: Sleep apnea in olivopontocerebellar degeneration: Treatment with trazodone. Ann Neurol 1988;23:399–401.

Sanchez-Ramos JR, Ortoll R, Paulson GW: Visual hallucinations associated with Parkinson's disease. Arch Neurol 1996;53:1265–1268.

Schapira AHV: Sleep attacks (sleep episodes) with pergolide. Lancet 2000;355:1332–1333.

Scholz E, Dichgans J: Treatment of drug-induced exogenous psychosis in parkinsonism with clozapine and fluperlapine. Eur Arch Psychiatry Neurol Sci 1985;235:60–64.

Schrag A, Jahanshahi M, Quinn N: How does Parkinson's disease affect quality of life? A comparison with quality of life in the general population. Mov Disord 2000;15:1112–1118.

Schrag A, Jahanshahi M, Quinn NP: What contributes to depression in Parkinson's disease? Psychol Med 2001;31:65–73.

Snider SR, Fahn S, Isgreen WP, Cote LJ: Primary sensory symptoms in parkinsonism. Neurology 1976;26:423–429.

Stein MB, Heuser IJ, Juncos JL, Uhde TW: Anxiety disorders in patients with Parkinson's disease [see comments]. Am J Psychiatry 1990;147:217–220.

Stocchi F, Carbone A, Inghilleri M, Monge A, et al: Urodynamic and neurophysiological evaluation in Parkinson's disease and multiple system atrophy. J Neurol Neurosurg Psychiatry 1997;62:507–511.

Strieder DJ, Baker WG, Baringer JR, Kazemi H: Chronic hypoventilation of central origin: A case with encephalitis lethargica and Parkinson's syndrome. Am Rev Respir Dis 1967;96:501–507.

Swinn L, Schrag A, Viswanathan R, et al: Sweating dysfunction in Parkinson's disease. Mov Disord 2003;18(12):1459–1463.

Swope DM: Preliminary report: Use of sildenafil to treat dyskinesias in patients with Parkinson's disease. Neurology 2000;54(suppl 3):A90–A91.

Tandberg E, Larsen JP, Karlsen K: Excessive daytime sleepiness and sleep benefit in Parkinson's disease: A community-based study. Mov Disord 1999;14:922–927.

Tesei S, Antonini A, Canesi M, et al: Tolerability of paroxetine in Parkinson's disease: A prospective study. Mov Disord 2000;15:986–989.

Van Hilten B, Hoff JI, Middelkoop HAM, et al: Sleep disruption in Parkinson's disease: Assessment by continuous activity monitoring. Arch Neurol 1994;51:922–928.

Van Laar T, de Vries JJ, Nakhosteen A, Leenders KL: Rivastigmine as anti-psychotic in patients with Parkinson's disease. Parkinsonism Relat Disord 2001;7(suppl):S73.

Voon V, Hassan K, Zurowski M, et al: Prospective prevalence of pathologic gambling and medication association in Parkinson disease. Neurology 2006;66(11):1750–1752.

Wakabayashi K, Takahashi H, Takeda E, et al: Parkinson's disease: The presence of Lewy bodies in Auerbach's and Meissner's plexuses. Acta Neuropathol 1988;76:217–221.

Wolters EC, Hurwitz TA, Mak E, et al: Clozapine in the treatment of parkinsonian patients with dopaminomimetic psychosis. Neurology 1990;40:832–834.

Wolters EC, Jansen ENH, Tuynman-Qua HG, Bergmans PLM: Olanzapine in the treatment of dopaminomimetic psychosis in patients with Parkinson's disease. Neurology 1996;47:1085–1087.

Wu JC, Iacono R, Ayman M, et al: Correlation of intellectual impairment in Parkinson's disease with FDG PET scan. Neuroreport 2000;11:2139–2144.

Zesiewicz TA, Helal M, Hauser RA: Sildenafil citrate (Viagra) for the treatment of erectile dysfunction in men with Parkinson's disease. Mov Disord 2000;15:305–308.

Zoldan J, Friedberg C, Livneh M, Melamed E: Psychosis in advanced Parkinson's disease: Treatment with ondansetron, a 5-HT3 receptor antagonist. Neurology 1995;45:1305–1308.

# Chapter 9

# Experimental Models and New, Emerging Therapies for Parkinson Disease

Parkinson disease (PD) is an age-related disorder that affects up to 1 in 500 people in the general population and 1 in 100 individuals over the age of 60 (Schoenberg, 1987). The prevalence of PD will rise as life expectancy increases, and the number of affected individuals will rise significantly over the next three decades. PD is caused primarily by the destruction of dopaminergic neurons in the zona compacta of the substantia nigra and the subsequent loss of caudate-putamen dopamine content leading to the onset of the cardinal symptoms of akinesia, rigidity, and tremor (Obeso et al., 2000). The three preceding chapters described current treatment (both medical and surgical) of the motor and nonmotor symptoms of PD. Here, the current treatment challenges are briefly outlined and the rationale for developing new therapies is explained.

Dopamine replacement therapy remains the mainstay of the treatment of PD. Levodopa is the most commonly employed agent, but there is increasing use of dopamine agonist drugs, such as ropinirole and pramipexole (Parkinson Study Group, 2000, 2004b; Rascol et al., 2000), and novel MAO B inhibitors, such as rasagiline (Rascol et al., 2005; Biglan et al., 2006). Early symptomatic control of PD disease is not problematic; rather, it is the long-term control of motor symptoms that remains difficult, as detailed in Chapter 6, coupled with the onset of side effects and a lack of effect of current therapies on nonmotor components of the illness (Jankovic, 1998), as discussed in Chapter 8. Chronic treatment of PD is associated with a loss of drug efficacy in the form of wearing-off and on-off phenomena (Jankovic, 2005a). In addition, involuntary movements appear in the form of dystonia and/or chorea; and hallucinations, psychosis, and dementia may occur. Dyskinesias and psychosis can become treatment-limiting and are thought to affect some 30% to 40% of all patients with PD (Ahlskog and Muenter, 2001). Long-term complications are a particular feature of the use of levodopa, and the current use of dopamine agonist drugs is based on their ability to control the early motor symptoms of PD without extensive priming of basal ganglia for the appearance of dyskinesia (Oertel, 2000; Parkinson Study Group, 2000; Rascol et al., 2000), although dyskinesia may appear at the expected rate once levodopa therapy is introduced (Rascol et al., 2006). Patients with PD also suffer from a range of motor and nonmotor problems, including bladder and bowel dysfunction, sweating, drooling, and, in particular, postural instability, that do not respond to dopaminergic therapy and consequently remain untreatable at this time (Jankovic, 1998; Chaudhuri et al., 2005, 2006; Stacy et al., 2005). The other major long-term treatment problem in PD is that all current therapy is aimed at symptomatic control while the pathology of the illness continues to advance. No currently available therapies have been proven to influence disease progression in either a neuroprotective or a neurorestorative manner (Schapira 2004; Jankovic, 2005b; Olanow and Jankovic, 2005).

Current research into PD is aimed both at developing neuroprotective therapies and at improving the symptomatic treatment of the illness by the production of a new generation of agents. The objective of this research is to produce drugs that are effective throughout the illness without loss of efficacy and that do not prime the basal ganglia for the production of dyskinesia or provoke established involuntary movements. In addition, such drugs should not provoke psychosis; they should avoid some of the acute peripheral side effects of dopaminergic therapies, such as nausea, vomiting, and hypertension; and they should have effects on the currently untreatable symptoms of PD, such as postural instability. In addition, it is hoped that novel agents for the treatment of PD will have neuroprotective effects, thus preventing or slowing the progression of disease. To achieve these ends, it is necessary to have effective experimental models of PD in which new agents can be evaluated before clinical studies are attempted. A number of models exist, and recent advances in the understanding of the genetic basis of familial PD have started to provide some transgenic and mutant models of the disorder. In this chapter, the value of experimental models for the development of new approaches to the treatment of PD will be assessed, together with their usefulness in evaluating new dopaminergic and nondopaminergic approaches to the treatment of PD.

## RODENT MODELS OF PARKINSON DISEASE

A range of rodent models of PD has existed for some time, and novel approaches based on genetic manipulation are under development. Early rodent models were based on the use of chemical depletion of dopamine or the use of toxins to destroy the nigrostriatal pathway. However, the increasing use of mutants and transgenics is providing a new generation of models, though they still require development and evaluation.

### Reserpine and α-Methyl-para-Tyrosine-Treated Rodents

The earliest approach to developing a model of PD relates to the use of drugs that either disrupt the storage of dopamine in presynaptic terminals or inhibit its synthesis (Marsden et al., 1975). Administration of reserpine to rodents disrupts the storage of monoamines in presynaptic vesicles (Carlsson et al., 1957) by inhibiting the vesicular monoamine transporter. The subsequent depletion of dopamine as well as norepinephrine and 5-HT produces an animal that is akinetic and hunched and that shows little exploratory activity. The effects of reserpine treatment can be reversed by the administration of levodopa and dopamine agonist drugs (Dolphin et al., 1976). Similarly, the administration of α-methyl-para-tyrosine (AMPT) as an inhibitor of tyrosine hydroxylase, the rate-limiting enzyme for dopamine formation, reduces dopamine levels but without affecting the norepinephrine or 5-HT content of the brain (Corrodi et al., 1970). Again, AMPT-treated animals show a reduction in spontaneous locomotion that can be reversed by the administration of levodopa and dopamine agonists (Costall and Naylor, 1975). Reserpine and AMPT have also been used in combination to doubly impair the synthesis and storage of dopamine and to ensure marked dopamine depletion and motor dysfunction. As a primary screen for novel antiparkinsonian agents, particularly those that affect dopaminergic systems, these models can be extremely useful. However, the use of AMPT and reserpine has a number of disadvantages. Neither agent selectively produces dopamine loss in the nigrostriatal pathway, and there is also a marked depletion in both the mesolimbic and mesocortical regions of brain, which are relatively spared in PD. Neither agent causes destruction of the nigrostriatal pathway; therefore, these agents do not mimic the disorder as it occurs in humans. Further, both reserpine and AMPT produce a reversible depletion of dopamine in the brain, and the timing of studies employing these agents is important, as it is critical to examine the effects of potential antiparkinsonian drugs at the time of maximal dopamine synthesis or storage inhibition (Haggendal and Lindqvist, 1964). Both agents also impair monoaminergic function in the periphery, and the use of reserpine is associated with changes in cardiovascular function and temperature control; it also induces marked diarrhea in rodents. Reserpine does, however, mimic PD by affecting norepinephrine and 5-HT levels as well as dopamine, whereas AMPT is selective for dopaminergic systems.

## Toxin-Based Models of Parkinson Disease in Rodents

The use of toxins that selectively destroy the nigrostriatal dopaminergic pathway is a common means of creating models of PD. Such models may utilize systemic toxin administration but commonly employ the stereotaxic injection of toxins directly into the nigrostriatal pathway.

The most commonly utilized and well-characterized model of PD is the unilateral 6-hydroxydopamine (6-OHDA) lesioned rat model, which has more recently been characterized in mice (Iancu et al., 2005). 6-OHDA is a toxin that is presumed to act through free radical mechanisms (Graham et al., 1978) and that is selectively taken up into and destroys catecholamine-containing neurons. This classic model was first developed during the 1960s and has been successfully employed for the routine screening of potential antiparkinsonian agents (Ungerstedt, 1971a, 1971b; Von Voigtlander and Moore, 1973). Unilateral injection of 6-OHDA either directly into the substantia nigra or into the medial forebrain bundle is the most frequently used procedure. This results in a subsequent degeneration of the nigrostriatal pathway in one hemisphere over a period of days, associated with the development of postsynaptic dopamine receptor supersensitivity in the denervated striatum. 6-OHDA is routinely used in combination with desipramine pretreatment to prevent the toxin from being taken up into and destroying noradrenergic fibers that also ascend in the medial forebrain bundle. 6-OHDA has also been directly injected into the striatum, where it appears to

undergo retrograde transport to the substantia nigra, causing a gradual dying back of dopaminergic neurons that has been proposed as a model of progression of PD (Przedborski et al., 1995). The latter could be useful both for the development of symptomatic treatments of PD and in detecting neuroprotective agents for this disorder.

Following 6-OHDA-induced destruction of the nigrostriatal pathway, animals exhibit an asymmetric motor response to the administration of directly or indirectly acting dopaminergic agonists in the form of rotational behavior (Reavill et al., 1983). Administration of directly acting dopamine agonists or of levodopa results in turning away from the side of the lesion (contraversive rotation), whereas indirectly acting dopaminomimetics act through the intact hemisphere and thus cause rotational response toward the side of the lesion (ipsiversive rotation). So this model not only shows responsiveness to dopaminergic drugs but also can indicate the mechanism through which they produce their effects. All currently used dopaminergic agents in the treatment of PD result in a rotational response in this model. It is an excellent and effective high-throughput screening system for the development of antiparkinsonian drugs. Unfortunately, 6-OHDA cannot be used to produce a bilateral lesion model, since such animals show adipsia and aphagia and rapidly waste. The major disadvantage of the 6-OHDA-lesioned rat is that false positives occur with drugs, such as the D1 receptor agonist SKF 38393, that induce rotation but are subsequently shown to be ineffective in either primate models of PD or the human disease (Setler et al., 1978; Nomoto et al., 1985; Braun et al., 1987). Recently, other components of the motor dysfunction induced by 6-OHDA have been explored, and gait disturbances resembling those that occur in PD have been identified (Metz et al., 2005). There has also been keen interest in the sensitization to levodopa that occurs on repeated drug treatment in 6-OHDA-lesioned rats and the occurrence of abnormal involuntary movements as potential models of motor complications in PD, particularly dyskinesia, although this remains disputed (Papa et al., 1994; Cenci et al., 2002; Monville et al., 2005). Interestingly, the testing environment that is used appears to be critical to detecting sensitization phenomena (Pinna et al., 2006).

The discovery of the selective nigral toxicity of 1-methyl-4-phenyl-1,2,3,6-tetrahydropyridine (MPTP) provided a major opportunity for the development of an effective model of PD by systemic toxin administration (Davis et al., 1979; Langston et al., 1983). The toxicity of MPTP is mediated by its active metabolite 1-methyl-4-phenyl-pyridinium species (MPP$^+$), which is produced as a result of the metabolism of MPTP by type B monoamine oxidase (MAO) in glial cells. MPP$^+$ is thought to act by inhibiting complex I of the mitochondrial respiratory chain following its selective uptake into dopaminergic neurons (Jenner and Marsden, 1993; Smeyne and Jackson-Lewis, 2005). However, recent studies suggest that other mechanisms might be responsible for its neurotoxicity (Lotharius and O'Malley, 2000; Nakamura et al., 2000). Unfortunately, most rodent species are insensitive to the actions of MPTP, with the exception of some specific strains of mice—for example, black C57 mice and Swiss Webster mice (Heikkila, 1985; Bradbury et al., 1986b; Mayer et al., 1986; Sonsalla and Heikkila, 1986; Giovanni et al., 1991). Even in these strains, large doses of MPTP are needed to produce a loss of dopamine content in the striatum, and not all studies show that the administration of MPTP is associated with nigral damage. Rather, MPTP can also exert a reversible reserpine-like action, thus depleting striatal dopamine content without any effect on nigral cell number. However, in the experiments in which mice have been successfully lesioned with MPTP, a model is produced in which dopaminergic agents are able to reverse the akinesia that is induced as a result of toxin treatment. The systemic administration of MPTP results in a bilateral degeneration of substantia nigra, thus more closely mimicking events that occur in PD. However, damage is selective to the nigrostriatal pathway, and there is no loss of norepinephrine or 5-HT content in the brain, as occurs in PD. Rather than using the systemic administration of MPTP, MPP+ can be stereotaxically injected into the brain in a manner similar to that of 6-OHDA (Perry et al., 2005). Indeed, direct intranigral injection of MPP+ causes the loss of dopaminergic neurons in the substantia nigra, presumably through its ability to inhibit mitochondrial function (Langston et al., 1984b; Cavalla et al., 1985; Heikkila et al., 1985; Bradbury et al., 1986a). However, some caution is required, since the intranigral administration of MPP+ can lead to nonselective toxicity on nigral neurons through its mitochondrial respiratory chain actions. As with 6-OHDA, the use of MPP+ is restricted to producing a unilateral lesion, since bilateral lesions induce adipsia and aphagia, and the animals have poor survival rates.

Another toxin-based model of PD resembles that produced by MPP+ in that it utilizes mitochondrial inhibition as the mechanism underlying cell death but allows for systemic toxin administration. Rotenone, like MPP+, is an inhibitor of mitochondrial complex I activity, and it is the active ingredient in extracts of derris, which are used as a natural herbicide. Although rotenone, in contrast to MPTP, does not require metabolic activation, its effect appears to be mediated through a mechanism that is dependent on the involvement of microglia (Gao et al., 2002a), and its toxicity is enhanced after glial cell activation induced by prior treatment with lipopolysaccharide (Ling et al., 2004). Betarbet and colleagues (2000) showed that the intravenous infusion of rotenone in rats causes the selective degeneration of the nigrostriatal pathway, accompanied by the formation of Lewy body–like inclusions. The ability of rotenone to produce bilateral damage in the rat might provide a further means of assessing potential drug activity, although the response of these animals to current antiparkinsonian agents has not been reported. A drawback of this model is that the generalized toxicity produced by rotenone through mitochondrial inhibition leads to a high degree of mortality. A further drawback is the finding that pathologic change is more widespread than was initially reported and that it more closely resembles multiple-system atrophy than PD (Hoglinger et al., 2003). It is possible, however, to use rotenone in a fashion similar to MPP+ by direct intranigral injection, thus avoiding its acute toxicity and diverse pathologic effects (Saravanan et al., 2005; Sindhu et al., 2005).

Another herbicide, paraquat, which is a structural analog of MPP+ has been shown to induce nigral cell degeneration on systemic administration (Brooks et al., 1999; Manning-Bog et al., 2002; Ossowska et al., 2005a). Long-term paraquat treatment has been proposed as producing slowly developing dysfunction of the nigrostriatal pathway in rats (Ossowska et al., 2005b). Previously, direct intranigral application of paraquat had been shown to cause damage to dopaminergic neurons (Liou et al., 1996, 2001), but it was thought that its charged structure would not permit its penetration through the blood-brain barrier (Naylor, 1995; Widdowson et al., 1996a, 1996b; Shimizu et al., 2001). However, repeated systemic injections of paraquat in mice induced dopaminergic cell death in the substantia nigra, and this was accompanied by the formation of proteinaceous inclusions (Manning-Bog et al., 2002, 2003). Paradoxically, however, there was no decline in striatal dopamine concentration, which requires some explanation, as it contrasts markedly with the loss that occurs in PD. In contrast, microinfusion of paraquat into the substantia nigra of rats induced nigral degeneration and a striatal dopamine deficiency, resulting in impaired motor function, which responded to treatment with apomorphine (Liou et al., 1996; 2001; Mollace et al., 2003).

A problem with toxin-based models of PD is that their mechanism of action might not reflect pathogenic events occurring in the substantia nigra. Recently, inhibition of the ubiquitin-proteasome system was proposed to undertake dopaminergic cell degeneration and Lewy body formation (McNaught and Olanow, 2003; McNaught et al., 2003). It is important to note that intranigral injections of the proteasomal inhibitor lactacystin caused selective loss of dopaminergic neurons that was accompanied by the formation of inclusions that were immunoreactive for ubiquitin and α-synuclein, as found with Lewy bodies (McNaught et al., 2002; Fornai et al., 2003). Recently, repeated systemic administration of another proteasomal inhibitor, PSI, has also been shown to induce selective degeneration of dopaminergic cells in the substantia nigra and progressive motor deficits, but it is important to note that pathologic changes also occurred in the raphe nuclei, locus coeruleus, and dorsal motor nucleus of the vagus, reflecting the wider pathology that occurs in PD (McNaught et al., 2004). The degeneration of neurons was accompanied by the formation of inclusions resembling Lewy bodies. This might provide an excellent novel model of PD that reflects both the pathology and the pathogenesis of the illness in humans. However, these initial results have proved difficult to reproduce in many other laboratories in either rats or primates (Kordower et al., 2006b; Manning-Bog et al., 2006; Schapira et al., 2006b). In another laboratory, consistently produced nigral cell death in rats accompanied by motor deficits following systemic administration of PSI was seen (Zeng et al., 2006), but not to the same extent as in the original report. Skepticism exists over the validity of the systemic proteasomal inhibition model, however, and time and additional studies will be needed to determine its reliability and reproducibility. On the other hand, stereotactic injection of lactacystin into the substantia nigra of mice appears to reliably produce progressive dopaminergic degeneration (Pan et al., 2006).

## Mutant, Transgenic, and Nonmammalian Models of Parkinson Disease

Increasingly, mutations and genetic modification of rodent species are being employed to provide useful models of neurodegenerative disorders, including PD. A number of mutant rodents, such as the Weaver mouse and the Wobbler mouse, have been proposed as showing behavioral, biochemical, and pathologic deficits that reflect those occurring in PD, but these proposals have subsequently been discounted. A spontaneous mutation in a rat strain (AS/AGU) has been proposed as a model of PD on the basis of evidence for progressive striatal dopamine loss accompanied by nigral dopaminergic cell degeneration (Payne et al., 2000). The rats develop motor dysfunction that appears to be reversed by levodopa. However, the motor abnormalities exhibited by the mutants do not resemble that of PD; rather, they exhibit a complex motor syndrome that is suggestive of pathology in other brain areas. The genetic basis of this model remains unknown, and at this time, its relevance to PD is unclear.

There has been recent interest in Nurr1 knockout mice as a model of PD. Nurr1 is a member of the nuclear receptor gene superfamily and is essential for the development of dopaminergic neurons (Backman et al., 1999; Sacchetti et al., 2001; Jankovic et al., 2005). In homozygous Nurr1 knockout mice, there are no dopaminergic neurons in the substantia nigra or in the ventral tegmental area, and this is accompanied by striatal dopamine depletion without any change in brain levels of 5-HT or norepinephrine. Theoretically, this would seem to provide a highly relevant mouse model of PD in relation to degeneration of the nigrostriatal tract (Zetterstrom et al., 1997; Le et al., 1999b; Witta et al., 2000). However, at this time, the drug responsiveness of these animals has not been reported, so its usefulness as a means of assessing drug action in PD remains unknown (Le et al., 1999a).

Expression of the homeobox gene Pitx3 and Nurr1 occurs shortly before the expression of tyrosine hydroxylase in midbrain dopaminergic neurons, but unlike Nurr1, Pitx3 expression is confined, at least in the brain, to mesencephalic dopaminergic neurons (Jankovic et al., 2005; Smidt and Burbach, 2007). In the naturally occurring mouse mutant Aphakia, there is Pitx3 deficiency, and this has been associated with selective loss of substantia nigra dopaminergic neurons and loss of the nigrostriatal pathway (van den Munckhof et al., 2003). These mice show motor deficits that are reversed by levodopa treatment (Hwang et al., 2005; van den Munckhof et al., 2006). They also show the same adaptive changes in striatal output pathways as occur after acute toxin-induced degeneration of the nigrostriatal pathway. It will be interesting to determine in future studies how closely these mice mimic idiopathic PD in humans.

Intense interest has centered on producing a transgenic model of PD related to the discovery of two mutant forms of α-synuclein arising from gene defects in familial PD (Polymeropoulos et al., 1996, 1997; Kruger et al., 1998). Overexpression of mutant α-synuclein in cell lines leads to increased apoptotic cell death in response to toxic stimuli (Ostrerova-Golts et al., 2000; Tabrizi et al., 2000; Zhou et al., 2000). However, to date, attempts to produce an α-synuclein transgenic mouse that closely resembles PD in terms of pathology, the presence of inclusions, and biochemical changes accompanied by motor deficits have been relatively unsuccessful. One problem associated with the production of an α-synuclein transgenic is that the wild-type α-synuclein that is found in mice is identical to one of the mutant forms associated with familial PD.

Production of an α-synuclein knockout mouse did not result in loss of nigral dopaminergic cell bodies, fibers, or synapses, and there was a normal dopamine release and reuptake in the striatum on electrical stimulation of dopaminergic neurons (Abeliovich et al., 2000). There were, however, a decrease in striatal dopamine levels and a decreased locomotor response to amphetamine; otherwise, these animals did not appear to have an impaired motor system. Null α-synuclein mice are also resistant to MPTP (Dauer et al., 2002). Overexpression of human wild-type α-synuclein in mice resulted in the progressive accumulation of α-synuclein and ubiquitin immunoreactive inclusions in the cortex, hippocampus, and substantia nigra (Masliah et al., 2000). While a loss of dopaminergic terminals occurred in the striatum, this was not accompanied by cell loss in the substantia nigra. These mice showed motor deficits on a rotarod, but again, the major pathology of PD was not apparent. Overexpression of a human mutant form of α-synuclein (A53T α-synuclein) resulted in widespread brainstem pathology that included nigral cell loss (van der Putten et al., 2000). However, pathology also occurred in motor neurons, but it was accompanied by Lewy body–type inclusions and by widespread gliosis. These mice showed impaired motor performance, but once more, the pathology and the biochemical deficits that occur do not replicate events in PD (van der Putten et al., 2000; Giasson et al., 2002). Attempts to produce transgenic mice models of PD by using other gene defects found in familial disease, such as parkin and DJ-1, have been equally unsuccessful (Kim et al., 2005; Perez and Palmiter, 2005).

There has, however, been one approach to producing a α-synuclein transgenic with characteristics similar to those of PD through the expression of human wild-type and mutant α-synuclein in *Drosophila* (Feany and Bender, 2000), although even this is disputed (Pesah et al., 2005). There is an adult-onset loss of dopaminergic neurons in the nervous system and in the eye accompanied by the occurrence of filamentous intraneuronal inclusions that contain α-synuclein. The flies exhibit motor dysfunction, which is improved by the administration of levodopa and both D1 and D2 agonist drugs (Pendleton et al., 2002). So this might be an effective model of PD that could have utility in understanding cell death but also has a role as a model for drug discovery.

Nonmammalian species might also have utility as models of PD. The nematode *Caenorhabditis elegans* possesses dopaminergic neurons and all fundamental machinery for dopamine synthesis, storage, and inactivation (Rand and Nonet, 1997; Nass et al., 2001). Exposure of *C. elegans* to 6-OHDA causes selective degeneration of dopamine neurons and blockade of the dopamine transporter proteins against cell death (Nass et al., 2002). These findings open the door to an elegant means of assessing mechanisms of dopaminergic cell death and neuroprotective strategies for PD in a simple organism.

Genetic modifications to produce nigral dopaminergic cell degeneration could also be feasible through the use of gene delivery by a viral vector. This approach has great utility because it allows the introduction of gene defects that are known to occur in PD into nigral cells of any species, thus avoiding the problems associated with the production of transgenic mice. Delivery of the gene for mutant α-synuclein has already been shown to result in dopaminergic cell death in rats and primates (Nakamura et al., 2000; Kirik et al., 2003; Yamada et al., 2004; Maingay et al., 2005), although once more, replication of the original findings has not proved to be universal. Although in its infancy, viral vector technology could become a valuable tool in generating models of PD that are progressive and reflect the pathogenic mechanisms that are involved. Equally valuable may be the use of RNAi silencing of the expression of proteins involved in neurodegeneration (Kock et al., 2006; Sapru et al., 2006)

## THE MPTP-TREATED PRIMATE MODEL OF PARKINSON DISEASE

The discovery of the selective nigral toxicity of MPTP created a highly appropriate model of PD when it became apparent that the toxin was effective in primates (Burns et al., 1983; Jenner et al., 1984; Langston et al., 1984a). Administration of MPTP to a range of primate species causes selective nigral cell loss accompanied by a decrease in caudate-putamen dopamine content and the onset of major motor symptoms of PD, such as akinesia, bradykinesia, and rigidity. Tremor is not a common component of the MPTP syndrome, and while postural tremor does occur, rest tremor characteristic of PD is seen only in specific primate species, such as the green monkey. MPTP only partially mimics events that occur in PD and, most important, does not provide an exact model of the disorder. Most studies involving MPTP utilize systemic administration of MPTP to produce bilateral motor deficits. However, some investigators prefer to use unilateral intra-carotid injection of MPTP to produce a unilateral model, which lessens the adverse effects of the toxin (Barone et al., 1987; Clarke et al., 1989; Eberling et al., 1998; Emborg-Knott and Domino, 1998). The study of the actions of drugs during the course of MPTP treatment of primates is utilized to investigate potential neurorestorative and neuroprotective therapies, whereas novel symptomatic therapies can be investigated following establishment of a nigral lesion.

It is the drug responsiveness of the MPTP-treated primate that makes it a useful tool in the drug discovery process for assessing novel compounds for the treatment of PD. Administration of levodopa plus carbidopa or dopamine agonist to MPTP-treated primates results in a reversal of the akinesia or bradykinesia that is measurable as an increase in locomotor activity (Arai et al., 1995). This is accompanied by a decrease in motor disabilities that can be assessed by using an observer-rated scoring system. In addition, the repeated administration of levodopa to drug-naïve MPTP-treated primates rapidly results in the appearance of marked dyskinesias that closely resemble those occurring in the long-term treatment of patients with PD (Bedard et al., 1986; Boyce et al., 1990; Arai et al., 1995; Pearce et al., 1995). The rapid appearance of dyskinesia is related to the severity of the nigral lesions in MPTP-treated primates, which lowers the threshold for dyskinesia induction by levodopa (Di Monte et al., 2000). However, dyskinesia has also been reported to occur after acute levodopa administration to normal squirrel monkeys and following high-dose chronic treatment in macaques (Pearce et al., 2001; Togasaki et al., 2001, 2005). The long-term administration of levodopa to MPTP-treated animals also results in a shortening of the drug's effect, thus mimicking the wearing-off effect that is seen in patient populations (Blanchet et al., 1996). Other phenomena associated with levodopa's action in PD can be observed. For example, following acute challenge with levodopa, beginning-of-dose worsening and end-of-dose deterioration are observed (Kuoppamaki et al., 2002). On chronic levodopa treatment, on-off and freezing episodes can also occur. This opens up the opportunity of using the model to study the mechanism underlying treatment-related complications and their avoidance.

## NOVEL DOPAMINERGIC APPROACHES TO THE TREATMENT OF PARKINSON DISEASE

The MPTP-treated primate and the 6-OHDA-lesioned rat respond to the administration of all currently used dopaminergic drugs for the treatment of PD, including levodopa, bromocriptine, pergolide, ropinirole, pramipexole, and cabergoline. So far, all actions of these compounds that occur in MPTP-treated primates (and to a large extent in the rat) have turned out to be highly predictive of drug action in humans. For this reason, other novel dopaminergic approaches are now being evaluated in these models for their utility in the treatment of PD.

The MPTP model has been utilized to assess the relative roles of drugs acting on specific dopamine receptor subtypes. Agents that are active on the D2-like family of receptors are all antiparkinsonian in the MPTP-treated primates but provoke established dyskinesia in these animals resulting from prior levodopa exposure, reflecting the response that occurs in patients with PD (Gomez-Mancilla and Bedard, 1991; Blanchet et al., 1993). Drugs acting on D1-like receptors, such as dihydrexidine and ABT 431, also exert antiparkinsonian activity in MPTP-treated primates (Taylor et al., 1991; Shiosaki et al., 1996). While they too will provoke established dyskinesia, this is less intense than occurs with D2 agonist drugs, although clinical data suggest that this is not reflected in their actions in humans (Rascol, Nutt, et al., 2001). Many other dopaminergic approaches to the treatment of PD are currently under investigation despite the many dopamine agonists that are already available. A highly selective D2 agonist, sumanirole, appeared promising from studies in MPTP-treated primates (McCall et al., 2005; Stephenson et al., 2005), but its clinical development has been halted. There has also been interest in mixed D1/D2 agonists that might exert greater antiparkinsonian activity than do drugs that stimulate either receptor population alone and interest in selective drugs that interact with D3 or D4 dopamine receptors (Millan et al., 2004; Silverdale et al., 2004).

There has also been interest in the potential use of partial dopamine agonists, such as SLV 308, in the treatment of PD. Partial agonists act as full agonists in the denervated striatum, thus promoting an antiparkinsonian response. But in the relatively intact mesolimbic and mesocortical systems, they would act as antagonists by competing for receptor occupation with dopamine. Such an effect might prevent or subdue psychotic episodes in patients with PD. In MPTP-treated primates, partial dopamine agonist drugs can be highly effective in reversing parkinsonian symptoms and do not induce significant dyskinesia or exacerbate that produced by levodopa (Johnston et al., 2000). A number of these compounds are now entering clinical evaluation for their utility in humans, including SLV 308, which is now in phase III trials in PD.

Novel dopamine reuptake blockers, such as brasofensine, NS 2330, and BTS 74-398, have been assessed in MPTP-treated primates (Hansard et al., 1998; Pearce et al., 2002). This class of drug increases locomotor activity and decreases motor disability but does so without provoking established involuntary movements. The mechanism by which dopamine reuptake blockers can separate actions of benefit in PD from those that result in a major side effect is not clear at this time but relates to enhancement of mesocortical and mesolimbic dopamine function rather than a direct effect on the nigrostriatal pathway. There is certainly a potential role for these compounds in the treatment of PD (Nutt et al., 2004). However, clinical evaluation of brasofensine, NS 2330, and BTS 74-398 in PD all failed to show antiparkinsonian activity. This raises the concern that the MPTP-treated primate model of PD might not be predictive of clinical effect for this class of compound (Bara-Jimenez et al., 2004; Wu and Frucht, 2005).

Studies in the MPTP-treated primate are also used to assess routes of drug delivery for existing and novel dopaminergic agents. In particular, transdermal application of dopaminergic agents is being employed to produce more continuous dopaminergic stimulation and longer periods of mobility during the waking day. Studies in MPTP-treated primates have shown agents such as PHNO and N-0437 to be highly effective by application to the skin and by delivery from transdermal patches (Loschmann et al., 1989; Rupniak et al., 1989). This route of administration transforms drugs with relatively short half-lives following oral or systemic administration into agents that can act throughout a 24-hour period or longer. This route of administration would be exceptionally useful in treating PD, provided that tolerance does not develop as a result of constant receptor stimulation. On the basis of studies carried out in MPTP-treated primates, transdermal patches for PD have been studied in clinical investigations. However, PHNO incorporated into a transdermal patch did not produce an antiparkinsonian effect, although there was a reduction in the amount of levodopa required to maintain mobility (Coleman et al., 1989). The amount of drug flux across the skin might not have been sufficient to produce plasma/brain levels of PHNO needed to produce antiparkinsonian activity. However, studies incorporating the aminotetralin derivative N-0923 (rotigotine) into a patch not only led to a reduction in levodopa usage (Hutton et al., 2001) but also showed a dose-response antiparkinsonian effect produced by the drug when used alone (Fahn and Parkinson Study Group, 2001; Guldenpfennig et al., 2005). The ergot derivatives lisuride and proterguride are also under development for transdermal use in PD (Woitalla et al., 2004; Hofmann et al., 2006; Schurad et al., 2006). Microemulsion of apomorphine may also allow its transdermal administration and reduce motor scores in PD (Priano et al., 2004). Similarly, the subcutaneous implantation of polymer rods impregnated with apomorphine that is slowly released over many months produces antiparkinsonian effects in MPTP-treated primates but with little risk of dyskinesia (Bibbiani et al., 2005). Even transdermal administration of levodopa could become feasible, and this route of treatment might have significant utility in the future.

Other routes of drug delivery in PD may also have utility (Johnston et al., 2005). Rectal administration of drugs can avoid first-pass metabolism and be used following surgery or in PD patients in intensive care, but unfortunately, levodopa is not absorbed through the rectal mucosa (Eisler et al., 1981). Direct duodenal and jejunal infusion of levodopa is being tested using a new commercial packaging of levodopa known as Duodopa and now available in Europe. (Nilsson et al., 2001; Nyholm et al., 2005). Buccal or sublingual formulations or nasal or buccal sprays or inhalation can deliver drugs by means that avoid first-pass metabolism and overcome poor oral bioavailability and swallowing difficulties that occur in some patients with PD and to provide rapidly acting rescue medication. Recently, the pulmonary administration of apomorphine in PD has started clinical evaluation (Bartus et al., 2004). Water-soluble prodrugs of levodopa that are rapidly hydrolyzed have been tested by oral administration for this reason. These include levodopa methyl ester and levodopa ethyl ester, but while they produce a more rapid "on," they are not more effective or longer-acting than conventional levodopa (Steiger et al., 1991; Djaldetti et al., 2002a).

The ability of alternative routes of administration to overcome pharmacokinetic problems associated with specific drugs in PD has been emphasized by the use of subcutaneous and intravenous infusions of apomorphine. Apomorphine has a short duration of effect and poor oral bioavailability. By using infusions of apomorphine, a rapid, robust antiparkinsonian activity can be produced, significantly reducing refractory motor complications (Frankel et al., 1990; Manson et al., 2001).

## Dopamine Agonists and Continuous Dopaminergic Stimulation

The ability of levodopa and dopamine agonist drugs to induce dyskinesia in MPTP-treated primates has been used to study the factors that affect dyskinesia induction and treatment strategies that will avoid or reverse priming for involuntary movements (Jenner, 2000a). In animals with marked nigral denervation, dopamine agonist drugs used clinically to treat PD, such as bromocriptine, pergolide, cabergoline, pramipexole, and ropinirole, induce less dyskinesia than occurs with levodopa (Bedard et al., 1986; Grondin et al., 1996; Pearce et al., 1998; Jenner, 2000a; Maratos et al., 2003). Such studies strongly suggest that the early treatment of PD with dopamine agonist drugs would be less likely to provoke involuntary movements than starting therapy with levodopa. The effects that are observed in MPTP-treated primates have been validated by a series of long-term clinical studies of the early use of dopamine agonists as monotherapy for the treatment of PD (Rinne et al., 1998; Parkinson Study Group, 2000; Rascol et al., 2000; Oertel et al., 2006). Thus, in studies lasting up to 5 years, the use of ropinirole, pramipexole, pergolide, and cabergoline resulted in a low incidence of involuntary movements. Even when rescue with levodopa was required, the incidence of dyskinesia was lower than that produced by levodopa monotherapy. This was also confirmed by studies in MPTP-treated common marmosets, in which administration of ropinirole and levodopa in an agonist-dominant combination produced less dyskinesia than did an equivalent antiparkinsonian dose of levodopa (Maratos et al., 2001).

The evaluation of the studies undertaken in MPTP-treated primates has strongly suggested that levodopa is far more able to induce dyskinesia in these animals than are dopamine agonist drugs. However, this appears to be dependent on the nature of the receptor stimulation that is induced by dopamine agonists because there is some correlation between the duration of antiparkinsonian action and dyskinesia induction (Bedard et al., 1997) Thus, short-acting dopamine agonist drugs, including levodopa, that produce pulsatile stimulation of dopamine receptors appear more able to induce dyskinesia than do long-acting dopamine agonist drugs that produce a more continuous motor response. This has led to the concept of continuous dopaminergic stimulation as a means of avoiding dyskinesia (Olanow et al., 2000; Stocchi and Olanow, 2004). Continuous dopaminergic stimulation has been supported by studies in MPTP-treated primates of the administration of a number of drugs that are short-acting on acute subcutaneous injection but that can be given by subcutaneous infusion or transdermal application. Key experiments indicating the benefit of continuous dopaminergic stimulation involved the use of a short-acting D2 agonist and a short-acting D1 agonist (Blanchet et al., 1995). When these drugs were administered repeatedly by subcutaneous injection to MPTP-treated monkeys, both induced a marked incidence of dyskinesia. However, when the same drugs were administered by continuous subcutaneous infusion using osmotic minipumps, a much lower incidence of dyskinesia was observed. This suggests that the manner in which dopamine agonist drugs are administered is critical to the way in which dyskinesia induction occurs and to the incidence and intensity of involuntary movements. Similarly, for apomorphine and rotigotine, among others, dyskinesia induction is markedly reduced on continuous drug delivery compared to acute pulsatile treatment.

However, while continuous dopaminergic stimulation provides an important concept for defining the clinical treatment of PD, it has many flaws and does not explain many aspects of dyskinesia induction in either MPTP-treated primates or patients with PD. For example, the correlation between the duration of effect of dopamine agonist drugs examined in MPTP-treated primates and the occurrence of dyskinesia is not perfect. When the effects of repeated administration of equieffective doses of levodopa, pergolide, and apomorphine in MPTP-treated primates were studied, both pergolide and apomorphine induced less dyskinesia than levodopa did (Maratos et al., 2003). However, the duration of effect of these drugs is very different, with pergolide acting for some 8 to 9 hours, while apomorphine has a duration of only 1 to 2 hours. Although continuous dopaminergic stimulation might be a key component of the process that determines whether dyskinesia does or does not appear, it is not the only factor that dictates dyskinesia induction. It also does not entirely explain why levodopa is not only the most effective drug for treating all stages of PD but also the most likely drug to induce dyskinesia. Nor does it explain why younger patients are more likely to develop dyskinesias than are older patients with levodopa therapy (see Chapter 6).

A further potential factor affecting the occurrence of dyskinesia is the role of D1 and D2 receptors. Drugs that act on both D1 and D2 drugs can induce dyskinesia. But in most of the studies undertaken in MPTP-treated primates, dopamine agonists that are selective for either D1 or D2 receptors have been compared with levodopa, which presumably affects both receptor subtypes. There is synergy between the antiparkinsonian effects of selective D1 and D2 agonists, and the same could be true for dyskinesia induction (Carlson et al., 1987; Hu and White, 1994). Indeed, the intensity of dyskinesia produced by equieffective doses of the selective D2 agonists bromocriptine and ropinirole is less marked than that seen with the D1/D2 agonists pergolide and apomorphine (Maratos et al., 2003).

## A Strategy for Avoiding Dyskinesia Induction with Levodopa

In humans, the occurrence of dyskinesia seems to be related to the total exposure to levodopa (Agid et al., 1985). There is little doubt that treatment of patients with higher doses of levodopa leads to a greater incidence and intensity of dyskinesia than does treatment with lower doses of levodopa, as is clearly shown by the ELLDOPA study (Parkinson Study Group, 2004c). The concept of continuous dopaminergic stimulation suggests that if levodopa were delivered in a manner that avoided pulsatile stimulation, then it should avoid dyskinesia induction in the same manner as dopamine agonists when used as early monotherapy for PD.

Recent studies have evaluated the effects of levodopa dose, frequency of drug administration, and brain exposure to pulsatile levodopa administration on the genesis of dyskinesia in otherwise drug-naïve MPTP-treated primates (Smith et al., 2003). Administration of levodopa (12.5 mg/kg twice daily) plus a peripheral decarboxylase inhibitor produced a pulsatile stimulation of locomotor activity and reversal of motor disability. The motor response was significantly greater than that with twice-daily administration of a low dose (6.25 mg/kg) of levodopa. Thus, as expected, there is a dose relationship between the amount of levodopa administered and the improvement in motor performance that is observed. However, over a period of 30 days, twice-daily administration of the higher dose of levodopa resulted in the rapid onset of dyskinesia, which was more severe than was observed with the low dose of levodopa. So there is also a dose relationship between pulsatile exposure to levodopa and the induction of involuntary movements.

The effect of potentiating the effects of pulsatile administration of levodopa using the peripheral catechol-O-methyltransferase (COMT) inhibitor entacapone was also examined (Smith et al., 2003). The effects of the low dose of levodopa (6.25 mg/kg) plus a peripheral decarboxylase inhibitor given twice daily for 30 days to otherwise drug-naïve MPTP-treated primates were compared with the effects of administration of the same dose of levodopa combined with the administration of entacapone. The effect of entacapone on antiparkinsonian activity was to increase locomotor activity and to improve motor disability but in a pulsatile manner equivalent to that produced by the high dose of levodopa. The effect of potentiating the pulsatile actions of levodopa was to increase the intensity and severity of dyskinesia. This reflects an increased exposure of the brain to levodopa due to inhibition of its peripheral breakdown. With the concurrent use of COMT inhibitors, the amount of levodopa, and hence dopamine, entering the brain is increased as a result of COMT inhibition, such that there is increased brain exposure.

So does more continuous administration of levodopa produce less dyskinesia? In a recent study using MPTP-treated primates, the effects of repeated administration of pulsatile levodopa treatment (12.5 mg/kg orally plus carbidopa 12.5 mg/kg orally twice daily) with and without entacapone were compared with the effects of continuous treatment produced by using the same total daily dose of levodopa

(6.25 mg/kg orally plus carbidopa 6.25 mg/kg orally four times daily) with and without entacapone (Smith et al., 2005). Perhaps surprisingly, administration of continuous levodopa with entacapone resulted in a greater antiparkinsonian effect than was seen with the other treatments while inducing less intense dyskinesia of shorter duration. Consequently, the use of COMT inhibitors with more continuous administration of levodopa is being evaluated in a clinical study (STRIDE-PD) to determine whether it can be used in a similar manner in early PD to avoid or reduce the incidence or intensity of involuntary movements.

## Priming for Dyskinesia

Once dyskinesia induction occurs as a result of levodopa administration to MPTP-treated primates or to patients with PD, a priming of basal ganglia has occurred such that each administration of either levodopa or a dopamine agonist drug will induce the same involuntary movements. The induction of dyskinesia by levodopa seems to be a persistent if not irreversible process in MPTP-treated primates, since even after prolonged periods without exposure to dopaminergic drugs, such animals show involuntary movements on a single acute challenge. In patients with PD, priming might be partially reversible, but the situation is far from clear. The MPTP-treated primate, in conjunction with clinical investigations, has been used to study whether dopamine agonists might reverse the priming of basal ganglia produced by levodopa. A major problem is that the mechanisms responsible for priming for dyskinesia are poorly understood but might involve glutamatergic system in a manner associated with long-term depression or alterations in synaptic morphology so as to alter corticostriatal glutamatergic connectivity (Metman et al., 2000; Picconi et al., 2005). Dyskinesia is classically associated with an imbalance between the direct and indirect striatal output pathways, and there is considerable evidence from research on MPTP-treated primates to show the manner in which these output systems are affected by levodopa and dopamine agonist drugs (Morissette et al., 1999; Zeng et al., 2000). However, the duration of the biochemical changes that are observed is too short to explain the prolonged persistence of the priming process for dyskinesia, and the changes probably have more to do with the expression of involuntary movements than with the underlying pathogenic nature of priming. It is largely thought that only levodopa primes for dyskinesia induction and that dopamine agonists do not. This is clearly not an absolute distinction, as both in MPTP-treated primates and in PD, dopamine agonists still induce dyskinesia, though to a lesser extent than occurs with levodopa. More important, studies in MPTP-treated primates have shown that while dopamine agonists do not themselves lead to the appearance of marked dyskinesia, as soon as exposure to levodopa occurs, severe dyskinesia becomes apparent, showing that agonists do prime basal ganglia in the same way as levodopa does but that they do not lead to its expression (Smith et al., 2006; Jackson et al., 2007). A similar situation may exist in PD in patients who initially receive dopamine agonist monotherapy but who are then treated with levodopa.

As a consequence of the lack of knowledge about priming, there are currently no therapeutic strategies that can be used in patients with late-stage PD with disabling dyskinesia to reverse the cause of the involuntary movements. It is usual to adjust the levels of levodopa to minimize the dyskinesias without aggravating parkinsonian symptoms too much. However, a reduction in the intensity of dyskinesia can occur on continuous intravenous infusion of levodopa or the continuous subcutaneous or intravenous infusion of apomorphine (Frankel et al., 1990; Mouradian et al., 1990; Manson et al., 2001). In addition, switching patients who are on optimal doses of levodopa to high-dose pergolide treatment can lead to a reduction in dyskinesia intensity (Facca and Sanchez-Ramos, 1996). This evidence suggests that moving from pulsatile to continuous dopaminergic stimulation of dopamine receptors can reverse the process that is responsible for priming, although it is also likely that a less potent drug (e.g., a dopamine agonist) is less likely to cause dyskinesias. Similarly, in MPTP-treated primates that are primed with levodopa to exhibit dyskinesia, switching to the administration of the long-acting D2 agonist cabergoline for 6 to 8 weeks leads to a significant decrease in dyskinesia intensity associated with only minor reductions in antiparkinsonian activity (Hadj et al., 2000). In other studies, MPTP-treated primates that were dyskinetic in response to levodopa treatment showed an immediate decrease in dyskinesia intensity when switched to an equivalent antiparkinsonian dose of ropinirole or piribedil (Smith et al., 2006; Jackson et al., 2007).

These studies suggest not only that dopamine agonists are useful as an adjunct to levodopa in patients exhibiting wearing-off and other long-term motor complications as they have been classically employed but also that dopamine agonists have a use in early monotherapy in PD in the avoidance of dyskinesia. The latest data suggest that, in addition, they could have a role to play in late-stage disease in which switching from optimal levodopa dosage to a long-acting dopamine agonist might be a useful strategy in depriming patients who have disabling dyskinesia.

# NONDOPAMINERGIC APPROACHES TO THE TREATMENT OF PARKINSON DISEASE

For the past 40 years, the treatment of PD has been based on dopamine replacement therapy. Recently, the potential of a range of nondopaminergic neuronal targets within the striatum and other nuclei of basal ganglia through which motor activity has been explored (Brotchie, 1998; Jenner, 2000b; Brown et al., 2002; Johnston and Brotchie, 2004, 2006; Brotchie, 2005; Johnston et al., 2005; Fox et al., 2006; Schapira et al., 2006a). An entire range of novel approaches to the treatment of PD based on nondopaminergic drugs is now under active investigation and clinical development. Some of these are detailed here (Box 9-1).

## Glutamate Antagonists (Box 9-2)

Overactivity of glutamatergic mechanisms is thought to contribute to the motor symptoms of PD and to the occurrence of levodopa-induced dyskinesia. In particular, there is an overactivity of the subthalamic nucleus–GPi/SNr glutamate pathway in PD and probably also increased activity of the

Box 9-1 Nondopaminergic approaches to treatment

Glutamate antagonists
Cannabinoids
Opiates
Adrenergic antagonists
Serotonergic agonists
Antiepileptics
Muscarinics
Nicotinics
GABAergics

corticostriatal glutamate input (Bergman et al., 1990, 1994; Meshul et al., 1999; Greenamyre, 2001). Both NMDA and AMPA receptor antagonists have direct antiparkinsonian activity and synergize with levodopa and dopamine agonist drugs (Klockgether and Turski, 1990; Klockgether et al., 1991; Kelsey et al., 2004). These findings have been somewhat controversial, but a study involving reserpine-treated rats suggested that NMDA antagonists that are selective for the NR2B receptor possess antiparkinsonian activity (Nash et al., 1999). It has also been suggested that NMDA antagonists might improve response fluctuations in PD on the basis of their ability to prevent a decrease in the duration of response to levodopa seen on repeated administration to 6-OHDA-lesioned rats (Wessell et al., 2004). The clinical utility of this approach is shown by the finding that the NMDA antagonist remacemide improves motor scores and reduces "off" time in fluctuating PD patients who are receiving concurrent dopaminergic medication (Greenamyre et al., 1994). The glutamate antagonist riluzole, which acts through blockade of sodium channels, appears effective in experimental models of PD, but surprisingly, in clinical evaluation, its effects have been limited (Jankovic and Hunter, 2002; Braz et al., 2004).

NMDA antagonists have also been shown to control dyskinesia. Thus, both amantadine and LY 235959 can suppress dyskinesia in MPTP-treated primates produced by levodopa administration without adversely affecting the antiparkinsonian response to levodopa (Papa and Chase, 1996; Blanchet et al., 1998). Amantadine has been similarly shown to suppress involuntary movements in dyskinetic PD patients (Verhagen et al., 1998). If more selective glutamate antagonists can be produced for use in humans that do not adversely

affect glutamatergic function elsewhere in brain, then these could be useful clinical tools. Clinical trials evaluating newer glutamate antagonists are either actively ongoing or in the planning stages.

## Adenosine Antagonists

The A2a adenosine receptor has a highly selective localization to the indirect striatal output pathway (Svenningsson et al., 1997) (Box 9-3). It controls acetylcholine and GABA release in the striatum through presynaptic receptors on cholinergic interneurons and on recurrent collaterals on the striato-GPe GABAergic pathway (Mori and Shindou, 2000; Richardson and Kurokawa, 2000) (Box 9-4). A2a receptors are also located presynaptically on the terminals of the striato-GPe GABAergic pathway in the globus pallidus and again alter GABA release (Ochi et al., 2000). They may also modulate glutamatergic input in the striatum from the cortex (Nash and Brotchie, 2000). As such, they provide an important target for PD (Hauser and Schwarzschild, 2005; Jenner, 2005; Schwarzschild et al., 2006). A range of A2a antagonists, including KF 17837, KW 6002, SCH 58261, and ST 1535, all reverse motor deficits in a range of rodent models (Hauber et al., 2001; Pinna et al., 2001; Wardas et al., 2001). Most A2a antagonists have little or no effect alone in 6-OHDA lesioned rats but are able to potentiate the effects of a threshold dose of levodopa to induce contralateral rotation (Pinna et al., 2005a, 2005b; Rose et al., 2007). In MPTP-treated primates, KW 6002 and ST 1535 produce a modest increase in locomotor activity but a more substantial reversal of motor disability (Kanda et al., 2000; Rose et al., 2006) (Box 9-5). However, with KW 6002, this is not accompanied by the appearance of dyskinesias in animals that have been primed for the appearance of involuntary movements and that would exhibit dyskinesia when challenged with a dopaminergic agonist (Kanda et al., 1998). A2a antagonists therefore might be useful in patients with PD who have been treated previously with levodopa but now have incapacitating involuntary movements. Initial clinical studies with KW 6002 (istradephylline) showed it to be antiparkinsonian in patients receiving suboptimal infusions of levodopa (Sherzai et al., 2002) and to reduce "off" time in patients receiving oral levodopa therapy though, surprisingly, at the expense of an increase in nontroublesome dyskinesia (Hauser et al., 2003). Subsequent phase III clinical studies have not been so impressive, but these were undertaken in patients with wearing-off who were receiving optimal dopaminergic

Box 9-2 Glutamate antagonists and Parkinson disease

NMDA, AMPA, and metabotropic receptor antagonists improve motor function in reserpinized rats, 6-OHDA-lesioned rats, and MPTP-treated primates.
NMDA, AMPA, and metabotropic receptor antagonists also enhance the effects of levodopa and prevent the onset of wearing-off in 6-OHDA-lesioned rats.
NMDA and AMPA antagonists reduce dyskinesia in MPTP-treated primates.
Amantadine reduces dyskinesia in patients with PD.

Box 9-3 Adenosine receptors

| Subtypes | $A_{2a}$ Receptors in the Brain |
|---|---|
| $A_1$ inhibit adenylate cyclase | Localized to basal ganglia |
| $A_{2a}$ and $A_{2b}$ stimulate adenylate cyclase | Abundant in the striatum |
| $A_3$ inhibit adenylate cyclase | Localized to medium spiny GABAergic neurons of indirect output pathway |

**Box 9-4** Adenosine antagonists and Parkinson disease

Suppress GABAergic transmission in the striatum.
Enhance GABAergic transmission in the globus pallidus.
Modulate GABA and acetylcholine release.
Increase striatal glutamate outflow.
Dimerize with $D_2$ receptors.
Dimerize with glutamate receptors.

**Box 9-6** 5-HT agonists/antagonists and Parkinson disease

$5-HT_{2C}$ antagonists improve motor symptoms in 6-OHDA-lesioned rats.
$5-HT_{1A}$ agonist tandospirone alleviates dyskinesia in PD.
$5-HT_{1A}$ agonist sarizotan reduces dyskinesia in MPTP-treated primates but failed in a clinical trial.
Also may improve wearing-off in PD.

medication with no allowance for a reduction in levodopa intake.

A2a antagonists may also have utility in preventing priming for dyskinesia. Thus, in unilateral 6-OHDA-lesioned mice, the sensitization produced by repeated administration of levodopa was not observed in mice with an A2a receptor knockout (Fredduzzi et al., 2002). In addition, blockade of A2a receptors or knockout of the A2a receptor impairs the induction of long-term potentiation, a process that has been associated with priming for dyskinesia (d'Alcantara et al., 2001). Recently, in MPTP-treated primates, KW 6002 was found to delay the appearance of dyskinesia when coadministered with apomorphine (Bibbiani et al., 2003). In a similar investigation, KW 6002 administered with levodopa to MPTP-treated primates improved motor function compared to that seen with levodopa alone without worsening dyskinesia induction (unpublished data). No studies with a levodopa-sparing strategy have yet been undertaken in MPTP-treated primates.

## 5-HT Agonists and Antagonists (Box 9-6)

The basal ganglia receive a significant 5-HT neuronal input from the raphe nuclei, and many types of 5-HT receptors are present in the striatum and other basal ganglia nuclei. There is a long history of serotonergic modulation of dopaminergic-mediated motor function, but this has yet to be exploited in the treatment of PD. Increasing 5-HT transmission by blocking serotonin reuptake with fluoxetine in both MPTP-treated primates and patients with PD can suppress levodopa-induced dyskinesia (Gomez-Mancilla and Bedard, 1993; Durif et al., 1995), although overall, this remains an area of controversy. The major problem might be in determining which of the multiple 5-HT 1-7 receptors might be an appropriate target.

**Box 9-5** Antiparkinsonian actions of A2a antagonists in nonhuman primates

Increase locomotor activity and reduce motor disability in MPTP-treated primates.
Produce additive effects with levodopa and dopamine agonists.
Increase antiparkinsonian activity in MPTP-treated primates with minor enhancement of dyskinesia using optimal levodopa therapy.
Delay onset of dyskinesia in MPTP-treated primates by sparing levodopa.

$5-HT_{1A}$ receptors act as autoreceptors controlling the release of serotonin as well as dopamine derived from levodopa by decarboxylation in 5-HT neurons (Santiago et al., 1998; Yamato et al., 2001). In 6-OHDA-lesioned rats, the $5-HT_{1A}$ agonist sarizotan did not produce rotational behavior but prevented the shortening of response to levodopa that occurs with chronic administration (Bibbiani et al., 2001). In MPTP-treated monkeys, sarizotan had no antiparkinsonian effect alone or in combination with levodopa but blocked the dyskinesias provoked by levodopa treatment (Bibbiani et al., 2001). However, in patients with PD, the $5-HT_{1A}$ agonist tandospirone suppressed dyskinesia in 50% of patients but caused a worsening of parkinsonian features in the rest (Kannari et al., 2002). Indeed, despite an apparent suppression of dyskinesia without worsening of parkinsonism with sarizotan in phase II clinical trials in PD, the drug failed in subsequent phase III evaluation, in which a reduction of dosage led to no effect on dyskinesia or on motor symptoms (Olanow et al., 2004; Goetz et al., 2007). The effects of $5-HT_{1A}$ agonists have been difficult to assess, as most also alter dopaminergic function. However, a recent study in MPTP-treated primates showed that a selective $5-HT_{1A}$ agonist, 8-OHDPAT, only suppressed dyskinesia with a worsening of motor disability (Iravani, Tayarani-Binazir, et al., 2006). This suggests that this approach might not have utility in PD, although $5-HT_{1A}$ may also exert neuroprotective actions (Bezard et al., 2006).

Other receptor subtypes may also be inappropriate targets, since in a series of experiments in MPTP-treated monkeys, $5-HT_{1B/D}$ receptor agonists and antagonists had no effect when administered alone or in combination with levodopa or when given to animals exhibiting levodopa-induced dyskinesia (Jackson et al., 2004).

## Cholinergic and Anticholinergic Drugs (Box 9-7)

The manipulation of cholinergic function within the basal ganglia is an established approach to treating PD that has been largely overlooked. Interneurons within the striatum are largely cholinergic, and there is significant cholinergic input into most nuclei of the basal ganglia from the pedunculopontine nucleus (Woolf and Butcher, 1986). Currently, anticholinergic drugs acting on muscarinic receptors are used to treat mild symptoms of PD, particularly tremor (Parkes et al., 1987), but there has been no recent evaluation of their potential therapeutic role in the illness. Anticholinergics are viewed as old drugs that have low efficacy and well-documented

Box 9-7 Cholinergic drugs and Parkinson disease

Intimately involved in control of movement.
Anticholinergics can improve motor deficits and
  manipulate dyskinesia in MPTP-treated primates.
The effect of nicotinic agonists is unclear.

side effects. However, acute dystonic reactions induced by neuroleptic drugs can be reversed by the administration of anticholinergic agents, and in idiopathic torsion dystonia, high-dose anticholinergic therapy might reduce the involuntary movements (Fahn, 1983; Burke et al., 1986; Parkes et al., 1987). In addition, nicotinic receptors are present within the striatum, most notably on the terminals of dopaminergic terminals that stimulate dopamine release (Rowell et al., 1987). For this reason, the ability of cholinergic agonists and antagonists to manipulate motor symptoms in MPTP-treated primates and to alter components of dyskinesia in levodopa-primed animals was re-evaluated (Banerji et al., 1996). Surprisingly, anticholinergics were highly effective in reversing motor deficits in MPTP-treated animals, contrary to the expectations based on their clinical reputation. Administration of muscarinic antagonists to MPTP-treated, levodopa-primed animals induced some chorea but no dystonia, whereas the administration of muscarinic agonists produced some dystonia but no chorea. In animals that were challenged with levodopa to induce dyskinesia, the coadministration of anticholinergics reduced the dystonic component at the expense of remaining chorea, whereas cholinergic agonists decreased chorea leaving the dystonic elements. In contrast, the administration of nicotine to MPTP-treated animals had no effect on basal motor disability alone; it did not induce dyskinetic symptoms in levodopa-primed animals, and it did not alter the ability of levodopa to induce dyskinesia (Banerji et al., 1996). However, it might be necessary to act on specific nicotinic receptor subtypes located in the basal ganglia for motor effects to be observed. Indeed, the nicotinic agonist SIB-1508Y induces rotational behavior in 6-OHDA-lesioned rats (Cosford et al., 1996). It is also claimed to potentiate the effects of levodopa in MPTP-treated primates and to exert a mild antiparkinsonian effect when given alone (Pope-Coleman et al., 1996), although these actions were not replicated. In addition, SIB-1508Y might improve cognitive function in MPTP-treated animals and improve object retrieval performance (Van-Velson et al., 1997; Schneider et al., 1998).

The ability of manipulation of muscarinic receptors to alter the components of dyskinesia suggests a central role for these neurons in the mediation of involuntary movements. However, the currently used anticholinergic agents are nonselective for the muscarinic receptor subtypes within the basal ganglia (Di Chiara et al., 1994; Kawaguchi et al., 1995; Rodriguez-Puertas et al., 1997). There might be a case for producing more selective agents to determine the effects of occupation of striatal muscarinic receptors on the control of PD and the expression of dyskinesia. Similarly, recent studies suggest that targeting nicotinic receptor subtypes could be a novel approach to the treatment of PD (Quik and Kulak, 2002; Quik et al., 2005; Quik and McIntosh, 2006).

## Opioid Antagonists

Mu, delta, and kappa opioid receptors are present within the output regions of basal ganglia and are well placed to manipulate motor function. Indeed, alterations in enkephalin and dynorphin in the indirect and direct output pathways occur in PD (Morissette et al., 1999; Zeng et al., 2000), and as a result of levodopa treatment (Rodriguez-Puertas et al., 1997), and opioid binding is altered in patients with PD who exhibit dyskinesia (Piccini et al., 1997). In MPTP-treated primates, opioid receptor antagonists reduce levodopa-induced dyskinesia in the order mu = delta > kappa (Henry et al., 2001). However, the clinical evidence for the utility of this approach is mixed with reports of both inhibition and no effect on levodopa-induced dyskinesia in PD (Trabucchi et al., 1982; Sandyk and Snider, 1986; Vermeulen et al., 1995). The situation might be even more complex, as there are both clinical and laboratory data showing a reduction of levodopa-induced dyskinesia by opioid agonists (Vermeulen et al., 1995; Berg et al., 1999).

## α-Adrenergic Antagonists (Box 9-8)

$\alpha\text{-}_{2C}$ receptors are present on the cell bodies of medium spiny output neurons from the striatum and in the GPe, Gpi, and SNr and might be involved in the control of motor function (Unnerstall et al., 1984; Scheinin et al., 1994; Rosin et al., 1996; Kulatunga et al., 1997; Holmberg et al., 1999). They might be the target site of innervation from the locus coeruleus or respond to noradrenaline formed from levodopa/dopamine. Indeed, there is considerable evidence of a functional interaction between dopaminergic and noradrenergic systems in the control of motor behaviors.

The $\alpha_2$ antagonist idazoxan reduces levodopa-induced dyskinesia in MPTP-treated primates (Colpaert et al., 1991; Henry et al., 1999; Grondin et al., 2000). Interestingly, in the same model, idazoxan did not inhibit apomorphine-induced dyskinesia, suggesting mechanistic differences between the ways in which these drugs induce involuntary movements (Fox et al., 2001). Other facets of the pharmacologic actions of idazoxan could also be important; studies in 6-OHDA-lesioned rats suggest a serotonergic component to its motor actions (Srinivasan and Schmidt, 2004). Recently, another $\alpha_2$ antagonist, fipamezole, was reported to show a reduction in levodopa-induced dyskinesia while extending its duration of action in MPTP-treated primates (Savola et al., 2003), although this has been difficult to reproduce.

Box 9-8 $\alpha_2$-Adrenergic antagonists and Parkinson disease

Idazoxan enhances the antiparkinsonian actions of
  levodopa and reduces dyskinesia in MPTP treated
  primates.
Fipamezole also extends levodopa's action and
  decreases dyskinesia in 6-OHDA-lesioned rats
  and MPTP-treated primates.
Idazoxan was active in a phase II clinical trial
  and fipamezole was effective in a phase II
  proof of principle study.

The clinical benefit to be derived from this approach is currently unclear. Idazoxan reduced levodopa-induced dyskinesia in a phase II clinical study in PD (Peyro-Saint-Paul et al., 1996; Rascol, Arnulf, et al., 2001), but no effect was found in a phase III investigation. This could have resulted more from trial design than from drug failure. Indeed, the antidepressant mirtazapine, whose principal action is $\alpha_2$ receptor antagonism, has also been reported to decrease levodopa-induced dyskinesia in PD (Pact and Giduz, 1999). Fipamezole was found to decrease dyskinesia and to extend the duration of effect of levodopa in an early small phase II study in PD, but subsequent clinical investigations have not been undertaken. Consequently, the clinical utility of this drug class remains unresolved.

## Cannabinoid Drugs

A final potential means of manipulating basal ganglia function is through cannabinoid receptors. CB-1 receptors are located on the terminals of striato-GPe neurons in the Gpi, and stimulation of these receptors enhances GABAergic transmission in GPe by inhibiting GABA reuptake (Mailleux et al., 1992; Maneuf et al., 1996). Studies in rodents indicate complex interactions with a range of neurotransmitters in basal ganglia and suggest that dosing issues might affect behavioral outcomes (Gonzalez et al., 2006). There have been case reports of cannabis ingestion improving parkinsonian features, although these were not borne out by controlled evaluation (Carroll et al., 2004). However, the cannabinoid receptor agonist nabilone reduces levodopa-induced dyskinesia in patients with PD (Sieradzan et al., 2001). The role of cannabinoid drugs is currently confused, however, since both cannabinoid antagonists and antagonists have been reported to have antidyskinetic effects in MPTP-treated primates (Brotchie, 2000).

## Summary

Therefore, nondopaminergic approaches could overcome some of the problems associated with the chronic treatment of PD using dopamine replacement therapy, but there has yet to be a major breakthrough in this area, and no such treatment strategy has had effectiveness even close to that of levodopa. Furthermore, it is likely that all these novel approaches will bring their own range of side effects. Another concern is how predictive the MPTP model is of clinical efficacy of nondopaminergic drugs in PD compared to its ability to detect effects of dopaminergic agents. Perhaps too many nondopaminergic drugs appear to be effective (Silverdale et al., 2005; Gomez-Ramirez et al., 2006), and this is not always backed up by clinical experience. One example of this may be the apparent effectiveness of levetiracetam (Bezard et al., 2004; Hill et al., 20004a, 2004b) in suppressing dyskinesia in MPTP-treated primates compared to its sedative effects in patients with PD (Lyons and Pahwa, 2006).

## NEUROPROTECTIVE APPROACHES TO THE TREATMENT OF PARKINSON DISEASE

All current treatments for PD are aimed at control of the motor symptoms of the illness, but these treatments mask the underlying advance of pathology. Currently, no drugs are available that have been definitively shown to slow or stop disease progression. A number of agents that were previously investigated have failed to live up to expectations in clinical trials based on effects in vitro and in vivo experimental models (Fahn and Sulzer, 2004; Olanow and Jankovic, 2005; Anderson et al., 2006; Hirsch, 2006; Jankovic, 2006; Lang, 2006; Poewe, 2006; Waldmeier et al., 2006). These include the type B MAO inhibitor selegiline, vitamin E, riluzole, glial-derived neurotrophic factor (GDNF), immunophilins, GAPDH inhibitors, JNK kinase inhibitors, and perhaps dopamine agonists (but see later). Selegiline was proposed as a potential neuroprotective agent on the basis of extensive preclinical data, but because of its mild symptomatic effect in clinical studies (Parkinson Study Group, 1989), this conclusion remains controversial (Shoulson, 1998; Djaldetti et al., 2002b). Recent reports suggest that there is no overall change in disease progression with selegiline but that there is some gain with respect to delaying the onset of freezing episodes (Shoulson et al., 2002) and the onset of wearing-off (Palhagen et al., 2006). The effective dose of selegiline remains uncertain, since in in vitro experiments, selegiline inhibits the neuroprotective actions of its metabolite, desmethylselegiline, which is considered to be the active moiety (Mytilineou et al., 1997). In addition, the action of selegiline could be compromised by its metabolism to amphetamine derivatives. In laboratory studies, selegiline prevented oxidative stress, excitotoxicity, and apoptosis and exerted neurotrophic activity (Mytilineou and Cohen, 1985; Tatton and Greenwood, 1991; Ansari et al., 1993). These actions would seem highly relevant to pathogenic mechanisms occurring in PD (see Chapter 5). The ability of selegiline to prevent the nuclear translocation of glyceraldehyde 3-phosphate dehydrogenase to the nucleus by binding to the tetrameric form and preventing dimer formation has been highlighted as the mechanism by which selegiline might be effective in a wide range of models of neuronal death. Other MAO inhibitors are currently under clinical development for both symptomatic and neuroprotective use in PD (Jenner, 2004). The selective type B MAO inhibitor rasagiline, which has symptomatic activity in patients with early PD (Parkinson Study Group, 2002a, 2005), has potential neuroprotective actions due to antiapoptotic properties (Goggi et al., 2000; Maruyama et al., 2002). Rasagiline is more potent than selegiline and is not metabolized to amphetamine derivatives. Like selegiline, it inhibits apoptosis and prevents glyceraldehyde 3-phosphate dehydrogenase translocation. An initial clinical study also suggests some disease-modifying activity (Parkinson Study Group, 2004a).

On the basis of the binding of selegiline to the tetrameric form of glyceraldehyde 3-phosphate dehydrogenase, a tricyclic analog TCH346 (CGP 3466B) was described that does not inhibit either type A or type B MAO or produce improvement in experimental models of PD. TCH346 prevents apoptosis and prevents the intracellular accumulation and nuclear translocation of glyceraldehyde 3-phosphate dehydrogenase (Waldmeier et al., 2006). It prevents the toxicity of 6-OHDA and MPP$^+$ to primary fetal ventral mesencephalon cultures and the toxicity of the complex I inhibitor rotenone. It is important to note that TCH346 prevents MPTP toxicity to dopaminergic cells in SNc in mice and monkeys despite not inhibiting MAO activity. However, TCH346 failed to alter disease progression in a phase II clinical study in PD (Olanow et al., 2006). The doses that were employed might not have been appropriate, partially because preclinical studies showed evidence of a bell-shaped dose response curve. Nevertheless, this raises the question about the predictive nature of the experimental models that have been used to assess potential neuroprotective activity (Waldmeier et al., 2006).

Many potential neuroprotective agents are detected through their actions in cell culture using cell lines or primary neuronal cultures. However, the environment is artificial and can be modified to produce a variety of outcomes. Media tend to be low in antioxidants and to contain excessive amounts of iron, thus promoting a pro-oxidant situation. Both in vitro and in vivo, there is heavy reliance on the use of toxin-based models (6-OHDA, MPP+, MPTP, rotenone), which could have mechanisms of action that are unrelated to pathogenic events occurring in PD. For example, MPTP toxicity involves mitochondrial dysfunction, oxidative stress, excitoxicity, and nitric oxide toxicity, leading to apoptotic cell death. Many compounds have been shown to inhibit MPTP toxicity in rodents and primates. These include MAO inhibitors, dopamine reuptake blockers, glutamate antagonists, nitric oxide synthase inhibitors, antioxidants, iron chelators, and a wide variety of other molecules. There are no data to show that any of these approaches has clinical significance to the progression of PD. For example, the sodium channel blocker riluzole, which reduces glutamate release, exhibits neuroprotective effects against both MPTP and 6-OHDA toxicity in rodents and against MPTP toxicity in primates (Boireau et al., 1994a, 1994b; Barneoud et al., 1996; Bezard et al., 1998; Obinu et al., 2002). However, riluzole treatment did not reduce the rate of disease progression in PD.

Other approaches to neuroprotection involve attempts to inhibit specific components of the cell death cascade. Inhibitors of c-jun N-terminal kinase prevent apoptotic cell death. CEP-1347, CEP-11004, and SP600125 protect against 6-OHDA toxicity in neonatal rats and MPTP toxicity in mice (Saporito et al., 1999; Ganguly et al., 2004; Wang et al., 2004). MPTP activates c-jun N-terminal kinase and its upstream regulatory kinase, and this was prevented by CEP-1347 (Saporito et al., 2000). Systemically active caspase inhibitors prevent MPTP toxicity in mice associated with prevention of increases in caspase 8 and 9 in the midbrain (Yang et al., 2004). Whether such approaches to inhibiting neuronal loss at a single point in the sequence of events occurring in PD will work remains to be determined. However, CEP 1347 has failed in a phase II/III evaluation for neuroprotection in PD.

On the basis of the mitochondrial complex I defects that occur in PD, bioenergetic approaches to neuroprotection are being assessed. Coenzyme Q10, creatinine, carnitine, ginkgo biloba, and α-lipoic acid have all been proposed as potentially effective on the basis of preclinical studies. Of these, coenzyme Q10 has been the most intensely investigated both as a cofactor for complex I and as an antioxidant (Beal, 2004). Coenzyme Q10 prevents MPTP toxicity in mice (Beal et al., 1998). In PD, the redox state of coenzyme Q10 is altered in platelets, and its levels correlate with activity of complex I and complex II/III in mitochondria (Shults et al., 1997; Gotz et al., 2000; Sohmiya et al., 2004). Coenzyme Q10 has been examined with patients with PD, but it is unclear whether the results are due to neuroprotective or symptomatic benefit (Shults et al., 1998, 2002, 2004; Muller et al., 2003). Whether neuroprotection occurs with higher doses remains to be evaluated.

Some of the approaches to neuroprotection deserve special mention, as they have bearing on pharmacologic treatments, which could also be of symptomatic benefit in the treatment of PD. In addition, it is worthwhile to examine the role played by glial cells, as opposed to neurons, in disease progression.

## Adenosine Antagonists

There is a large literature on the role that adenosine plays in neurodegeneration. Adenosine A2a antagonists have been shown to be neuroprotective in a range of models of stroke and cerebral ischemia but, more recently, have been examined in experimental models of PD. Caffeine consumption has been associated with a decreased risk of developing PD (Ascherio et al., 2001; Morelli and Wardas, 2001), and caffeine protects against MPTP toxicity in mice through an A2a receptor–mediated mechanism (Chen et al., 2001b). Unlike its locomotor stimulant actions, which show tolerance on repeated administration, there is no tolerance to the neuroprotective actions of caffeine (Xu et al., 2002). The A2a antagonist KW 6002 protected against the nigral cell induced by 6-OHDA in rats and the loss of dopaminergic terminals produced by MPTP treatment of mice (Ikeda et al., 2002). The neurotoxic effects of MPTP in mice were also prevented by the A2a antagonist CSC and by the knockout of A2a receptors (Chen et al., 2001a). The mechanisms responsible for these effects are unknown but might relate to inhibition of glutamate release or to the deactivation of glial cells and a decrease in cytokine release (Obinu et al., 2002). Indeed, the A2a antagonist SCH 58261 in low doses protects against the excitotoxicity of quinolinic acid through a presynaptic mechanism that inhibits glutamate release (Chen et al., 2001a).

## Nicotinic Agonists

One of the few consistent findings in PD has been the decreased risk of developing the illness associated with cigarette smoking (Popoli et al., 2002). Indeed, nicotine and nicotinic agonists protect against a range of toxic insults in a dose-dependent manner that is blocked by nicotinic antagonists such as mecamylamine (Kaneko et al., 1997; Hernan et al., 2001). Administration of nicotine or cigarette smoke inhibits MPTP toxicity in mice, but there is controversy over these findings (Janson et al., 1988; Donnelly-Roberts et al., 1996). Other studies suggest that either there is no protection against MPTP and 6-OHDA toxicity or that nicotine enhances MPTP-induced damage (Carr and Rowell, 1990; Behmand and Harik, 1992; Janson et al., 1992; Hadjiconstantinou et al., 1994; Blum et al., 1996). The dose of nicotine that is employed appears to be critical, since low but not high doses of nicotine protected against 6-OHDA toxicity in rats (Ferger et al., 1998). The higher doses of nicotine led to receptor desensitization and a loss of protective activity. The mechanisms that are responsible for the neuroprotective effects of nicotine remain unclear at this time and require further investigation (Quik, 2004).

One reason for the controversy over effect might be related to the receptor subtype involved, and the nigrostriatal pathway expresses a wide range of nicotinic receptor subunits. Both the α4/β2 and α7 receptor subtypes have been implicated in neuroprotection, while other studies suggest that non-α7 subunits are involved and that knockout of the α4 subunit in mice removes the neuroprotective effect of nicotine against 6-OHDA toxicity. Recently, α6 subunits have been associated with both potential symptomatic and neuroprotective effects of nicotinic agonists in MPTP-treated primates (Quik and Kulak, 2002; Quik et al., 2005, 2006).

## Dopamine Agonists

Currently under investigation is the ability of dopamine agonist drugs to slow early disease progression (Schapira 2002; Schapira et al., 2006a). In a range of in vitro and in vivo experimental models, dopamine agonist drugs exert a range of activities, including the trapping of free radical species and the prevention of toxic insults to cells (Ogawa et al., 1994; Nishibayashi et al., 1996; Gu et al., 2004). This seems to be a universal property of dopamine agonists, but there is currently dispute as to whether it is mediated through dopamine receptors and whether there is D2 or D3 receptor involvement or whether other mechanisms are involved (Le et al., 2000; Joyce et al., 2003; Gu et al., 2004). The latter would seem more likely, since dopamine agonists appear to be active in models of neuronal destruction—for example, spinal motor neuron axotomy, which does not involve dopaminergic neurons or dopaminergic mechanisms (Iwasaki et al., 1996; Sethy et al., 1997). In addition, for compounds with a chiral center, such as pramipexole, neuroprotective activity is found in the enantiomer that is inactive as a dopamine agonist (Gu et al., 2004). Pramipexole and rotigotine have also been shown to be effective in blocking the toxicity of MPTP to nigral dopaminergic cells in primates (Iravani, Haddon, et al., 2006; Scheller et al., 2007). There are now clinical data based on single-photon-emission computed tomography and positron emission tomography analyses that suggest that pramipexole (CALM-PD), ropinirole (REAL-PET), and pergolide (PELMOPET) might slow the progression of PD or that levodopa might hasten it (Parkinson Study Group, 2002b; Whone et al., 2003). However, the interpretation of these studies is unclear, as no placebo group was included, and the possibility exists that levodopa could have a pharmacologic effect on dopa decarboxylase and dopamine transporter to influence these neuroimaging studies. It is also unlikely that levodopa exerts any adverse effects on the basis of the results of the ELLDOPA study (Fahn 2006). At present, it is not possible to differentiate between a positive neuroprotective effect of dopamine agonists and a potential neurotoxic effect of levodopa, but on the basis of imaging, there appears to be a disease-modifying effect because the addition of levodopa to subjects who are already taking pramipexole does not alter the improved imaging from pramipexole alone (Parkinson Study Group, 2002b).

## Glial Cell Activation

Glial cells might also play a role in the pathology of PD, since a reactive microgliosis accompanies nigral cell degeneration. Activated glial cells secrete a range of cytokines, nitric oxide, glutamate, and reactive oxygen species, all of which can be potentially toxic to dopaminergic neurons while at the same decreasing their secretion of trophic factors that are normally essential for the maintenance of neuronal integrity (Hirsch et al., 1998; McNaught and Jenner, 1999). Indeed, the activation of astrocytes with lipopolysaccharide causes them to become toxic when mixed with primary dopaminergic mesencephalic cultures. In addition, the injection or infusion of lipopolysaccharide into the rat substantia nigra leads to the selective destruction of dopaminergic neurons (Castano et al.,

1998; McNaught and Jenner, 2000). This process is associated with glial cell activation and with the induction of inducible nitric-oxide synthase (iNOS) in glial cells (Gao et al., 2002b). The toxicity of lipopolysaccharide to dopaminergic neurons can be at least partially prevented by an iNOS inhibitor, suggesting a key role for nitric oxide or peroxynitrite in the pathogenic process (Iravani et al., 2002). It is important to note that blockade of microglial cell activation by the antibiotic minocycline protects mice against MPTP toxicity, emphasizing the key role played by microglia in dopaminergic cell death (Du et al., 2001; Wu et al., 2002). Further evidence for microglial involvement in nigral cell death is shown by the neuroinflammation that occurs during 6-OHDA-induced toxicity (Cicchetti et al., 2002). This might be highly significant, given the recent finding that treatment with nonsteroidal anti-inflammatory drugs (NSAIDs) protects against the risk of developing PD, although this is disputed (Ton et al., 2006). Interestingly, MPTP toxicity in rodents is prevented by both aspirin and some selective cyclooxygenase inhibitors, again suggesting a role for inflammatory mechanisms, although these effects do not appear to be mediated through prostaglandin mechanisms (Aubin et al., 1998; Teismann and Ferger, 2001).

## Summary

All of the previous discussion reflects only some of the approaches that are being used to develop a neuroprotective therapy for PD (Johnston and Brotchie, 2004). This is a field that will continue to expand and mature over the coming years. However, it is also an area with many presumptions and many unknowns. Some of the potential pitfalls are assumptions (1) that PD is a single disorder and that patient populations are homogeneous, (2) that cell death is initiated at the same point in individual patients, (3) that interfering at a single point in the cell death cascade will be neuroprotective, (4) that preventing cell death in substantia nigra will reflect a neuroprotective effect in other areas of brain that show pathology in PD, and (5) that current models of PD truly reflect the pathogenic processes.

At this time, the primary cause of nigral cell death remains unknown, making the selection of drugs as neuroprotectants an empirical process (Meissner et al., 2004). The failure of animal models to predict clinically effective neuroprotective agents is worrying and echoes the problems that have been encountered in translating to humans the effects found in models of stroke. There is a need to develop new models of PD that reflect relevant pathogenic events such as Lewy body formation and glial cell activation. Clinical endpoints for neuroprotectant studies need to be developed, and it is essential to establish biomarkers of the disease (Michell et al., 2004). There also might be a need to rethink the way in which novel approaches to neurodegenerative disease are developed for use in humans (Lansbury, 2004).

# NEURORESTORATIVE APPROACHES TO THE TREATMENT OF PARKINSON DISEASE

In addition to attempts to stop or slow the progression of PD, there is considerable interest in trying to use neurorestorative techniques to reverse the damage inflicted by the illness. The use of fetal cell transplantation has continued for some time and may produce benefit in some patients, although there is a concern over the induction of disabling dyskinesia (Freed et al., 2001; Olanow et al., 2003). A major drawback to fetal cell transplantation is the availability of the material required, and it is currently hoped that new approaches to xenotransplantation (Duan et al., 2001) or to the development of techniques for promoting the transformation of stem cells into an endless supply of dopaminergic neurons could overcome such problems (Bjorklund, 2005; Pluchino et al., 2005; Snyder and Olanow, 2005; Taylor and Minger, 2005; Dass et al., 2006; Soderstrom et al., 2006). Autologous grafting might provide a means of providing donor tissue. Grafted sympathetic neurons appear to increase dopamine formation in patients with PD (Nakao et al., 2004). Stereotaxic implantation of human retinal pigment epithelial cells attached to gelatin microcarriers (Spheramine) improves motor deficits in 6-OHDA-lesioned rats and MPTP-treated primates and decreases "off" motor symptoms in patients with PD (Watts et al., 2003; Bakay et al., 2004). Cotransplantation of carotid body and ventral mesencephalic cells has been suggested as an approach that improves functional recovery in 6-OHDA lesioned rats (Shukla et al., 2004). Implantation of embryonic stem cells or derived dopamine neurons into the rat striatum leads to the development of normal midbrain dopaminergic neurons and reduces motor abnormalities in 6-OHDA-lesioned rats (Bjorklund et al., 2002; Kim et al., 2002; Park et al., 2003; Baier et al., 2004; Cho et al., 2006; Kim et al., 2006). Cell therapies, including those using stem cells, as a treatment for PD face a long journey full of scientific—not to mention ethical and political—obstacles and challenges. Among the many scientific challenges is the problem of unregulated growth of the implanted stem cells, including tumorigenesis, survivability, immugenicity, supply, and cost. It is difficult to make any predictions at this time as to whether cell transplantation will play an important role in the future treatment of PD, but the reader is referred to some thoughtful reviews on this topic (Roitberg et al., 2004; Smidt and Burbach, 2007).

There also has been considerable interest in the ability of neurotrophic factors, such as brain-derived neurotrophic factor, GDNF, and sonic hedgehog, to repair the damaged nigrostriatal system in PD (Lindsay et al., 1993; Dass et al., 2002; Tsuboi et al., 2002; Hurtado-Lorenzo et al., 2004). Immunophilin-like drugs have also been proposed as being potentially useful in producing trophic actions in PD (Steiner et al., 1997; Costantini et al., 1998, 2001). However, there has been continuing controversy over whether immunophilins produce neurotrophic effects (Harper et al., 1999), and to date, studies of immunophilin in MPTP-treated primates and in PD have been disappointing.

The study of GDNF has been extensive and appeared to be one of the promising approaches to a neurorestorative approach to the treatment of PD. GDNF was effective in preventing or reversing nigral cell degeneration or motor deficits in 6-OHDA-lesioned rats and MPTP-treated primates (Hoffer et al., 1994; Kearns and Gash, 1995; Sauer et al., 1995; Bowenkamp et al., 1996; Gash et al., 1996; Winkler et al., 1996; Miyoshi et al., 1997; Zhang et al., 1997). At least in the intrastriatal 6-OHDA-lesioned rat model, it was necessary to inject GDNF into the striatum to preserve dopamine terminals with no effect of intranigral or intraventricular administration of GDNF (Kirik et al., 2000). Preservation of dopaminergic neurons also occurs when GDNF is infused into the ventricular system following intrastriatal 6-OHDA administration and in aged and MPTP-treated primates (Kirik et al., 2001; Grondin et al., 2002, 2003). Similarly, intraventricular injection of GDNF is effective in MPTP-treated common marmosets that had previously been exposed to levodopa to induce involuntary movements (Costa et al., 2001). GDNF reduced basal motor disability without affecting the antiparkinsonian action of levodopa. However, GDNF diminished the intensity of dyskinesia produced by levodopa while increasing the number of tyrosine hydroxylase-positive cells in the substantia nigra (Iravani et al., 2001). Indeed, it might be that there is linkage between the neuroprotective/neurorestorative effects of levodopa and its ability to reverse dyskinesia, since the intensity of involuntary movements is related to the degree of striatal denervation. GDNF can also improve the functional response to fetal ventral mesencephalon implants in 6-OHDA-lesioned rats (Chaturvedi et al., 2003).

However, a clinical study of GDNF injections into the ventricular system in PD patients showed no effect on motor symptoms and was associated with weight loss and parathesias (Nutt et al., 2003). A subsequent study employing continuous infusions of GDNF directly into the putamen apparently resulted in symptomatic benefit associated with improvements in 18F-dopa PET scans (Gill et al., 2003). Unfortunately, not only did recent double-blind clinical investigation using striatal infusion of GDNF fail but immunologic reactions were uncovered as well (Lang et al., 2006). Coupled to the discovery of cerebellar pathology in a primate toxologic study (Oiwa et al., 2006), although this might not occur in humans (Chebrolu et al., 2006; Slevin et al., 2006), the further development of GDNF protein infusions looks uncertain. However, other approaches might still prove to be useful.

A general problem with the delivery of neurotrophic factors is that these large proteins do not penetrate the blood-brain barrier and must be administered by invasive intracerebral administration. GDNF can be loaded into microspheres and implanted into the striatum, thereby removing the necessity for repeated application (Gouhier et al., 2002). This approach can protect against 6-OHDA toxicity in rats. Similarly, the intrastriatal grafting of aggregates of the Zuckerkandl organ, which express GDNF, induces functional recovery in 6-OHDA-lesioned rats (Espejo et al., 2001). In addition, astrocytes transfected with the gene for GDNF production, using a retroviral vector and transplanted into the striatum of mice, protected against the neurotoxic effects of 6-OHDA (Cunningham and Su, 2002). Indeed, adenoviral, adeno-associated, lentiviral, herpes simplex virus, or equine infectious anemia virus vectors expressing GDNF can prevent or reverse the effects of 6-OHDA lesions in rats and MPTP toxicity in primates (Bilang-Bleuel et al., 1997; Mandel et al., 1999; Kordower et al., 2000; Kozlowski et al., 2000; Palfi et al., 2002; Eslamboli et al., 2003; Azzouz et al., 2004; Monville et al., 2004). Although still invasive, the use of a viral vector delivering GDNF could provide benefit over many years if gene expression is maintained and can overcome some of the problems associated with the use of the protein itself. A highly promising approach appears to be the use of a viral vector to produce GDNF-secreting cells that can then be encapsulated in a plastic polymer and implanted in the brain (Ahn et al., 2005; Sajadi et al., 2006). Using this approach produced improvements in motor function in 6-OHDA-lesioned rats. A reservation with such approaches might be that long-term expression of GDNF can downregulate

TH expression in the substantia nigra (Rosenblad et al., 2003). Also, while preventing 6-OHDA- and MPTP-induced nigral degeneration, lentiviral delivery of GDNF did not protect against A30P mutant α-synuclein-initiated toxicity (Lo et al., 2004) and so might not be as effective in patients with PD as was seen in animal models of the disorder.

An interesting alternative to GDNF is the use of neurturin (CERE-120), which is a member of the same trophic family but does not seem to be associated with the same toxicologic or immunologic problems. CERE-120 delivered to the basal ganglia using an AAV viral vector produces long-term protein production and protects against 6-OHDA-induced nigrostriatal damage in rats and against MPTP toxicity in primates (Horger et al., 1998; Rosenblad et al., 1999; Fjord-Larsen et al., 2005; Kordower et al., 2006a). In a phase I study in patients with PD, viral vector delivery of neurturin appeared safe and apparently resulted in an improvement in motor function. Phase II studies have been initiated, and the results will be important in determining whether this type of approach will be viable in PD, although long-term safety and problems associated with dyskinesia or other motor complications will need to be assessed. Even if successful, all such approaches focusing on the restoration of nigrostriatal function and motor symptoms of PD will not deal with components of the illness that arise from pathology in other brain regions or the problems of nondopamine nonmotor symptoms of PD.

Other approaches that might have both neuroprotective and neurorestorative function include AL-108 (Allon Therapeutics), an intranasally formulated eight-amino-acid peptide that has been shown to protect neurons against numerous toxins and cellular stresses. Another technology that might have therapeutic implications in PD involves the utilization of zinc finger DNA binding proteins (ZFPs). Each finger recognizes a three-base-pair triplet of DNA and can be designed to recognize particular triplet sequences. "Fingers" can then be linked together to recognize larger sequences and can be used as the DNA recognition domain of engineered ZFP transcription factors, which can mimic a natural mode of gene regulation and can be used to activate certain genes, such as the GDNF gene (Sangamo BioSciences, Inc., Richmond, California).

## CONCLUDING REMARKS

The future direction of the treatment of PD is likely to move into neuroprotective areas to prevent the onset and progression of cell death. It is also clear that nondopaminergic approaches to symptomatic treatment are likely to become prevalent in the treatment of the disease by bypassing the damaged motor system and acting on cell surface receptors in other target areas within the basal ganglia. Eventually, it might well become possible to replace damaged neurons in the parkinsonian brain and to reverse the damage occurring to cells by the use of a variety of novel molecular biology-based approaches and gene therapy.

## References

Abeliovich A, Schmitz Y, Farinas I, et al: Mice lacking alpha-synuclein display functional deficits in the nigrostriatal dopamine system. Neuron 2000;25:239–252.

Agid Y, Bonnet AM, Ruberg M, Javoy-Agid F: Pathophysiology of L-dopa-induced abnormal involuntary movements. Psychopharmacology Suppl 1985;2:145–159.

Ahlskog JE, Muenter MD: Frequency of levodopa-related dyskinesias and motor fluctuations as estimated from the cumulative literature. Mov Disord 2001;16:448–458.

Ahn YH, Bensadoun JC, Aebischer P, et al: Increased fiber outgrowth from xeno-transplanted human embryonic dopaminergic neurons with co-implants of polymer-encapsulated genetically modified cells releasing glial cell line-derived neurotrophic factor. Brain Res Bull 2005;66:135–142.

Anderson DW, Bradbury KA, Schneider JS: Neuroprotection in Parkinson models varies with toxin administration protocol. Eur J Neurosci 2006;24:3174–3182.

Ansari KS, Yu PH, Kruck TP, Tatton WG: Rescue of axotomized immature rat facial motoneurons by R(−)-deprenyl: Stereospecificity and independence from monoamine oxidase inhibition. J Neurosci 1993;13:4042–4053.

Arai N, Isaji M, Miyata H, et al: Differential effects of three dopamine receptor agonists in MPTP-treated monkeys. J Neural Transm Park Dis Dement Sect 1995;10:55–62.

Ascherio A, Zhang SM, Hernan MA, et al: Prospective study of caffeine consumption and risk of Parkinson's disease in men and women. Ann Neurol 2001;50:56–63.

Aubin N, Curet O, Deffois A, Carter C: Aspirin and salicylate protect against MPTP-induced dopamine depletion in mice. J Neurochem 1998;71:1635–1642.

Azzouz M, Ralph S, Wong LF, et al: Neuroprotection in a rat Parkinson model by GDNF gene therapy using EIAV vector. Neuroreport 2004;15:985–990.

Backman C, Perlmann T, Wallen A, et al: A selective group of dopaminergic neurons express Nurr1 in the adult mouse brain. Brain Res 1999;851:125–132.

Baier PC, Schindehutte J, Thinyane K, et al: Behavioral changes in unilaterally 6-hydroxy-dopamine lesioned rats after transplantation of differentiated mouse embryonic stem cells without morphological integration. Stem Cells 2004;22:396–404.

Bakay RA, Raiser CD, Stover NP, et al: Implantation of Spheramine in advanced Parkinson's disease (PD). Front Biosci 2004;9:592–602.

Banerji T, Pearce RK, Jackson MJ, Marsden CD: Cholinergic manipulation of L-DOPA-induced dyskinesias in the MPTP-treated common marmoset (Callithrix jacchus). Br J Pharmacol 1996;117:24.

Bara-Jimenez W, Dimitrova T, Sherzai A, et al: Effect of monoamine reuptake inhibitor NS 2330 in advanced Parkinson's disease. Mov Disord 2004;19:1183–1186.

Barneoud P, Mazadier M, Miquet JM, et al: Neuroprotective effects of riluzole on a model of Parkinson's disease in the rat. Neuroscience 1996;74:971–983.

Barone P, Bankiewicz KS, Corsini GU, et al: Dopaminergic mechanisms in hemiparkinsonian monkeys. Neurology 1987;37:1592–1595.

Bartus RT, Emerich D, Snodgrass-Belt P, et al: A pulmonary formulation of L-dopa enhances its effectiveness in a rat model of Parkinson's disease. J Pharmacol Exp Ther 2004;310:828–835.

Beal MF: Mitochondrial dysfunction and oxidative damage in Alzheimer's and Parkinson's diseases and coenzyme Q10 as a potential treatment. J Bioenerg Biomembr 2004;36:381–386.

Beal MF, Matthews RT, Tieleman A, Shults CW: Coenzyme Q10 attenuates the 1-methyl-4-phenyl-1,2,3,tetrahydropyridine (MPTP) induced loss of striatal dopamine and dopaminergic axons in aged mice. Brain Res 1998;783:109–114.

Bedard PJ, Di Paolo T, Falardeau P, Boucher R: Chronic treatment with L-DOPA, but not bromocriptine induces dyskinesia in MPTP-parkinsonian monkeys: Correlation with [3H]spiperone binding. Brain Res 1986;379:294–299.

Bedard PJ, Gomez-Mancilla B, Blanchet P, et al: Dopamine agonists as the first line therapy of parkinsonism in MPTP monkeys. In

Olanow CW (ed): Beyond the Decade of the Brain: Dopamine Agonists in Early Parkinson's Disease. Kent, England, Wells Medical Ltd, 1997, pp 101–113.

Behmand RA, Harik SI: Nicotine enhances 1-methyl-4-phenyl-1,2,3,6-tetrahydropyridine neurotoxicity. J Neurochem 1992;58:776–779.

Berg D, Becker G, Reiners K: Reduction of dyskinesia and induction of akinesia induced by morphine in two parkinsonian patients with severe sciatica. J Neural Transm 1999;106:725–728.

Bergman H, Wichmann T, DeLong MR: Reversal of experimental parkinsonism by lesions of the subthalamic nucleus. Science 1990;249:1436–1438.

Bergman H, Wichmann T, Karmon B, DeLong MR: The primate subthalamic nucleus: II. Neuronal activity in the MPTP model of parkinsonism. J Neurophysiol 1994;72:507–520.

Betarbet R, Sherer TB, MacKenzie G, et al: Chronic systemic pesticide exposure reproduces features of Parkinson's disease. Nat Neurosci 2000;3:1301–1306.

Bezard E, Gerlach I, Moratalla R, et al: 5-HT1A receptor agonist-mediated protection from MPTP toxicity in mouse and macaque models of Parkinson's disease. Neurobiol Dis 2006;23:77–86.

Bezard E, Hill MP, Crossman AR, et al: Levetiracetam improves choreic levodopa-induced dyskinesia in the MPTP-treated macaque. Eur J Pharmacol 2004;485:159–164.

Bezard E, Stutzmann JM, Imbert C, et al: Riluzole delayed appearance of parkinsonian motor abnormalities in a chronic MPTP monkey model. Eur J Pharmacol 1998;356:101–104.

Bibbiani F, Costantini LC, Patel R, Chase TN: Continuous dopaminergic stimulation reduces risk of motor complications in parkinsonian primates. Exp Neurol 2005;192:73–78.

Bibbiani F, Oh JD, Chase TN: Serotonin 5-HT1A agonist improves motor complications in rodent and primate parkinsonian models. Neurology 2001;57:1829–1834.

Bibbiani F, Oh JD, Petzer JP, et al: A2A antagonist prevents dopamine agonist-induced motor complications in animal models of Parkinson's disease. Exp Neurol 2003;184:285–294.

Biglan KM, Schwid S, Eberly S, et al: Rasagiline improves quality of life in patients with early Parkinson's disease. Mov Disord 2006;21:616–623.

Bilang-Bleuel A, Revah F, Colin P, et al: Intrastriatal injection of an adenoviral vector expressing glial-cell-line-derived neurotrophic factor prevents dopaminergic neuron degeneration and behavioral impairment in a rat model of Parkinson disease. Proc Natl Acad Sci U S A 1997;94:8818–8823.

Bjorklund A: Cell therapy for Parkinson's disease: Problems and prospects. Novartis Found Symp 2005;265:174–186.

Bjorklund LM, Sanchez-Pernaute R, Chung S, et al: Embryonic stem cells develop into functional dopaminergic neurons after transplantation in a Parkinson rat model. Proc Natl Acad Sci U S A 2002;99:2344–2349.

Blanchet P, Bedard PJ, Britton DR, Kebabian JW: Differential effect of selective D-1 and D-2 dopamine receptor agonists on levodopa-induced dyskinesia in 1-methyl-4-phenyl-1,2,3,6-tetrahydropyridine-exposed monkeys. J Pharmacol Exp Ther 1993;267:275–279.

Blanchet PJ, Calon F, Martel JC, et al: Continuous administration decreases and pulsatile administration increases behavioral sensitivity to a novel dopamine D2 agonist (U-91356A) in MPTP-exposed monkeys. J Pharmacol Exp Ther 1995;272:854–859.

Blanchet PJ, Grondin R, Bedard PJ: Dyskinesia and wearing-off following dopamine D1 agonist treatment in drug-naive 1-methyl-4-phenyl-1,2,3,6-tetrahydropyridine-lesioned primates. Mov Disord 1996;11:91–94.

Blanchet PJ, Konitsiotis S, Chase TN: Amantadine reduces levodopa-induced dyskinesias in parkinsonian monkeys. Mov Disord 1998;13:798–802.

Blum M, Wu G, Mudo G, et al: Chronic continuous infusion of (−)nicotine reduces basic fibroblast growth factor messenger RNA levels in the ventral midbrain of the intact but not of the 6-hydroxydopamine-lesioned rat. Neuroscience 1996;70:169–177.

Boireau A, Dubedat P, Bordier F, et al: Riluzole and experimental parkinsonism: Antagonism of MPTP-induced decrease in central dopamine levels in mice. Neuroreport 1994a;5:2657–2660.

Boireau A, Miquet JM, Dubedat P, et al: Riluzole and experimental parkinsonism: Partial antagonism of MPP(+)-induced increase in striatal extracellular dopamine in rats in vivo. Neuroreport 1994b; 5:2157–2160.

Bowenkamp KE, David D, Lapchak PL, et al: 6-hydroxydopamine induces the loss of the dopaminergic phenotype in substantia nigra neurons of the rat: A possible mechanism for restoration of the nigrostriatal circuit mediated by glial cell line-derived neurotrophic factor. Exp Brain Res 1996;111:1–7.

Boyce S, Clarke CE, Luquin R, et al: Induction of chorea and dystonia in parkinsonian primates. Mov Disord 1990;5:3–7.

Bradbury AJ, Costall B, Domeney AM, et al: 1-methyl-4-phenylpyridine is neurotoxic to the nigrostriatal dopamine pathway. Nature 1986a;319:56–57.

Bradbury AJ, Costall B, Jenner PG, et al: The effect of 1-methyl-4-phenyl-1,2,3,6-tetrahydropyridine (MPTP) on striatal and limbic catecholamine neurones in white and black mice: Antagonism by monoamine oxidase inhibitors. Neuropharmacology 1986b;25: 897–904.

Braun A, Fabbrini G, Mouradian MM, et al: Selective D-1 dopamine receptor agonist treatment of Parkinson's disease. J Neural Transm 1987;68:41–50.

Braz CA, Borges V, Ferraz HB: Effect of riluzole on dyskinesia and duration of the on state in Parkinson disease patients: A double-blind, placebo-controlled pilot study. Clin Neuropharmacol 2004;27:25–29.

Brooks AI, Chadwick CA, Gelbard HA, et al: Paraquat elicited neurobehavioral syndrome caused by dopaminergic neuron loss. Brain Res 1999;823:1–10.

Brotchie JM: Adjuncts to dopamine replacement: A pragmatic approach to reducing the problem of dyskinesia in Parkinson's disease. Mov Disord 1998;13:871–876.

Brotchie JM: The neural mechanisms underlying levodopa-induced dyskinesia in Parkinson's disease. Ann Neurol 2000;47:S105–S112.

Brotchie JM: Nondopaminergic mechanisms in levodopa-induced dyskinesia. Mov Disord 2005;20:919–931.

Brown T, de Groote C, Brotchie J: Recent advances in the treatment of L-DOPA-induced dyskinesia. IDrugs 2002;5:454–468.

Burke RE, Fahn S, Marsden CD: Torsion dystonia: A double-blind, prospective trial of high-dosage trihexyphenidyl. Neurology 1986; 36:160–164.

Burns RS, Chiueh CC, Markey SP, et al: A primate model of parkinsonism: Selective destruction of dopaminergic neurons in the pars compacta of the substantia nigra by N-methyl-4-phenyl-1,2,3,6-tetrahydropyridine. Proc Natl Acad Sci U S A 1983;80: 4546–4550.

Carlson JH, Bergstrom DA, Walters JR: Stimulation of both D1 and D2 dopamine receptors appears necessary for full expression of postsynaptic effects of dopamine agonists: A neurophysiological study. Brain Res 1987;400:205–218.

Carlsson A, Lindqvist M, Magnusson T: 3,4-Dihydroxyphenylalanine and 5-hydroxytryptophan as reserpine antagonists. Nature 1957;180:1200.

Carr LA, Rowell PP: Attenuation of 1-methyl-4-phenyl-1,2,3,6-tetrahydropyridine-induced neurotoxicity by tobacco smoke. Neuropharmacology 1990;29:311–314.

Carroll CB, Bain PG, Teare L, et al: Cannabis for dyskinesia in Parkinson disease: A randomized double-blind crossover study. Neurology 2004;63:1245–1250.

Castano A, Herrera AJ, Cano J, Machado A: Lipopolysaccharide intranigral injection induces inflammatory reaction and damage in nigrostriatal dopaminergic system. J Neurochem 1998;70: 1584–1592.

Cavalla D, Hadjiconstantinou M, Laird HE, Neff NH: Intra-cerebroventricular administration of 1-methyl-4-phenyl-1,2,3,6-tetrahydropyridine (MPTP) and its metabolite 1-methyl-4-phenylpyridinium ion (MPP+) decrease dopamine and increase acetylcholine in the mouse neostriatum. Neuropharmacology 1985;24:585–586.

Cenci MA, Whishaw IQ, Schallert T: Animal models of neurological deficits: How relevant is the rat? Nat Rev Neurosci 2002;3:574–579.

Chaturvedi RK, Agrawal AK, Seth K, et al: Effect of glial cell line-derived neurotrophic factor (GDNF) co-transplantation with fetal ventral mesencephalic cells (VMC) on functional restoration in 6-hydroxydopamine (6-OHDA) lesioned rat model of Parkinson's disease: Neurobehavioral, neurochemical and immunohistochemical studies. Int J Dev Neurosci 2003;21:391–400.

Chaudhuri KR, Healy DG, Schapira AH: Non-motor symptoms of Parkinson's disease: Diagnosis and management. Lancet Neurol 2006;5:235–245.

Chaudhuri KR, Yates L, Martinez-Martin P: The non-motor symptom complex of Parkinson's disease: A comprehensive assessment is essential. Curr Neurol Neurosci Rep 2005;5:275–283.

Chebrolu H, Slevin JT, Gash DA, et al: MRI volumetric and intensity analysis of the cerebellum in Parkinson's disease patients infused with glial-derived neurotrophic factor (GDNF). Exp Neurol 2006;198:450–456.

Chen JF, Moratalla R, Impagnatiello F, et al: The role of the D(2) dopamine receptor (D(2)R) in A(2A) adenosine receptor (A(2A)R)-mediated behavioral and cellular responses as revealed by A(2A) and D(2) receptor knockout mice. Proc Natl Acad Sci U S A 2001a;98:1970–1975.

Chen JF, Xu K, Petzer JP, et al: Neuroprotection by caffeine and A(2A) adenosine receptor inactivation in a model of Parkinson's disease. J Neurosci 2001b;21:RC143.

Cho YH, Kim DS, Kim PG, et al: Dopamine neurons derived from embryonic stem cells efficiently induce behavioral recovery in a Parkinsonian rat model. Biochem Biophys Res Commun 2006;341:6–12.

Cicchetti F, Brownell AL, Williams K, et al: Neuroinflammation of the nigrostriatal pathway during progressive 6-OHDA dopamine degeneration in rats monitored by immunohistochemistry and PET imaging. Eur J Neurosci 2002;15:991–998.

Clarke CE, Boyce S, Robertson RG, et al: Drug-induced dyskinesia in primates rendered hemiparkinsonian by intracarotid administration of 1-methyl-4-phenyl-1,2,3,6-tetrahydropyridine (MPTP). J Neurol Sci 1989;90:307–314.

Coleman RJ, Temlett JA, Nomoto N, et al: The antiparkinsonian effects of transdermal +PHNO. In Quinn NP, Jenner P (eds): Disorders of Movement, Clinical, Pharmacological and Physiological Aspects. New York, Academic Press, 1989, pp 147–156.

Colpaert FC, Degryse AD, Van Craenenendonck HV: Effects of an alpha 2 antagonist in a 20-year-old Java monkey with MPTP-induced parkinsonian signs. Brain Res Bull 1991;26:627–631.

Corrodi H, Fuxe K, Hamberger B, Ljungdahl A: Studies on central and peripheral noradrenaline neurons using a new dopamine-(beta)-hydroxylase inhibitor. Eur J Pharmacol 1970;12:145–155.

Cosford ND, Bleicher L, Herbaut A, et al: (S)-(−)-5-ethynyl-3-(1-methyl-2-pyrrolidinyl)pyridine maleate (SIB-1508Y): A novel anti-parkinsonian agent with selectivity for neuronal nicotinic acetylcholine receptors. J Med Chem 1996;39:3235–3237.

Costa S, Iravani MM, Pearce RK, Jenner P: Glial cell line-derived neurotrophic factor concentration dependently improves disability and motor activity in MPTP-treated common marmosets. Eur J Pharmacol 2001;412:45–50.

Costall B, Naylor RJ: Actions of dopaminergic agonists on motor function. Adv Neurol 1975;9:285–297.

Costantini LC, Chaturvedi P, Armistead DM, et al: A novel immunophilin ligand: Distinct branching effects on dopaminer-gic neurons in culture and neurotrophic actions after oral administration in an animal model of Parkinson's disease. Neurobiol Dis 1998;5:97–106.

Costantini LC, Cole D, Chaturvedi P, Isacson O: Immunophilin ligands can prevent progressive dopaminergic degeneration in animal models of Parkinson's disease. Eur J Neurosci 2001;13:1085–1092.

Cunningham LA, Su C: Astrocyte delivery of glial cell line-derived neurotrophic factor in a mouse model of Parkinson's disease. Exp Neurol 2002;174:230–242.

d'Alcantara P, Ledent C, Swillens S, Schiffmann SN: Inactivation of adenosine A2A receptor impairs long term potentiation in the accumbens nucleus without altering basal synaptic transmission. Neuroscience 2001;107:455–464.

Dass B, Iravani MM, Jackson MJ, et al: Behavioural and immunohistochemical changes following supranigral administration of sonic hedgehog in 1-methyl-4-phenyl-1,2,3,6-tetrahydropyridine-treated common marmosets. Neuroscience 2002;114:99–109.

Dass B, Olanow CW, Kordower JH: Gene transfer of trophic factors and stem cell grafting as treatments for Parkinson's disease. Neurology 2006;66:S89–S103.

Dauer W, Kholodilov N, Vila M, et al: Resistance of alpha-synuclein null mice to the parkinsonian neurotoxin MPTP. Proc Natl Acad Sci U S A. 2002;99(22):14524–14529.

Davis GC, Williams AC, Markey SP, et al: Chronic Parkinsonism secondary to intravenous injection of meperidine analogues. Psychiatry Res 1979;1:249–254.

Di Chiara G, Morelli M, Consolo S: Modulatory functions of neurotransmitters in the striatum: ACh/dopamine/NMDA interactions. Trends Neurosci 1994;17:228–233.

Di Monte DA, McCormack A, Petzinger G, et al: Relationship among nigrostriatal denervation, parkinsonism, and dyskinesias in the MPTP primate model. Mov Disord 2000;15:459–466.

Djaldetti R, Inzelberg R, Giladi N, et al: Oral solution of levodopa ethylester for treatment of response fluctuations in patients with advanced Parkinson's disease. Mov Disord 2002a;17:297–302.

Djaldetti R, Ziv I, Melamed E: The effect of deprenyl washout in patients with long-standing Parkinson's disease. J Neural Transm 2002b;109:797–803.

Dolphin AC, Jenner P, Marsden CD: The relative importance of dopamine and noradrenaline receptor stimulation for the restoration of motor activity in reserpine or alpha-methyl-p-tyrosine pre-treated mice. Pharmacol Biochem Behav 1976;4:661–670.

Donnelly-Roberts DL, Xue IC, Arneric SP, Sullivan JP: In vitro neuroprotective properties of the novel cholinergic channel activator (ChCA), ABT-418. Brain Res 1996;719:36–44.

Du Y, Ma Z, Lin S, et al: Minocycline prevents nigrostriatal dopaminergic neurodegeneration in the MPTP model of Parkinson's disease. Proc Natl Acad Sci U S A 2001;98:14669–14674.

Duan WM, Westerman M, Flores T, Low WC: Survival of intrastriatal xenografts of ventral mesencephalic dopamine neurons from MHC-deficient mice to adult rats. Exp Neurol 2001;167:108–117.

Durif F, Vidailhet M, Bonnet AM, et al: Levodopa-induced dyskinesias are improved by fluoxetine. Neurology 1995;45:1855–1858.

Eberling JL, Jagust WJ, Taylor S, et al: A novel MPTP primate model of Parkinson's disease: Neurochemical and clinical changes. Brain Res 1998;805:259–262.

Eisler T, Eng N, Plotkin C, Calne DB: Absorption of levodopa after rectal administration. Neurology 1981;31(2):215–217.

Emborg-Knott ME, Domino EF: MPTP-Induced hemiparkinsonism in nonhuman primates 6-8 years after a single unilateral intracarotid dose. Exp Neurol 1998;152:214–220.

Eslamboli A, Cummings RM, Ridley RM, et al: Recombinant adeno-associated viral vector (rAAV) delivery of GDNF provides protection against 6-OHDA lesion in the common marmoset monkey (Callithrix jacchus). Exp Neurol 2003;184:536–548.

Espejo EF, Gonzalez-Albo MC, Moraes JP, et al: Functional regeneration in a rat Parkinson's model after intrastriatal grafts of glial cell line-derived neurotrophic factor and transforming growth factor beta1-expressing extra-adrenal chromaffin cells of the Zuckerkandl's organ. J Neurosci 2001;21:9888–9895.

Facca A, Sanchez-Ramos J: High-dose pergolide monotherapy in the treatment of severe levodopa-induced dyskinesias. Mov Disord 1996;11:327–329.

Fahn S: High dosage anticholinergic therapy in dystonia. Neurology 1983;33:1255–1261.

Fahn S: A new look at levodopa based on the ELLDOPA study. J Neural Transm Suppl 2006;70:419–426.

Fahn S, Parkinson Study Group: Rotigotine transdermal system (SPM-962) is safe and effective as monotherapy in early Parkinson's disease (PD). Parkinsonism Relat Disord 2001;7:S55.

Fahn S, Sulzer D: Neurodegeneration and neuroprotection in Parkinson disease. NeuroRx 2004;1:139–154.

Feany MB, Bender WW: A Drosophila model of Parkinson's disease. Nature 2000;404:394–398.

Ferger B, Spratt C, Earl CD, et al: Effects of nicotine on hydroxyl free radical formation in vitro and on MPTP-induced neurotoxicity in vivo. Naunyn Schmiedebergs Arch Pharmacol 1998;358:351–359.

Fjord-Larsen L, Johansen JL, Kusk P, et al: Efficient in vivo protection of nigral dopaminergic neurons by lentiviral gene transfer of a modified Neurturin construct. Exp Neurol 2005;195:49–60.

Fornai F, Lenzi P, Gesi M, et al: Fine structure and biochemical mechanisms underlying nigrostriatal inclusions and cell death after proteasome inhibition. J Neurosci 2003;23:8955–8966.

Fox SH, Henry B, Hill MP, et al: Neural mechanisms underlying peak-dose dyskinesia induced by levodopa and apomorphine are distinct: Evidence from the effects of the alpha(2) adrenoceptor antagonist idazoxan. Mov Disord 2001;16:642–650.

Fox SH, Lang AE, Brotchie JM: Translation of nondopaminergic treatments for levodopa-induced dyskinesia from MPTP-lesioned nonhuman primates to phase IIa clinical studies: Keys to success and roads to failure. Mov Disord 2006;21:1578–1594.

Frankel JP, Lees AJ, Kempster PA, Stern GM: Subcutaneous apomorphine in the treatment of Parkinson's disease. J Neurol Neurosurg Psychiatry 1990;53:96–101.

Fredduzzi S, Moratalla R, Monopoli A, et al: Persistent behavioral sensitization to chronic L-DOPA requires A2A adenosine receptors. J Neurosci 2002;22:1054–1062.

Freed CR, Greene PE, Breeze RE, et al: Transplantation of embryonic dopamine neurons for severe Parkinson's disease. N Engl J Med 2001;344:710–719.

Ganguly A, Oo TF, Rzhetskaya M, et al: CEP11004, a novel inhibitor of the mixed lineage kinases, suppresses apoptotic death in dopamine neurons of the substantia nigra induced by 6-hydroxydopamine. J Neurochem 2004;88:469–480.

Gao HM, Hong JS, Zhang W, Liu B: Distinct role for microglia in rotenone-induced degeneration of dopaminergic neurons. J Neurosci 2002a;22:782–790.

Gao HM, Jiang J, Wilson B, et al: Microglial activation-mediated delayed and progressive degeneration of rat nigral dopaminergic neurons: Relevance to Parkinson's disease. J Neurochem 2002b; 81:1285–1297.

Gash DM, Zhang Z, Ovadia A, et al: Functional recovery in parkinsonian monkeys treated with GDNF. Nature 1996;380:252–255.

Giasson BI, Duda JE, Quinn SM, et al: Neuronal alpha-synucleinopathy with severe movement disorder in mice expressing A53T human alpha-synuclein. Neuron 2002;34:521–533.

Gill SS, Patel NK, Hotton GR, et al: Direct brain infusion of glial cell line-derived neurotrophic factor in Parkinson disease. Nat Med 2003;9:589–595.

Giovanni A, Sieber BA, Heikkila RE, Sonsalla PK: Correlation between the neostriatal content of the 1-methyl-4-phenylpyridinium species and dopaminergic neurotoxicity following 1-methyl-4-phenyl-1,2,3,6-tetrahydropyridine administration to several strains of mice. J Pharmacol Exp Ther 1991;257:691–697.

Goetz CG, Damier P, Hicking C, et al: Sarizotan as a treatment for dyskinesias in Parkinson's disease: A double-blind placebo-controlled trial. Mov Disord 2007;22(2):179–186.

Goggi J, Theofilopoulos S, Riaz SS, et al: The neuronal survival effects of rasagiline and deprenyl on fetal human and rat ventral mesencephalic neurones in culture. Neuroreport 2000;11:3937–3941.

Gomez-Mancilla B, Bedard PJ: Effect of D1 and D2 agonists and antagonists on dyskinesia produced by L-dopa in 1-methyl-4-phenyl-1,2,3,6-tetrahydropyridine-treated monkeys. J Pharmacol Exp Ther 1991;259:409–413.

Gomez-Mancilla B, Bedard PJ: Effect of nondopaminergic drugs on L-dopa-induced dyskinesias in MPTP-treated monkeys. Clin Neuropharmacol 1993;16:418–427.

Gomez-Ramirez J, Johnston TH, Visanji NP, et al: Histamine H3 receptor agonists reduce L-dopa-induced chorea, but not dystonia, in the MPTP-lesioned nonhuman primate model of Parkinson's disease. Mov Disord 2006;21:839–846.

Gonzalez S, Scorticati C, Garcia-Arencibia M, et al: Effects of rimonabant, a selective cannabinoid CB1 receptor antagonist, in a rat model of Parkinson's disease. Brain Res 2006;1073–1074:209–219.

Gotz ME, Gerstner A, Harth R, et al: Altered redox state of platelet coenzyme Q10 in Parkinson's disease. J Neural Transm 2000;107: 41–48.

Gouhier C, Chalon S, Aubert-Pouessel A, et al: Protection of dopaminergic nigrostriatal afferents by GDNF delivered by microspheres in a rodent model of Parkinson's disease. Synapse 2002;44:124–131.

Graham DG, Tiffany SM, Bell WR Jr., Gutknecht WF: Autoxidation versus covalent binding of quinones as the mechanism of toxicity of dopamine, 6-hydroxydopamine, and related compounds toward C1300 neuroblastoma cells in vitro. Mol Pharmacol 1978; 14:644–653.

Greenamyre JT: Glutamatergic influences on the basal ganglia. Clin Neuropharmacol 2001;24:65–70.

Greenamyre JT, Eller RV, Zhang Z, et al: Antiparkinsonian effects of remacemide hydrochloride, a glutamate antagonist, in rodent and primate models of Parkinson's disease. Ann Neurol 1994;35: 655–661.

Grondin R, Cass WA, Zhang Z, et al: Glial cell line-derived neurotrophic factor increases stimulus-evoked dopamine release and motor speed in aged rhesus monkeys. J Neurosci 2003;23:1974–1980.

Grondin R, Goulet M, Di Paolo T, Bedard PJ: Cabergoline, a long-acting dopamine D2-like receptor agonist, produces a sustained antiparkinsonian effect with transient dyskinesias in parkinsonian drug-naive primates. Brain Res 1996;735:298–306.

Grondin R, Hadj TA, Doan VD, et al: Noradrenoceptor antagonism with idazoxan improves L-dopa-induced dyskinesias in MPTP monkeys. Naunyn Schmiedebergs Arch Pharmacol 2000;361: 181–186.

Grondin R, Zhang Z, Yi A, et al: Chronic, controlled GDNF infusion promotes structural and functional recovery in advanced parkinsonian monkeys. Brain 2002;125:2191–2201.

Gu M, Iravani MM, Cooper JM, et al: Pramipexole protects against apoptotic cell death by non-dopaminergic mechanisms. J Neurochem 2004;91:1075–1081.

Guldenpfennig WM, Poole KH, Sommerville KW, Boroojerdi B: Safety, tolerability, and efficacy of continuous transdermal dopaminergic stimulation with rotigotine patch in early-stage idiopathic Parkinson disease. Clin Neuropharmacol 2005;28: 106–110.

Hadj Tahar A, Gregoire L, Bangassoro E, Bedard PJ: Sustained cabergoline treatment reverses levodopa-induced dyskinesias in parkinsonian monkeys. Clin Neuropharmacol 2000;23:195–202.

Hadjiconstantinou M, Hubble JP, Wemlinger TA, Neff NH: Enhanced MPTP neurotoxicity after treatment with isoflurophate or cholinergic agonists. J Pharmacol Exp Ther 1994;270:639–644.

Haggendal J, Lindqvist M: Brain monoamine levels and behaviour during long-term administration of reserpine. Int J Neuropharmacol 1964;3:59–64.

Hansard MJ, Smith LA, Jackson MJ, et al: The antiparkinsonian ability of Bupropion in MPTP-treated common marmosets. Brit J Pharmacol 1998;125:373–380.

Harper S, Bilsland J, Young L, et al: Analysis of the neurotrophic effects of GPI-1046 on neuron survival and regeneration in culture and in vivo. Neuroscience 1999;88:257–267.

Hauber W, Neuscheler P, Nagel J, Muller CE: Catalepsy induced by a blockade of dopamine D1 or D2 receptors was reversed by a concomitant blockade of adenosine A(2A) receptors in the caudate-putamen of rats. Eur J Neurosci 2001;14:1287–1293.

Hauser RA, Hubble JP, Truong DD: Randomized trial of the adenosine A(2A) receptor antagonist istradefylline in advanced PD. Neurology 2003;61:297–303.

Hauser RA, Schwarzschild MA: Adenosine A2A receptor antagonists for Parkinson's disease: Rationale, therapeutic potential and clinical experience. Drugs Aging 2005;22:471–482.

Heikkila RE: Differential neurotoxicity of 1-methyl-4-phenyl-1,2,3,6-tetrahydropyridine (MPTP) in Swiss-Webster mice from different sources. Eur J Pharmacol 1985;117:131–133.

Heikkila RE, Nicklas WJ, Duvoisin RC: Dopaminergic toxicity after the stereotaxic administration of the 1-methyl-4-phenylpyridinium ion (MPP+) to rats. Neurosci Lett 1985;59:135–140.

Henry B, Fox SH, Crossman AR, Brotchie JM: Mu- and delta-opioid receptor antagonists reduce levodopa-induced dyskinesia in the MPTP-lesioned primate model of Parkinson's disease. Exp Neurol 2001;171:139–146.

Henry B, Fox SH, Peggs D, et al: The alpha2-adrenergic receptor antagonist idazoxan reduces dyskinesia and enhances antiparkinsonian actions of L-dopa in the MPTP-lesioned primate model of Parkinson's disease. Mov Disord 1999;14:744–753.

Hernan MA, Zhang SM, Rueda-deCastro AM, et al: Cigarette smoking and the incidence of Parkinson's disease in two prospective studies. Ann Neurol 2001;50:780–786.

Hill MP, Brotchie JM, Crossman AR, et al: Levetiracetam interferes with the L-dopa priming process in MPTP-lesioned drug-naive marmosets. Clin Neuropharmacol 2004a;27:171–177.

Hill MP, Ravenscroft P, Bezard E, et al: Levetiracetam potentiates the antidyskinetic action of amantadine in the 1-methyl-4-phenyl-1,2,3,6-tetrahydropyridine (MPTP)-lesioned primate model of Parkinson's disease. J Pharmacol Exp Ther 2004b;310:386–394.

Hirsch EC: How to judge animal models of Parkinson's disease in terms of neuroprotection. J Neural Transm Suppl 2006;(70):255–260.

Hirsch EC, Hunot S, Damier P, Faucheux B: Glial cells and inflammation in Parkinson's disease: A role in neurodegeneration? Ann Neurol 1998;44:S115–S120.

Hoffer BJ, Hoffman A, Bowenkamp K, et al: Glial cell line-derived neurotrophic factor reverses toxin-induced injury to midbrain dopaminergic neurons in vivo. Neurosci Lett 1994;182:107–111.

Hofmann C, Penner U, Dorow R, et al: Lisuride, a dopamine receptor agonist with 5-HT2B receptor antagonist properties: Absence of cardiac valvulopathy adverse drug reaction reports supports the concept of a crucial role for 5-HT2B receptor agonism in cardiac valvular fibrosis. Clin Neuropharmacol 2006;29:80–86.

Hoglinger GU, Feger J, Prigent A, et al: Chronic systemic complex I inhibition induces a hypokinetic multisystem degeneration in rats. J Neurochem 2003;84:491–502.

Holmberg M, Scheinin M, Kurose H, Miettinen R: Adrenergic alpha2C-receptors reside in rat striatal GABAergic projection neurons: Comparison of radioligand binding and immunohistochemistry. Neuroscience 1999;93:1323–1333.

Horger BA, Nishimura MC, Armanini MP, et al: Neurturin exerts potent actions on survival and function of midbrain dopaminergic neurons. J Neurosci 1998;18:4929–4937.

Hu XT, White FJ: Loss of D1/D2 dopamine receptor synergisms following repeated administration of D1 or D2 receptor selective antagonists: Electrophysiological and behavioral studies. Synapse 1994;17:43–61.

Hurtado-Lorenzo A, Millan E, Gonzalez-Nicolini V, et al: Differentiation and transcription factor gene therapy in experimental parkinson's disease: Sonic hedgehog and Gli-1, but not Nurr-1, protect nigrostriatal cell bodies from 6-OHDA-induced neurodegeneration. Mol Ther 2004;10:507–524.

Hutton JT, Metman LV, Chase TN, et al: Transdermal dopaminergic D(2) receptor agonist therapy in Parkinson's disease with N-0923 TDS: A double-blind, placebo-controlled study. Mov Disord 2001; 16:459–463.

Hwang DY, Fleming SM, Ardayfio P, et al: 3,4-dihydroxyphenylalanine reverses the motor deficits in Pitx3-deficient aphakia mice: Behavioral characterization of a novel genetic model of Parkinson's disease. J Neurosci 2005;25:2132–2137.

Iancu R, Mohapel P, Brundin P, Paul G: Behavioral characterization of a unilateral 6-OHDA-lesion model of Parkinson's disease in mice. Behav Brain Res 2005;162:1–10.

Ikeda K, Kurokawa M, Aoyama S, Kuwana Y: Neuroprotection by adenosine A2A receptor blockade in experimental models of Parkinson's disease. J Neurochem 2002;80:262–270.

Iravani MM, Costa S, Jackson MJ, et al: GDNF reverses priming for dyskinesia in MPTP-treated, L-DOPA-primed common marmosets. Eur J Neurosci 2001;13:597–608.

Iravani MM, Haddon CO, Cooper JM, et al: Pramipexole protects against MPTP toxicity in non-human primates. J Neurochem 2006;96:1315–1321.

Iravani MM, Kashefi K, Mander P, et al: Involvement of inducible nitric oxide synthase in inflammation-induced dopaminergic neurodegeneration. Neuroscience 2002;110:49–58.

Iravani MM, Tayarani-Binazir K, Chu WB, et al: In 1-methyl-4-phenyl-1,2,3,6-tetrahydropyridine-treated primates, the selective 5-hydroxytryptamine 1a agonist (R)-(+)-8-OHDPAT inhibits levodopa-induced dyskinesia but only with increased motor disability. J Pharmacol Exp Ther 2006;319:1225–1234.

Iwasaki Y, Ikeda K, Shiojima T, et al: Deprenyl and pergolide rescue spinal motor neurons from axotomy-induced neuronal death in the neonatal rat. Neurol Res 1996;18:168–170.

Jackson MJ, Al-Barghouthy G, Pearce RK, et al: Effect of 5-HT1B/D receptor agonist and antagonist administration on motor function in haloperidol and MPTP-treated common marmosets. Pharmacol Biochem Behav 2004;79:391–400.

Jackson MJ, Smith LA, Al-Barghouthy G, et al: Decreased expression of l-dopa-induced dyskinesia by switching to ropinirole in MPTP-treated common marmosets. Exp Neurol 2007;204:162–170.

Jankovic J: Therapeutic strategies in parkinson's disease. Parkinson's Dis Mov Disord 1998;10:191–220.

Jankovic J: Motor fluctuations and dyskinesias in Parkinson's disease: Clinical manifestations. Mov Disord 2005a;20(suppl 11):S11–S16.

Jankovic J: Progression of Parkinson disease: Are we making progress in charting the course? Arch Neurol 2005b;62:351–352.

Jankovic J: An update on the treatment of Parkinson's disease. Mt Sinai J Med 2006;73:682–689.

Jankovic J, Chen S, Le W-D: The role of Nurr1 in the development of dopaminergic neurons and Parkinson's disease. Prog Neurobiol 2005;77:128–138.

Jankovic J, Hunter C: A double-blind, placebo-controlled and longitudinal study of riluzole in early Parkinson's disease. Parkinsonism Relat Disord 2002;8:271–276.

Janson AM, Fuxe K, Goldstein M: Differential effects of acute and chronic nicotine treatment on MPTP-(1-methyl-4-phenyl-

1,2,3,6-tetrahydropyridine) induced degeneration of nigrostriatal dopamine neurons in the black mouse. Clin Investig 1992;70: 232–238.

Janson AM, Fuxe K, Sundstrom E, et al: Chronic nicotine treatment partly protects against the 1-methyl-4-phenyl-2,3,6-tetrahydropyridine-induced degeneration of nigrostriatal dopamine neurons in the black mouse. Acta Physiol Scand 1988;132:589–591.

Jenner P: Factors influencing the onset and persistence of dyskinesia in MPTP-treated primates. Ann Neurol 2000a;47:S90–S99.

Jenner P: Pathophysiology and biochemistry of dyskinesia: Clues for the development of non-dopaminergic treatments. J Neurol 2000b;247(suppl 2):1143–1150.

Jenner P: Preclinical evidence for neuroprotection with monoamine oxidase-B inhibitors in Parkinson's disease. Neurology 2004;63: S13–S22.

Jenner P: Istradefylline, a novel adenosine A2A receptor antagonist, for the treatment of Parkinson's disease. Expert Opin Investig Drugs 2005;14:729–738.

Jenner P, Marsden CD: MPTP-Induced parkinsonism: A model of parkinson's disease and its relevance to the disease process. Parkinson's Dis Mov Disord 1993;4:55–75.

Jenner P, Rupniak NM, Rose S, et al: 1-Methyl-4-phenyl-1,2,3,6-tetrahydropyridine-induced parkinsonism in the common marmoset. Neurosci Lett 1984;50:85–90.

Johnston LC, Smith LA, Rose S, Jenner P: The novel dopamine D2 receptor partial agonist, SLV-308, reverses motor disability in MPTP-lesioned common marmosets (Callithrix jacchus). Br J Pharmacol 2000;133, 134P.

Johnston TH, Brotchie JM: Drugs in development for Parkinson's disease. Curr Opin Investig Drugs 2004;5:720–726.

Johnston TH, Brotchie JM: Drugs in development for Parkinson's disease: An update. Curr Opin Investig Drugs 2006;7:25–32.

Johnston TH, Fox SH, Brotchie JM: Advances in the delivery of treatments for Parkinson's disease. Expert Opin Drug Deli 2005; 2:1059–1073.

Joyce JN, Presgraves S, Renish L, et al: Neuroprotective effects of the novel D3/D2 receptor agonist and antiparkinson agent, S32504, in vitro against 1-methyl-4-phenylpyridinium (MPP+) and in vivo against 1-methyl-4-phenyl-1,2,3,6-tetrahydropyridine (MPTP): A comparison to ropinirole. Exp Neurol 2003;184: 393–407.

Kanda T, Jackson MJ, Smith LA, et al: Adenosine A2A antagonist: A novel antiparkinsonian agent that does not provoke dyskinesia in parkinsonian monkeys. Ann Neurol 1998;43:507–513.

Kanda T, Jackson MJ, Smith LA, et al: Combined use of the adenosine A(2A) antagonist KW-6002 with L-DOPA or with selective D1 or D2 dopamine agonists increases antiparkinsonian activity but not dyskinesia in MPTP-treated monkeys. Exp Neurol 2000;162: 321–327.

Kaneko S, Maeda T, Kume T, et al: Nicotine protects cultured cortical neurons against glutamate-induced cytotoxicity via alpha7-neuronal receptors and neuronal CNS receptors. Brain Res 1997; 765:135–140.

Kannari K, Kurahashi K, Tomiyama M, et al: Tandospirone citrate, a selective 5-HT1A agonist, alleviates L-DOPA-induced dyskinesia in patients with Parkinson's disease [in Japanese]. No To Shinkei 2002;54:133–137.

Kawaguchi Y, Wilson CJ, Augood SJ, Emson PC: Striatal interneurones: Chemical, physiological and morphological characterization. Trends Neurosci 1995;18:527–535.

Kearns CM, Gash DM: GDNF protects nigral dopamine neurons against 6-hydroxydopamine in vivo. Brain Res 1995;672:104–111.

Kelsey JE, Mague SD, Pijanowski RS, et al: NMDA receptor antagonists ameliorate the stepping deficits produced by unilateral medial forebrain bundle injections of 6-OHDA in rats. Psychopharmacology (Berl) 2004;175:179–188.

Kim JH, Auerbach JM, Rodriguez-Gomez JA, et al: Dopamine neurons derived from embryonic stem cells function in an animal model of Parkinson's disease. Nature 2002;418:50–56.

Kim RH, Smith PD, Aleyasin H, et al: Hypersensitivity of DJ-1-deficient mice to 1-methyl-4-phenyl-1,2,3,6-tetrahydropyrindine (MPTP) and oxidative stress. Proc Natl Acad Sci U S A 2005;102: 5215–5220.

Kim SU, Park IH, Kim TH, et al: Brain transplantation of human neural stem cells transduced with tyrosine hydroxylase and GTP cyclohydrolase 1 provides functional improvement in animal models of Parkinson disease. Neuropathology 2006;26:129–140.

Kirik D, Annett LE, Burger C, et al: Nigrostriatal alpha-synucleinopathy induced by viral vector-mediated overexpression of human alpha-synuclein: A new primate model of Parkinson's disease. Proc Natl Acad Sci U S A 2003;100:2884–2889.

Kirik D, Georgievska B, Rosenblad C, Bjorklund A: Delayed infusion of GDNF promotes recovery of motor function in the partial lesion model of Parkinson's disease. Eur J Neurosci 2001;13:1589–1599.

Kirik D, Rosenblad C, Bjorklund A: Preservation of a functional nigrostriatal dopamine pathway by GDNF in the intrastriatal 6-OHDA lesion model depends on the site of administration of the trophic factor. Eur J Neurosci 2000;12:3871–3882.

Klockgether T, Turski L: NMDA antagonists potentiate antiparkinsonian actions of L-dopa in monoamine-depleted rats. Ann Neurol 1990;28:539–546.

Klockgether T, Turski L, Honore T, et al: The AMPA receptor antagonist NBQX has antiparkinsonian effects in monoamine-depleted rats and MPTP-treated monkeys. Ann Neurol 1991;30: 717–723.

Kock N, Allchorne AJ, Sena-Esteves M, et al: RNAi blocks DYT1 mutant torsinA inclusions in neurons. Neurosci Lett 2006;395: 201–205.

Kordower JH, Emborg ME, Bloch J, et al: Neurodegeneration prevented by lentiviral vector delivery of GDNF in primate models of Parkinson's disease. Science 2000;290:767–773.

Kordower JH, Herzog CD, Dass B, et al: Delivery of neurturin by AAV2 (CERE-120)-mediated gene transfer provides structural and functional neuroprotection and neurorestoration in MPTP-treated monkeys. Ann Neurol 2006a;60:706–715.

Kordower JH, Kanaan NM, Chu Y, et al: Failure of proteasome inhibitor administration to provide a model of Parkinson's disease in rats and monkeys. Ann Neurol 2006b;60:264–268.

Kozlowski DA, Connor B, Tillerson JL, et al: Delivery of a GDNF gene into the substantia nigra after a progressive 6-OHDA lesion maintains functional nigrostriatal connections. Exp Neurol 2000;166: 1–15.

Kruger R, Kuhn W, Muller T, et al: Ala30Pro mutation in the gene encoding alpha-synuclein in Parkinson's disease. Nat Genet 1998; 18:106–108.

Kulatunga M, Scheinin M, Kotti T, et al: Coexistence of $a_{2c}$-adrenoceptor immunoreactivity with GABA, calbindin D28K and parvalbumin immunoreactivity in rat striatal neurons. Soc Neuroscience 1997;23:586.

Kuoppamaki M, Al Barghouthy G, Jackson M, et al: Beginning-of-dose and rebound worsening in MPTP-treated common marmosets treated with levodopa. Mov Disord 2002;17:1312–1317.

Lang AE: Neuroprotection in Parkinson's disease: And now for something completely different? Lancet Neurol 2006;5:990–991.

Lang AE, Gill S, Patel NK, et al: Randomized controlled trial of intraputamenal glial cell line-derived neurotrophic factor infusion in Parkinson disease. Ann Neurol 2006;59:459–466.

Langston JW, Ballard P, Tetrud JW, Irwin I: Chronic Parkinsonism in humans due to a product of meperidine-analog synthesis. Science 1983;219:979–980.

Langston JW, Forno LS, Rebert CS, Irwin I: Selective nigral toxicity after systemic administration of 1-methyl-4-phenyl-1,2,5,6-tetrahydropyrine (MPTP) in the squirrel monkey. Brain Res 1984a; 292:390–394.

Langston JW, Irwin I, Langston EB, Forno LS: 1-Methyl-4-phenylpyridinium ion (MPP+): Identification of a metabolite of MPTP, a toxin selective to the substantia nigra. Neurosci Lett 1984b;48:87–92.

Lansbury PT Jr: Back to the future: The "old-fashioned" way to new medications for neurodegeneration. Nat Med 2004;10(suppl): S51–S57.

Le W, Conneely OM, He Y, et al: Reduced Nurr1 expression increases the vulnerability of mesencephalic dopamine neurons to MPTP-induced injury. J Neurochem 1999a;73:2218–2221.

Le W, Conneely OM, Zou L, et al: Selective agenesis of mesencephalic dopaminergic neurons in Nurr1-deficient mice. Exp Neurol 1999b; 159:451–458.

Le WD, Jankovic J, Xie W, Appel SH: Antioxidant property of pramipexole independent of dopamine receptor activation in neuroprotection. J Neural Transm 2000;107:1165–1173.

Lindsay RM, Altar CA, Cedarbaum JM, et al: The therapeutic potential of neurotrophic factors in the treatment of Parkinson's disease. Exp Neurol 1993;124:103–118.

Ling Z, Chang QA, Tong CW, et al: Rotenone potentiates dopamine neuron loss in animals exposed to lipopolysaccharide prenatally. Exp Neurol 2004;190:373–383.

Liou HH, Chen RC, Chen TH, et al: Attenuation of paraquat-induced dopaminergic toxicity on the substantia nigra by (−)-deprenyl in vivo. Toxicol Appl Pharmacol 2001;172:37–43.

Liou HH, Chen RC, Tsai YF, et al: Effects of paraquat on the substantia nigra of the wistar rats: Neurochemical, histological, and behavioral studies. Toxicol Appl Pharmacol 1996;137:34–41.

Lo BC, Deglon N, Pralong W, Aebischer P: Lentiviral nigral delivery of GDNF does not prevent neurodegeneration in a genetic rat model of Parkinson's disease. Neurobiol Dis 2004;17:283–289.

Loschmann PA, Chong PN, Nomoto M, et al: Stereoselective reversal of MPTP-induced parkinsonism in the marmoset after dermal application of N-0437. Eur J Pharmacol 1989;166:373–380.

Lotharius J, O'Malley KL: The parkinsonism-inducing drug 1-methyl-4-phenylpyridinium triggers intracellular dopamine oxidation: A novel mechanism of toxicity. J Biol Chem 2000;275:38581–38588.

Lyons KE, Pahwa R: Efficacy and tolerability of levetiracetam in Parkinson disease patients with levodopa-induced dyskinesia. Clin Neuropharmacol 2006;29:48–153.

Mailleux P, Parmentier M, Vanderhaeghen JJ: Distribution of cannabinoid receptor messenger RNA in the human brain: An in situ hybridization histochemistry with oligonucleotides. Neurosci Lett 1992;143:200–204.

Maingay M, Romero-Ramos M, Kirik D: Viral vector mediated overexpression of human alpha-synuclein in the nigrostriatal dopaminergic neurons: A new model for Parkinson's disease. CNS Spectr 2005;10:235–244.

Mandel RJ, Snyder RO, Leff SE: Recombinant adeno-associated viral vector-mediated glial cell line-derived neurotrophic factor gene transfer protects nigral dopamine neurons after onset of progressive degeneration in a rat model of Parkinson's disease. Exp Neurol 1999;160:205–214.

Maneuf YP, Nash JE, Crossman AR, Brotchie JM: Activation of the cannabinoid receptor by delta 9-tetrahydrocannabinol reduces gamma-aminobutyric acid uptake in the globus pallidus. Eur J Pharmacol 1996;308:161–164.

Manning-Bog AB, McCormack AL, Li J, et al: The herbicide paraquat causes up-regulation and aggregation of alpha-synuclein in mice: Paraquat and alpha-synuclein. J Biol Chem 2002;277:1641–1644.

Manning-Bog AB, McCormack AL, Purisai MG, et al: Alpha-synuclein overexpression protects against paraquat-induced neurodegeneration. J Neurosci 2003;23:3095–3099.

Manning-Bog AB, Reaney SH, Chou VP, et al: Lack of nigrostriatal pathology in a rat model of proteasome inhibition. Ann Neurol 2006;60:256–260.

Manson AJ, Hanagasi H, Turner K, et al: Intravenous apomorphine therapy in Parkinson's disease: Clinical and pharmacokinetic observations. Brain 2001;124:331–340.

Maratos EC, Jackson MJ, Pearce RK, et al: Both short- and long-acting D-1/D-2 dopamine agonists induce less dyskinesia than L-DOPA in the MPTP-lesioned common marmoset (Callithrix jacchus). Exp Neurol 2003;179:90–102.

Maratos EC, Jackson MJ, Pearce RK, Jenner P: Antiparkinsonian activity and dyskinesia risk of ropinirole and L-DOPA combination therapy in drug naive MPTP-lesioned common marmosets (Callithrix jacchus). Mov Disord 2001;16:631–641.

Marsden CD, Duvoisin RC, Jenner P, et al: Relationship between animal models and clinical parkinsonism. Adv Neurol 1975;9:165–175.

Maruyama W, Takahashi T, Youdim M, Naoi M: The anti-Parkinson drug, rasagiline, prevents apoptotic DNA damage induced by peroxynitrite in human dopaminergic neuroblastoma SH-SY5Y cells. J Neural Transm 2002;109:467–481.

Masliah E, Rockenstein E, Veinbergs I, et al: Dopaminergic loss and inclusion body formation in alpha-synuclein mice: Implications for neurodegenerative disorders. Science 2000;287:1265–1269.

Mayer RA, Walters AS, Heikkila RE: 1-Methyl-4-phenyl-1,2,3,6-tetrahydropyridine (MPTP) administration to C57-black mice leads to parallel decrements in neostriatal dopamine content and tyrosine hydroxylase activity. Eur J Pharmacol 1986;120:375–377.

McCall RB, Lookingland KJ, Bedard PJ, Huff RM: Sumanirole, a highly dopamine D2-selective receptor agonist: In vitro and in vivo pharmacological characterization and efficacy in animal models of Parkinson's disease. J Pharmacol Exp Ther 2005;314:1248–1256.

McNaught KS, Belizaire R, Isacson O, et al: Altered proteasomal function in sporadic Parkinson's disease. Exp Neurol 2003;179:38–46.

McNaught KS, Bjorklund LM, Belizaire R, et al: Proteasome inhibition causes nigral degeneration with inclusion bodies in rats. Neuroreport 2002;13:1437–1441.

McNaught KS, Jenner P: Altered glial function causes neuronal death and increases neuronal susceptibility to 1-methyl-4-phenylpyridinium- and 6-hydroxydopamine-induced toxicity in astrocytic/ventral mesencephalic co-cultures. J Neurochem 1999;73:2469-2476.

McNaught KS, Jenner P: Dysfunction of rat forebrain astrocytes in culture alters cytokine and neurotrophic factor release. Neurosci Lett 2000;285:61–65.

McNaught KS, Olanow CW: Proteolytic stress: A unifying concept for the etiopathogenesis of Parkinson's disease. Ann Neurol 2003; 53(suppl 3):S73–S84.

McNaught KS, Perl DP, Brownell AL, Olanow CW: Systemic exposure to proteasome inhibitors causes a progressive model of Parkinson's disease. Ann Neurol 2004;56:149–162.

Meissner W, Hill MP, Tison F, et al: Neuroprotective strategies for Parkinson's disease: Conceptual limits of animal models and clinical trials. Trends Pharmacol Sci 2004;25:249–253.

Meshul CK, Emre N, Nakamura CM, et al: Time-dependent changes in striatal glutamate synapses following a 6-hydroxydopamine lesion. Neuroscience 1999;88:1–16.

Metman LV, Konitsiotis S, Chase TN: Pathophysiology of motor response complications in Parkinson's disease: Hypotheses on the why, where, and what. Mov Disord 2000;15:3–8.

Metz GA., Tse A, Ballermann M, et al: The unilateral 6-OHDA rat model of Parkinson's disease revisited: an electromyographic and behavioural analysis. Eur J Neurosci 2005;22:735–744.

Michell AW, Lewis SJ, Foltynie T, Barker RA: Biomarkers and Parkinson's disease. Brain 2004;127:1693–1705.

Millan MJ, Di Cara B, Hill M, et al: S32504, a novel naphtoxazine agonist at dopamine D3/D2 receptors: II. Actions in rodent, primate, and cellular models of antiparkinsonian activity in comparison to ropinirole. J Pharmacol Exp Ther 2004;309:921–935.

Miyoshi Y, Zhang Z, Ovadia A, et al: Glial cell line-derived neurotrophic factor-levodopa interactions and reduction of side effects in parkinsonian monkeys. Ann Neurol 1997;42:208–214.

Mollace V, Iannone M, Muscoli C, et al: The role of oxidative stress in paraquat-induced neurotoxicity in rats: Protection by non peptidyl superoxide dismutase mimetic. Neurosci Lett 2003;335:163–166.

Monville C, Torres EM, Dunnett SB: Validation of the l-dopa-induced dyskinesia in the 6-OHDA model and evaluation of the effects of selective dopamine receptor agonists and antagonists. Brain Res Bull 2005;68:16–23.

Monville C, Torres E, Thomas E, et al: HSV vector-delivery of GDNF in a rat model of PD: Partial efficacy obscured by vector toxicity. Brain Res 2004;1024:1–15.

Morelli M, Wardas J: Adenosine A(2a) receptor antagonists: Potential therapeutic and neuroprotective effects in Parkinson's disease. Neurotox Res 2001;3:545–556.

Mori A, Shindou T: Physiology of adenosine receptors in the striatum regulation of striatal projection neurons. In Kase H, Richardson PJ, Jenner P (eds): Adenosine Receptors and Parkinson's Disease. New York, Academic Press, 2000, pp 107–128.

Morissette M, Grondin R, Goulet M, et al: Differential regulation of striatal preproenkephalin and preprotachykinin mRNA levels in MPTP-lesioned monkeys chronically treated with dopamine D1 or D2 receptor agonists. J Neurochem 1999;72:682–692.

Mouradian MM, Heuser IJ, Baronti F, Chase TN: Modification of central dopaminergic mechanisms by continuous levodopa therapy for advanced Parkinson's disease. Ann Neurol 1990;27:18–23.

Muller T, Buttner T, Gholipour AF, Kuhn W: Coenzyme Q10 supplementation provides mild symptomatic benefit in patients with Parkinson's disease. Neurosci Lett 2003;341:201–204.

Mytilineou C, Cohen G: Deprenyl protects dopamine neurons from the neurotoxic effect of 1-methyl-4-phenylpyridinium ion. J Neurochem 1985;45:1951–1953.

Mytilineou C, Radcliffe PM, Olanow CW: L-(−)-desmethylselegiline, a metabolite of selegiline [L-(−)-deprenyl], protects mesencephalic dopamine neurons from excitotoxicity in vitro. J Neurochem 1997;68:434–436.

Nakamura K, Bindokas VP, Marks JD, et al: The selective toxicity of 1-methyl-4-phenylpyridinium to dopaminergic neurons: The role of mitochondrial complex I and reactive oxygen species revisited. Mol Pharmacol 2000;58:271–278.

Nakao N, Shintani-Mizushima A, Kakishita K, Itakura T: The ability of grafted human sympathetic neurons to synthesize and store dopamine: A potential mechanism for the clinical effect of sympathetic neuron autografts in patients with Parkinson's disease. Exp Neurol 2004;188:65–73.

Nash JE, Brotchie JM: A common signaling pathway for striatal NMDA and adenosine A2a receptors: Implications for the treatment of Parkinson's disease. J Neurosci 2000;20:7782–7789.

Nash JE, Hill MP, Brotchie JM: Antiparkinsonian actions of blockade of NR2B-containing NMDA receptors in the reserpine-treated rat. Exp Neurol 1999;155:42–48.

Nass R, Hall DH, Miller DM III, Blakely RD: Neurotoxin-induced degeneration of dopamine neurons in Caenorhabditis elegans. Proc Natl Acad Sci U S A 2002;99:3264–3269.

Nass R, Miller DM, Blakely RD: C. elegans: A novel pharmacogenetic model to study Parkinson's disease. Parkinsonism Relat Disord 2001;7:185–191.

Naylor RJ: Further evidence that the blood/brain barrier impedes paraquat entry into the brain. Hum Exp Toxicol 1995;14:587–594.

Nilsson D, Nyholm D, Aquilonius SM: Duodenal levodopa infusion in Parkinson's disease: Long-term experience. Acta Neurol Scand 2001;104(6):343–348.

Nishibayashi S, Asanuma M, Kohno M, et al: Scavenging effects of dopamine agonists on nitric oxide radicals. J Neurochem 1996;67:2208–2211.

Nomoto M, Jenner P, Marsden CD: The dopamine D2 agonist LY 141865, but not the D1 agonist SKF 38393, reverses parkinsonism induced by 1-methyl-4-phenyl-1,2,3,6-tetrahydropyridine (MPTP) in the common marmoset. Neurosci Lett 1985;57:37–41.

Nutt JG, Burchiel KJ, Comella CL, et al: Randomized, double-blind trial of glial cell line-derived neurotrophic factor (GDNF) in PD. Neurology 2003;60:69–73.

Nutt JG, Carter JH, Sexton GJ: The dopamine transporter: Importance in Parkinson's disease. Ann Neurol 2004;55:766–773.

Nyholm D, Remahl AIMN, Dizdar N, et al: Duodenal levodopa infusion monotherapy vs oral polypharmacy in advanced Parkinson disease. Neurology 2005;64(2):216–223.

Obeso JA, Olanow CW, Nutt JG: Levodopa motor complications in Parkinson's disease. Trends Neurosci 2000;23:S2–S7.

Obinu MC, Reibaud M, Blanchard V, et al: Neuroprotective effect of riluzole in a primate model of Parkinson's disease: Behavioral and histological evidence. Mov Disord 2002;17:13–19.

Ochi M, Koga K, Kurokawa M, et al: Systemic administration of adenosine A(2A) receptor antagonist reverses increased GABA release in the globus pallidus of unilateral 6-hydroxydopamine-lesioned rats: A microdialysis study. Neuroscience 2000;100:53–62.

Oertel WH: Pergolide vs L-DOPA (PELMOPET). Mov Disord 2000;15:S4.

Oertel WH, Wolters E, Sampaio C, et al: Pergolide versus levodopa monotherapy in early Parkinson's disease patients: The PELMOPET study. Mov Disord 2006;21:343–353.

Ogawa N, Tanaka K, Asanuma M, et al: Bromocriptine protects mice against 6-hydroxydopamine and scavenges hydroxyl free radicals in vitro. Brain Res 1994;657:207–213.

Oiwa Y, Nakai K, Itakura T: Histological effects of intraputaminal infusion of glial cell line-derived neurotrophic factor in Parkinson disease model macaque monkeys. Neurol Med Chir (Tokyo) 2006;46:267–275.

Olanow CW, Damier P, Goetz CG, et al: Multicenter, open-label, trial of sarizotan in Parkinson disease patients with levodopa-induced dyskinesias (the SPLENDID Study). Clin Neuropharmacol 2004;27:58–62.

Olanow CW, Goetz CG, Kordower JH, et al: A double-blind controlled trial of bilateral fetal nigral transplantation in Parkinson's disease. Ann Neurol 2003;54:403–414.

Olanow CW, Jankovic J: Neuroprotective therapy in Parkinson's disease and motor complications: A search for a pathogenesis-targeted, disease-modifying strategy. Mov Disord 2005;20(suppl 11):S3–S10.

Olanow CW, Schapira AH, Lewitt PA, et al: TCH346 as a neuroprotective drug in Parkinson's disease: A double-blind, randomised, controlled trial. Lancet Neurol 2006;5:1013–1020.

Olanow CW, Schapira AH, Rascol O: Continuous dopamine-receptor stimulation in early Parkinson's disease. Trends Neurosci 2000;23:117–126.

Ossowska K, Wardas J, Kuter K, et al: Influence of paraquat on dopaminergic transporter in the rat brain. Pharmacol Rep 2005a;57:330–335.

Ossowska K, Wardas J, Smialowska M, et al: A slowly developing dysfunction of dopaminergic nigrostriatal neurons induced by long-term paraquat administration in rats: An animal model of preclinical stages of Parkinson's disease? Eur J Neurosci 2005b; 22:1294–1304.

Ostrerova-Golts N, Petrucelli L, Hardy J, et al: The A53T alpha-synuclein mutation increases iron-dependent aggregation and toxicity. J Neurosci 2000;20:6048–6054.

Pact V, Giduz T: Mirtazapine treats resting tremor, essential tremor, and levodopa-induced dyskinesias. Neurology 1999;53:1154.

Palfi S, Leventhal L, Chu Y, et al: Lentivirally delivered glial cell line-derived neurotrophic factor increases the number of striatal dopaminergic neurons in primate models of nigrostriatal degeneration. J Neurosci 2002;22:4942–4954.

Palhagen S, Heinonen E, Hagglund J, et al: Selegiline slows the progression of the symptoms of Parkinson disease. Neurology 2006; 66:1200–1206.

Pan T, Kondo S, Zhu W, et al: Enhancement of autophagy and neuroprotection of rapamycin in lactacystin-induced injury of dopaminergic neurons in vitro. Mov Disord 2006;21:S505.

Papa SM, Chase TN: Levodopa-induced dyskinesias improved by a glutamate antagonist in Parkinsonian monkeys. Ann Neurol 1996;39:574–578.

Papa SM, Engber TM, Kask AM, Chase TN: Motor fluctuations in levodopa treated parkinsonian rats: Relation to lesion extent and treatment duration. Brain Res 1994;662:69–74.

Park S, Kim EY, Ghil GS, et al: Genetically modified human embryonic stem cells relieve symptomatic motor behavior in a rat model of Parkinson's disease. Neurosci Lett 2003;353:91–94.

Parkes D, Jenner P, Rushton D, Marsden D: Neurological Disorders. London, Springer Verlag, 1987.

Parkinson Study Group: Effect of deprenyl on the progression of disability in early Parkisnon's disease. N Engl J Med 1989;321: 1364–1371.

Parkinson Study Group: Pramipexole vs levodopa as initial treatment for Parkinson's disease. JAMA 2000;284:1931–1938.

Parkinson Study Group: Dopamine transporter brain imaging to assess the effects of pramipexole vs levodopa on Parkinson's disease progression. JAMA 2002a;287:1653–1661.

Parkinson Study Group: A controlled trial of rasagiline in early Parkinson disease: The TEMPO Study. Arch Neurol 2002b;59: 1937–1943.

Parkinson Study Group: A controlled, randomized, delayed start study of rasagiline in early Parkinson disease. Arch Neurol 2004a; 61(4):561–566.

Parkinson Study Group: Levodopa and the progression of Parkinson's disease. N Engl J Med 2004b;351(24):2498–2508.

Parkinson Study Group: Pramipexole vs levodopa as initial treatment for Parkinson's disease. Arch Neurol 2004c;61:1044–1053.

Parkinson Study Group: A randomized placebo-controlled trial of rasagiline in levodopa-treated patients with Parkinson disease and motor fluctuations: The PRESTO study. Arch Neurol 2005; 62:241–248.

Payne AP, Campbell JM, Russell D, et al: The AS/AGU rat: A spontaneous model of disruption and degeneration in the nigrostriatal dopaminergic system. J Anat 2000;196(pt 4):629–633.

Pearce RK, Banerji T, Jenner P, Marsden CD: De novo administration of ropinirole and bromocriptine induces less dyskinesia than L-dopa in the MPTP-treated marmoset. Mov Disord 1998;13: 234–241.

Pearce RK, Heikkila M, Linden IB, Jenner P: L-dopa induces dyskinesia in normal monkeys: Behavioural and pharmacokinetic observations. Psychopharmacology (Berl) 2001;156:402–409.

Pearce RK, Jackson M, Smith L, et al: Chronic L-DOPA administration induces dyskinesias in the 1-methyl-4-phenyl-1,2,3, 6-tetrahydropyridine-treated common marmoset (Callithrix jacchus). Mov Disord 1995;10:731–740.

Pearce RK, Smith LA, Jackson MJ, et al: The monoamine reuptake blocker brasofensine reverses akinesia without dyskinesia in MPTP-treated and levodopa-primed common marmosets. Mov Disord 2002;17:877–886.

Pendleton RG, Parvez F, Sayed M, Hillman R: Effects of pharmacological agents upon a transgenic model of Parkinson's disease in Drosophila melanogaster. J Pharmacol Exp Ther 2002;300: 91–96.

Perez FA, Palmiter RD: Parkin-deficient mice are not a robust model of parkinsonism. Proc Natl Acad Sci U S A 2005;102:2174–2179.

Perry JC, Hipolide DC, Tufik S, et al: Intra-nigral MPTP lesion in rats: Behavioral and autoradiography studies. Exp Neurol 2005; 195:322–329.

Pesah Y, Burgess H, Middlebrooks B, et al: Whole-mount analysis reveals normal numbers of dopaminergic neurons following misexpression of alpha-synuclein in Drosophila. Genesis 2005;41:154–159.

Peyro-Saint-Paul H, Rascol O, Blin O, et al: A pilot study of idazoxan, an alpha$_2$ antagonist, in Parkinson's disease. Mov Disord 1996; 11(suppl 1):116.

Piccini P, Weeks RA, Brooks DJ: Alterations in opioid receptor binding in Parkinson's disease patients with levodopa-induced dyskinesias. Ann Neurol 1997;42:720–726.

Picconi B, Pisani A, Barone I, et al: Pathological synaptic plasticity in the striatum: Implications for Parkinson's disease. Neurotoxicology 2005;26:779–783.

Pinna A, Fenu S, Morelli M: Motor stimulant effects of the adenosine A2A receptor antagonist SCH 58261 do not develop tolerance after repeated treatments in 6-hydroxydopamine-lesioned rats. Synapse 2001;39:233–238.

Pinna A, Pontis S, Morelli M: Expression of dyskinetic movements and turning behaviour in subchronic L-DOPA 6-hydroxydopamine-treated rats is influenced by the testing environment. Behav Brain Res 2006;171:175–178.

Pinna A, Volpini R, Cristalli G, Morelli M: New adenosine A2A receptor antagonists: Actions on Parkinson's disease models. Eur J Pharmacol 2005a;512:157–164.

Pinna A, Wardas J, Simola N, Morelli M: New therapies for the treatment of Parkinson's disease: Adenosine A2A receptor antagonists. Life Sci 2005b;77:3259–3267.

Pluchino S, Zanotti L, Deleidi M, Martino G: Neural stem cells and their use as therapeutic tool in neurological disorders. Brain Res Brain Res Rev 2005;48:211–219.

Poewe W: The need for neuroprotective therapies in Parkinson's disease: A clinical perspective. Neurology 2006;66:S2–S9.

Polymeropoulos MH, Higgins JJ, Golbe LI, et al: Mapping of a gene for Parkinson's disease to chromosome 4q21-q23. Science 1996; 274:229–232.

Polymeropoulos MH, Lavedan C, Leroy E, et al: Mutation in the alpha-synuclein gene identified in families with Parkinson's disease. Science 1997;276:2045–2047.

Pope-Coleman A, Lloyd GK, Schneider JS: The nicotinic receptor agonist SIB-1508Y potentiates L-dopa responses in parkinsonian monkeys. Soc Neurosci Abstr 1996;22:217.

Popoli P, Pintor A, Domenici MR, et al: Blockade of striatal adenosine A2A receptor reduces, through a presynaptic mechanism, quinolinic acid-induced excitotoxicity: Possible relevance to neuroprotective interventions in neurodegenerative diseases of the striatum. J Neurosci 2002;22:1967–1975.

Priano L, Albani G, Brioschi A, et al: Transdermal apomorphine permeation from microemulsions: A new treatment in Parkinson's disease. Mov Disord 2004;19:937–942.

Przedborski S, Levivier M, Jiang H, et al: Dose-dependent lesions of the dopaminergic nigrostriatal pathway induced by intrastriatal injection of 6-hydroxydopamine. Neuroscience 1995;67:631–647.

Quik M: Smoking, nicotine and Parkinson's disease. Trends Neurosci 2004;27:561–568.

Quik M, Kulak JM: Nicotine and nicotinic receptors: Relevance to Parkinson's disease. Neurotoxicology 2002;23:581–594.

Quik M, McIntosh JM: Striatal alpha6* nicotinic acetylcholine receptors: Potential targets for Parkinson's disease therapy. J Pharmacol Exp Ther 2006;316:481–489.

Quik M, Parameswaran N, McCallum SE, et al: Chronic oral nicotine treatment protects against striatal degeneration in MPTP-treated primates. J Neurochem 2006;98:1866–1875.

Quik M, Vailati S, Bordia T, et al: Subunit composition of nicotinic receptors in monkey striatum: Effect of treatments with 1-methyl-4-phenyl-1,2,3,6-tetrahydropyridine or L-DOPA. Mol Pharmacol 2005;67:32–41.

Rand JB, Nonet ML: Neurotransmitter assignments for specific neurons. In Riddle DL, Blumenthal T, Meyer BJ, Priess JR (eds): C. elegans II. New York, Cold Spring Harbor Laboratory Press, 1997, pp 611–643.

Rascol O, Arnulf I, Peyro-Saint-Paul H, et al: Idazoxan, an alpha-2 antagonist, and L-DOPA-induced dyskinesias in patients with Parkinson's disease. Mov Disord 2001;16(4):708–713.

Rascol O, Brooks DJ, Korczyn AD, et al: A five-year study of the incidence of dyskinesia in patients with early Parkinson's disease who were treated with ropinirole or levodopa. 056 Study Group. N Engl J Med 2000;342:1484–1491.

Rascol O, Brooks DJ, Korczyn AD, et al: Development of dyskinesias in a 5-year trial of ropinirole and L-dopa. Mov Disord 2006;21:1844–1850.

Rascol O, Brooks DJ, Melamed E, et al: Rasagiline as an adjunct to levodopa in patients with Parkinson's disease and motor fluctuations (LARGO, Lasting effect in Adjunct therapy with Rasagiline Given Once daily, study): A randomised, double-blind, parallel-group trial. Lancet 2005;365:947–954.

Rascol O, Nutt JG, Blin O, et al: Induction by dopamine D1 receptor agonist ABT-431 of dyskinesia similar to levodopa in patients with Parkinson disease. Arch Neurol 2001;58:249–254.

Reavill C, Jenner P, Marsden CD: Differentiation of dopamine agonists using drug-induced rotation in rats with unilateral or bilateral 6-hydroxydopamine destruction of ascending dopamine pathways. Biochem Pharmacol 1983;32:865–870.

Richardson PJ, Kurokawa M: Regulation of neurotransmitter release in basal ganglia by adenosine receptor agonists and antagonists in vitro and in vivo. In Kase H, Richardson PJ, Jenner P (eds): Adenosine receptors and Parkinson's disease. New York, Academic Press, 2000, pp 129–148.

Rinne UK, Bracco F, Chouza C, et al: Early treatment of Parkinson's disease with cabergoline delays the onset of motor complications: Results of a double-blind levodopa controlled trial. The PKDS009 Study Group. Drugs 1998;55(suppl 1):23–30.

Rodriguez-Puertas R, Pascual J, Vilaro T, Pazos A: Autoradiographic distribution of M1, M2, M3, and M4 muscarinic receptor subtypes in Alzheimer's disease. Synapse 1997;26:341–350.

Roitberg B, Urbaniak K, Emborg M: Cell transplantation for Parkinson's disease. Neurol Res 2004;26(4):355–362.

Rose S, Jackson MJ, Smith LA, et al: The novel adenosine A2a receptor antagonist ST1535 potentiates the effects of a threshold dose of L-DOPA in MPTP treated common marmosets. Eur J Pharmacol 2006;546:82–87.

Rose S, Ramsay CN, Jenner P: The novel adenosine A2a antagonist ST1535 potentiates the effects of a threshold dose of l-dopa in unilaterally 6-OHDA-lesioned rats. Brain Res 2007;1133(1):110–114.

Rosenblad C, Georgievska B, Kirik D: Long-term striatal overexpression of GDNF selectively downregulates tyrosine hydroxylase in the intact nigrostriatal dopamine system. Eur J Neurosci 2003;17:260–270.

Rosenblad C, Kirik D, Devaux B, et al: Protection and regeneration of nigral dopaminergic neurons by neurturin or GDNF in a partial lesion model of Parkinson's disease after administration into the striatum or the lateral ventricle. Eur J Neurosci 1999;11:1554–1566.

Rosin DL, Talley EM, Lee A, et al: Distribution of alpha 2C-adrenergic receptor-like immunoreactivity in the rat central nervous system. J Comp Neurol 1996;372:135–165.

Rowell PP, Carr LA, Garner AC: Stimulation of [3H]dopamine release by nicotine in rat nucleus accumbens. J Neurochem 1987;49:1449–1454.

Rupniak NM, Tye SJ, Jennings CA, et al: Antiparkinsonian efficacy of a novel transdermal delivery system for (+)-PHNO in MPTP-treated squirrel monkeys. Neurology 1989;39:329–335.

Sacchetti P, Mitchell TR, Granneman JG, Bannon MJ: Nurr1 enhances transcription of the human dopamine transporter gene through a novel mechanism. J Neurochem 2001;76:1565–1572.

Sajadi A, Bensadoun JC, Schneider BL, et al: Transient striatal delivery of GDNF via encapsulated cells leads to sustained behavioral improvement in a bilateral model of Parkinson disease. Neurobiol Dis 2006;22:119–129.

Sandyk R, Snider SR: Naloxone treatment of L-dopa-induced dyskinesias in Parkinson's disease. Am J Psychiatry 1986;143:118.

Santiago M, Matarredona ER, Machado A, Cano J: Influence of serotoninergic drugs on in vivo dopamine extracellular output in rat striatum. J Neurosci Res 1998;52:591–598.

Saporito MS, Brown EM, Miller MS, Carswell S: CEP-1347/KT-7515, an inhibitor of c-jun N-terminal kinase activation, attenuates the 1-methyl-4-phenyl tetrahydropyridine-mediated loss of nigrostriatal dopaminergic neurons in vivo. J Pharmacol Exp Ther 1999;288:421–427.

Saporito MS, Thomas BA, Scott RW: MPTP activates c-Jun NH(2)-terminal kinase (JNK) and its upstream regulatory kinase MKK4 in nigrostriatal neurons in vivo. J Neurochem 2000;75:1200–1208.

Sapru MK, Yates JW, Hogan S, et al: Silencing of human alpha-synuclein in vitro and in rat brain using lentiviral-mediated RNAi. Exp Neurol 2006;198:382–390.

Saravanan KS, Sindhu KM, Mohanakumar KP: Acute intranigral infusion of rotenone in rats causes progressive biochemical lesions in the striatum similar to Parkinson's disease. Brain Res 2005;1049:147–155.

Sauer H, Rosenblad C, Bjorklund A: Glial cell line-derived neurotrophic factor but not transforming growth factor beta 3 prevents delayed degeneration of nigral dopaminergic neurons following striatal 6-hydroxydopamine lesion. Proc Natl Acad Sci U S A 1995;92:8935–8939.

Savola JM, Hill M, Engstrom M, et al: Fipamezole (JP-1730) is a potent alpha2 adrenergic receptor antagonist that reduces levodopa-induced dyskinesia in the MPTP-lesioned primate model of Parkinson's disease. Mov Disord 2003;18:872–883.

Schapira AH: Neuroprotection and dopamine agonists. Neurology 2002;58:S9–S18.

Schapira AH: Disease modification in Parkinson's disease. Lancet Neurol 2004;3:362–368.

Schapira AH, Bezard E, Brotchie J, et al: Novel pharmacological targets for the treatment of Parkinson's disease. Nat Rev Drug Discov 2006a;5:845–854.

Schapira AH, Cleeter MW, Muddle JR, et al: Proteasomal inhibition causes loss of nigral tyrosine hydroxylase neurons. Ann Neurol 2006b;60:253–255.

Scheinin M, Lomasney JW, Hayden-Hixson DM, et al: Distribution of alpha 2-adrenergic receptor subtype gene expression in rat brain. Brain Res Mol Brain Res 1994;21:133–149.

Scheller D, Chan P, Li Q, et al: Rotigotine treatment partially protects from MPTP toxicity in a progressive macaque model of Parkinson's disease. Exp Neurol 2007;203(2):415–422.

Schneider JS, Van Velson M, Menzaghi F, Lloyd GK: Effects of the nicotinic acetylcholine receptor agonist SIB-1508Y on object retrieval performance in MPTP-treated monkeys: Comparison with levodopa treatment. Ann Neurol 1998;43:311–317.

Schoenberg BS: Descriptive epidemiology of Parkinson's disease: Disease distribution and hypothesis formulation. Adv Neurol 1987;45:277–283.

Schurad B, Horowski R, Jahnichen S, et al: Proterguride, a highly potent dopamine receptor agonist promising for transdermal administration in Parkinson's disease: Interactions with alpha(1)-, 5-HT(2)- and H(1)-receptors. Life Sci 2006;78:2358–2364.

Schwarzschild MA, Agnati L, Fuxe K, et al: Targeting adenosine A2A receptors in Parkinson's disease. Trends Neurosci 2006;29:647–654.

Sethy VH, Wu H, Oostveen JA, Hall ED: Neuroprotective effects of the dopamine agonists pramipexole and bromocriptine in 3-acetylpyridine-treated rats. Brain Res 1997;754:181–186.

Setler PE, Sarau HM, Zirkle CL, Saunders HL: The central effects of a novel dopamine agonist. Eur J Pharmacol 1978;50:419–430.

Sherzai A, Bara-Jimenez W, Gillespie M, et al: Adenosine A2a antagonist treatment of Parkinson's disease. Neurology 2002;58:A667.

Shimizu K, Ohtaki K, Matsubara K, et al: Carrier-mediated processes in blood-brain barrier penetration and neural uptake of paraquat. Brain Res 2001;906:135–142.

Shiosaki K, Jenner P, Asin KE, et al: ABT-431: The diacetyl prodrug of A-86929, a potent and selective dopamine D1 receptor agonist: In vitro characterization and effects in animal models of Parkinson's disease. J Pharmacol Exp Ther 1996;276:150–160.

Shoulson I: DATATOP: A decade of neuroprotective inquiry. Parkinson Study Group. Deprenyl and tocopherol antioxidative therapy of parkinsonism. Ann Neurol 1998;44:S160–S166.

Shoulson I, Oakes D, Fahn S, et al: Impact of sustained deprenyl (selegiline) in levodopa-treated Parkinson's disease: A randomized placebo-controlled extension of the deprenyl and tocopherol antioxidative therapy of parkinsonism trial. Ann Neurol 2002;51:604–612.

Shukla S, Agrawal AK, Chaturvedi RK, et al: Co-transplantation of carotid body and ventral mesencephalic cells as an alternative approach towards functional restoration in 6-hydroxydopamine-lesioned rats: Implications for Parkinson's disease. J Neurochem 2004;91:274–284.

Shults CW, Beal MF, Fontaine D, et al: Absorption, tolerability, and effects on mitochondrial activity of oral coenzyme Q10 in parkinsonian patients. Neurology 1998;50:793–795.

Shults CW, Flint BM, Song D, Fontaine D: Pilot trial of high dosages of coenzyme Q10 in patients with Parkinson's disease. Exp Neurol 2004;188:491–494.

Shults CW, Haas RH, Passov D, Beal MF: Coenzyme Q10 levels correlate with the activities of complexes I and II/III in mitochondria from parkinsonian and nonparkinsonian subjects. Ann Neurol 1997;42:261–264.

Shults CW, Oakes D, Kieburtz K, et al: Effects of coenzyme Q10 in early Parkinson disease: Evidence of slowing of the functional decline. Arch Neurol 2002;59:1541–1550.

Sieradzan KA, Fox SH, Hill M, et al: Cannabinoids reduce levodopa-induced dyskinesia in Parkinson's disease: A pilot study. Neurology 2001;57:2108–2111.

Silverdale MA, Nicholson SL, Crossman AR, Brotchie JM: Topiramate reduces levodopa-induced dyskinesia in the MPTP-lesioned marmoset model of Parkinson's disease. Mov Disord 2005;20:403–409.

Silverdale MA, Nicholson SL, Ravenscroft P, et al: Selective blockade of D(3) dopamine receptors enhances the anti-parkinsonian properties of ropinirole and levodopa in the MPTP-lesioned primate. Exp Neurol 2004;188:128–138.

Sindhu KM, Saravanan KS, Mohanakumar KP: Behavioral differences in a rotenone-induced hemiparkinsonian rat model developed following intranigral or median forebrain bundle infusion. Brain Res 2005;1051:25–34.

Slevin JT, Gash DM, Smith C D, et al: Unilateral intraputaminal glial cell line-derived neurotrophic factor in patients with Parkinson disease: Response to 1 year each of treatment and withdrawal. Neurosurg Focus 2006;20:E1.

Smeyne RJ, Jackson-Lewis V: The MPTP model of Parkinson's disease. Brain Res Mol Brain Res 2005;134:57–66.

Smidt MP, Burbach JP: How to make a mesodiencephalic dopaminergic neuron. Nat Rev Neurosci 2007;8(1):21–32.

Smith LA, Jackson MJ, Al-Barghouthy G, et al: Multiple small doses of levodopa plus entacapone produce continuous dopaminergic stimulation and reduce dyskinesia induction in MPTP-treated drug-naive primates. Mov Disord 2005;20:306–314.

Smith LA, Jackson MJ, Hansard MJ, et al: Effect of pulsatile administration of levodopa on dyskinesia induction in drug-naive MPTP-treated common marmosets: Effect of dose, frequency of administration, and brain exposure. Mov Disord 2003;18:487–495.

Smith LA, Jackson MJ, Johnston L, et al: Switching from levodopa to the long-acting dopamine D2/D3 agonist piribedil reduces the expression of dyskinesia while maintaining effective motor activity in MPTP-treated primates. Clin Neuropharmacol 2006;29:112–125.

Snyder BJ, Olanow CW: Stem cell treatment for Parkinson's disease: An update for 2005. Curr Opin Neurol 2005;18:376–385.

Soderstrom K, O'Malley J, Steece-Collier K, Kordower JH: Neural repair strategies for Parkinson's disease: Insights from primate models. Cell Transplant 2006;15:251–265.

Sohmiya M, Tanaka M, Tak NW, et al: Redox status of plasma coenzyme Q10 indicates elevated systemic oxidative stress in Parkinson's disease. J Neurol Sci 2004;223:161–166.

Sonsalla PK, Heikkila RE: The influence of dose and dosing interval on MPTP-induced dopaminergic neurotoxicity in mice. Eur J Pharmacol 1986;129:339–345.

Srinivasan J, Schmidt WJ: The effect of the alpha2-adrenoreceptor antagonist idazoxan against 6-hydroxydopamine-induced Parkinsonism in rats: Multiple facets of action? Naunyn Schmiedebergs Arch Pharmacol 2004;369:629–638.

Stacy M, Bowron A, Guttman M, et al: Identification of motor and nonmotor wearing-off in Parkinson's disease: Comparison of a patient questionnaire versus a clinician assessment. Mov Disord 2005;20:726–733.

Steiger MJ, Stocchi F, Carta A, et al: The clinical efficacy of oral levodopa methyl ester solution in reversing afternoon "off" periods in Parkinson's disease. Clin Neuropharmacol 1991;14:241–244.

Steiner JP, Hamilton GS, Ross DT, et al: Neurotrophic immunophilin ligands stimulate structural and functional recovery in neurodegenerative animal models. Proc Natl Acad Sci U S A 1997;94:2019–2024.

Stephenson DT, Meglasson MD, Connell MA, et al: The effects of a selective dopamine D2 receptor agonist on behavioral and pathological outcome in 1-methyl-4-phenyl-1,2,3,6-tetrahydropyridine-treated squirrel monkeys. J Pharmacol Exp Ther 2005;314:1257–1266.

Stocchi F, Olanow CW: Continuous dopaminergic stimulation in early and advanced Parkinson's disease. Neurology 2004;62:S56–S63.

Svenningsson P, Hall H, Sedvall G, Fredholm BB: Distribution of adenosine receptors in the postmortem human brain: An extended autoradiographic study. Synapse 1997;27:322–335.

Tabrizi SJ, Orth M, Wilkinson JM, et al: Expression of mutant alpha-synuclein causes increased susceptibility to dopamine toxicity. Hum Mol Genet 2000;9:2683–2689.

Tatton WG, Greenwood CE: Rescue of dying neurons: A new action for deprenyl in MPTP parkinsonism. J Neurosci Res 1991;30:666–672.

Taylor H, Minger SL: Regenerative medicine in Parkinson's disease: Generation of mesencephalic dopaminergic cells from embryonic stem cells. Curr Opin Biotechnol 2005;16:487–492.

Taylor JR, Lawrence MS, Redmond DE Jr, et al: Dihydrexidine, a full dopamine D1 agonist, reduces MPTP-induced parkinsonism in monkeys. Eur J Pharmacol 1991;199:380–391.

Teismann P, Ferger B: Inhibition of the cyclooxygenase isoenzymes COX-1 and COX-2 provide neuroprotection in the MPTP-mouse model of Parkinson's disease. Synapse 2001;39:167–174.

Togasaki DM, Protell P, Tan LC, et al: Dyskinesias in normal squirrel monkeys induced by nomifensine and levodopa. Neuropharmacology 2005;48:398–405.

Togasaki DM, Tan L, Protell P, et al: Levodopa induces dyskinesias in normal squirrel monkeys. Ann Neurol 2001;50:254–257.

Ton TG, Heckbert SR, Longstreth WT Jr, et al: Nonsteroidal anti-inflammatory drugs and risk of Parkinson's disease. Mov Disord 2006;21:964–969.

Trabucchi M, Bassi S, Frattola L: Effect of naloxone on the "on-off" syndrome in patients receiving long-term levodopa therapy. Arch Neurol 1982;39:120–121.

Tsuboi K, Shults CW: Intrastriatal injection of sonic hedgehog reduces behavioral impairment in a rat model of Parkinson's disease. Exp Neurol 2002;173:95–104.

Ungerstedt U: Postsynaptic supersensitivity after 6-hydroxy-dopamine induced degeneration of the nigro-striatal dopamine system. Acta Physiol Scand Suppl 1971a;367:69–93.

Ungerstedt U: Striatal dopamine release after amphetamine or nerve degeneration revealed by rotational behaviour. Acta Physiol Scand Suppl 1971b;367:49–68.

Unnerstall JR, Kopajtic TA, Kuhar MJ: Distribution of alpha 2 agonist binding sites in the rat and human central nervous system: Analysis of some functional, anatomic correlates of the pharmacologic effects of clonidine and related adrenergic agents. Brain Res 1984;319:69–101.

van den Munckhof P, Gilbert F, Chamberland M, et al: Striatal neuroadaptation and rescue of locomotor deficit by L-dopa in aphakia mice, a model of Parkinson's disease. J Neurochem 2006;96:160–170.

van den Munckhof P, Luk KC, Ste-Marie L, et al: Pitx3 is required for motor activity and for survival of a subset of midbrain dopaminergic neurons. Development 2003;130:2535–2542.

van der Putten H, Wiederhold KH, Probst A, et al: Neuropathology in mice expressing human alpha-synuclein. J Neurosci 2000;20:6021–6029.

Van-Velson M, Tinker J, Lloyd GK, et al: The nicotinic receptor agonist SIB-1508Y, but not levodopa, improves cognition in chronic MPTP-treated monkeys with and without motor disability. Soc Neurosci Abstr 1997;23:1898.

Verhagen ML, Del Dotto P, van den MP, et al: Amantadine as treatment for dyskinesias and motor fluctuations in Parkinson's disease. Neurology 1998;50:1323–1326.

Vermeulen RJ, Drukarch B, Sahadat MC, et al: Morphine and naltrexone modulate D2 but not D1 receptor induced motor behavior in MPTP-lesioned monkeys. Psychopharmacology (Berl) 1995;118:451–459.

Von Voigtlander PF, Moore KE: Turning behavior of mice with unilateral 6-hydroxydopamine lesions in the striatum: Effects of apomorphine, L-DOPA, amanthadine, amphetamine and other psychomotor stimulants. Neuropharmacology 1973;12:451–462.

Waldmeier P, Bozyczko-Coyne D, Williams M, Vaught JL: Recent clinical failures in Parkinson's disease with apoptosis inhibitors underline the need for a paradigm shift in drug discovery for neurodegenerative diseases. Biochem Pharmacol 2006;72:1197–1206.

Wang W, Shi L, Xie Y, et al: SP600125, a new JNK inhibitor, protects dopaminergic neurons in the MPTP model of Parkinson's disease. Neurosci Res 2004;48:195–202.

Wardas J, Konieczny J, Lorenc-Koci E: SCH 58261, an A(2A) adenosine receptor antagonist, counteracts parkinsonian-like muscle rigidity in rats. Synapse 2001;41:160–171.

Watts RL, Raiser CD, Stover NP, et al: Stereotaxic intrastriatal implantation of human retinal pigment epithelial (hRPE) cells attached to gelatin microcarriers: A potential new cell therapy for Parkinson's disease. J Neural Transm Suppl 2003;215–227.

Wessell RH, Ahmed SM, Menniti FS, et al: NR2B selective NMDA receptor antagonist CP-101,606 prevents levodopa-induced motor response alterations in hemi-parkinsonian rats. Neuropharmacology 2004;47:184–194.

Whone AL, Watts RL, Stoessl AJ, et al: Slower progression of Parkinson's disease with ropinirole versus levodopa: The REAL-PET study. Ann Neurol 2003;54:93–101.

Widdowson PS, Farnworth MJ, Simpson MG, Lock EA: Influence of age on the passage of paraquat through the blood-brain barrier in rats: A distribution and pathological examination. Hum Exp Toxicol 1996a;15:231–236.

Widdowson PS, Farnworth MJ, Upton R, Simpson MG: No changes in behaviour, nigro-striatal system neurochemistry or neuronal cell death following toxic multiple oral paraquat administration to rats. Hum Exp Toxicol 1996b;15:583–591.

Winkler C, Sauer H, Lee CS, Bjorklund A: Short-term GDNF treatment provides long-term rescue of lesioned nigral dopaminergic neurons in a rat model of Parkinson's disease. J Neurosci 1996;16:7206–7215.

Witta J, Baffi JS, Palkovits M, et al: Nigrostriatal innervation is preserved in Nurr1-null mice, although dopaminergic neuron precursors are arrested from terminal differentiation. Brain Res Mol Brain Res 2000;84:67–78.

Woitalla D, Muller T, Benz S, et al: Transdermal lisuride delivery in the treatment of Parkinson's disease. J Neural Transm Suppl 2004;(68):89–95.

Woolf NJ, Butcher LL: Cholinergic systems of the rat brain: III. Projections from the pontomesencephalic tegmentum to the thalamus, tectum, basal ganglia and basal forebrain. Brain Res Bull 1986;16:603–637.

Wu DC, Jackson-Lewis V, Vila M, et al: Blockade of microglial activation is neuroprotective in the 1-methyl-4-phenyl-1,2,3,6-tetrahydropyridine mouse model of Parkinson disease. J Neurosci 2002;22:1763–1771.

Wu SS, Frucht SJ: Treatment of Parkinson's disease: What's on the horizon? CNS Drugs 2005;19:23–743.

Xu K, Xu YH, Chen JF, Schwarzschild MA: Caffeine's neuroprotection against 1-methyl-4-phenyl-1,2,3,6-tetrahydropyridine toxicity shows no tolerance to chronic caffeine administration in mice. Neurosci Lett 2002;322:13–16.

Yamada M, Iwatsubo T, Mizuno Y, Mochizuki H: Overexpression of alpha-synuclein in rat substantia nigra results in loss of dopaminergic neurons, phosphorylation of alpha-synuclein and activation of caspase-9: Resemblance to pathogenetic changes in Parkinson's disease. J Neurochem 2004;91:451–461.

Yamato H, Kannari K, Shen H, et al: Fluoxetine reduces L-DOPA-derived extracellular DA in the 6-OHDA-lesioned rat striatum. Neuroreport 2001;12:1123–1126.

Yang L, Sugama S, Mischak RP, et al: A novel systemically active caspase inhibitor attenuates the toxicities of MPTP, malonate, and 3NP in vivo. Neurobiol Dis 2004;17:250–259.

Zeng BY, Bukhatwa S, Hikima A, et al: Reproducible nigral cell loss after systemic proteasomal inhibitor administration to rats. Ann Neurol 2006;60:248–252.

Zeng BY, Pearce RK, MacKenzie GM, Jenner P: Alterations in pre-proenkephalin and adenosine-2a receptor mRNA, but not pre-protachykinin mRNA correlate with occurrence of dyskinesia in normal monkeys chronically treated with L-DOPA. Eur J Neurosci 2000;12:1096–1104.

Zetterstrom RH, Solomin L, Jansson L, et al: Dopamine neuron agenesis in Nurr1-deficient mice. Science 1997;276:248–250.

Zhang Z, Miyoshi Y, Lapchak PA, et al: Dose response to intraventricular glial cell line-derived neurotrophic factor administration in parkinsonian monkeys. J Pharmacol Exp Ther 1997;282:1396–1401.

Zhou W, Hurlbert MS, Schaack J, et al: Overexpression of human alpha-synuclein causes dopamine neuron death in rat primary culture and immortalized mesencephalon-derived cells. Brain Res 2000;866:33–43.

# Chapter 10

# Parkinsonism-Plus Syndromes and Secondary Parkinsonian Disorders

Most patients who are referred to specialized movement disorder clinics with hypokinetic disorders are diagnosed clinically as having Parkinson disease (PD) (Table 10-1) (Jankovic et al., 2000). The second most common group of parkinsonian patients is categorized clinically as having parkinsonism-plus disorders and pathologically as having multiple-system degenerations (Fahn, 1977; Jankovic, 1989; Stacy and Jankovic, 1992; Jankovic et al., 2000; Litvan et al., 2003). There is, however, a growing body of evidence to support the emerging classification of neurodegenerative disorders according to pathogenetic mechanisms into (1) amyloidoses (e.g., Alzheimer disease, or AD), (2) ubiquitin-proteasome disorders (e.g., PD, parkin PD), (3) synucleinopathies (e.g., PD, multiple-system atrophy, or MSA), (4) tauopathies (e.g., frontotemporal dementia [FTD] with parkinsonism, or FTDP; progressive supranuclear palsy, or PSP; corticobasal degeneration, or CBD), (5) polyglutamine expansion diseases (e.g., Huntington disease, spinocerebellar atrophies [SCAs]), and (6) prion diseases (e.g., Creutzfeldt-Jakob disease). As the current understanding of the mechanisms of these diseases advances, refinements in this classification and new categories of disease will undoubtedly emerge. Besides parkinsonian findings, patients with these disorders exhibit additional ("plus") features. For example, supranuclear ophthalmoparesis typifies patients with PSP; dysautonomia and ataxia are typically present in MSA; laryngeal stridor occurs in striatonigral degeneration (SND); a combination of apraxia, cortical myoclonus, and "alien hand" occurs in CBD; dementia occurs in AD or dementia with Lewy bodies (DLB); and dementia coupled with motor neuron disease occurs in parkinsonism-dementia-amyotrophic lateral sclerosis complex of Guam (Table 10-2). As there are no biologic markers for any of these disorders, the diagnostic criteria are based on the presence of certain clinical features and neuropathologic confirmation (Cummings, 2003; Litvan et al., 2003). Rarely, psychogenic causes have been implicated in the pathogenesis of parkinsonism (Lang et al., 1995). This chapter focuses only on the sporadic (nongenetic) forms of multisystem degenerations. The secondary and heredodegenerative causes of parkinsonism are covered elsewhere in this book and in other reviews.

## PROGRESSIVE SUPRANUCLEAR PALSY

### Clinical Features and Natural History

First described by Steele, Richardson, and Olszewski (Steele et al., 1964; Steele, 1972) in 1964, progressive supranuclear palsy (PSP) has become a well-characterized, distinct clinical-pathologic entity (Jankovic et al., 1990; Golbe, 1993; Collins et al., 1995; Litvan, 1998b). The first volume solely devoted to PSP was published in 1993 (Litvan and Agid, 1993), and a summary of the 1999 "First Brainstorming Conference on PSP" was published (Litvan et al., 2000). The diagnosis of PSP should be considered in any patient with progressive parkinsonism and disturbance of ocular motility (Jankovic, 1984a; Maher and Lees, 1986; Jankovic, Friedman, et al., 1990; Friedman et al., 1992; Cardoso and Jankovic, 1994).

PSP is considered to be a sporadic disorder, but familial PSP has been reported (Brown et al., 1993; de Yebenes et al., 1995; Tetrud et al., 1996; Rojo et al., 1999). The supranuclear ophthalmoparesis was not well documented in the familial cases, and the presence of atypical features, such as early cognitive decline in the family reported by Brown and colleagues (1993) and the relatively early age at onset (53 years) in the de Yebenes and colleagues (1995) kindred, suggested that these families had a neurodegenerative disorder that was distinct from idiopathic PSP. Furthermore, no linkage to the *tau* gene has been identified in any of these families, although linkage to 1q31.1 has been demonstrated in one large Spanish family (Ros et al., 2005).

In a review of 126 PSP patients, unsteadiness of gait, frequent falling, monotonous speech, loss of eye contact, slowness of movement and of mentation, sloppy eating habits, and nonspecific visual difficulty were the most typical presenting features (Jankovic, Friedman, et al., 1990). The earliest and most disabling symptom of PSP usually relates to gait and balance impairment, as a result of which patients frequently fall and sustain injuries. The average period from onset of symptoms to the first fall in PSP is 16.8 months, as compared to 108 months in PD, 42 months in MSA, 54 months in dementia with Lewy bodies, and 40.8 months in vascular parkinsonism (Williams et al., 2006). The marked instability is presumably a result of visual-vestibular impairment, axial rigidity, and bradykinesia (Jankovic, Friedman, et al., 1990). Using computerized posturography, Ondo and colleagues (2000) demonstrated that measures of balance impairment can reliably differentiate between PSP and PD even in early stages of the disease. In contrast to the short and shuffling steps, stooped posture, narrow base, and flexed knees that are typically seen in PD, PSP patients have a stiff and broad-based gait, with a tendency to have their knees (and trunk) extended and arms slightly abducted. Instead of turning en bloc, they tend to pivot, which further compromises their balance (Video 10-1). Some PSP patients may present with the syndrome of pure akinesia, also referred to by some as motor blocks (Matsuo et al., 1991; Giladi et al., 1992; Riley et al., 1994) and gait ignition failure (Atchison et al., 1993; Nutt et al., 1993), which is manifested chiefly by akinesia of gait (start hesitation, freezing, motor blocks, festination, disequilibrium with frequent falling), marked impairment of speech (stuttering, stammering, hypophonia), handwriting difficulty (micrographia), and eyelid motor disturbance (blepharospasm, eyelid freezing) without rigidity, tremor, or dementia and without response to levodopa. Primary progressive freezing gait may be the initial

Table 10-1 Categorization of parkinsonism

| Parkinsonism | n = 7564 |
|---|---|
| Parkinson disease | 5410 (71.5%) |
| Progressive supranuclear palsy | 381 (5.0%) |
| Multiple-system atrophy (SDS, SND, OPCA) | 349 (4.6%) |
| Vascular | 265 (3.5%) |
| Drug-induced | 227 (4.4%) |
| Corticobasal ganglionic degeneration | 143 (3.0%) |
| Hemiparkinsonism-hemiatrophy | 81 (1.0 %) |
| Gait disorders | 187 (2.4%) |
| Other | 521 (6.9%) |

Based on a combined database of all new patients evaluated in the Movement Disorders Clinic at Baylor College of Medicine, Houston (n = 4334) and Columbia University Medical Center, New York (n = 3230).
OPCA, olivopontocerebellar atrophy; SDS, Shy-Drager syndrome; SND, striatonigral degeneration.

and main presentation of PSP, although some of these patients also have evidence of pallidonigroluysian degeneration, CBD, and diffuse Lewy body disease (Factor et al., 2006). In addition to PSP, frontal gait disorder may be the initial manifestation of AD and CBD (Rossor et al., 1999). Although the PSP gait appears ataxic, the patients usually do not exhibit prominent cerebellar findings. The uncompensated loss of postural reflexes and motor blocks (freezing), especially on turning, coupled with a peculiar lack of insight into the difficulties with equilibrium (possibly secondary to frontal lobe dysfunc-

tion) leads to frequent falling. This is often present even in the early stages of the disease and helps to differentiate PSP from PD (Litvan, Mangone, et al., 1996). Although a rating scale specifically modified to assess motor function in PSP has been proposed, the motor subscale of the Unified Parkinson's Disease Rating Scale has been found to reliably assess most aspects of PSP (Cubo et al., 2000).

Along with postural instability, supranuclear ophthalmoparesis typically manifested by paralysis of downgaze is the most important distinguishing sign of PSP (Litvan, Campbell, et al., 1997) (Video 10-2). The predictability of these two features with regard to the final pathologic diagnosis was confirmed by a clinical-pathologic study of 24 autopsy-proven cases of PSP (Litvan, Agid, et al., 1996). About one third of PSP patients complain of blurred vision, diplopia, and eye discomfort, but most eventually lose their ability to read or maintain eye contact (Friedman et al., 1992). Involuntary persistence of ocular fixation is a typical, though rarely mentioned, feature of PSP. Other oculomotor abnormalities that are seen in patients with PSP include impairment of saccades, optokinetic nystagmus, and the presence of square wave jerks (Rascol et al., 1991). In early stages of PSP, patients might have only mild limitation of voluntary downgaze and inability to converge, but slowing of horizontal and vertical saccades (also demonstrated by optokinetic nystagmus) appears to be the earliest oculomotor sign of PSP (Video 10-3). One study compared saccades, optokinetic nystagmus, and other ophthalmologic signs in six patients with PSP compared to PD and normal controls (Garbutt et al., 2004). All PSP patients showed slowing of vertical saccade and quick phase of nystagmus; square wave jerks were more frequent and larger during fixation; vertical optokinetic nystagmus showed impaired slow

Table 10-2 Parkinsonism-plus syndromes: Differential diagnosis

| | PD | PSP | MSA-P | MSA-C | CBD | DLB | PDACG |
|---|---|---|---|---|---|---|---|
| Bradykinesia | + | + | + | ± | + | ± | + |
| Rigidity | + | + | + | + | + | ± | + |
| Gait disturbance | + | + | + | + | + | ± | + |
| Tremor | + | − | − | ± | ± | − | + |
| Ataxia | − | − | − | + | − | − | ± |
| Dysautonomia | ± | ± | ± | ± | − | ± | ± |
| Dementia | ± | + | − | − | ± | + | + |
| Dysarthria/dysphagia | ± | + | + | + | + | ± | + |
| Dystonia | ± | ± | ± | − | + | − | − |
| Eyelid apraxia | − | + | ± | − | ± | − | ± |
| Limb apraxia | − | − | − | − | + | ± | − |
| Motor neuron disease | − | − | ± | − | − | − | + |
| Myoclonus | ± | − | ± | ± | + | ± | − |
| Neuropathy | − | − | − | ± | − | − | − |
| Oculomotor deficit | − | + | − | + | + | ± | ± |
| Sleep impairment | ± | ± | ± | ± | − | ± | − |
| Asymmetric findings | + | − | ± | − | + | − | − |
| Levodopa response | + | ± | ± | ± | − | − | − |
| Levodopa dyskinesia | + | − | ± | − | − | − | − |
| Family history | ± | − | − | − | − | − | − |
| Putaminal T2 hypointensity | − | ± | + | + | − | − | − |
| Lewy bodies | + | − | ± | ± | ± | + | − |

CBD, cortical-basal ganglionic degeneration; DLB, dementia with Lewy bodies; MSA-C, multiple system atrophy, predominantly cerebellar; MSA-P, multiple-system atrophy, predominantly cerebellar; PD, Parkinson disease; PDACG, parkinsonism-dementia-amyotrophic lateral sclerosis complex of Guam; PSP, progressive supranuclear palsy.

wave response, and quick phases were slowed and combined with square wave jerks. Deficient generation of the motor command by midbrain burst neurons has been suggested as the primary mechanism for the slow vertical saccades (Bhidayasiri et al., 2001). Slowing of vertical saccades might help to differentiate PSP from other parkinsonian disorders, including PD, MSA, and CBD, although some slowing of vertical saccades can be seen occasionally also in these parkinsonian disorders (Vidailhet et al., 1994; Rivaud-Péchoux et al., 2000; Bhidayasiri et al., 2001). In addition to slow vertical saccades, bilateral impairment of the antisaccade task (the patient is instructed to look in the direction opposite to the visual stimulus) correlates well with frontal lobe dysfunction in PSP (Vidailhet et al., 1994) and other neurodegenerative and frontal lobe disorders (Condy et al., 2004; Munoz and Everling, 2004; Zee and Lasker, 2004). Abnormalities in antisaccades imply a dysfunction of the dorsolateral prefrontal cortex and the superior colliculus (Condy et al., 2004). Later, limitation of vertical and then lateral eye movements follows. The ophthalmoparesis can be overcome by the oculocephalic (doll's eye) maneuver (Video 10-4; see also Videos 10-1 and 10-2), but with disease progression and brainstem involvement, vestibulo-ocular reflexes can be lost, suggesting additional nuclear involvement (Ishino et al., 1973).

Several clinical-pathologic studies have attempted to establish criteria that separate PSP from other, related disorders. In 60 cases of patients clinically diagnosed with PSP, 47 (78%) of which were pathologically proven, false-positive diagnoses included PD combined with cortical Lewy body pathology or AD, MSA, CBD, Pick disease, motor neuron disease, cerebrovascular disease, and FTD (Osaki et al., 2004). The application of NINDS and other criteria improved the accuracy of initial clinical diagnosis only marginally. On the basis of an analysis of 103 pathologically confirmed consecutive cases of PSP, Williams and colleagues (2005) divided PSP into two categories: Richardson syndrome, characterized by the typical features described in the original report, and PSP-P, in which the clinical features overlap with PD and the course is more benign. The mean 4R-tau/3R-tau ratio of the isoform composition of insoluble tangle-tau isolated from the pons was significantly higher in Richardson syndrome (2.84) than in PSP-P syndrome (1.63). Further studies are needed to confirm or refute this classification.

Pathologically documented cases of PSP without ophthalmoparesis have been reported (Davis et al., 1985; Collins et al., 1995; Daniel et al., 1995). When PSP patients with ophthalmoparesis were compared with those without ophthalmoparesis, no differences in the pathology of the two groups were noted, and there was no correlation between the severity of clinical symptoms and degenerative changes (Daniel et al., 1995). In another pathologic study, brains of PSP patients with gaze palsy compared with those without gaze palsy had twofold greater loss of neurons in the substantia nigra reticulata (SNr) (Halliday et al., 2000). Since SNr projects to the superior colliculi, degeneration of SNr might contribute to the limitation of eye movements. Supranuclear ophthalmoparesis may also occur in DLB (Lewis and Gawel, 1990; Fearnley et al., 1991; De Bruin et al., 1992; Daniel et al., 1995; Brett et al., 2002), CBD (Gibb et al, 1990), postencephalitic parkinsonism, prion disease, Wernicke encephalopathy, dorsal midbrain syndrome, paraneoplastic syndrome, progressive subcortical gliosis, Whipple disease (Jankovic, 1986; Simpson et al., 1995;

Averbuch-Heller et al., 1999), Niemann-Pick and Gaucher disease (Shulman et al., 1995; Uc et al., 2000), Kufor-Rakeb syndrome (Hampshire et al., 2001), primary pallidal degeneration, and other disorders (Calabrese and Hadfield, 1991).

Pseudobulbar symptoms in PSP patients are characterized chiefly by dysarthria, dysphagia, and "emotional incontinence" (Video 10-5). Rigidity, bradykinesia, and hypertonicity of the facial muscles produce deep facial folds and typical worried or astonished facial expressions (Jankovic, 1984b). The worried appearance is partly due to contraction of the procerus (and possibly corrugator) muscle, the so-called "procerus signs" (Romano and Colosimo, 2001) (see Videos 10-1 and 10-2). Speech in PSP is characterized by a spastic, hypernasal, hypokinetic, ataxic, monotonous, low-pitched dysarthria (Kluin et al., 1993) (see Videos 10-1, 10-4, and 10-5). The speech rate may be slow or fast, and some patients have severe palilalia and stuttering. An "apraxia of phonation" has been reported in one patient who was aphonic except during periods of excitement or during sleep (Jankovic, 1984b). In contrast, some patients have almost continuous involuntary vocalizations, including loud groaning, moaning, humming, and grunting sounds (Jankovic, Friedman, et al., 1990). Progressive dysphagia causes most patients to modify their diet, and some eventually need a feeding gastrostomy to maintain adequate nutrition. As a result of chewing difficulties, inability to look down, and poor hand coordination, PSP patients are often described as "sloppy eaters."

In a review of dystonia in pathologically proven cases of PD, MSA, and PSP, Rivest and colleagues (1990) found dystonia to be an uncommon feature, noted in only 15 of 118 (13%) cases. They regarded the frequently reported neck extension as a form of axial rigidity rather than dystonia. In another study, the increased neck muscle tone was thought to have features of both dystonia (tonic shortening reaction) and rigidity (antagonist muscle contraction indicative of increased tonic stretch reflex) (Tanigawa et al., 1998). Neck extension, although often noted in published reports, is actually an uncommon sign in PSP. Indeed, neck flexion, usually associated with MSA (Quinn, 1994), can occasionally be seen in PSP (Daniel et al., 1995). In contrast to the typical presence of neck rigidity, truncal muscle tone is only slightly increased, and distal limbs may actually seem hypotonic (Tanigawa et al., 1998). In some patients, however, distal dystonia can be seen (Barclay and Lang, 1997). Although PSP is usually a symmetric disorder, dystonia represents an occasional exception in that unilateral dystonia may be present, particularly in the more advanced stages of the disease. The most common form of dystonia in PSP is blepharospasm. In one study, 29% of patients had involuntary orbicularis oculi contractions producing blepharospasm, and over one third had "apraxia" of eyelid opening, eyelid closure, or both (Friedman et al., 1992). Although some (Lepore and Duvoisin, 1985) have hypothesized that these lid abnormalities are due to involuntary supranuclear inhibition of levator palpebrae, others have drawn attention to the similarity of this disorder of eyelid motor control and the parkinsonian phenomenon of sudden transient freezing, hence suggesting the term *lid freezing* (Jankovic, 1995a). Other terms that are used to describe this condition include *pretarsal blepharospasm* (Elston, 1992) and *focal eyelid dystonia* (Krack and Marion, 1994). In one study of 83 patients with PSP, 38 (46%) had some form of dystonia, 22 (24%) had blepharospasm, 22 (27%) had limb dystonia, and

14 (17%) had axial dystonia (Barclay and Lang, 1997). Sometimes, spontaneous arm levitation, a well-recognized sign in CBD, is also seen in patients with PSP and may be wrongly attributed to dystonia (Barclay et al., 1999).

In their original monograph, Steele, Richardson, and Olszewski (1964) indicated that mild dementia was present during early stages of the disease. Although some investigators have reported severe cognitive impairment in this population (Pillon and Dubois, 1993), others have attributed these deficits, at least in part, to poor visual processing (Fisk et al., 1982; Rafal et al., 1988; Jankovic, Friedman, et al., 1990; Daniel et al., 1995). Despite a relative preservation of short-term memory, cognitive slowing, impairment of executive (goal-directed) functions, and subcortical dementia with deficits in tasks requiring sequential movements, conceptual shifts, and rapid retrieval of verbal knowledge are typically present in patients with PSP (Johnson et al., 1991; Pillon and Dubois, 1993; Litvan, Paulsen, et al., 1998). The memory disturbance that is found in patients with PSP is similar to that of patients with PD and Huntington disease, but it is markedly different from that of patients with AD (et al., 1994). The apathy, with or without depression, and other hypoactive behaviors that are typically seen in PSP have been attributed to a dysfunction in the frontal cortex and associated circuitry (Litvan, Paulsen, et al., 1998). This is contrast to Huntington disease, in which behaviors such as agitation, anxiety, and irritability have been related to hyperactivity of the medial and orbitofrontal cortical circuitry. Sparing of olfactory function in PSP, in contrast to that in PD, is another clinical difference between the two neurodegenerative disorders (Doty et al., 1993). Litvan, Mega, and colleagues (1996) studied the neuropsychiatric aspects of PSP in 22 patients and found that apathy occurred in 91%, disinhibition in 36%, dysphoria in 18%, anxiety in 18%, and irritability in fewer than 9%. Another sign of frontal lobe dysfunction in PSP is the "applause sign" (*signe de l'applaudissement*), which probably represents a perseveration of automatic behavior (Dubois et al. 1995, 2005) (Video 10-6). This  sign, characteristically present in patients with PSP (but also present in some patients with FTD with parkinsonism and CBD), is manifested by persistence (perseveration) of clapping after the patient is instructed to clap consecutively three times as quickly as possible.

After idiopathic PSP, the most common cause of PSP is a multi-infarct state. Multi-infarct or vascular PSP can be difficult to differentiate clinically from the more common idiopathic variety (Dubinsky and Jankovic, 1987; Stern et al., 1989; Winikates and Jankovic, 1994). In addition to a much higher frequency of stroke risk factors and abnormal imaging studies, the vascular PSP patients are more likely to have asymmetric and predominantly lower-body involvement, cortical and pseudobulbar signs, dementia, and bowel and bladder incontinence (Winikates and Jankovic, 1994). The concept of vascular PSP is supported by the observation by Ghika and Bogousslavsky (1997), who found that 81.0% of patients with clinically diagnosed PSP had hypertension. A clinical-pathologic study of four patients who were clinically diagnosed with PSP but found to have vascular PSP at autopsy showed that vascular PSP is characterized by asymmetric signs, falls within 1 year of onset, and vascular lesions on magnetic resonance imaging (MRI) (Josephs et al., 2002). In addition, three of the four patients carried the H2 tau haplotype, whereas 93.7% of patients with idiopathic PSP carry the H1 tau haplotype (78.4% of controls carry

this haplotype) (see later). Reported causes of secondary PSP include exposure to organic solvents (McCrank et al., 1989), paraneoplastic syndrome (Jankovic, 1985), mesencephalic tumor (Siderowf et al., 1998), surgery on the aorta (Mokri et al., 2004), and other rare and often unsubstantiated causes.

The relentlessly progressive course of PSP leads to death, usually from aspiration, within 10 years of onset in the majority of cases. In one clinical-pathologic study of 24 patients with PSP, the median survival from onset was 5.6 years, and this was shorter in men and in patients who experienced falls during the first year of symptoms and who had early dysphagia or supranuclear palsy (Litvan, Mangone, et al. 1996; Litvan, 2003).

In another clinical-pathologic study involving 16 cases of PSP, Birdi and colleagues (2002) found the mean survival time to be 8.6 years (range: 3 to 24), and the mean age at death was 72.3 years (range: 60 to 89). The early onset, presence of falls, slowness, and early downward gaze palsy correlated with rapid disease progression (Santacruz et al., 1998). In a review of 187 cases, those with early bulbar features had around 5 years less life expectancy than did those who had no or late bulbar features (Nath et al., 2003). Similar to other series, the median survival in this study was 5.7 years. Since this figure is based on deceased cases, it might be too pessimistic because slowly progressive cases are still being followed. In another study of 50 PSP patients, Goetz and colleagues (2003) found the median survival from the onset of first symptoms to be 7.9 years (6.5 years in the 21 patients who were followed to death).

## Epidemiology

About 6% of all parkinsonian patients who are evaluated in a specialized clinic fulfill the clinical criteria for PSP (see Table 10-1). On the basis of a medical record review of the Rochester Epidemiology Project, the average annual incidence rate has been estimated to be 5.3 new cases per 100,000 person-years (Bower et al., 1997). The prevalence, after age adjustment to the U.S. population, has been estimated to be 1.39 per 100,000 (Golbe et al., 1988). In a review of computerized records of 15 general practices in and around London, Schrag and colleagues (1999) found an age-adjusted prevalence for PSP of 6.4 per 100,000. In other studies carried out in the United Kingdom, the prevalence of PSP ranged from 1 to 6.5 per 100,000 (Nath et al., 2001). Similar to the European studies, a prevalence of 5.82 per 100,000 has been reported in Yonago, Japan (Kawashima et al., 2004).

Like PD, PSP occurs more often in men, but its onset at a mean age of 63 years is about 10 years later than the typical onset of PD. Although no well-designed epidemiologic studies have been performed in PSP, one case-control study found that PSP patients were more likely to live in areas of relatively sparse population (Davis et al., 1988). Another study by the same investigators failed to identify any risk factor, except for low likelihood of completing at least 12 years of education, that would differentiate patients with PSP from a matched control population (Golbe et al., 1996).

## Neurodiagnostic Studies

Electrophysiologic studies have been helpful in documenting other abnormalities, such as sleep difficulties and seizures. Polysomnographic evaluation of 10 patients with moderate to severe PSP revealed marked sleep abnormalities; all had significant periods (2 to 6 hours) of insomnia (Aldrich et al., 1989). Sleep problems were correlated with worsening dementia. Another study showed marked reduction in percentage of REM sleep (Montplaisir et al., 1997). The same study also showed frontal electroencephalogram (EEG) slowing in patients with PSP. In a review of 62 patients seen over a 9-year period, Nygaard and colleagues (1989) noted seizures in 7 patients and suggested a higher-than-expected frequency of seizures in this population. This has not been our observation, but the relatively high frequency of seizures reported by Nygaard and colleagues (1989) might have been secondary to cortical infarcts. Abnormalities in motor and frontal sensory evoked potentials have been found in 8 of 13 patients with the clinical diagnosis of PSP (Abbruzzese et al., 1991).

The typical findings on computed tomography or MRI scans of patients with PSP include generalized and brainstem, particularly midbrain, atrophy (Stern et al., 1989; Soliveri et al., 1999). Measuring the anteroposterior diameter of the suprapontine midbrain, Warmuth-Metz and colleagues (2001) found that, in contrast to PD patients (mean 18.5 mm), PSP patients had a significantly lower diameter (13.4 mm) on axial T2-weighted MRI, and as a result, the authors concluded that this finding reliably differentiates between PD and PSP and recommended that this evaluation "should be incorporated into the diagnostic criteria for PSP." In another study, utilizing midsagittal MRI, the average midbrain area of patients with PSP was 56 mm², which was significantly smaller than that of patients with PD (103 mm²) or MSA-P (97.2 mm²), and this parameter, particularly the ratio of the area of the midbrain to the area of the pons, was found to reliably differentiate among the three disorders (Oba et al., 2005). On the midsagittal view of the MRI, as a result of atrophy of the rostral midbrain tegmentum, the most rostral midbrain, the midbrain tegmentum, the pontine base, and the cerebellum appear to correspond to the bill, head, body, and wing, respectively, of a hummingbird (Kato et al., 2003) or penguin (Oba et al., 2005). The "hummingbird sign" was demonstrated in all 8 MRI scans of PSP patients but not in any of the 12 scans of PD patients or 10 scans of normal controls (Kato et al., 2003). The "morning glory sign"—a peculiar MRI finding of midbrain atrophy with concavity of the lateral margin of the midbrain tegmentum, resembling the lateral margin of the morning glory flower—is observed in PSP patients with supranuclear gaze palsy (Adachi et al., 2004). Using diffusion-weighted MRI (DWI-MRI), Seppi and colleagues (2003) were able to differentiate between PSP and PD with 90% sensitivity and 100% specificity, but this technique could not differentiate between PSP and MSA. Using diffusion tensor imaging and voxel based morphometry in PSP, Padovani and colleagues (2006) provided evidence of both grey and white matter degeneration even in early stages of PSP. Through the use of voxel-based morphometry in 15 patients with clinically proven PSP and 14 with CBD, distinct patterns of atrophy were observed that differentiated between the two disorders with 93% accuracy (Boxer et al., 2006). CBD patients had a marked asymmetric (L > R) pattern of atrophy involving premotor cortex, superior parietal lobules, and striatum, whereas PSP was characterized by atrophy of the midbrain, pons, thalamus, and striatum.

Stroke risk factors and a multi-infarct state on computed tomography or MRI have been noted in patients with PSP

with a higher frequency than in those with PD (Dubinsky and Jankovic, 1987). One etiology for a subgroup of PSP might be small vessel disease producing subcortical ischemia with reduction of regional cerebral blood flow, cerebral hypometabolism, and a multi-infarct state. MRIs in patients with PSP, MSA, and other parkinsonian syndromes have been associated with putaminal hypointensity on T2-weighted MRI, but this finding is less consistently noted in PSP than in the other parkinsonism-plus syndromes (Drayer et al., 1989; Stern et al., 1989). In one study, PSP could be differentiated from MSA by the presence of marked atrophy and hyperintensity of the midbrain as well as atrophy of the frontal and temporal lobes (Schrag et al., 2000) (Fig. 10-1). The "eye of the tiger" sign on brain MRI, typically associated with neurodegeneration with brain iron accumulation type 1 (NBIA-1), formerly Hallervorden-Spatz disease (see later), has also been reported in PSP (Davie et al., 1997). PSP is associated with dorsal midbrain atrophy, and as a result of degeneration of superior colliculi, the floor of the third ventricle is flattened on sagittal MRI images (Savoiardo et al., 1994).

Positron emission tomography (PET) scanning has revealed decreased metabolic activity in the caudate, putamen, and prefrontal cortex (Foster et al., 1988; Goffinet et al., 1989; Blin et al., 1990), but the earliest sign of PSP appears to be decreased glucose metabolism in the midbrain (Mishina et al., 2004). Uptake of ¹⁸F-dopa is usually reduced in PSP but may be normal in early stages (Bhatt et al., 1991). This suggests that the parkinsonian findings in early PSP are related more to postsynaptic receptor changes than to a loss of presynaptic dopamine terminals. In another study, ¹⁸F-dopa uptake was markedly reduced in the caudate as well as in the anterior and posterior putamen of PSP patients (Brooks, Ibanez et al., 1990).

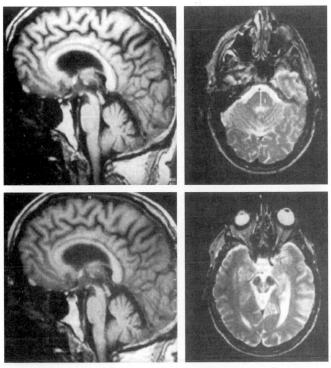

Figure 10-1 Typical findings of reduced midbrain diameter in patients with PS (*bottom*) as compared to normal controls (*top*).

In contrast, the uptake was reduced only in the posterior putamen in PD patients. Similarly, dopamine transporter, imaged by [¹¹C]-WIN PET, showed a relatively uniform reduction involving the entire striatum, whereas patients with PD had involvement chiefly of the posterior putamen (Ilgin et al., 1999). F-dopa and F-deoxyglucose PET were abnormal in 5 (33%) individuals among 15 subjects at risk of familial PSP, even though they did not (yet) exhibit any symptoms (Piccini et al., 2001). Using ¹¹C-raclopride as a D2 ligand, Brooks and colleagues (1992) showed a 24% reduction in D2 density in the caudate and a 9% reduction in the putamen of patients with PSP. A discriminant analysis of striatal 18F-dopa PET studies indicates that this technique can reliably differentiate between PD and PSP, but it is less accurate in differentiating between PD and MSA (Burn et al., 1994). By using [¹¹C]diprenorphine, significantly reduced opioidergic binding has been demonstrated in both caudate and putamen, whereas the binding is essentially normal in PD and reduced in the putamen but not the caudate in SND (Burn et al., 1995). The cortical muscarinic acetylcholine receptors, as measured by PET and [¹¹C]N-methyl-4-piperidyl benzilate, were found to be normal in a series of patients with PSP (Asahina et al., 1998). Using [¹²³I]β-CIT SPECT, Pirker and colleagues (2000) showed marked reduction of striatal binding in PD, PSP, MSA, and CBD, but the pattern of abnormality (reduction in overall binding and asymmetry) did not allow a differentiation among the various disorders.

## Neuropathology and Neurochemistry

The motor, neurobehavioral, and neuro-ophthalmic findings seen in patients with PSP reflect marked neuronal degeneration in the basal nucleus of Meynert, pallidum, subthalamic nucleus, superior colliculi, mesencephalic tegmentum, SNpc and SNpr, locus coeruleus, red nucleus, reticular formation, vestibular nuclei, cerebellum, and spinal cord (Steele et al., 1964; Steele, 1972; Zweig et al., 1987; Juncos et al., 1991; Jellinger and Bancher, 1993; Hardman et al., 1997a, 1997b). In addition, in contrast to PD, both the globus pallidus internus (GPi) and externus (GPe) are markedly affected in PSP, and this may contribute to thalamic inhibition and some of the parkinsonian features (Hardman and Halliday, 1999a, 1999b). Along with the degeneration of the SNpc and the pedunculopontine tegmental nucleus, the glutamatergic caudal intralaminar thalamic nuclei are involved in both PSP and PD (Henderson et al., 2000). Atrophy of the superior cerebellar peduncle has been found to be a frequent finding in the brains of patients with PSP, and this correlates with the duration of the disease (Tsuboi et al., 2003b). In one pathologic study, marked atrophy of the GPi differentiated PSP from PD and DLB (Cordato et al., 2000). Although bladder dysfunction has not been considered a prominent feature in patients with PSP, the finding of neuronal loss in Onuf's nucleus in patients with PSP suggests that bladder function should be carefully evaluated in patients with PSP (Scaravilli et al., 2000).

On the basis of a workshop sponsored by the National Institutes of Health, the following neuropathologic criteria were proposed: (1) high-density neurofibrillary tangles (NFTs) and neuropil threads in the basal ganglia and brainstem and (2) tau-positive astrocytes or their processes in areas of involvement (Hauw et al., 1994; Litvan, Agid, et al., 1996). Using rather crude pathologic criteria, De Bruin and Lees

(1994) demonstrated that the clinical manifestations of PSP can vary considerably. They reviewed 90 cases reported in the literature between 1951 and 1992 that met the following two criteria: subcortical neurofibrillary degeneration and exclusion of other recognized nosologic entities. There were 51 men and 34 women (in 5 cases, the gender was not specified), with an average age at onset of 62 years and mean age at death of 67 years. The most common symptoms were unsteady gait (70.7%), stiffness (67.4%), slurred speech (67.4%), falls (60.6%), dysphagia (57.3%), and blurring of vision (21%). Vertical gaze palsy was the most common sign but was noted in only 68.5% of all cases, followed by bradykinesia in 67.4%, dysarthria in 67.4%, rigidity in 58.4%, axial dystonia in 48.3%, segmental dystonia in 20.2%, and tremor in 16.8%.

Microscopic examination reveals NFTs, granulovacuolar degeneration, gliosis, and rare Lewy bodies (Steele et al., 1964; Steele, 1972; De Bruin and Lees, 1994). One pathologic study showed no evidence of increased Lewy bodies in PSP (Tsuboi et al., 2001). The NFTs in PSP differ from those seen in AD and other neurodegenerative disorders in that PSP tangles consist of 15-nm straight tubules rather than 20- to 24-nm-wide paired helical filaments (PHFs) (Joachim et al., 1987; Jellinger and Bancher, 1993; Dickson, 1997). PHFs are composed of the microtubule-associated protein tau (MAPT) in a hyperphosphorylated state (Goedert et al., 1996). In contrast to the other neurodegenerative diseases with tau pathology, such as AD, Pick disease, CBD, and the parkinsonism-dementia complex of Guam, which are characterized by flame-shaped NFTs, the NFTs in PSP are predominantly of the globose type. The tau-containing astrocytic inclusions ("tufted astrocytes") are more common in the basal ganglia and the brainstem of PSP, whereas they are more common in the cortex of brains of CBD. Tau inclusions in PSP oligodendrocytes are described as "coiled bodies." Tsuboi and colleagues (2003a) showed that APOE ε4 is a risk factor for Alzheimer-type pathology in PSP.

The clinical and pathologic overlap between PSP, CBD, and AD provides evidence that these disorders are closely related, although the absence of amyloid deposits in PSP and CBD suggests a clear difference between the two disorders and AD (Feany and Dickson, 1996; Litvan et al., 1999; Rossor et al., 1999; Boeve, Lang, et al., 2003; Wakabayashi et al., 2004; Galpern and Lang, 2006). Among 180 cases of clinically diagnosed PSP that came to autopsy, only 137 (36%) met the pathologic criteria for PSP (Josephs and Dickson, 2003). The other diagnoses included CBD, MSA, diffuse Lewy body disease (DLBD), and Creutzfeldt-Jakob disease (CJD). The following features were seen more frequently in non-PSP cases than in PSP cases: tremor, psychosis, early dementia, asymmetric findings, absence of H1 haplotype, and presence of APOE ε4. The various disorders can be differentiated by a careful histologic examination. For example, the tau in NFTs of AD shows marked ubiquitin immunoreactivity, whereas the NFT-tau from PSP does not (Flament et al., 1991; Shin et al., 1991). While the abnormal tau in AD consists chiefly of 55-, 64-, and 68–kDa forms, the PSP tau consists only of 64- and 68-kDa forms (Conrad et al., 1997). PSP and CBD also share pathologic tau doublet (64 and 69 kDa) as well as the predominance of 4R tau isoforms with argyrophilic grain disease, a late-onset dementia in which pathologically aggregated tau proteins are found in limbic structures in the shape of distinct argyrophilic grains and coiled bodies (Tolnay et al., 2002; Liang et al., 2005).

Cdk5, a kinase that is physiologically involved in the phosphorylation of tau protein, is overexpressed in PSP brains (Borghi et al., 2002). PSP and CBD also overlap with FTD in clinical, pathologic, biochemical, and genetic aspects (Boeve, Lang, et al., 2003). Tuft-shaped astrocytes seem to be more indicative of PSP than CBD, with prominent tuft-shaped astrocytes in the precentral gyrus and premotor cortex, caudate, putamen and globus pallidus, red nucleus, and superior colliculus in PSP brains (Hattori et al., 2003). The histopathologic features of PSP also overlap closely with those of postencephalitic parkinsonism (Litvan, Jankovic, et al., 1998) and the parkinsonism-dementia complex of Guam, but the pallidum and the subthalamic nucleus are usually spared in the former, and the cortex seems to be more involved in the latter. Rarely, cases with clinical presentation nearly identical to that of PSP have been reported to have the pathologic picture of pallidonigroluysial atrophy (Kosaka et al., 1981). In one study, 54% of pathologically proven cases of PSP had coexistent AD and PD, providing evidence for overlap between these neurodegenerative disorders (Gearing et al., 1994). Calbindin-D$_{28k}$ immunoreactivity, normally found in the medium-sized neurons and neuropil of the striatal matrix, GP, and SNpr, is reduced in the GP of patients with PSP (and in the striatum and SNpr of patients with SND) (Ito et al., 1992). This finding suggests that calcium cytotoxicity might play a role in the marked neuronal degeneration that is found in these structures.

Molecular misreading of the ubiquitin-B (*UBB*) gene results in a dinucleotide deletion in ubiquitin-B mRNA, which in turn leads to accumulation of the mutant protein ubiquitin-B+1 in AD, Pick disease, FTD, PSP, and argyrophilic grain disease but not in synucleinopathies (PD or MSA) (Fischer et al., 2003). This finding provides evidence that the ubiquitin-proteasome system is impaired in these tauopathies and that ubiquitin-B+1 protein serves as a marker for these diseases. Unique haplotype in 17q21, found in 16% of Spanish as well as American PSP patients but not in any of the controls, provides further evidence that PSP is a form of a tauopathy (Pastor et al., 2004). Better understanding of the molecular pathways that are altered in various neurodegenerative disorders could be helpful in differential diagnosis based on postmortem examination of brain tissue. Using microarray technology in substantia nigra (SN) samples from six patients with PD, two patients with PSP, one patient with FTDP, and five controls, Hauser and colleagues (2005) found 142 genes that were differentially expressed in PD cases and controls, 96 in the combination of PSP-FTDP, and 12 genes that were common to all three disorders.

## Pathogenesis

The marked reduction in striatal D2 receptors in PSP, demonstrated by PET studies, has also been documented in postmortem studies (Ruberg et al., 1993). In contrast to the D2 receptors, the striatal D1 receptors are spared (Pierot et al., 1988; Pascual et al., 1992). Biochemical studies show that in addition to degeneration of the nigrostriatal dopaminergic system, the cholinergic and GABAergic systems seem to be particularly affected. Cholinergic neurons have been found to degenerate in the Edinger-Westphal nucleus, the rostral interstitial nucleus of Cajal (possibly contributing to the extensor nuchal rigidity), the medial longitudinal fasciculus (contributing to vertical gaze palsy), the superior colliculus, and the pedunculopontine nucleus (Zweig et al., 1987; Juncos et al., 1991). Using the technique of an in situ hybridization of GAD$_{67}$ messenger RNA, Levy and colleagues (1995) demonstrated 50% to 60% reduction in the number of neurons expressing GAD$_{67}$ messenger RNA in the caudate nucleus, ventral striatum, and both segments of the GP in three brains of patients with PSP. They suggest that the marked destruction of the basal ganglia output nuclei might explain the poor response to dopaminergic therapy in this disorder.

The most striking neurochemical abnormality found in PSP brains is a marked reduction in striatal dopamine, dopamine receptor density, choline acetyl transferase activity, and loss of nicotinic, rather than muscarinic, cholinergic receptors in the basal forebrain (Young, 1985; Pierot et al., 1988; Ruberg et al., 1993). Normal dopamine levels in the nucleus accumbens suggest that the mesolimbic system is relatively spared. Because of the relative sparing of the mesocorticolimbic dopaminergic system in contrast to the severe degeneration of the mesostriatal system, some investigators have suggested that the primary site of pathology in PSP is the striatum and that the changes observed in the SN are simply a result of a retrograde degeneration (Ruberg et al., 1993). The cholinergic neurons are, however, also markedly affected and may be primarily involved in PSP. The cholinergic innervation of the thalamus is particularly affected, and this finding helps to differentiate PSP from PD (Shinotoh et al., 1999). Also, reduction in acetylcholine vesicular transporter has been found to differentiate PSP from other types of neurodegenerative disorders (Suzuki et al., 2002). Suzuki and colleagues (2002) were able to correlate reductions in acetylcholine vesicular transporter and choline acetyl transferase activity in the striatum of postmortem brains of patients with PSP, but choline acetyl transferase was also significantly reduced in the inferior frontal cortex. Glutamate has been found to be increased in the striatum, pallidum, nucleus accumbens, and occipital and temporal cortex. In contrast to PD, glutathione was found to be increased in the SN of PSP patients (Perry et al., 1988). The observation that multiple neurotransmitters, particularly dopamine and acetylcholine, are affected in PSP suggests that PSP is not a primary neurotransmitter disease but a disorder in which multiple subpopulations of neurons degenerate for yet unknown reason.

The cause of PSP is unknown, but oxidative damage, mitochondrial dysfunction, and abnormal protein (e.g., tau) processing have received the most attention (Albers and Augood, 2001). Decreased rates of adenosine triphosphate production were found in a preliminary study of muscle mitochondria function in patients with PSP, suggesting impaired mitochondrial respiratory chain activity in PSP (Di Monte et al., 1994). Further support for mitochondrial defect in PSP was later provided by additional studies. Using cybrid lines expressing mitochondrial genes, Swerdlow and colleagues (2000) found a 12.4% decrease in complex I activity ($P < .005$) in cybrid (cytoplasmic hybrid) cells but no change in complex IV activity. Cybrid cells also had significantly increased levels of several antioxidant enzymes. This study suggests a mtDNA-encoded electron transport chain enzyme defect in PSP. Further evidence for a defect in mitochondrial oxidative metabolism is the finding of significantly reduced levels of phosphocreatine and Mg$^{2+}$ and increased levels of adenosine diphosphate and inorganic phosphate using phosphorus magnetic resonance spectroscopy of the brain and calf muscle in five PSP patients

(Martinelli et al., 2000). Rats that are exposed systemically and chronically to annonacin, a lipophilic mitochondrial complex I inhibitor extracted from tropical fruit plants, have been shown to produce neurodegeneration resembling PSP, providing further evidence of mitochondrial dysfunction in PSP (Champy et al., 2004). Another potential animal model of PSP is a transgenic mouse that expresses wild-type human tau driven by the astrocyte-specific glial fibrillary acidic protein promoter (Forman et al., 2005). These transgenic mice accumulate tau in astrocytes, similar to what occurs in PSP, leading to focal neuronal degeneration. Using proton magnetic resonance spectroscopic imaging, Tedeschi and colleagues (1997) found a reduced N-acetylaspartate/creatine-phospho-creatine ratio in the brainstem, centrum semiovale, and frontal and precentral cortex and N-acetylaspartate/choline in the lentiform nucleus in patients with PSP.

Recent studies have drawn attention to abnormal phosphorylation of tau proteins as an important mechanism of neurodegeneration in PSP. *Tau* exon 10 + 16 mutation in *tau* gene (MAPT, IVS10, C-U, +16) was found in a case of young-onset (age 40 years) of PSP phenotype with neuropathologic features of FTD (Morris et al., 2003). Tau is phosphorylated by serine, threonine, and tyrosine kinases, and this phosphorylation might lead to abnormal aggregation. The relationship between abnormalities in tau and PSP is described in detail in the section on tauopathies.

## Treatment

Although in the early stages, mild improvement in parkinsonian symptoms may be noted with levodopa or dopamine agonists (e.g., pergolide, pramipexole), most PSP patients fail to reach and maintain any meaningful improvement with these drugs (Jankovic, 1983; Litvan and Chase, 1993; Nieforth and Golbe, 1993; Jankovic, 1994; Weiner et al., 1999). The most likely reason is that in PSP, there is a marked loss of the postsynaptic receptors, particularly the D2 receptors, secondary to the loss of the postsynaptic striatal neurons (Pierot et al., 1988). Idazoxan, an experimental potent and selective α-2 presynaptic inhibitor that increases norepinephrine (NE) transmission, was shown in a double-blind crossover study to improve motor function in nine PSP patients (Ghika et al., 1991). Physostigmine has been shown to have variable clinical effects on cognitive deficits (Blin et al., 1995). Furthermore, PSP patients have been found to be unusually sensitive to cholinergic blockade with anticholinergic drugs (Litvan et al., 1994); therefore, these drugs should be avoided in patients with PSP. On the other hand, the cholinergic drug donepezil has not been found to be beneficial in a placebo-controlled trial of 21 patients with PSP, and it might actually worsen motor function (Litvan, Phipps, et al., 2001). Other drugs, including methysergide and amitriptyline, although anecdotally reported to be beneficial, have been generally disappointing (Newman, 1985). Zolpidem, a GABA agonist and a short-acting hypnotic drug, was found to improve moderately voluntary saccadic eye movements and motor function in a small (*n* = 10) group of patients with PSP as compared to a placebo (Daniele et al., 1999). Blepharospasm, with or without eyelid freezing, and other forms of focal dystonias, can be effectively treated with botulinum toxin injections (Jankovic and Brin, 1991; Jankovic, 2004) (Video 10-7). Electroconvulsive therapy, while helpful in some patients with PD, markedly exacerbated motor and mental symptoms in one patient with PSP (Hauser and Trehan, 1994). Cricopharyngeal myotomy is almost never performed, but severe dysphagia in advanced stages of the disease often necessitates the placement of a feeding gastrostomy. There is no evidence, however, that tube feeding prevents aspiration (Finucane et al., 1999).

Only symptomatic therapy has been used thus far, albeit with disappointing results, but it is hoped that better understanding of the pathogenesis of neuronal degeneration in PSP will lead to more effective, hypothesis-driven therapeutic interventions. It is possible, for example, that since cross-linking of tau protein by transglutaminase stabilized tau filaments into NFTs, inhibitors of transglutaminase may prevent the formation of NFTs and may have a neuroprotective effect on the disease (Zemaitaitis et al., 2000). For example, drugs such as valproic acid that inhibit abnormal phosphorylation of the tau protein by blocking the enzyme GSK-3β (also known as tau protein kinase I) might possibly exert neuroprotective effects (Chen et al., 1999). By limiting tau phosphorylation, valproate would be expected to prevent the disturbed microtubule function, disrupted intracellular protein trafficking, formation of NFTs, and neuronal death. Valproate might also prevent elevations of intracellular calcium, increase levels of the antiapoptotic protein Bcl-2, and act as a histone deacetylase inhibitor (which might interfere with apoptosis) (Phiel et al., 2001). Other kinase inhibitors, such as lithium, noscovitine, and olomoucine, might play a role as potential therapeutic strategies in PSP. (See Appendix 10-1.)

# MULTIPLE-SYSTEM ATROPHY

## Clinical Features and Natural History

Historically, the first case that James Parkinson described in his 1817 "Essay on the Shaking Palsy" had associated autonomic features and might have been the first case of MSA. First coined by Graham and Oppenheimer in 1969 (Graham and Oppenheimer, 1969), the term *multiple-system atrophy* describes a syndrome characterized clinically by parkinsonism, dysautonomia, and other features previously reported as Shy-Drager syndrome (SDS), SND, and sporadic olivopontocerebellar atrophy (OPCA). The term *Shy-Drager syndrome* is still occasionally used in the literature, particularly by some American clinicians, as a tribute to Dr. Shy, a neurologist from University of Pennsylvania and Columbia University, and Dr. Drager, a urologist at Baylor College of Medicine, who first drew attention to this disorder in 1960 (Shy and Drager, 1960). In their initial report, Shy and Drager described two men who presented with symptoms of orthostatic syncope, impotence, and bladder dysfunction. They later developed parkinsonian features, including gait disturbance, mild tremor, dysarthria, constipation, and bowel and bladder incontinence. In addition to the combination of parkinsonism and autonomic failure, patients with SDS also frequently manifest cerebellar (60%) and pyramidal signs (50%). Other features described by Shy and Drager as part of the "full syndrome," such as rectal incontinence, fasciculations, and iris atrophy, are seen rarely. The term *striatonigral degeneration* was introduced in the 1960s by Adams, Van Bogaert, and Van de Eecken (Aotsuka and Paulson, 1993). In an attempt to characterize SND, Gouider-Khouja and colleagues (1995) used the following clinical criteria: (1) onset after 40 years; (2)

disease duration less than 10 years; (3) parkinsonian syndrome poorly responsive or unresponsive to levodopa; (4) autonomic failure; and (5) absence of family history, dementia, apraxia, supranuclear ophthalmoplegia, and "detectable focal lesions on neuroimaging study." Dejerine and Thomas (1900) introduced the term *olivopontocerebellar atrophy* to describe a group of heterogeneous disorders characterized clinically by the combination of progressive parkinsonism and cerebellar ataxia and pathologically by neuronal loss in the ventral pons, inferior olives, and cerebellar cortex (Berciano, 1992). OPCA may be inherited, usually in an autosomal-dominant pattern (Currier and Subramony, 1993; Rosenberg, 1995), but only the sporadic OPCAs are included in the classification of MSA (Berciano, 1992; Gilman and Quinn, 1996; Wenning, Colosimo, et al., 2004). A rating scale, the Unified Multiple System Atrophy Rating Scale, that assesses all important symptoms and signs of MSA has been developed and validated against related rating scales, such as the Unified Parkinson's Disease Rating Scale and the International Cooperative Ataxia Rating Scale (Wenning, Tison, et al., 2004).

The discovery by Papp and colleagues (1989) that the pathologic hallmark shared by all three disorders is the presence of filamentous α-synuclein containing glial cytoplasmic inclusions (GCI) led to the recognition that these disorders are manifestations of the same pathologic process. MSA has therefore been redefined as a sporadic, progressive, adult-onset disorder characterized clinically by autonomic dysfunction (MSA-A), parkinsonism (MSA-P), and cerebellar ataxia (MSA-C) in any combination (American Academy of Neurology, 1996; Consensus Committee of the AAS and AAN, 1996; Gilman et al., 1998; Gilman, 2002; Osaki et al., 2002; Watanabe et al., 2002). Until the mid-1990s, the literature still used the terms *SND* and *OPCA*, and these terms are still used when appropriate.

Fearnley and Lees (1990) reviewed 10 patients, ranging in age from 47 to 50 years, with autopsy-proven SND (MSA-P). Five of these patients were misdiagnosed as having PD, largely because of good response to levodopa. Features that were helpful in differentiating SND from other parkinsonian disorders included early-onset falling, severe dysarthria and dysphonia, excessive snoring and sleep apnea, respiratory stridor, hyperreflexia, and extensor plantar responses. Cerebellar or pyramidal tract signs were present in two patients each, while autonomic symptoms were present in seven. Duration of illness ranged from 3 to 8 years, and no difference in survival was seen in levodopa responders compared to non–levodopa responders. In another series, tremor was found in only 6% of SND patients and in 71% of PD patients; the predominant features were rigidity and hypokinesia, present at onset in 84% of all SND (MSA-P) patients (Van Leeuwen and Perquin, 1988). Besides lack of tremor, the symmetric onset of SND (MSA-P) is sometimes helpful in differentiating SND from PD, although 6 of 10 patients described by Fearnly and Lees (1990) had asymmetric onset. In a study comparing 16 patients with pathologically proven MSA of the SND (MSA-P) variety with PD and PSP, a set of clinical criteria reliably differentiated MSA from PD but not from PSP (Colosimo et al., 1995). In addition to cerebellar and pyramidal signs, early instability with falls, and relative preservation of cognition, the following features were more typically present in MSA than in PD: autonomic dysfunction (69% versus 5%),

absence of rest tremor (87% versus 40%), rapid progression (mean disease duration 7.1 years versus 13.6 years), and poor or unsustained response to levodopa (31% versus 0%). In contrast to other reports, only 43.7% of the MSA patients in this series had a symmetric onset. As in PD, PSP, and other subcortical neurodegenerative disorders, the cognitive deficit in SND consists chiefly of mild impairment of memory and executive functions, which has been attributed to "inefficient planning of memory processes" and "frontal lobe like syndrome related to a dysfunction of the supervisory attentional system" (Pillon, Gouider-Khouja, et al., 1995).

MSA appears to be more common in men than in women, with symptoms first beginning in the sixth decade; death usually occurs 7 to 8 years after the initial symptoms and approximately 4 years after the onset of neurologic impairment (McLeod and Tuck, 1987a, 1987b). In a review of 188 pathologically proven cases of MSA, 28% patients had involvement of all four systems (parkinsonism, cerebellar dysfunction, corticospinal signs, and dysautonomia); 18% had the combination of parkinsonism, pyramidal, and autonomic findings; 11% had parkinsonian, cerebellar, and autonomic findings; another 11% had parkinsonism and dysautonomia; 10% had only parkinsonism; and parkinsonism was absent in 11% of all cases (Quinn, 1994). The clinical features and natural history of MSA were analyzed in 100 cases with probable MSA; of which 14 were confirmed at autopsy (Wenning, Shlomo, et al., 1994). The population consisted of 67 men and 33 women, with a median age at onset of 53 years (range: 33 to 76). Autonomic symptoms were present at onset in only 41% of the patients, but 97% developed autonomic dysfunction during the course of the disease. Whereas impotence was the most frequent autonomic symptom in males, urinary incontinence predominated in women. Some evidence of orthostatic hypotension was present in 68% of patients, but severe orthostatic hypotension was noted in only 15%. In contrast to PD and other parkinsonian disorders in which the latency to onset of orthostatic hypotension is usually several years, patients with MSA usually develop symptomatic orthostatic hypotension within the first year after onset of symptoms (Wenning et al., 1999), and urinary dysfunction may occur even earlier (Sakakibara et al., 2000a, 2000b). Parkinsonism was the predominant motor disorder in SND, while gait ataxia was the usual presentation of the OPCA type of MSA. Tremor was present in only 29% and was typical "pill-rolling" in only 9%. Although 29% of all patients had initial good or excellent response to levodopa, this benefit was usually short-lived; only 13% maintained a good response to levodopa. Facial dystonia (often asymmetric) was a typical levodopa-induced complication in patients with MSA. In another study of 16 autopsy-proven cases of MSA, Litvan, Goetz, and colleagues (1997) identified early severe autonomic failure, absence of cognitive impairment, early cerebellar symptoms, and early gait problems as the best predictors of the diagnosis of MSA. In a study designed to validate the clinical criteria for MSA, Litvan, Booth, and colleagues (1998) found that the accuracy was best when at least six of the following eight features were present: sporadic adult onset, dysautonomia, parkinsonism, pyramidal signs, cerebellar signs, no levodopa response, no cognitive dysfunction, and no downward gaze palsy. Wenning and colleagues (1997) examined the clinical features of 203 pathologically proven cases of MSA reported in 108 publications. The male:female ratio was 1.3:1, dysautonomia was present in 74%, parkinsonism in 87%, cerebellar ataxia in 54%, and pyramidal signs in 49%. The progression and prognosis were analyzed in 230 Japanese patients with MSA; the median time from onset to aid-requiring walking, confinement to wheelchair, bedridden state, and death were 3, 5, 8, and 9 years, respectively (Watanabe et al., 2002). MSA-P patients had more rapid deterioration than MSA-C patients. When patients present with parkinsonism alone, without other evidence of MSA, their MSA might be difficult to differentiate from PD during the first 6 years (Albanese et al., 1995). In one study, the following features were found to be the best predictors of MSA: dysautonomia, poor response to levodopa, speech or bulbar dysfunction, falls, and absence of dementia and of levodopa-induced confusion (Wenning et al., 2000). It should be noted, however, that pure autonomic failure (PAF) might herald the onset not only of MSA but also of PD and DLB (Kaufmann et al., 2004; Mabuchi et al., 2005). In PAF, orthostatic hypotension and sudomotor dysfunction followed by constipation are the typical initial symptoms, whereas in MSA, the initial presentation usually consists of urinary problems, followed by sudomotor dysfunction or orthostatic hypotension, with subsequent progression to respiratory dysfunction (Mabuchi et al., 2005).

Prior to reclassification of sporadic OPCA as MSA-C, there were many attempts to characterize the different forms of OPCA. Approximately one quarter of patients with sporadic OPCA, particularly those with older-onset ataxia, develop parkinsonian features and evolve into MSA-C (Gilman et al., 2000). Berciano (1992) reviewed 133 (68 familial and 65 sporadic) pathologically proven cases of OPCA. While there was a nearly 2:1 male preponderance in familial OPCA, no gender difference was found in the sporadic form. Age at onset was more variable in this disorder than in the other parkinsonism-plus syndromes, ranging from infancy to 66 years. Cerebellar ataxia was the presenting symptom in 73% of all patients; 8.2% began with parkinsonian symptoms, and the remainder presented with nonspecific symptoms. Dementia, gaze impairment, dysarthria, dysphagia, incontinence, and upper and lower motor neuron signs usually become apparent within a few years after onset. In one large Japanese family with OPCA, the oculomotor abnormalities consisted of limitation of upgaze and convergence, horizontal gaze nystagmus, relative sparing of pupil reactivity, and loss of vestibulo-ocular responses (Shimizu et al., 1990). Autopsy of one patient in this series revealed degeneration of the oculomotor nucleus with sparing of the Edinger-Westphal nucleus. Neuropsychological evaluation in patients with clinically diagnosed OPCA revealed emotionality, anxiety, and a tendency toward depression without cognitive decline (Brent et al., 1990). Other studies, however, noted some degree of dementia in up to 80% of patients (Berciano, 1992).

While this review focuses on the sporadic forms of OPCA, it is worth pointing out that the classification of familial cerebellar ataxias has been markedly facilitated by the discoveries of specific mutations associated with the different phenotypes. Of the autosomal-dominant cerebellar ataxias with known genetic defects, SCA1, SCA2, SCA3, Machado-Joseph disease (Kawaguchi et al., 1994; Lu et al., 2004), SCA21, and dentato-rubral-pallidoluysian atrophy (Komure et al., 1995; Warner et al., 1995) are associated with extrapyramidal features, including parkinsonism (Rosenberg, 1995). Young-onset, levodopa-responsive parkinsonism may be the presentation of

SCA2 and may precede the onset of ataxia by 25 years (Furtado et al., 2002; Lu at el, 2002; Payami et al., 2003; Furtado et al., 2004; Lu et al., 2004). Although rarely pathologic features of sporadic MSA are found in the autosomal-dominant form of SCA (Gilman, Sima, et al., 1996), the typical sporadic MSA is genetically distinct from the inherited forms of SCA and OPCA (Bandmann et al., 1997). These disorders should be differentiated from cortical cerebellar atrophy and SCA, in which cerebellar signs are unaccompanied by autonomic features (Bürk et al., 1996; Dürr et al., 1996; Gilman and Quinn, 1996; Hammans, 1996; Osaki et al., 2002). Pathologically, there might be some similarities between the central disorders, including the presence of GCI in rare cases of SCA, but the spinal cord is usually more atrophied in SCA than in MSA. Some features of MSA overlap with the syndrome of fragile X–associated tremor/ataxia syndrome caused by permutations of the fragile X mental retardation 1 gene (*FMR1*), and fragile X–associated tremor/ataxia syndrome may be a rare cause of MSA (Biancalana et al., 2005).

Movement disorders other than parkinsonism that are seen in patients with MSA include dystonia, stimulus-sensitive cortical myoclonus, hemiballism, and chorea, unrelated to dopaminergic therapy (Chen et al., 1992; Steiger et al., 1992; Salazar et al., 2000). Dystonia is relatively rare in MSA patients (Rivest et al., 1990), but in one study, 46% of patients with MSA were found to have dystonia, particularly if anterocollis is considered a form of cervical dystonia (Boesch et al., 2002). Although dystonia is frequently considered to be a cause of the MSA-associated anterocollis, the mechanism of progressive neck flexion, so characteristic of MSA, particularly MSA-P, may be multifactorial. In some cases, the neck flexion has been attributed to neck extensor weakness as part of "dropped head" syndrome associated with axial myopathy (Suarez and Kelly, 1992; Oerlemans and de Visser, 1998; Askmark et al., 2001), motor neuron disease (Gourie-Devi et al., 2003), or other causes. Neck flexion, however, is not unique to MSA and can also be seen in patients with otherwise typical PD (Djaldetti et al., 1999). In some cases of PD, more frequently than in MSA, the axial postural abnormality may lead to severe flexion of the trunk, the so-called bent spine syndrome, or camptocormia (Umapathi et al., 2002; Azher and Jankovic, 2005). Another abnormal posture frequently encountered in MSA is the "Pisa syndrome," which is characterized by the leaning of the body to one side (reminiscent of the leaning Tower of Pisa) (Ashour and Jankovic, 2006) (Video 10-8).  Besides anterocollis, another form of dystonia that is relatively frequently encountered in patients with MSA is facial and oromandibular dystonia associated with levodopa therapy. As was noted earlier in the chapter, inspiratory stridor may be a variant of laryngeal dystonia (Merlo et al., 2002). In addition to action myoclonus (see Video 10-8), focal reflex myoclonus, induced by pinprick, may be seen in MSA patients (Clouston et al., 1996; Salazar et al., 2000). This form of myoclonus has a longer latency than that seen in patients with CBD (see later). In 9 of 11 patients with MSA and myoclonic tremulous movements, jerk-locked averaging technique showed premyoclonic potential, suggesting that the jerk-like movements represent a form of cortical myoclonus (Okuma et al., 2005).

Although dysautonomia is a cardinal feature of MSA, this neurodegenerative disorder should be differentiated from PAF, which has no central component (Mathias, 1997). Autonomic dysfunction is essential for the diagnosis of MSA, and in many cases of MSA, autonomic failure, particularly impotence, precedes other neurologic symptoms or signs by several years. In contrast to PD associated with dysautonomia, in which there is growing evidence of peripheral, particularly myocardial (Goldstein et al., 2002), sympathetic denervation, the peripheral autonomic system appears to be spared in MSA; in fact, some persistence of central autonomic tone might be responsible for the frequently observed supine hypertension in MSA (Parikh et al., 2002). The "cold hands" sign, manifested by a cold, dusky, violaceous appearance of the hands, is another characteristic feature of MSA (Klein et al., 1997). Some patients have the "cold feet" sign (Video 10-9). Liquid meal, consisting chiefly of glucose and milk, markedly reduces blood pressure in patients with MSA but not in those with PD (Thomaides et al., 1993) (see Video 10-9). Respiratory disturbance, including severe obstructive sleep apnea, and vocal cord paralysis with stridor may be found in more advanced stages of the disease (Munschauer et al., 1990). Inspiratory stridor due to the paradoxical movement of the vocal cords (also known as Gerhardt syndrome) has been described in MSA (Eissler et al., 2001). The observation that stridor improves with botulinum toxin injections into the adductor laryngeal muscles suggests that this symptom of MSA could be due to focal laryngeal dystonia (Merlo et al., 2002). The occurrence of nocturnal or daytime stridor carries a poor prognosis, particularly when it is associated with central hypoventilation (Silber and Levine, 2000). Occasionally, however, vocal cord abductor paralysis can be seen even in the initial stages of the disease, and it has been associated with nocturnal sudden death (Isozaki et al., 1996). Early diagnosis can be made by laryngoscopy during sleep. Impaired hypoxic ventilatory response has been reported in patients with MSA, and in one study, this feature helped to differentiate MSA-C from idiopathic late-onset cerebellar ataxia (Tsuda et al., 2002).

## Natural History

The natural history of MSA has been the subject of several recent studies. In contrast to the approximately 1.5% annual decline in Unified Parkinson's Disease Rating Scale III noted in patients with PD (Jankovic and Kapadia, 2001), the average annual decline in MSA-P is 28.3% (Seppi et al., 2005). Since most of the studies were based on pathologically proven cases, the prognosis in these series has been worse than otherwise predicted. In one study of 59 patients with MSA that included 25 with SDS, 24 with OPCA, and 10 with SND, the survival rate was poorest in those with SDS, followed by those with SND and OPCA (Saito et al., 1994). On the basis of a meta-analysis of 433 reported cases of MSA, Ben-Shlomo and colleagues (1997) found survival to range from 0.5 to 24 years (mean: 6.2 years), and cerebellar features were associated with marginally better survival. In one study of 100 patients clinically diagnosed with probable MSA (14 of whom were pathologically confirmed), nearly half of all the patients were markedly disabled or wheelchair bound within 5 years after onset, and the median survival was 9.5 years (Wenning, Shlomo, et al., 1994) (Fig. 10-2). In another study, the investigators analyzed 35 pathologically confirmed cases of MSA and confirmed a direct correlation between severity of disease and nigrostriatal cell loss (Wenning et al., 1995). Although marked degeneration in the olivopontocerebellar system, particularly the cerebellar vermis, was noted in 88% of the brains, the cere-

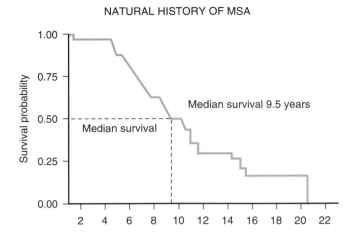

**NATURAL HISTORY OF MSA**

Figure 10-2 A survival curve indicating the progression of patients with MSA.

bellar pathology did not correlate with the presence of cerebellar signs. Although some authors have suggested that the earlier and the more severe the involvement of the autonomic nervous system, the poorer the prognosis (Saito et al., 1994), this has not been confirmed by other studies (Ben-Shlomo et al., 1997). MSA patients usually die from aspiration, sleep apnea, or cardiac arrhythmia.

## Epidemiology

The average annual incidence rate for MSA has been estimated to be 3.0 new cases per 100,000 person-years. (Bower et al., 1997), and the age-adjusted prevalence has been estimated at 4.4 per 100,000 (Schrag et al., 1999). Some studies have shown that, like PD, smoking is significantly less frequent in patients with MSA, and farming is an independent risk factor for MSA (Vanacore et al., 2005).

## Neurodiagnostic Studies

In addition to tests of autonomic function, patterns of plasma levels of catecholamines and their metabolites may be helpful in differentiating the various forms of autonomic failures (Cohen et al., 1987; Goldstein et al., 1989; Polinsky, 1993; Mathias, 1995; American Academy of Neurology, 1996; Parikh et al., 2002). These studies are designed primarily to localize the site of autonomic impairment and include investigation of neurogenic bladder (Fowler, 1996), sphincter electromyography (EMG) (Stocchi et al., 1997), and other investigations designed to test the integrity of the autonomic nervous system. Neurogenic sphincter electromyography, however, can also be seen in other disorders, including PD, PSP, Huntington disease, and a variety of common urologic problems (Colosimo et al., 1999; Giladi et al., 2000; Vodusek, 2001). Although anorectal dysfunction does not differentiate MSA from PD, external anal sphincter electromyography denervation is a very sensitive measure of anorectal dysfunction (Tison et al., 2000), and this abnormality occurs much earlier in MSA than in PD (Stocchi et al., 2000). Patients with SDS show a deficit in the central component of the baroreflex, whereas peripheral sympathetic pathways are affected primarily in the syndrome of

PAF. While the peripheral sympathetic neurons are spared in MSA, there is some evidence that they lack the normal preganglionic activation (Parikh et al., 2002). Furthermore, the relatively well-preserved sympathetic tone is probably responsible for the supine hypertension that is seen in most patients with MSA. In neurogenic orthostatic hypotension, the rise in NE levels is minimal or absent despite a marked drop in blood pressure after either head-up tilt or an upright position. Clonidine has been found to increase growth hormone in normal controls, patients with PAF, and patients with PD but not patients with MSA (Thomaides et al., 1992; Kimber et al., 1997). Whether this clonidine-GH test can reliably differentiate between MSA and PD, as Kimber and colleagues (1997) suggested, awaits further clinical-pathologic studies. Using PET scan technology to measure 6-[$^{18}$F]fluoro-dopamine-derived radioactivity in the myocardium, Goldstein and colleagues found normal rates of cardiac spillover of NE and normal production of levodopa, dihydroxyphenyl-glycol, and dihydroxyphenylacetic acid suggestive of intact cardiac sympathetic terminals in patients with SDS (Goldstein et al., 1997). This is in contrast to absent radioactivity in patients with PAF, indicating loss of postganglionic sympathetic terminals in this peripheral autonomic disorder. The value of this test in diagnosing MSA has been questioned (Mathias, 1997), however, since both sympathetic and parasympathetic failure have been associated with MSA. Neurochemical changes seen in MSA are similar to those present in PAF, and some suggest that MSA represents a central progression from PAF (McLeod and Tuck, 1987a, 1987b). Pharmacologically, these two conditions may be distinguished by supine and standing plasma NE levels. In PAF, both standing and supine NE levels are low, while in MSA, only the standing value is diminished. Besides decreased NE, acetylcholine and cerebrospinal fluid (CSF) acetylcholinesterase levels are also reduced (Polinsky et al., 1989). This is consistent with the notion that postganglionic sympathetic neurons are intact in MSA but their function is markedly impaired in PAF.

In a study comparing polysomnograms of seven patients with SDS with those of seven control patients, significant obstructive sleep apnea without oxygen desaturation was seen in four of the five nontracheotomized SDS patients; three of these patients later died suddenly during sleep (Munschauer et al., 1990). In a more recent study, Plazzi and colleagues (1997) demonstrated that 90% of MSA patients experience some form of REM sleep behavioral disorder (RBD). Using [$^{11}$C]DTBZ PET and [$^{123}$I]iodobenzovesamicol single-photon emission computed tomography (SPECT), Gilman, Koeppe, and colleagues (2003) showed that RBD in patients with MSA correlates with nigrostriatal dopaminergic deficit. Furthermore, obstructive sleep apnea in MSA is related to a thalamic cholinergic deficit, possibly owing to decreased pontine cholinergic projections (Gilman, Chervin, et al., 2003). While somatosensory, visual, and auditory evoked responses are often abnormal, motor evoked potentials are usually normal (Abele et al., 2000). In one study, 73% of patients with SDS had abnormal brainstem auditory evoked responses (Sinatra et al., 1988).

Neuroimaging, specifically designed to assess putaminal integrity, may prove helpful in differentiating MSA from PD and in predicting levodopa response (Drayer et al., 1989; Stern et al., 1989). MRI in patients with SDS sometimes reveals areas of decreased signal bilaterally in the posterolateral putamen on T2-weighted images (Pastakia et al., 1986). Although increased levels of iron may contribute to this hypointensity, reactive microgliosis and astrogliosis may also play an important role. In addition to striatal (putaminal) hypointensity on T2-weighted MRI scans, a characteristic finding in patients with MSA, particularly MSA-P, is the slit-hyperintensity in the lateral margin of the putamen (Savoiardo et al., 1994). This abnormality was found in 17 of 28 (61%) of patients with clinically diagnosed MSA (Konagaya et al., 1994). Although not all MSA patients with this slit-hyperintensity had parkinsonism, none of the 25 patients with clinically diagnosed PD demonstrated this finding on MRI. Although hyperintense putaminal rim is quite specific for MSA, putaminal hypointensity was not found to be a useful discriminator in one study (Schrag et al., 1998). Using DWI-MRI, Schocke and colleagues (2002) found that regional apparent diffusion coefficient values are increased in the putamen of patients with MSA, and this evidence of striatal degeneration apparently reliably differentiates MSA from PD. Ghaemi and colleagues (2002) found that both multitracer PET and three-dimensional MRI-based volumetry are very sensitive measures and that they reliably differentiate MSA from PD by demonstrating decreased putaminal volume, glucose metabolism, and postsynaptic D2 receptor density in patients with MSA. These techniques, when applied to the imaging of the midbrain, did contribute additional gain in diagnostic accuracy. In one study, however, the typical "hot cross bun" sign in the pons was present on MRI in 63% of patients (Watanabe et al., 2002). This study also drew attention to the involvement of the cortex in MSA. T2*-weighted gradient echo was more sensitive in demonstrating hypointense putaminal changes than T2-weighted fast spin echo MRI (Kraft et al., 2002) (Fig. 10-3). A diagnostic algorithm based on brain MRIs has been proposed (Bhattacharya et al., 2002). Using proton magnetic resonance spectroscopy, Davie and colleagues (1995) showed a significant reduction in the N-acetylaspartate (NAA)/creatine ratio from the lentiform nucleus in six of seven patients with MSA and in only one of nine patients with PD. Similar abnormalities were found in some patients with OPCA and most likely reflect regional neuronal loss. Further studies are needed to determine whether this technique can reliably differentiate between MSA and PD. Brain parenchyma sonography has been used in one study to differentiate PD from atypical parkinsonism, mostly MSA (Walter et al., 2003). The investigators found that 24 of 25 (96%) patients with PD exhibited hyperechogenicity, whereas only 2 of 23 (9%) patients with atypical parkinsonism showed a similar pattern. They concluded that brain parenchyma sonography might be highly specific in differentiating between PD and atypical parkinsonism. Computed tomography and MRI scans in patients with OPCA (MSA-C) typically show pancerebellar and brainstem atrophy, enlarged fourth ventricle and cerebellopontine angle cisterns, and demyelination of transverse pontine fibers on T2-weighted MRI images (Berciano, 1992). Although the MRI findings in MSA are highly specific, they have low sensitivity (Schrag et al., 2000). In a cross-sectional study of 15 MSA-P patients and 17 PD patients matched for age and disease duration, there were lower activity ratios of striatal to frontal uptake on IBZM-SPECT; and on diffusion-weighted imaging (DWI), there were similar differences in the regional apparent diffusion coefficients (rADC). The findings from DWI were more accurate when compared to IBZM-SPECT based on the higher specificity, predictive accuracy,

MULTIPLE-SYSTEM ATROPHY

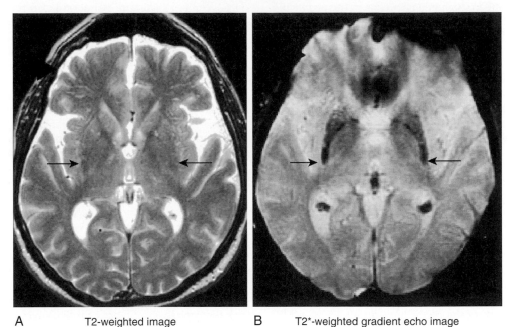

| A | T2-weighted image | B | T2*-weighted gradient echo image |

Figure 10-3 Typical MRI findings in patients with MSA. **A**, Axial T2-weighted image in a patient with MSA, signal intensity: putamen = pallidum. **B**, T2*-weighted GE image: marked hypointensity in the putamen compared with the pallidum.

and positive predictive values of both the methods. Further studies using DWI validating these changes with disease progression are needed (Seppi et al., 2004).

PET scanning has revealed decreased striatal and frontal lobe metabolism (De Volder et al., 1989; Brooks, Ibanez, et al., 1990; Eidelberg et al., 1993) and a reduction in D2 receptor density in the striatum (Brooks et al., 1992; Antonini et al., 1997). Using [18F]fluorodeoxyglucose, [18F]fluorodopa, and [11C]raclopride (RACLO) PET scans, Antonini and colleagues (1997) showed that the combination of [18F]fluorodeoxyglucose and [11C]raclopride scans reliably differentiated between MSA and PD, but [18F]fluorodopa PET scans could not distinguish between the different forms of parkinsonism. In a study of three patients with SDS, the two with more advanced stages of the disease showed reduced 18F-6-fluorodopa uptake, indicating nigrostriatal dysfunction (Bhatt et al., 1990). Gilman and colleagues (1999) found significantly reduced specific binding to the type 2 vesicular monoamine transporter using PET and [11C]dihydrotetrabenazine as a type 2 vesicular monoamine transporter ligand in striatal monoaminergic presynaptic terminal of patients with MSA. PET scans in patients with MSA-C show a reduced metabolic rate in the brainstem and cerebellum (Gilman, 2002), and these changes can be detected even before the onset of extrapyramidal features (Gilman, Frey, et al., 1996). A study of 10 patients with the sporadic OPCA form of MSA showed that the 18F-fluorodopa uptake was reduced by a mean of 21% in the putamen, and 11C-diprenorphine uptake was reduced by a mean of 22% (Rinne et al., 1995). Although the authors suggest that these findings support "subclinical" nigrostriatal dysfunction, all of the patients were clinically impaired, and some were disabled by severe ataxia and autonomic dysfunction. The reduced 11C-diprenorphine uptake suggests that in addition to involvement of the nigrostriatal projection, some MSA patients have a loss of intrinsic striatal neurons that contain presynaptic and postsynaptic mu, kappa, and delta opioid receptors.

Besides neuroimaging, transcranial ultrasonography has been reported to provide high diagnostic yield in differentiating PD from atypical parkinsonian disorders. Sonographic studies in 102 patients with PD, 34 with MSA, and 21 with PSP found marked unilateral or bilateral hyperechogenicity in 89% of 88 patients with PD, 25% of 32 patients with MSA-P, and 39% of 18 patients with PSP (Behnke et al., 2005).

## Neuropathology and Neurochemistry

The spectrum of pathologic changes in MSA includes cell loss, gliosis, and demyelination in the striatum (caudate and putamen), SN, locus coeruleus, inferior olives, pontine nuclei, dorsal vagal nuclei, Purkinje cells of the cerebellum, intermediolateral cell columns, and Onuf's nucleus of the caudal spinal cord. Involvement of at least three of these areas, including the putamen and SN, is required for the pathologic diagnosis of MSA (Quinn, 1994; Ito et al., 1996). In one pathologic study of 100 MSA cases (46 men and 54 women), 34% were categorized as SND, 17% were categorized as OPCA (MSA-C), and the reminder (49%) had a mixed pathology (Ozawa et al., 2004). On the basis of the distribution of GCIs and correlation of the clinicopathologic changes, the study showed that GCIs might be contributing to neuronal damage in the MSA-C type more than the MSA-P type, suggesting the possibility of different mechanisms of cell death in the subtypes of MSA. The brunt of the pathology in MSA brains is in the dorsolateral portion of the striatum and ventrolateral portion of the globus pallidus and SN, and the degree of response to levodopa seems to correlate inversely with the severity of the striatal efferent involvement (Ito et al., 1996). The putamen is the most prominently affected, with neuronal cell loss and deposition of iron, producing brownish pigmentation (O'Brien et al., 1990). Cholinergic neurons in the pedunculopontine nucleus and laterodorsal tegmentum and noradrenergic neurons in the locus coeruleus have been found to be markedly depleted in the brains of patients with MSA, whereas the serotonergic rostral raphe neurons are well preserved (Benarroch et al., 2002). Lewy bodies or NFTs are not common. Using calcineurin immunostaining, Goto and colleagues (1996) found marked neuronal loss, particularly in the caudal and lateral portion of the putamen, with corresponding degeneration of the GPi, GPe, and ventrolateral portion of the SNr. The same group (Goto et al., 1990b) noted selective degeneration of the met-enkephalin-containing neurons in the putamen and GPe, with relative preservation of the caudate nucleus. Previous studies have noted low levels of dopamine and increased activity of dopamine β-hydroxylase, the NE-synthesizing enzyme, in the midbrain. Vasomotor impairment in SND has been attributed to selective loss of tyrosine hydroxylase-immunoreactive neurons in the A1 and A2 regions of the medulla oblongata (Malessa et al., 1990). Calbindin-D$_{28k}$ immunoreactivity in the striatal projection system is markedly decreased in the brains of patients with SND (Ito et al., 1992) and in Purkinje cells of the cerebellum in patients with MSA (Wüllner et al., 2000). Reduced calcium-binding capacity in these neurons might affect the bcl-2 family of proteins and lead to apoptosis of selected neuronal regions not only in PD but also in other neurodegenerative diseases, such as MSA. The small myelinated fibers innervating the vocal cord are lost in nearly all patients with MSA, but when the large myelinated fibers of the recurrent laryngeal nerve become affected, as is seen in some patients with SND, vocal cord paralysis becomes evident and may be life-threatening (Hayashi et al., 1997).

The fundamental pathologic changes in OPCA (MSA-C), whether familial or sporadic, are a loss of Purkinje cells in the cerebellar cortex, particularly in the vermis, and degeneration of the olivopontine nuclei (Wenning et al., 1996). In addition to cerebellar atrophy, SN degeneration and depigmentation, neuronal loss in other brainstem nuclei, and demyelination of corticospinal tracts and posterior columns are seen (Koeppen et al., 1986; Matsuo et al., 1998). One clinical-pathologic study found a strong correlation between the frequency of neuronal cytoplasmic inclusions exclusively found in the pontine nucleus and the severity of olivopontocerebellar degeneration. The immunohistochemical and ultrastructural features of the neuronal inclusions were identical to those of the glial inclusions (Yokoyama et al., 2001). Detailed morphometric and biochemical studies of OPCA brains correlated reductions in aspartic and glutamic acid with Purkinje cell loss in the cerebellar cortex and with neuronal cell loss in the inferior olives (aspartic acid) (Bebin et al., 1990). In addition, quisqualate receptors appear to be decreased, while quinolinic acid metabolism is increased (Makoweic et al., 1990; Kish et al., 1991). The increased quinolinic acid phosphoribosyl-transferase activity in OPCA has been interpreted as a compensatory mechanism designed to protect quinolinic acid–sensitive granule cells (Kish et al., 1991). In addition, low glutamate dehydrogenase activity has been found in most, but not all, studies; however, this defect probably is not disease-specific (Berciano, 1992; Kostic et al., 1989). In a study of 14 brains of patients with OPCA, Kish and colleagues (1992) found a 53% reduction in dopamine in the putamen, 35% in the caudate, and 31% in the nucleus accumbens. Only two patients had severe neuronal loss in SN and a corresponding dopamine depletion in the

striatum. Mitochondrial deoxyribonucleic acid abnormalities have been postulated to be important in the pathogenesis of OPCA in some patients (Truong et al., 1990). A mitochondrial DNA G11778 mutation has been identified in a family with levodopa-responsive parkinsonism and multisystem degeneration (Simon et al., 1999).

Degeneration of the catecholaminergic neurons in the intermediate reticular formation of the rostral ventrolateral medulla seems to correlate well with autonomic failure in patients with MSA (Benarroch et al., 1998, 2000). The medial spiny neurons that give rise to both the direct pathway from the striatum to the GPi and the indirect pathway from the striatum to the GPe are affected. Gliosis, however, seems to be much more prevalent in GPe than in GPi. Upregulation of D1 receptors, determined by dopamine-stimulated adenylyl cyclase, has been demonstrated in brains of patients with PD as compared to PSP and MSA ($n = 10$ each); it is actually reduced in MSA (Tong et al., 2004). While the median CSF concentration of the neurotransmitter metabolites 5-hydroxyindolacetic acid and 3-methoxy-4-hydroxyphenylethyleneglycol was reduced significantly (49% to 70%) in MSA compared to PD, several brain-specific proteins (tau, neuron-specific enolase, myelin basic protein) were elevated (130% to 230%) in MSA compared with those in PD (Abdo et al., 2004). Although a combination of CSF tau and 3-methoxy-4-hydroxyphenylethyleneglycol significantly discriminated PD from MSA, it is too early to recommend routine use of CSF in differentiating these two disorders.

The discovery in 1989 by Papp and Lantos (Papp et al., 1989) of the characteristic histologic marker, the GCIs, led to improved characterization of MSA as a clinical-pathologic entity. These inclusions are particularly concentrated in the oligodendrogliocytes and have been found in all autopsied brains of patients with SDS, SND, and sporadic OPCA. This shared pathologic feature strongly argues in support of the notion that these three disorders should be regarded as variants of the same disease entity, namely, MSA (Kato and Nakamura, 1990; Arima et al., 1992; Murayama et al., 1992; Papp and Lantos, 1992; Lantos and Papp, 1994; Quinn, 1994; Wenning, Quinn, et al., 1994). GCI, argyophilic, perinuclear inclusions with a diameter varying from 4 μm to 20 μm are found particularly in the oligodendrogliocytes in the supplementary motor cortex, anterior central gyrus, putamen, pallidum, basal pons, and medullary reticular formation. They are composed of 20- to 30-nm straight tubules, and they contain ubiquitin, tau protein, α- and β-tubulin, MAP-5, αB-crystallin, and α-synuclein. Several studies have documented the presence of α-synuclein in the GCI (Spillantini et al., 1998; Tu et al., 1998; Wakabayashi et al., 1998), but the significance of this finding is uncertain (Mezey et al., 1998). Although very characteristic of MSA, GCIs have rarely been found in other disorders, such as CBD, PSP, and autosomal-dominant spinocerebellar ataxia (Gilman, Sima, et al., 1996). The characteristics and distribution of the inclusions, however, may be slightly different from the typical GCIs that are seen in MSA. Originally, α-synuclein was identified as the precursor protein for the non-Aβ component (**NAC**) of Alzheimer of amyloid plaques, and these plaques have been found to contain fragments of the α-synuclein protein (NAC precursor protein, or NACP). NACP/α-synuclein accumulates not only in Lewy bodies but also as small granules in neurons and as diffuse deposits in the neuronal process in PD brains (Shoji et al., 2000). In addition, NACP accumulates in cortical astrocytes. The distribution and cell type of NACP accumulation are similar in DLB, but in MSA, NACP accumulates chiefly in the oligodendroglia and olivary neurons. α-Synuclein is selectively and extensively phosphorylated at serine 129, especially by casein kinase 1 and 2, in various synucleinopathies, including MSA (Fujiwara et al., 2002). Recently, p39 immunoreactive GCIs have been reported as the hallmark of GCI in MSA (Honjyo et al., 2001). A cdk5 (cyclin-dependent kinase) activator in oligodendrocytes, p39 induces formation of GCI in the oligodendrocytes. Midkine, a neurotrophic factor, has also been identified in the GCI, indicating a rescue of neurons via oligode (Burn and Jaros, 2001). Only 10% of the MSA cases are found to have Lewy bodies (Ozawa et al., 2004). A significant correlation has been found between the frequency of GCIs, severity of neuronal cell loss, and disease duration (Ozawa et al., 2004).

Using antibodies against certain components of myelin basic protein, several investigators found evidence of extensive myelin degeneration in MSA, thus supporting the notion of widespread oligodendroglial dysfunction in MSA (Castellani, 1998; Matsuo et al., 1998). Other studies found evidence of apoptosis in the glia, but not neurons, of MSA brains (Probst-Cousin et al., 1998). Furthermore, microglial activation involving translocation of NF-kappB/Rel A to the nucleus was found to be particularly prominent in affected brain regions (Schwarz et al., 1998).

In addition to the typical findings in the brain, there is a marked loss of neurons in the lateral horns of the spinal cord, but these pathologic changes correlate poorly with dysautonomia (Gray et al., 1988). Substance P–like immunoreactivity was markedly decreased in laminae I + II of the fourth thoracic and third lumbar spinal cord segments in 10 of 11 SDS patients, and all had a decrease in small and large myelinated fibers in the fourth thoracic ventral roots (Tomokane et al., 1991).

## Pathogenesis

The cause of MSA is unknown, and genetic factors probably do not play an important role. Recent findings link MSA to PD and related neurodegenerative disorders as "α-synucleinopathies" (Jaros and Burn, 2000; Galvin et al., 2001). While many studies have investigated the putative role of environmental toxins in the pathogenesis of idiopathic PD, the possible role of such toxins in MSA has received little attention. Ten patients whose clinical features were consistent with MSA and in whom toxins were suspected to play an etiologic role were investigated (Hanna et al., 1999). One patient with pathologically confirmed MSA was exposed to high concentrations of various toxins, including formaldehyde, malathion, and diazinon. The other MSA patients had a history of heavy exposure to various agents, such as n-hexane, benzene, methyl-isobutyl-ketone, and pesticides. The pathologic case revealed extensive advanced glial changes, including GCIs, which were seen particularly in the deep cerebellar white matter, brainstem, cortex (superior frontal, insula, and hippocampus), and putamen. Additionally, there was notable neuronal cell loss with depigmentation of the SN and locus coeruleus. Although a cause-and-effect relationship cannot be proven, these cases suggest that environmental toxins could play a role in the pathogenesis of some cases of MSA. The inverse relationship between PD and smoking has also been found with MSA but not with PSP (Vanacore et al., 2000). Although there is no experimental model of MSA, intraperitoneal injection of 3-acetylpyridine in rats produces neurochemical and histologic changes that are consistent with OPCA (Deutch et al., 1989). In addition to causing degeneration of the nigrostriatal dopaminergic pathway, this neurotoxin causes degeneration of the climbing fibers, which normally originate in the inferior olive and terminate in the cerebellum. Transgenic mice overexpressing human wild-type α-synuclein in oligodendrocytes exhibit many of the features of MSA (Yazawa et al., 2005).

## Treatment

About two thirds of patients with MSA respond to levodopa. Parkinsonian symptoms accompanying SDS are difficult to treat, because dopaminergic drugs frequently exacerbate the already prominent symptoms of orthostatic hypotension. The addition of liberal salt, fludrocortisone, and elastic stockings can improve standing blood pressures (Mathias and Kimber, 1998). However, parkinsonian patients have difficulty putting on elastic stockings, such as the Jobst stockings. In addition, physical maneuvers such as leg-crossing and squatting can alleviate orthostatic lightheadedness (Van Lieshout et al., 1992). In a double-blind, placebo-controlled study of 97 patients with various causes of autonomic failure, including 18 patients with SDS and 22 patients with PD, midodrine, a peripheral α-adrenergic agonist, has been found to be effective in the treatment of orthostatic hypotension (Jankovic, Gilden, et al., 1993; Jankovic, Rajput, et al., 1993). The safety and efficacy of midodrine were later confirmed by a larger controlled study involving a total of 171 patients with orthostatic hypotension (Low et al., 1997). Wright and colleagues (1998) showed dose-dependent increases in standing systolic blood pressure with midodrine in patients with MSA. In patients with neurally mediated recurrent syncope, midodrine reduced frequency of syncope from 67% (8 of 12) to 17% (2 of 12) when compared to placebo (Kaufmann et al., 2002). The most frequent side effects associated with the drug included piloerection, scalp pruritus, urinary retention, and supine hypertension. The effects of subcutaneous injections of octreotide, a somatostatin analog, were tested in a group of nine patients with MSA (Bordet et al., 1995). The drug improved orthostatic hypotension, and it allowed patients to maintain an upright posture for a longer period of time as compared to a placebo. Although this modest improvement was attributed to a release of NE by octreotide during maintenance of erect posture, no increase in plasma NE levels could be demonstrated. Other agents that are used to increase standing blood pressure include indomethacin, ibuprofen, pseudoephedrine and other sympathomimetics, caffeine and dihydroergotamine, yohimbine, and NE precursors, such as 3,4-dihydroxyphenyl serine (McLeod and Tuck, 1987a, 1987b; Polinsky, 1993; Senard et al., 1993; Freeman et al., 1999). All of these are of limited value, however, because of lack of efficacy or untoward side effects. Because fludrocortisone and midodrine, particularly when combined with liberal salt intake, increase the risk of supine hypertension, patients should be instructed to place their beds in the reverse Trendelenburg position. The use of nighttime nitroglyceride or clonidine patches has been suggested for the treatment of supine hypertension, but these measures are not always successful.

Bladder problems, particularly urinary retention and incontinence, are relatively common and often troublesome manifestations of MSA (Scientific Committee of the First International Consultation on Incontinence, 2000). Increased urinary frequency due to overactive bladder is less common and often improves with 5 mg of antimuscarinic oxybutynin

(Ditropan) three to four times per day and 2 mg of tolterodine (Detrol) three times per day. The latter drug may be better tolerated because it has eight times less affinity for the salivary gland, thus having much lower frequency of dry mouth. Use of 0.4 mg of the α-blocker tamsulosin (Flomax) twice a day may be effective if the urinary frequency is associated with benign prostatic hypertrophy; this condition must be excluded prior to the use of antimuscarinic agents. Prazosin and moxisylyte are specific antagonists of bladder α-adrenergic receptors. In a controlled study done in 49 patients, there was improvement in symptoms in 47.6% in the prazosin group and 53.6% in the moxisylyte group. Orthostatic hypotension was seen in about 23% in the prazosin group and 11% in the moxisylyte group. More than 35% of patients had reduction in residual volume, and there was improvement in urinary urgency, frequency, and incontinence. The dosage used was 1 mg of prazosin and 10 mg of moxisylyte three times a day in an oral form (Sakakibara et al., 2000a, 2000b). Sildenafil citrate (Viagra) has been found to be safe and effective in the treatment of erectile dysfunction associated with PD, but it may unmask orthostatic hypotension in patients with MSA (Zesiewicz et al., 2000; Hussain et al., 2001).

Despite the marked involvement of the striatum, many patients with MSA improve with levodopa, at least initially (Fearnley and Lees, 1990). Although patients with MSA often respond to dopaminergic therapy (levodopa or apomorphine), in contrast to those with PD, the MSA patients may experience dyskinesias without concomitant improvement in motor functioning (Hughes, Colosimo, et al., 1992). The levodopa-induced dyskinesias that are seen in MSA patients seem to be more dystonic, often involving the face rather than the choreic or stereotypic movements that are characteristically seen in patients with PD. Furthermore, MSA patients do not seem to notice a recurrence of parkinsonian symptoms until several days after levodopa withdrawal. In one study, only four of eight patients with MSA had a moderate response to levodopa; in contrast, all eight control patients with PD had a consistently good response to levodopa (Parati et al., 1993). Ataxia, present in patients with the OPCA type of MSA, does not respond to pharmacologic therapy and has to be treated by physical means, such as a cane or a walker. In a study of 20 patients with MSA, Iranzo and colleagues (2000) found vocal cord abduction dysfunction in 14 (70%); and in 3 of 3 patients, continuous positive airway pressure completely eliminated laryngeal stridor, obstructive apnea, and hemoglobin desaturation. In another study, continuous positive airway pressure effectively ameliorated nocturnal stridor in 13 patients with MSA (Iranzo et al., 2004). Tracheostomy or other airway restoration techniques must sometimes be performed in patients who have vocal cord abductor paralysis (Isozaki et al., 1996). Stridor has been reported to improve with botulinum toxin injections into the adductor laryngeal muscles (Merlo et al., 2002). (See Appendix 10-1.)

# CORTICOBASAL GANGLIONIC DEGENERATION

## Clinical Features and Natural History

In 1968, Rebeiz and colleagues (1968) reported three patients of Irish descent with parkinsonism, myoclonus, supranuclear palsy, and apraxia who were found at autopsy to have "corti-

codentatonigral degeneration with neuronal achromasia." The full spectrum of clinical manifestations of this complex neurodegenerative disorder was not fully recognized until recently. Since cerebellar deficit is not a feature of the disorder, the term *corticobasal ganglionic degeneration* has been used to describe the predominant involvement of the cortex and the basal ganglia; the term *corticobasal degeneration* is also used, particularly in the European literature (Mahapatra et al., 2004). The most striking features of CBD include marked asymmetry of involvement; focal rigidity and dystonia with or without contractures; and hand, limb, gait, and speech apraxia (Video 10-10). In addition, some patients manifest coarse rest and action tremor, cortical-type focal myoclonus (see Video 10-8), and parkinsonism, and in some cases cognitive decline may precede these classic features (Bergeron et al., 1998). Other features include cortical sensory deficit, language and speech alterations (Özsancak et al., 2000), frontal lobe symptomatology, depression, apathy, irritability, and agitation (Litvan, Cummings, et al., 1998).

The asymmetric onset differentiates CBD from most other neurodegenerative disorders, and some patients who have been categorized as having "asymmetric cortical degenerative syndrome" (Caselli et al., 2000) might have CBD. In a study of 14 patients with pathologically confirmed CBD, Wenning and colleagues (1998) found that asymmetric hand clumsiness was the most common presenting symptom, noted at onset in 50% of the patients. At the time of the first neurologic visit, about 3 years after onset, the following signs were present: unilateral limb rigidity (79%), bradykinesia (71%), ideomotor apraxia (64%), postural imbalance (45%), unilateral limb dystonia (43%), and cortical dementia (36%). The mean age at onset was $63 \pm 7.7$ years; the mean duration of symptoms from onset to death was $7.9 \pm 0.7$ years (range: 2.5 to 12.5). Patients with early bradykinesia, frontal syndrome, and two of the following three—tremor, rigidity, and bradykinesia—had a poor prognosis. These clinical features are similar to those described earlier by Rinne, Lee, and colleagues (1994), who reviewed 36 patients (20 females and 16 males), with a mean age at onset of $60.9 \pm 9.7$ years (range: 40 to 76). In the patients reported by Riley and colleagues (1990), the mean age at onset was 60 years (range: 51 to 71), and men were more commonly affected than women (3:2). Two patients died 7 and 10 years after disease onset. In a series of 147 cases collected from eight centers, the following features were most common: parkinsonism (100%), higher cortical dysfunction (93%), dyspraxia (82%), gait disorder (80%), dystonia (71%), tremor (55%), myoclonus (55%), alien limb (42%), cortical sensory loss (33%), dementia (25%) (Kompoliti et al., 1998).

The typical features of CBD can be categorized into movement disorders (akinesia, rigidity, postural instability, limb dystonia, cortical myoclonus, and postural/intention tremor) and cortical signs, such as cortical sensory loss, apraxias (ideational and ideomotor) (see Video 10-10), and the alien limb phenomenon (Video 10-11) (Riley et al., 1990; Rinne, Lee, et al., 1994). Ideomotor apraxia, possibly secondary to involvement of the supplementary motor area and characterized by not knowing "how to do it" (as opposed to not knowing "what to do" in ideational apraxia), is the most typical form of apraxia (Leiguarda et al., 1994; Leiguarda and Marsden, 2000). This apraxia may improve with tactile stimulation, such as the use of the appropriate tool (Graham et al., 1999). Using the De Renzi ideomotor apraxia test, Soliveri and colleagues (2005) compared limb apraxia in patients with CBD ($n = 24$) and PSP ($n = 25$). They found that "awkwardness errors," conceptually appropriate but clumsily executed actions because of impaired fine finger motility, were the most common apraxic error in patients with CBD, followed by spatial errors, characterized by incorrect orientation or trajectory of the arm, hand, or digits in space or in relation to the body. Sequence errors, incorrect sequences of actions or inappropriate repetition of movements, were least impaired in CBD. The order of impairment was reversed in patients with PSP. Overall, apraxia was more frequent and more severe in patients with CBD than in those with PSP. Limb contractures, often preceded by the alien hand phenomenon, are more common in this condition than in the other parkinsonism-plus syndromes (Doody and Jankovic, 1992; Leiguarda et al., 1994; Leiguarda and Marsden, 2000). This anterior or motor alien hand syndrome must be differentiated from sensory or posterior syndrome associated with a lesion in the thalamus, splenium of corpus callosum, and temporal-occipital lobe (Hakan et al., 1998). In autopsy-proven cases of CBD, the following were found to be the best predictors of the diagnosis of CBD: limb dystonia, ideomotor apraxia, myoclonus, and asymmetric akinetic-rigid syndrome with late onset of gait or balance disturbance (Litvan, Agid, Goetz, et al., 1997; Wenning et al., 1998). In some cases of CBD, the alien hand phenomenon is associated with spontaneous arm levitation. The latter has also been described in PSP (Barclay et al., 1999). In one study of 66 patients diagnosed clinically with CBD, 39 (59%) had dystonia (Vanek and Jankovic, 2001).

Neurologic examination often reveals asymmetric apraxia, oculomotility disturbance particularly manifested by impaired convergence and vertical and horizontal gaze palsy, bulbar impairment, focal myoclonus, mirror movements, hyperreflexia, Babinski sign, but no ataxia. In contrast to PSP, the vertical saccades are only slightly impaired in CBD and usually involve only upward gaze; furthermore, there is a marked increase in horizontal saccade latency in CBD, which correlates well with an "apraxia score" (Vidailhet et al., 1994. Focal myoclonus, usually involving one arm, present at rest and exacerbated by voluntary movement or in response to sensory stimulation, resembles typical cortical myoclonus but differs in several features. In contrast to the typical reflex cortical myoclonus, which is characterized by long latency (50 msec in the hand), enlarged somatosensory evoked responses (SEP), and cortical discharge preceding the movement, the reflex myoclonus associated with CBD is usually not associated with enlarged SEP and has a shorter latency from stimulus to jerk (40 msec) (Thompson et al., 1994). This suggests that the characteristic short-latency reflex myoclonus in CBD represents enhancement of a direct sensory-cortical pathway, whereas the more typical reflex cortical myoclonus involves abnormal sensorimotor cortical relays (Strafella et al., 1997). Using transcranial magnetic stimulation, Valls-Solé and colleagues (2001) found evidence of enhanced excitability, or reduced inhibition, in the motor area of the hemisphere contralateral to the alien hand sign in patients with CBD. [$^{18}$F]fluorodeoxyglucose PET scanning in patients with CBD and upper limb apraxia showed marked hypometabolism in the superior parietal lobule and supplementary motor area (Peigneux et al., 2001).

Despite the finding of "dementia as the most common presentation" of CBD (Grimes et al., 1999), in our experience, dementia is a late feature of CBD. Although apraxia and aphasia are common, semantic memory is usually well preserved (Graham et al., 2003a, 2003b). The full spectrum of clinical features typically seen in CBD can also be present in patients with documented Pick disease, but the latter disorder is usually dominated by cognitive, behavioral, and language disturbances, such as primary progressive aphasia (PPA) and semantic dementia (Kertesz et al., 1994; Bond Chapman et al., 1997; Litvan, Agid, Sastrj, et al., 1997; Hodges, 2001; Rossor, 2001; Graham et al., 2003b; Kertesz and Munoz, 2003). Maurice Ravel, the well-known French composer, was thought to have PPA, which later evolved to right hand apraxia and other features of CBD (Amaducci et al., 2002). Neuropsychological testing in patients with CBD typically shows deficits in frontal-striatal-parietal cognitive domains, including attention/concentration, executive functions, verbal fluency, praxis, language, and visuospatial functioning (Pillon, Blin, et al., 1995). Patients also typically exhibit impaired graphesthesia and may present with visuospatial dysfunction (Tang-Wai et al., 2003). This profile depends on which hemisphere is primarily affected. Usually characterized by word-finding disturbances (anomia), this language disorder then evolves into impairment of the grammatical structure (syntax) and comprehension (semantics) (Mesulam, 2003). In one study of 10 patients with PPA who were followed prospectively until they became nonfluent or mute, Kertesz and Munoz (2003) found that at autopsy, all had evidence of FTD: CBD in 4, Pick body dementia in 3, and tau and synuclein negative ubiquinated inclusions of the motor neuron disease in 3. Although no mutations were found in the *tau* gene in 25 patients with PPA, there was a significant overrepresentation of the tau H1/H1 genotype, also found in PSP and CBD (Mesulam, 2003; Sobrido et al., 2003). Imaging studies have shown that PPA is often associated with atrophy in the left frontotemporal region, and other areas such as the fusiform and precentral gyri and intrapariatal sulcus are activated, possibly as a compensatory neuronal strategy (Sonty et al., 2003). These and other studies provide evidence that PPA is related to dissociation with respect to grammatical and working memory aspects of sentence processing within the left frontal cortex (Grossman, 2002).

PPA is sometimes confused with the syndrome of slowly progressive anarthria that is seen in the late anterior opercular syndrome (see later), but in the latter syndrome, there is no associated language or cognitive deficit. The majority of patients with CBD have been found to have aphasia (e.g., anomic, Broca, and transcortical motor aphasia) (Frattali et al., 2000) with phonologic (e.g., spelling) impairment even without clinically observable aphasia (Graham et al., 2003b). Another disorder that progresses rapidly to a nonambulatory state and muteness is motor neuron disease–inclusion body dementia (MND-ID) (Josephs et al., 2003; Kleiner-Fisman et al., 2004). This entity, a subtype of FTD, which is confirmed only pathologically, usually begins in the patient's mid-40s and shares some features of CBD. Typically, the patients have early dysphagia suggestive of bulbar palsy but without fasciculations. Pathologically, the brain shows severe caudate atrophy, with intracytoplasmic inclusions that stain with antibodies against heavy and light subunits of neurofilaments and against ubiquitin. Families with clinical features of Pick disease and the pathologic picture of CBD have been described (Brown et al., 1996). In contrast, apraxia and parkinsonism, if present, are usually late findings in Pick disease, whereas personality changes, aggressive behavior, disinhibition, cognitive deficits, elements of Klüver-Bucy syndrome, and other features of FTD are common (Cherrier and Mendez, 1999; Nasreddine et al., 1999). CBD is probably most frequently confused with PSP, chiefly because of the overlapping oculomotor findings. The CBD patients, however, have much more marked asymmetry in their motor deficits, less severe ophthalmoparesis, and more prominent apraxia and myoclonus (see Table 10-2). The neuropsychological studies show a pattern of deficits that is different from that seen in PSP or AD. When 21 patients with CBD were compared with a group of patients with AD, the CBD patients performed significantly better than the AD patients on tests of immediate and delayed recall of verbal material, whereas the AD patients (with or without extrapyramidal symptoms) performed better on tests of praxis, finger-tapping speed, and motor programming (Massman et al., 1996). The CBD and AD groups all displayed prominent deficits on tests of sustained attention/mental control and verbal fluency and exhibited mild deficits on confrontation naming. The CBD patients endorsed significantly more depressive symptoms on the Geriatric Depression Scale. A similar neuropsychological pattern was demonstrated in another study of 15 patients with CBD (Pillon, Blin, et al., 1995). The spectrum of neuropsychological deficits in CBD is broadening (Bergeron et al., 1997). Some patients with clinical presentation consistent with FTD have been found to have CBD at autopsy (Mathuranath et al., 2000b).

## Neurodiagnostic Studies

Computed tomography scans were abnormal in 14 of the 15 patients in one series; 8 had asymmetric parietal lobe atrophy corresponding to the most affected side, and 6 had bilateral parietal atrophy (Riley et al., 1990). Asymmetric frontoparietal atrophy helps to differentiate CBD from PSP (Soliveri et al., 1999). Another radiographic abnormality that is occasionally encountered in CBD is the "eye of the tiger" sign on brain MRI, characteristically seen in NBIA-1 (formerly Hallervorden-Spatz disease) (Molinuevo et al., 1999). One patient with typical CBD clinically was found to have basal ganglia calcification, similar to that of Fahr disease, on MRI (Manyam et al., 2001; Brodaty et al., 2002; Warren et al., 2002; Oliveira et al., 2004). In a clinical-radiologic study of 8 patients with CBD compared to 36 controls, Yamauchi and colleagues (1998) found atrophy of the corpus callosum, especially the middle portion, which correlated with cognitive impairment and cerebral cortical metabolism measured by [18]F-fludeoxyglucose PET. Despite these reported abnormalities, no specific neuroimaging picture of CBD has emerged, and there is no correlation between antemortem MRI and pathologically confirmed CBD (Josephs et al., 2004). PET scans show reduced [[18]F]fluorodopa uptake in the caudate and putamen and markedly asymmetric cortical hypometabolism, especially in the superior temporal and inferior parietal lobe (Eidelberg et al., 1991; Sawle et al., 1991; Blin et al., 1992). In one study, [[123]I]β-CIT SPECT showed marked asymmetry in reduced striatal binding in patients with CBD, as in PD, but this did not allow reliable differentiation between PD, PSP, MSA, and CBD (Pirker et al., 2000). In two CBD patients with myoclonus, SEP showed a reduced N20 amplitude but without giant SEP (Brunt et al., 1995). Although the other neurophysiologic studies were consistent with cortical reflex myoclonus, the unusual absence of SEP may be explained either by cortical parietal atrophy or by pathologic hyperexcitability of the motor cortex due to a loss of inhibitory input from the sensory cortex (Lu et al., 1998).

## Neuropathology and Neurochemistry

Despite marked asymmetry in clinical findings, autopsy studies show predominantly bilateral atrophy of the precentral gyrus without significant asymmetry of neuropathologic changes (Cordato et al., 2001). Pathologic features in this disease include neuronal degeneration in the precentral and postcentral cortical areas, degeneration of the basal ganglia, including the SN, and the presence of achromatic neural inclusions seen not only in the cortex but also in the thalamus, subthalamic nucleus, red nucleus, and SN (Gibb et al., 1990; Lippa et al., 1991; Lowe et al., 1992; Kumar et al., 2002). These ballooned (chromatolytic, achromasic) neurons show strong diffuse cytoplasmic immunoreactivity with anti-αB crystallin, a protein that is homologous with the small cell stress proteins. They also show weak, diffuse immunoreactivity with antiubiquitin (not present in swollen neurons in the infarcted brain). While ballooned neurons are not specific for CBD, tau-containing distal astrocytic processes producing "astrocytic plaques" have been suggested by Feany and Dickson (1996) to be a distinctive pathologic feature of CBD. These cortical plaques, which are amyloid- and microglia-negative, represent clusters of miliary-like tau-positive structures within the distal processes of the astrocytes. Abnormal phosphorylation of tau is not specific for CBD; it can be seen in a variety of neurodegenerative disorders. In the CBD brain, however, tau accumulates as two 64- and 68-kDA polypeptides that are not recognized by antibodies specific to the adult tau sequences encoded by exons 3 and 10 of the *tau* gene (Bergeron et al., 1998; Kumar et al., 2002). In contrast to the 80-nm periodicity of twisted filaments in AD, the periodicity is about 290 nm in CBD. Tau immunostains usually show granular neuronal deposits, neuropil threads, and glial inclusions. In addition, NFTs and Pick bodies, spherical cortical intraneuronal inclusions, are usually present in the cortical areas but, in contrast to Pick disease, not in the hippocampus. Another characteristic finding of CBD is the presence of corticobasal inclusions, which consist of fibrillary or homogeneous basophilic inclusions. Neuronal inclusions in CBD are found predominantly in cortical pyramidal and nonpyramidal neurons and may have a distinctive perinuclear, coiled filamentous appearance. In addition to the different distribution, the Pick bodies of Pick disease and the Pick-like bodies of CBD have distinct staining characteristics. While Pick bodies are strongly argentophilic with Bodian and Bielschowsky stains but negative with the Gallyas stain, the Pick-like bodies of CBD stain with Gallyas stain but are not strongly argentophilic. Furthermore, typical Pick bodies usually do not stain with the anti-tau antibody 12E8, which detects phosphorylation at SER 262/356, while the CBD inclusions are recognized by the 12E8 antibody. Astrocytic plaques, different from thorn-shaped astrocytes that are typically seen in PSP, are also typically present in the brains of patients with CBD. In addition, coiled bodies, ubiquitin-negative, tau-immunoreactive inclusions and oligodendroglial inclusions that consist of filaments coiled around a nucleus and extend into the proximal part of the cell process are also typically present in CBD. These inclusions are found not only in CBD but also in PSP and Pick disease; they are particularly numerous in CBD and PSP.

The apparent overlap in clinical and pathologic features between CBD, PSP, and Pick disease needs clarification from further pathologic studies (Kosaka et al., 1991; Lang et al., 1994; Mori et al., 1994; Jendroska et al., 1995; Schneider et al., 1997; Boeve et al., 1999; Cordato et al., 2001; Boeve, Lang, et al., 2003). In one study of 13 patients with clinically diagnosed CBD, pathologic examination found evidence of CBD in 7 patients; AD in 2 patients; and PSP, Pick disease, CJD, and nonspecific neurodegenerative disorder in 1 patient each (Boeve et al., 1999). This indicates marked pathologic heterogeneity and argues for a need to examine the brain before the diagnosis of CBD can be confirmed. Asymmetric parietofrontal cortical degeneration was the most consistent pathologic abnormality in this autopsy series.

A relationship between CBD, Pick disease, and PSP is suggested by the presence of ballooned neurons and nigral basophilic inclusions, which are usually present in all three disorders. Although these disorders are clinically and pathologically similar, there are some distinguishing pathologic features. While "parietal Pick disease" has been reported, the vast majority of pathologically documented Pick cases exhibit degenerative changes predominantly in the frontotemporal distribution with "knife-edge" atrophy of the gyri. In addition, ballooned neurons and Pick bodies, strongly argentophilic and homogeneously ubiquitinated intraneuronal inclusions, are typically present in Pick disease. However, neither of the two histologic hallmarks is absolutely required for the neuropathologic diagnosis of Pick disease (Growdon and Primavera, 2000). Kertesz and colleagues (1994) proposed the concept of "Pick complex" for certain focal cortical degenerations such as PPA (with or without amyotrophic lateral sclerosis, or ALS), frontal lobe dementia, and CBD. He and his colleagues (Kertesz et al., 2000b) later suggested that there is a clinical and pathologic overlap between CBD, FTD, and PPA.

Dopamine concentration was reduced in the CBD brains throughout the striatum and SN when compared with age-matched controls (Riley et al., 1990).

## Treatment

To date, no effective treatment for CBD has been found, although myoclonus may improve with clonazepam, and painful rigidity and dystonia may improve with botulinum toxin injections (Jankovic and Brin, 1991). Dopaminergic drugs are rarely, if ever, effective. Although levodopa rarely provides any improvement in patients with CBD (Kompoliti et al., 1998), levodopa-induced dyskinesia has been reported in rare autopsy-proven cases (Frucht et al., 2000). Rehabilitation has been reported to improve ideomotor apraxia following stroke, but it is not known whether similar strategies improve apraxia associated with CBD (Hanna-Pladdy et al., 2003).

## PARKINSONISM-DEMENTIA SYNDROMES

### Clinical Aspects

Cognitive impairment is common in parkinsonian disorders, and characteristic psychological profiles can differentiate PD from atypical parkinsonian syndromes (Pillon et al., 1996;

Litvan, 1998a; Emre, 2003). Significant dementia occurs in approximately 20% of patients with PD, particularly later in the course of the illness (Braak et al., 2005). In one prospective study, the incidence of dementia was 19% over 54 months of observation (Biggins et al., 1992). Patients with PD have nearly twice the risk for developing dementia as controls have (Marder et al., 1995), and siblings of demented PD patients have an increased risk for AD (Marder et al., 1999). Poor performance on tests of verbal fluency appears to be predictive of incipient dementia in patients who are in early phases of PD (Jacobs et al., 1995). Cognitive decline seems to be more prominent in patients with older onset and the postural instability with dysfunctional gait form of PD (Jankovic, McDermott, et al., 1990; Biggins et al., 1992; Galasko et al., 1994a). In addition to the Mini-Mental State Examination (Dufouil et al., 2000), other tests have been developed and validated to assess the cognitive (e.g., the Addenbrooke's Cognitive Examination) (Mathuranath et al., 2000a) and frontal lobe function (e.g., the Frontal Assessment Battery) (Dubois et al., 2000) in patients with dementia with or without parkinsonism. About 15% to 45% of patients with AD develop parkinsonism, and the presence of such motor impairment markedly increases the burden on the patient and increases the cost of patient care (Murman et al., 2003). Except for tremor, parkinsonian and other motor signs increase during the course of the disease (Scarmeas et al., 2004).

In addition to the expected Lewy bodies in the SN, patients with parkinsonism and dementia have cortical pathology, including Lewy bodies in the neocortex, the density correlating with the severity of dementia (Hurtig et al., 2000). Diffuse Lewy body disease is the most common pathologic finding in patients with PD who later develop dementia (Apaydin et al., 2002). But Braak and colleagues (2005), in their detailed clinical-pathologic studies, attribute cognitive decline in PD to "the cumulative effects of the progressive PD pathology," although cognitively impaired PD patients also had a greater degree of AD pathology than did those who were cognitively unimpaired.

Extrapyramidal signs have been reported in about one third of patients with AD (Chen et al., 1991), and their presence correlates with greater cognitive impairment and worse prognosis as compared to AD patients without extrapyramidal signs (Funkenstein et al., 1993; Merello et al., 1994; Stern et al., 1994; Clark et al., 1997; Kurlan et al., 2000; Wilson et al., 2003). Using [$^{11}$C]β-CFT PET scans to image striatal dopamine reuptake site, Rinne and colleagues (1998) showed a significant reduction in the dopamine transporter in patients with AD, and the reduction correlated with the severity of the extrapyramidal symptoms. Pathologically, the parkinsonian signs in AD correlate best with the presence of NFTs rather than Lewy bodies in the SN (Liu et al., 1997). Other studies have shown that AD patients with parkinsonism have PD-like pathology in their SN (Burns et al., 2005). In a prospective clinicopathologic study by the Consortium to Establish a Registry for Alzheimer's Disease (CERAD), 16 (20.5%) of the 78 cases of AD had coexistent PD pathology (Hulette et al., 1995). Research into molecular, cellular, and genetic mechanisms of AD will undoubtedly provide insight not only into AD but also into other neurodegenerative disorders. Current research has been focusing on the role of the amyloid-β (Aβ) amyloid precursor protein (APP) in the pathogenesis of AD. Elevated levels of APP have been found to correlate with cognitive decline (Näslund et al., 2000). For example, mice expressing mutations in the *APP* gene develop Aβ deposits, and this process is accelerated by coexpression of mutant senilin genes and by apolipoprotein E (Emilien et al., 2000). In addition to the gene mutation in 21q21.2 that produces mutant *APP* and is responsible for early-onset AD, mutations in other genes (e.g., 1q41,12p, 14q24.3, and 19q13.2) affect the formation of Aβ. Currently, the most sensitive and specific biologic markers for AD are reduced levels of Aβ42 amyloid protein and sulfatide and increased levels of tau and phosphorylated tau in the CSF. Although they are considered valid diagnostic markers, analysis of these molecules has not had an important impact on the diagnosis of AD (Irizarry et al., 2003).

Consensus guidelines for the clinical and pathologic diagnosis of DLB have been proposed (McKeith et al., 1996; Hohl et al., 2000; Lopez et al., 2002; McKeith et al., 2005). These criteria have been reformulated by the Consortium on DLB by adding the presence of extrapyramidal signs (McKeith et al., 1996; Mega et al., 1996). In addition to progressive cognitive decline, two of the following criteria are required for the diagnosis of probable DLB (one for a "possible" diagnosis): (1) fluctuating cognition with pronounced variations in attention and alertness; (2) recurrent, typically well-formed, visual hallucinations; and (3) motor features of parkinsonism. Supportive features, not required for the diagnosis, include repeated falls, syncope, transient loss of consciousness, neuroleptic sensitivity, systematized delusions, and hallucinations in other modalities. Using these clinical criteria in 18 cases of pathologically diagnosed AD, the authors found 100% specificity with high interrater reliability (Mega et al., 1996). In a review of 31 pathologically proven cases of DLB, Louis and colleagues (1997) found that the presence of myoclonus, absence of rest tremor, no response to levodopa, or no perceived need to treat with levodopa was highly predictive of the diagnosis of DLB. REM sleep behavior disorder has been described at onset in a group of patients with DLB (Boeve et al., 1998), and REM sleep behavior disorder and depression were added as additional features that are supportive of the diagnosis of DLB during the second DLB workshop (McKeith et al., 1999).

Dementia with Lewy bodies (DLB), considered by some as a variant of AD or an overlap between AD and PD, is now well recognized, but its clinical and pathologic criteria have not yet been fully defined (Burkhardt et al., 1988; Crystal et al., 1990; Sage and Mark, 1993; McKeith et al., 1994; McKeith et al., 1996; Mega et al., 1996; Litvan, MacIntyre, et al., 1998; Gomez-Isla et al., 1999; Verghese et al., 1999; Lopez et al., 2002; Pompeu and Growdon, 2002; McKeith et al., 2005). Also referred to variably as diffuse Lewy body disease, senile dementia of Lewy body type, and Lewy body variant of AD, DLB has emerged as the second most common cause of degenerative dementia in the elderly. Although it is usually a sporadic disorder, few families with DLB have been described (Tsuang et al., 2002). Differentiation of AD and DLB on clinical findings alone can be difficult. Crystal and colleagues (1990) reviewed the course of six patients with DLB, three with AD, and one with PD with autopsy-confirmed diagnosis and found that DLB patients were more likely to have gait impairment, rigidity, and resting tremor early in the course of the illness. In another study of 30 patients with DLB, psychosis and dementia were often found to precede parkinsonism (Burkhardt et al., 1988). Agitation, hallucinations, delusions, and abnormal EEGs were more common in the DLB than in the AD patients (Burkhardt et al., 1988). Complex visual hallucinations, even in the early stages of the disease, are particularly characteristic of DLB (Manford and Andermann, 1998). Visual hallucinations in DLB seem to correlate with the presence of Lewy bodies in the temporal lobe (Harding et al., 2002). In a study of 15 patients (14 men) diagnosed at the Mayo Clinic with RBD, all had clear histories of dream enactment behavior, and 10 had RBD confirmed by polysomnography; the neuropathologic diagnoses were LBD in 12 patients (neocortical in 11 and limbic in 1) and MSA in 3 patients (Boeve, Lang, et al., 2003). The clinical and pathologic literature therefore suggests that when associated with a neurodegenerative disorder, RBD tends to occur in certain disorders (e.g., DLB, PD, and MSA) and rarely if ever occurs in others (e.g., PSP, CBD, AD, FTD). In another study, the authors showed that in the setting of dementia or parkinsonism, the presence of RBD often reflects synucleinopathy (Boeve, Silber, et al., 2003). No differences were found with respect to age, gender, or disease progression between autopsy-proven cases of AD and DLB (Gibb, Luthert, et al., 1989). On neurologic examination, rigidity, bradykinesia, and action tremor were more frequent in the DLB patients, while impairment of upgaze was surprisingly more common in the AD group. Fluctuations, particularly when associated with disturbed arousal and disorganized speech, are very characteristic of DLB and serve to differentiate it from AD (Ferman et al., 2004). Although DLB patients might not respond as well to levodopa as do those with typical PD, many do obtain satisfactory improvement with levodopa and benefit from chronic treatment (Bonelli et al., 2004).

Differentiation between DLB and the other parkinsonism-plus syndromes, particularly PSP, can be particularly difficult when a patient with parkinsonism and dementia is also found to have oculomotor disturbance, as has been noted in some patients with DLB (Lewis and Gawel, 1990). Since orthostatic hypotension and other autonomic symptoms can be seen in DLB, this disorder may at times be difficult to differentiate from MSA (Thaisetthawatkul et al., 2004). In contrast to AD, in which urinary incontinence usually occurs late in the course of the dementia, urinary incontinence may precede severe cognitive decline in DLB (Del-Ser et al., 1996). The relationship between AD and other dementing disorders such as DLB, CBD, and Pick disease is illustrated by the observation of rapidly progressive aphasia, apraxia, dementia, myoclonus, and parkinsonism in an autopsy-proven case of AD (Wojcieszek et al., 1994). Medial temporal lobe atrophy (MTA) on MRI failed to differentiate between DLB and AD, although the latter had more severe MTA (Barber et al., 1999).

Until a disease-specific biologic marker that differentiates the various neurodegenerative disorders is identified, the clinical categorization of the various dementing diseases will continue to present a diagnostic challenge. In this regard, the study of various risk markers might provide clues to the pathogenesis of the various disorders. The frequency of the APOE ε4 allele, a major risk factor for AD, in nondemented controls is 10% to 15% (Roses, 1995). The finding that the frequency of APOE ε4 allele was increased to a similar extent in autopsy-proven cases of AD and the Lewy body variant of AD (40% and 29%, respectively) (Galasko et al., 1994b) and that APOE ε4 allele is strongly associated with increased neuritic plaques in both disorders (Olichney et al., 1996) suggests that the two disorders are related and that they are different from

DLB, in which the frequency of the APOE ε4 allele was significantly lower (6.2%). The frequency of the APOE ε4 genotype did not differ between demented and nondemented patients with clinically diagnosed PD and was similar to that in controls, thus suggesting that the PD-related dementia is pathogenetically different from that of AD (Koller et al., 1995). Mutations in the β-synuclein gene have recently been linked to cases of DLB (Ohtake et al., 2004).

# FRONTOTEMPORAL DEMENTIAS

The FTDs, along with PSP, CBD, Pick disease, and other neurodegenerative disorders, are examples of an emerging group of neurologic disorders that are referred to as tauopathies (Box 10-1). The prototype tauopathy is an inherited parkinsonism-dementia disorder, initially described as the Wilhelmsen-Lynch disease (disinhibition-dementia-parkinsonism-amyotrophy complex), linked initially by Lynch and colleagues (1994) to a locus on 17q21–q22. Another family with autosomal-dominant parkinsonism-dementia was later described by Muenter and colleagues (1998). Clinically, the affected individuals had young-onset, rapidly progressive, levodopa-responsive parkinsonism and mild dysautonomia, later associated with dementia. Some members of the family had isolated postural tremor, phenomenologically identical to essential tremor. Pathologically, the brains showed features similar to those of primary PD. Subsequently other families with the hereditary parkinsonism-dementia have been described, and the disorder is now referred to as frontotemporal dementia and parkinsonism linked to chromosome 17 (FTDP-17) (Lendon et al., 1998; Poorkaj et al., 1998; Stevens et al., 1998; Cherrier and Mendez, 1999; Foster, 1995; Nasreddine et al., 1999; van Swieten et al., 1999; Spillantini and Goedert, 2000; Yasuda et al., 2000; Lee et al., 2001; McKhann et al., 2001; Morris et al., 2001). In a study of nine British families with pathologically and genetically proven FTD, disinhibition was the most common presenting symptom, followed by frontal dysexecutive symptoms, apathy, impairment of episodic memory, and depression (Janssen et al., 2002). Subsequently, essentially all patients develop personality and behavioral changes, memory impairment, language deficits, ritualistic behavior, hyperphagia, hyperorality,

**Box 10-1** Classification of tauopathies

**3R Tauopathies**
Pick disease (PiD)

**4R Tauopathies**
Progressive supranuclear palsy
Corticobasal degeneration
Argyrophilic grain disease

**3R and 4R Tauopathies**
Tangle-predominant dementia

**Dementia Lacking Distinctive Histopathology (No Inclusions)**

**Dementia with Motor Neuron Disease-Type Inclusions (FTD-MND)**

parkinsonism, and neuroleptic sensitivity. Stereotypies, such as rubbing and self-injurious behavior, similar to those seen in patients with autism and mental retardation, are also characteristically seen in patients with FTD (Mendez et al., 2005).

The following diagnostic criteria for FTD were formulated by an international group of clinical and basic scientists (McKhann et al., 2001):

1. The development of behavioral or cognitive deficits manifested by either:
   a. early and progressive change in personality, characterized by difficulty in modulating behavior, often resulting in inappropriate responses or activities, or
   b. early and progressive changes in language, characterized by problems with expression or severe naming difficulty and problems with word meaning.
2. The deficits in 1a and 1b cause significant impairment in social or occupational functioning and represent a significant decline from previous level of functioning.
3. The course is characterized by gradual onset and continuing decline in function.
4. Other causes are excluded.

Several studies have demonstrated that 11% to 50% of all patients with familial FTD have mutations in the *tau* gene (Morris et al., 2001). The majority of testing for the various mutations in the *MAPT* gene is done on a research basis, but information about commercially available testing can be found at http://www.genetests.org. Furthermore, the presence of tau pathologic findings (neuronal loss and glial tau deposition) strongly predicts the presence of tau mutation, whereas FTD with ubiquitin inclusions or with neuronal loss and spongiosis essentially excludes mutation in tau. The neuropathologic examination shows tau-positive neuronal and glial inclusions (Lantos et al., 2002).

FTDP-17 joins a growing list of tauopathies such as AD, Pick disease, PSP, CBD, ALS-dementia complex (lytico-bodig disease of Guam), pallidopontonigral degeneration, Niemann-Pick disease type C, Gertmann-Straussler-Sheinker disease with tangles, prion protein amyloid angiopathy, familial multiple-system tauopathy, hereditary-dysphasic-disinhibition-dementia, and familial progressive subcortical gliosis (Lee and Trojanowski, 1999; Morris, Lees, et al., 1999; Hutton, 2001; Kuzuhara et al., 2001). Although FTDP-17 is heterogeneous in its presentation, typical clinical features include personality changes (withdrawal, apathy, depression, aggressive behavior, alcoholism, excessive craving of sweets, childishness, apathy, abulia, Klüver-Bucy syndrome, hypersexuality, and other evidence of disinhibition), defective executive functions (e.g., drawing to command), language deficits eventually leading to muteness, seizures (Sperfeld et al., 1999), pyramidal signs, and amyotrophy. Parkinsonian features include bradykinesia, rigidity, and gait difficulty, but there is usually no tremor and no response to levodopa. The age at onset is usually in the sixth and seventh decades, but the symptoms can begin as early as age 27 and as late as age 75. The family history suggests autosomal-dominant inheritance. There are two major phenotypes of FTDP-17: Type 1 (late age at onset, dementia, cortical pathology, missense mutations) and Type 2 (earlier onset, parkinsonism, basal ganglia pathology). Besides the tau locus, there are probably other genetic loci in which mutations can produce a clinical-pathologic phenotype that is similar to that of FTD-17 (Kertesz et al., 2000b). Reduction in striatal dopamine transporter correlates with the severity of parkinsonian symptoms in patients with FTDP-17 (Rinne et al., 2002).

Although FTD is relatively common, only a small percentage of these patients have an autosomal-dominant FTDP-17, caused by a coding or intronic mutation in the *tau* gene. After sequencing the *tau* gene, located in the 17q21.11 locus, Hutton (1999) and colleagues (1998) found three missense mutations and three mutations in the 5′ splice site of exon 10. This results in increased usage of the 5′ splice, causing an increase in exon 10 messenger RNA, consequently increasing the portion of tau containing four microtubule-binding repeats. Three types of mutations in the *tau* gene have been subsequently identified: intronic mutations in a presumed stem-loop splice site that alters expression of tau isoforms, missense mutations in sites that bind microtubules, and missense mutations in or near phosphorylation sites. The numerous mutations that have been identified in the microtubule-binding domain of the *tau* gene are localized to the following areas: exon 9 (Gly272Val), exon 10 (Pro301Leu), and exon 12 (Val337Met) or in the splice region immediately following exon 10. Mutations outside of exon 10 and its flanking region tend to result in AD-like pathology (NFTs consisting of PHF made up of all six isoforms of tau). Exon 10 mutations results in a four-repeat tau pattern, typically seen in PSP and FTDP-17, in which the ratio is at least 3:1 in favor of the four-repeat tau. About 30 different mutations have been identified in more than 60 separately ascertained families. One of the earliest families identified, a large American family with pallidopontonigral degeneration (Wszolek et al., 1995), has been found to have *N279K* mutation in exon 10 (Clark et al., 1998). This, the third most common mutation, is characterized by rapidly progressive, levodopa-nonresponsive, parkinsonism-predominant phenotype with supranuclear palsy (Tsuboi, Baker, et al., 2002). A novel mutation, consisting of a C-to-T transition at position +12 of the intron following exon 10, has also been described (Yasuda et al., 2000). This resulted clinically in FTD; pathologically, the brains of patients with this disorder had tau aggregates in degenerating neurons and glia with overproduction of tau isoforms with four microtubule-binding repeats. Thus, instead of the normal 1:1 ratio of the three-repeat and four-repeat isoforms, the brains of patients with FTDP-17 have an increased proportion of exon 10+ mRNA and a corresponding increase in the proportion of four-repeat tau. Intronic mutations, however, also destabilize a stem-loop structure that sequesters the 5′ splice downstream of exon 10 in tau pre-mRNA, leading to increases in U1 snRNP binding and in splicing between exons 10 and 11. As a result of the altered structure, the 5′ splice site mutations increase recognition of exon 10 by the U1 snRNP splicing factor, increasing the proportion of exon 10+ mRNA and four-repeat tau (Hutton, 2000). Thus, mutations close to the 5′ splice site appear to disrupt a stem-loop-type secondary structure in the tau pre-mRNA around the exon-intron junction and eventually lead to abnormal aggregation of the tau protein. An extended tau haplotype (H1), known to be associated with PSP, has been found to interact with the ε2 allele of APOE to increase the risk of FTD (Verpillat et al., 2002).

Mutations in exons 9, 10, 12, and 13 of MAPT are associated with prominent dementia, whereas intronic and exonic mutations are associated with overproduction of four-repeat tau and predominant parkinsonism-plus phenotype. The phenotypic variation related to the type of mutation is illustrated by one study, which found that the average age at onset of symptoms was greatest in patients with the R406W mutation (59.2 years) as compared with the other mutations: P301L (51.4 years), G272B (47.6 years), and delta-K280 (53 years) (van Swieten et al., 1999). The R406W mutation was also associated with a longer duration of illness and later development of mutism. The presenting symptoms, such as disinhibition, loss of initiative, and obsessive-compulsive behavior did not seem to differ between the four tau mutations. Additional studies are needed to explain the intrafamilial variation or differences in genotype. Expression of human tau containing the most common FTDP-17 mutation (P301L) in transgenic mice results in motor and behavioral deficits similar to those in human tauopathies, along with formation of NFTs and Pick body–like neuronal inclusions in the amygdala, hippocampus, brainstem, cerebellum, and basal ganglia (Lewis et al., 2000). Further studies in humans as well as in mouse and drosophila models of tauopathies will undoubtedly provide greater insight into the phenotypic variability of tauopathies and clarify the question of whether the observed tau aggregates are the cause or the result of neurodegeneration (de Silva and Farrer, 2002). Clinicopathologic studies have shown that FTDs that are manifested chiefly by behavioral symptoms and semantic dementia have a broad specific range of pathologic changes, whereas those associated with motor neuron disease have predominantly ubiquitinated inclusions; parkinsonism and apraxia are associated with corticobasal pathology, and nonfluent aphasia predicted Pick bodies (Hodges et al., 2004).

These disorders not only have in common genetic abnormalities in the *tau* gene but also overlap in neuropathologic abnormalities (Munoz et al., 2003; Goldman et al., 2004). The human gene that encodes MAPT occupies over 100 kb on chromosome 17q21 and contains 16 exons (Lee et al., 2001). Tau is a low-molecular-weight protein that has a number of functions, including stabilization of polymerization of microtubules in the brain, facilitating axonal transport, and contributing to cytoskeletal stability (Buee et al., 2000). In certain disorders, such as PSP, AD, CBD, and Pick disease (tauopathies), the normally soluble tau protein becomes hyperphosphorylated and forms ordered filamentous assemblies; these deposits of filamentous tau are the characteristic pathologic features of tauopathies. Alternative splicing of tau mRNA from 11 of the 16 exons produces six tau isoforms ranging in size from 352 to 441 amino acids. These three- and four-carboxy-terminal tandem repeat forms are further differentiated by tau isoforms without (0N) or with either 29 (1N) or 58 (2N) amino acid inserts located on the N-terminal half; an additional 31 amino acid insert is located on the C-terminal half. Inclusion of the latter, which is encoded by exon 10 of the *tau* gene, gives rise to the three isoforms with four microtubule-binding repeats each; the other three isoforms have three repeats each. While all six tau isoforms are found in the abnormal filaments in AD, only four-repeat tau isoforms are found in PSP and CBD, and there is a preponderance of three-repeat isoforms in Pick disease. Splicing, a process in which introns are excised and the remaining exons are joined together to generate mRNA, is regulated in part by unique proteins, such as the neuro-oncologic ventral antigen 1 (NOVA-1) (Dredge et al., 2001). The six major tau protein isoforms that are found in the normal adult brain are generated by alternative splicing of exons 2, 3, and 10; exons 9 to 12 encode four microtubule-binding domains that are imperfect repeats of 31 or 32 amino acid residues. Exon 10 encodes the second of four microtubule-binding domains in the C-terminal half of the protein. Alternative splicing of exon 10 generates isoforms with either four or three microtubule-binding domains; the inclusion of exon 10 results in isoforms with four repeats, and the exclusion of exon 10 results in three repeats. Mutations in the splice-donor site of exon 10 lead to increased incorporation of exon 10 and therefore an increase in levels of four-repeat tau. The presence of three or four microtubule-binding repeats in the C-terminal region depends on whether E10 is spliced out or in (Goedert et al., 1998). The tau protein occurs in equal proportions of two isoforms, one with three repeats and the other with four repeats of microtubule-binding peptide domain, but the 1N-insert tau isoform is more abundant than the 0N isoform.

There are four tau microtubule-binding domains localized to the C-terminus of the protein. In the longest isoform, there are 79 serine and threonine sites to accept phosphorylation, about 30 of these sites being phosphorylated under normal circumstances (Buee et al., 2000). Overall tau phosphorylation is high during brain development but declines after birth. Abnormally high levels of tau phosphorylation in adult brains are associated with a variety of neurodegenerative disorders (Brich et al., 2003). A new proteinopathy, termed *neuronal intermediate filaments inclusion disease*, has been described with the identification of the novel intermediate filament protein α-internexin (DeKosky and Ikonomovic, 2004). This is the fourth of the phosphorylated neurofilament proteins that have been found to accumulate in various degenerative disorders; the others include light, medium, and heavy neurofilament triplet proteins (Cairns et al., 2004). The clinical phenotype is very similar to that of other FTDs. Different N-terminally cleaved tau fragments have been found in brains of patients with PSP and CBD; a 33-kDa band predominated in the low-molecular-weight tau fragments in PSP, whereas two closely related bands of approximately 37 kDa predominated in CBD (Arai et al., 2004). This suggests that the two disorders have different proteolytic processing of abnormal tau. Some, but not all (e.g., AD), diseases characterized by tau phosphorylation are associated with mutations in the *tau* gene. These sites flank the microtubule-binding domains. Since phosphorylation decreases microtubule binding, regulating tau phosphorylation might be of therapeutic value in neurodegenerative disorders associated with an abnormality of tau, including PSP. A number of serine- and threonine-protein kinases, including glycogen synthase kinase 3β (GSK-3β), cyclin-dependent kinases 2 (cdk2), and 5 (cdk 5), have been identified as possible regulators of tau phosphorylation (Buee et al., 2000). Valproate has been found to inhibit these protein kinases regulating phosphorylation of tau, including GSK-3β (Mora et al., 1998), suggesting that it might have a modifying effect on the course of PSP.

The role of tau in neurodegeneration is unknown, but one hypothesis suggests that the hyperphosphorylated tau loses its affinity for microtubules and becomes resistant to proteases, thus leading to aggregation. Tau is also the main component of NFTs, and tau pathology is observed in neurons, C4d-positive oligodendrocytes, and glial fibrillary acidic protein–positive and CD44-positive astrocytes (Ikeda et al., 1998). Another hypothesis suggests that under oxidative conditions, the cystein 322 residue on tau forms intermolecular bridges between tau proteins (Schweers et al., 1995). Tau immunoblot-

ting has shown that four-repeat tau predominates in insoluble fractions of NFTs from PSP brains, particularly the basal ganglia (Sergeant et al., 1999). Although case-control studies have failed to show that family history is a significant risk factor, research involving the *tau* gene suggests that certain polymorphisms or mutations in this gene increase an individual's susceptibility to PSP, but the penetrance of this "risk allele" is low. The genetic association between PSP and an intronic short tandem repeat polymorphism within the *tau* gene indicates that tau is a candidate gene for PSP. In a family with phenotypically heterogeneous PSP, Stanford and colleagues (2000) found a novel mutation in the *tau* gene that does not change the amino acid sequence in the tau protein, but it causes a 4.8-fold increase in the splicing of exon 10, disrupting the RNA stem loop and resulting in a tau that contains four microtubule-binding repeats. In another report, after screening 96 PSP patients for MAPT for mutations, Poorkaj and colleagues (2002) found a single point mutation, which they concluded caused PSP by a gain-of-function mechanism.

There is growing evidence that mRNA for a tau protein isoform that contributes to NFTs is overexpressed in the brainstem of patients with PSP but not in patients with AD. Chambers and colleagues (1999) showed that, compared to control brains, PSP brains had elevated levels of four microtubule-binding domains (4R) mRNA in the brainstem but not in frontal or cerebellar cortex. They found that the regional distribution of the increases in 4R tau mRNA expression in PSP correlated with the selective vulnerability for NFT in the disease, and they concluded, "The genetic as well as pathologic studies have provided powerful evidence that overexpression of 4R tau isoforms plays an important role in the formation of NFTs and in the pathogenesis of PSP and that PSP is a repeat tauopathy." One mutation, located in exon 10 of the *tau* gene, results in a 4.8-fold increase in the splicing of exon 10, resulting in tau with four microtubule-binding repeats (Stanford et al., 2000). The *tau* genetic markers associated with PSP are therefore probably related to a defect within an intron yet to be sequenced. Zemaitaitis and colleagues (2000) have hypothesized that "transglutaminase-induced cross-linking may be a factor contributing to the abnormal polymerization and stabilization of tau in straight and PHFs leading to NFT formation in neurodegenerative diseases, including PSP and AD." Atypical PSP was found to be due to homozygosity for the delN296 mutation in the *tau* gene (Pastor et al., 2001).

An association of a particular *tau* genetic marker with PSP was initially reported by Conrad and colleagues (1997). In their study, they found that 95% of 22 PSP patients were homozygous for the A0 tau allele, whereas only half of controls and AD patients were homozygous for this particular allele. In another study, Morris, Janssen, and colleagues (1999) found the A0 allele in 91% and the A0/A0 genotype in 84% of patients with PSP and in 73% (allele) and 53% (genotype) of controls ($P < .001$ and $P < .01$, respectively). The A0 allele and A0/A0 genotype were more frequent in patients with PSP than in controls, but this is also true for asymptomatic relatives of patients with PSP (Hoenicka et al., 1999). This finding, suggesting that PSP is associated with a genetic alteration in *tau*, is further supported by the demonstration that the tau $a_1$ allele and the tau $a_1a_1$ genotype are overrepresented in patients with PSP and that the tau polymorphism is in linkage disequilibrium with the PSP disease locus using a disease model of recessive inheritance (Higgins et al., 1998). Although some studies have demonstrated an increased frequency of the A0 allele and the A0/A0 genotype in PSP versus controls (Bennett et al., 1998; Oliva et al., 1998), this finding could not be confirmed in Japanese patients (Conrad et al., 1998). Furthermore, this finding does not seem to be specific for PSP, and a higher frequency of the A0/A0 genotype has also been demonstrated in PD (Pastor et al., 2000). Other studies showed that the H1 haplotype (93.7% versus 78.4%) and the H1/H1 genotype (87.5% versus 62.8%) are significantly overrepresented in patients with PSP compared to controls (Baker et al., 1999). In addition to the overrepresentation of the H1 haplotype, other genotypes have been found (e.g., extended, 670 Kb, haplotype H1E) to be overrepresented, thus suggesting that changes in the tau gene could increase the genetic susceptibility to PSP (Pastor et al., 2002). Both H1 and H1/H1 are also overrepresented in CBD compared to controls, strongly supporting the conclusion that PSP and CBD are genetically and pathologically related. This suggests a common pathogenic mechanism involving *tau* dysfunction, although other risk factors must be present to explain the divergent clinical and pathologic presentation (Houlden et al., 2001). The observation that the haplotype that is overrepresented in PSP is the common tau haplotype present in a homozygous form in about 55% of normal white individuals suggests that the *tau* gene is a susceptibility gene for PSP but that other genetic and environmental factors must play an important role in the pathogenesis of this neurodegenerative disorder. Some studies, however, failed to demonstrate that the H1 haplotype has a major influence on the biochemical or pathologic phenotype of PSP (Liu et al., 2001), and neither H1/H1 nor A0/A0 genotype predicts the prognosis of PSP (Litvan, Baker, et al., 2001).

Subsequently, other "susceptibility" haplotypes have been identified in PSP patients (Higgins, 1999; Pastor and Tolosa, 2002). In a follow-up study of 52 patients with PSP and 54 age-matched controls, Higgins and colleagues (2000), found that an extended 5′-tau haplotype consisting of four single nucleotide polymorphisms (SNPs) in tau exons 1, 4A, and 8 has a 98% sensitivity and a 67% specificity, suggesting that this susceptibility haplotype is a sensitive marker for sporadic PSP. The four SNPs formed two homozygous 5′-tau haplotypes (HapA and HapC) or a heterozygous genotype. Fifty-one (98%) patients with PSP had HapA haplotype, same as H1 haplotype found originally by Hutton's group (Baker et al., 1999), whereas only 33% of controls had the same haplotype. While the tau mutations in FTD and parkinsonism linked to chromosome 17 (FTDP-17) (see later) affect microtubule-binding domains of the C-terminus of the tau protein, the PSP variants affect domains that interact with the neural plasma membrane. The clinically typical PSP is most likely associated with the tau PSP susceptibility genotype (H1/H1) and doublet tau protein pattern (64 and 69kDa) (Morris et al., 2002).

There are only two common extended haplotypes, H1 and H2, that cover the entire *tau* gene. In certain neurodegenerative disorders, termed *tauopathies*, this normal ratio is altered: NFTs found in PSP, CBD, and FTDP-17 (see later) contain only four-repeat tau isoforms, whereas NFTs in AD contain all six, and those in Pick disease contain only three isoforms. Other tauopathies include postencephalitic parkinsonism and ALS-dementia-parkinsonism syndrome. It has been proposed that an increase in the available pool of free tau, not bound to microtubules, leads to NFT formation. An increase in the 4R tau isoform mRNA has been demonstrated in PSP. Furthermore, phosphorylated tau protein is unable to interact with the microtubules. Free unbound tau protein can form tau polymers via crosslinking by transglutaminase. These insoluble complexes become resistant to proteolysis and can eventually accumulate and lead to neurodegeneration. If this hypothesis is correct, transglutaminase inhibitors, such as cystamine and monodansyl cadaverine, could potentially have a neuroprotective effect in these neurodegenerative disorders.

It is possible that the four-repeat tau leads to a pathologic increase in tau aggregation, as has been noted not only in FTDP-17 but also in other neurodegenerative diseases such as PSP (Chambers et al., 1999; Stanford et al., 2000). *Tau* gene mutation has been associated with early dementia and PSP-like syndrome (Soliveri et al., 2003). Despite identical missense mutations in the *tau* gene involving exon 10, various family members exhibit marked clinical and genetic heterogeneity, suggesting the influence of additional environmental and/or genetic factors (Bird et al., 1999). Biochemically and pathologically confirmed Pick disease also has been associated with mutations in the *tau* gene (Neumann et al., 2001). The unifying theme of all these tauopathes is that the mutated tau cannot interact with microtubules, thus inappropriately freeing the mutant tau, resulting in an accumulation of the aberrant tau.

Even though genetically engineered mice that make no tau seem healthy, an animal model that reproduces neuronal tau pathology is now available. These transgenic mice of human tau with four tubulin-binding repeats (4R) containing three missense mutations associated with FTD-17, G272V, P301L, and R406W develop intracellular filaments composed of hyperphosphorylated 4R tau mainly concentrated in the apical dendrites and distributed in the cortex, hippocampus, and basal forebrain (Lim et al., 2001). This and other models (Lewis et al., 2000) can be used to study the effects of oxidative stress or toxins to clarify the role of tau pathology in neurodegeneration.

Besides tauopathies (PSP, CBD, Pick disease, dementia pugilistica, FTDP-17, postencephalitic parkinsonism, and ALS-dementia-parkinsonism syndrome) (Fig. 10-4), there are synucleinopathies (PD, MSA, DLB, and neurodegeneration with brain iron accumulation type 1, NBIA). There is growing evidence, however, that tau and α-synuclein affect each other, which might explain the overlap in clinical and pathologic features of the two types of neurodegenerative disease (Lee et al., 2004). Some patients with ALS-dementia-parkinsonism of Guam (ADPG) have been found to have both tau and synuclein inclusions. Genomewide analysis, however, has not identified any mutations in patients with ADPG (Morris et al., 2004). An X-linked dystonia parkinsonism that is seen almost exclusively in male adults with maternal roots from the Philippine island of Panay may, in addition to dystonia (intermittent twisting referred to as Lubag, sustained posturing referred to as Wa-eg) and parkinsonism with bradykinesia and shuffling gait (referred to as Sud-sud), manifest a wide spectrum of movement disorders. These include tremor, myoclonus, chorea, and myorhythmia. One form of FTD, associated with ALS, has been linked to chromosome 9q21–q22 (Hosler et al., 2000). Other genes in which mutations have been associated with FTD include those coding for "charged multivesicular body protein 2B" (CHMP2B), DJ-1, other proteins, such as valosin, synuclein, TDP-43, and prion protein (Rowland, 2006).

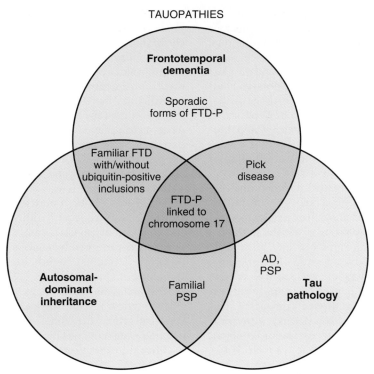

TAUOPATHIES

Figure 10-4 Overlap between different tauopathies.

## Neurodiagnostic Studies

There are no diagnostic studies, including PET scans, that can reliably differentiate between PD, AD, and DLB (Tyrell et al., 1990). PET metabolic studies in patients with FTDP-17 show marked frontal hypoactivity. Using SPECT to image [123I]iodobenzovesamicol, Kuhl and colleagues (1996) have found that, in contrast to nondemented PD patients, those who have coexistent dementia have extensive cortical reduction in the binding of this cholinergic marker, suggesting that the integrity of the cholinergic neurons is impaired in demented PD patients in a pattern similar to that of early AD.

In one series of 37 AD patients, concentrations of CSF homovanillic acid and biopterin were noted to be significantly lower in the AD patients with extrapyramidal signs than in the group without extrapyramidal signs matched for age and dementia severity (Kaye et al., 1988). It is not yet clear whether apolipoprotein E genotyping will be useful in the differential diagnosis of the parkinsonism-dementia syndrome (Roses, 1995).

## Neuropathology and Neurochemistry

The development of new immunocytochemical staining techniques using antibodies directed against ubiquitin, a highly conserved protein that is produced by cells in response to stress, has dramatically improved the identification of Lewy bodies. A ubiquitin-like epitope of PHFs is also present in Lewy bodies and may represent a common link between Lewy bodies and NFTs (Dickson et al., 1989). About one third of patients with AD have both cortical and SN Lewy bodies at autopsy (Forstl et al., 1992; Galasko et al., 1994a), and essentially all patients with PD have Lewy bodies in the cortex (Hughes, Ben-Shlomo, et al., 1992). Patients with DLB, however, seem to have a greater neuronal loss in the SN, substan-

tia innominata, and locus coeruleus and have lower cortical choline acetyltransferase levels than do the AD patients (Gibb, Luthert, et al., 1989). In addition to the diffuse distribution of Lewy bodies throughout the basal forebrain, brainstem, and hypothalamus, the lack of NFTs in DLB helps to differentiate it from AD (Burkhardt et al., 1988; Gibb, Mountjoy, et al., 1989). Though Gibb, Mountjoy, and colleagues (1989) found no Lewy bodies in the hippocampus or cortex in AD, Burkhardt and colleagues (1988) reported "Lewy-like" bodies in the limbic system and neocortex. Others report different antigenic components of the Lewy body in DLB and PD, tau protein being present only in the dementing disorder (Galloway et al., 1989). Pathologic changes in AD have been well characterized: Neuritic plaques containing β-amyloid protein have been demonstrated in both sporadic and familial AD; and NFTs consist of the PHF tau. The abnormal phosphate substitution is thought to interfere with normal neurotubule formation (Kosic, 1991). The NFTs in AD are found predominantly in the hippocampus, but extrapyramidal signs are more likely associated with the presence of NFTs in SN (Gibb, Mountjoy, et al., 1989). Tabaton and colleagues (1988) noted antigenic similarities between the tangles of PSP and AD when they were derived from neurons of similar populations and postulated that anatomic location, rather than disease specificity, was the determining factor for antigenicity. In a study contrasting PD dementia and AD, de la Monte and colleagues (1989) found similar reductions in the cross-sectional areas of the globus pallidus-putamen; but greater cell loss was noted in the amygdala of PD dementia brains, while AD was associated with prominent cortical atrophy. However, the relative frequencies of Lewy bodies, neuritic plaques, and NFTs were not discussed.

In contrast to PD, no reductions in dopamine transporter sites, tyrosine hydroxylase, and D2 autoreceptors were found in the SN of patients with AD or AD-parkinsonism (Murray et al., 1995). The brains of patients with pure AD, however, had loss of dopamine transporter sites in the nucleus accumbens, and those with AD-parkinsonism had additional loss, particularly in the rostral caudate and putamen. Since bradykinesia and rigidity, but not tremor, are usually the chief parkinsonian features of AD-parkinsonism, the observed biochemical alterations are consistent with the hypothesis that the presence of tremor correlates with dopamine depletion in the caudal, rather than rostral, caudate nucleus. The pathologic findings suggest that in AD-parkinsonism, the loss of dopaminergic striatal terminals is not simply a reflection of nigral dopaminergic neuronal loss.

The tauopathies are neurodegenerative disorders that are manifested pathologically by neuronal and glial inclusions consisting of hyperphosphorylated, insoluble tau. The mutated tau presumably prevents proper binding to the microtubules, which could either destabilize the microtubules, interfering with axoplasmic transport, or lead to an excess of free-floating, toxic tau. In vitro experiments have shown that four repeats preferentially form into straight-filament NFTs. All the identified mutations appear to destabilize the self-aggregating stem loop structure at the exon 10 splice site, leading to overproduction of four (rather than three) repeat isoforms of tau (Morris, Lees, et al., 1999). The four-repeat tau is insoluble, and it aggregates to form neuronal and glial inclusions. These inclusions contain "twisted ribbon" filaments rather than the PHFs and straight filaments that are typically observed in AD (Poorkaj et al., 1998; Hutton, 1999; Hutton, 2000). In contrast, missense mutations outside exon 10, which affect all tau isoforms, result in neuronal inclusions that consist of both three- and four-repeat tau, with morphology similar to that of AD. In addition to the abnormal tau, brains of patients with FTDP-17 have pronounced frontotemporal atrophy, neuronal loss, gliosis, granulovacuolar degeneration, and cortical spongiform changes. Silver-positive, spheroidal enlargements of the presynaptic terminals have been found within the neuropil of the vulnerable regions (Zhou et al., 1998). These neuropil spheroids are immunopositive cytoskeletal proteins, including tau, and probably represent dystrophic changes associated with retrograde degeneration.

There are many disorders that resemble AD-parkinsonism clinically but that can be differentiated from pure AD only at autopsy. These include not only DLB, as discussed previously, but also Pick disease, CJD, and sporadic or familial progressive subcortical gliosis (Lanska et al., 1994).

NBIA-1, formerly known as Hallervorden-Spatz disease, is an autosomal-recessive disorder characterized by dystonia, parkinsonism, dementia, and brain iron accumulation (Thomas and Jankovic, 2003). Because of Julius Hallervorden's terrible past and his shameless involvement in active euthanasia during World War II (Shevell, 2003), the eponym carrying his name has been replaced by the new term *NBIA-1*. Characterized by childhood-onset progressive rigidity, dystonia, choreoathetosis, spasticity, optic nerve atrophy, and dementia, NBIA-1 has also been associated in some cases with acanthocytosis (Racette et al., 2001; Thomas and Jankovic, 2003). NBIA-1 can present as an adult-onset parkinsonism-dystonia-dementia syndrome (Jankovic et al., 1985). Linkage analyses initially localized the *NBIA-1* gene on 20p12.3–p13; subsequently, 7-bp deletion and various missense mutations were identified in the coding sequence of gene *PANK2*, which codes for pantothenate kinase (Taylor et al., 1996; Zhou et al., 2001; Hayflick et al., 2003)—

hence the term *pantothenate kinase-associated neurodegeneration*. Pantothenate kinase is an essential regulatory enzyme in coenzyme A biosynthesis. It has been postulated that as a result of phosphopantothenate deficiency, cystein accumulates in the globus pallidus of brains of patients with NBIA-1. It undergoes rapid auto-oxidation in the presence of nonheme iron, which normally accumulates in the GPi and SN, generating free radicals that are locally neurotoxic. Interestingly, atypical subjects were found to be compound heterozygotes for certain mutations for which classic subjects were homozygous. Most, but not all, patients with NBIA-1 phenotype have mutations in the *PANK2* gene (Thomas and Jankovic, 2003). On the basis of an analysis of 123 patients from 98 families with NBIA-1, Hayflick and colleagues (2003) found that "classic Hallervorden-Spatz syndrome" was associated with *PANK2* mutation in all cases and one third of "atypical" cases (late onset, slowly progressive disorder characterized by palilalia, dysarthria, dystonia, perseverative behavior and movements, freezing, and dementia) had the mutations within the *PANK2* gene. Those who had the *PANK2* mutation were more likely to have dysarthria and psychiatric symptoms, and all had the typical "eye-of-the-tiger" abnormality on MRI with a specific pattern of hyperintensity within the hypointense GPi.

Other disorders that are associated with abnormal brain iron accumulation include PD, MSA, AD, Huntington disease, human immunodeficiency encephalopathy, neuroferritinopathy (caused by a mutation in the gene coding for ferritin light polypetide on chromosome 19q13.3) (Curtis et al., 2001), and aceruloplasminemia (caused by mutations in the gene coding ceruloplasmin (Miyajima et al., 2002; Nittis and Gitlin, 2002). A novel mutation in the ferritin light chain gene was reported in a French Canadian family with Dutch ancestry manifested chiefly by atypical postural instability with dysfunctional gait, parkinsonism with blepharospasm and oromandibular dystonia, and putaminal hyperintensity on T2-weighted MRI (Mancuso et al., 2005).

## Treatment

Although the parkinsonian features might improve with dopaminergic therapy, there is little that one can do to improve the cognitive deficit. With the introduction of cholinesterase inhibitors such as donepezil (Aricept) and rivastigmine (Exelon), it is possible that cognition, orientation, and language function will improve, leading to a meaningful improvement in function. Rivastigmine inhibits not only acetylcholinesterase but also butyrylcholinesterase, which, in contrast to its relative absence in the normal brain, accounts for 40% of cholinergic activity in the cortex and 60% in the hippocampus in AD brains. In a randomized, double-blind, placebo-controlled, multicenter study of 120 patients with probable DLB, McKeith and colleagues (2000) found the drug to be safe and to effectively ameliorate apathy, anxiety, delusions, and hallucinations. The efficacy of cholinesterase inhibitors in DLB has been attributed to relative preservation of cortical muscarinic M1 receptors. In addition to the usual side effects of cholinesterase inhibitors, such as nausea, vomiting, anorexia, and weight loss, four patients noted emergent tremor without a significant worsening of Unified Parkinson's Disease Rating Scale. Hallucinations, a frequent complication of dopaminergic drug therapy, may be controlled with clozapine, but potentially serious side effects, including agranulocytosis, require weekly monitoring of the white blood cells (Kahn et al., 1991; Chacko et al., 1993). Olanzapine (Zyprexa), another atypical neuroleptic, has been reported to exert an antipsychotic effect similar to that of clozapine but without the risk of agranulocytosis (Wolters et al., 1996). In several studies, however, olanzapine was associated with exacerbation of parkinsonian motor disability (Ondo et al., 2002b). Quetiapine fumarate (Seroquel), a dibenzothiazepine that blocks not only D1 and D2 receptors but also 5-HT$_{1A}$ and 5-HT$_2$ receptors, has also been found to have a beneficial effect in PD patients with hallucinations described previously with the other atypical neuroleptics (Fernandez et al., 1999). Indeed, quetiapine is our drug of choice for psychosis in patients with PD, followed by clozapine and olanzapine.

# PARKINSONISM–DEMENTIA–AMYOTROPHIC LATERAL SCLEROSIS COMPLEX OF GUAM

## Clinical Aspects

The combination of parkinsonism, dementia, and motor neuron disease was first noted in a population of Guam, where it is known as lytico-bodig (Hirano et al., 1961), and the associated dementia is known among the Chamorros, the native inhabitants of Guam, as *Mariana dementia* (Galasko et al., 2002). In a review of 363 Chamorro and 3 Filipino immigrants with this disease, men were affected twice as frequently as women, but no differences in age of onset (57 years) or death (62 years) were seen between the genders (Zhang et al., 1990). Besides parkinsonism, supranuclear ocular motility disorder has been reported in all 37 patients in one series (Lepore et al., 1988)  (Video 10-12). Patients with parkinsonism usually present later than those with ALS, possibly because patients presenting with motor neuron disease do not survive long enough to develop extrapyramidal symptoms (Zhang et al., 1990; Rowland and Shneider, 2001). Furthermore, basal ganglia signs might be masked by the motor neuron disease. Environmental etiology of the parkinsonism-dementia-ALS complex of Guam (PDACG) is suggested not only by its restricted geographic distribution but also by its declining incidence (Galasko et al., 2002). Among 194 Chamorros evaluated between 1997 and 2000, Galasko and colleagues (2002) found 10 with ALS, 11 with PD, 90 with parkinsonism-dementia complex, and 83 with late-life dementia. They suggest that the rapid decline in incidence of these disorders in Guam strongly supports the role of environmental factors in their pathogenesis. In a report of 13 patients diagnosed with motor neuron disease who exhibited some clinical features of coexistent parkinsonism, Qureshi and colleagues (1996) suggested that motor neuron disease and parkinsonism have common pathogenetic mechanisms because the onset of the two disorders was closely temporarily related.

Another geographically determined PSP-like disorder was described in 1999 by Caparros-Lefebvre and colleagues (1999) on the Caribbean island of Guadeloupe. The case-control survey found that the disease is associated with the use of two indigenous plants that contain the mitochondrial complex I and dopaminergic neuronal toxins reticuline and corxime (Hoglinger et al., 2003): *Annona muricata* (synonyms: soursop, corossol, guanbana, graviola, and sweetsop) and custard apple (considered to be one of the foods containing annonaceous benzyltetrahydroisoquinoline alkaloids that might be responsible for the neurotoxicity leading to these geographically specific tauopathies [Steele et al., 2002]), which is associated in some cases with unusual asymptomatic retinopathy (Campbell et al., 1993; Jano-Edward et al., 2002). A similar clinical syndrome has been reported in Afro-Caribbean and Indian immigrants in England who regularly consumed imported Annonaceae products (Chaudhuri et al., 2000). The Guadeloupean parkinsonism was later characterized as a PSP-like tauopathy, although no mutation of the *tau* gene was found (Caparros-Lefebvre et al., 2002; Steele et al., 2002). It has been postulated that the high prevalence of atypical parkinsonism resembling PSP on the island of Guadeloupe is related to consumption of Annonaceae fruit and teas that contain high levels of mitochondrial complex I inhibitors such as benzyltetrahydroisoquinolines (TIQs, reticuline) and tetrahydroprotoberverine (corexime). In addition to Guam and Guadeloupe, another geographic area where ALD-dementia-parkinsonism complex has been identified is the Kii peninsula of Japan (Kuzuhara et al., 2001). Although the *tau* gene failed to show any mutations, an analysis of insoluble protein extracted from the brain of one of the affected family members showed a 60-, 64-, 68-kDa triple, suggesting that this disorder might be a variant of a tauopathy. While no mutations in the *tau* gene have been identified, Poorkaj and colleagues (2001) suggested that the *tau* gene might be a modifying gene because of linkage disequilibrium between PDACG and certain tau polymorphisms.

## Neurodiagnostic Studies

PET scanning in patients with the parkinsonian form of this disease reveals decreased presynaptic [$^{18}$F]fluorodopa uptake similar to that in patients with PD, while those with ALS have a picture intermediate between that of PD and that of control populations, suggesting a preclinical lesion (Snow et al., 1990). Reduced [$^{18}$F]fluorodopa uptake on PET scans of patients with advanced ALS has provided evidence in support of basal ganglia involvement in ALS.

## Neuropathology and Neurochemistry

The increased frequency of this neurodegenerative disorder on the island of Guam suggests a possible environmental etiology (Hirano et al., 1961). The neurotoxins methyl-azoxymethanol β-D-glucoside (cycasin) and β-N-methylamino-L-alanine, compounds that are found in the cycad plant and are believed to be in high concentrations in flour made from this plant, produce a similar spectrum of neurologic decline in monkeys (Spencer et al., 1987; Kisby et al., 1992). However, an analysis of the β-N-methylamino-L-alanine content of cycad flour suggests that the quantities of β-N-methylamino-L-alanine that are normally consumed by the inhabitants of the endemic areas were not sufficient to produce neurologic toxicity (Duncan et al., 1990). Cox and Sacks (2002) have hypothesized that the consumption of flying foxes by the Chamorro people might have generated sufficiently high cumulative doses of plant neurotoxins (Banack and Cox, 2003; Cox et al., 2003). The Chamorro eat flying foxes (*Pteropus mariannus*) boiled in coconut cream at ceremonial feasts. The bats eat the seeds of cycad trees (*Cycas micronesia*), which contain neurotoxin β-N-methylamino-L-alanine. Flying foxes, like the disease, are now rare. Other hypotheses concerning abnormalities in mineral metabolism and hypomagnesemia or hypocalcemia have also been suggested, but supporting evidence is lacking (Garruto and Yase, 1986; Ahlskog et al., 1995).

Pathologically, this condition resembles AD more than PD. Tau-containing NFTs are present, particularly in the hippocampus (Gilbert et al., 1988; Shankar et al., 1989) and other brain and spinal cord areas (Matsumoto et al., 1990). Beta-amyloid protein-containing NFTs have been identified in the brains of patients with PDACG (Ito et al., 1991). Immunohistochemical studies of autopsied brains of patients with PDACG showed marked reduction in the number of dopaminergic neurons in both the lateral and medial SN (Goto et al., 1990a). Despite marked reduction of nigrostriatal dopamine concentration, the striatal output system was well preserved, and glutamate, GABA, choline acetyltransferase, and serotonin were spared. One study provided evidence for nigrostriatal dopaminergic dysfunction in patients with familial ALS, but patients without the copper/zinc superoxide dismutase mutations were more likely to have the abnormality than were those with the mutation (Przedborski et al., 1996). This suggests that the mutation is more cytotoxic to motor neurons than to the dopaminergic neurons.

## HEREDODEGENERATIVE PARKINSONISM

Parkinsonism may be an associated feature or the dominant clinical feature in some heredodegenerative disorders, as listed in Box 10-2. Most of these disorders are discussed elsewhere.

## SECONDARY PARKINSONISM

Parkinsonism, the clinical syndrome that is manifested chiefly by tremor, bradykinesia, rigidity, and postural instability, may be the sole manifestation of a disorder, such as PD; it may be a component of a more complex disorder such as one of the multiple-system degenerations or heredodegenerations; or it may result from pharmacologic, physiologic, or pathologic abnormalities with different etiologies (see Box 10-2). Although the "secondary" parkinsonian disorders are produced by different mechanisms, they all seem to produce parkinsonian symptoms by interfering with normal dopaminergic production or transmission. Only the most important secondary types of parkinsonism are reviewed here.

### Infections

An exposure to an infectious agent, such as the one (or more) responsible for the 1917 to 1928 pandemic of encephalitis lethargica (von Economo encephalitis), has long been recognized as a cause of parkinsonism (Krusz et al., 1987, Calne and Lees, 1988; Takahashi and Yamada, 1999; Dale et al., 2004). Indeed, postencephalitic parkinsonism was once thought to be the primary cause of PD (Litvan, Jankovic, et al., 1998). The clinical presentation often involved fever, somnolence, ophthalmoplegia, and CSF lymphocytic pleocytosis (50 to 100 lymphocytes). About 40% of the affected individuals died during the acute illness. Parkinsonism occurred in 50% of the survivors within 5 years and 80% within 10 years. In addition to the typical parkinsonian features, which were usually levodopa

responsive, there were many other neurologic and movement disorders that helped to differentiate this postencephalitic syndrome from idiopathic PD. The accompanying features included oculogyric crises, blepharospasm, palilalia, and various hyperkinesias such as dystonia, chorea, tics, and hiccups.

The pathologic finding of the acute disorder consisted chiefly of midbrain and periventricular inflammation. The delayed-onset movement disorder was characterized by marked depletion of neurons in the SN and NFTs in the residual neurons (Litvan, Jankovic, et al., 1998). No virus was ever documented as the cause of postencephalitic parkinsonism, but there has been a recent reemergence of interest in the influenza A virus as a possible etiologic agent. This virus displays preferential tropism to the brainstem (especially the nigral neurons), cerebellum, and limbic system, and it produces changes (e.g., phosphorylation of cytoskeletal proteins and alterations in intermediate filaments) that could lead to the formation of Lewy bodies (Takahashi and Yamada, 1999). The mechanism of the latency between the acute illness and the subsequent development of parkinsonism has never been elucidated. The syndrome of postencephalitic parkinsonism, however, serves as a model for other delayed-onset movement disorders (Saint Hilaire et al., 1991; Scott and Jankovic, 1996).

Sporadic cases of postencephalitic parkinsonism have been reported since the 1917 to 1928 pandemic (Howard and Lees, 1987). Japanese encephalitis not only may involve the cortex, thalamus, brainstem, and spinal cord but also in some cases may be associated pathologically with predominant involvement of the SN and clinically with otherwise typical parkinsonism (Pradham et al., 1999). West Nile encephalitis has been associated with tremor, myoclonus, and parkinsonism during the acute illness with complete recovery in some patients (Sejvar et al., 2003). The case of a 21-year-old man with viral encephalitis involving the SN and a review of the world's literature of similar cases were reported (Savant et al., 2003). More recently, West Nile encephalitis involving the SN has been increasingly recognized as a cause of acute parkinsonism (Bosanko et al., 2003). When it affects other brainstem areas and the spinal cord, West Nile infection can present as acute poliomyelitis (Agamanolis et al., 2003). Dale and colleagues (2004) described 20 patients with the clinical picture of encephalitis lethargica; in 55%, the onset was preceded by pharyngitis. MRI showed inflammatory changes in the deep gray matter in 40% of patients. Laboratory investigation suggested poststreptococcal etiology in that ASO was elevated in 65% of patients and Western immunoblotting showed that 95% of the patients had autoantibodies reactive against human basal ganglia antigens, compared to 2% to 4% of these antibodies in controls ($n = 173$, $P < .0001$). One case that was examined at autopsy showed striatal encephalitis with perivenous B- and T-lymphocytic infiltration. The methodology of the study and the specificity of the antibodies, however, have been questioned (Vincent, 2004). Other infectious causes of parkinsonism include human immunodeficiency virus and associated infections (Nath et al., 1987).

### Prion Diseases

The elegant studies of Prusiner and his collaborators have drawn attention to a group of disorders known as *prion diseases*, and because of their growing scientific importance as

**Box 10-2** Classification of parkinsonism

### I. Primary (Idiopathic) Parkinsonism
- Parkinson disease
- Juvenile parkinsonism (Ishikawa and Miyatake, 1995)

### II. Multiple System Degenerations (Parkinsonism-Plus)
- Progressive supranuclear palsy
- Multiple-system atrophy
- Striatonigral degeneration
- Olivopontocerebellar atrophy
- Shy-Drager syndrome
- Lytico-bodig or parkinsonism-dementia-ALS complex of Guam
- Corticobasal ganglionic degeneration
- Progressive pallidal atrophy (primary pallidal degeneration)
- Parkinsonism-dementia complex
- Pallidopyramidal disease (Remy et al., 1995)

### III. Heredodegenerative Parkinsonism
- Hereditary juvenile dystonia-parkinsonism (Ishikawa and Miyatake, 1995)
- Autosomal-dominant Lewy body disease (Wszolek et al., 1995)
- Huntington disease (Jankovic and Ashizawa, 1995)
- Wilson disease (Thomas et al., 1995)
- Hereditary ceruloplasmin deficiency (Morita et al., 1995)
- Hallervorden-Spatz disease (Jankovic et al., 1985; Hayflick et al., 2003)
- Spinocerebellar ataxia type 2 (Shan et al., 2001)
- Machado-Joseph disease, spinocerebellar ataxia type 3 (Tuite et al., 1995)
- Familial amyotrophy-dementia-parkinsonism (Majoor-Krakauer et al., 1994)
- Disinhibition-dementia-parkinsonism-amyotrophy-complex (DDPAC) (Lynch et al., 1994)
- Parkinsonism-depression-weight-loss-central hypoventilation (Tsuboi, Wszolek, et al., 2002)
- Gerstmann-Strausler-Scheinker disease
- Familial progressive subcortical gliosis (FPSG) (Lanska et al., 1994)
- Lubag (X-linked dystonia-parkinsonism) (Wilhelmsen et al., 1991)
- Familial basal ganglia calcification (bilateral striopallidodentate calcinosis; Fahr disease) (Manyam et al., 2001; Brodaty et al., 2002; Oliveira et al., 2004)
- Mitochondrial cytopathies with striatal necrosis
- Juvenile neuronal ceroid lipofuscinosis (Åberg et al., 2000)
- Juvenile parkinsonism with neuronal intranuclear inclusion (O'Sullivan et al., 2000)
- Familial parkinsonism with peripheral neuropathy
- Parkinsonian-pyramidal syndrome (Nisipeanu et al., 1994)
- Neuroacanthocytosis (Rinne et al., 1994)
- Hereditary hemochromatosis (Nielsen et al., 1995; Costello et al., 2004)
- Parkinsonism and kinetic tremor associated with premutation in the fragile X gene
- (FRM1) (Hagerman et al., 2001; Jacquemont et al., 2003)
- Autosomal-dominant striatal degeneration with dysarthria and gait disorder
- (5q13–5q14) (Kuhlenbaummer et al., 2004)

### IV. Secondary (Acquired, Symptomatic) Parkinsonism
- Infectious: postencephalitic, AIDS, SSPE, CJD, prion diseases
- Drugs: dopamine receptor–blocking drugs (antipsychotic, antiemetic drugs), reserpine, tetrabenazine, α-methyl-dopa, lithium, flunarizine, cinnarizine, ecstasy (MDMA)
- (Mintzer et al., 1999)
- Toxins: 1-methyl-4-phenyl 1,2,3,6-tetrahydropyridine, CO, Mn, Hg, $CS_2$, cyanide (Rosenow et al., 1995), methanol, ethanol, organophosphates (Bhatt et al., 1999)
- Vascular: multi-infarct, Binswanger disease, Sjögren syndrome
- Trauma: pugilistic encephalopathy
- Other: parathyroid abnormalities, hypothyroidism, hepatocerebral degeneration (Burkhard et al., 2003), alcohol-induced coma and respiratory acidosis with bilateral pallidal lesions (Kuoppamaki et al., 2005), brain tumor, brain stem astrocytoma (Cicarelli et al., 1999), paraneoplastic, normal pressure hydrocephalus (NPH), noncommunicating hydrocephalus, syringomesencephalia, hemiatrophy-hemiparkinsonism, wasp sting, peripherally induced tremor and parkinsonism, and psychogenic

---

well as their potential impact on public health, Prusiner was awarded the 1997 Nobel Prize for Medicine (Prusiner, 1997, 2001; Glatzel et al., 2005). These transmissible spongiform encephalopathies, some of which are associated with parkinsonian features, consist of four conditions: (1) CJD and its variant (see later), (2) kuru (Kompoliti et al., 1999), (3) Gerstmann-Sträussler-Scheinker (GSS) disease, and (4) familial or sporadic fatal insomnia (Haywood, 1997; Gambetti and Parchi, 1999; Mastrianni et al., 1999; Collins et al., 2004). CJD can present with rapidly progressive parkinsonism, often accompanied by dementia, myoclonus, and gait disorder (Shinobu et al., 1999). In a series of 232 cases of sporadic CJD

that was shown to be experimentally transmitted, cognitive decline was present in 100%, myoclonus in 78%, cerebellar signs in 71%, pyramidal signs in 62%, and extrapyramidal signs, including parkinsonism, in 56% (Brown et al., 1994). Prominent amyotrophy is also occasionally present in patients with CJD (Worrall et al., 2000). Periodic EEG was recorded in only 60% of the cases, and this pattern was rarely present in the familial cases. Periodic complexes are relatively specific for CJD, with only a 9% false positive rate (Steinhoff et al., 2004). On the basis of a study involving 300 cases of sporadic CJD the authors proposed a classification of six phenotypic variants with a variable degree of rapidly progressive dementia, myoclonus, ataxia, insomnia, and typical EEG (Parchi et al., 1999). The "new-variant" CJD, caused by bovine spongiform encephalopathy prions, differs dramatically from the more common sporadic form in that the patients' age is usually in the twenties, about three or four decades earlier than that in the sporadic disease, and many patients present with prominent affective symptoms, including dysphoria, irritability, anxiety, apathy, loss of energy, insomnia, and social withdrawal. Symptoms that are typically seen in the sporadic disease, such as cognitive impairment, dysarthria, gait abnormalities, and myoclonus, are late features.

A definite diagnosis of these disorders can be made only by examination of the brain tissue, but one study showed that neuron-specific enolase can be a potentially useful biochemical marker for CJD (Zerr et al., 1995). Diagnostic criteria for sporadic CJD include immunohistochemistry with antibodies against the prion protein (Kretzschmar et al., 1996). When the CSF of 58 patients with definite or probable CJD was examined and compared with that of 29 control subjects, the level was significantly higher in the former group ($P < .001$), and when a cutoff of 35 ng/mL was used, the optimum sensitivity was 80%, and specificity was 92%. More recently, two studies have detected two disease-specific proteins, p130/131, in the CSF of patients with CJD (Hsich et al., 1996; Zerr et al., 1996). Several studies showed that the presence of 14-3-3 protein in the CSF improved the diagnosis of CJD (Poser et al., 1999; Aksamit, 2003). Although the sensitivity of this test may be as high as 97% and its specificity may be as high as 87% (Lemstra et al., 2000; Castellani et al., 2004), particularly in the classic variety of sporadic CJD, some studies have found the sensitivity to be as low as 53% (Geschwind et al., 2003). False positives include stroke, meningoencephalitis, vasculitis, paraneoplastic disorders, FTD, and AD (Chapman et al., 2000). When added to the diagnostic criteria, the presence of 14-3-3 protein in the CSF markedly increased the sensitivity of diagnostic criteria and increased the estimated incidence of CJD (Brandel et al., 2000; Zerr et al., 2000). Subsequent studies, however, showed that the 14-3-3 test does not differentiate between CJD and other neurodegenerative disorders associated with dementia (Burkhard et al., 2001). In addition to the positive 14-3-3 immunoassay, over 70% of patients with the new variant of CJD who were homozygous for methionine at codon 129 of the prion protein gene had bilateral pulvinar high signal on MRI (Will et al., 2000). More recently, CSF tau-protein assay by enzyme-linked immunosorbent assay, already readily available in routine laboratories, has been found to have a 92% positive predictive value in diagnosing CJD; 74 of 77 patients with probable CJD had tau protein greater than 1300 pg/mL, whereas only 2 of 28 patients with AD had such high levels, and the percentage was even lower in those with other dementias (Otto et al., 2002). The National Prion Disease Pathology Surveillance Center at Case Western Reserve University offers, free of charge, a variety of diagnostic tests, including Western blots on frozen brain tissue to detect protease-resistant PrP, immunohistochemical tests for PrP on fixed tissue, analysis of DNA extracted from blood or brain tissue for PRNP, and analysis of CSF for 14-3-3 protein. Parchi and colleagues (1999) classified the six types of CJD according to homozygosity or heterozygosity of methionine (M) and valine (V) at codon 129 of the prion protein gene: The MM1 and MV1 correlate with the phenotype of classic sporadic CJD (rapidly progressive dementia with periodic EEG), whereas others are more atypical, with slower progression and young age at onset (VV1) or ataxia (MV2 and VV2).

Imaging can also be very helpful in the diagnosis of CJD. DWI-MRI has the highest sensitivity for the detection of signal intensity abnormalities in CJD. Increased signal intensity is typically seen bilaterally in the striatum, thalamus, and cortex ("cortical ribbon") (Murata et al., 2002; Mendez et al., 2003; Tschampa et al., 2003; Shiga et al., 2004). In an analysis of 19 reported cases of CJD with DWI-MRI lesions, CSF protein 14-3-3 was negative in 6 cases and positive in 2 others (Mendez et al., 2003). The authors concluded that "multifocal cortical and subcortical hyperintensities confined to gray matter regions in DWI-MRI may be a more useful noninvasive diagnostic marker for CJD than CSF protein 14-3-3." Furthermore, high T2W signal in the basal ganglia correlated with VV or MV codon 129 genotypes (Meissner et al., 2004).

The prion diseases appear to be related to an abnormal metabolism of a normal cellular constituent, the prion protein (PrP), which is normally encoded by a gene on the short arm of chromosome 20 (Haywood, 1997; Prusiner, 1997). When the normal PrP$^c$ protein, which has an α-helical structure, undergoes a conformational change to a β-pleated structure, the resulting abnormal PrP$^{sc}$ (Sc = scrapie) isoform leads to development of the disease. There is growing evidence that the fundamental process in prion propagation involves seeded aggregation of misfolded host proteins (Collinge, 2005). A substantial percentage of patients with sporadic or iatrogenic CJD share methionine or valine homozygosity in codon 129, indicating increased susceptibility of this population. In sporadic CJD, an increase of relative risk for CJD with codon 129 genotypes (Met/Met:Val/Val:Met/Va) was assessed at 11:4:1. The molecular strain characteristics of nvCJD are clearly different from those of previously recognized human prion strains but closely resembled those seen in bovine spongiform encephalopathy. None of the patients with nvCJD had mutations in the *PRNP* gene, but all so far reported have been methionine homozygotes at codon 129.

Point missense mutations and insertional mutations have also been instructive in classifying familial CJD. In other human prion diseases, mutations causing familial forms of disease have been identified. In Gerstmann-Strassler-Scheinker disease, *PRNP* mutations were found in codons 102, 117, 198, and 217. In FFI, a *PRNP* mutation is present in codon 178. Clinicopathologic diversity of FFI overlaps widely with CJD, and it has been proposed that molecular diagnostics (*PRNP* mutation at codon 178, polymorphism at codon 129) might separate those two entities. Point mutations in the prion protein gene segregate with the familial prion diseases. For example, a mutation at codon 210, coupled with some genetic and environmental factors, is associated with CJD (Pocchiari et al., 1993). The risk of developing CJD in Libyan Jews with the *PRNP* gene codon 200 point mutation is virtually 100% by age 80 years (Chapman et al., 1994; Goldfarb and Brown, 1995). A mutation in codon 200 accounts for three geographic clusters that have been described in Slovakia and in Chile. Insertional mutations of additional copies of an octapeptide (24 to 216 base pairs) in the *PRNP* gene have been described in CJD patients worldwide.

Mutations in the prion protein gene (*PRNP*) have been found not only in patients with CJD but also in fatal familial insomnia and Gerstmann-Sträussler-Scheinker disease, manifested by autosomal-dominantly inherited progressive ataxia and dementia

(Panegyres et al., 2001). Prion protein abnormalities, however, do not seem to be associated with either idiopathic parkinsonism or with MSA (Jendroska et al., 1994). The area of experimental therapeutics of CJD and other transmissible spongiform encephalopathies is an emerging branch of basic science research that is soon to be translated into clinical trials. Some novel therapies that are currently being tested in experimental animals include a variety of anti-infectious agents, immunomodulating drugs, compounds designed to eliminate misfolded membrane-bound prion proteins, and neutralizing antibodies (Brown, 2002). Detection of pathologic PrP^sc in the olfactory epithelium in nine patients with sporadic CJD but not in any controls suggests that the olfactory pathway might be the route of infection by the prions; this finding suggests that olfactory biopsy might be of diagnostic importance (Zanusso et al., 2003).

There is no treatment for CJD, but there might be some rationale for using the antimalarial drug quinacrine because of its protease resistance of PrP peptide aggregates, although there is little hope that this drug will significantly alter the natural course of the fatal disease (Barret et al., 2003). Flupirtine, a centrally acting nonopioid analgesic antiapoptotic drug, was found to have beneficial effects on cognitive functioning of patients with CJD (Otto et al., 2002).

## Drugs

Although drug-induced parkinsonism might be the most common form of parkinsonism, it is not commonly encountered in movement disorder clinics (see Table 10-1). Parkinsonian symptoms and findings, often indistinguishable from those seen in patients with PD, may be evident within the first few days of neuroleptic therapy; nearly all cases become evident within 3 months after initiation of treatment (Hardie and Lees, 1988; Jankovic, 1995c). In addition, chronically treated patients may develop parkinsonian findings when the dose of a neuroleptic is increased. The prevalence of neuroleptic-induced parkinsonism has been reported to range from 10% to 60% of patients treated with antipsychotics. Advanced age, female gender, and possibly genetic predisposition, such as the presence of essential tremor, have been identified as potential risk factors. About one third of all patients referred to a large movement disorder clinic with drug-induced movement disorders, such as tardive dyskinesia, have parkinsonian findings (Jankovic, 1995c). While two thirds of all patients recover within 7 weeks after stopping the offending drug, the symptoms may persist for more than 18 months. In one study, 11% of patients who recovered from neuroleptic-induced parkinsonism were later found to have the characteristic pathologic findings of PD at autopsy (Rajput et al., 1982). This suggests that parkinsonism that persists even after the offending drug is withdrawn may represent subclinical, latent PD. Evidence for persistent dysfunction in patients with drug-induced parkinsonism has been provided by the demonstration of reduced [$^{18}$F]fluorodopa uptake in some patients and by depression of platelet mitochondrial complex I activity (Burkhardt et al., 1993; Burn and Brooks, 1993). In a study of 20 patients with drug-induced parkinsonism, 11 had abnormal β-CIT SPECT scans that indicated underlying nigrostriatal deficiency, which suggested that even though the patients were taking neuroleptics, their parkinsonism may have been due to exacerbation of underlying PD (Lorberboym et al., 2006). There were no differences in clinical features

between the 11 patients who had abnormal SPECT scans and the 9 patients who had normal scans.

## Toxins

Knowledge of the mechanisms and treatment of parkinsonism has expanded dramatically as a result of the discovery that the neurotoxin 1-methyl-4-phenyl-1,2,3,6-tetrahydropyridine (MPTP) can induce parkinsonism (Langston et al., 1983; Bloem et al., 1990). MPTP can produce parkinsonism in animals (particularly primates) and humans that can be clinically indistinguishable from idiopathic PD. In contrast to PD, which affects chiefly the putamen, however, MPTP impairs dopaminergic function in both the caudate and putamen (Snow et al., 2000).

There are several other toxins that can cause parkinsonism, but only carbon monoxide and manganese are reviewed here. Carbon monoxide exposure can result in acute intoxication, which is associated with about a 35% mortality rate, progressive akinetic-mute state, or delayed-relapsing encephalopathy (Sohn et al., 2000). The latter syndrome usually develops after a 3-week recovery period. The delayed relapsing type of carbon monoxide sequelae is characterized by slow, short-stepped gait; start hesitation; freezing; body bradykinesia; and rigidity but little or no tremor. In addition, these patients often develop akinetic mutism and other peculiar behaviors. They usually do not improve with levodopa. In a review of 8 patients with progressive sequelae and 23 patients with the delayed relapsing sequelae, Lee and Marsden (1994) could not identify any reliable predictors of eventual outcome following acute intoxication. During a 1-year follow-up, 50% of the patients with the progressive type of carbon monoxide encephalopathy died, and another 50% remained severely disabled; some developed contractures in the advanced stages (Lee and Marsden, 1994). Of the patients with the delayed relapsing type of carbon monoxide sequelae, 61% subsequently improved, and 13% died. Delayed-onset parkinsonism has been documented not only after carbon monoxide poisoning but also after anoxia, trauma, and other brain injuries (Bhatt et al., 1993; Scott and Jankovic, 1996; Li et al., 2000).

Because certain metals, such as iron, copper, and manganese, can facilitate oxidative reactions, there is growing interest in these transitional metals in the pathogenesis of neurodegenerative disorders. Manganese was first reported to cause a parkinsonian syndrome in 1837, only 20 years after James Parkinson described the disease that now bears his name (Calne et al., 1994). Since that time, there have been many reports of manganese intoxication causing psychiatric problems ("manganese madness"), usually followed in a few months by motor symptoms. These consist of dystonia, parkinsonism, retropulsion, and a characteristic gait called cock-walk, which is manifested by walking on the toes with elbows flexed and the spine erect. There is usually no tremor, and the motor deficits rarely improve with levodopa therapy. Manganese intoxication has been reported in miners, smelters, welders, workers involved in the manufacture of dry batteries, chronic accidental ingestion of potassium permanganate, and incorrect concentration of manganese in parenteral nutrition. Welders with PD were found to have their onset of PD on the average 17 years earlier than a control population of PD patients, suggesting that welding, possibly by causing manganese toxicity, is a risk factor for PD (Racette et al., 2001). Besides welding and manganese mining, manganese toxicity may occur with long-term parental nutrition. Although it has been postulated that manganese causes parkinsonism because of pallidal damage, some studies, including β-CIT SPECT scans, indicate a presynaptic form of parkinsonism associated with a reduction in striatal dopamine transporter (Kim et al., 2002). Manganese intoxication has been suggested as a possible cause of some of the neurologic abnormalities and abnormal MRI imaging (abnormal signal hyperintensity in the globus pallidus and SN on T1-weighted images) associated with chronic liver failure (Hauser et al., 1994; Racette et al., 2005). The abnormal imaging studies and the lack of response to levodopa are consistent with the pathologic findings in humans and experimental primates of marked neuronal loss and gliosis in the globus pallidus and SNr (Olanow et al., 1996). Despite a growing number of publications, there is little evidence that welding causes manganese-induced parkinsonism or PD (Jankovic, 2005; Kieburtz and Kurlan, 2005). The associated marked accumulation of iron and aluminum suggests that oxidant stress plays an important role in manganese neurotoxicity. One piece of evidence that has been used to link welding with manganese-induced parkinsonism is the occasional report of increased T1 basal ganglia signal on MRI of the brain (Sadek et al., 2003; Josephs et al., 2005). In one report from the Mayo Clinic, eight male career welders with such MRI findings exhibited parkinsonism (three patients), myoclonus and limited cognitive impairment (two patients), vestibular-auditory dysfunction (two patients), and minor subjective cognitive impairment, anxiety, and sleep apnea (one patient) (Josephs et al., 2005). The broad spectrum of clinical manifestations, however, argues against a direct cause-and-effect relationship. In contrast to PD, fluorodopa PET scans are normal in patients with manganese parkinsonism (Lu et al., 1994), and raclopride (D2 receptor) binding is only slightly reduced in the caudate but is normal in the putamen (Shinotoh et al., 1997). Beta-CIT SPECT scans, however, may be abnormal, indicating degeneration of presynaptic dopaminergic terminals in some patients with manganese parkinsonism (Kim et al., 2002).

There are other toxins, such as certain hydrocarbons (Pezzoli et al., 2000) and organophosphates (Bhatt et al., 1999), that have been implicated in the pathogenesis of parkinsonian syndromes. Many of the cases are complicated by legal issues; therefore, it is not always easy to prove a cause-and-effect relationship. If the parkinsonian syndrome occurs in a cluster, then it is more likely that the putative toxin is responsible.

## Vascular

Parkinsonism due to strokes or other vascular causes has been described, but the clinical correlates of vascular parkinsonism have not been fully characterized. Winikates and Jankovic (1998) compared a group of patients who satisfied the clinical, radiographic, or pathologic criteria for vascular parkinsonism with a group of patients with PD to determine which clinical variables differentiate these two forms of parkinsonism. Patients with vascular parkinsonism were older, were more likely to present with gait difficulty than with tremor, and were less likely to respond to levodopa than were patients with PD. Vascular patients were also significantly more likely to have predominant lower-body involvement, postural instability, a history of falling, dementia, corticospinal findings,

incontinence, and pseudobulbar affect. "Lower-body" parkinsonism, a condition in which upper-body motor function is relatively preserved while gait is markedly impaired, has previously been linked to multiple lacunar infarctions (Fitzgerald and Jankovic, 1989). Only about one third of patients with vascular parkinsonism respond to levodopa (Demirkiran et al., 2001). A clinical-pathologic study of 17 patients concluded that vascular disease per se can cause parkinsonism without invoking coexistent neurodegenerative disease (Zijlmans et al., 2004a). Binswanger disease, a form of leukoencephalopathy caused by hypoxia-ischemia of distal watershed periventricular territories associated with aging, hyperviscosity, and increased fibrinogen levels (Roman, 1999), can rarely present as levodopa-responsive parkinsonism (Mark et al., 1995). Alternatively, about 10% of patients with small deep infarcts and white matter lesions have been found to have a parkinsonian syndrome (van Zagten et al., 1998). It is possible that some of the familial forms of vascular parkinsonism represent the entity CADASIL, an autosomal-dominant arteriopathy associated with stroke and dementia, caused by mutations in the *Notch3* gene on chromosome 19p13.2 (Joutel et al., 2000; Wang et al., 2000). Because of multiple mutations, patients who are suspected to have this syndrome should first be screened for mutations in exons 4, 5, and 6, and if the tests are negative, a skin biopsy should be carried out searching for thickened basal lamina distorted by irregular deposits of granular osmophilic material, coupled with MRI T2 scanning (Markus et al., 2002). Vascular parkinsonism has also been described in Moyamoya (Tan et al., 2003). A substantial number of patients with vascular parkinsonism improve with levodopa, particularly those with vascular lesions in or close to the nigrostriatal pathway (Zijlmans et al., 2004b). About one third of patients with vascular parkinsonism, particularly those who respond to levodopa and do not have vertical gaze palsy or freezing, have a transient improvement in their gait after removal of 35 to 40 mL of CSF (Ondo et al., 2002a).

## Trauma

Although no definite link between trauma and PD can be established, there is convincing evidence for the concept of posttraumatic parkinsonism (Factor and Weiner, 1991; Goetz and Stebbins, 1991; Stern, 1991; Jankovic, 1994). Parkinsonism is a rare complication of a single trauma to the head unless the injury is severe enough to result in a comatose or vegetative state or causes a penetrating injury to the brainstem or a subdural hematoma with compression of the brainstem. However, parkinsonism is a well-recognized sequela of repeated head trauma, such as is seen in the "punch-drunk" syndrome or pugilistic dementia in boxers. In addition to typical parkinsonian symptoms, other neurologic consequences of boxing include dementia, paranoia, loss of inhibitions, and bradyphrenia. One of the reasons for the initial underrecognition of boxer's parkinsonism and other progressive neurologic problems has been the long latency, lasting several years or even decades, between cessation of competitive boxing and the development of neurologic symptoms and signs. The evidence indicates that it is the number of bouts (and presumably repetitive subconcussive blows) rather than the number of knockouts that correlates best with the development of chronic brain damage (Lampert and Hardman, 1984). A study of 86 amateur boxers found no evidence of cognitive impairment, suggesting that only a small minority of boxers have brain damage (Butler et al., 1993).

Most of the blows to the head that boxers sustain result in rotational (angular) acceleration, which can cause not only subdural hematoma, petechial hemorrhages, and diffuse axonal injury to the long fiber tracts but also injury to the medial temporal cortex and rostral brainstem, particularly the SN. Marked neuronal degeneration, especially in the lateral and intermediate cell groups, depigmentation, gliosis, and NFTs have been well documented in the SN of boxers' brains (Lampert and Hardman, 1984). Although initial pathologic studies of brains of boxers with dementia pugilistica emphasized the presence of numerous NFTs without plaques, subsequent reexamination of the brains with immunocytochemical methods has provided evidence that the β-amyloid protein present in brains of patients with AD is also present in the boxers' brains and that dementia pugilistica and AD share common pathogenic mechanisms (Roberts et al., 1990). One study showed increased severity of neurologic deficits in boxers with the APOE ε4 allele, suggesting that genetic predisposition may play a role in the neurologic impairments associated with chronic traumatic brain injury (Jordan et al., 1997).

Parkinsonism can result not only from injury to the central nervous system but also from peripheral trauma (Cardoso and Jankovic, 1995). In 21 patients, the onset of movement disorder began within 2 months after injury; in 6 patients, the tremor started 3 to 5 months after the trauma; and the onset was delayed by 1 year in 1 patient. The mean age at onset of the movement disorder was 46.5 ± 14.1 years. Among the parkinsonian patients, high-dose levodopa failed to ameliorate the symptoms in 4 of the 10 patients, and the others had only modest improvement. None of the patients achieved spontaneous remission; in 19 patients, the movement disorder worsened or remained unchanged. The PET scans showed decreased fluorodopa uptake in the striatum of three patients who were tested, and the raclopride binding in the striatum was symmetric and slightly increased in two of the three patients. While it is possible that the parkinsonism in these patients occurred by chance alone, the young age at onset, the anatomic and temporal relationship to severe local injury, and the atypical clinical and pharmacologic features suggest that peripherally induced parkinsonism should be added to the growing list of peripherally induced movement disorders.

## Hemiparkinsonism-Hemiatrophy

Hemiparkinsonism-hemiatrophy syndrome is a rare form of secondary parkinsonism that usually begins in the third or fourth decade; it is characterized by unilateral body atrophy and ipsilateral parkinsonian findings, dystonia, slow progression, and poor response to levodopa (Jankovic, 1988; Giladi et al., 1990). Contralateral cortical hemiatrophy is usually present, and there is often a history of perinatal asphyxia (Scott and Jankovic, 1996). In contrast to a presynaptic involvement in PD, PET studies have provided evidence of presynaptic and postsynaptic nigrostriatal dopaminergic dysfunction in patients with hemiparkinsonism-hemiatrophy syndrome (Przedborski et al., 1994). One patient with hemiparkinsonism-hemiatrophy was found to

have a mutation in the *parkin* gene on chromosome 6 (Pramstaller et al., 2002).

## Normal Pressure Hydrocephalus

Normal pressure hydrocephalus (NPH) should be considered in the differential diagnosis of all patients with progressive gait disturbance and other parkinsonian features (Curran and Lang, 1994; Vanneste, 2000). Since the CSF pressure is not always normal and the disorder seems to be quite heterogeneous in terms of age at onset and clinical presentation, the term *chronic hydrocephalus* has been proposed (Bret et al., 2002). The gait and parkinsonian features associated with NPH include short steps, wide base, stiff legs, start hesitation, and freezing ("magnetic gait"). In contrast to other parkinsonian disorders associated with freezing, the gait of patients with NPH usually does not improve with visual clues (Lai and Jankovic, 1995). In addition to the characteristic gait disturbance, NPH patients frequently exhibit bradykinesia, flexed posture, and loss of postural reflexes as well as cognitive decline and urinary incontinence. In contrast to those with PD, patients with NPH have near normal leg function in supine and sitting positions, and they tend to have less tremor. Some patients with NPH may later develop PD (Curran and Lang, 1994). Shunting may be considered for patients with NPH in whom gait disturbance precedes mental impairment and in whom the mental impairment is of recent origin and mild. Other predictors of favorable outcome after shunting include a known cause of NPH, absence of white matter lesions on MRI, a substantial clinical improvement after CSF tap, 50% occurrence of B-wave on intracranial pressure recording, and resistance to CSF outflow of at least 18 Hg/mL per minute during CSF infusion test.

Patients with short history, a known cause of hydrocephalus, predominant gait disorder, and imaging studies suggestive of hydrodynamic hydrocephalus without cortical atrophy and without white matter involvement, are considered the best candidates for shunting, and 50% to 70% experience substantial improvement after surgery (Vanneste, 2000). NPH is sometimes difficult to differentiate from vascular parkinsonism or subcortical arteriosclerotic encephalopathy (SAE). The CSF sulfatide concentration was markedly increased in patients with arteriosclerotic encephalopathy (mean: 766 nmol/L, range: 300 to 3800 nmol/L), and this test distinguished between patients with arteriosclerotic encephalopathy and those with NPH with a sensitivity of 74% and a specificity of 94%, making it an important diagnostic marker (Tullberg et al., 2000). Obstructive hydrocephalus, with or without aqueductal stenosis, can also result in parkinsonism that may respond to levodopa (Jankovic et al., 1986; Zeidler et al., 1998; Racette et al., 2004). Most patients with disabling symptoms of hydrocephalus-associated parkinsonism require ventriculoperitoneal shunting.

## Other

It is beyond the scope of this review to discuss all other causes of parkinsonism. Brain tumors and gliomatosis cerebri, even when they spare basal ganglia, may cause parkinsonism (Krauss et al., 1995; Cicarelli et al., 1999; Pohle and Krauss, 1999; Tagliati et al., 2000). Other causes of parkinsonism include paraneoplastic degeneration of the SN manifested by parkinsonism and dystonia (Golbe et al., 1989), central pontine and extrapontine myelinolysis (Seiser et al., 1998), wasp sting (Leopold et al., 1999), Sjögren syndrome (Walker et al., 1999), and others.

Parkinsonism and pyramidal signs associated with speech and orofacial apraxia slowly progressing to anarthria and muteness without other language or cognitive deficits should suggest the possibility of late anterior opercular syndrome (Broussolle et al., 1996; Bakar et al., 1998). This syndrome resembles Foix-Chavany-Marie syndrome, also known as Worster-Drought syndrome (Christen et al., 2000), which is characterized by bilateral facioglossopharyngomasticatory paresis (pseudobulbar palsy) associated with bilateral lesions in the frontal and parietal opercula. The anterior opercular syndrome is a severe form of pseudobulbar palsy in which patients with bilateral lesions of the perisylvian cortex or subcortical connections become completely mute. These patients can follow commands involving the extremities but not the cranial nerves; for example, they might be unable to open or close their eyes or mouth or smile voluntarily, yet they smile when amused, yawn spontaneously, and even utter cries in response to emotional stimuli. The syndrome is usually seen in patients who have had multiple strokes, but rare cases of progressive disease, as in the syndrome of primary progressive anarthria, may occur. A related cheiro-oral syndrome (sensory disturbance in one hand and the ipsilateral oral corner) has been associated with rostral brainstem lesions. Similar to CBD, imaging studies usually show markedly asymmetric (L > R) cortical atrophy and reduced metabolism, especially involving the posterior inferior frontal lobe, particularly the operculum (the cerebral cortex and subcortical white matter covering the insula). One of our patients with this syndrome also exhibited pseudobulbar palsy, vertical ophthalmoparesis, and postural instability similar to that of PSP. Supranuclear ophthalmoparesis has been described in some previously reported cases of the anterior opercular syndrome. Some of the cases that came to autopsy showed focal frontal (particularly left opercular) cortical atrophy with spongiform changes in layers II and III and SN degeneration without Lewy bodies. Although this syndrome is considered to be due to some yet unknown neurodegeneration, phenotypically similar cases have been documented to be due to herpes simplex encephalitis (McGrath et al., 1997), cortical infarcts, trauma, meningitis, benign epilepsy of childhood with rolandic spikes, and developmental dysplasia (Weller, 1993). Parkinsonism, frontal dementia, peripheral neuropathy, neurogenic bladder, and upper motor neuron signs have been described in adult polyglucosan body disease (Robertson et al., 1998). A single point mutation in mitochondrial 12SrRNA has recently been reported to be associated with parkinsonism, deafness, and neuropathy (Thyagarajan et al., 2000). Encephalopathy and parkinsonism have been reported in children with leukemia who have been treated with bone marrow transplantation, amphotericin, immunosuppressants, and total body irradiation (Mott et al., 1995). Juvenile parkinsonism, often characterized by prominent gait and balance difficulties, dystonia, and improvement after sleep, may occur sporadically or as an autosomal-recessive disorder (Ishikawa and Miyatake, 1995; Ishikawa and Tsuji, 1996; Shimoda-Matsubayashi et al., 1997). Some causes of secondary parkinsonism in childhood were reviewed by Pranzatelli and colleagues (1994). Although the heredogenerations are reviewed elsewhere, some of the genetic forms of parkinsonism with known genetic defects are listed in Box 10-2.

# References

Abbruzzese G, Tabaton M, Dall'Agata D, Favale E: Motor and sensory evoked potentials in progressive supranuclear palsy. Mov Disord 1991;6:49–54.

Abdo WF, De Jong D, Hendriks JC, et al: Cerebrospinal fluid analysis differentiates multiple system atrophy from Parkinson's disease. Mov Disord 2004;19:571–579.

Abele M, Schulz JB, Bürk K, et al: Evoked potentials in multiple system atrophy (MSA). Acta Neurol Scand 2000;101:111–115.

Åberg L, Liewenedahl K, Nikkinen P, et al: Decreased striatal dopamine transporter density in JCNL patients with parkinsonian symptoms. Neurology 2000;54:1069–1074.

Adachi M, Kawanami T, Ohshima H, et al: Morning glory sign: A particular MR finding in progressive supranuclear palsy. Magn Reson Med Sci 2004;3:125–132.

Agamanolis DP, Leslie MJ, Caveny EA, et al: Neuropathological findings in West Nile virus encephalitis: A case report. Ann Neurol 2003;54:547–551.

Ahlskog JE, Waring SC, Kurland LT, et al: Guamanian neurodegenerative disease: Investigation of the calcium metabolism/heavy metal hypothesis. Neurology 1995;45:1340–1344.

Aksamit AJ: Cerebrospinal fluid 14-3-3 protein. Variability of sporadic Creutzfeldt-Jakob disease, laboratory standards, and quantitation. Arch Neurol 2003;60:803–804.

Albanese A, Colosimo C, Bentivoglio AR, et al: Multiple system atrophy presenting as parkinsonism: Clinical features and diagnostic criteria. J Neurol Neurosurg Psychiatry 1995;59:144–151.

Albers DS, Augood SJ: New insights into progressive supranuclear palsy. Trends Neurosci 2001;24:347–353.

Aldrich MS, Foster NL, White RF, et al: Sleep abnormalities in progressive supranuclear palsy. Ann Neurol 1989;25:577–581.

Amaducci L, Grassi E, Boller F: Maurice Ravel and right-hemisphere musical creativity: Influence of disease on his last musical works? Eur J Neurol 2002;9:75–82.

American Academy of Neurology: Assessment: Clinical autonomic testing report of the Therapeutics and Technology Assessment Subcommittee of the American Academy of Neurology. Neurology 1996;46:673–680.

Antonini A, Leenders KL, Vontobel P, et al: Complementary PET studies of striatal neuronal function in the differential diagnosis between multiple system atrophy and Parkinson's disease. Brain 1997;120:2187–2195.

Aotsuka A, Paulson GW: Striatonigral degeneration. In Stern MB, Koller WC (eds): Parkinsonian Syndromes. New York, Marcell Dekker, 1993, pp 33–42.

Apaydin H, Ahlskog JE, Parisi JE, et al: Parkinson disease neuropathology: Later-developing dementia and loss of the levodopa response. Arch Neurol 2002;59:102–112.

Arai T, Ikeda K, Akiyama H, et al: Identification of amino-terminally cleaved tau fragments that distinguish progressive supranuclear palsy from corticobasal degeneration. Ann Neurol 2004;55:72–79.

Arima K, Murayama S, Mukoyama M, Inose T: Immunocytochemical and ultrastructural studies and oligodendroglial cytoplasmic inclusions in multiple system atrophy: 1. Neuronal cytoplasmic inclusions. Acta Neuropathologica 1992;83:454–460.

Asahina M, Suhara T, Shinotoh H, et al: Brain muscarinic receptors in progressive supranuclear palsy and Parkinson's disease: A positron emission tomographic study. J Neurol Neurosurg Psychiatry 1998;65:155–163.

Ashour R, Jankovic J: Joint and skeletal deformities in Parkinson's disease, multiple system atrophy, and progressive supranuclear palsy. Mov Disord 2006; 21(11):1856–1863.

Askmark H, Edebol Eeg-Olofsson K, Johnsson A, et al: Parkinsonism and neck extensor myopathy: A new syndrome or coincidental findings. Arch Neurol 2001;58:232–237.

Atchison PR, Thompson PD, Frackowiak SJ, Marsden CD: The syndrome of gait ignition failure: A report of six cases. Mov Disord 1993;8:285–292.

Averbuch-Heller L, Paulson GW, Daroff RB, Leigh RJ: Whipple's disease mimicking progressive supranuclear palsy: The diagnostic value of eye movement recording. J Neurol Neurosurg Psychiatry 1999;66:532–535.

Azher SN, Jankovic J: Camptocormia: Pathogenesis, classification, and response to therapy. Neurology 2005;65:355–359.

Bakar M, Kirshner HS, Niaz F: The opercular-subopercular syndrome: Four cases with review of the literature. Behavioural Neurology 1998;11:97–103.

Baker M, Litvan I, Houlden H, et al: Association of an extended haplotype in the tau gene with progressive supranuclear palsy. Hum Mol Genet 1999;8:711–715.

Banack SA, Cox PA: Biomagnification of cycad neurotoxins in flying foxes: Implications for ALS-PDC in Guam. Neurology 2003;61:387–389.

Bandmann O, Sweeney MG, Daniel SE, et al: Multiple-system atrophy is genetically distinct from identified inherited causes of spinocerebellar degeneration. Neurology 1997;49:1598–1604.

Barber R, Gholkar A, Scheltens P, et al: Medial temporal lobe atrophy on MRI in dementia with Lewy bodies. Neurology 1999;52:1153–1158.

Barclay CL, Bergeron C, Lang AE: Arm levitation in progressive supranuclear palsy. Neurology 1999;52:879–882.

Barclay CL, Lang AE: Dystonia in progressive supranuclear palsy. J Neurol Neurosurg Psychiatry 1997;62:352–356.

Barret A, Tagliavini F, Forloni G, et al: Evaluation of quinacrine treatment for prion diseases. J Virol 2003;77:8462–8469.

Bebin EM, Bebin J, Currier RD, et al: Morphometric studies in dominant olivopontocerebellar atrophy. Arch Neurol 1990;47:188–196.

Behnke S, Berg D, Naumann M, Becker G: Differentiation of Parkinson's disease and atypical parkinsonian syndromes by transcranial ultrasound. J Neurol Neurosurg Psychiatry 2005;76:423–425.

Benarroch EE, Schmeichel AM, Parisi JE: Involvement of the ventrolateral medually in parkinsonism with autonomic failure. Neurology 2000;54:963–968.

Benarroch EE, Schmeichel AM, Parisi JE: Depletion of mesopontine cholinergic and sparing of raphe neurons in multiple system atrophy. Neurology 2002;59:944–946.

Benarroch EE, Smithson II, Low PA, Parisi JE: Depletion of catecholaminergic neurons of the rostral ventrolateral medulla in multiple system atrophy with autonomic failure. Ann Neurol 1998;43:156–163.

Bennett P, Bonifati V, Bonuccelli U, et al: Direct genetic evidence for involvement of tau in progressive supranuclear palsy. Neurology 1998;51:982–985.

Ben-Shlomo Y, Wenning GK, Tison F, Quinn NP: Survival of patients with pathologically proven multiple system atrophy: A meta-analysis. Neurology 1997;48:484–493.

Berciano J: Olivopontocerebellar atrophy. In Jankovic J, Tolosa E (eds): Parkinson's Disease and Movement Disorders, 3rd ed. Baltimore, Williams & Wilkins, 1992, pp 263–296.

Bergeron C, Davis A, Lang AE: Corticobasal ganglionic degeneration and progressive supranuclear palsy presenting with cognitive decline. Brain Pathology 1998;8:355–365.

Bergeron C, Pollanen MD, Weyer L, et al: Unusual clinical presentation of cortical-basal ganglionic degeneration. Ann Neurol 1997;40:893–900.

Bhatt MH, Elias MA, Mankodi AK: Acute and reversible parkinsonism due to organophospate pesticide intoxication: Five cases. Neurology 1999;52:1467–1471.

Bhatt MH, Obeso JA, Marsden CD: Time course of postanoxic akinetic-rigid and dystonic syndromes. Neurology 1993;43:314–317.

Bhatt MH, Snow BJ, Martin WRW, et al: Positron emission tomography in Shy-Drager syndrome. Ann Neurol 1990;28:101–103.

Bhatt MH, Snow BJ, Martin WRW, et al: Positron emission tomography in supranuclear palsy. Arch Neurol 1991;48:389–391.

Bhattacharya K, Saadia D, Eisenkraft B, et al: Brain magnetic resonance imaging in multiple-system atrophy and Parkinson disease. Arch Neurol 2002;59:835–842.

Bhidayasiri R, Riley DA, Somers JT, et al: Pathophysiology of slow vertical saccades in progressive supranuclear palsy. Neurology 2001;57:2070–2077.

Biancalana V, Toft M, Le Ber I, et al: FMR1 premutations associated with fragile X-associated tremor/ataxia syndrome in multiple system atrophy. Arch Neurol 2005;62:962–966.

Biggins CA, Boyd JI, Harrop FM, et al: A controlled, longitudinal study of dementia in Parkinson's disease. J Neurol Neurosurg Psychiatry 1992;55:566–571.

Bird TD, Nochlin D, Poorkaj P, et al: A clinical pathological comparison of three families with frontotemporal dementia and identical mutations in the tau gene (P301L). Brain 1999;122:741–756.

Birdi S, Rajput AH, Fenton M, et al: Progressive supranuclear palsy diagnosis and confounding features: Report on 16 autopsied cases. Mov Disord 2002;17:1255–1264.

Blin J, Baron JC, Dubois B, et al: Positron emission tomography in progressive supranuclear palsy. Arch Neurol 1990;47:747–752.

Blin J, Mazetti P, Mazoyer B, et al: Does the enhancement of cholinergic neurotransmission influence brain glucose kinetics and clinical symptomatology in progressive supranuclear palsy. Brain 1995;118:1485–1495.

Blin J, Vidailet MJ, Pillon B, et al: Corticobasal degeneration: Decreased and asymmetrical glucose consumption as studied with PET. Mov Disord 1992;7:348–354.

Bloem BR, Irwin I, Buruma OJS, et al: The MPTP model: Versatile contributions to the treatment of idiopathic Parkinson's disease. J Neurol Sci 1990;97:273–293.

Boesch SM, Wenning GK, Ransmayr G, Poewe W: Dystonia in multiple system atrophy. J Neurol Neurosurg Psychiatry 2002;72:300–303.

Boeve BF, Lang AE, Litvan I: Corticobasal degeneration and its relationship to progressive supranuclear palsy and frontotemporal dementia. Ann Neurol 2003;54:S15–S19.

Boeve BF, Maraganore DM, Parisi JE, et al: Pathological heterogeneity in clinically diagnosed corticobasal degeneration. Neurology 1999;53:795–800.

Boeve BF, Silber MH, Ferman TJ, et al: REM sleep behavior disorder and degenerative dementia: An association likely reflecting Lewy body disease. Neurology 1998;51:363–370.

Boeve BF, Silber MH, Parisi JE, et al: Synucleinopathy pathology and REM sleep behavior disorder plus dementia or parkinsonism. Neurology 2003;61:40–45.

Bond Chapman S, Rosenberg R, Weiner MF, Shobe A: Autosomal dominant progressive syndrome of motor-speech loss without dementia. Neurology 1997;49:1298–1306.

Bonelli SB, Ransmayr G, Steffelbauer M, et al: L-dopa responsiveness in dementia with Lewy bodies, Parkinson disease with and without dementia. Neurology 2004;63:376–378.

Bordet R, Behhadjali J, Destee A, et al: Octreotide effects on orthostatic hypotension in patients with multiple system atrophy: A controlled study of acute administration. Clin Neuropharmacol 1995;18:83–89.

Borghi R, Giliberto L, Assini A, et al: Increase of cdk5 is related to neurofibrillary pathology in progressive supranuclear palsy. Neurology 2002;58:589–592.

Bosanko CM, Gilroy J, Wang A-M, et al: West Nile virus encephalitis involving the substantia nigra. Arch Neurol 2003;60:1448–1452.

Bower JH, Maraganore DM, McDonnell SK, Rocca WA: Incidence of progressive supranuclear palsy and multiple system atrophy in Olmsted County, Minnesota, 1976–1990. Neurology 1997;49:1284–1288.

Boxer AL, Geschwind MD, Belfor N, et al: Patterns of brain atrophy that differentiate corticobasal degeneration syndrome from progressive supranuclear palsy. Arch Neurol 2006;63:81–86.

Braak H, Rub U, Jansen Steur EN, et al: Cognitive status correlates with neuropathologic stage in Parkinson disease. Neurology 2005; 64:1404–1410.

Brandel J-P, Delasnerie-Lauprêtre N, Laplance J-L, et al: Diagnosis of Creutzfeldt-Jakob disease: Effect of clinical criteria on incidence estimates. Neurology 2000;54:1095–1099.

Brent S, Giordani B, Gilman S, et al: Neuropsychological changes in olivopontocerebellar atrophy. Arch Neurol 1990;47:997–1002.

Bret P, Guyotat J, Chazal J: Is normal pressure hydrocephalus a valid concept in 2002? A reappraisal in five questions and proposal for a new designation of the syndrome as "chronic hydrocephalus." J Neurol Neurosurg Psychiatry 2002;73:9–12.

Brett FM, Henson C, Staunton H: Familial diffuse Lewy body disease, eye movement abnormalities, and distribution of pathology. Arch Neurol 2002;59:464–467.

Brich J, Shie FS, Howell BW, et al: Genetic modulation of tau phosphorylation in the mouse. J Neurosci 2003;23:187–192.

Brodaty H, Mitchell P, Luscombe G, et al: Familial idiopathic basal ganglia calcification (Fahr's disease) without neurological, cognitive and psychiatric symptoms is not linked to the IBGC1 locus on chromosome 14q. Hum Genet 2002;110:8–14.

Brooks DJ, Ibanez V, Sawle GV, et al: Differing patterns of striatal 18F-dopa uptake in Parkinson's disease, multiple system atrophy, and progressive supranuclear palsy. Ann Neurol 1990;28:547–555.

Brooks DJ, Ibanez V, Sawle GV, et al: Striatal D2 receptor status in patients with Parkinson's disease, striatonigral degeneration, and progressive supranuclear palsy, measured with 11C-raclopride and positron emission tomography. Ann Neurol 1992;31:184–192.

Brooks DJ, Salmon EP, Mathias CJ, et al: The relationship between locomotor disability, autonomic dysfunction, and integrity of the striatonigral dopaminergic system in patients with multiple system atrophy, pure autonomic failure and Parkinson's disease, studied with PET. Brain 1990;113:1539–1552.

Broussolle E, Backchine S, Tommasi M, et al: Slowly progressive anarthria with late anterior opercular syndrome: A variant form of frontal cortical atrophy syndrome. J Neurol Sci 1996;144:44–58.

Brown J, Lantos PL, Penelope Roques, et al: Familial dementia with swollen achromatic neurons and corticobasal inclusion bodies: A clinical and pathological study. J Neurol Sci 1996;135:21–30.

Brown J, Lantos P, Stratton M, et al: Familial progressive supranuclear palsy. J Neurol Neurosurg Psychiatry 1993;56:473–476.

Brown P: Drug therapy in human and experimental transmissible spongiform encephalopathy. Neurology 2002;58:1720–1725.

Brown P, Gibbs CJ, Rodgers-Johnson P, et al: Human spongiform encephalopathy: The National Institutes of Health series of 300 cases of experimentally transmitted disease. Ann Neurol 1994;35: 513–529.

Brunt ERP, van Weerden TW, Pruim J, et al: Unique myoclonic pattern in corticobasal degeneration. Mov Disord 1995;10: 132–142.

Buee L, Bussiere T, Buee-Scherrer V, et al: Tau protein isoforms, phosphorylation and role in neurodegenerative disorders. Brain Res Brain Res Rev 2000;33: 95–130.

Bürk K, Abele M, Fetter M, et al: Autosomal dominant cerebellar ataxia: Clinical features and MRI in families with SCA1, SCA2 and SCA3. Brain 1996;119:1497–1506.

Burkhard PR, Delavelle J, Du Pasquier R, Spahr L: Chronic parkinsonism associated with cirrhosis: A distinct subset of acquired hepatocerebral degeneration. Arch Neurol 2003;60:521–528.

Burkhard PR, Sanchez J-C, Landis T, Hochstrasser DF: CSF detection of the 14-3-3 protein in unselected patients with dementia. Neurology 2001;56:1528–1533.

Burkhardt C, Kelly JP, Lim Y-H, et al: Neuroleptic medications inhibit complex I of the electron transport chain. Ann Neurol 1993;33: 512–517.

Burkhardt CR, Filley CM, Kleinschmidt-DeMasters, et al: Diffuse Lewy body disease and progressive dementia. Neurology 1988;38: 1520–1528.

Burn DJ, Brooks DJ: Nigral dysfunction in drug-induced parkinsonism. Neurology 1993;43:552–556.

Burn DJ, Jaros E: Multiple system atrophy: Cellular and molecular pathology. Mol Pathol 2001;54:419–426.

Burn DJ, Rinne JO, Quinn NP, et al: Striatal opioid receptor binding in Parkinson's disease, striatonigral degeneration and Steele-Richardson-Olszweski syndrome: A [11C]diprenorphine PET study. Brain 1995;118:951–958.

Burn DJ, Sawle GV, Brooks DJ: Differential diagnosis of Parkinson's disease, multiple system atrophy, and Steele-Richardson-Olszewski syndrome: Discriminant analysis of striatal 18F-dopa PET data. J Neurol Neurosurg Psychiatry 1994;57:278–284.

Burns JM, Galvin JE, Roe CM, et al: The pathology of the substantia nigra in Alzheimer disease with extrapyramidal signs. Neurology 2005;64:1397–1403.

Butler RJ, Forsythe WI, Beverly DW, Adams LM: A prospective controlled investigation of the cognitive effects of amateur boxing. J Neurol Neurosurg Psychiatry 1993;56:1055–1061.

Cairns NJ, Grossman M, Arnold SE, et al: Clinical and neuropathologic variation in neuronal intermediate filament inclusion disease. Neurology 2004;63:1376–1384.

Calabrese VP, Hadfield MG: Parkinsonism and extraocular motor abnormalities with unusual neuropathological findings. Mov Disord 1991;6:257–260.

Calne DB, Chu N-S, Huan CC, et al: Manganism and idiopathic parkinsonism: Similarities and differences. Neurology 1994;44: 1583–1586.

Calne DB, Lees AJ: Late progression of post-encephalitic Parkinson's syndrome. Can J Neurol Sci 1988;15:135–138.

Campbell RJ, Steele JC, Cox TA, et al: Pathologic findings in the retinal pigment epitheliopathy associated with the amyotrophic lateral sclerosis/parkinsonism-dementia complex of Guam. Ophthalmology 1993;100:37–42.

Caparros-Lefebvre D, Elbaz A, Caribbean Parkinsonism Study Group: Possible relation of atypical parkinsonism in the French West Indies with consumption of tropical plants: A case-control study. Lancet 1999;354:281–286.

Caparros-Lefebvre D, Sergeant N, Lees A, et al: Guadeloupean parkinsonism: A cluster of progressive supranuclear palsy-like tauopathy. Brain 2002;125:801–811.

Cardoso F, Jankovic J: Progressive supranuclear palsy. In Calne DB (ed): Neurodegenerative Diseases. Philadelphia, WB Saunders, 1994, pp 769–786.

Cardoso F, Jankovic J: Peripherally-induced tremor and parkinsonism. Arch Neurol 1995;52:263–270.

Caselli RJ: Focal and asymmetric cortical degenerative syndromes. Adv Neurol 2000;82:35–51.

Castellani R: Multiple system atrophy: Clues from inclusions. Am J Pathol 1998;153:671–676.

Castellani RJ, Colucci M, Xie Z, et al: Sensitivity of 14-3-3 protein test varies in subtypes of sporadic Creutzfeldt-Jakob disease. Neurology 2004;63:436–442.

Chacko RC, Hurley R, Jankovic J: Clozapine use in diffuse Lewy body disease. J Neuropsychiatry Clin Neurosci 1993;5:206–208.

Chambers CB, Lee JM, Troncoso JC, et al: Overexpression of four-repeat tau mRNA isoforms in progressive supranuclear palsy but not in Alzheimer's disease. Ann Neurol 1999;46:325–332.

Champy P, Hoglinger GU, Feger J, et al: Annonacin, a lipophilic inhibitor of mitochondrial complex I, induces nigral and striatal neurodegeneration in rats: Possible relevance for atypical parkinsonism in Guadeloupe. J Neurochem 2004;88:63–69.

Chapman J, Ben-Israel J, Goldhammer Y, et al: The risk of developing Creutzfeldt-Jakob disease in subjects with the PRNP gene codon 200 point mutation. Neurology 1994;44:1683–1686.

Chapman T, McKeel DW, Morris JC: Misleading results with the 14-3-3 assay for the diagnosis of Creutzfeldt-Jakob disease. Neurology 2000;55:1396–1397.

Chaudhuri KR, Hu MT, Brooks DJ: Atypical parkinsonism in Afro-Caribbean and Indian origin immigrants to the UK. Mov Disord 2000;15:18–23.

Chen G, Huang LD, Jiang YM, Manji HK: The mood-stabilizing agent valproate inhibits the activity of glycogen synthase kinase-3. J Neurochem 1999;72:1327–1330.

Chen JY, Stern Y, Sano M, Mayeux R: Cumulative risks of developing extrapyramidal signs, psychosis, or myoclonus in the course of Alzheimer's disease. Arch Neurol 1991;48:1141–1143.

Chen R, Ashby P, Lang AE: Stimulus-sensitive myoclonus in akinetic-rigid syndromes. Brain 1992;115:1875–1888.

Cherrier MM, Mendez M: Pick's disease: An introduction and review of the literature. Neurologist 1999;5:57–62.

Christen HJ, Hanefeld F, Kruse E, et al: Foix-Chavany-Marie (anterior operculum) syndrome in childhood: A reappraisal of Worster-Drought syndrome. Dev Med Child Neurol 2000;42:122–132.

Cicarelli G, Pellecchia MT, Maiuri F, Barone P: Brain stem cystic astrocytoma presenting with "pure" parkinsonism. Mov Disord 1999;14:364–365.

Clark CM, Ewbank D, Lerner A, et al: The relationship between extrapyramidal signs and cognitive performance in patients with Alzheimer's disease enrolled in the CERAD study. Neurology 1997;49:70–75.

Clark LN, Poorkaj P, Wszolek Z, et al: Pathogenic implications of mutations in the tau gene in pallido-ponto-nigral degeneration and related neurodegenerative disorders linked to chromosome 17. Proc Natl Acad Sci U S A 1998;95:13103–13107.

Clouston PD, Lim CL, Fung V, et al: Brainstem myoclonus in a patient with non-dopa-responsive parkinsonism. Mov Disord 1996;11:404–410.

Cohen J, Low P, Fealey R, et al: Somatic and autonomic function in progressive autonomic failure and multiple system atrophy. Ann Neurol 1987;22:692–699.

Collinge J: Molecular neurology of prion disease. J Neurol Neurosurg Psychiatry 2005;76:906–919.

Collins SJ, Ahlskog JE, Parisi JE, Maraganore DM: Progressive supranuclear palsy: Neuropathological based diagnostic clinical criteria. J Neurol Neurosurg Psychiatry 1995;58:167–173.

Collins SJ, Lawson VA, Masters CL: Transmissible spongiform encephalopathies. Lancet 2004;563:51–61.

Colosimo C, Albanese A, Hughes AJ, et al: Some specific clinical features differentiate multiple system atrophy (striatonigral variety) from Parkinson's disease. Arch Neurol 1995;52:294–298.

Colosimo C, Romano S, Inghilleri M, Chaudhuri KR: Sphincter EMG abnormalities in Parkinson's disease. Park Rel Disord 1999;5:S37.

Condy C, Rivaud-Pechoux S, Ostendorf F, et al: Neural substrate of antisaccades: Role of subcortical structures. Neurology 2004;63:1571–1578.

Conrad C, Amano N, Andreadis A, et al: Differences in a dinucleotide repeat polymorphism in the tau gene between Caucasian and Japanese populations: Implication for progressive supranuclear palsy. Neurosci Lett 1998;250:135–137.

Conrad C, Andreadis A, Trojanowski JQ, et al: Genetic evidence for the involvement of τ in progressive supranuclear palsy. Ann Neurol 1997;41:277–281.

Consensus Committee of the American Autonomic Society (AAS) and the American Academy of Neurology (AAN): Consensus statement on the definition of orthostatic hypotension, pure autonomic failure, and multiple system atrophy. Neurology 1996;46:1470.

Cordato NJ, Halliday GM, Harding AJ, et al: Regional brain atrophy in progressive supranuclear palsy and Lewy body disease. Ann Neurol 2000;47:718–728.

Cordato NJ, Halliday GM, McCann H, et al: Corticobasal syndrome with tau pathology. Mov Disord 2001;16:656–667.

Costello DJ, Walsh SL, Harrington HJ, Walsh CH: Concurrent hereditary haemochromatosis and idiopathic Parkinson's disease: A case report series. J Neurol Neurosurg Psychiatry 2004;75:631–633.

Cox P, Sacks OW: Cycad neurotoxins, consumption of flying foxes, and ALS-PDC disease in Guam. Neurology 2002;58:956–959.

Cox PA, Banack SA, Murch SJ: Biomagnification of cyanobacterial neurotoxins and neurodegenerative disease among the Chamorro people of Guam. Proc Natl Acad Sci U S A 2003;100:13380–13383.

Crystal HA, Dickson DW, Lizardi JE, et al: Antemortem diagnosis of diffuse Lewy body disease. Neurology 1990;40:1523–1528.

Cubo E, Stebbins GT, Golbe LI, et al: Application of the Unified Parkinson's Disease Rating Scale in Progressive Supranuclear Palsy: Factor analysis of the motor scale. Mov Disord 2000;15:276–279.

Cummings JL: Toward a molecular neuropsychiatry of neurodegenerative diseases. Ann Neurol 2003;54:147–154.

Curran T, Lang AE: Parkinsonian syndromes associated with hydrocephalus: Case reports, a review of the literature, and pathophysiological hypotheses. Mov Disord 1994;9:508–520.

Currier RD, Subramony SH: Distinguishing between the adult ataxias. In Lechtenberg R (ed): Handbook of Cerebellar Diseases. New York, Marcel Dekker, 1993, pp 337–344.

Curtis AR, Fey C, Morris CM, et al: Mutation in the gene encoding ferritin light polypeptide causes dominant adult-onset basal ganglia disease. Nat Genet 2001;28:350–354.

Dale RC, Church AJ, Surtees RA, et al: Encephalitis lethargica syndrome: 20 new cases and evidence of basal ganglia autoimmunity. Brain 2004;127:21–33.

Daniel SE, De Bruin VMS, Lees AJ: The clinical and pathological spectrum of Steele-Richardson-Olszweski syndrome (progressive supranuclear palsy): A reappraisal. Brain 1995;118:759–770.

Daniele A, Moro E, Bentivoglio AR: Zolpidem in progressive supranuclear palsy. N Engl J Med 1999;341:543–544.

Davie CA, Barker GJ, Machado C, et al: Proton magnetic resonance spectroscopy in Steele-Richardson-Olszewski syndrome. Mov Disord 1997;12:767–771.

Davie CA, Wenning GK, Barker GJ, et al: Differentiation of multiple system atrophy from idiopathic Parkinson's disease using proton magnetic resonance spectroscopy. Ann Neurol 1995;37:204–210.

Davis PH, Bergeron C, McLaughlin DR: Atypical presentation of progressive supranuclear palsy. Ann Neurol 1985;17:337–343.

Davis PH, Golbe LI, Duvoisin RC, Schoenberg BS: Risk factors for progressive supranuclear palsy. Neurology 1988;38:1546–1552.

De Bruin VMS, Lees AJ: Subcortical neurofibrillary degeneration presenting as Steele-Richardson-Olszewski and other related syndromes: A review of 90 pathologically verified cases. Mov Disord 1994;9: 381–389.

De Bruin VMS, Lees AJ, Daniel SE: Diffuse Lewy body disease presenting with supranuclear gaze palsy, parkinsonism, and dementia: A case report. Mov Disord 1992;7:355–358.

Dejerine J, Thomas A: L'atrophie olivo-ponto-cérébelleuse. Nouv Iconogr Salpêt 1900;330:370.

DeKosky ST, Ikonomovic MD: NIFID: A new molecular pathology with a frontotemporal dementia phenotype. Neurology 2004;63: 1348–1349.

de la Monte SM, Wells SE, Hedley-Whyte ET, Growdon JH: Neuropathological distinction between Parkinson's dementia and Parkinson's plus Alzheimer's disease. Ann Neurol 1989;26: 309–320.

Del-Ser T, Munoz DG, Hachinski V: Temporal pattern of cognitive decline and incontinence is different in Alzheimer's disease and diffuse Lewy body disease. Neurology 1996;46:682–686.

Demirkiran M, Bozdemir H, Sarica Y: Vascular parkinsonism: A distinct, heterogenous clinical entity. Acta Neurol Scand 2001;104: 63–67.

de Silva R, Farrer M: Tau neurotoxicity without the lesions: A fly challenges a tangled web. Trends Neurosci 2002;25:327–329.

Deutch AY, Rosin DL, Goldstein M, Roth RH: 3-Acetylpyridine-induced degeneration of the nigrostriatal dopamine system: An animal model of olivopontocerebellar atrophy-associated parkinsonism. Exp Neurol 1989;105:1–9.

De Volder AG, Francart J, Laterre C, et al: Decreased glucose utilization in the striatum and frontal lobe in probable striatonigral degeneration. Ann Neurol 1989;26:239–247.

de Yebenes JG, Sarasa JL, Daniel SE, Lees AJ: Familial progressive supranuclear palsy. Description of a pedigree and review of the literature. Brain 1995;118:1095–1104.

Dickson DW: Neurodegenerative diseases with cytoskeletal pathology: A biochemical classifiaction. Ann Neurol 1997;42:541–544.

Dickson DW, Crystal H, Mattiace LA, et al: Diffuse Lewy body disease: Light and electron microscopic immunocytochemistry of senile plaques. Acta Neuropathol 1989;78:572–584.

Di Monte DA, Harati Y, Jankovic J, et al: Muscle mitochondrial ATP production in progressive supranuclear palsy. J Neurochem 1994;62:1631–1634.

Djaldetti R, Mosberg-Galili R, Sroka H, et al: Camptocormia (bent spine) in patients with Parkinson's disease: Characterization and possible pathogenesis of an unusual phenomenon. Mov Disord 1999;14:443–447.

Doody RS, Jankovic J: The alien hand and related signs. J Neurol Neurosurg Psychiatry 1992;55:806–810.

Doty RL, Golbe LI, McKeown DA, et al: Olfactory testing differentiates between progressive supranuclear palsy and idiopathic Parkinson's disease. Neurology 1993;43:962–965.

Drayer BP, Olanow W, Burger P, et al: Parkinson plus syndrome: Diagnosis using high field MR imaging of brain iron. Radiology 1989;159:493–498.

Dredge BK, Polydorides AD, Darnell RB: The splice of life: Alternative splicing and neurological disease. Nat Rev Neurosci 2001;2:43–50.

Dubinsky RM, Jankovic J: Progressive supranuclear palsy and multi-infarct state. Neurology 1987;37:570–576.

Dubois B, Defontaines B, Deweer B, et al: Cognitive and behavioral changes in patients with focal lesions of the basal ganglia. Adv Neurol 1995;65:29–41.

Dubois B, Slachevsky A, Litvan I, Pillon B: The FAB: A frontal assessment battery at bedside. Neurology 2000;55:1621–1626.

Dubois B, Slachevsky A, Pillon B, et al: "Applause sign" helps to discriminate PSP from FTD and PD. Neurology 2005;64:2132–2133.

Dufouil C, Clayton D, Brayne C, et al: Population norms for the MMSE in the very old: Estimates based on longitudinal data. Neurology 2000;55:1609–1613.

Duncan MW, Steele JC, Kopin IJ, Markey SP: 2-Amino-3-(methyl-amino) propanoic acid (BMAA) in cycad flour: An unlikely cause of amyotrophic lateral sclerosis and parkinsonism-dementia complex of Guam. Neurology 1990;40:767–772.

Dürr A, Stevanin G, Cancel G, et al: Spinocerebellar ataxia 3 and Machado-Joseph disease: Clinical, molecular, and neuropathological features. Ann Neurol 1996;39:490–499.

Eidelberg D, Dhawan V, Moeller JR, et al. The metabolic landscape of cortico-basal ganglionic degeneration: Regional asymmetries studied with positron emission tomography. J Neurol Neurosurg Psychiatry 1991;54:856–862.

Eidelberg D, Takikawa S, Moeller JR, et al: Striatal hypometabolism distinguishes striatonigral degeneration from Parkinson's disease. Ann Neurol 1993;33:518–527.

Eissler M, Holocher R, Lindenstrauss M, et al: Autonomic dysfunction with nocturnal dyspnea (Gerhart-syndrome) in a patient with multiple system atrophy. Med Lin 2001;96:626–631.

Elston JS: A new variant of blepharospasm. J Neurol Neurosurg Psychiatry 1992;55:369–371.

Emilien G, Maloteaux J-M, Beyreuther K, Masters CL: Alzheimer disease: Mouse models pave the way for therapeutic opportunities. Arch Neurol 2000;57:176–181.

Emre M: What causes mental dysfunction in Parkinson's disease? Mov Disord 2003;18(suppl 6):S63–S71.

Factor SA, Higgins DS, Qian J: Primary progressive freezing gait: A syndrome with many causes. Neurology 2006;66:411–414.

Factor SA, Weiner WJ: Prior history of head trauma in Parkinson's disease. Mov Disord 1991;3:30–36.

Fahn S: Secondary parkinsonism. In Goldensohn ES, Appel SH (eds): Scientific Approaches to Clinical Neurology. Philadelphia, Lea & Febiger, 1977, pp 1159–1189.

Feany MB, Dickson DW: Neurodegenerative disorders with extensive tau pathology: A comparative study and review. Ann Neurol 1996;40:139–148.

Fearnley JM, Lees AJ: Striatonigral degeneration. Brain 1990;113:1823–1842.

Fearnley JM, Revesz T, Brooks DJ, et al: Diffuse Lewy body disease presenting with unusual supranuclear gaze palsy. J Neurol Neurosurg Psychiatry 1991;54:159–161.

Ferman TJ, Smith GE, Boeve BF, et al: DLB fluctuations: Specific features that reliably differentiate DLB from AD and normal aging. Neurology 2004;62:181–187.

Fernandez HH, Friedman JH, Jacques C, Rosenfeld M: Quetiapine for the treatment of drug-induced psychosis in Parkinson's disease. Mov Disord 1999;14:484–487.

Finucane TE, Christmas C, Travis K: Tube feeding in patients with advanced dementia: A review of the evidence. JAMA 1999;282:1365–1370.

Fischer DF, De Vos RA, Van Dijk R, et al: Disease-specific accumulation of mutant ubiquitin as a marker for proteasomal dysfunction in the brain. FASEB J 2003;17:2014–2024.

Fisk JD, Goodale MA, Burkhart MA, et al: Progressive supranuclear palsy: The relationship between oculomotility dysfunction and psychological test performance. Neurology 1982;32:698–705.

Fitzgerald PM, Jankovic J: Lower body parkinsonism: Evidence for vascular etiology. Mov Disord 1989;4:249–260.

Flament S, Delacourte A, Verny M, et al: Abnormal tau-proteins in progressive supranuclear palsy: Similarities and differences with neurofibrillary degeneration of the Alzheimer type. Acta Neuropathol 1991;81:591–596.

Forman MS, Lal D, Zhang B, et al: Transgenic mouse model of tau pathology in astrocytes leading to nervous system degeneration. J Neurosci 2005;25:3539–3550.

Forstl H, Burns A, Levy R, et al: Neurologic signs in Alzheimer's disease: Results of prospective clinical and neuropathological study. Arch Neurol 1992;49:1038–1042.

Foster NL: Frontotemporal dementia with parkinsonism linked to chromosome 17 (FTDP-17): A clinician's guide. Neurologist 1995:213–221.

Foster NL, Gilman S, Berent S, et al: Cerebral hypometabolism in progressive supranuclear palsy studied with positron emission tomography. Ann Neurol 1988;24:399–406.

Fowler CJ: Investigation of the neurogenic bladder. J Neurol Neurosurg Psychiatry 1996;60:6–13.

Frattali CM, Grafman J, Patronas N, et al: Language disturbances in corticobasal degeneration. Neurology 2000;54:990–992.

Freeman R, Landsberg L, Young J: The treatment of neurogenic orthostatic hypotension with 3,4-DL-threo-dihydrophenylserine. Neurology 1999;53:2151–2157.

Friedman DI, Jankovic J, McCrary JA: Neuro-ophthalmic findings in progressive supranuclear palsy. J Clin Neuroophthalmol 1992;12:104–109.

Frucht S, Fahn S, Chin S, et al: Levodopa-induced dyskinesias in autopsy-proven cortical-basal ganglionic degeneration. Mov Disord 2000;15:340–343.

Fujiwara H, Hasegawa M, Dohmae N, et al: Alpha-synuclein is phosphorylated in synucleinopathy lesions. Nat Cell Biol 2002;4:160–164.

Funkenstein HH, Albert MS, Cook NR, et al: Extrapyramidal signs and other neurologic findings in clinically diagnosed Alzheimer's disease. Arch Neurol 1993;50:51–56.

Furtado S, Farrer M, Tsuboi Y, et al: SCA-2 presenting as parkinsonism in an Alberta family: Clinical, genetic, and PET findings. Neurology 2002;59:1625–1627.

Furtado S, Payami H, Lockhart PJ, et al: Profile of families with parkinsonism-predominant spinocerebellar ataxia type 2 (SCA2). Mov Disord 2004;19:622–629.

Galasko D, Hansen LA, Katzman R, et al: Clinical-neuropathological correlations in Alzheimer's disease and related dementias. Arch Neurol 1994a;51:888–895.

Galasko D, Saitoh T, Xia Y, et al: The apolipoprotein E allele ε4 is overrepresented in patients with the Lewy body variant of Alzhemier's disease. Neurology 1994b;44:1950–1951.

Galasko D, Salmon DP, Craig UK, et al: Clinical features and changing patterns of neurodegenerative disorders on Guam, 1997–2000. Neurology 2002;58:90–97.

Galloway PG, Bergeron C, Perry G: The presence of tau distinguishes Lewy bodies of diffuse Lewy body disease from those of idiopathic Parkinson's disease. Neurosci Lett 1989;100:6–9.

Galpern WR, Lang AE: Interface between tauopathies and synucleinopathies: A tale of two proteins. Ann Neurol 2006;59:449–458.

Galvin JE, Lee VMY, Trojanowski JQ: Synucleinopathies: Clinical and pathological implications. Arch Neurol 2001;58:186–190.

Gambetti P, Parchi P: Insomnia in prion diseases: Sporadic and familial. N Engl J Med 1999;340:1675–1676.

Garbutt S, Riley DE, Kumar AN, et al: Abnormalities of optokinetic nystagmus in progressive supranuclear palsy. J Neurol Neurosurg Psychiatry 2004;75:1386–1394.

Garruto RM, Yase Y: Neurodegenerative disorders of the western Pacific: The search for mechanisms of pathogenesis. Trends Neurosci 1986;9:368–371.

Gearing M, Olson DA, Watts RL, Mirra SS: Progressive supranuclear palsy: Neuropathologic and clinical heterogeneity. Neurology 1994;44:1015–1024.

Geschwind MD, Martindale J, Miller D, et al: Challenging the clinical utility of the 14-3-3 protein for the diagnosis of sporadic Creutzfeldt-Jakob disease. Arch Neurol 2003;60:813–816.

Ghaemi M, Hilker R, Rudolf J, et al: Differentiating multiple system atrophy from Parkinson's disease: Contribution of striatal and midbrain MRI volumetry and multi-tracer PET imaging. J Neurol Neurosurg Psychiatry 2002;73:517–523.

Ghika J, Bogousslavsky J: Presymptomatic hypertension is a major feature in the diagnosis of progressive supranuclear palsy. Arch Neurol 1997;54:1104–1108.

Ghika J, Tennis M, Hoffman E, et al: Idazoxan treatment in progressive supranuclear palsy. Neurology 1991;41:986–991.

Gibb WRG, Luthert PJ, Janota I, Lantos PL: Cortical Lewy body dementia: Clinical features and classification. J Neurol Neurosurg Psychiatry 1989;52:185–189.

Gibb WRG, Luthert PJ, Marsden CD: Clinical and pathological features of corticobasal degeneration. Adv Neurol 1990;53:51–54.

Gibb WRG, Mountjoy CQ, Mann DMA, Lees AJ: The substantia nigra and ventral tegmental area in Alzheimer's disease and Down's syndrome. J Neurol Neurosurg Psychiatry 1989;52:193–196.

Giladi N, Burke RE, Kostic V, et al: Hemiparkinsonism-hemiatrophy syndrome. Neurology 1990;40:1731–1734.

Giladi N, McMahon D, Przedborski S, et al: Motor blocks in Parkinson's disease. Neurology 1992;42:333–339.

Giladi N, Simon ES, Korczyn AD, et al: Anal sphincter EMG does not distinguish between multiple system atrophy and Parkinson's disease. Muscle Nerve 2000;23:731–734.

Gilbert JJ, Kish SJ, Chang L-J, et al: Dementia, parkinsonism and motor neuron disease: Neurochemical and neuropathological correlates. Ann Neurol 1988;24:688–691.

Gilman S: Multiple system atrophy. In Jankovic J, Tolosa E (eds): Parkinson's Disease and Movement Disorders, 4th ed. Philadelphia, Lippincott Williams & Wilkins, 2002, pp 170–184.

Gilman S, Chervin RD, Koeppe RA, et al: Obstructive sleep apnea is related to a thalamic cholinergic deficit in MSA. Neurology 2003;61:35–39.

Gilman S, Frey KA, Koeppe RA, et al: Decreased striatal monoaminergic terminals in olivopontocerebellar atrophy and multiple system atrophy demonstrated with positron emission tomography. Ann Neurol 1996;40:885–892.

Gilman S, Koeppe RA, Chervin RD, et al: REM sleep behavior disorder is related to striatal monoaminergic deficit in MSA. Neurology 2003;61:29–34.

Gilman S, Koeppe RA, Junck L, et al: Decreased striatal monoaminergic terminal in multiple system atrophy detected with positron emission tomography. Ann Neurol 1999;45:769–777.

Gilman S, Little R, Johanns J, et al: Evolution of sporadic olivopontocerebellar atrophy into multiple system atrophy. Neurology 2000;55:527–532.

Gilman S, Low PA, Quinn N, et al: Consensus statement on the diagnosis of multiple system atrophy. J Auton Nerv Syst 1998;74:189–192.

Gilman S, Quinn NP: The relationship of multiple system atrophy to sporadic olivopontocerebellar atrophy and other forms of idiopathic late-onset cerebellar atrophy. Neurology 1996;46:1197–1199.

Gilman S, Sima AAF, Junck L, et al: Spinocerebellar ataxia type I with multiple system degeneration and glial cytoplasmic inclusions. Ann Neurol 1996;39:241–255.

Glatzel M, Stoeck K, Seeger H, et al: Human prion diseases: Molecular and clinical aspects. Arch Neurol 2005;62:545–552.

Goedert M, Jakes R, Spillantini MG, et al: Assembly of microtubule-associated protein tau into Alzheimer-like filaments induced by sulphated glycoaminoglycans. Nature 1996;383:550–553.

Goedert M, Spillantini MG, Davies SW: Filamentous nerve cell inclusions in neurodegenerative diseases. Curr Opin Neurobiol 1998;8:619–632.

Goetz CG, Leurgans S, Lang AE, Litvan I: Progression of gait, speech and swallowing deficits in progressive supranuclear palsy. Neurology 2003;60:917–922.

Goetz CG, Stebbins GT: Effects of head trauma from motor vehicle accidents on Parkinson's disease. Ann Neurol 1991;29:191–193.

Goffinet AM, De Volder AG, Gillian C, et al: Positron tomography demonstrates frontal lobe hypometabolism in progressive supranuclear palsy. Ann Neurol 1989;25:131–139.

Golbe LI: Progressive supranuclear palsy. In Stern MB, Koller WC (eds): Parkinsonian Disorders. New York, Marcel Dekker, 1993, pp 227–248.

Golbe LI, Miller DC, Duvoisin RC: Paraneoplastic degeneration of the substantia nigra with dystonia and parkinsonism. Mov Disord 1989;4:147–152.

Golbe LI, Rubin RS, Cody RP, et al: Follow-up study of risk factors in progressive supranuclear palsy. Neurology 1996;47:148–154.

Golbe LI, Farrell TM, Davis PH: Case-control study of early life dietary factors in Parkinson's disease. Arch Neurol 1988;45:1350–1353.

Goldfarb LG, Brown P: The transmissible spongiform encephalopathies. Ann Rev Med 1995;46:57–65.

Goldman JS, Farmer JM, Van Deerlin VM, et al: Frontotemporal dementia: Genetics and genetic counseling dilemmas. Neurologist 2004;10:227–234.

Goldstein DS, Holmes C, Cannon RO, et al: Sympathetic cardioneuropathy in dysautonomias. N Engl J Med 1997;336:696–702.

Goldstein DS, Holmes CS, Dendi R, et al: Orthostatic hypotension from sympathetic denervation in Parkinson's disease. Neurology 2002;58:1247–1255.

Goldstein DS, Polinsky RJ, Garty M, et al: Patterns of plasma levels of catechols in neurogenic orthostatic hypotension. Ann Neurol 1989;26:558–563.

Gomez-Isla T, Growdon WB, McNamara M, et al: Clinicopathologic correlates in temporal cortex in dementia with Lewy bodies. Neurology 1999;53:2003–2009.

Goto S, Hirano A, Matsumoto S: Immunohistochemical study of the striatal efferents and nigral dopaminergic neurons in parkinsonism-dementia complex on Guam in comparison with those in Parkinson's and Alzheimer's disease. Ann Neurol 1990a;27:520–527.

Goto S, Hirano A, Matsumoto S: Met-enkephalin immunoreactivity in the basal ganglia in Parkinson's disease and striatonigral degeneration. Neurology 1990b;40:1051–1056.

Goto S, Matsumoto S, Ushio Y, Hirano A: Subregional loss of putaminal efferents to the basal ganglia output nuclei may cause parkinsonism in striatonigral degeneration. Neurology 1996;47:1032–1036.

Gouider-Khouja N, Vidailhet M, Bonnet A-M, et al: "Pure" striatonigral degeneration and Parkinson's disease: A comparative clinical study. Mov Disord 1995;10:288–294.

Gourie-Devi M, Nalini A, Sandhya S: Early or late appearance of "dropped head syndrome" in amyotrophic lateral sclerosis. J Neurol Neurosurg Psychiatry 2003;74:683–686.

Graham JG, Oppenheimer DR: Orthostatic hypotension and nicotinic sensitivity in a case of multiple system atrophy. J Neurol Neurosurg Psychiatry 1969;32:28–34.

Graham NL, Bak T, Hodges JR: Corticobasal degeneration as a cognitive disorder. Mov Disord 2003a;18:1224–1232.

Graham NL, Bak T, Patterson K, Hodges JR: Language function and dysfunction in corticobasal degeneration. Neurology 2003b;61:493–499.

Graham NL, Zeman A, Young AW, et al: Dyspraxia in a patient with corticobasal degeneration: The role of visual and tactile inputs. J Neurol Neurosurg Psychiatry 1999;67:334–344.

Gray F, Vincent D, Hauw JJ: Quantitative study of lateral horn cells in 15 cases of multiple system atrophy. Acta Neuropath 1988;75: 513–520.

Grimes DA, Lang AE, Bergeron CB: Dementia as the most common presentation of cortical-basal ganglionic degeneration. Neurology 1999;53:1969–1974.

Grossman M: Progressive aphasic syndromes: Clinical and theoretical advances. Curr Opin Neurol 2002;15:409–413.

Growdon JH, Primavera JM: Case 11-2000. N Engl J Med 2000;342:1110–1117.

Hagerman RJ, Leehey M, Heinrichs W, et al: Intention tremor, parkinsonism, and generalized brain atrophy in male carriers of fragile X. Neurology 2001;57:127–130.

Hakan A, Buonanno SF, Price BH, et al: Sensory alien hand syndrome: Case report and review of the literature. J Neurol Neurosurg Psychiatry 1998;65:366–369.

Halliday GM, Hardman CD, Cordato NJ, et al: A role for the substantia nigra pars reticulata in the gaze palsy of progressive supranuclear palsy. Brain 2000;123:724–732.

Hammans SR: The inherited ataxias and the new genetics. J Neurol Neurosurg Psychiatry 1996;61:327–332.

Hampshire DJ, Roberts E, Crow Y, et al: Kufor-Rakeb syndrome, pallido-pyramidal degeneration with supranuclear upgaze paresis and dementia, maps to 1p36. J Med Genet 2001;38:680–682.

Hanna P, Jankovic J, Kilkpatrick J: Multiple system atrophy: The putative causative role of environmental toxins. Arch Neurol 1999;56:90–94.

Hanna-Pladdy B, Heilman KM, Foundas AL: Ecological implications of ideomotor apraxia: Evidence from physical activities of daily living. Neurology 2003;60:487–490.

Hardie RJ, Lees AJ: Neuroleptic-induced Parkinson's syndrome: Clinical features and results of treatment with levodopa. J Neurol Neurosurg Psychiatry 1988;51:850–854.

Harding AJ, Broe GA, Halliday GM: Visual hallucinations in Lewy body disease relate to Lewy bodies in the temporal lobe. Brain 2002;125:391–403.

Hardman CD, Halliday GM: The external globus pallidus in patients with Parkinson's disese and progressive supranuclear palsy. Mov Disord 1999a;14:626–633.

Hardman CD, Halliday GD: The internal globus pallidus is affected in progressive supranuclear palsy and Parkinson's disease. Exp Neurol 1999b;158:135–142.

Hardman CD, Halliday GM, McRitchie DA, et al: Progressive supranuclear palsy affects both the substantia nigra pars compacta and reticulata. Exp Neurol 1997a;144:183–192.

Hardman CD, Halliday GM, McRitchie DA, Morris JGL: The subthalamic nucleus in Parkinson's disease and progressive supranuclear palsy. J Neuropath Exp Neurol 1997b;56:132–142.

Hattori M, Hashizume Y, Yoshida M, et al: Distribution of astrocytic plaques in the corticobasal degeneration brain and comparison with tuft-shaped astrocytes in the progressive supranuclear palsy brain. Acta Neuropathol (Berl) 2003;106:143–149.

Hauser MA, Li YJ, Xu H, et al: Expression profiling of substantia nigra in Parkinson disease, progressive supranuclear palsy, and frontotemporal dementia with parkinsonism. Arch Neurol 2005;62:917–921.

Hauser RA, Trehan R: Initial experience with electroconvulsive therapy for progressive supranuclear palsy. Mov Disord 1994;9:467–469.

Hauser RA, Zesiewicz TA, Rosemurgy AS, et al: Manganese intoxication and chronic liver failure. Ann Neurol 1994;36:871–875.

Hauw JJ, Daniel SE, Dickson D, et al: Preliminary NINDS neuropathologic criteria for Steele-Richardson-Olszewski syndrome (progressive supranuclear palsy). Neurology 1994;44:2015–2019.

Hayashi M, Isozaki E, Oda M, et al: Loss of large myelineated fibres of the recurrent laryngeal nerve in patients with multiple system atrophy and vocal cord palsy. J Neurol Neurosurg Psychiatry 1997;62:234–238.

Hayflick SJ, Westaway SK, Levinson B, et al: Genetic, clinical, and radiographic delineation of Hallervorden-Spatz syndrome. N Engl J Med 2003;348:33–40.

Haywood AM: Transmissible spongiform encephalopathies. N Engl J Med 1997;337:1821–1828.

Henderson JM, Carpenter K, Cartwright H, Halliday GM: Loss of thalamic intralaminar nuclei in progressive supranuclear palsy and Parkinson's disease: Clinical and therapeutic implications. Brain 2000;123:1410–1421.

Higgins JJ: Mutational analysis of the tau gene in progressive supranuclear palsy. Neurology 1999;53:1421–1424.

Higgins JJ, Golbe LI, De Biase A, et al: An extended 5′-tau susceptibility haplotype in progressive supranuclear palsy. Neurology 2000;55:1364–1367.

Higgins JJ, Litvan I, Pho LT, et al: Progressive supranuclear palsy is in linkage disequilibrium with the τ and not the α-synuclein gene. Neurology 1998;50:270–273.

Hirano A, Kurland LT, Krooth RS, Lessell LS: Parkinsonism-dementia complex, and endemic disease on the island of Guam. Clinical features: II. Pathologic features. Brain 1961;84:642–661, 662–679.

Hodges JR: Frontotemporal dementia (Pick's disease): Clinical features and assessment. Neurology 2001;56(suppl 4):S6–S10.

Hodges JR, Davies RR, Xuereb JH, et al: Clinicopathological correlates in frontotemporal dementia. Ann Neurol 2004;56:399–406.

Hoenicka J, Perez M, Perez-Tur J, et al: The tau gene A0 allele and progressive supranuclear palsy. Neurology 1999;53:1219–1225.

Hoglinger GU, Feger J, Prigent A, et al: Chronic systemic complex I inhibition induces a hypokinetic multisystem degeneration in rats. J Neurochem 2003;84:491–502.

Hohl U, Tiraboschi P, Hansen LA, et al: Diagnostic accuracy of dementia with Lewy bodies. Arch Neurol 2000;57:347–351.

Honjyo Y, Kawamoto Y, Nakamura S, et al: P39 immunoreactivity in glial cytoplasmic inclusions in brains with multiple system atrophy. Acta Neuropathol 2001;101:190–194.

Hosler BA, Siddique T, Sapp PC, et al: Linkage of familial amyotrophic lateral sclerosis with frontotemporal dementia to chromosome 9q21-q22. JAMA 2000;284:1664–1669.

Houlden H, Baker M, Morris HR, et al: Corticobasal degeneration and progressive supranuclear palsy share a common tau haplotype. Neurology 2001;56:1702–17056.

Howard RS, Lees AJ: Encephalitis lethargica: A report of four recent cases. Brain 1987;110:19–33.

Hsich G, Kennedy K, Gibbs CJ, et al: The 14-3-3 brain protein in cerebrospinal fluid as a marker for transmissible spongiform encephalopathies. N Engl J Med 1996;335:924–930.

Hughes AJ, Ben-Shlomo Y, Daniel SE, Lees AJ: What features improve the accuracy of clinical diagnosis in Parkinson's disease: A clinical pathological study. Neurology 1992;42:1142–1146.

Hughes AJ, Colosimo C, Kleedorfer B, et al: The dopaminergic response in multiple system atrophy. J Neurol Neurosurg Psychiatry 1992;55:1009–1013.

Hulette C, Mirra S, Wilkinson W, et al: The Consortium to Establish a Registry for Alzheimer's Disease (CERAD): IX. A prospective cliniconeuropathological study of Parkinson's features in Alzheimer's disease. Neurology 1995;45:1991–1995.

Hurtig HI, Trojanowski JQ, Galvin J, et al: Alpha-synuclein cortical Lewy bodies correlate with dementia in Parkinson's disease. Neurology 2000;54:1916–1921.

Hussain IF, Brady CM, Swinn MJ, et al: Treatment of erectile dysfunction with sildenafil citrate (Viagra) in parkinsonism due to Parkinson's disease or multiple system atrophy with observations on orthostatic hypotension. J Neurol Neurosurg Psychiatry 2001;71:371–374.

Hutton M: Missense and splicing mutations in tau associated with FTDP-17: Multiple pathogenic mechanisms. Neuroscience 1999;2:73–82.

Hutton M: "Missing" tau mutation identified. Ann Neurol 2000;47: 417–418.

Hutton M: Missense and splice site mutations in tau associated with FTDP-17: Multiple pathogenic mechanisms. Neurology 2001;56 (suppl 4):S21–S25.

Hutton M, Lendon C, Rizzu P, et al: Association of missense and 5′-splice-site mutations in tau with the inherited dementia FTDP-17. Nature 1998;393:702–705.

Ikeda K, Akiyama H, Arai T, Nishimura T: Glial tau pathology in neurodegenerative diseases: Their nature and comparison with neuronal tangles. Neurobiol Aging 1998;19(suppl 1):S85–S91.

Ilgin N, Zubieta J, Reich SG, et al: PET imaging of the dopamine transporter in progressive supranuclear palsy and Parkinson's disease. Neurology 1999;52:1221–1226.

Iranzo A, Santamaria J, Tolosa E, et al: Continuous positive air pressure eliminates nocturnal stridor in multiple system atrophy. Lancet 2000;356:1329–1330.

Iranzo A, Santamaria J, Tolosa E, et al: Long-term effect of CPAP in the treatment of nocturnal stridor in multiple system atrophy. Neurology 2004;63:930–932.

Irizarry MC: A turn of the sulfatide in Alzheimer's disease. Ann Neurol 2003;54:7–8.

Ishikawa A, Miyatake T: A family with hereditary juvenile dystonia-parkinsonism. Mov Disord 1995;10:482–488.

Ishikawa A, Tsuji S: Clinical analysis of 17 patients in 12 Japanese families with autosomal-recessive type juvenile parkinsonism. Neurology 1996;47:160–166.

Ishino H, Higashi H, Kuroda S, et al: Motor nuclear involvement in progressive supranuclear palsy. J Neurol Sci 1973;22:235–241.

Isozaki E, Naito A, Horiuchi S, et al: Early diagnosis and stage classification of vocal cord abductor paralysis in patients with multiple system atrophy. J Neurol Neurosurg Psychiatry 1996;60:399–402.

Ito H, Goto S, Sakamoto S, Hirano A: Calbindin-D$_{28k}$ in the basal ganglia of patients with parkinsonism. Ann Neurol 1992;32:543–550.

Ito H, Hirano A, Yen SH, Kato S: Demonstration of beta-amyloid protein-containing neurofibrillary tangles in parkinsonism-dementia complex on Guam. Neuropathol Appl Neurobiol 1991;17:365–373.

Ito H, Kusaka H, Matsumoto S, Imai T: Striatal efferent involvement and its correlation to levodopa efficacy in patients with multiple system atrophy. Neurology 1996;47:1291–1299.

Jacobs DM, Marder K, Cote LJ, et al: Neuropsychological characteristics of preclinical dementia in Parkinson's disease. Neurology 1995;45:1691–1696.

Jacquemont S, Hagerman RJ, Leehey M, et al: Fragile X premutation tremor/ataxia syndrome: Molecular, clinical, and neuroimaging correlates. Am J Hum Genet 2003;72:869–878.

Jankovic J: Controlled trial of pergolide mesylate in Parkinson's disease and progressive supranuclear palsy. Neurology 1983;33: 505–507.

Jankovic J: Apraxia of eyelid opening in progressive supranuclear palsy. Ann Neurol 1984a;15:115.

Jankovic J: Progressive supranuclear palsy: Clinical and pharmacologic update. Neurol Clin 1984b;2:473–486.

Jankovic J: Progressive supranuclear palsy: Paraneoplastic effect of bronchial carcinoma. Neurology 1985;35:446–447.

Jankovic J: Whipple's disease of the central nervous system in AIDS. N Engl J Med 1986;31:1029–1030.

Jankovic J: Hemiparkinsonism and hemiatrophy. Neurology 1988;38: 1815.

Jankovic J: Parkinson's plus syndromes. Mov Disord 1989;4:S95–S119.

Jankovic J: Posttraumatic movement disorders: Central and peripheral mechanisms. Neurology 1994;44:2008–2014.

Jankovic J: Apraxia of eyelid opening or eyelid freezing. Mov Disord 1995a;10:686–687.

Jankovic J: Parkinsonian syndromes. In Kurlan R (ed): Treatment of Movement Disorders. Philadelphia, JB Lippincott, 1995b, pp 95–114.

Jankovic J: Tardive syndromes and other drug-induced movement disorders. Clin Neuropharmacol 1995c;18:197–214.

Jankovic J: Dystonia: Medical therapy and botulinum toxin. In Fahn S, Hallett M, DeLong DR (eds): Dystonia 4: Advances in Neurology, vol 94. Philadelphia, Lippincott Williams & Wilkins, 2004, pp 275–283.

Jankovic J: Searching for a relationship between manganese and welding, and Parkinson's disease. Neurology 2005;64: 2021–2028.

Jankovic J, Ashizawa T. Huntington's disease. In Appel SH (ed): Current Neurology, vol 15. Chicago, Mosby Year Book, 1995 pp 29–60.

Jankovic J, Brin MF: Therapeutic uses of botulinum toxin. N Engl J Med 1991;324:1186–1194.

Jankovic J, Friedman DI, Pirozzolo FJ, McCrary JA: Progressive supranuclear palsy: Motor, neurobehavioral, and neuro-ophthalmic findings. Adv Neurol 1990;53:293–304.

Jankovic J, Gilden JL, Hiner BC, et al: Neurogenic orthostatic hypotension: A double-blind placebo-controlled study with midodrine. Am J Med 1993;95:38–48.

Jankovic J, Kapadia AS: Functional decline in Parkinson's disease. Arch Neurol 2001;58:1611–1615.

Jankovic J, Kirkpatrick JB, Blomquist KA, et al: Late-onset Hallervorden-Spatz disease presenting as familial parkinsonism. Neurology 1985;35:227–234.

Jankovic J, McDermott M, Carter J, et al: Variable expression of Parkinson's disease: A baseline analysis of the DATATOP cohort. Neurology 1990;40:1529–1534.

Jankovic J, Newmark M, Peter P: Parkinsonism and aquired hydrocephalus. Mov Disord 1986;1:59–64.

Jankovic J, Rajput A, Golbe L, Goodman JC: What is it? Case 1, 1993: Parkinsonism, dysautonomia, ophthalmoparesis. Mov Disord 1993;8:525–532.

Jankovic J, Rajput AH, McDermott MP, Perl DP: The evolution of diagnosis in early Parkinson disease. Arch Neurol 2000;57:369–372.

Jano-Edward JP, Steele JC, Wresch R, et al: Guam retinal pigment epitheliopathy (GRPE) and the amyotrophic lateral sclerosis/Parkinsonism-Dementia Complex (ALS/PDC): The association of two unusual diseases of Guam and possible clue to the etiology of tauopathy. Mov Disord 2002;17(suppl 5):S253.

Janssen JC, Warrington EK, Morris HR, et al: Clinical features of frontotemporal dementia due to the intronic tau 10$^{(+16)}$ mutation. Neurology 2002;58:1161–1168.

Jaros E, Burn DJ: The pathogenesis of multiple system atrophy: Past, present, and future. Mov Disord 2000;15:784–788.

Jellinger KA, Bancher C: Neuropathology. In Litvan I, Agid Y (eds): Progressive Supranuclear Palsy: Clinical and Research Approaches. Oxford, UK, Oxford University Press, 1993, pp 44–88.

Jendroska K, Hoffmann O, Schelosky L, et al: Absence of disease related prion protein in neurodegenerative disorders presenting with Parkinson's syndrome. J Neurol Neurosurg Psychiatry 1994;57:1249–1251.

Jendroska K, Rossor MN, Mathias CJ, et al: Morphological overlap between corticobasal degeneration and Pick's disease: A clinicopathological report. Mov Disord 1995;10:111–114.

Joachim CL, Morris JH, Kosik KS, Selkoe DJ: Tau antisera recognize neurofibrillary tangles in a range of neurodegenerative disorders. Ann Neurol 1987;22:514–520.

Johnson R, Litvan I, Grafman J: Progressive supranuclear palsy: Altered sensory processing leads to degraded cognition. Neurology 1991;41:1257–1262.

Jordan BD, Relin NR, Ravdin LD, et al: Apolipoprotein E ε4 associated with chronic traumatic brain injury in boxing. JAMA 1997;278:136–140.

Josephs KA, Ahlskog JE, Klos KJ, et al: Neurologic manifestations in welders with pallidal MRI T1 hyperintensity. Neurology 2005;64: 2033–2039.

Josephs KA, Dickson DW: Diagnostic accuracy of progressive supranuclear palsy in the Society for Progressive Supranuclear Palsy brain bank. Mov Disord 2003;18:1018–1026.

Josephs KA, Holton JL, Rossor MN, et al: Neurofilament inclusion body disease: A new proteinopathy? Brain 2003;126:2291–2303.

Josephs KA, Ishizawa T, Tsuboi Y, et al: A clinicopathological study of vascular progressive supranuclear palsy: A multi-infarct disorder presenting as progressive supranuclear palsy. Arch Neurol 2002;59:1597–1601.

Josephs KA, Tang-Wai DF, Edland SD, et al: Correlation between antemortem magnetic resonance imaging findings and pathologically confirmed corticobasal degeneration. Arch Neurol 2004; 61:1881–1884.

Joutel A, Dodick DD, Parisi JE, et al: De novo mutation in the Notch3 gene causing CADASIL. Ann Neurol 2000;47:388–391.

Juncos JL, Hirsch EC, Malessa S, et al: Mesencephalic cholinergic nuclei in progressive supranuclear palsy. Neurology 1991;41:25–30.

Kahn N, Freeman A, Juncos JL, et al: Clozapine is beneficial for psychosis in Parkinson's disease. Neurology 1991;41:1699–1700.

Kato N, Arai K, Hattori T: Study of the rostral midbrain atrophy in progressive supranuclear palsy. J Neurol Sci 2003;210:57–60.

Kato S, Nakamura H: Cytoplasmic argyophilic inclusions in neurons of pontine nuclei in patients with olivopontocerebellar atrophy: Immunohistochemical and ultrastructural studies. Acta Neuropath (Berlin) 1990;79:584–594.

Kaufmann H, Nahm K, Purohit D, Wolfe D: Autonomic failure as the initial presentation of Parkinson disease and dementia with Lewy bodies. Neurology 2004;63:1093–1095.

Kaufmann H, Saadia D, Voustianiouk A: Midodrine in neurally mediated syncope: A double-blind, randomized, crossover study. Ann Neurol 2002;52:342–345.

Kawaguchi Y, Okamoto T, Taniwaki M, et al: CAG expansions in a novel gene from Machado-Joseph disease at chromosome 14q32.1. Nat Genet 1994;8:221–228.

Kawashima M, Miyake M, Kusumi M, et al: Prevalence of progressive supranuclear palsy in Yonago, Japan. Mov Disord 2004;19: 1239–1240.

Kaye JA, May C, Daly E, et al: Cerebrospinal fluid monoamine markers are decreased in dementia of the Alzheimer type with extrapyramidal features. Neurology 1988;38:554–557.

Kertesz A, Hudson L, Mackenzie RA, et al: The pathology and nosology of primary progressive aphasia. Neurology 1994;44:2065–2072.

Kertesz A, Kawarai T, Rogaeva E, et al: Familial frontotemporal dementia with ubiquitin-positive, tau-negative inclusions. Neurology 2000a;54:818–827.

Kertesz A, Martinez-Lage P, Davidson W, et al: The corticobasal degeneration syndrome overlaps progressive aphasia and frontotemporal dementia. Neurology 2000b;55:1368–1375.

Kertesz A, Munoz DG: Primary progressive aphasia and Pick complex. J Neurol Sci 2003;206:97–107.

Kieburtz K, Kurlan R: Welding and Parkinson disease: Is there a bond? Neurology 2005;64:2001–2003.

Kim Y, Kim J-M, Kim J-W, et al: Dopamine transporter density is decreased in parkinsonian patients with a history of manganese exposure: What does it mean? Mov Disord 2002;17:568–572.

Kimber J, Watson L, Mathias CJ: Distinction of idiopathic Parkinson's disease from multiple-system atrophy by stimulation of growth-hormone release with clonidine. Lancet 1997;349:1877–1881.

Kisby GE, Ellison M, Spencer PS: Content of the neurotoxins cycasin (methylazoxymethanol β-D-glucoside) and BMAA (β-N-methyl-amino-L-alanine) in cycad flour prepared by Guam Chamorros. Neurology 1992;42:1336–1340.

Kish SJ, Du F, Parks DA, et al: Quinolinic acid catabolism is increased in cerebellum of patients with dominantly inherited olivopontocerebellar atrophy. Ann Neurol 1991;29:100–104.

Kish SJ, Robitaille Y, El-Awar M, et al: Striatal monoamine neurotransmitters and metabolites in dominantly inherited olivopontocerebellar atrophy. Neurology 1992;42:1573–1577.

Klein C, Brown R, Wenning G, Quinn N: The "cold hands sign" in multiple system atrophy. Mov Disord 1997;12:514–518.

Kleiner-Fisman G, Lang AE, Bergeron C, et al: Rapidly progressive behavioral changes and parkinsonism in a 68-year-old man. Mov Disord 2004;19:534–543.

Kluin KJ, Foster N, Berent S, Gilman S: Perceptual analysis of speech disorders in progressive supranuclear palsy. Neurology 1993;43: 563–566.

Koeppen AH, Mitzen EJ, Hans MC, Barron KD: Olivopontocerebellar atrophy; immunocytochemical and Golgi observations. Neurology 1986;36:1478–1488.

Koller WC, Glatt SL, Hubble JP, et al: Apolipoprotein E genotypes in Parkinson's disease with and without dementia. Ann Neurol 1995;37:242–245.

Kompoliti K, Goetz CG, Boeve BF, et al: Clinical presentation and pharmacologic therapy in corticobasal degeneration. Arch Neurol 1998;55:957–961.

Kompoliti K, Goetz CG, Gajdusek DC, Cubo E: Movement disorders in Kuru. Mov Disord 1999;14:800–804.

Komure O, Sano A, Nishino N, et al: DNA analysis in hereditary dentatorubral-pallidolusian atrophy: Correlation between CAG repeat length and phenotypic variation and the molecular basis of anticipation. Neurology 1995;45:143–149.

Konagaya M, Konagaya Y, Iida M: Clinical and magnetic resonance imaging study of extrapyramidal symptoms in multiple system atrophy. J Neurol Neurosurg Psychiatry 1994;57:1528–1531.

Kosaka K, Ikeda K, Kobayashi K, Mehraein P: Striatopallidonigral degeneration in Pick's disease: A clinicopathological study of 41 cases. J Neurol 1991;238:151–160.

Kosaka K, Matsushita R, Oyanagi S, et al: Pallido-nigral-luysial atrophy with massive appearance of corpora amylacea in the CNS. Acta Neuropath (Berlin) 1981;53:169–172.

Kosic KS: Alzheimer's plaques and tangles: Advances on both fronts. Trends Neurosci 1991;14:218–221.

Kostic VS, Mojsilvoc LJ, Stojanovic M: Degenerative neurological disorders associated with a deficiency of glutamate dehydrogenase. J Neurol 1989;236:111–116.

Krack P, Marion MH: "Apraxia of lid opening." A focal eyelid dystonia: Clinical study of 32 patients. Mov Disord 1994;9: 610–615.

Kraft E, Trenkwalder C, Auer DP: T2*-weighted MRI differentiates multiple system atrophy from Parkinson's disease. Neurology 2002;59:1265–1267.

Krauss JK, Paduch T, Mundinger F, Seeger W: Parkinsonism and rest tremor secondary to supratentorial tumours sparing the basal ganglia. Acta Neurochir 1995;133:22–29.

Kretzschmar HA, Ironside JW, DeArmond SJ, Tateishi J: Diagnostic criteria for sporadic Creutzfeldt-Jakob disease. Arch Neurol 1996;53:913–920.

Krusz JC, Koller WC, Ziegler DK: Historical review: Abnormal movements associated with epidemic encephalitis lethargica. Mov Disord 1987;2:137–141.

Kuhl DE, Minoshima S, Fessler JA, et al: In vivo mapping of cholinergic terminals in normal aging, Alzheimer's disease, and Parkinson's disease. Ann Neurol 1996;40:399–410.

Kuhlenbaumer G, Ludemann P, Schirmacher A, et al: Autosomal dominant striatal degeneration (ADSD): Clinical description and mapping to 5q13-5q14. Neurology 2004;62:2203–2208.

Kumar R, Bergeron C, Lang AE: Corticobasal degeneration. In Jankovic J, Tolosa E (eds): Parkinson's Disease and Movement Disorders, 4th ed. Philadelphia, Lippincott Williams & Wilkins, 2002, pp 185–198.

Kuoppamaki M, Rothwell JC, Brown RG, et al: Parkinsonism following bilateral lesions of the globus pallidus: Performance on a variety of motor tasks shows similarities with Parkinson's disease. J Neurol Neurosurg Psychiatry 2005;76:482–490.

Kurlan R, Richard IH, Papka M, Marshall F: Movement disorders in Alzheimer's disease: More rigidity of definitions needed. Mov Disord 2000;15:24–29.

Kuzuhara S, Kokubo Y, Sasaki R, et al: Familial amyotrophy lateral sclerosis and parkinsonism-dementia complex of the Kii peninsula of Japan: Clinical and neuropathological study and tau analysis. Ann Neurol 2001;49:501–511.

Lai E, Jankovic J: Gait disorders. In Gilman S, Goldstein GW, Waxman SG (eds): Neurobase. La Jolla, Calif, Arbor Publishing, 1995.

Lampert PW, Hardman JM: Morphological changes in brains of boxers. JAMA 1984;251:2676–2679.

Lang AE, Bergeron C, Pollanen MS, Ashby P: Parietal Pick's disease mimicking cortical-basal ganglionic degeneration. Neurology 1994;44:1436–1440.

Lang AE, Koller WC, Fahn S: Psychogenic parkinsonism. Arch Neurol 1995;52:802–810.

Langston JW, Ballard PA, Tetrud JW, Irwin I: Chronic parkinsonism in humans due to a product of meperidine analogue synthesis. Science 1983;219:979–980.

Lanska DJ, Currier RD, Cohen M, et al: Familial progressive subcortical gliosis. Neurology 1994;44:1633–1643.

Lantos PL, Cairns NJ, Khan MN, et al: Neuropathologic variation in frontotemporal dementia due to the intronic tau 10$^{(+16)}$ mutation. Neurology 2002;58:1169–1175.

Lantos PL, Papp MI: Cellular pathology of multiple system atrophy: A review. J Neurol Neurosurg Psychiatry 1994;57:129–133.

Lee MS, Marsden CD: Neurological sequelae following carbon monoxide poisoning: Clinical course and outcome according to the clinical types and brain computed tomography scan findings. Mov Disord 1994;9:550–558.

Lee VM, Giasson BI, Trojanowski JQ: More than just two peas in a pod: Common amyloidogenic properties of tau and alpha-synuclein in neurodegenerative diseases. Trends Neurosci 2004;27:129–134.

Lee VM, Goedert M, Trojanowski JQ: Neurodegenerative tauopathies. Annu Rev Neurosci 2001;24:1121–1159.

Lee VM-Y, Trojanowski JQ: Neurodegenerative tauopathies: Human disease and transgenic mouse models. Neuron 1999;24:507–510.

Leiguarda R, Lees AJ, Merello M, et al: The nature of apraxia in corticobasal degeneration. J Neurol Neurosurg Psychiatry 1994;57:455–459.

Leiguarda RC, Marsden CD: Limb apraxias. Higher-order disorders of sensorimotor integration. Brain 2000;123:860–879.

Lemstra AW, van Meegen MT, Vreyling JP, et al: 14-3-3 testing in diagnosing Creutzfeldt-Jakob disease: A prospective study of 112 patients. Neurology 2000;55:514–516.

Lendon CL, Lynch T, Norton J, et al: Hereditary dysphasic disinhibition dementia: A frontotemporal dementia linked to 17q21-22. Neurology 1998;50:1546–1555.

Leopold N, Bara-Jimenez W, Hallett M: Parkinsonism after a wasp sting. Mov Disord 1999;14:122–127.

Lepore FE, Duvoisin RC: "Apraxia" of eyelid opening: An involuntary levator inhibition. Neurology 1985;35:423–427.

Lepore FE, Steele JC, Cox TA, et al: Supranuclear disturbances of ocular motility in Lytico-Bodig. Neurology 1988;38:1849–1853.

Levy R, Ruberg M, Herrero MT, et al: Alterations of GABAergic neurons in the basal ganglia of patients with progressive supranuclear palsy: An in situ hybridization study of GAD$_{67}$ messenger RNA. Neurology 1995;45:127–134.

Lewis AJ, Gawel MJ: Diffuse Lewy body disease with dementia and oculomotor dysfunction. Mov Disord 1990;5:143–147.

Lewis J, McGowan E, Rockwood J, et al: Neurofibrillary tangles, amyotrophy and progressive motor disturbance in mice expressing mutant (P301L) tau protein. Nat Genet 2000;25:402–405.

Li JY, Lai PH, Chen CY, et al: Postanoxic parkinsonism: Clinical, radiologic, and pathologic correlation. Neurology 2000;55:591–593.

Liang TW, Forman MS, Duda JE, et al: Multiple pathologies in a patient with a progressive neurodegenerative syndrome. J Neurol Neurosurg Psychiatry 2005;76:252–255.

Lim F, Hernandez F, Lucas JJ, et al: FTDP-17 mutations in tau transgenic mice provoke lysosomal abnormalities and tau filaments in forebrain. Mol Cell Neurosci 2001;18:702–714.

Lippa CF, Cohen R, Smith TW, Drachman DA: Primary progressive aphasia with focal neuronal achromasia. Neurology 1991;41:882–886.

Litvan I: Parkinsonism-dementia syndromes. In Jankovic J, Tolosa E (eds): Parkinson's Disease and Movement Disorders, 3rd ed. Baltimore, Williams & Wilkins, 1998a, pp 819–836.

Litvan I: Progressive supranuclear palsy revisited. Acta Neurol Scand 1998b;98:74–84.

Litvan I: Update on epidemiological aspects of progressive supranuclear palsy. Mov Disord 2003;18(suppl 6):S43–S50.

Litvan I, Agid Y (eds): Progressive Supranuclear Palsy. Clinical and Research Approaches. Oxford, UK, Oxford University Press, 1993.

Litvan I, Agid Y, Goetz C, et al: Accuracy of the clinical diagnosis of corticobasal degeneration: A clinicopathologic study. Neurology 1997;48:119–125.

Litvan I, Agid Y, Jankovic J, et al: Accuracy of clinical criteria for the diagnosis of progressive supranuclear palsy (Steele-Richardson-Olszewski syndrome). Neurology 1996;46:922–930.

Litvan I, Agid Y, Sastrj N, et al: What are the obstacles for an accurate clinical diagnosis of Pick's disease? A clinicopathologic study. Neurology 1997;49:62–69.

Litvan I, Baker M, Hutton M: Tau genotype: No effect on onset, symptom severity, or survival in progressive supranuclear palsy. Neurology 2001;57:138–140.

Litvan I, Bhatia KP, Burn DJ, et al: SIC Task Force appraisal of clinical diagnostic criteria for parkinsonian disorders. Mov Disord 2003;18:467–486.

Litvan I, Blesa R, Clark K, et al: Pharmacological evaluation of the cholinergic system in progressive supranuclear palsy. Ann Neurol 1994;36:55–61.

Litvan I, Booth V, Wenning GK, et al: Retrospective application of a set of clinical diagnostic criteria for the diagnosis of multiple system atrophy. J Neural Transm 1998;105:217–227.

Litvan I, Campbell G, Mangone CA, et al: Which clinical features differentiate progressive supranuclear palsy (Steele-Richardson-Olszewski syndrome) from related disorders? A clinipathological study. Brain 1997;120:65–74.

Litvan I, Chase TN: Traditional and experimental therapeutic approaches. In Litvan I, Agid Y (eds): Progressive Supranuclear Palsy: Clinical and Research Approaches. Oxford, UK, Oxford University Press, 1993, pp 254–269.

Litvan I, Cummings JL, Mega M: Neuropsychiatric features of corticobasal degeneration. J Neurol Neurosurg Psychiatry 1998;65:717–721.

Litvan I, Dickson DW, Buttner-Ennever JA, et al: Research goals in progressive supranuclear palsy. Mov Disord 2000;15:446–458.

Litvan I, Goetz C, Jankovic J, et al: What is the accuracy of the clinical diagnosis of multiple system atrophy? A clinicopathological study. Arch Neurol 1997;54:937–944.

Litvan I, Grimes DA, Lang AE, et al: Clinical features differentiating patients with postmortem confirmed progressive supranuclear palsy and corticobasal degeneration. J Neurol 1999;246 (suppl 2): 1–5.

Litvan I, Jankovic J, Goetz CG, et al: Accuracy of the clinical diagnosis of postencephalitic parkinsonism: A clinicopathologic study. Eur J Neurol 1998;5:451–457.

Litvan I, MacIntyre A, Goetz CG, et al: Accuracy of the clinical diagnosis of Lewy body disease, Parkinson's disease, and dementia with Lewy bodies: A clinicopathologic study. Arch Neurol 1998;55:969–978.

Litvan I, Mangone CA, McKee A, et al: Natural history of progressive supranuclear palsy (Steele-Richardson-Olszewski) and clinical predictors of survival: A clinicopathological study. J Neurol Neurosurg Psychiatry 1996;60:615–620.

Litvan I, Mega MS, Cummings JL, Fairbanks L: Neuropsychiatric aspects of progressive supranuclear palsy. Neurology 1996;47: 1184–1189.

Litvan I, Paulsen JS, Mega MS, Cummings JL: Neuropsychiatric assessment of patients with hyperkinetic and hypokinetic movement disorders. Arch Neurol 1998;55:1313–1319.

Litvan I, Phipps M, Phar VL, et al: Randomized placebo-controlled trial of donepezil in patients with progressive supranuclear palsy. Neurology 2001;57:467–473.

Liu W-K, Le TV, Adamson J, et al: Relationship of the extended tau haplotype to tau biochemistry and neuropathology in progressive supranuclear palsy. Ann Neurol 2001;50:494–502.

Liu Y, Stern Y, Chun MR, et al: Pathological correlates of extrapyramidal signs in Alzheimer's disease. Ann Neurol 1997;41:368–374.

Lopez OL, Becker JT, Kaufer DI, et al: Research evaluation and prospective diagnosis of dementia with Lewy bodies. Arch Neurol 2002;59:43–46.

Lorberboym M, Treves TA, Melamed E, et al: [123I]-FP/CIT SPECT imaging for distinguishing drug-induced parkinsonism from Parkinson's disease. Mov Disord 2006;21:510–514.

Louis ED, Klatka LA, Liu Y, Fahn S: Comparison of extrapyramidal features in 31 pathologically confirmed cases of diffuse Lewy body disease and 34 pathologically confirmed cases of Parkinson's disease. Neurology 1997;48:376–380.

Low PA, Gilden JL, Freeman R, et al: Efficacy of midodrine vs placebo in neurogenic orthostatic hypotension: A randomized, double-blind multicenter study. JAMA 1997;277:1046–1051.

Lowe J, Errington DR, Lenox G, et al: Ballooned neurons in several neurodegenerative diseases and stroke contain αB crystallin. Neuropathol Appl Neurobiol 1992;18:341–350.

Lu C-S, Huang C-C, Chu N-S, Calne DB: Levodopa failure in chronic manganism. Neurology 1994;44:1600–1602.

Lu C-S, Ikeda A, Terada K, et al: Electrophysiological studies of early stage corticobasal degeneration. Mov Disord 1998;13:140–146.

Lu C-S, Wu Chou Y-H, Kuo P-C, et al: The parkinsonian phenotype of spinocerebellar ataxia type 2. Arch Neurol 2004;61:35–38.

Lu C-S, Wu Chou Y-H, Yen T-C, et al: Dopa-responsive parkinsonism phenotype of spinocerebellar ataxia type 2. Mov Disord 2002;17:1046–1051.

Lynch T, Sano M, Marder KS, et al: Clinical characteristics of a family with chromosome 17-linked disinhibition-dementia-parkinsonism-amyotrophy complex. Neurology 1994;44:1878–1884.

Mabuchi N, Hirayama M, Koike Y, et al: Progression and prognosis in pure autonomic failure (PAF): Comparison with multiple system atrophy. J Neurol Neurosurg Psychiatry 2005;76:947–952.

Mahapatra RK, Edwards MJ, Schott JM, Bhatia KP: Corticobasal degeneration. Lancet Neurol 2004;3:736–743.

Maher ER, Lees AJ: The clinical features and natural history of Steele-Richardson-Olszewski (progressive supranuclear palsy). Neurology 1986;36:1005–1008.

Majoor-Krakauer D, Ottman R, Johnson WG, Rowland LP: Familial aggregation of amyotrophic lateral sclerosis, dementia, and Parkinson's disesase: Evidence of shared genetic susceptibility. Neurology 1994;44:1872–1877.

Makoweic RL, Albin RL, Cha JJ, et al: Two types of quisqualate receptors are decreased in human olivopontocerebellar atrophy cerebellar cortex. Brain Res 1990;523:309–312.

Malessa S, Hirsch EC, Cervera P, et al: Catecholaminergic systems in the medulla oblongata in parkinsonian syndromes. Neurology 1990;40:1739–1743.

Mancuso M, Davidzon G, Kurlan RM, et al: Hereditary ferritinopathy: A novel mutation, its cellular pathology, and pathogenetic insights. J Neuropathol Exp Neurol 2005;64:280–294.

Manford M, Andermann F: Complex visual hallucinations: Clinical and neurobiological insights. Brain 1998;121:1819–1840.

Manyam BV, Walters AS, Narla KR: Bilateral striopallidal calcinosis: Clinical characteristics of patients seen in a registry. Mov Disord 2001;16:258–264.

Marder K, Tang M-X, Alfaro B, et al: Risk of Alzheimer's disease in relatives of Parkinson's disease patients with and without dementia. Neurology 1999;52:719–724.

Marder K, Tang M-X, Cote L, et al: The frequency and associated risk factors for dementia in patients with Parkinson's disease. Arch Neurol 1995;52:695–701.

Mark MH, Sage JI, Walters AS, et al: Binswanger's disease presenting as levodopa-responsive Parkinson's disease: Clinicopathological study of three cases. Mov Disord 1995;10:450–454.

Markus HS, Martin RJ, Simpson MA, et al: Diagnostic strategies in CADASIL. Neurology 2002;59:1134–1138.

Martinelli P, Scaglione C, Lodi S, et al: Defects of brain and skeletal muscle bioenergetics in progressive supranuclear palsy shown in vivo by phosphorus magnetic resonance spectroscopy. Mov Disord 2000;15:889–893.

Massman PJ, Kreiter KT, Jankovic J, Doody RS: Neuropsychological functioning in cortico-basal ganglionic degeneration: Differentiation from Alzheimer's disease. Neurology 1996;36:720–726.

Mastrianni JA, Nixon R, Layzer R, et al: Prion protein conformation in a patient with sporadic fatal insomnia. N Engl J Med 1999;340:1630–1638.

Mathias CJ: Orthostatic hypotension: Causes, mechanisms, and influencing factors. Neurology 1995;45(suppl 5):S6–S11.

Mathias CJ: Autonomic disorders and their recognition. N Engl J Med 1997;336:721–724.

Mathias CJ, Kimber JR: Treatment of postural hypotension. J Neurol Neurosurg Psychiatry 1998;65:285–289.

Mathuranath PS, Nestor PJ, Berrior GE, et al: A brief cognitive test battery to differentiate Alzheimer's disease and frontotemporal dementia. Neurology 2000a;55:1613–1620.

Mathuranath PS, Xuereb JH, Bak T, Hodges JR: Corticobasal ganglionic degeneration and/or frontotemporal dementia? A report of two overlap cases and review of literature. J Neurol Neurosurg Psychiatry 2000b;68:304–312.

Matsumoto S, Hirano A, Goto S: Spinal cord neurofibrillary tangle of Guamanian amyotrophic lateral sclerosis and parkinsonism-dementia complex. Neurology 1990;40:975–979.

Matsuo A, Akiguchi I, Lee GC, et al: Myelin degeneration in multiple system atrophy detected by unique antibodies. Am J Pathol 1998;153:735–744.

Matsuo H, Takashima H, Kishikawa M, et al: Pure akinesia: An atypical manifestation of progressive supranuclear palsy. J Neurol Neurosurg Psychiatry 1991;54:397–400.

McCrank E, Rabheru K: Four cases of progressive supranuclear palsy in patients exposed to organic solvents. Can J Psychiatry 1989;34:934–935.

McGrath NM, Anderson NE, Hope JKA, et al: Anterior opercular syndrome, caused by herpes simplex encephalitis. Neurology 1997;49:494–497.

McKeith IG, Del Ser T, Spano PF, et al: Efficacy of rivastigmine in dementia with Lewy bodies: A randomized, double-blind, placebo-controlled international study. Lancet 2000;356:2031–2036.

McKeith IG, Dickson DW, Lowe J, et al: Diagnosis and management of dementia with Lewy bodies: Third report of the DLB Consortium. Neurology 2005;65:1863–1872.

McKeith IG, Fairbairn AF, Bothwell RA, et al: An evaluation of the predictive validity and inter-rater reliability of clinical diagnostic criteria for senile dementia of Lewy body type. Neurology 1994;44:872–877.

McKeith IG, Galasko D, Kosaka K, et al: Consensus guidelines for the clinical and pathological diagnosis of dementia with Lewy bodies (DLB): Report of the consortium on DLB international workshop. Neurology 1996;47:113–124.

McKeith IG, Perry EK, Perry RH, et al: Report of the second dementia with Lewy body international workshop: Diagnosis and treatment. Neurology 1999;53:902–905.

McKhann GM, Ambert SA, Grossman M, et al: Clinical and pathological diagnosis of frontotemporal dementia: Report of the Work Group on Frontotemporal Dementia and Pick's disease. Arch Neurol 2001;58:1803–1809.

McLeod JG, Tuck RR: Disorders of the autonomic nervous system: 1. Pathophysiology and clinical features. Ann Neurol 1987a;21:419–430.

McLeod JC, Tuck RR: Disorders of the autonomic nervous system: 2. Investigation and treatment. Ann Neurol 1987b;21:519–529.

Mega MS, Masterman DL, Benson F, et al: Dementia with Lewy bodies: Reliability and validity of clinical and pathological criteria. Neurology 1996;47:1403–1409.

Meissner B, Kohler K, Kortner K, et al: Sporadic Creutzfeldt-Jakob disease: Magnetic resonance imaging and clinical findings. Neurology 2004;63:45–56.

Mendez MF, Shapira JS, Miller BL: Stereotypical movements and frontotemporal dementia. Mov Disord 2005;20:742–745.

Mendez OE, Shang J, Jungreis CA, Kaufer DI: Diffusion-weighted MRI in Creutzfeldt-Jakob disease: A better diagnostic marker than CSF protein 14-3-3? J Neuroimaging 2003;13:147–151.

Merello M, Sabe L, Teson A, et al: Extrapyramidalism in Alzheimer's disease: Prevalence, psychiatric, and neuropsychological correlates. J Neurol Neurosurg Psychiatry 1994;57:1503–1509.

Merlo IM, Occhini A, Pacchetti C, Alfonsi E: Not paralysis, but dystonia causes stridor in multiple system atrophy. Neurology 2002;58:649–652.

Mesulam MM: Primary progressive aphasia: A language based dementia. N Engl J Med 2003;349:1535–1542.

Mezey E, Dehejia A, Harta G, et al: Alpha synuclein in neurodegenerative disorders: Murderer or accomplice? Nature Med 1998;4:755–757.

Mintzer S, Hickenbottom S, Gilman S: Parkinsonism after taking ecstasy. N Engl J Med 1999;340:1443.

Mishina M, Ishii K, Mitani K, et al: Midbrain hypometabolism as early diagnostic sign for progressive supranuclear palsy. Acta Neurol Scand 2004;110:128–135.

Miyajima H: Genetic disorders affecting proteins of iron and copper metabolism: Clinical implications. Intern Med 2002;41:762–769.

Mokri B, Ahlskog JE, Fulgham JR, Matsumoto JY: Syndrome resembling PSP after surgical repair of ascending aorta dissection or aneurysm. Neurology 2004;62:971–973.

Molinuevo JL, Munoz E, Valldeoriola F, Tolosa E: The eye of the tiger sign in cortico-basal ganglionic degeneration. Mov Disord 1999;14:169–171.

Montplaisir J, Petit D, Decary A: Sleep and quantitative EEG in patients with progressive supranuclear palsy. Neurology 1997;49:999–1003.

Mora A, Gonzalez-Polo RA, Fuentes JM, et al: Different mechanisms of protection against apoptosis by valproate and Li+. Eur J Biochem 1998;266:886–891.

Mori H, Nishimura M, Namba Y, Oda M: Corticobasal degeneration: A disease with widespread appearance of abnormal tau and neurofibrillary tangles, and its relation to progressive supranuclear palsy. Acta Neuropathol (Berl) 1994;88:113–121.

Morita H, Ikeda S, Yamamoto K, et al: Hereditary ceruloplasmin deficiency with hemosiderosis: A clinicopathological study of a Japanese family. Ann Neurol 1995;37:646–656.

Morris HR, Gibb G, Katzenschlager R, et al: Pathological, clinical and genetic heterogeneity in progressive supranuclear palsy. Brain 2002;125:969–975.

Morris HR, Janssen JC, Bandmann O, et al: The tau A0 polymorphism in progressive supranuclear palsy and related neurodegenerative diseases. J Neurol Neurosurg Psychiatry 1999;66:665–667.

Morris HR, Khan MN, Janssen JC, et al: The genetic and pathological classification of familial frontotemporal dementia. Arch Neurol 2001;58:1813–1816.

Morris HR, Lees AJ, Wood NW: Neurofibrillary tangle parkinsonsian disorders: Tau pathology and tau genetics. Mov Disord 1999;14:731–736.

Morris HR, Osaki Y, Holton J, et al: Tau exon 10 +16 mutation FTDP-17 presenting clinically as sporadic young onset PSP. Neurology 2003;61:102–104.

Morris HR, Steele JC, Crook R, et al: Genome-wide analysis of the parkinsonism-dementia complex of Guam. Arch Neurol 2004;61:1889–1897.

Mott SH, Packer RJ, Vezina LG, et al: Encephalopathy with parkinsonian features in children following bone marrow transplantations and high-dose amphotericin B. Ann Neurol 1995;37:810–814.

Muenter MD, Forno LS, Hornykiewcz O, et al: Hereditary form of parkinsonism-dementia. Ann Neurol 1998;43:768–781.

Munoz DG, Dickson DW, Bergeron C, et al: The neuropathology and biochemistry of frontotemporal dementia. Ann Neurol 2003;54:S24–S28.

Munoz DP, Everling S: Look away: The anti-saccade task and the voluntary control of eye movement. Nat Rev Neurosci 2004;5:218–228.

Munschauer FE, Loh L, Bannister R, Newsom-Davis J: Abnormal respiration and sudden death during sleep in multiple system atrophy with autonomic failure. Neurology 1990;40:677–679.

Murata T, Shiga Y, Higano S, et al: Conspicuity and evolution of lesions in Creutzfeldt-Jakob disease at diffusion-weighted imaging. AJNR Am J Neuroradiol 2002;23:1164–1172.

Murayama S, Arima K, Nakazato Y, et al: Immunocytochemical and ultrastructural studies of neuronal and oligodendroglial cytoplasmic inclusions in multiple system atrophy: 2. Oligodendroglial cytoplasmic inclusions. Acta Neuropathologica 1992;84:32–38.

Murman DL, Kuo SB, Powell MC, Colenda CC: The impact of parkinsonism on costs of care in patients with AD and dementia with Lewy bodies. Neurology 2003;61:944–949.

Murray AM, Weihmueller FB, Marshal JF, et al: Damage to dopamine systems differs between Parkinson's disease and Alzheimer's disease with parkinsonism. Ann Neurol 1995;37:300–312.

Näslund J, Haroutunian V, Mohs R, et al: Correlation between elevated levels of amyloid β-peptide in the brain and cognitive decline. JAMA 2000;283:1571–1577.

Nasreddine ZS, Loginov M, Clark LN, et al: From genotype to phenotype: A clinical, pathological, and biochemical investigation of frontotemporal dementia and parkinsonism (FTDP-17) caused by the P301L tau mutation. Ann Neurol 1999;45:704–715.

Nath A, Jankovic J, Pettigrew C: Movement disorders and AIDS. Neurology 1987;37–41.

Nath U, Ben-Shlomo Y, Thomson RG, et al: The prevalence of progressive supranuclear palsy (Steele-Richardson-Olszewski syndrome) in the UK. Brain 2001;124:1438–1449.

Nath U, Ben-Shlomo Y, Thomson RG, et al: Clinical features and natural history of progressive supranuclear palsy: A clinical cohort study. Neurology 2003;60:910–916.

Neumann M, Schulz-Schaeffer W, Crother A, et al: Pick's disease associated with the novel tau gene mutation K369I. Ann Neurol 2001;50:503–513.

Newman GC: Treatment of progressive supranuclear palsy with tricyclic antidepressants. Neurology 1985;35:1189–1193.

Nieforth KA, Golbe LI: Retrospective study of drug response in 87 patients with progressive supranuclear palsy. Clin Neuropharmacol 1993;16:338–346.

Nielsen JE, Jensen NL, Krabbe K: Hereditary haemochromatosis: A case of iron accumulation in the basal ganglia associated with a parkinsonian syndrome. J Neurol Neurosurg Psychiatry 1995;59: 318–321.

Nisipeanu P, Kuritzky A, Korczyn AD: Familial levodopa-responsive parkinsonian-pyramidal syndrome. Mov Disord 1994;9:673–675.

Nittis T, Gitlin JD: The copper-iron connection: Hereditary aceruloplasminemia. Semin Hematol 2002;39:282–289.

Nutt JG, Marsden CD, Thompson PD: Human walking and higher-level gait disorders, particularly in the elderly. Neurology 1993;43:268–279.

Nygaard TG, Duvoisin RC, Manocha M, Chokroverty S: Seizures in progressive supranuclear palsy. Neurology 1989;39:138–140.

Oba H, Yagishita A, Terada H, et al: New and reliable MRI diagnosis for progressive supranuclear palsy. Neurology 2005;64:2050–2055.

O'Brien C, Sung JH, McGeachie RE, Lee MC: Striatonigral degeneration: Clinical, MRI, and pathologic correlation. Neurology 1990;40:710–711.

Oerlemans WGH, de Visser M: Dropped head syndrome and bent spine syndrome: Two separate clinical entities or different manifestations of axial myopathy? J Neurol Neurosurg Psychiatry 1998; 65:258–259.

Ohtake H, Limprasert P, Fan Y, et al: Beta-synuclein gene alterations in dementia with Lewy bodies. Neurology 2004;63:805–811.

Okuma Y, Fujishima K, Miwa H, et al: Myoclonic tremulous movements in multiple system atrophy are a form of cortical myoclonus. Mov Disord 2005;20:451–456.

Olanow CW, Good PF, Shinotoh H, et al: Manganese intoxication in the rhesus monkey: A clinical, imaging, pathologic, and biochemical study. Neurology 1996;46:492–498.

Olichney JM, Hansen LA, Galasko D, et al: The apolipoprotein E ε4 allele is associated with increased neuritic plaques and cerebral amyloid angiopathy in Alzheimer's disease and Lewy body variant. Neurology 1996;47:190–196.

Oliva R, Tolosa E, Ezquerra M, et al: Significant changes in the tau A0 and A3 alleles in progressive supranuclear palsy and improved genotyping by silver detection. Arch Neurol 1998;55:1122–1124.

Oliveira JR, Spiteri E, Sobrido MJ, et al: Genetic heterogeneity in familial idiopathic basal ganglia calcification (Fahr disease). Neurology 2004;63:2165–2167.

Ondo W, Warrior D, Overby A, et al: Computerized posturography in progressive supranuclear palsy: Comparison with Parkinson's disease and normal controls. Arch Neurol 2000;57:1464–1469.

Ondo WG, Chan LL, Levy JK: Vascular parkinsonism: Clinical correlates predicting motor improvement after lumbar puncture. Mov Disord 2002a;17:91–97.

Ondo WG, Hunter C, Vuong KD, Jankovic J: Olanzapine treatment for dopaminergic-induced hallucinations. Mov Disord 2002b;17:1031–1035.

Osaki Y, Ben-Shlomo Y, Lees AJ, et al: Accuracy of clinical diagnosis of progressive supranuclear palsy. Mov Disord 2004;19:181–189.

Osaki Y, Wenning GK, Daniel SE, et al: Do published criteria improve clinical diagnostic accuracy in multiple system atrophy? Neurology 2002;59:1486–1491.

O'Sullivan JD, Hanagasi H, Daniel SE, et al: Neuronal intranuclear inclusion disease and juvenile parkinsonism. Mov Disord 2000;15:990–995.

Otto M, Wiltfang J, Cepek L, et al: Tau protein and 14-3-3 protein in the differential diagnosis of Creuzfeldt-Jakob disease. Neurology 2002;58:192–197.

Ozawa T, Paviour D, Quinn NP, et al: The spectrum of pathological involvement of the striatonigral and olivopontocerebellar systems in multiple system atrophy: Clinicopathological correlations. Brain 2004;127:2657–2671.

Özsancak C, Auzou P, Hannequin D: Dysarthria and orofacial apraxia in corticobasal degeneration. Mov Disord 2000;15:905–910.

Padovani A, Borroni B, Brambati SM, et al: Diffusion tensor imaging and voxel based morphometry study in early progressive supranuclear palsy. J Neurol Neurosurg Psychiatry 2006;77:457–463.

Panegyres PK, Toufexis K, Kakulas BA, et al: A new PRNP mutation (G131V) associated with Gerstmann-Sträussler-Scheinker disease. Arch Neurol 2001;58:1899–1902.

Papp M, Lantos P: Accumulation of tubular structures in oligodendroglial and neuronal cells as the basic alteration in multiple system atrophy. J Neurol Sci 1992;107:172–182.

Papp MI, Khan JE, Lantos PL: Glial cytoplasmic inclusions in the CNS of patients with multiple system atrophy (striatonigral degeneration, olivopontocerebellar atrophy and Shy-Drager syndrome). J Neurol Sci 1989;94:79–100.

Parati EA, Fetoni V, Germiniani GC, et al: Response to L-DOPA in multiple system atrophy. Clin Neuropharmacol 1993;16:139–144.

Parchi P, Hiese A, Capellari S, et al: Classification of sporadic Creutzfeldt-Jakob disease based on molecular and phenotypic analysis of 300 subjects. Ann Neurol 1999;46:224–233.

Parikh SM, Diedrich A, Biaggioni I, Robertson D: The nature of the autonomic dysfunction in multiple system atrophy. J Neurol Sci 2002;200:1–10.

Pascual J, Berciano J, Grijalba B, et al: Dopamine D1 and D2 receptors in progressive supranuclear palsy: An autoradiographic study. Ann Neurol 1992;32:703–707.

Pastakia B, Polinsky R, Di Chiro G, et al: Multiple system atrophy (Shy-Drager syndrome): MR imaging. Radiology 1986;159:499–502.

Pastor P, Ezquerra M, Munoz E, et al: Significant association between the tau gene A0/A0 genotype and Parkinson's disease. Ann Neurol 2000;47:242–245.

Pastor P, Ezquerra M, Perez JC, et al: Novel haplotypes in 17q21 are associated with progressive supranuclear palsy. Ann Neurol 2004;56:249–258.

Pastor P, Ezquerra M, Tolosa E, et al: Further extension of the H1 haplotype associated with progressive supranuclear palsy. Mov Disord 2002;17:550–556.

Pastor P, Pastor E, Carnero C, et al: Familial atypical progressive supranuclear palsy associated with homozygosity for the delN296 mutation in the tau gene. Ann Neurol 2001;49:263–267.

Pastor P, Tolosa E: Progressive supranuclear palsy: Clinical and genetic aspects. Curr Opin Neurol 2002;15:429–437.

Payami H, Nutt J, Gancher S, et al: SCA2 may present as levodopa-responsive parkinsonism. Mov Disord 2003;18:425–429.

Peigneux P, Salmon E, Garraux G, et al: Neural and cognitive bases of upper limb apraxia in corticobasal degeneration. Ann Neurol 2001;57:1259–1268.

Perry TL, Hansen S, Jones K: Brain amino acids and glutathione in progressive supranuclear palsy. Neurology 1988;38:943–946.

Pezzoli G, Canesi M, Antonini A, et al: Hydrocarbon exposure and Parkinson's disease. Neurology 2000;55:667–673.

Phiel CJ, Zhang F, Huang EY, et al: Histone deacetylase is a direct target of valproic acid, a potent anticonvulsant, mood stabilizer, and teratogen. J Biol Chem 2001;276: 36734–36741.

Piccini P, de Yebenez J, Lees AJ, et al: Familial progressive supranuclear palsy: Detection of subclinical cases using [18]F-dopa and [18]fluorodeoxyglucose positron emission tomography. Arch Neurol 2001;58:1846–1851.

Pierot L, Desnos L, Blin J, et al: D1 and D2-type dopamine receptors in patients with Parkinson's disease and progressive supranuclear palsy. J Neurol Sci 1988;86:291–306.

Pillon B, Blin J, Vidailhet M, et al: The neuropsychological pattern of corticobasal degeneration: Comparison with progressive supranuclear palsy and Alzheimer's disease. Neurology 1995;45:1477–1483.

Pillon B, Deweer B, Michon A, et al: Are explicit memory disorders of progressive supranuclear palsy related to damage to striatofrontal circuits? Comparison with Alzheimer's, Parkinson's and Huntington's diseases. Neurology 1994;44:1264–1270.

Pillon B, Dubois B: Cognitive and behavioral impairments. In Litvan I, Agid Y (eds): Progressive Supranuclear Palsy: Clinical and Research Approaches. Oxford, UK, Oxford University Press, 1993, pp 223–239.

Pillon B, Dubois B, Agid Y: Testing cognition may contribute to the diagnosis of movement disorders. Neurology 1996;46:329–334.

Pillon B, Gouider-Khouja N, Deweer B, et al: Neuropsychological pattern of striatonigral degeneration: Comparison with Parkinson's disease and progressive supranuclear palsy. J Neurol Neurosurg Psychiatry 1995;58:174–178.

Pirker W, Asebaum S, Bencsits G, et al: [$^{123}$I]β-CIT SPECT in multiple system atrophy, progressive supranuclear palsy, and corticobasal degeneration. Mov Disord 2000;15:1158–1167.

Plazzi G, Corsini R, Provini F, et al: REM sleep behavior disorders in multiple system atrophy. Neurology 1997;48:1094–1097.

Pocchiari M, Salvatore M, Cutruzzola F, et al: A new point mutation of the prion protein gene in Creutzfeldt-Jakob disease. Ann Neurol 1993;34:802–807.

Pohle T, Krauss JK: Parkinsonism in children resulting from mesencephalic tumors. Mov Disord 1999;14:842–846.

Polinsky RJ: Shy-Drager syndrome. In Jankovic J, Tolosa E (eds): Parkinson's Disease and Movement Disorders, 2nd ed. Baltimore, Williams & Wilkins, 1993, pp 191–204.

Polinsky RJ, Holmes KV, Brown RT, Weise V: CSF acetylcholinesterase levels are reduced in multiple system atrophy with autonomic failure. Neurology 1989;39:40–44.

Pompeu FM Growdon JH: Diagnosing dementia with Lewy bodies. Arch Neurol 2002;59:29–30.

Poorkaj P, Bird TD, Wijsman E, et al: Tau is a candidate gene for chromosome 17 frontotemporal dementia. Ann Neurol 1998;43:815–825.

Poorkaj P, Muma NA, Zhukareva V, et al: An R5L tau mutation in a subject with a progressive supranuclear palsy phenotype. Ann Neurol 2002;52:511–516.

Poorkaj P, Tsuang D, Wijsman E, et al: Tau as a susceptibility gene for amyotrophic lateral sclerosis-parkinsonism dementia complex of Guam. Arch Neurol 2001;58:1871–1878.

Poser S, Mollenhauer B, Kraub A, et al: How to improve the clinical diagnosis of Creutzfeldt-Jakob disease. Brain 1999;122:2345–2351.

Pradham S, Pandley N, Shashank S, et al: Parkinsonism due to predominant involvement of substantia nigra in Japanese encephalitis. Neurology 1999;53:1781–1786.

Pramstaller PP, Kunig G, Leenders K, et al: Parkin mutations in a patient with hemiparkinsonism-hemiatrophy: A clinical-genetic and PET study. Neurology 2002;58:808–810.

Pranzatelli MR, Mott SH, Pavlakis SG, et al: Clinical spectrum of secondary parkinsonism in childhood: A reversible disorder. Pediatr Neurol 1994;10:131–140.

Probst-Cousin S, Rickert CH, Schmid KW, Gullotta F: Cell death mechanisms in multiple system atrophy. J Neuropathol Exp Neurol 1998;57:814–821.

Prusiner SB: Prion diseases and the BSE crisis. Science 1997;278:245–251.

Prusiner SB: Shattuck lecture: Neurodegenerative disease and prions. N Engl J Med 2001;344:1516–1551.

Przedborski S, Dhawan V, Donaldson DM, et al: Nitrostriatal dopaminergic function in familial amyotrophic lateral sclerosis patients with and without copper/zinc superoxide dismutase mutations. Neurology 1996;47:1546–1551.

Przedborski S, Giladi N, Takikawa S, et al: Metabolic topography of the hemiparkinsonism-hemiatrophy syndrome. Neurology 1994;44:1622–1628.

Quinn N: Multiple system atrophy. In Marsden CD, Fahn S (eds): Movement Disorders, 3rd ed. Oxford, UK, Butterworth-Heinemann, 1994, pp 262–281.

Qureshi A, Wilmont G, Diphenia B, et al: Motor neuron disease with parkinsonism. Arch Neurol 1996;53:987–991.

Racette BA, Antenor JA, McGee-Minnich L, et al: [(18)F]FDOPA PET and clinical features in parkinsonism due to manganism. Mov Disord 2005;20:492–496.

Racette BA, Esper GJ, Antenor J, et al: Pathophysiology of parkinsonism due to hydrocephalus. J Neurol Neurosurg Psychiatry 2004;75:1617–1619.

Racette BA, McGee-Minnich L, Moerlein SM, et al: Welding-related parkinsonism: Clinical features, treatment, and pathophysiology. Neurology 2001;56:8–13.

Rafal RD, Posner MI, Friedman D, et al: Orienting of visual attention in progressive supranuclear palsy. Brain 1988;111:267–280.

Rajput A, Rozdilsky B, Hornykiewicz O, et al: Reversible drug-induced parkinsonism: Clinicopathologic study of two cases. Arch Neurol 1982;39:644–646.

Rascol O, Sabatini U, Simonetta-Moreau M, et al: Square wave jerks in parkinsonian syndromes. J Neurol Neurosurg Psychiatry 1991;54:599–602.

Rebeiz JJ, Kolodny EH, Richardson EP: Corticodentatonigral degeneration with neuronal achromasia. Arch Neurol 1968;18:20–23.

Remy P, Hosseini H, Degos J-D, et al. Striatal dopaminergic denervation in pallidopyramidal disease demonstrated by positron emission tomography. Ann Neurol 1995;38:954–956.

Riley DE, Fogt N, Leigh RJ: The syndrome of "pure akinesia" and its relationship to progressive supranuclear palsy. Neurology 1994;44:1025–1029.

Riley DE, Lang AE, Lewis A, et al: Cortical-basal ganglionic degeneration. Neurology 1990;40:1203–1212.

Rinne JO, Burn DJ, Mathias CJ, et al: Positron emission tomography studies on the dopaminergic system and striatal opioid binding in the olivopontocerebellar atrophy variant of multiple system atrophy. Ann Neurol 1995;37:568–573.

Rinne JO, Daniel SE, Scaravilli F, et al: The neuropathological features of neuroacanthocytosis. Mov Disord 1994;9:297–304.

Rinne JO, Laine M, Kaasinen V, et al: Striatal dopamine transporter and extrapyramidal symptoms in frontotemporal dementia. Neurology 2002;58:1489–1493.

Rinne JO, Lee MS, Thompson PD, Marsden CD: Corticobasal degeneration: A clinical study of 36 cases. Brain 1994;117:1183–1196.

Rinne JO, Sahlberg N, Ruottinen H, et al: Striatal uptake of the dopamine reuptake ligand [$^{11}$C]β-CFT is reduced in Alzheimer's disease assessed by positron emission tomography. Neurology 1998;50:152–156.

Rivaud-Péchoux S, Vidailhet M, Gallouedec G, et al: Longitudinal ocular motor study in corticobasal degeneration and progressive supranuclear palsy. Neurology 2000;54:1029–1032.

Rivest J, Quinn N, Marsden CD: Dystonia in Parkinson's disease, multiple system atrophy, and progressive supranuclear palsy. Neurology 1990;40:1571–1578.

Roberts GW, Allsop D, Bruton C: The occult aftermath of boxing. J Neurol Neurosurg Psychiatry 1990;53:373–378.

Robertson NP, Wharton S, Anderson J, Scolding NJ: Adult polyglucosan body disease associated with an extrapyramidal syndrome. J Neurol Neurosurg Psychiatry 1998;65:788–790.

Rojo A, Pernaute RS, Fontán A, et al: Clinical genetics of familial progressive supranuclear palsy. Brain 1999;122:1233–1245.

Roman GC: New insight into Binswanger disease. Arch Neurol 1999;56:1061–1062.

Romano S, Colosimo C. Procerus sign in progressive supranuclear palsy. Neurology 2001;57:1928.

Ros R, Gomez Garre P, Hirano M, et al: Genetic linkage of autosomal dominant progressive supranuclear palsy to 1q31.1. Ann Neurol 2005;57:634–641.

Rosenberg RN: Autosomal dominant cerebellar phenotypes: The genotype has settled the issue. Neurology 1995;45:1–5.

Rosenow F, Herholz K, Lanfermann H, et al: Neurological sequelae of cyanide intoxication: The pattern of clinical, magnetic resonance imaging, and positron emission tomography findings. Ann Neurol 1995;38:825–828.

Roses AD: Apolipoprotein E genotyping in the differential diagnosis, not prediction, of Alzheimer's disease. Ann Neurol 1995;38:6–14.

Rossor MN: Pick's disease: A clinical overview. Neurology 2001;56 (suppl 4):S3–S5.

Rossor MN, Tyrrell PJ, Warrington EK, et al: Progressive frontal gait disturbance with atypical Alzheimer's disease and corticobasal degeneration. J Neurol Neurosurg Psychiatry 1999;67:345–352.

Rowland LP: Frontotemporal dementia, chromosome 17, and progranulin. Ann Neurol 2006;60:275–277.

Rowland LP, Shneider NA: Amyotrophic lateral sclerosis. N Engl J Med 2001;344:1688–1700.

Ruberg M, Hirsch E, Javoy-Agid F: Neurochemistry. In Litvan I, Agid Y (eds): Progressive Supranuclear Palsy. Clinical and Research Approaches. Oxford, UK, Oxford University Press, 1993, pp 89–109.

Sadek AH, Rauch R, Schulz PE: Parkinsonism due to manganism in a welder. Int J Toxicol 2003;22:393–401.

Sage JJ, Mark MH: Diffuse Lewy body disease. In Stern MB, Koller WC (eds): Parkinsonian Disorders, New York, Marcel Dekker, 1993, pp 393–411.

Saint Hilaire M-H, Burke RE, Bressman SB, et al: Delayed-onset dystonia due to perinatal or early childhood asphyxia. Neurology 1991;41:216–222.

Saito Y, Matsuoka Y, Takahashi A, Ohno Y: Survival of patients with multiple system atrophy. Int Med 1994; 33:321–325.

Sakakibara R, Hattori T, Uchiyama T, et al: Are alpha-blockers involved in lower urinary tract dysfunction in multiple system atrophy? A comparison of prazosin and moxisylyte. J Auton Nerv Syst 2000a;79:191–195.

Sakakibara R, Hattori T, Uchiyama T, et al: Urinary dysfunction and orthostatic hypotension in multiple system atrophy: Which is the more common and earlier manifestation? J Neurol Neurosurg Psychiatry 2000b;68:65–69.

Salazar G, Valls-Solle J, Marti M, et al: Postural and action myoclonus in patients with parkinsonian type multiple system atrophy. Mov Disord 2000;15:77–83.

Santacruz P, Uttl B, Litvan I, Grafman J: Progressive supranuclear palsy: A survey of the disease course. Neurology 1998;50:1637–1647.

Savant CS, Singhal BS, Jankovic J, et al: Substantia nigra lesions in viral encephalitis. Mov Disord 2003;18:213–216.

Savoiardo M, Girotti F, Strada L, Ciceri E: Magnetic resonance imaging in progressive supranuclear palsy and other parkinsonian disorders. J Neurol Transm 1994;42(suppl):93–110.

Sawle GV, Brooks DJ, Marsden CD, Frackowiak SJ: Corticobasal degeneration. Brain 1991;114:541–556.

Scaravilli T, Pramstaller PP, Salerno A, et al: Neuronal loss in Onuf's nucleus in three patients with progressive supranuclear palsy. Ann Neurol 2000;48:97–101.

Scarmeas N, Hadjigeorgiou GM, Papadimitriou A, et al: Motor signs during the course of Alzheimer disease. Neurology 2004;63:975–982.

Schneider JA, Watts RL, Gearing M, et al: Corticobasal degeneration: Neuropathologic and clinical heterogeneity. Neurology 1997;48:959–969.

Schocke MF, Seppi K, Esterhammer R, et al: Diffusion-weighted MRI differentiates the Parkinson variant of multiple system atrophy from PD. Neurology 2002;58:575–580.

Schrag A, Ben-Shlomo Y, Quinn NP: Prevalence of progressive supranuclear palsy and multiple system atrophy: A cross-sectional study. Lancet 1999;354:1771–1775.

Schrag A, Good CD, Miszkiel K, et al: Differentiation of atypical parkinsonian syndromes with routine MRI. Neurology 2000;54:697–702.

Schrag A, Kingsley D, Phatouros C, et al: Clinical usefulness of magnetic resonance imaging in mutiple system atrophy. J Neurol Neurosurg Psychiatry 1998;65:65–71.

Schwarz SC, Seufferlein T, Liptay S, et al: Microglial activation in multiple system atrophy: A potential role for NF-kappa B/rel proteins. Neuroreport 1998;9:3029–3032.

Schweers O, Mandelkow E, Biernat J, et al: Oxidation of cystein-322 in the repeat domain of microtubule-associated protein tau controls the in vitro assembly of paired helical filaments. Proc Natl Acad Sci U S A 1995;92:8463–8467.

Scientific Committee of the First International Consultation on Incontinence: Assessment and treatment of urinary incontinence. Lancet 2000;355:2153–2158.

Scott B, Jankovic J: Delayed-onset progressive movement disorders. Neurology 1996;46:68–74.

Seiser A, Schwarz S, Aichinger-Steiner MM, et al: Parkinsonism and dystonia in central and extrapontine myelinolysis. J Neurol Neurosurg Psychiatry 1998;65:119–121.

Sejvar JJ, Haddad MB, Tierney BC, et al: Neurologic manifestations and outcome of West Nile virus infection. JAMA 2003;290:511–515.

Senard JM, Rascol O, Durrieu G, et al: Effects of yohimbine on plasma catecholamine levels in orthostatic hypotension related to Parkinson disease or multiple system atrophy. Clin Neuropharmacol 1993; 16:70–76.

Seppi K, Schocke MF, Donnemiller E, et al: Comparison of diffusion-weighted imaging and [123I]IBZM-SPECT for the differentiation of patients with the Parkinson variant of multiple system atrophy from those with Parkinson's disease. Mov Disord 2004;19: 1438–1445.

Seppi K, Schocke MF, Esterhammer R, et al: Diffusion-weighted imaging discriminates progressive supranuclear palsy from PD, but not from the parkinson variant of multiple system atrophy. Neurology 2003;60:922–927.

Seppi K, Yekhlef F, Diem A, et al: Progression of parkinsonism in multiple system atrophy. J Neurol 2005;252:91–96.

Sergeant N, Wattez A, Delacourte A: Neurofibrillary degeneration in progressive supranuclear palsy and corticobasal degeneration: Tau pathologies with exclusively "exon 10" isoforms. J Neurochem 1999;72:1243–1249.

Shan DE, Soong B-W, Sun C-M, et al: Spinocerebellar ataxia type 2 presenting as familial levodopa-responsive parkinsonism. Ann Neurol 2001;50:812–815.

Shankar SK, Yanagihara R, Garruto RM, et al: Immunocyto-chemical characterization of neurofibrillary tangles in amyotrophic lateral sclerosis and parkinsonism-dementia complex of Guam. Ann Neurol 1989;25:146–151.

Shiga Y, Miyazawa K, Sato S, et al: Diffusion-weighted MRI abnormalities as an early diagnostic marker for Creutzfeldt-Jakob disease. Neurology 2004;63:443–449.

Shevell M: Hallervorden and history. N Engl J Med 2003;348(1):3–4.

Shimizu N, Takiyama Y, Mizuno Y, et al: Characteristics of oculomotility disorders of a family with Joseph's disease. J Neurol 1990; 237:393–397.

Shimoda-Matsubayashi S, Hattaori T, Matsumine H, et al: Mn SOD activity and protein in a patient with chromosome 6-linked autosomal recessive parkinsonism in comparison with Parkinson's disease and conrol. Neurology 1997;49:1257–1262.

Shin R-W, Kitamoto T, Tateishi J: Modified tau is present in younger nondemented persons: A study of subcortical nuclei in Alzheimer's disease and progressive supranuclear palsy. Acta Neuropathol 1991;81:617–623.

Shinobu LA, Budzik RF, Frosch MP: Case 28-1999. N Engl J Med 1999;341:901–908.

Shinotoh H, Namba H, Yamaguchi M, et al: Positron emission tomographic measurement of acetycholinesterase activity reveals differential loss of ascending cholinergic systems in Parkinson's disease and progressive supranuclear palsy. Ann Neurol 1999;46: 62–69.

Shinotoh H, Snow BJ, Chu N-S, et al: Presynaptic and postsynaptic striatal dopaminergic function in patients with manganese intoxication: A positron emission tomography study. Neurology 1997;48:1053–1056.

Shoji M, Harigaya Y, Sasaki A, et al: Accumulation of NACP/α-synuclein in Lewy bodies and multiple system atrophy. J Neurol Neurosurg Psychiatry 2000;68:605–608.

Shulman LM, Lang AE, Jankovic J, et al: Case 1, 1995: Psychosis, dementia, chorea, ataxia, and supranuclear gaze dysfunction. Mov Disord 1995;10:257–262.

Shy GM, Drager GA: A neurological syndrome associated with orthostatic hypotension: A clinical-pathological study. Arch Neurol 1960;2:511–527.

Siderowf AD, Galetta SL, Hurtig HI, Liu GT: Posey and Spiller and progressive supranuclear palsy: An incorrect attribution. Mov Disord 1998;13:170–174.

Silber MH, Levine S: Stridor and death in multiple system atrophy. Mov Disord 2000;15:699–704.

Simon DK, Pulst SM, Sutton JP, et al: Familial multisystem degeneration with parkinsonism associated with the 11778 mitochondrial DNA mutation. Neurology 1999;53:1787–1793.

Simpson DA, Wishnow R, Gargulinski RB, Pawlak AM: Oculofacial-skeletal myorhythmia in central nervous system Whipple's disease: Additional case and review of the literature. Mov Disord 1995;10:195–200.

Sinatra MG, Baldini SM, Baiocco F, Carenini L: Auditory brainstem response patterns in familial and sporadic olivopontocerebellar atrophy. Eur Neurol 1988;28:288–290.

Snow BJ, Peppard RF, Guttman M, et al: Positron emission tomographic scanning demonstrates a presynaptic dopaminergic lesion in Lytico-Bodig. Arch Neurol 1990;47:870–874.

Snow BJ, Vingerhoets FJG, Langston JW, et al: Pattern of dopaminergic loss in the striatum of humans with MPTP induced parkinsonism. J Neurol Neurosurg Psychiatry 2000;68:313–316.

Sobrido MJ, Abu-Khalil A, Weintraub S, et al: Possible association of the tau H1/H1 genotype with primary progressive aphasia. Neurology 2003;60:862–864.

Sohn YH, Jeong Y, Kim H, et al: The brain lesion responsible for parkinsonism after carbon monoxide poisoning. Arch Neurol 2000;57:1214–1218.

Soliveri P, Monza D, Paridi D, et al: Cognitive and magnetic resonance imaging aspects of corticobasal degeneration and progressive supranuclear palsy. Neurology 1999;53:502–507.

Soliveri P, Piacentini S, Girotti F: Limb apraxia in corticobasal degeneration and progressive supranuclear palsy. Neurology 2005;64: 448–453.

Soliveri P, Rossi G, Monza D, et al: A case of dementia parkinsonism resembling progressive supranuclear palsy due to mutation in the tau protein gene. Arch Neurol 2003;60:1454–1456.

Sonty SP, Mesulam MM, Thompson CK, et al: Primary progressive aphasia: PPA and the language network. Ann Neurol 2003;53: 35–49.

Spencer PS, Nunn PB, Hugon JS, et al: Guam amyotrophic lateral sclerosis-parkinsonism and dementia linked to a plant excitant neurotoxin. Science 1987;237:517–522.

Sperfeld AD, Collatz MB, Baier H, et al: FTDP-17: An early-onset phenotype with parkinsonism and epileptic seizures caused by a novel mutation. Ann Neurol 1999;46:708–715.

Spillantini MG, Crowther RA, Jakes R, et al: Filamentous alpha-synuclein inclusions link multiple system atrophy with Parkinson's disease and dementia with Lewy bodies. Neurosci Lett 1998;251:205–208.

Spillantini MG, Goedert M: Tau mutations in familial frontotemporal dementia. Brain 2000;123:857–859.

Stacy M, Jankovic J: Differential diagnosis of Parkinson's disease and the parkinsonism plus syndromes. Neurol Clin 1992;10:341–359.

Stanford PM, Halliday GM, Brooks WS, et al: Progressive supranuclear palsy pathology caused by a novel silent mutation in exon 10 of the tau gene. Expansion of the disease phenotype caused by tau gene mutations. Brain 2000;123:880–893.

Steele JC: Progressive supranuclear palsy. Brain 1972;95:693–704.

Steele JC, Caparros-Lefebvre D, Lees AJ, Sacks OW: Progressive supranuclear palsy and its relation to pacific foci of the parkinsonism-dementia complex and Guadeloupean parkinsonism. Parkinsonism Relat Disord 2002;9:39–54.

Steele JC, Richardson JC, Olszewski J: Progressive supranuclear palsy: A heterogeneous degeneration involving the brainstem, basal ganglia and cerebellum with vertical gaze and pseudobulbar palsy, nuchal dystonia and dementia. Arch Neurol 1964;10:333–359.

Steiger MJ, Pires M, Searavilli F, et al: Hemiballism and chorea in a patient with parkinsonism due to a multisystem degeneration. Mov Disord 1992;7:71–77.

Steinhoff BJ, Zerr I, Glatting M, et al: Diagnostic value of periodic complexes in Creutzfeldt-Jakob disease. Ann Neurol 2004;56:702–708.

Stern MB: Head trauma as a risk factor for Parkinson's disease. Mov Disord 1991;6:95–97.

Stern MB, Braffman BH, Skolnick BE, et al: Magnetic resonance imaging in Parkinson's disease and parkinsonian syndromes. Neurology 1989;39:1524–1526.

Stern Y, Albert M, Brandt J, et al: Utility of extrapyramidal signs and psychosis as predictors of cognitive and functional decline, nursing home admission, and death in Alzheimer's disease: Prospective analyses from the Predictors Study. Neurology 1994; 44:2300–2307.

Stevens M, van Duijn CM, Kamphorst W, et al: Familial aggregation in frontotemporal dementia. Neurology 1998;50:1541–1545.

Stocchi F, Badiali D, Vacca L, et al: Anorectal function in multiple system atrophy and Parkinson's disease. Mov Disord 2000;15:71–76.

Stocchi F, Carbone A, Inghiller M, et al: Urodynamic and neurophysiologic evaluation in Parkinson's disease and multiple system atrophy. J Neurol Neurosurg Psychiatry 1997;62:507–511.

Strafella A, Ashby P, Lang AE: Reflex myoclonus in cortical-basal ganglionic degeneration involves a transcortical pathway. Mov Disord 1997;12:360–369.

Suarez GA, Kelly JJ: The dropped head syndrome. Neurology 1992;42:1625–1627.

Suzuki M, Desmond TJ, Albin RL, Frey KA: Cholinergic vesicular transporters in progressive supranuclear palsy. Neurology 2002;58:1013–1018.

Swerdlow RH, Golbe LI, Parks JK, et al: Mitochondrial dysfunction in cybrid lines expressing mitochondrial genes from patients with progressive supranuclear palsy. J Neurochem 2000;75:1681–1684.

Tabaton M, Perry G, Autilio-Gambetti P, et al: Influence of neuronal location on antigenic properties of neurofibrillary tangles. Ann Neurol 1988;23:604–610.

Tagliati M, Perl DP, Drayer B, Olanow CW: Progressive dementia and gait disorder in a 78 year old woman. J Neurol Neurosurg Psychiatry 2000;68:526–531.

Takahashi M, Yamada T: Influenza A virus and Parkinson's disease. NeuroScience News 1999;2:93–102.

Tan EK, Chan LL, Yu GX, et al: Vascular parkinsonism in moyamoya: Microvascular biopsy and imaging correlates. Ann Neurol 2003;54:836–840.

Tang-Wai DF, Josephs KA, Boeve BF, et al: Pathologically confirmed corticobasal degeneration presenting with visuospatial dysfunction. Neurology 2003;61:1134–1135.

Tanigawa A, Komiyama A, Hasegawa O: Truncal muscle tonus in progressive supranuclear palsy. J Neurol Neurosurg Psychiatry 1998; 64:190–196.

Taylor TD, Litt M, Kramer P, et al: Homozygosity mapping of Hallervorden-Spatz syndrome 20p12.3-p13. Nat Genet 1996;14: 479–481.

Tedeschi G, Litvan I, Bonavita S, et al: Proton magnetic resonance spectroscopic imaging in progressive supranuclear palsy, Parkinson's disease and corticobasal degeneration. Brain 1997;120:1541–1552.

Tetrud JW, Golbe LI, Forno LS, Farmer PM: Autopsy-proven progressive supranuclear palsy in two siblings. Neurology 1996;46: 931–934.

Thaisetthawatkul P, Boeve BF, Benarroch EE, et al: Autonomic dysfunction in dementia with Lewy bodies. Neurology 2004;62:1804–1809.

Thomaides T, Chaudhuri RK, Maule S, et al: Growth hormone response to clonidine in central and peripheral primary autonomic failure. Lancet 1992;340:263–266.

Thomaides T, Bleasdale-Barr K, Chaudhuri KR, et al: Cardiovascular and hormonal responses to liquid food challenge in idiopathic Parkinson's disease, multiple system atrophy, and pure autonomic failure. Neurology 1993;43:900–904.

Thomas GR, Forbes JR, Roberts EA, et al. The Wilson disease gene: Spectrum of mutations and their consequences. Nat Genet 1995;9:210–217.

Thomas M, Jankovic J: Parkinson-plus syndromes. In Noseworthy J (ed): Neurological Therapeutics: Principles and Practice. London, Martin Dunitz, 2003, pp 2483–2504.

Thompson PD, Day BL, Rothwell JC, et al: The myoclonus in corticobasal degeneration: Evidence for two forms of cortical reflex myoclonus. Brain 1994;117:1197–1208.

Thyagarajan D, Bressman S, Bruno C, et al: A novel mitochondrial 12SrRNA point mutation in parkinsonism, deafness, and neuropathy. Ann Neurol 2000;48:730–736.

Tison F, Arne P, Sourgen C, et al: The value of external anal sphincter electromyography for diagnosis of multiple system atrophy. Mov Disord 2000;15:1148–1157.

Tolnay M, Sergeant N, Ghestem A, et al: Argyrophilic grain disease and Alzheimer's disease are distinguished by their different distribution of tau protein isoforms. Acta Neuropathol 2002;104: 425–434.

Tomokane NT, Kitamoto T, Tateishi J, Sato Y: Immunohistochemical quantification of substance P in spinal dorsal horns of patients with multiple system atrophy. J Neurol Neurosurg Psychiatry 1991;54:535–541.

Tong J, Fitzmaurice PS, Ang LC, et al: Brain dopamine-stimulated adenylyl cyclase activity in Parkinson's disease, multiple system atrophy, and progressive supranuclear palsy. Ann Neurol 2004; 55:125–129.

Truong DD, Harding AE, Scaravilli F, et al: Movement disorders in mitochondrial myopathies. Mov Disord 1990;5:109–117.

Tschampa HJ, Murtz P, Flacke S, et al: Thalamic involvement in sporadic Creutzfeldt-Jakob disease: A diffusion-weighted MR imaging study. AJNR Am J Neuroradiol 2003;24:908–915.

Tsuang DW, Dalan AM, Eugenio CJ, et al: Familial dementia with Lewy bodies: A clinical and neuropathological study of 2 families. Arch Neurol 2002;59:1622–1630.

Tsuboi Y, Ahlskog JE, Apaydin H, et al: Lewy bodies are not increased in progressive supranuclear palsy compared with normal controls. Neurology 2001;57:1675–1678.

Tsuboi Y, Baker M, Hutton ML, et al: Clinical and genetic studies of families with the tau N279K mutation (FTDP-17). Neurology 2002;59:1791–1793.

Tsuboi Y, Josephs KA, Cookson N, Dickson DW: APOE E4 is a determinant for Alzheimer type pathology in progressive supranuclear palsy. Neurology 2003a;60:240–245.

Tsuboi Y, Slowinski J, Josephs KA, et al: Atrophy of superior cerebellar peduncle in progressive supranuclear palsy. Neurology 2003b;60:1766–1769.

Tsuboi Y, Wszolek ZK, Kusuhara T, et al: Japanese family with parkinsonism, depression, weight loss, and central hypoventilation. Neurology 2002;58:1025–1030.

Tsuda T, Onodera H, Okabe S, et al: Impaired chemosensitivity to hypoxia is a marker of multiple system atrophy. Ann Neurol 2002;52:367–371.

Tu P-H, Galvin JE, Baba M, et al: Glial cytoplasmic inclusions in white matter oligodenrocytes of multiple system atrophy brain contain insoluble α-synuclein. Ann Neurol 1998;44:415–422.

Tuite PJ, Rogaeva EA, St. George-Hyslop PH, Lang AE: Dopa-responsive parkinsonism phenotype of Machado-Joseph disease: Confirmation of 14q CAG expansion. Ann Neurol 1995;38: 684–687.

Tullberg M, Mansson JE, Fredman P, et al: CSF sulfatide distinguishes between normal pressure hydrocephalus and subcortical arteriosclerotic encephalopathy. J Neurol Neurosurg Psychiatry 2000;69:74–81.

Tyrell PJ, Sawle GV, Ibanez V, et al: Clinical and positron emission tomographic studies in the "extrapyramidal syndrome" of dementia of the Alzheimer type. Arch Neurol 1990;47:1318–1323.

Uc EY, Wenger DA, Jankovic J: Niemann-Pick disease type C: Two cases and review of literature. Mov Disord 2000;15:1199–1203.

Umapathi T, Chaudry V, Cornblath D, et al: Head drop and camptocormia. J Neurol Neurosurg Psychiatry 2002;73:1–7.

Valls-Solé J, Tolosa E, Marti MJ, et al: Examination of motor output pathways in patients with corticobasal ganglionic degeneration using transcranial magnetic stimulation. Brain 2001;124:1131–1137.

Vanacore N, Bonifati V, Fabbrini G, et al: Smoking habits in multiple system atrophy and progressive supranuclear palsy. Neurology 2000;54:114–119.

Vanacore N, Bonifati V, Fabbrini G, et al: Case-control study of multiple system atrophy. Mov Disord 2005;20:158–163.

Vanek Z, Jankovic J: Dystonia in corticobasal degeneration. Mov Disord 2001;16:252–257.

Van Leeuwen RB, Perquin WVM: Striatonigral degeneration. Clin Neurol Neurosurg 1988;90:121–124.

Van Lieshout JJ, Harkel ADJ, Wieling W: Physical maneuvers for combating orthostatic dizziness in autonomic failure. Lancet 1992; 339:897–898.

Vanneste JA: Diagnosis and management of normal-pressure hydrocephalus. J Neurol 2000;247:5–14.

van Swieten JC, Stevens M, Rosso SM, et al: Phenotypic variation in hereditary frontotemporal dementia with tau mutations. Ann Neurol 1999;46:617–626.

van Zagten M, Lodder J, Kessels F: Gait disorder and parkinsonian signs in patients with stroke related to small deep infarcts and white matter lesions. Mov Disord 1998;13:89–95.

Verghese J, Crystal HA, Disckson DW, Lipton RB: Validity of clinical criteria for the diagnosis of dementia with Lewy bodies. Neurology 1999;53:1974–1982.

Verpillat P, Camuzat A, Hannequin D, et al: Association between the extended tau haplotype and frontotemporal dementia. Arch Neurol 2002;59:935–939.

Vidailhet M, Rivaud S, Gouider-Khouja N, et al: Eye movements in parkinsonian syndromes. Ann Neurol 1994;35:420–426.

Vincent A: Encephalitis lethargica: Part of a spectrum of post-streptococcal autoimmune diseases? Brain 2004;127:2–3.

Vodusek DB: Sphincter EMG and differential diagnosis of multiple system atrophy. Mov Disord 2001;16:600–607.

Wakabayashi K, Hayashi S, Kakita A, et al: Accumulation of alpha-synuclein/NACP is a cytopathological feature common to Lewy body disease and multiple system atrophy. Acta Neuropathol 1998;96:445–452.

Wakabayashi K, Takahashi H: Pathological heterogeneity in progressive supranuclear palsy and corticobasal degeneration. Neuropathology 2004;24:79–86.

Walker RH, Spiera H, Brin MF, Olanow CW: Parkinsonism associated with Sjögren's syndrome: Three cases and review of the literature. Mov Disord 1999;14:262–268.

Walter U, Niehaus L, Probst T, et al: Brain parenchyma sonography discriminates Parkinson's disease and atypical parkinsonian syndromes. Neurology 2003;60:74–77.

Wang T, Sharma SD, Fox N, et al: Description of simple test for CADASIL disease and determination of mutation frequencies in sporadic ischemic stroke and dementia patients. J Neurol Neurosurg Psychiatry 2000;69:652–654.

Warmuth-Metz M, Naumann M, Csoti I, Solymosi L: Measurement of the midbrain diameter on routine magnetic resonance imaging: A simple and accurate method of differentiating between Parkinson disease and progressive supranuclear palsy. Arch Neurol 2001;58:1076–1079.

Warner TT, Williams LD, Walker RWH, et al: A clinical and molecular genetic study of dentatorubropallidoluysian atrophy in four families. Ann Neurol 1995;37:452–459.

Warren JD, Mummery CJ, Al-Din AS, et al: Corticobasal degeneration syndrome with basal ganglia calcification: Fahr's disease as a corticobasal look-alike? Mov Disord 2002;17:563–567.

Watanabe H, Saito Y, Terao S, et al: Progression and prognosis in multiple system atrophy: An analysis of 230 Japanese patients. Brain 2002;125:1070–1083.

Weiner WJ, Minagar A, Shulman LM: Pramipexole in progressive supranuclear palsy. Neurology 1999;52:873–874.

Weller M: Anterior opercular cortex lesions cause dissociated lower cranial nerve palsies and anarthria but no aphasia: Foix-Chavany-Marie syndrome and "automatic voluntary dissociation" revisited. J Neurol 1993;240:199–208.

Wenning GK, Ben-Shlomo Y, Hughes A, et al: What clinical features are most useful to distinguish definite multiple system atrophy from Parkinson's disease. J Neurol Neurosurg Psychiatry 2000; 68:434–440.

Wenning GK, Ben-Shlomo Y, Magalhaes M, et al: Clinicopathological study of 35 cases of multiple system atrophy. J Neurol Neurosurg Psychiatry 1995;58:160–166.

Wenning GK, Colosimo C, Geser F, Poewe W: Multiple system atrophy. Lancet Neurol 2004;3:93–103.

Wenning GK, Litvan I, Jankovic J, et al: Natural history and survival of 14 patients with corticobasal degeneration confirmed at postmortem examination. J Neurol Neurosurg Psychiatry 1998;64: 184–189.

Wenning GK, Quinn N, Magalhaes M, et al: "Minimal change" multiple system atrophy. Mov Disord 1994;9:161–166.

Wenning GK, Scherfler C, Granata R, et al: Time course of symptomatic orthostatic hypotension and urinary incontinence in patients with postmortem confirmed parkinsonian syndromes: A clinicopathological study. J Neurol Neurosurg Psychiatry 1999;67: 620–623.

Wenning GK, Shlomo YB, Magalhaes M, et al: Clinical features and natural history of multiple system atrophy: An analysis of 100 cases. Brain 1994;117:835–845.

Wenning GK, Tison F, Elliot L, et al: Olivopontocerebellar pathology in multiple system atrophy. Mov Disord 1996;11:157–162.

Wenning GK, Tison F, Seppi K, et al: Development and validation of the Unified Multiple System Atrophy Rating Scale (UMSARS). Mov Disord 2004;19:1391–1402.

Wenning GK, Tison F, Shlomo BY, et al: Multiple system atrophy: A review of 203 pathologically proven cases. Mov Disord 1997;12: 133–147.

Wilhelmsen KC, Weeks DE, Nygaard TG, et al: Genetic mapping of "lubag" (X-linked dystonia-parkinsonism) in a Filipino kindred to the pericentromeric region of the X-chromosome. Ann Neurol 1991;29:124–131.

Will RG, Zeidler M, Stewart GE, et al: Diagnosis of new variant Creutzfeldt-Jakob disease. Ann Neurol 2000;47:575–582.

Williams DR, de Silva R, Paviour DC, et al: Characteristics of two distinct clinical phenotypes in pathologically proven progressive supranuclear palsy: Richardson's syndrome and PSP-parkinsonism. Brain 2005;128:1247–1258.

Williams DR, Watt HC, Lees AJ: Predictors of falls and fractures in bradykinetic rigid syndromes: A retrospective study. J Neurol Neurosurg Psychiatry 2006;77:468–473.

Wilson RS, Schneider JA, Bienias JL, et al: Parkinsonianlike signs and risk of incident Alzheimer disease in older persons. Arch Neurol 2003;60:539–544.

Winikates J, Jankovic J: Vascular progressive supranuclear palsy. J Neural Transm 1994;42(suppl):189–201.

Winikates J, Jankovic J: Clinical correlates of vascular parkinsonism. Arch Neurol 1999;56:98–102.

Wojcieszek J, Lang AE, Jankovic J, et al: Case 1, 1994: Rapidly progressive aphasia, apraxia, dementia, myoclonus, and parkinsonism. Mov Disord 1994;9:358–366.

Wolters EC, Jansen ENH, Tuynman-Qua, Bergmans S: Olanzapine in the treatment of dopaminomimetic psychosis in patients with Parkinson's disease. Neurology 1996;47:1085–1087.

Worrall BB, Rowland LP, Chin SS-M, Mastrianni JA: Amyotrophy in prion diseases. Arch Neurol 2000;57:33–38.

Wszolek ZK, Pfeiffer B, Fukgham JR, et al: Western Nebraska family (family D) with autosomal dominant parkinsonism. Neurology 1995;45:502–505.

Wüllner U, Weller M, Kornhuber J, et al: Altered expression of calcium- and apoptosis-regulating proteins in multiple system atrophy Purkinje cells. Mov Disord 2000;15:269–275.

Yamauchi H, Fukuyama H, Nagahama Y, et al: Atrophy of the corpus callosum, cortical hypometabolism, and cognitive impairment in corticobasal degeneration. Arch Neurol 1998;55:609–614.

Yasuda M, Takamatsu J, D'Souza I, et al: A novel mutation at position +12 in the intron following exon 10 of the tau gene in familial frontotemporal dementia (FTD-Kumamoto). Ann Neurol 2000; 47:422–429.

Yazawa I, Giasson BI, Sasaki R, et al: Mouse model of multiple system atrophy alpha-synuclein expression in oligodendrocytes causes glial and neuronal degeneration. Neuron 2005;45:847–859.

Yokoyama T, Kusunoki JI, Hasegawa K, et al: Distribution and dynamic process of neuronal cytoplasmic inclusion (NCI) in MSA: Correlation of the density of NCI and the degree of involvement of the pontine nuclei. Neuropathology 2001;21:145–154.

Young A: Progressive supranuclear palsy: Postmortem chemical analysis. Ann Neurol 1985;18:521–522.

Zanusso G, Ferrari S, Cardone F, et al: Detection of pathologic prion protein in the olfactory epithelium in sporadic Creutzfeldt-Jakob disease. N Engl J Med 2003;348:711–719.

Zee DS, Lasker AG: Antisaccades: Probing cognitive flexibility with eye movements. Neurology 2004;63:1554.

Zeidler M, Dorman PJ, Ferguson IT, Bateman DE: Parkinsonism associated with obstructive hydrocephalus due to idiopathic aqueductal stenosis. J Neurol Neurosurg Psychiatry 1998;657–659.

Zemaitaitis MO, Lee JM, Troncoso JC, Muma NA: Transglutaminase-induced cross-linking of tau proteins in progressive supranuclear palsy. J Neuropath Exp Neurology 2000;59:983–989.

Zerr I, Bodemer M, Otto M, et al: Diagnosis of Creutzfeldt-Jakob disease by two-dimensional gel electrophoresis of cerebrospinal fluid. Lancet 1996;348:846–849.

Zerr I, Bodemer M, Räcker S, et al: Cerebrospinal fluid concentration of neuron-specific enolase in diagnosis of Creutzfeldt-Jakob disease. Lancet 1995;345:1609–1610.

Zerr I, Pocchiari M, Collins S, et al: Analysis of EEG and CSF 14-3-3 proteins as aids to the diagnosis of Creuzfeldt-Jakob disease. Neurology 2000;55:811–815.

Zesiewicz TA, Helal M, Hauser RA: Sildenafil citrate (Viagra) for the treatment of erectile dysfunction in men with Parkinson's disease. Mov Disord 2000;15:305–308.

Zhang Z, Anderson DW, Lavine L, Mantel N: Patterns of acquiring parkinsonism-dementia complex of Guam. Arch Neurol 1990;47: 1019–1024.

Zhou L, Miller BL, McDaniel CH, et al: Frontotemporal dementia: Neuropil spheroids and presynaptic terminal degeneration. Ann Neurol 1998;44:99–109.

Zhou B, Westaway SK, Levinson B, et al: A novel pantothenate kinase gene (PANK2) is defective in Hallervorden-Spatz syndrome. Nat Genet 2001;28:345–349.

Zijlmans JC, Daniel SE, Hughes AJ, et al: Clinicopathological investigation of vascular parkinsonism, including clinical criteria for diagnosis. Mov Disord 2004a;19:630–640.

Zijlmans JC, Katzenschlager R, Daniel SE, Lees AJ: The L-dopa response in vascular parkinsonism. J Neurol Neurosurg Psychiatry 2004b;75:545–547.

Zweig RM, Whitehouse PJ, Casanova MF, et al: Loss of pedunculopontine neurons in progressive supranuclear palsy. Ann Neurol 1987;22:18–25.

## APPENDIX 10-1

### Patient Organizations

**Society for Progressive Supranuclear Palsy**
Executive Plaza III
11350 McCormick Road, Suite 906
Hunt Valley, Maryland 21031
Website: http://www.psp.org

*SDS/MSA Support Group Websites*

http://www.shy-drager.com/news.htm
http://www.msaweb.co.uk
http://groups.yahoo.com/group/shydrager
http://www.emedicine.com/neuro/topic671.htm

## Chapter 11

# Gait Disorders
## Pathophysiology and Clinical Syndromes

Gait is a fundamental skill. It permits movement from place to place, and as anthropologists are fond of pointing out, the fact that humans do it on two legs frees up the arms for other skilled tasks. The ability to walk is basic to quality of life. However, walking on two legs is a difficult motor task involving the ability to balance and execute a complex motor program at the same time. Many neurologic diseases, including many movement disorders, affect gait, and gait impairment becomes an important aspect of the disorder. Conversely, the nature of the gait disorder, of course, can be a clue to the diagnosis of the movement disorder. This chapter first briefly reviews the physiology of balance and gait and then considers the different gait disorders.

## BALANCE

It is important to distinguish between balance and stance. Stance is the posture of standing. It is normally upright on two legs with a distance between the feet approximately equal to pelvic width. An example of abnormal stance would be the stooped posture seen in Parkinson disease. Balance is the ability to maintain stance without falling or excessive lurching (Benvenuti, 2001). If balance is poor, people sometimes modify their stance. The most common manifestation is increasing the distance between the feet to widen the base of support (BOS).

From standard Newtonian physics, for an object to maintain its position, its center of mass (COM) must be over its BOS. In the case of a human standing, the COM is generally somewhere in the abdomen, and the BOS is the area between and including the feet. Since the BOS is relatively small and the COM is relatively high above the BOS, it does take considerable skill to maintain the BOS above the COM. Recently, it has been recognized that the ability to remain upright cannot be explained best by just the simple need to maintain the BOS above the COM. That is a static requirement, and the body or body parts are constantly moving. This movement must be taken into account. A dynamic model of balance includes consideration of the velocity of COM (Pai et al., 1998). The general principle is that the balance mechanisms of the body (such as the postural muscles) must be able to counteract any large velocities of the COM, even if the COM is currently over the BOS, since if they cannot, the COM will soon be beyond the BOS.

The body is constantly moving, and this movement is called sway. Each body part can have its own movement, but the important "summary" of these movements would be the movement of the COM for the reasons already described. Neurologists are used to doing a visual analysis of sway, but this is not very exact, of course. Instrumental methods have been developed. The position of the COM can be estimated, although this is generally somewhat difficult. The position of the different body parts can be determined with video methods, and if their individual masses are estimated, the COM can be calculated. This is generally done only in research laboratories. An alternative method, generally called posturography, comes from the ability to record forces that the body exerts on the floor with devices called force plates (Kaufman et al., 2001). The devices measure force in three directions—vertical, forward/backward, and side to side—and the two-dimensional center of action of the forward/backward and side-to-side force is called the center of pressure (COP). In the static situation, the COM is directly over the COP. Movements of the COM cause deviance of the matching of the COM and COP, but if the movements are small and slow, the deviance is not much. For this reason, sway is often measured with movements of the COP.

Generally, it is thought that more sway means less good balance. This is often, but not always, true. In some circumstances, because their balance is bad, patients stiffen up, voluntarily or involuntarily, and the sway might decrease. This might be true in Parkinson disease, for example (Panzer et al., 1990). When a patient is "off," balance is poor and patients are very stiff, often swaying little. When the patient is "on," balance is better, the patient is more relaxed, and sway might increase. Sway markedly increases with dyskinesias (characteristic of the on state and good balance). In most circumstances, however, increased sway does indeed indicate poor balance, and posturography can be employed to make this assessment quantitatively. A more sure way of assessing balance is to find out what happens with a perturbation to stance. If patients can remain upright, then balance is good; if they fall, balance is defective. This is the logic of the pull test.

The pull test is done by having the patient stand and having the investigator stand behind the patient and give a sudden pull backward. The patient is told to maintain balance. The top level of ability is to deal with the perturbation by body movements without moving the feet. A second-level ability is to maintain balance by taking a timely step backward. Failure, of course, is a fall, and that is the reason that the test is a pull rather than a push: The patient can fall into the examiner. Balance is virtually always better in the forward direction than the backward direction. With poor balance, patients tend to fall backward. All the reasons for this are not clear, but one reason is likely that when a person is standing, the COM is closer to the back of the foot than the front. In any event, because of this, the pull test is often done only in the backward direction.

Good balance depends on good motor control abilities but also good sensory feedback about what the exact body position and velocity are at any time. Feedback comes from vision, proprioception, and vestibular sensation. When one sensory modality is impaired, the others generally can compensate. When two modalities are impaired, there is more of a

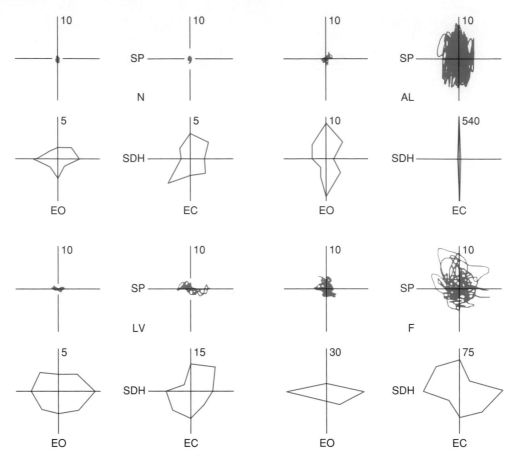

**Figure 11-1** Examples of posturography, the path of the COP while standing. In each part of the figure, SP is the sway path and SDH is the sway direction histogram. The upper left (*N*) is the normal pattern; the upper right (*AL*) is from a cerebellar patient with anterior lobe dysfunction; the lower left (*LV*) is from a cerebellar patient with lower vermis dysfunction; the lower right (*F*) is from a patient with Friedreich ataxia. (Reprinted with permission from Diener HC, Dichgans J, Bacher M, Gompf B: Quantification of postural sway in normals and patients with cerebellar diseases. Electroencephalogr Clin Neurophysiol 1984;57:134–142.)

problem. This is the source for the popular Romberg test. Sway is assessed when the eyes are closed. If there is a problem with proprioception, in the absence of vision, sway will be increased.

Abnormalities in posturography have been reported in many disorders. The best studies have examined cerebellar disturbances (Diener et al., 1984; Gatev et al., 1996); the findings are reviewed in detail in Chapter 2 and illustrated as an example here (Fig. 11-1).

## GAIT

Human gait is a complex, rhythmic, cyclic movement (Winter, 1991). The movements are generated to some extent by a locomotor generator in the spinal cord, but they are under control by supraspinal mechanisms. The spinal cord generator can produce only simple, primitive stepping and react to perturbations in stereotypic fashion (Burke, 2001). Supraspinal mechanisms are required for a person to go in desired directions, with desired velocities, and to deal well with perturbations. An important supraspinal control center is the mesencephalic locomotor region, which includes the pedunculopontine nucleus. The pedunculopontine nucleus is

an important integrator of activity from basal ganglia, cerebellum, and motor cortex and projects to reticular nuclei in the brainstem. The fastigial nucleus of the cerebellum also seems important (Mori et al., 2001). Supraspinal control signals are conveyed to the spinal cord by reticulospinal and vestibulospinal tracts.

A number of terms that are useful in describing gait are defined here:

Stance phase: When the foot is on the floor.

Swing phase: When the foot is in the air.

Stance time: The time that the foot is on the floor, measured as the time between heel strike and toe or heel off, whichever is last.

Swing time: The time that the foot is in the air, measured as the time between toe off and heel strike.

Cadence: The number of steps per minute.

Step length: The distance advanced by one foot compared to the position of the other.

Stride length: The sum of two consecutive step lengths or the distance advanced by one foot compared to its prior position.

Step time: The time between heel strike of one foot to the subsequent heel strike of the contralateral foot.

Gait cycle: One complete cycle of events, often considered the time between two consecutive heel strikes of the same foot. Hence, a gait cycle would begin at the beginning of stance phase of one foot, go through stance and swing, and end at the end of swing (which is the beginning of the next stance phase).

Stride time: The time for a full gait cycle.

Average gait velocity: The stride length divided by the stride time.

A gait cycle for the right leg is illustrated in Figure 11-2. Note that the gait cycle for the left leg is not exactly 180 degrees out of phase. For this reason, and because the stance phase is longer than the swing phase, there are several periods when both feet are on the ground; these are called double support. (In normal walking, there are no periods of simultaneous swing—that is, no "flying"—but this can occur with running.) With normal gait, when the foot contacts the ground, the heel contacts first, and then the foot rotates to flat, with the heel as the point of rotation. When the foot leaves the floor for swing, the foot rotates over the toe, and the heel leaves the ground first.

The joint angles of a normal gait cycle are illustrated in Figure 11-3. The ankle shows a brief plantar flexion at heel strike, followed by a gentle dorsiflexion in stance as the body moves over the foot. The ankle then shows a brisk plantar flexion, producing push-off lasting from heel off to toe off. During swing, there is a dorsiflexion of the ankle to avoid hitting the toe on the ground and to prepare for heel strike. The knee shows a slight flexion during stance and a more pronounced flexion during swing. The hip extends in stance and flexes during swing.

Muscle activities during gait are illustrated in Figure 11-4. During the gait cycle, the triceps surae (gastrocnemius-soleus) is active primarily at the end of stance to push off for the swing phase. The tibialis anterior muscle is active in the beginning of stance to slow the plantarflexion of the foot so that the foot does not slap onto the floor. This muscle is active again during swing to produce the dorsiflexion of the ankle mentioned previously.

## Gait Initiation

The initiation of gait is a special problem (Elble et al., 1994). Not only does it pose a unique biomechanical problem; it also causes some patients particular difficulty. The task is to get the body moving forward and to get the first foot off the ground into a "swing phase." In quiet standing, there is a very slight tonic activation of the triceps surae. This prevents the body from falling forward, since the COM is anterior to the ankle joints. The first event is a diminution of activity in the triceps surae muscles, more prominent on the side of the leg that will become the stance leg for the first step. This by itself would cause the body to start moving forward, rotating around the ankle. Then the tibialis anterior muscles contract, which actively rotates the body forward around the ankle. These events get the body moving.

The next set of events is like a ministep. The leg that will become the stance leg briefly flexes slightly at the knee and hip, just as it does in a swing phase. This helps to drive the COP toward the swing leg. Then the swing leg makes a large burst of electromyographic activity in the triceps surae, producing the push-off force for the swing phase. This force,

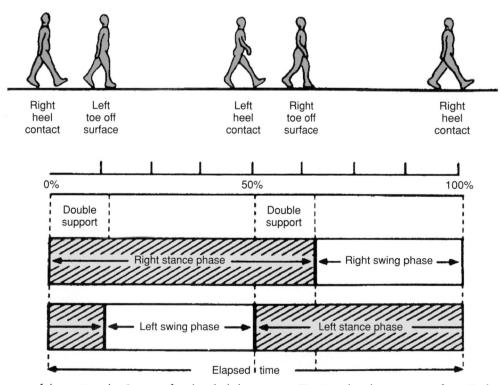

**Figure 11-2** Diagram of the gait cycle. See text for detailed description. (Reprinted with permission from Sudarsky L: Geriatrics: Gait disorders in the elderly. N Engl J Med 1990;322:1441–1446.)

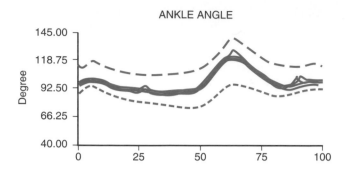

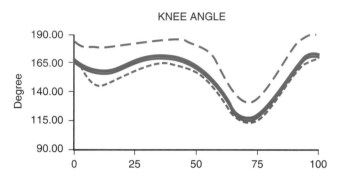

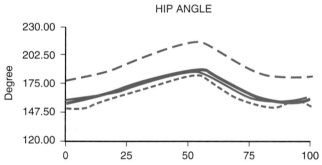

**Figure 11-3** Changes of the ankle, knee, and hip angles during a full gait cycle beginning with the start of stance phase. The solid lines are multiple trials from a single, normal subject showing the excellent reproducibility from cycle to cycle. The dashed lines are the normal limits from a group of 10 normal subjects. (Modified from Palliyath S, Hallett M, Thomas SL, Lebiedowska MK: Gait in patients with cerebellar ataxia. Mov Disord 1998;13:958–964.)

coupled with a slight abduction of the hip, drives the COP toward the stance leg, which it accepts as it serves a full stance function during the swing of the other leg.

## GAIT DISORDERS

### Epidemiology

Gait problems are a major neurologic problem, particularly in the elderly (Sudarsky, 2001). In the elderly population, the common causes for problems are stroke, peripheral neuropathy, brain or spinal cord trauma, and Parkinson disease. The term *senile gait* is sometimes used, but it likely does not exist as a

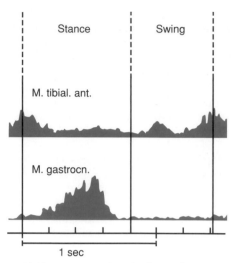

**Figure 11-4** EMG activity in the tibialis and gastrocnemius muscles during a full gait cycle. The figure shows rectified activity in a normal subject. (Modified from Conrad B, Meinck HM, Benecke R: Motor patterns in human gait: Adaptation to different modes of progression. In Bles W, Brandt T [eds]: Disorders of Posture and Gait. Amsterdam. Elsevier Science Publishers., 1986, pp 53–67.)

distinct entity. Multiple medical problems accumulate with age, including visual difficulties and arthritis, that become additive.

Sudarsky evaluated a series of patients who were referred for an unknown gait disorder (Sudarsky, 1997). After careful neurologic evaluation, he was able to make a diagnosis in most (Table 11-1). The most common entities were sensory deficits, myelopathy, multiple infarcts, parkinsonism, and unknown.

## Evaluation of Gait

Of course, the gait itself should be observed, but special attention should be paid to different aspects, such as the nature of the steps, including the stride length and cadence, deviations

**Table 11-1** Frequency of etiologies of neurologically referred undiagnosed gait disorders

| Etiology | Percent |
| --- | --- |
| Sensory deficits | 18.3% |
| Myelopathy | 16.7% |
| Multiple infarcts | 15.0% |
| Unknown | 14.2% |
| Parkinsonism | 11.7% |
| Cerebellar degeneration | 6.7% |
| Hydrocephalus | 6.7% |
| Psychogenic | 3.3% |
| Other | 7.5% |

"Other" etiologies included metabolic encephalopathy, antidepressant and sedative drugs, toxic disorders, brain tumor, and subdural hematoma.

Reprinted with permission from Sudarsky L: Clinical approaches to gait disorders of aging. In Masdeu J, Sudarsky L, Wolfson L (eds): Gait Disorders of Aging: Falls and Therapeutic Strategies. Philadelphia, Lippincott-Raven, 1997, pp 147–158.

from the direction of progression, the width of the feet from each other during periods of double support, the variability of the stepping, and the angular movements at the joints. Any stiffness of motion should be noted. Additionally, the ability to initiate stepping and the ability to turn should be noted. In looking for more subtle abnormalities, individuals can be asked to walk a straight line, heel to toe. In the case of dystonia, the patients might be asked to walk backward to determine whether this improves the performance. Balance should be assessed as well, with observation of quiet standing with eyes open and eyes closed and performance of the pull test. Of course, it is critical to evaluate patients for non-neurologic features such as arthritis, limitation of motion, pain (antalgic gait), and asymmetries of leg length.

A number of important observations have implications for the differential diagnosis (Nutt et al., 1993):

Weakness: Weakness should ordinarily be noted on general neurologic examination. Depending on the muscles that are affected, certain patterns will be identified, such as steppage and waddling, which are described further later. Weakness is commonly due to neuropathy or myopathy.

Dysmetria of stepping: Steps that are abnormal by virtue of being of the wrong length or direction and that are also highly variable. This is characteristic of ataxia and chorea. Ataxia looks mostly clumsy, while chorea often has a dancing quality.

Stiffness or rigidity: This is characterized by reduction of joint movement. It is seen with spasticity, parkinsonism, and dystonia.

Veering: Deviations from a direct line of progression are due to either vestibular or cerebellar disorders.

Freezing: Freezing is also known as motor blocks and is characterized by lack of movement, with the feet looking as though they are glued to the floor. Patients often look as though they are trying to move, but they cannot. This might be due to inability to generate sufficient postural shifting to initiate forward movement (Elble et al., 1996). Freezing can occur in trying to initiate gait, in which circumstance it has also been called start hesitation. Freezing can also interrupt walking, and in this circumstance, it is sometimes precipitated by a sensory stimulus such as a doorway, the ring of a doorbell, or a traffic light changing color. Curiously, sensory stimuli can also be used to improve freezing. They appear to act in this regard by providing external triggers for movement. In addition to the absence of movement, another form of freezing is characterized by rapid side-to-side shifting of weight but no lifting of the feet and no forward progression. This has been called slipping clutch syndrome. In this situation, physiologic studies show cocontraction activity in antagonist muscles, apparently not permitting effective forward movement (Yanagisawa et al., 2001). Freezing is very common in idiopathic Parkinson disease but is also seen in other parkinsonian states, such as progressive supranuclear palsy, vascular parkinsonism, and normal pressure hydrocephalus. It seems less common in multiple-system atrophy and drug-induced parkinsonism (Giladi, 2001).

Marche à petit pas: Walking with very short, often shuffling, steps. This is most typical of a multi-infarct state but can be seen with parkinsonism.

Festination: This is when short steps become progressively more rapid. This extension of marche à petit pas is also characteristic of parkinsonism. The stepping may even become much more rapid than normal. This can also be called a propulsive gait.

## Anatomic/Physiologic Classification

Gait disorders, like gait itself, are very complex. This chapter follows the classification of Nutt, Marsden, and Thompson, proposed in 1993, since that has been the most commonly used (Nutt et al., 1993). Some more recent refinements have been suggested (Jankovic et al., 2001; Nutt, 2001).

### LOWEST LEVEL

The lowest level refers to elemental disorders such as those resulting from muscle, nerve, or root disorders. This would also include the consequences of sensory deficits, such as peripheral neuropathy, vestibular disorder, or visual disorder. Severe sensory loss can produce a gait similar to that of cerebellar ataxia; these patients have particular difficulty walking in the dark. An example is the GALOP syndrome, characterized by gait "ataxia" and peripheral neuropathy associated with a monoclonal IgM specific for galopin, a central nervous system white matter antigen (Alpert, 2004).

One set of examples relates to disturbances generated by particular patterns of weakness. For example, the steppage gait is the result of a foot drop. The hip and knee have to be excessively flexed to bring the leg up high enough that the toes do not scrape the floor. Another example is the waddling gait, in which weakness of the hip abductors leads to dropping of the pelvis toward the swing leg and compensatory lean toward the stance leg.

### MIDDLE LEVEL

The middle level refers to central nervous system disorders arising from standard parts of the motor system.

#### Hemiparetic Gait

Owing to a unilateral lesion of the corticospinal tract, most commonly seen with stroke, there is a stiff extended leg that circumducts during swing with scraping of the toe (Video 11-1). Typically, of course, there should be some weakness in a pyramidal distribution and increased reflexes. The earliest sign might be reduced knee flexion during swing (Kerrigan et al., 2001).

Treatment of the spasticity might be useful, but this must be done carefully, since without spasticity, the leg might collapse and not provide support. Oral agents or intrathecal baclofen can be used. Botulinum toxin directed to the triceps surae has been used very successfully, particularly in the setting of cerebral palsy (Simpson, 1997; Flett et al., 1999).

#### Paraparetic Gait

Paraparetic gait is a bilateral hemiparetic gait and shows stiffness of both legs with scissoring (excessive hip adduction) (Video 11-2). Conditions in which this is prominent include spinal cord injury, hereditary spastic paraparesis, and primary lateral sclerosis.

### Stiff-Legged Gait

Stiff-legged gait includes the spastic syndromes of hemiparetic and paraparetic and also the disorder that is seen with the stiff-person syndrome (Video 11-3). There is particular stiffness of the spine with hyperlordosis, but all joints of the lower extremity will have reduced range of motion as well.

### Ataxic Gait

Patients with cerebellar ataxia have difficulty with motor control by virtue of dysmetria, dyssynergia, variability of performance, and poor balance. All these features contribute to their disorder of gait. Clinically, the gait is characterized by irregularity of stepping, in direction, distance, and timing. Patients may lurch in different directions. Stability of upright stance is poor, and patients may fall. Just as with standing balance, the base, or distance between the feet, is said to be broad (Video 11-4).

Palliyath and colleagues (1998) studied the gait pattern in 10 patients with cerebellar degenerations. Gait at natural speed was studied by using a video-based kinematic data acquisition system for measuring body movements. Patients showed a reduced step and stride length with a trend to reduced cadence. Heel off time, toe off time, and time of peak flexion of the knee in swing were all delayed. Range of rotation of ankle, knee, and hip were all reduced, but only ankle range of rotation reached significance. Multijoint coordination was impaired, as indicated by a relatively greater delay of plantar flexion of the ankle compared with flexion of the knee and a relatively late knee flexion compared with hip flexion at the onset of swing. The patients also showed increased variability of almost all measures. While some of the deviations from normal were due simply to the slowness of walking, the gait pattern of patients with cerebellar degeneration showed incoordination similar to that previously described for their multijoint limb motion. A wide base was not seen in this study, but it was seen in another study (Hudson and Krebs, 2000).

Patients with essential tremor have a mild gait abnormality that is ataxic in type (Stolze et al., 2001b). This forms part of the evidence that essential tremor results from cerebellar dysfunction.

### Parkinsonian Gait

Parkinson patients often have a stooped posture and stand and walk on a narrow base (Morris et al., 2001a, 2001b). Sometimes there is marked flexion of the trunk, called camptocormia, a condition also seen in dystonia and in psychogenic conditions (Azher and Jankovic, 2005). Balance is poor. Patients have short, shuffling steps (marche à petit pas) and this can be associated with festination. They turn en bloc, and important associated signs are lack of armswing and tremor of the hands. Freezing is common and can occur both in the "off" and "on "states. Freezing is seen in about a quarter of patients by 4 years after diagnosis (Rascol et al., 2000).

Gait speed in Parkinson disease is slow. If trying to walk faster, patients increase step rate proportionately more than stride length (compared with normals) (Morris et al., 1994, 1998). Electromyography studies have illuminated the pathophysiology (Albani et al., 2003).

Variability of stride length is a gait feature that has been associated with falls. Stride time and variability were studied in patients with Parkinson disease and compared with other clinical measures (Schaafsma et al., 2003). Variability was independent of tremor, rigidity, and bradykinesia but somewhat responsive to levodopa. Gait variability markedly increases with a simultaneous cognitive task, and this certainly would make patients more prone to falls (Hausdorff et al., 2003a). Patients with more freezing also have more variability, suggesting that this might be a factor in the etiology of freezing (Hausdorff et al., 2003b). Abnormalities of electromyographic pattern have been described (Nieuwboer et al., 2004).

Treatment of the parkinsonism with dopaminergic therapy or deep brain stimulation improves gait but often not as much as it improves other motor symptoms (Lubik et al., 2006). Parkinsonian gait can also be improved by rhythmic visual or auditory clues (Suteerawattananon et al., 2004). Physical therapy can help but might have only a short-term benefit (Ellis et al., 2005).

Freezing is generally difficult to treat, but "off" freezing might well improve with dopaminergic medication. "On" freezing is a particularly difficult problem and might even respond to lowering the dopaminergic medication. It was suggested that botulinum toxin might improve gait freezing (Giladi et al., 2001), but this has not been confirmed in a double-blind trial (Wieler et al., 2005).

### Dystonic Gait

An early common manifestation of dystonic gait is inversion of the foot with walking. The great toe can be flexed or extended. It is an action dystonia and would not be present at rest. As the dystonia worsens, there can be more abnormal posturing of the legs, trunk, and arms. Sometimes, there is so much abnormal movement that the gait looks like the dancing gait of chorea. The disorder is task specific, so walking backward might be much better than walking forward, and running can be spared (Video 11-5). Dystonic gaits can look very unusual, and care is needed to distinguish them from psychogenic. Camptocormia—flexion of the spine—is one such abnormal posture in which a principal differential diagnosis is psychogenic.

### Choreic Gait

Choreic gait is often called dancing gait and represents the superimposition of chorea on the locomotor movements. Stepping is also uncoordinated and appears dysmetric, like an ataxic gait (Video 11-6).

### Bouncing Gait (Myoclonus)

When myoclonus affects stance and gait, it gives rise to a characteristic bouncing (Video 11-7). The appearance is due more to frequent negative myoclonus than positive myoclonus.

### HIGHEST LEVEL

The highest-level disorders come from malfunction of the cerebral hemispheres and include disorders arising from psychiatric origin, including cautious gait and psychogenic gait. These disorders are not completely distinct from each other; patients may have characteristics of more than one or may progress from one to another (Jankovic et al., 2001; Nutt, 2001; Thompson, 2001).

## Subcortical Disequilibrium

Subcortical disequilibrium is a severe impairment of balance (Masdeu, 2001). The disorder arises from dysfunction at midbrain, basal ganglia, or thalamic levels and is often a feature of parkinsonism-plus disorders. It has been called thalamic astasia. This entity, by its etiology, is really misplaced and belongs in the middle-level category. Perhaps it really represents a combined basal ganglionic and cerebellar balance disorder.

The next three conditions—frontal disequilibrium, isolated gait ignition failure, and frontal gait disorder—are frequently difficult to separate from each other and might be considered varied presentations of a frontal lobe dysfunction of gait (Fig. 11-5).

## Frontal Disequilibrium

Frontal disequilibrium is also characterized by a loss of balance but is accompanied by disordered stepping that is difficult to describe. Some have called the stepping disorder apraxia (Gerstman and Schilder, 1926), and others have called it ataxia (Bruns, 1892). The concept of apraxia comes from the observation that leg movements that are not related to walking seem reasonably good. It is also associated with frontal lobe signs, and it is this feature that suggests the frontal origin.

## Isolated Gait Ignition Failure

Isolated gait ignition failure is a particular difficulty in initiating and sustaining locomotion. The patient experiences freezing, especially in getting started. The term *primary progressive freezing gait* has been used (Factor et al., 2002). Balance can be good, and while steps begin short, they gradually increase in amplitude. Thus, patients might say that they walk normally once they get started. This gradual increase differs from festination in that with festination, the stepping is never really normal looking.

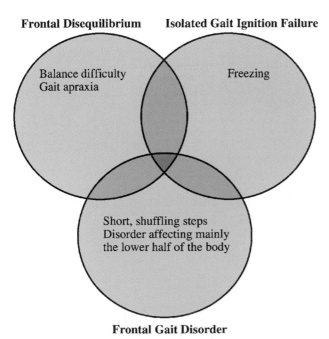

**Frontal Disequilibrium**　　　**Isolated Gait Ignition Failure**

Balance difficulty
Gait apraxia

Freezing

Short, shuffling steps
Disorder affecting mainly
the lower half of the body

**Frontal Gait Disorder**

Figure 11-5 Relationship of the three different types of higher-level gait disorders arising from frontal lobe dysfunction. See text for more detail.

## Frontal Gait Disorder

Patients with frontal gait disorder at first look as though they have a parkinsonian gait, with short, shuffling steps; poor balance; initiation failure; and hesitations on turns (Video 11-8).  Differentiating features are a more upright stance, lack of tremor, frontal lobe signs, and apparent involvement of only the lower part of the body (Thompson, 2001). This last feature gives rise to the term *lower half parkinsonism* or *lower body parkinsonism*. The disorder can evolve to a frontal disequilibrium with the difficult-to-describe stepping disorder. The disorder does not respond to levodopa.

As has been noted, frontal disequilibrium, isolated gait ignition failure, and frontal gait disorder often overlap. Their etiologies are also similar and include subcortical arteriosclerotic encephalopathy (Binswanger disease), multi-infarct state, anterior cerebral artery stroke, normal pressure hydrocephalus, Pick disease, Alzheimer disease, frontotemporal dementia, subdural hematoma, brain tumor, multiple sclerosis, progressive supranuclear palsy, and corticobasal degeneration (Thompson, 2001). The gait in normal pressure hydrocephalus has been the most studied. These patients have freezing and gait apraxia. Quantitative gait studies show decreased stride length and reduced foot floor clearance (Stolze et al., 2000, 2001a).

In the series of 30 patients reported by Factor and colleagues (2002) under the name *primary progressive freezing gait*, they found a clinically distinct progressive neurologic disorder that primarily affected gait, initially resulting in freezing and later in postural instability. A wheelchair-bound state often developed within 5 years. It was accompanied by other parkinsonian features, particularly bradykinesia, but was unresponsive to dopaminergic medications. Because of its stereotyped manner, they suggested that it be considered a specific entity within the parkinsonism-plus disorders.

Another classification of frontal gait disorders has been proposed: three main types based on presumptive sites of anatomic damage. These are (1) ignition apraxia, in which damage is predominantly in the supplementary motor area and its connections, with good responses to external clues; (2) equilibrium apraxia, in which damage is predominantly in the premotor area in its connections, with poor responses to external cues; and (3) mixed gait apraxia (Liston et al., 2003). The authors of this proposal studied 13 patients with cerebral multi-infarct states and higher-level gait disorder and diagnosed 7 with ignition apraxia and 6 with equilibrium apraxia.

## Cautious Gait

This is a common disorder, especially in the elderly or with patients who have already experienced a fall for some reason. The term *space phobia* has been used. Patients become cautious because of anxiety that they will fall. The gait is like what it would be for normal people who are walking on ice. There is a wide base with slow, short steps; turns are en bloc. Arms are tense. Patients try to find support, and when they have it, there is marked improvement. These individuals do not have overt freezing or shuffling.

## Psychogenic Gait

A gait disorder is a common way for psychogenic movement disorders to present (Lempert et al., 1991; Hayes et al., 1999; Bhatia, 2001; Morris et al., 2006) (Video 11-9). This is also called astasia-abasia or acrobatic gait. There are unusual patterns of stance and gait, often inconsistent, often dramatic, with lurching but only rarely falls (and then without patients hurting themselves). Sudden knee buckling without falling is a common pattern (Lempert et al., 1991). Extreme slow motion can be seen, and there is a sense that energy is being wasted. Camptocormia is one of the patterns that is commonly psychogenic. Careful observation will show that the person typically demonstrates excellent balance. There might well be wide fluctuations over short periods of time. As with other psychogenic movement disorders, positive psychiatric features are frequent and can be important in making a clear diagnosis. A possible clue to this is a suffering or strained facial expression, with accompanying moaning and hyperventilation (Lempert et al., 1991).

It was mentioned earlier but is worth noting again at this point that disorders of gait are often multifactorial, particularly in the elderly. It is useful to continue searching for etiologies even after one has been identified. This is certainly true of psychogenic gait, since many of these patients have organic neurologic disturbances.

## THERAPEUTIC CONSIDERATIONS

As with other aspects of movement disorders, etiologic considerations come first. Is there a treatable neuropathy? Can vision be improved? Parkinson disease can be treated, as can normal pressure hydrocephalus. The second consideration would be symptomatic treatments. Physical therapy can help with strengthening exercises or practice with elemental coordinations. There is a variety of walking aids, from canes to walkers. There are weighted walkers and rolling walkers that help in special circumstances. It is also critical to know when to suggest that the patient no longer should be trying to walk without assistance. Falls are potentially disastrous, with broken hips and subdural hematomas as possible consequences.

## Acknowledgment

This chapter is the work of the U.S. government and is not copyrighted.

## References

Albani G, Sandrini G, Kunig G, et al: Differences in the EMG pattern of leg muscle activation during locomotion in Parkinson's disease. Funct Neurol 2003;18:165–170.

Alpert JN: GALOP syndrome: Case report with 7-year follow-up. South Med J 2004;97:410–412.

Azher SN, Jankovic J: Camptocormia: Pathogenesis, classification, and response to therapy. Neurology 2005;65:355–359.

Benvenuti F: Physiology of human balance. Adv Neurol 2001;87:41–51.

Bhatia KP: Psychogenic gait disorders. Adv Neurol 2001;87:251–254.

Bruns L: Uber storugen des gleichgewichtes bei stirnhirntumoren. Dtsch Med Wochensch 1892;18:138–140.

Burke RE: The central pattern generator for locomotion in mammals. Adv Neurol 2001;87:11–24.

Conrad B, Meinck HM, Benecke R: Motor patterns in human gait: Adaptation to different modes of progression. In Bles W, Brandt T (eds): Disorders of Posture and Gait. Amsterdam, Elsevier, 1986, pp 53–67.

Diener HC, Dichgans J, Bacher M, Gompf B: Quantification of postural sway in normals and patients with cerebellar diseases. Electroencephalogr Clin Neurophysiol 1984;57:134–142.

Elble RJ, Cousins R, Leffler K, Hughes L: Gait initiation by patients with lower-half parkinsonism. Brain 1996;119(pt 5):1705–1716.

Elble RJ, Moody C, Leffler K, Sinha R: The initiation of normal walking. Mov Disord 1994;9:139–146.

Ellis T, de Goede CJ, Feldman RG, et al: Efficacy of a physical therapy program in patients with Parkinson's disease: A randomized controlled trial. Arch Phys Med Rehabil 2005;86:626–632.

Factor SA, Jennings DL, Molho ES, Marek KL: The natural history of the syndrome of primary progressive freezing gait. Arch Neurol 2002;59:1778–1783.

Flett PJ, Stern LM, Waddy H, et al: Botulinum toxin A versus fixed cast stretching for dynamic calf tightness in cerebral palsy. J Paediatr Child Health 1999;35:71–77.

Gatev P, Thomas S, Lou J-S, et al: Effects of diminished and conflicting sensory information on balance in patients with cerebellar deficits. Mov Disord 1996;11:654–664.

Gerstmann J, Schilder P: Uber eine besondere gangstorieng bei stirn-hirnerkankhungen. Wien Med Wschr 1926;76:97–107.

Giladi N: Freezing of gait: Clinical overview. Adv Neurol 2001;87:191–197.

Giladi N, Gurevich T, Shabtai H, et al: The effect of botulinum toxin injections to the calf muscles on freezing of gait in parkinsonism: A pilot study. J Neurol 2001;248:572–576.

Hausdorff JM, Balash J, Giladi N: Effects of cognitive challenge on gait variability in patients with Parkinson's disease. J Geriatr Psychiatry Neurol 2003a;16:53–58.

Hausdorff JM, Schaafsma JD, Balash Y, et al: Impaired regulation of stride variability in Parkinson's disease subjects with freezing of gait. Exp Brain Res 2003b;149:187–194.

Hayes MW, Graham S, Heldorf P, et al: A video review of the diagnosis of psychogenic gait: Appendix and commentary. Mov Disord 1999;14:914–921.

Hudson CC, Krebs DE: Frontal plane dynamic stability and coordination in subjects with cerebellar degeneration. Exp Brain Res 2000;132:103–113.

Jankovic J, Nutt JG, Sudarsky L: Classification, diagnosis, and etiology of gait disorders. Adv Neurol 2001;87:119–133.

Kaufman KR, Shaughnessy WJ, Noseworthy JH: Use of motion analysis for quantifying movement disorders. Adv Neurol 2001;87:71–81.

Kerrigan DC, Karvosky ME, Riley PO: Spastic paretic stiff-legged gait: Joint kinetics. Am J Phys Med Rehabil 2001;80:244–249.

Lempert T, Brandt T, Dieterich M, Huppert D: How to identify psychogenic disorders of stance and gait: A video study in 37 patients. J Neurol 1991;238:140–146.

Liston R, Mickelborough J, Bene J, Tallis R: A new classification of higher level gait disorders in patients with cerebral multi-infarct states. Age Ageing 2003;32:252–258.

Lubik S, Fogel W, Tronnier V, et al: Gait analysis in patients with advanced Parkinson disease: Different or additive effects on gait induced by levodopa and chronic STN stimulation. J Neural Transm 2006;113(2):163–173.

Masdeu JC: Central disequilibrium syndromes. Adv Neurol 2001;87:183–189.

Mori S, Matsuyama K, Mori F, Nakajima K: Supraspinal sites that induce locomotion in the vertebrate central nervous system. Adv Neurol 2001;87:25–40.

Morris JG, Mark de Moore G, Herberstein M: Psychogenic gait: An example of deceptive signaling. In Hallett M, Fahn S, Jankovic J, et al (eds): Psychogenic Movement Disorders: Neurology and Neuropsychiatry. Lippincott Williams & Wilkins, Philadelphia, 2006, pp 69–75.

Morris M, Iansek R, Matyas T, Summers J: Abnormalities in the stride length-cadence relation in parkinsonian gait. Mov Disord 1998;13:61–69.

Morris ME, Huxham F, McGinley J, et al: The biomechanics and motor control of gait in Parkinson disease. Clin Biomech (Bristol, Avon) 2001a;16:459–470.

Morris ME, Huxham FE, McGinley J, Iansek R: Gait disorders and gait rehabilitation in Parkinson's disease. Adv Neurol 2001b;87: 347–361.

Morris ME, Iansek R, Matyas TA, Summers JJ: Ability to modulate walking cadence remains intact in Parkinson's disease. J Neurol Neurosurg Psychiatry 1994;57:1532–1534.

Nieuwboer A, Dom R, De Weerdt W, et al: Electromyographic profiles of gait prior to onset of freezing episodes in patients with Parkinson's disease. Brain 2004;127:1650–1660.

Nutt JG: Classification of gait and balance disorders. Adv Neurol 2001;87:135–141.

Nutt JG, Marsden CD, Thompson PD: Human walking and higher-level gait disorders, particularly in the elderly. Neurology 1993;43: 268–279.

Pai YC, Rogers MW, Patton J, et al: Static versus dynamic predictions of protective stepping following waist-pull perturbations in young and older adults. J Biomech 1998;31:1111–1118.

Palliyath S, Hallett M, Thomas SL, Lebiedowska MK: Gait in patients with cerebellar ataxia. Mov Disord 1998;13:958–964.

Panzer VP, Zeffiro TA, Hallett M: Kinematics of standing posture associated with aging and Parkinson's disease. In Brandt T, Paulus W, Bles W, et al (eds): Disorders of Posture and Gait 1990. Stuttgart, Georg Thieme, 1990, pp 390–393.

Rascol O, Brooks DJ, Korczyn AD, et al: A five-year study of the incidence of dyskinesia in patients with early Parkinson's disease who were treated with ropinirole or levodopa: 056 Study Group. N Engl J Med 2000;342:1484–1491.

Schaafsma JD, Giladi N, Balash Y, et al: Gait dynamics in Parkinson's disease: Relationship to parkinsonian features, falls and response to levodopa. J Neurol Sci 2003;212:47–53.

Simpson DM: Clinical trials of botulinum toxin in the treatment of spasticity. Muscle Nerve Suppl 1997;6:S169–S175.

Stolze H, Kuhtz-Buschbeck JP, Drucke H, et al: Gait analysis in idiopathic normal pressure hydrocephalus: Which parameters respond to the CSF tap test? Clin Neurophysiol 2000;111:1678–1686.

Stolze H, Kuhtz-Buschbeck JP, Drucke H, et al: Comparative analysis of the gait disorder of normal pressure hydrocephalus and Parkinson's disease. J Neurol Neurosurg Psychiatry 2001a;70:289–297.

Stolze H, Petersen G, Raethjen J, et al: The gait disorder of advanced essential tremor. Brain 2001b;124:2278–2286.

Sudarsky L: Clinical approaches to gait disorders of aging. In Masdeu J, Sudarsky L, Wolfson L (eds): Gait Disorders of Aging: Falls and Therapeutic Strategies. Philadelphia, Lippincott-Raven, 1997, pp 147–158.

Sudarsky L: Gait disorders: Prevalence, morbidity, and etiology. Adv Neurol 2001;87:111–117.

Suteerawattananon M, Morris GS, Etnyre BR, et al: Effects of visual and auditory cues on gait in individuals with Parkinson's disease. J Neurol Sci 2004;219:63–69.

Thompson PD: Gait disorders accompanying diseases of the frontal lobes. Adv Neurol 2001;87:235–241.

Wieler M, Camicioli R, Jones CA, et al: Botulinum toxin injections do not improve freezing of gait in Parkinson disease. Neurology 2005;65:626–628.

Winter DA: The Biomechanics and Motor Control of Human Gait: Normal, Elderly and Pathological. Waterloo, United Kingdom, University of Waterloo Press, 1991.

Yanagisawa N, Hayashi R, Mitoma H: Pathophysiology of frozen gait in parkinsonism. Adv Neurol 2001;87:199–207.

# Chapter 12

# Stiffness Syndromes

Muscle stiffness may be the presenting symptom in many disorders of the motor nervous system and muscles (Box 12-1) (Rowland, 1985; Thompson, 1993, 1994; Brown and Marsden, 1999). Spasticity is the most classic, and the others must be distinguished from it. In this chapter, therefore, spasticity is considered first. Stiff-person syndrome, along with its variants, is perhaps the major entity confronting the movement disorder specialist, and it is considered next. Stiffness can arise not only from dysfunction of the central nervous system but also from disorders in which there is continuous muscle activity in which the pathology lies in the muscle, nerve, or anterior horn cell. These conditions are considered last.

Stiffness is assessed by the amount of force needed to get a movement. *Tone*, the more general clinical term, can be defined as the resistance to passive stretch of a joint. Normal tone is very low, and it is difficult to appreciate a decrease in tone, but some authorities say that they can detect a hypotonia in cerebellar dysfunction. Increased tone—hypertonia—is characteristic of several different states. Increased tone can come from three theoretical mechanisms: (1) altered mechanical properties of the muscle or joint, (2) background cocontraction of muscles acting on the joint, or (3) an increase in reflex response to the stretch opposing the movement (Hallett, 1999, 2000). A clear example of altered mechanical properties is contracture. Increased background contraction is often seen with difficulty in relaxation, such as commonly characterizes Parkinson disease. There are many different reflexes that can occur in response to stretch, and these can help to differentiate different states of hypertonia. In differentiating spasticity and rigidity, in simple terms, spasticity shows exaggerated short latency reflexes, and rigidity shows exaggerated long latency reflexes.

## SPASTICITY

Spasticity is a form of hypertonia with a number of characteristic features (Benecke et al., 2002; Sheean, 2002). The increased resistance to stretch is velocity sensitive; the faster the joint is moved, the more resistance there is. There may be a clasped-knife phenomenon in which the resistance increases and then suddenly gives way. There are also a number of other "positive" features, such as increased tendon jerks, clonus, increased flexor reflexes, spontaneous flexor spasms, and abnormal postures (spastic dystonia). Importantly, there are also "negative" features, including weakness (in a "pyramidal distribution"), fatigue, loss of coordination, and a decrease of some cutaneous reflexes. It can be noted that the increased stiffness can be valuable to a patient with significant weakness, as it might, for example, allow the patient to stand.

Loosely, neurologists usually say that spasticity arises from a lesion in the pyramidal tract or that it is from damage to the "upper motor neuron." The first seems false, and the second is vague. Supraspinal control of movement is complicated and consists of many tracts. Briefly, the fibers that go through the pyramid arise from the cortex and go to the spinal cord and can also be called the corticospinal tract (Wiesendanger, 1984; Davidoff, 1990). Approximately 30% of those fibers arise from the primary motor cortex; there are also significant contributions from the premotor cortex and sensory cortex. The fibers largely cross in the pyramid, but some remain uncrossed. Some terminate as monosynaptic projections onto alpha-motoneurons, and others terminate on interneurons, including those in the dorsal horn. Other cortical neurons project to basal ganglia, cerebellum, and brainstem, and these structures can also originate spinal projections. Particularly important is the reticular formation that originates several tracts with different functions (Nathan et al., 1996). The dorsal reticulospinal tract may have particular relevance for spasticity and is normally inhibitory onto the spinal cord (Takakusaki et al., 2001). In thinking about the cortical innervation of the reticular formation, it is possible to speak of a corticoreticulospinal tract. Lesions of the primary motor area alone and lesions of the pyramid alone do not cause spasticity (Sherman et al., 2000). It appears that premotor damage is necessary, and there is likely involvement of corticoreticulospinal pathways. Dysfunction of the dorsal reticulospinal tract will disinhibit the spinal cord and might give rise to the hyperexcitability that is characteristic of spasticity. The term *corticofugal syndrome* has been suggested to indicate that "spasticity" has important negative as well as positive features and that the lesions involve descending tracts other than the corticospinal tracts, but the term does not seem to have been commonly accepted (Thilmann, 1993).

The clinical and physiologic features of spasticity differ to some degree, depending on whether the lesion is cortical or spinal. Spasticity seen in hemiparesis differs from that seen with spinal cord lesions. For example, exaggeration of flexor reflexes is much more likely with spinal lesions. This certainly must come from the difference of the exact pattern of damage to the descending tracts.

The neurologic syndromes in which spasticity can be seen are numerous. These include stroke, spinal cord injury, brain trauma, cerebral palsy, and demyelinating illnesses such as multiple sclerosis. Spasticity can also be a part of degenerative disorders such as amyotrophic lateral sclerosis. In primary lateral sclerosis or hereditary spastic paraplegia, spasticity is the primary feature. A variety of degenerative movement disorders such as the ataxias often include some spasticity.

Clinical features of spasticity that help with the diagnosis, in addition to the velocity-dependent increased tone, include brisk tendon reflexes, the Babinski sign, Hoffman reflex (indicating brisk finger flexor reflexes), and loss of cutaneous abdominal reflexes. The negative features will often be seen as well, with weakness in the lower extremities of flexors more

Box 12-1 Causes of muscle stiffness, cramps, spasms, rigidity, or contracture

**Cerebral: Brainstem**
Encephalitis lethargica
Torsion dystonia
Akinetic-rigid syndromes

**Spinal Cord**
Stiff-person syndrome (also supraspinal abnormalities)
Toxins
    Tetanus
    Strychnine poisoning
    Black widow spider bite
Inflammatory myelitis
    Progressive encephalomyelitis with rigidity
    Subacute myoclonic spinal neuronitis
    *Borrelia burgdorferi* infection
Traumatic myelopathy
Spinal cord neoplasm (intrinsic)
Ischemic myelopathy
Spinal arteriovenous malformation
Cervical spondylotic myelopathy

**Peripheral Nerve**
Neuromyotonia (myokymia with impaired muscle relaxation)
    Idiopathic
    Isaacs syndrome
    Paraneoplastic syndrome
    Hereditary motor and sensory neuropathies
    Inflammatory neuropathies
    Toxic neuropathies
    Radiation plexopathies
    Paroxysmal ataxia and myokymia
Morvan syndrome (Morvan's fibrillary chorea)
Episodic ataxia type 1
Hereditary distal muscle cramps without neuropathy
Tetany (hypocalcemia, hypomagnesemia)
Cramps
    Postexertion

Dehydration/salt depletion
Pregnancy
Denervation (motor neuron disease, motor neuropathies)
Cause unknown

**Muscle**
Myotonic syndromes
    Myotonic dystrophy
    Myotonia congenita
    Paramyotonia congenita
Metabolic myopathies
    Myophosphorylase deficiency (McArdle disease)
    Phosphofructokinase deficiency
    $Ca^{2+}$ ATPase deficiency (Brody disease)
Inflammatory myopathies
    Polymyositis
Endocrine myopathies
    Hypothyroidism
    Addison disease
Congenital myopathies
    Stiff-spine syndrome
    Emery-Dreifuss muscular dystrophy
    Bethlem muscular dystrophy
Schwartz-Jampel syndrome
Other conditions presumed to be muscular in origin:
    Rippling muscle disease
    Rolling muscle disease

**Unknown Origin**
Satoyoshi syndrome

**Contracture**
Bone (ankylosis)
    Arthritis
    Ankylosing spondylitis
Soft tissue
    Volkmann ischemic contracture

than extensors and in the upper extremities of extensors more than flexors. In the clinical neurophysiology laboratory, there will be increased H reflexes, identified with an increase of the maximum amplitude H reflex compared to the M wave (muscle response to direct supramaximal stimulation of the nerve), called the H/M ratio (Hallett, 1999, 2000; Benecke et al., 2002). There is also a diminished decrease of the H reflex with vibration of the body part. Characteristics of the tonic stretch reflex can also be assessed for threshold and gain to stretches of varying velocity. In spasticity, there is some controversy, but both lowered velocity threshold and an increased gain have been found (Powers et al., 1988; Katz and Rymer, 1989; Thilmann et al., 1991; Ibrahim et al., 1993).

There are many methods for the treatment of spasticity, but this must be done carefully, as correction of the positive features might not be very helpful and, as was noted earlier, might even be detrimental. For many patients, the much more important aspects of their corticofugal syndrome are the negative features such as the weakness, and this cannot be dealt with easily. Increased tone can be improved with a variety of oral agents, including benzodiazepines, baclofen, and tizani-

dine (Krach, 2001; Abbruzzese, 2002). Baclofen can be given intrathecally by pump, and this can be much more efficacious, likely because of the ability to increase the dose at the target tissue without side effects (Ivanhoe et al., 2001; Albright et al., 2003). Tolperisone is a new drug for spasticity that has been evaluated in patients after stroke (Stamenova et al., 2005). Direct blockade of muscle contraction with agents such as phenol has been used for some time, and the introduction of botulinum toxin for this purpose has been welcomed with enthusiasm (Boyd and Hays, 2001; Moore, 2002; Barnes, 2003; Mancini et al., 2005). Surgical methods such as rhizotomy can also be used in some cases for symptomatic relief of severe spasticity (Lazorthes et al., 2002).

# STIFF-PERSON SYNDROME

Stiff-person syndrome (originally called stiff-man syndrome) (Box 12-2) consists of progressive fluctuating muscular rigidity (Moersch and Woltman, 1956; Blum and Jankovic, 1991; Thompson, 1993, 1994; Stayer and Meinck, 1998; Brown and

**Box 12-2** Criteria for the diagnosis of stiff-person syndrome

### Clinical
Gradual onset of aching and tightness of axial muscles
Slow progression; stiffness spreads from axial muscles to limbs (legs > arms)
Persistent contraction of thoracolumbar paraspinal and abdominal muscles
Abnormal hyperlordotic posture of lumbar spine
Board-like rigidity of abdominal muscles
Rigidity abolished by sleep
Stimulus-sensitive painful muscle spasms
No other abnormal neurologic signs
Intellect normal
Cranial muscles rarely (if ever) involved

### Neurophysiologic
Continuous motor unit activity at rest
EMG activity abolished by sleep, peripheral nerve block, or spinal or general anesthesia
Normal peripheral nerve conduction

### Normal Motor Unit Morphology
Disturbed exteroceptive reflexes and reciprocal inhibition
Exaggerated startle reflex

### Other Observations (of Uncertain Diagnostic Specificity)
Autoantibodies directed against GABAergic neurons, in particular glutamic acid decarboxylase
Increased CSF IgG and oligoclonal bands in some
Association with autoimmune endocrine disease (e.g., diabetes, pernicious anemia, vitiligo, hypothyroidism)
Epilepsy in 10%

Marsden, 1999; Levy et al., 1999; Thompson, 2001; Meinck and Thompson, 2002). Typically, the rigidity affects axial muscles of the back, abdomen, hips, and shoulders, causing excessive lordosis with prominent contraction of paraspinal muscles, a board-like abdomen, and stiffness of the legs on walking (Fig. 12-1) (Video 12-1; see also Video 1-32). Superimposed on this continuous stiffness are spasms provoked by excitement, anxiety, voluntary movement, sudden noise, or peripheral stimuli. These spasms can be intensely painful and forceful to the point of fracturing bones or dislocating joints. Voluntary movement can provoke similar spasms that can sometimes cause falls "like a wooden man."

The syndrome usually begins in the fourth and fifth decades and affects men and women equally. The onset of the illness is usually gradual, with increasing painful tightness, stiffness, clumsiness of the trunk and legs, and limitation of range of motion (Fig. 12-2). On examination, there is continuous muscular contraction of the paraspinal and abdominal muscles, but there are no other neurologic signs other than brisk reflexes. The illness is slowly progressive, with stiffness spreading from the trunk to the hip and then shoulder muscles, but the face and distal limbs are usually spared. Sphincter function is normal. While the onset of the disorder seems typically spontaneous, one case has been reported in which the onset appears to have been triggered by West Nile fever (Hassin-Baer et al., 2004). There has also been a report of a father and daughter, each with anti–glutamic acid decarboxylase (GAD)–positive stiff-person syndrome (Burns et al., 2003).

Electromyography shows continuous normal motor unit activity, despite attempted relaxation, with no signs of denervation and normal peripheral motor and sensory nerve conduction velocity. Other physiologic abnormalities include exaggerated, nonhabituating exteroceptive or cutaneomuscular reflexes, brainstem myoclonus, and an exaggerated startle

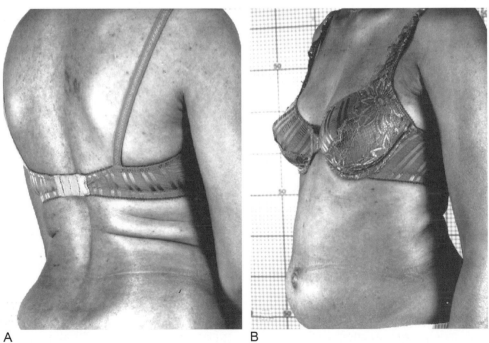

A B

**Figure 12-1** A patient with stiff-person syndrome. Note the marked lumbar lordosis (**A**) and the prominent abdomen (**B**). (Photos courtesy of Dr. M. Dalakas.)

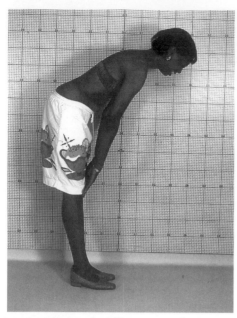

Figure 12-2 A patient with stiff-person syndrome attempting to bend forward. Note the limitation in bending forward. (See Color Plate 13.) (Photo courtesy of Dr. M. Dalakas.)

reflex ("jerking stiff-man") (Leigh et al., 1980; Meinck et al., 1983; Matsumoto et al., 1994; Meinck et al., 1995; Stayer and Meinck, 1998).

Insulin-dependent diabetes mellitus occurs in up to two thirds of patients. Diabetic ketoacidosis is the commonest cause of death in such patients. Other autoimmune endocrine diseases include thyroid disease, pernicious anemia, and vitiligo (Solimena et al., 1990). Epilepsy is said to occur in 10% of cases, although this is debatable.

A central origin for the spasms, rigidity, and continuous motor unit activity, perhaps in the spinal cord, is suggested by their disappearance after peripheral nerve block, sleep, and general anesthesia. Other neurophysiologic tests suggest that spinal motor neuron excitability is normal and that the condition is due to defective input of inhibitory pathways onto motoneurons. To test inhibitory spinal circuits in patients, Floeter and colleagues (1998) used H-reflexes to test reciprocal inhibition in the forearm and thigh, vibration-induced inhibition of flexor carpi radialis and soleus H-reflexes, recurrent inhibition, and nonreciprocal (1b) inhibition of soleus H-reflexes. Vibration-induced inhibition of H-reflexes was diminished in eight of nine patients tested, but the presynaptic period of reciprocal inhibition was normal in most patients. Both circuits are presumed to involve presynaptic inhibition and GABAergic interneurons. Presumed glycinergic circuits, including the first period of reciprocal inhibition and nonreciprocal (1b) inhibition, showed occasional abnormalities. Recurrent inhibition was normal in all five patients tested. It appears that some, but not all, populations of GABAergic neurons are affected. The involvement of presumptive glycinergic circuits in some patients could point to impairment of non-GABAergic neurons, unrecognized involvement of GABAergic neurons in these inhibitory circuits, or, more likely, alterations of supraspinal systems that exert descending control over spinal circuits. Studies of corti-

cal excitability with transcranial magnetic stimulation show decreased intracortical inhibition, likely due to loss of GABA-function at this level (Sandbrink et al., 2000). Direct measurement of GABA with magnetic resonance spectroscopy shows a deficiency in the sensorimotor cortex (Levy et al., 2005). Hyperexcitability of the brainstem has been demonstrated by increased R2 recovery in the blink reflex recovery curve (Molloy et al., 2002).

The significance of the association of insulin-dependent diabetes mellitus with stiff-person syndrome has been emphasized by the discovery of antibodies directed against GAD, the enzyme that is responsible for the synthesis of GABA, in both blood and cerebrospinal fluid (CSF) in 60% or more of patients (Solimena et al., 1990; Walikonis and Lennon, 1998). The great majority of these patients also have antibodies directed against pancreatic islet cells as well as gastric parietal cells and the thyroid. The anti-GAD antibodies are the same as those found in insulin-dependent diabetes mellitus, but it appears that the antibodies do have subtle differences (Lohmann et al., 2000). Currently, the best test is the radioimmunoassay for GAD65 (Walikonis and Lennon, 1998). Present evidence raises the possibility that the anti-GAD antibodies destroy GABAergic inhibitory mechanisms in the spinal cord (Raju et al., 2005), but alternatively, they might be secondary to some other process leading to an appropriate immunologic response. Anti-GAD antibodies have been demonstrated to block GABAergic neurotransmission in rat cerebellar slices (Ishida et al., 1999; Mitoma et al., 2000). One study reported that motor cortex excitability correlated with antibody levels, suggesting an etiologic role (Koerner et al., 2004). In a study of 18 patients with stiff-person syndrome and serum antibodies, all had high titers as well in the CSF, and 11 of 13 patients had an increased anti-GAD(65)-specific IgG index (Dalakas et al., 2001b). In the same study, the mean level of GABA in the CSF was found to be lower in patients than in controls. On the other hand, the levels of antibodies do not correlate with the severity of the disorder (Rakocevic et al., 2004).

Oligoclonal bands have been reported in the CSF in a number of cases (Meinck and Ricker, 1987; Williams et al., 1988; Meinck et al., 1994), and white matter lesions have been seen on brain magnetic resonance imaging. However, so far, no consistent pathology has been demonstrated in the few cases that have come to autopsy.

Stiff-person syndrome can also be seen in association with antiamphiphysin I antibodies in patients with breast cancer (Saiz et al., 1999; Wessig et al., 2003). Other neurologic disorders, such as sensory neuropathy, cerebellar ataxia and opsoclonus, may be present as well, and the syndrome can occur with other tumor types (Antoine et al., 1999). Another antibody in some cases is directed against 17-beta-hydroxysteroid dehydrogenase type 4 (Dinkel et al., 2002).

The treatment of this condition relies on a combination of benzodiazepines and baclofen in high dosage. These drugs may decrease the superimposed severe spasms but are not entirely effective in controlling the background sustained continuous muscle hyperactivity. Sodium valproate and tizanidine have also been reported to be of benefit (Meinck and Conrad, 1986; Stayer and Meinck, 1998). Intrathecal baclofen has been used (Silbert et al., 1995; Stayer et al., 1997; Stayer and Meinck, 1998). Occasionally patients have been reported to respond to steroid therapy (Blum and Jankovic, 1991), intravenous human immunoglobulin (IVIg) infusions (Khanlou and Eiger, 1999; Souza-Lima et al., 2000), and plasmaphoresis (Vicari et al., 1989; Blum and Jankovic, 1991; Brashear and Phillips, 1991; Hayashi et al., 1999), but others have gained no benefit from plasmaphoresis (Harding et al., 1989). A double-blind, placebo-controlled study documented the value of IVIg (Dalakas et al., 2001a). Another study has shown improvement in quality of life with IVIg (Gerschlager and Brown, 2002).

Progressive encephalomyelitis with rigidity, sometimes known as spinal interneuronitis, may present with clinical features similar to those of stiff-person syndrome. However, such patients go on to develop a relentless and progressive course, with the emergence of cranial nerve dysfunction producing bulbar symptoms and disorders of eye movement, along with cognitive impairment and long tract signs (Whiteley et al., 1976; Howell et al., 1979; Brown and Marsden, 1999; Gouider-Khouja et al., 2002). The condition may be isolated, or it may occur in the setting of neoplasia associated with the pathologic changes of paraneoplastic encephalomyelitis (Roobol et al., 1987; Bateman et al., 1990).

The condition can start at any age in adults. Initial symptoms may be those of pain, dysesthesia, or sensory loss in the limbs or weakness, stiffness, clumsiness, and rigidity. Extensor trunk spasm and/or brainstem myoclonus may be striking (Video 12-2; see also Video 1-31). The tendon reflexes often are absent, and the plantar responses are extensor. Nystagmus, opsoclonus, ophthalmoplegia, deafness, dysarthria, and dysphagia can occur. The illness usually leads to death within about 3 years. As in stiff-person syndrome, there is continuous motor unit activity, with particular involvement of trunk muscles, which disappears after a peripheral nerve or spinal nerve root block or general anesthesia. Electromyography (EMG) exploration can reveal evidence of denervation of muscles. A few patients have reticular reflex myoclonus. Some of these patients may also exhibit anti-GAD (Burn et al., 1991) or antineuronal (anti-Ri) antibodies (Casado et al., 1994). The CSF may contain a lymphocytic pleocytosis, elevated protein and immunoglobulin levels, and oligoclonal IgG bands. Magnetic resonance imaging may show brainstem atrophy and altered signal in the brainstem and spinal cord.

Pathologic examination has shown widespread encephalomyelitis with perivascular lymphocytic cuffing and infiltration, associated with neuronal loss throughout the brainstem and spinal cord, mainly involving interneurons.

As with stiff-person syndrome, treatment is with high doses of diazepam and baclofen. One case, with evidence of myelitis on spinal cord biopsy, improved on steroids (McCombe et al., 1989).

The relationship of progressive encephalomyelitis with rigidity to classic stiff-person syndrome, particularly in patients with anti-GAD antibodies, remains to be established (Brown and Marsden, 1999).

Spinal alpha rigidity is a related condition that results from isolation of spinal motor neurons from inhibitory interneuronal control (Gelfan and Tarlov, 1959). Examples have been described with trauma, cord vascular disease, cord tumors, and syringomyelia, as well as with myelitis. Most of these lesions have involved the cervical cord. Characteristically, there are stimulus-induced spasms, rigidity, and abnormal limb postures involving rigid adduction, extension, and internal rotation of the affected body parts. These postures are produced by continuous motor activity, which is not influenced by voluntary effort. In addition, there is wasting, weakness, and loss of tendon reflexes in the arms, with long tract signs in the legs.

A variant of stiff-person syndrome has been recognized, namely, "stiff leg" syndrome (Brown et al., 1997; Barker et al., 1998; Brown and Marsden, 1999; Fiol et al., 2001; Gurol et al., 2001; Bartsch et al., 2003). In contrast to classic stiff-person syndrome, in which continuous motor unit activity affects the back and thighs, patients with stiff-leg syndrome present with stiffness and painful spasms of one or both legs, which are rigid and dystonic. EMG findings are characteristic, with continuous motor unit activity at rest, spasms of repetitive grouped discharges, and abnormal cutaneomuscular reflexes. Anti-GAD antibodies are present in about 15% of cases. Whether this is a partial syndrome or a separate disorder is debated. The prognosis is generally relatively benign, with absence of other neurologic symptoms and signs for up to 16 years, but other cases can progress to the syndrome of progressive encephalomyelitis with rigidity (Gouider-Khouja et al., 2002).

Jerking stiff-man syndrome is another variant of stiff-person syndrome, with brainstem signs (Brown and Marsden, 1999). Brainstem myoclonus is characteristic; these may occur in paroxysms that compromise respiration. Again, anti-GAD antibodies may be present.

## SYNDROMES OF CONTINUOUS MUSCLE ACTIVITY

### Continuous Muscle Fiber Activity or Neuromyotonia

A variety of disorders of peripheral nerve origin may produce continuous muscle activity causing stiffness and cramps (Box 12-3). This condition has been described as continuous muscle fiber activity or Isaacs syndrome (Isaacs, 1961), neuromyotonia (Mertens and Zschocke, 1965), myokymia with impaired muscle relaxation (Gardner-Medwin and Walton, 1969), or pseudomyotonia and myokymia (Hughes and Matthews, 1969). This variable terminology reflects the overlap between the clinical and electromyographic use of terms such as *myokymia* (a wave-like rippling of muscle or motor unit discharges in doublets or triplets) and *neuromyotonia* (delayed muscle relaxation or high-frequency EMG discharges).

The characteristic and fairly stereotyped clinical picture of this condition is the gradual onset of muscle stiffness at rest, with continuous twitching (fasciculation) or rippling (myokymia) of muscles, with cramps following voluntary contractions due to delay in muscle relaxation (pseudomyotonia). Pain is rare, but muscle aching is common. The distribution of muscle contraction often is predominantly distal (in contrast to the axial involvement in stiff-person syndrome), producing a pseudo-tetany picture. However, proximal and cranial muscles can be affected. Involvement can be focal, as exemplified by one patient who presented with finger flexion that resembled focal hand dystonia (Jamora et al., 2006). The symptoms of muscle contraction, often accompanied by profuse sweating, persist during sleep and following peripheral nerve or spinal nerve root block or general anesthesia. The continuous muscle fiber activity is abolished by peripheral neuromuscular blockade with curare, indicating its origin at the neuromuscular junction.

**Box 12-3** Neuromyotonia

### Clinical

Gradual onset of muscle stiffness at rest
Continuous twitching (fasciculation) or rippling
  (myokymia)
Cramps and delayed relaxation (pseudomyotonia)
Mainly distal (carpopedal)
Sweating
Possible peripheral neuropathy
Treatment: carbamazepine, phenytoin, procainamide,
  plasmaphoresis

### Electromyography

Continuous motor unit activity
Persists in sleep and after nerve block
Fasciculations
Grouped high-frequency discharges
After discharges
Denervation changes
Nerve conduction studies abnormal

### Causes

Idiopathic (autoimmune, K+ channels of nerve membrane)
Paraneoplastic
Peripheral neuropathies
HMSN I and II
Inflammatory
Toxic
Radiation plexopathies

In many cases, there are clinical signs and electrophysiologic findings of a peripheral neuropathy. Muscles may be wasted and weak as well as exhibit rippling myokymia and fasciculations. Sometimes, there is muscular hypertrophy. Despite the pseudomyotonia, there is no percussion myotonia. The tendon reflexes are absent, and there may be appropriate sensory loss. The serum creatine phosphokinase is raised.

The condition can be inherited (Ashizawa et al., 1983; Auger et al., 1984) or sporadic (Isaacs, 1961; Gardner-Medwin and Walton, 1969), and it may occur as a result of a paraneoplastic process (Walsh, 1976; Lahrmann et al., 2001) or thymoma with acetylcholine receptor antibodies with or without myasthenia gravis (Halbach et al., 1987; Garcia-Merino et al., 1991) or be associated with many types of inherited (Vasilescu et al., 1984b; Hahn et al., 1991), inflammatory (Valenstein et al., 1978; Vasilescu et al., 1984a), or metabolic (Wallis et al., 1970; Vasilescu and Florescu, 1982) peripheral neuropathies. A case has been described in the setting of lupus (Taylor, 2005). A search for a remote neoplasm is required.

An autoimmune basis for neuromyotonia has been demonstrated in those with no obvious precipitating cause, on the basis of antibodies to specific nerve membrane voltage-gated potassium ion channels (Sinha et al., 1991; Shillito et al., 1995; Nagado et al., 1999; Hart, 2000; Hayat et al., 2000; Arimura et al., 2002; Vernino and Lennon, 2002; Lang and Vincent, 2003; Newsom-Davis et al., 2003).

Electrophysiologically, the hallmark of the syndrome is the presence of continuous motor unit activity that persists during sleep and usually following peripheral nerve block. This continuous muscle activity may originate in proximal nerve segments

(when distal nerve block suppresses activity), or distal segments (when nerve block has no effect). The motor unit activity often is increased by hyperventilation or ischemia. Fasciculations and grouped high-frequency discharges are evident on electromyography, with repetitive bursts of motor units of normal appearance (myokymia) (Fig. 12-3) and bizarre high-frequency (150 to 300 Hz) discharges (neuromyotonia) (Fig. 12-4). Prolonged high-frequency discharges following nerve stimulation, voluntary contraction, or muscle percussion are characteristic. Evidence of muscle denervation and reinnervation may be found, and measurement of peripheral nerve motor and sensory conduction may confirm the presence of peripheral neuropathy.

Carbamazepine and phenytoin can be successful in abolishing most of the symptoms of neuromyotonia and continuous muscle fiber activity. When the disorder is autoimmune, plasmapheresis may be effective (Hayat et al., 2000; Nakatsuji et al., 2000) as can IVIg (Alessi et al., 2000). Neuromyotonia without malignancy or peripheral neuropathy may prove to be relatively benign (Isaacs and Heffron, 1974; Wilton and Gardner-Medwin, 1990).

Morvan syndrome (Morvan's fibrillary chorea) is a disorder related to neuromyotonia (Kleopa et al., 2006). It is characterized by generalized myokymia, burning pain, cramping, weakness, pruritus, hyperhidrosis, weight loss, sleeplessness, and hallucinations (Madrid et al., 1996). Some cases are of unknown cause; others are associated with mercury intoxication, chrysotherapy, thymoma, and other remote neoplasms. In one case with thymoma, muscle histopathology disclosed chronic denervation and myopathic changes, and in vitro electrophysiology demonstrated both presynaptic and postsynaptic defects in neuromuscular transmission (Lee et al., 1998). Probably most cases are associated with increased antibodies to voltage-gated potassium channels (Liguori et al., 2001; Kleopa et al., 2006). Other serum antibodies, such as those to acetylcholine receptors, titin, and N-type calcium channels, can also be detected. Plasmapheresis (Liguori et al., 2001), thymectomy, and long-term immunosuppression may induce a dramatic resolution of symptoms.

Rippling muscle disease is an autosomal-dominant inherited disorder of skeletal muscle in which patients present with muscle cramps, pain, and stiffness, especially on exercise, and exhibit a characteristic lateral rolling movement of muscle after contraction and balling of muscle on percussion (Stephan et al., 1994; Vorgerd et al., 1999; Torbergsen, 2002). In one family with 11 affected members, muscle stiffness and myalgia were the most prominent symptoms (So et al., 2001). Muscle

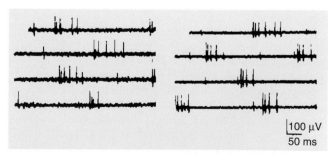

100 µV
50 ms

**Figure 12-3** Two examples of myokymic discharges as might be seen in patients with neuromyotonia. (Reprinted with permission from Kimura J: Electrodiagnosis in Diseases of Nerve and Muscle: Principles and Practice. Philadelphia, FA Davis, 1984.)

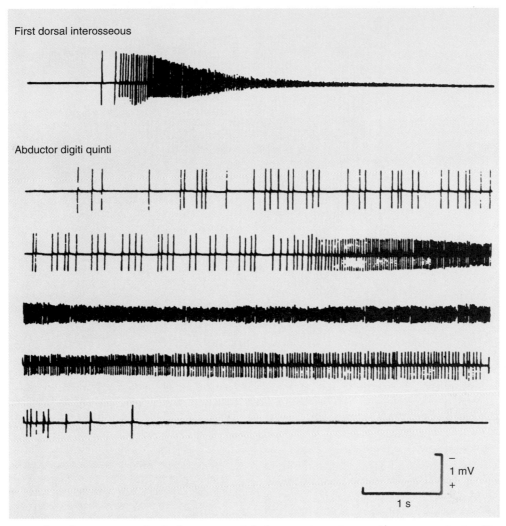

First dorsal interosseous

Abductor digiti quinti

1 mV

1 s

**Figure 12-4** Two examples of neuromyotonic discharges as might be seen in patients with neuromyotonia. (Reprinted with permission from the AAEM Glossary of Terms in Electromyography. Muscle Nerve 1987;10:G1–G60.)

rippling was present in only six affected family members, whereas persistent muscle contraction to muscle percussion was present in all affected adults. Curiously, EMG shows normal recruitment and motor unit potentials. One hypothesis is that the abnormal muscle contractions are evoked by "silent" action potentials traveling in the muscle's tubular system (Lamb, 2005). In a genetic study of five families, a genomewide linkage analysis identified a locus on chromosome 3p25 with missense mutations in *CAV3* (encoding caveolin 3) (Betz et al., 2001). Mutations in *CAV3* have also been described in limb-girdle muscular dystrophy type 1C (LGMD1C), again demonstrating that different phenotypes can come from mutations in the same gene (Sotgia et al., 2003; Woodman et al., 2004). A mutation in the same gene was found in a sporadic case of rippling muscle disease (Vorgerd et al., 2001). In two cases, this disorder preceded the development of myasthenia gravis and was improved with immunosuppression (Muller-Felber et al., 1999). Indeed, it does appear that rippling muscle disease can be immune-mediated without a mutation in the *CAV3* gene (Schulte-Mattler et al., 2005).

Myokymia is a feature of episodic ataxia type 1 (EA-1). In this disorder, the myokymia is prominent around the eyes or lips or in the fingers. See Chapters 22 and 23 for more details.

Schwartz-Jampel syndrome (chondrodystrophic myotonia) is a rare familial condition, usually occurring with an autosomal-recessive pattern of inheritance (Schwartz and Jampel, 1962; Taylor et al., 1972; Fowler et al., 1974; Fontaine et al., 1996) but occasionally as an autosomal-dominant trait (Pascuzzi et al., 1990; Spaans, 1991). The typical picture is of continuous muscle fiber activity and muscle stiffness, especially of the face, with an abnormal facial appearance (blepharophimosis, a small jaw and a puckered chin, and low-set ears), skeletal abnormalities (spondyloepiphyseal dysplasia) and short stature. Percussion myotonia may be present. The muscle stiffness is due to semi-continuous motor unit discharges, with high-frequency and after-discharges of muscle fibers (Fig. 12-5). These abnormalities persist after ischemia and curare (Spaans et al., 1990). An abnormality of muscle fiber sodium channels has been demonstrated (Lehmann-Horn et al., 1990). Procainamide abolishes such abnormal muscle activity (Lehmann-Horn et al., 1990). In a number of patients, a mutation in the gene for perlecan, the major proteoglycan of basement membranes, has been identified (Nicole et al., 2000; Arikawa-Hirasawa et al., 2002).

Satoyoshi syndrome (Satoyoshi, 1978) begins in childhood or adolescence with severe intermittent painful muscle spasms and twitches, twisting the body into abnormal postures. The

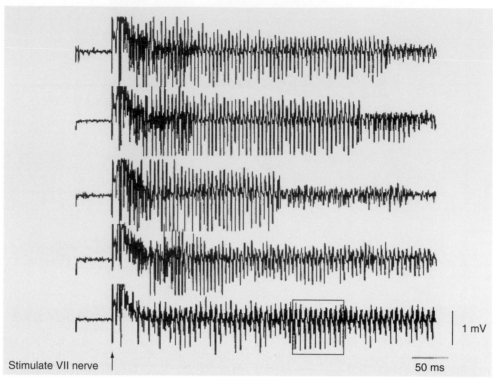

**Figure 12-5** An example of EMG discharge from a patient with Schwartz-Jampel syndrome. The discharge is triggered by stimulation of the seventh nerve. (Reprinted with permission from Thompson PD: Stiff people. In Marsden CD, Fahn S [eds]: Movement Disorders, vol 3. Oxford, UK, Butterworth-Heinemann, 1994, pp 373–405.)

spasms last up to a few minutes and occur frequently, up to hundreds of times per day. They are precipitated by movement or stimulation of the affected area. The cause is unknown. At the same time, complete alopecia and intestinal malabsorption with diarrhea develop. There also is metaphyseal dysplasia with growth retardation. It may also affect adults (Ikeda et al., 1998). One case had only unilateral manifestations (Uddin et al., 2002). Treatment with steroids can be effective (Wisuthsarewong et al., 2001; Endo et al., 2003), as can IVIg (Arita et al., 1996).

## Acknowledgment

This chapter is the work of the U.S. government and is not copyrighted. It has been extensively modified and updated from an original written by C. D. Marsden.

## References

Abbruzzese G: The medical management of spasticity. Eur J Neurol 2002;9(suppl 1):30–34, discussion 53–61.

Albright AL, Gilmartin R, Swift D, et al: Long-term intrathecal baclofen therapy for severe spasticity of cerebral origin. J Neurosurg 2003;98:291–295.

Alessi G, De Reuck J, De Bleecker J, Vancayzeele S: Successful immunoglobulin treatment in a patient with neuromyotonia. Clin Neurol Neurosurg 2000;102:173–175.

Antoine JC, Absi L, Honnorat J, et al: Antiamphiphysin antibodies are associated with various paraneoplastic neurological syndromes and tumors. Arch Neurol 1999;56:172–177.

Arikawa-Hirasawa E, Le AH, Nishino I, et al: Structural and functional mutations of the perlecan gene cause Schwartz-Jampel syndrome, with myotonic myopathy and chondrodysplasia. Am J Hum Genet 2002;70:1368–1375.

Arimura K, Sonoda Y, Watanabe O, et al: Isaacs' syndrome as a potassium channelopathy of the nerve. Muscle Nerve 2002;11(suppl):S55–S58.

Arita J, Hamano S, Nara T, Maekawa K: Intravenous gammaglobulin therapy of Satoyoshi syndrome. Brain Dev 1996;18:409–411.

Ashizawa T, Butler IJ, Harati Y, Roongta SM: A dominantly inherited syndrome with continuous motor neuron discharges. Ann Neurol 1983;13:285–290.

Auger RG, Daube JR, Gomez MR, Lambert EH: Hereditary form of sustained muscle activity of peripheral nerve origin causing generalized myokymia and muscle stiffness. Ann Neurol 1984;15:13–21.

Barker RA, Revesz T, Thom M, et al: Review of 23 patients affected by the stiff man syndrome: Clinical subdivision into stiff trunk (man) syndrome, stiff limb syndrome, and progressive encephalomyelitis with rigidity. J Neurol Neurosurg Psychiatry 1998;65:633–640.

Barnes M: Botulinum toxin: Mechanisms of action and clinical use in spasticity. J Rehabil Med 2003:56–59.

Bartsch T, Herzog J, Baron R, Deuschl G: The stiff limb syndrome: A new case and a literature review. J Neurol 2003;250:488–490.

Bateman DE, Weller RO, Kennedy P: Stiffman syndrome: A rare paraneoplastic disorder? J Neurol Neurosurg Psychiatry 1990;53:695–696.

Benecke R, Classen J, Dressler D: Tone and its disorders. In Brown WF, Bolton CF, Aminoff MJ (eds): Neuromuscular Function and Disease, vol 2. Philadelphia, WB Saunders, 2002, pp 1781–1801.

Betz RC, Schoser BG, Kasper D, et al: Mutations in CAV3 cause mechanical hyperirritability of skeletal muscle in rippling muscle disease. Nat Genet 2001;28:218–219.

Blum P, Jankovic J: Stiff-person syndrome: An autoimmune disease. Mov Disord 1991;6:12–20.

Boyd RN, Hays RM: Current evidence for the use of botulinum toxin type A in the management of children with cerebral palsy: A systematic review. Eur J Neurol 2001;8(suppl 5):1–20.

Brashear HR, Phillips LH, 2nd: Autoantibodies to GABAergic neurons and response to plasmapheresis in stiff-man syndrome. Neurology 1991;41:1588–1592.

Brown P, Marsden CD: The stiff man and stiff man plus syndromes. J Neurol 1999;246:648–652.

Brown P, Rothwell JC, Marsden CD: The stiff leg syndrome. J Neurol Neurosurg Psychiatry 1997;62:31–37.

Burn DJ, Ball J, Lees AJ, et al: A case of progressive encephalomyelitis with rigidity and positive antiglutamic acid decarboxylase antibodies [corrected]. J Neurol Neurosurg Psychiatry 1991;54:449–451.

Burns TM, Jones HR, Phillips LH 2nd, et al: Clinically disparate stiff-person syndrome with GAD65 autoantibody in a father and daughter. Neurology 2003;61:1291–1293.

Casado JL, Gil-Peralta A, Graus F, et al: Anti-Ri antibodies associated with opsoclonus and progressive encephalomyelitis with rigidity. Neurology 1994;44:1521–1522.

Dalakas MC, Fujii M, Li M, et al: High-dose intravenous immune globulin for stiff-person syndrome. N Engl J Med 2001a;345: 1870–1876.

Dalakas MC, Li M, Fujii M, Jacobowitz DM: Stiff person syndrome: Quantification, specificity, and intrathecal synthesis of GAD65 antibodies. Neurology 2001b;57:780–784.

Davidoff RA: The pyramidal tract. Neurology 1990;40:332–339.

Dinkel K, Rickert M, Moller G, et al: Stiff-man syndrome: Identification of 17 beta-hydroxysteroid dehydrogenase type 4 as a novel 80-kDa antineuronal antigen. J Neuroimmunol 2002;130: 184–193.

Endo K, Yamamoto T, Nakamura K, et al: Improvement of Satoyoshi syndrome with tacrolimus and corticosteroids. Neurology 2003; 60:2014–2015.

Fiol M, Cammarota A, Rivero A, et al: Focal stiff-person syndrome. Neurologia 2001;16:89–91.

Floeter MK, Valls-Sole J, Toro C, et al: Physiologic studies of spinal inhibitory circuits in patients with stiff-person syndrome. Neurology 1998;51:85–93.

Fontaine B, Nicole S, Topaloglu H, et al: Recessive Schwartz-Jampel syndrome (SJS): Confirmation of linkage to chromosome 1p, evidence of genetic homogeneity and reduction of the SJS locus to a 3-cM interval. Hum Genet 1996;98:380–385.

Fowler WM, Jr, Layzer RB, Taylor RG, et al: The Schwartz-Jampel syndrome: Its clinical, physiological and histological expressions. J Neurol Sci 1974;22:127–146.

Garcia-Merino A, Cabello A, Mora JS, Liano H: Continuous muscle fiber activity, peripheral neuropathy, and thymoma. Ann Neurol 1991;29:215–218.

Gardner-Medwin D, Walton JN: Myokymia with impaired muscular relaxation. Lancet 1969;1:127–130.

Gelfan S, Tarlov IM: Interneurons and rigidity of spinal origin. J Physiol (Lond) 1959;146:594–617.

Gerschlager W, Brown P: Effect of treatment with intravenous immunoglobulin on quality of life in patients with stiff-person syndrome. Mov Disord 2002;17:590–593.

Gouider-Khouja N, Mekaouar A, Larnaout A, et al: Progressive encephalomyelitis with rigidity presenting as a stiff-person syndrome. Parkinsonism Relat Disord 2002;8:285–288.

Gurol ME, Ertas M, Hanagasi HA, et al: Stiff leg syndrome: Case report. Mov Disord 2001;16:1189–1193.

Hahn AF, Parkes AW, Bolton CF, Stewart SA: Neuromyotonia in hereditary motor neuropathy. J Neurol Neurosurg Psychiatry 1991;54:230–235.

Halbach M, Homberg V, Freund HJ: Neuromuscular, autonomic and central cholinergic hyperactivity associated with thymoma and acetylcholine receptor-binding antibody. J Neurol 1987;234:433–436.

Hallett M: Electrophysiologic evaluation of movement disorders. In Aminoff MJ (ed): Electrodiagnosis in Clinical Neurology. New York, Churchill Livingstone, 1999, pp 365–380.

Hallett M: Electrodiagnosis in movement disorders. In Levin KH, Lüders HO (eds): Comprehensive Clinical Neurophysiology. Philadelphia, WB Saunders, 2000, pp 281–294.

Harding AE, Thompson PD, Kocen RS, et al: Plasma exchange and immunosuppression in the stiff man syndrome. Lancet 1989;2: 915.

Hart IK: Acquired neuromyotonia: A new autoantibody-mediated neuronal potassium channelopathy. Am J Med Sci 2000;319:209–216.

Hassin-Baer S, Kirson ED, Shulman L, et al: Stiff-person syndrome following West Nile fever. Arch Neurol 2004;61:938–941.

Hayashi A, Nakamagoe K, Ohkoshi N, et al: Double filtration plasma exchange and immunoadsorption therapy in a case of stiff-man syndrome with negative anti-GAD antibody. J Med 1999;30:321–327.

Hayat GR, Kulkantrakorn K, Campbell WW, Giuliani MJ: Neuromyotonia: Autoimmune pathogenesis and response to immune modulating therapy. J Neurol Sci 2000;181:38–43.

Howell DA, Lees AJ, Toghill PJ: Spinal internuncial neurones in progressive encephalomyelitis with rigidity. J Neurol Neurosurg Psychiatry 1979;42:773–785.

Hughes RC, Matthews WB: Pseudo-myotonia and myokymia. J Neurol Neurosurg Psychiatry 1969;32:11–14.

Ibrahim IK, Berger W, Trippel M, Dietz V: Stretch-induced electromyographic activity and torque in spastic elbow muscles: Differential modulation of reflex activity in passive and active motor tasks. Brain 1993;116(4):971–989.

Ikeda K, Satoyoshi E, Kinoshita M, et al: Satoyoshi's syndrome in an adult: A review of the literature of adult onset cases. Intern Med 1998;37:784–787.

Isaacs H: A syndrome of continuous muscle-fibre activity. J Neurol Neurosurg Psychiatry 1961;24:319–325.

Isaacs H, Heffron JJ: The syndrome of "continuous muscle-fibre activity" cured: Further studies. J Neurol Neurosurg Psychiatry 1974;37:1231–1235.

Ishida K, Mitoma H, Song SY, et al: Selective suppression of cerebellar GABAergic transmission by an autoantibody to glutamic acid decarboxylase. Ann Neurol 1999;46:263–267.

Ivanhoe CB, Tilton AH, Francisco GE: Intrathecal baclofen therapy for spastic hypertonia. Phys Med Rehabil Clin N Am 2001;12: 923–938, viii–ix.

Jamora RDG, Umapathi T, Tan LCS: Finger flexion resembling focal dystonia in Isaacs' syndrome. Parkinsonism Relat Disord 2006; 12:61–63.

Katz RT, Rymer WZ: Spastic hypertonia: Mechanisms and measurement. Arch Phys Med Rehabil 1989;70:144–155.

Khanlou H, Eiger G: Long-term remission of refractory stiff-man syndrome after treatment with intravenous immunoglobulin. Mayo Clin Proc 1999;74:1231–1232.

Kleopa KA, Elman LB, Lang B, et al: Neuromyotonia and limbic encephalitis sera target mature Shaker-type K+ channels: Subunit specificity correlates with clinical manifestations. Brain 2006:129: 1570–1584.

Koerner C, Wieland B, Richter W, Meinck HM: Stiff-person syndromes: Motor cortex hyperexcitability correlates with anti-GAD autoimmunity. Neurology 2004;62:1357–1362.

Krach LE: Pharmacotherapy of spasticity: Oral medications and intrathecal baclofen. J Child Neurol 2001;16:31–36.

Lahrmann H, Albrecht G, Drlicek M, et al: Acquired neuromyotonia and peripheral neuropathy in a patient with Hodgkin's disease. Muscle Nerve 2001;24:834–838.

Lamb GD: Rippling muscle disease may be caused by "silent" action potentials in the tubular system of skeletal muscle fibers. Muscle Nerve 2005;31:652–658.

Lang B, Vincent A: Autoantibodies to ion channels at the neuromuscular junction. Autoimmun Rev 2003;2:94–100.

Lazorthes Y, Sol JC, Sallerin B, Verdie JC: The surgical management of spasticity. Eur J Neurol 2002;9(suppl 1):35–41; discussion: 53–61.

Lee EK, Maselli RA, Ellis WG, Agius MA: Morvan's fibrillary chorea: A paraneoplastic manifestation of thymoma. J Neurol Neurosurg Psychiatry 1998;65:857–862.

Lehmann-Horn F, Iaizzo PA, Franke C, et al: Schwartz-Jampel syndrome: II. Na+ channel defect causes myotonia. Muscle Nerve 1990;13:528–535.

Leigh PN, Rothwell JC, Traub M, Marsden CD: A patient with reflex myoclonus and muscle rigidity: "jerking stiff-man syndrome." J Neurol Neurosurg Psychiatry 1980;43:1125–1131.

Levy LM, Dalakas MC, Floeter MK: The stiff-person syndrome: An autoimmune disorder affecting neurotransmission of gamma-aminobutyric acid. Ann Intern Med 1999;131:522–530.

Levy LM, Levy-Reis I, Fujii M, Dalakas MC: Brain gamma-aminobutyric acid changes in stiff-person syndrome. Arch Neurol 2005;62:970–974.

Liguori R, Vincent A, Clover L, et al: Morvan's syndrome: Peripheral and central nervous system and cardiac involvement with antibodies to voltage-gated potassium channels. Brain 2001;124: 2417–2426.

Lohmann T, Hawa M, Leslie RD, et al: Immune reactivity to glutamic acid decarboxylase 65 in stiffman syndrome and type 1 diabetes mellitus [see comments]. Lancet 2000;356:31–35.

Madrid A, Gil-Peralta A, Gil-Neciga E, et al: Morvan's fibrillary chorea: Remission after plasmapheresis. J Neurol 1996;243:350–353.

Mancini F, Sandrini G, Moglia A, et al: A randomised, double-blind, dose-ranging study to evaluate efficacy and safety of three doses of botulinum toxin type A (Botox) for the treatment of spastic foot. Neurol Sci 2005;26:26–31.

Matsumoto JY, Caviness JN, McEvoy KM: The acoustic startle reflex in stiff-man syndrome. Neurology 1994;44:1952–1955.

McCombe PA, Chalk JB, Searle JW, et al: Progressive encephalomyelitis with rigidity: A case report with magnetic resonance imaging findings. J Neurol Neurosurg Psychiatry 1989;52:1429–1431.

Meinck HM, Benecke R, Kuster S, Conrad B: Cutaneomuscular (flexor) reflex organization in normal man and in patients with motor disorders. Adv Neurol 1983;39:787–796.

Meinck HM, Conrad B: Neuropharmacological investigations in the stiff-man syndrome. J Neurol 1986;233:340–347.

Meinck HM, Ricker K: Long-standing "stiff-man" syndrome: A particular form of disseminated inflammatory CNS disease? J Neurol Neurosurg Psychiatry 1987;50:1556–1557.

Meinck HM, Ricker K, Hulser PJ, et al: Stiff man syndrome: Clinical and laboratory findings in eight patients. J Neurol 1994;241: 157–166.

Meinck HM, Ricker K, Hulser PJ, Solimena M: Stiff man syndrome: Neurophysiological findings in eight patients. J Neurol 1995;242: 134–142.

Meinck HM, Thompson PD: Stiff man syndrome and related conditions. Mov Disord 2002;17:853–866.

Mertens H-G, Zschocke S: Neuromyotonie. Klin Wochenschr 1965; 43:917–925.

Mitoma H, Song S, Ishida K, et al: Presynaptic impairment of cerebellar inhibitory synapses by an autoantibody to glutamate decarboxylase. J Neurol Sci 2000;175:40–44.

Moersch FP, Woltman HW: Progressive fluctuating muscular rigidity and spasm ("stiff-man" syndrome): Report of a case and some observations in 13 other cases. Mayo Clinic Proc 1956;31:421–427.

Molloy FM, Dalakas MC, Floeter MK: Increased brainstem excitability in stiff-person syndrome. Neurology 2002;59:449–451.

Moore AP: Botulinum toxin A (BoNT-A) for spasticity in adults: What is the evidence? Eur J Neurol 2002;9(suppl 1):42–47; discussion: 53–61.

Muller-Felber W, Ansevin CF, Ricker K, et al: Immunosuppressive treatment of rippling muscles in patients with myasthenia gravis. Neuromuscul Disord 1999;9:604–607.

Nagado T, Arimura K, Sonoda Y, et al: Potassium current suppression in patients with peripheral nerve hyperexcitability. Brain 1999;122:2057–2066.

Nakatsuji Y, Kaido M, Sugai F, et al: Isaacs' syndrome successfully treated by immunoadsorption plasmapheresis. Acta Neurol Scand 2000;102:271–273.

Nathan PW, Smith M, Deacon P: Vestibulospinal, reticulospinal and descending propriospinal nerve fibres in man. Brain 1996;119(6): 1809–1833.

Newsom-Davis J, Buckley C, Clover L, et al: Autoimmune disorders of neuronal potassium channels. Ann N Y Acad Sci 2003;998: 202–210.

Nicole S, Davoine CS, Topaloglu H, et al: Perlecan, the major proteoglycan of basement membranes, is altered in patients with Schwartz-Jampel syndrome (chondrodystrophic myotonia). Nat Genet 2000;26:480–483.

Pascuzzi RM, Gratianne R, Azzarelli B, Kincaid JC: Schwartz-Jampel syndrome with dominant inheritance. Muscle Nerve 1990;13: 1152–1163.

Powers RK, Marder-Meyer J, Rymer WZ: Quantitative relations between hypertonia and stretch reflex threshold in spastic hemiparesis. Ann Neurol 1988;23:115–124.

Raju R, Foote J, Banga JP: Analysis of GAD65 autoantibodies in stiff-person syndrome patients. J Immunol 2005;175:7755–7762.

Rakocevic G, Raju R, Dalakas MC: Anti-glutamic acid decarboxylase antibodies in the serum and cerebrospinal fluid of patients with stiff-person syndrome: Correlation with clinical severity. Arch Neurol 2004;61:902–904.

Roobol TH, Kazzaz BA, Vecht CJ: Segmental rigidity and spinal myoclonus as a paraneoplastic syndrome. J Neurol Neurosurg Psychiatry 1987;50:628–631.

Rowland LP: Cramps, spasms and muscle stiffness. Rev Neurol 1985; 141:261–273.

Saiz A, Dalmau J, Butler MH, et al: Anti-amphiphysin I antibodies in patients with paraneoplastic neurological disorders associated with small cell lung carcinoma. J Neurol Neurosurg Psychiatry 1999;66:214–217.

Sandbrink F, Syed NA, Fujii MD, et al: Motor cortex excitability in stiff-person syndrome. Brain 2000;123:2231–2239.

Satoyoshi E: A syndrome of progressive muscle spasm, alopecia, and diarrhea. Neurology 1978;28:458–471.

Schulte-Mattler WJ, Kley RA, Rothenfusser-Korber E, et al: Immune-mediated rippling muscle disease. Neurology 2005;64:364–367.

Schwartz O, Jampel RS: Congenital blepharophimosis associated with a unique generalized myopathy. Arch Ophthamol 1962;68:52–57.

Sheean G: The pathophysiology of spasticity. Eur J Neurol 2002;9(suppl 1):3–9; discussion: 53–61.

Sherman SJ, Koshland GF, Laguna JF: Hyper-reflexia without spasticity after unilateral infarct of the medullary pyramid. J Neurol Sci 2000;175:145–155.

Shillito P, Molenaar PC, Vincent A, et al: Acquired neuromyotonia: Evidence for autoantibodies directed against K+ channels of peripheral nerves. Ann Neurol 1995;38:714–722.

Silbert PL, Matsumoto JY, McManis PG, et al: Intrathecal baclofen therapy in stiff-man syndrome: A double-blind, placebo-controlled trial. Neurology 1995;45:1893–1897.

Sinha S, Newsom-Davis J, Mills K, et al: Autoimmune aetiology for acquired neuromyotonia (Isaacs' syndrome). Lancet 1991;338: 75–77.

So YT, Zu L, Barraza C, et al: Rippling muscle disease: Evidence for phenotypic and genetic heterogeneity. Muscle Nerve 2001;24: 340–344.

Solimena M, Folli F, Aparisi R, et al: Autoantibodies to GABA-ergic neurons and pancreatic beta cells in stiff-man syndrome. N Engl J Med 1990;322:1555–1560.

Sotgia F, Woodman SE, Bonuccelli G, et al: Phenotypic behavior of caveolin-3 (R26Q), a mutant associated with hyperCKemia, distal myopathy, and rippling muscle disease. Am J Physiol Cell Physiol 2003;285:C1150–C1160.

Souza-Lima CF, Ferraz HB, Braz CA, et al: Marked improvement in a stiff-limb patient treated with intravenous immunoglobulin. Mov Disord 2000;15:358–359.

Spaans F: Schwartz-Jampel syndrome with dominant inheritance. Muscle Nerve 1991;14:1142–1144.

Spaans F, Theunissen P, Reekers AD, et al: Schwartz-Jampel syndrome: I. Clinical, electromyographic, and histologic studies. Muscle Nerve 1990;13:516–527.

Stamenova P, Koytchev R, Kuhn K, et al: A randomized, double-blind, placebo-controlled study of the efficacy and safety of tolperisone in spasticity following cerebral stroke. Eur J Neurol 2005;12: 453–461.

Stayer C, Meinck HM: Stiff-man syndrome: An overview. Neurologia 1998;13:83–88.

Stayer C, Tronnier V, Dressnandt J, et al: Intrathecal baclofen therapy for stiff-man syndrome and progressive encephalomyelopathy with rigidity and myoclonus. Neurology 1997;49:1591–1597.

Stephan DA, Buist NR, Chittenden AB, et al: A rippling muscle disease gene is localized to 1q41: Evidence for multiple genes. Neurology 1994;44:1915–1920.

Takakusaki K, Kohyama J, Matsuyama K, Mori S: Medullary reticulospinal tract mediating the generalized motor inhibition in cats: Parallel inhibitory mechanisms acting on motoneurons and on interneuronal transmission in reflex pathways. Neuroscience 2001;103:511–527.

Taylor PW: Isaacs' syndrome (autoimmune neuromyotonia) in a patient with systemic lupus erythematosus. J Rheumatol 2005;32: 757–758.

Taylor RG, Layzer RB, Davis HS, Fowler WM, Jr: Continuous muscle fiber activity in the Schwartz-Jampel syndrome. Electroencephalogr Clin Neurophysiol 1972;33:497–509.

Thilmann AF: Spasticity: History, definitions, and usage of the term. In Thilmann AF, Burke DJ, Rymer WZ (eds): Spasticity: Mechanisms and Management. Berlin, Springer-Verlag, 1993, pp 1–5.

Thilmann AF, Fellows SJ, Garms E: The mechanism of spastic muscle hypertonus: Variation in reflex gain over the time course of spasticity. Brain 1991;114(pt 1A):233–244.

Thompson PD: Stiff muscles. J Neurol Neurosurg Psychiatry 1993; 56:121–124.

Thompson PD: Stiff people. In Marsden CD, Fahn S (eds): Movement Disorders, vol 3. Oxford, UK, Butterworth-Heinemann, 1994, pp 373–405.

Thompson PD: The stiff-man syndrome and related disorders. Parkinsonism Relat Disord 2001;8:147–153.

Torbergsen T: Rippling muscle disease: A review. Muscle Nerve 2002;11(suppl):S103–S107.

Uddin AB, Walters AS, Ali A, Brannan T: A unilateral presentation of "Satoyoshi syndrome." Parkinsonism Relat Disord 2002;8:211–213.

Valenstein E, Watson RT, Parker JL: Myokymia, muscle hypertrophy and percussion "myotonia" in chronic recurrent polyneuropathy. Neurology 1978;28:1130–1134.

Vasilescu C, Alexianu M, Dan A: Muscle hypertrophy and a syndrome of continuous motor unit activity in prednisone-responsive Guillain-Barre polyneuropathy. J Neurol 1984a;231:276–279.

Vasilescu C, Alexianu M, Dan A: Neuronal type of Charcot-Marie-Tooth disease with a syndrome of continuous motor unit activity. J Neurol Sci 1984b;63:11–25.

Vasilescu C, Florescu A: Peripheral neuropathy with a syndrome of continuous motor unit activity. J Neurol 1982;226:275–282.

Vernino S, Lennon VA: Ion channel and striational antibodies define a continuum of autoimmune neuromuscular hyperexcitability. Muscle Nerve 2002;26:702–707.

Vicari AM, Folli F, Pozza G, et al: Plasmapheresis in the treatment of stiff-man syndrome. N Engl J Med 1989;320:1499.

Vorgerd M, Bolz H, Patzold T, et al: Phenotypic variability in rippling muscle disease. Neurology 1999;52:1453–1459.

Vorgerd M, Ricker K, Ziemssen F, et al: A sporadic case of rippling muscle disease caused by a de novo caveolin-3 mutation. Neurology 2001;57:2273–2277.

Walikonis JE, Lennon VA: Radioimmunoassay for glutamic acid decarboxylase (GAD65) autoantibodies as a diagnostic aid for stiff-man syndrome and a correlate of susceptibility to type 1 diabetes mellitus. Mayo Clin Proc 1998;73:1161–1166.

Wallis WE, Van Poznak A, Plum F: Generalized muscular stiffness, fasciculations, and myokymia of peripheral nerve origin. Arch Neurol 1970;22:430–439.

Walsh JC: Neuromyotonia: An unusual presentation of intrathoracic malignancy. J Neurol Neurosurg Psychiatry 1976;39:1086–1091.

Wessig C, Klein R, Schneider MF, et al: Neuropathology and binding studies in anti-amphiphysin associated stiff-person syndrome. Neurology 2003;61:195–198.

Whiteley AM, Swash M, Urich H: Progressive encephalomyelitis with rigidity. Brain 1976;99:27–42.

Wiesendanger M: Pyramidal tract function and the clinical "pyramidal syndrome." Hum Neurobiol 1984;2:227–234.

Williams AC, Nutt JG, Hare T: Autoimmunity in stiff man syndrome. Lancet 1988;2:222.

Wilton A, Gardner-Medwin D: 21-year follow-up of myokymia with impaired muscle relaxation. Lancet 1990;336:1138–1139.

Wisuthsarewong W, Likitmaskul S, Manonukul J: Satoyoshi syndrome. Pediatr Dermatol 2001;18:406–410.

Woodman SE, Sotgia F, Galbiati F, et al: Caveolinopathies: Mutations in caveolin-3 cause four distinct autosomal dominant muscle diseases. Neurology 2004;62:538–543.

# Hyperkinetic Disorders

## Chapter 13

# Dystonia
## Phenomenology, Classification, Etiology, Pathology, Biochemistry, and Genetics

*In the course of the last five years I have repeatedly observed an affliction, whose meaning and classification caused great difficulties. When examining the first cases I was trying to decide between a diagnosis of hysteria, and idiopathic bilateral athetosis; but then I soon realized that neither of these diagnoses was appropriate, and that this was a new condition, or at least a new type of condition.*

*... The disease has something quite unique; namely the severe tonic cramps, particularly in the neck, head and the proximal sections of the extremities. The unique "torqued" gait is practically pathological. The prognosis is bad. All therapeutic attempts are as of yet unsuccessful. ...*

*During my efforts to delineate the methodology of the disease through an incisive name, I have selected the titles dysbasia lordotica progressiva and dystonia musculorum deformans and would prefer the latter.*

Hermann Oppenheim, 1911, from his
description of generalized dystonia

## HISTORICAL HIGHLIGHTS

In 1908, Schwalbe published his dissertation on a family with three affected children who are now recognized to have had primary generalized dystonia (Schwalbe, 1908). An English translation of Schwalbe's paper is available (Truong and Fahn, 1988). Three years later, Oppenheim (1911) described the same disorder and coined the word *dystonia* to indicate that in this disorder, there would be hypotonia on one occasion and tonic muscle spasms on another, usually but not exclusively elicited on volitional movements. Oppenheim called this syndrome by two different names: *dystonia musculorum deformans* and *dysbasia lordotica progressiva*. The first name relates to the spasms and to the postural deformities that develop in these children; the second name emphasizes the dromedary gait and the progressive nature of the illness. Oppenheim described muscle spasms; bizarre walking with bending and twisting of the torso; rapid, sometimes rhythmic jerking movements; and progression of symptoms leading eventually to sustained fixed postural deformities.

Oppenheim, however, failed to recognize the inherited nature of the disorder, which was emphasized by Flatau and Sterling (1911) later that year; they suggested the name *progressive torsion spasm*, which perhaps would have been the preferred, according to the full syndrome recognized today. The word *dystonia*, however, was immediately adopted by neurologists and has been used to describe both a distinctive motor phenomenology and a clinical syndrome in which these motoric features are present. Over time, different meanings were used for *dystonia* (for historical details, see Fahn et al., 1987). To clarify the definition, an ad hoc committee of the Dystonia Medical Research Foundation considered the clinical features described by Oppenheim (1911), Flatau and Sterling (1911), and other early observers and developed the following definition: *Dystonia is a syndrome of sustained muscle contractions, frequently causing twisting and repetitive movements or abnormal postures* (Fahn et al., 1987; Fahn, 1988). To emphasize the twisting quality of the abnormal movements and postures, the term *torsion* is often placed in front of the word *dystonia*. Such twisting is one feature that distinguishes dystonic movements from those of other dyskinesias, such as chorea, and distinguishes dystonic postures from other syndromes of increased muscle tone, such as rigidity, stiff-person syndrome, and neuromyotonia (Fahn, 1999). Exceptions to twisting are around joints that do not allow such torsion. Thus, dystonia involving the jaw, focusing on the temporomandibular joint, are jaw-opening and jaw-closing dystonias, rarely lateral jaw dystonia, but not twisting of the jaw.

The early observers described dystonia as a specific disease entity, but by the next decade, dystonia was recognized to be a feature in other neurologic disorders, such as Wilson disease and cerebral palsy, and following encephalitis. Soon, dystonia as a specific entity (today known as primary dystonia) was lost. It was Herz (1944a, 1944b, 1944c) who, in a masterful series of three papers, resurrected torsion dystonia as a specific neurologic entity as well as its presence within other neurologic diseases, who described the motor phenomenology and compared the duration of its contractions with those of chorea and athetosis, who utilized the analysis of cinematography to distinguish these differences in various movement disorders, and who showed the characteristic simultaneous contractions of agonist and antagonist muscles in dystonia. Another major pioneer in dystonia was Zeman (1970), who, along with his colleagues (Zeman and Dyken, 1967; Zeman et al., 1959, 1960), carried out the first epidemiologic study, emphasized the autosomal-dominant pattern of inheritance, described the focal dystonias as formes frustes of generalized dystonia, and found the pathologic anatomy to be normal in primary torsion dystonia (PTD). Still, patients with dystonia were often considered to be hysterical—that is, to have a psychogenic disorder and not an organic one, as Lesser and Fahn (1978) pointed out, often with tragic consequences, as described in Cooper's book (1976). Better awareness of the organic nature of dystonia, both generalized and focal (for torticollis and writer's cramp were often considered hysterical), began to come about with the holding and publication of the first international symposium on dystonia (Eldridge and Fahn, 1976). The final proof came with the discovery of the gene locus for Oppenheim dystonia (Ozelius et al., 1989) and the discovery that dystonia in the Ashkenazi Jewish population was inherited in an autosomal-dominant pattern (Bressman et al., 1989).

Other important events in the development of an understanding of dystonia are the formation of the Dystonia Medical Research Foundation in 1976, the creation of four international symposia on dystonia with their subsequent publications (Eldridge and Fahn, 1976; Fahn et al., 1988; Fahn, Marsden, et al., 1998; Fahn et al., 2004), and the investigations of clinical and molecular genetics that are leading to the discovery of the mutated genes and clarifying the classification and clinical features of the dystonias (Bressman et al., 1989; Ozelius et al., 1989, 1997; Nygaard et al., 1993; Bressman, de Leon, et al., 1994; Ichinose et al., 1994). The advances in genetics have led to a better etiologic classification of the dystonias (Fahn, Bressman, et al., 1998) and to the labeling of many of the dystonias using a *DYT* classification, as displayed in Box 13-1.

A number of reviews covering the historical aspects are available to which the reader is referred for more details than are provided in this chapter (Fahn, 1984b, 1989c, 1990; Fahn and Marsden, 1987; Fahn et al., 1987, 1988; Rothwell and Obeso, 1987; Tsui and Calne, 1995; Jankovic and Fahn, 1998). A collection of historical photographs about dystonia is available for perusal (Goetz et al., 2001).

Perhaps the greatest advances in dystonia in the past 10 years have been the continual unraveling of an increasing number of distinct genetic forms of dystonia based on gene mapping and cloning. In turn, this has led to the beginning of molecular biology research in the dystonias and a more comprehensive classification of the dystonias based on etiology. The first genetic form of dystonia whose gene was mapped was the form described by Oppenheim (1911), which he called dystonia musculorum deformans and which is now called Oppenheim dystonia (Fahn, Bressman, et al., 1998) and also *DYT1* dystonia (because the mapped gene was given that designation). The gene for Oppenheim dystonia has been identified and cloned, but not before the gene responsible for another genetic form of dystonia was identified, namely, dopa-responsive dystonia *(DYT5)*, or DRD, caused by a mutation in the gene for the enzyme guanosine triphosphate (GTP) cyclohydrolase I. As genes are being mapped, the clinicians are able to use this information to better define the clinical features of each genetic type. Box 13-1 lists the currently known genetic designations for the dystonias. The newest gene identified is that for NA-K-ATPase responsible for rapid-onset dystonia-parkinsonism (RDP) *(DYT12)* (de Carvalho Aguiar et al., 2004). The official nomenclature committee has labeled 15 *DYTs* but omitted other genetic forms of dystonia, which are listed after the first 15. Moreover, clinical neurologists usually consider *DYT8*, *DYT9*, and *DYT10* to be part of the category of movement disorders known as paroxysmal dyskinesias and not within the dystonia category.

A number of other dystonias are known to be genetic but have not received a *DYT* classification. Two new families with suspected *DYT2* dystonia were reported (Khan et al., 2003; Moretti et al., 2005). Siblings from two families with consanguinity developed autosomal-recessive childhood-onset generalized dystonia. Gene studies for other forms of dystonia were negative.

The gene causing lubag (*DYT3*) involves a multiple transcript system (Nolte et al., 2003). It is not possible to say which mutant protein (and there may be up to six from this mutation) is actually responsible for the disease.

De Carvalho Aguiar and colleagues (2004) reported the identification of missense mutations in the gene for the Na$^+$/K$^+$-ATPase $\alpha$3 subunit (*ATP1A3*) as a cause of RDP (*DYT12*).

A fuller description of the phenotype of *DYT13* (craniocervical-brachial dystonia) has been reported in the only known family with this disorder (Bentivoglio et al., 2004). Age at onset ranged from 5 to 43 years. Onset occurred either in the craniocervical region or in the upper limbs. Progression was mild, and the disease course was benign in most affected individuals; generalization occurred in only two cases. There was no anticipation of age at onset or of disease severity through generations. Most subjects presented with jerky, myoclonic-like dystonic movements of the neck or shoulders. *DYT13* is an autosomal-dominant disease, with incomplete penetrance (58%).

Two independent studies searched for mutations in the $\varepsilon$-sarcoglycan gene in patients with familial and sporadic myoclonus-dystonia and did not find any (Han et al., 2003; Valente et al., 2003). This finding, plus the report of one family having a mutation on a different chromosome, 18p11 (*DYT15*), provides additional evidence for genetic heterogeneity in myoclonus-dystonia.

The association with a polymorphism in the D5 receptor gene (DRD5) for primary focal dystonias could not be confirmed in German and French patients (Sibbing et al., 2003) but was seen in Italian patients (Brancati et al., 2003).

Box 13-1  Genetic classification of the dystonias

*DYT1* = 9q34, torsinA, AD, young-onset, limb-onset (Oppenheim dystonia) (Ozelius et al., 1997)

*DYT2* = AR, unconfirmed (Gimenez-Roldan et al., 1988; Khan et al., 2003; Moretti et al., 2005)

*DYT3* = Xq13.1, lubag in Filipino males (X-linked dystonia-parkinsonism), a multiple transcript system (Müller et al., 1994; Nolte et al., 2003)

*DYT4* = a whispering dysphonia family (Parker et al., 1985)

*DYT5* = 14q22.1, GTP cyclohydrolase-1, AD (known as dopa-responsive dystonia) (Ichinose et al., 1994); (also tyrosine hydroxylase deficiency = 11p11.5, AR, can respond to levodopa) (Knappskog et al., 1995)

*DYT6* = 8p21–q22, AD, mixed type, in the Mennonite/Amish population (Almasy et al., 1997)

*DYT7* = 18p, AD, familial torticollis, but localization is now in doubt (Leube et al., 1996)

*DYT8* = 2q33–q35, AD, paroxysmal nonkinesigenic dyskinesia (PNKD) (FDP1) (Mount-Rebak) (Fink et al., 1996; Fouad et al., 1996)

*DYT9* = 1p21, AD, paroxysmal dyskinesia with spasticity (CSE) (Auburger et al., 1996)

*DYT10* = 16p11.2–q12.1, AD, paroxysmal kinesigenic dyskinesia (PKD) (Tomita et al., 1999) (another PKD on 16q13–q22.1) (Valente et al., 2000) (also PED with infantile convulsions on 16p12–q11.2 (Szepetowski et al., 1997)

*DYT11* = 7q21–q23, ε-sarcoglycan, AD, myoclonus-dystonia (Zimprich et al., 2001)

*DYT12* = 19q, Na-K-ATPase, AD, rapid-onset dystonia-parkinsonism (Kramer et al., 1999; de Carvalho Aguiar et al., 2004)

*DYT13* = 1p36.13–p36.32, AD, cranial-cervical-brachial (Valente et al., 2001; Bentivoglio et al., 2004)

*DYT14* = 14q13, AD, DRD (Grotzsch et al., 2002)

*DYT15* = 18p11, AD, myoclonus-dystonia (Grimes et al., 2002)

**Disorders Not Labeled as *DYT* but in Which Dystonia and Sometimes Other Neurologic Features Are Present**

Deafness-dystonia (Mohr-Tranebjaerg syndrome), X-linked recessive (Jin et al., 1999; Koehler et al., 1999; Tranebjaerg et al., 2000). Torticollis and writer's cramp also seen in female carriers (Swerdlow and Wooten, 2001); faulty assembly of the DDP1/TIMM8a–TIMM13 complex (Roesch et al., 2002)

Mental retardation, seizures, and infantile spasms, X-linked recessive (Stromme et al., 2002). Some also with dystonia.

Aromatic amino acid decarboxylase deficiency; AR (Swoboda et al., 2003)

6-Pyruvoyltetrahydropterin synthase deficiency, AR (Hyland et al., 1998)

Pterin-4a-carbinolamine dehydratase deficiency, AR (Hyland et al., 1998)

Dihydropteridine reductase deficiency; AR (Hyland et al., 1998)

Sepiapterin reductase deficiency; AR (Blau et al., 2001; Neville et al., 2005)

Neurodegeneration with brain iron accumulation Type 1 (formerly called Hallervorden-Spatz syndrome), pantothenate kinase deficiency, AR, 20p12.3–p13 (Taylor et al., 1996; Zhou et al., 2001); recently renamed as pantothenate kinase–associated neurodegeneration (PKAN) (Hayflick et al., 2003).

Neuroferritinopathy, 19q13.3, ferritin light polypeptide, AD (Curtis et al., 2001; Mir et al., 2005)

Familial torticollis, dopamine D5 receptor gene as a susceptibility factor (Placzek et al., 2001)

Familial blepharospasm, dopamine D5 receptor gene as a susceptibility factor (Misbahuddin et al., 2002)

---

The autosomal-recessive disorder of early-onset cerebellar ataxia with oculomotor apraxia associated with a mutation of the aprataxin gene on chromosome 9p13 can also cause generalized dystonia (Sekijima et al., 2003). Adult-onset craniocervical dystonia preceded ataxia in a case with SCA-1 (Wu et al., 2004).

Some patients with adult-onset dystonia have been found to have a missense mutation in the mitochondrial complex I gene (Simon et al., 2003). In addition to dystonia, spasticity and core-type myopathy are present.

## PHENOMENOLOGY OF DYSTONIC MOVEMENTS

With few exceptions, the four clinically unifying, consistent, and predominant features of dystonic contractions are (1) their relatively long duration (compared to myoclonus and chorea), although short-duration contractions can occur in dystonia; (2) their simultaneous contractions of agonists and antagonists; (3) their resulting in a twisting of the affected body part; and (4) their continual contractions of the same muscle groups (called patterned movements; see Chapter 1). One exception to the twisting nature of dystonia is that dystonias in facial muscles are rarely twisting; they are patterned and involve sustained contractions of the forehead, eyelids, and lower face. As it turns out, twisting facial muscles that move the mouth to one side or the other or back and forth to each side are usually psychogenic (see Chapter 26).

Although the durations of the patterned contractions are usually more sustained than those of chorea, sometimes they can be very short. The range from very short to very prolonged contractions results in the appearance of a wide range in the speed of the patterned dystonic movements from rapid to slow. The movements can be so fast that they have the appearance of repetitive myoclonic jerking. The term *myoclonic dystonia* had been applied to such dystonia (Davidenkow, 1926; Obeso et al., 1983; Kurlan et al., 1988; Quinn et al., 1988), and the rapid jerks may respond to alcohol (Quinn et al., 1988). In some families, the phenomenology of the combination of myoclonus and dystonia is a major feature, and these families are genetically distinct from those of the originally described PTD (i.e., Oppenheim dystonia) (Wahlström et al., 1994) and have been called by different names: initially *dystonia-myoclonus* (Fahn, Bressman, et al., 1998) but now *myoclonus-dystonia* (Klein et al., 1999; Nygaard et al., 1999). The relationship of familial myoclonus-dystonia and hereditary essential myoclonus, which can also include patients with some dystonic features, is not clear (Fahn and Sjaastad, 1991; Quinn, 1996) but will soon be settled, as the identification of a gene (ε-sarcoglycan) for myoclonus-dystonia has been discovered (Zimprich et al., 2001).

 Primary dystonia almost always begins by affecting a single part of the body; this is focal dystonia (Video 13-1). Most patients' dystonia remains as a focal dystonia without spreading to other parts of the body. However, even within that single body part, multiple muscles can be affected. Thus, in  patients with dystonia of the neck (cervical dystonia, or torticollis), a combination of muscles is involved (Video 13-2). Moreover, even if the neck is postured to a stable position, there can be changes in muscle contraction patterns that can be detected with electromyographic recordings (Munchau, Filipovic, et al., 2001). In a sizable minority of patients, dystonia that starts in one body part can spread to involve other parts of the body. Most often, the spread is to contiguous body parts; hence, the spread is from focal dystonia to segmental dystonia. As a general rule, the younger the age at onset, the more likely it is that the dystonia will spread; for example, childhood onset with leg involvement usually leads to eventual generalized dystonia (Marsden et al., 1976; Fahn, 1986; Greene et al., 1995). Regardless of genetic etiology, the phenotypes of primary dystonias are affected by age at onset, with a caudal-to-rostral change in the site of onset as a function of age (O'Riordan et al., 2004). The severity of dystonia can be quantified by using clinical rating scales for generalized dystonia and the various focal dystonias (Burke et al., 1985; Fahn, 1989a; Comella et al., 1997, 2003).

Dystonic movements are almost always aggravated during voluntary movement. The appearance of dystonic movements with voluntary movement is referred to as action dystonia. Primary dystonia commonly begins with a specific action dystonia; that is, the abnormal movements appear with a special action (i.e., a task-specific action) and are not present at rest, in contrast to secondary dystonias, which are more likely to begin with dystonia at rest (Svetel et al., 2004). For example, a child who develops primary dystonia might have the initial symptom in one leg but only when walking forward. It could be absent when the child runs or walks backward (Video 13-3). Other common examples are the task-specific dystonias that are seen with writing (writer's cramp) (Video 13-4), playing a musical instrument (musician's cramp) (Video 13-5), chewing (Video 13-6), and speaking, including auctioneering (Scolding et al., 1995). Often, these task-specific dystonias produce occupational disability; for example, musicians usually no longer can play their instrument professionally. Robert Schumann's career as a pianist was impaired, probably because of musician's cramp (de Yebenes, 1995). Musician's cramp and other occupational cramps can occur in any part of body that is engaged in repetitive, highly skilled tasks. Embouchure (the pattern of lip, jaw, and tongue muscles used to control the flow of air into a mouthpiece) dystonia has been seen in horn and woodwind players. Patients with

embouchure dystonia can be separated into several groups, including embouchure tremor, involuntary lip movements, and jaw closure (Frucht et al., 2001). The dystonia can spread to other oral tasks, often producing significant disability. Focal task-specific tremors might be a form of focal dystonia rather than a manifestation of essential tremor (Soland et al., 1996b). Several reviews of musician's cramps were presented at an international symposium on dystonia (Brandfonbrener and Robson, 2004; Charness and Schlaug, 2004; Frucht, 2004; Jabusch and Altenmuller, 2004; Pesenti et al., 2004).

As the dystonic condition progresses, less specific voluntary motor actions of the involved limb can bring out the dystonic movements. In the previous example, the affected leg might also activate the dystonia when it is tapping the floor. With further evolution, actions in other parts of the body can induce dystonic movements of the involved leg, so-called overflow. Talking is the most common mechanism for causing overflow dystonia in other body parts. Such activation of involuntary movements by talking is also particularly common with levodopa-induced dyskinesias and in cerebral palsy. With still further worsening, the affected limb can develop dystonic movements while it is at rest. Eventually, the leg can have sustained posturing. Thus, dystonia at rest is usually a more severe form than pure action dystonia.

Much less common than action dystonia or overflow dystonia is the reverse phenomenon—that is, for dystonia at rest to be improved by talking or by other voluntary active movements, so-called paradoxical dystonia (Fahn, 1989b). With paradoxical dystonia, the patient is usually observed moving the affected or a nonaffected body part (see Video 1-52). The patient does this to obtain relief of the dystonia. When the paradoxical dystonia involves the trunk, the observer can easily mistake the patient's moving about as being due to restlessness or akathisia, which is the most common differential diagnosis  (Video 13-7). The focal dystonia that is most commonly decreased by voluntary motor activity is blepharospasm (Fahn et al., 1985). About 60% of patients with blepharospasm obtain relief when talking; about 40% worsen with talking.

Dystonia usually is present continually throughout the day whenever the affected body part is in use and, as a sign of more severity, also when the body part is at rest. Dystonic movements tend to increase with fatigue, stress, and emotional states; they tend to be suppressed with relaxation, hypnosis, and sleep (Fish et al., 1991). Dystonia may be precipitated or exacerbated by pregnancy (dystonia gravidarum) (Lim et al., 2006).Unless it is extremely severe, dystonia often disappears with deep sleep. For patients who appear to have persistent postural abnormalities that cannot be overcome by manual manipulation, it might be necessary to put them to sleep with anesthesia to determine whether a contracture is already present. Propofol anesthesia, however, does not entirely suppress dystonia because recurrences occur even under deep propofol anesthesia (Zabani and Vaghadia, 1996).

One of the characteristic and almost unique features of dystonic movements is that they can often be diminished by tactile or proprioceptive "sensory tricks" (*geste antagoniste*). Thus, touching the involved body part or an adjacent body part can often reduce the muscle contractions (Video 13-8). For example, patients with torticollis will often place a hand on the chin or side of the face to reduce nuchal contractions (see Video 13-2), and orolingual dystonia is often helped by touching the lips or placing an object in the mouth (Blunt et al., 1994). In a study of

50 patients with cervical dystonia who were known to have at least one sensory trick, 54% of them had two to five different tricks, and 82% had a reduction of head deviation by at least 30%, with a mean of 60% (Muller et al., 2001). In cervical dystonia, applying the trick when the head is in a neutral or even contralateral position was most effective, while no reduction of muscle activity occurs during trick application at the maximum dystonic head position (Schramm et al., 2004). Sometimes, a mechanical device can be utilized therapeutically, especially for cervical dystonia (Krack et al., 1998) (Video 13-9). Greene and Bressman (1998) found that in some patients with torsion dystonia, simply thinking about a sensory trick or task affects the dystonia in the same way as actually performing the activity. A positron emission tomography (PET) study has shown that the sensory trick brings about a normalization of the abnormal cortical physiology that is seen in dystonia and results in increasing activation of the ipsilateral superior and inferior parietal lobule and decreasing activity of the contralateral supplementary motor area and the primary sensorimotor cortex (Naumann et al., 2000). The presence of a sensory trick is not specific for primary dystonias; it can sometimes occur in secondary dystonias, including psychogenic dystonia (Munhoz and Lang, 2004).

Pain is uncommon in dystonia except in cervical dystonia; 75% of patients with cervical dystonia (spasmodic torticollis) have pain (Chan et al., 1991). The pain perception threshold appears to be lower in patients with primary cervical dystonia (Lobbezoo et al., 1996). Dystonia in most parts of the body rarely is accompanied by pain; when it is, it is not clear whether the pain is due to painful contractions of muscles or some other factor. The high incidence of pain in cervical dystonia appears to be due to muscle contractions because this pain is usually relieved by injections of botulinum toxin (Greene et al., 1990). It is believed that the posterior cervical muscles are rich in pain fibers and that continual contraction of these muscles results in pain. On the other hand, because no correlation was found between the severity of motor signs and pain, some investigators hypothesize that central mechanisms are also involved (Kutvonen et al., 1997). Quality of life is negatively affected with cervical dystonia (Camfield et al., 2002). It has been difficult to explain fixed painful postural torticollis following trauma, but recent analysis indicates that many of these cases appear to be psychogenic (Sa et al., 2003). Fixed dystonia in other parts of the body is also usually associated with a peripheral injury and overlaps with chronic regional pain syndrome (reflex sympathetic dystrophy); many of these individuals fulfill strict criteria for a somatoform disorder or psychogenic dystonia (Schrag et al., 2004).

Patients with PTD sometimes have rhythmic movements, particularly in the arms (Video 13-10) and neck, manifested as a tremor (Yanagisawa et al., 1972; Jankovic and Fahn, 1980). In one survey, 68% of patients with cervical dystonia had head tremor (Pal et al., 2000). Two basic types of tremors are seen in dystonic patients: an accompanying postural/action tremor that resembles essential tremor or enhanced physiologic tremor and a tremor that is a rhythmic expression of rapid dystonic movements (Yanagisawa and Goto, 1971). The latter can usually be distinguished from the former by showing that the tremor appears only when the affected body part is placed in a position of opposition to the major direction of pulling by the abnormal dystonic contractions and disappears when the body part is positioned where the dystonia wants to place it (see Video 1-86). Dystonic tremor appears to be less regular than essential tremor (Jedynak et al., 1991). Sometimes, it is very difficult to distinguish between the two types, particularly with writing tremor and cervical tremor. Primary writing tremor can sometimes represent task-specific dystonia or task-specific essential tremor (Cohen et al., 1987; Rosenbaum and Jankovic, 1988; Elble et al., 1990). A family history of tremor (and stuttering) is increased in PTD (Fletcher et al., 1991a).

Although accompanying essential tremor is recognized in patients with dystonia (Lou and Jankovic, 1991), there is uncertainty as to how common this occurrence is. Tremor of the hands can be seen fairly often in patients with cervical dystonia (spasmodic torticollis) (Couch, 1976). Deuschl and colleagues (1997) analyzed this tremor in 55 patients with cervical dystonia. The mean amplitudes of postural tremor were only slightly higher than those of the controls and much smaller than those found in classic essential tremor; analytic measurements showed evidence of physiologic tremor mechanisms only. In another study, arm tremor in patients with cervical dystonia was found to develop either before or simultaneously with onset of the torticollis; such temporal relationships do not correspond to either dystonic tremor or tremor in the presence of dystonia (Munchau, Schrag, et al., 2001).

Tics are another type of involuntary movement that appears to occur more commonly in patients with dystonia than in the general population (Shale et al., 1986; Stone and Jankovic, 1991).

Although this is rare, some children and adolescents with primary and secondary dystonia can develop a crisis of sudden marked increase in the severity of dystonia, which has been called dystonic storm (Dalvi et al., 1998) and *status dystonicus* (Manji et al., 1998). It can cause rhabdomyolysis and myoglobinuria, with a threat of death by renal failure (Jankovic and Penn, 1982; Paret et al., 1995). Placing the patient in an intensive-care unit and narcotizing him or her with barbiturates is usually necessary to treat this crisis. Intrathecal baclofen might be necessary if the dystonic storm persists and continues to be present when the patient is allowed to awaken (Jankovic and Penn, 1982; Dalvi et al., 1998). More recently, pallidotomy or pallidal stimulation has been utilized in place of intrathecal baclofen.

A case of orthostatic hemidystonia has been reported (Sethi et al., 2002). The patient developed hemidystonia on arising from the sitting position. It was due to poor vascular perfusion in the contralateral frontoparietal cortex and was the result of occlusion of the contralateral internal carotid artery and near-total occlusion of the ipsilateral internal carotid artery.

Dystonia patients are relatively free of psychopathology, as measured in patients with writer's cramp (Sheehy and Marsden, 1982) and blepharospasm (Scheidt et al., 1996). However, a recent study reports a prevalence of obsessive-compulsive disorder in 20% of patients with primary focal dystonias (Cavallaro et al., 2002). Attentional-executive cognitive deficits have been found in patients with primary dystonia by using the Cambridge Neuropsychological Test Automated Battery (Scott et al., 2003) but not by using a host of other tests (Jahanshahi et al., 2003). Obsessive-compulsive disorder and alcohol dependence are not uncommon in individuals who carry the *DYT11* gene for myoclonus-dystonia (Saunders-Pullman et al., 2002), and the *DYT1* gene has been associated with an increase in depression, whether the person is a manifesting or nonmanifesting carrier (Heiman et al., 2004).

Isolated foot dystonia following exercise in adults is sometimes seen as the first symptom of Parkinson disease. This has now been verified in a patient with neuroimaging by using dopamine transporter single photon emission computed tomography. Dystonia may be the presenting or dominant feature of many parkinsonian disorders besides Parkinson disease (Jankovic, 2005; Ashour and Jankovic, 2006).

## EPIDEMIOLOGY

Zeman and his colleagues (Zeman and Dyken, 1967; Zeman et al., 1959, 1960) carried out the first epidemiologic study in dystonia in the population of the state of Indiana and emphasized the autosomal dominant pattern of inheritance in PTD. They considered only generalized dystonia to be PTD and viewed other types as formes fruste. Today, those other forms are viewed as focal and segmental dystonia and as part of the spectrum of PTD. An epidemiologic study of PTD in the population living in Rochester, Minnesota, found the prevalence of generalized PTD to be 3.4 per 100,000 population and the prevalence of focal dystonia to be 30 per 100,000 (Nutt et al., 1988). In a study of dystonia in Israel, Zilber and colleagues (1984) estimated the prevalence of generalized dystonia among Jews of Eastern European ancestry to be 1 per 15,000, or 6.8 per 100,000, which is double the prevalence in the general population of Rochester. However, the recent analysis by Risch and colleagues (1995) indicates that the frequency in the Ashkenazi Jewish population is much higher (between 1 per 6000 and 1 per 2000), and they suggest that the Ashkenazi population with PTD descends from a limited group of founders of the *DYT1* mutation. These investigators also have traced the origin of the mutation to the northern part of the historic Jewish Pale of settlement (Lithuania and Byelorussia) approximately 350 years ago. In Japan, the *DYT1* mutation was looked for in 178 patients with various forms of dystonia and was found in 6 (3.4%) (Matsumoto et al., 2001)

and phenotypically resembled Oppenheim dystonia seen in other populations.

In Japan, the prevalence of focal dystonias was found to be 6.12 (Nakashima et al., 1995) and 10.1 (Matsumoto et al., 2003) per 100,000 population, which is considerably lower than the 30 per 100,000 found by Nutt and colleagues (1988) in Rochester, Minnesota. In the north of England, the prevalence of focal dystonias was found to be 12 per 100,000, and the prevalence of generalized dystonia was found to be 1.6 per 100,000 (Duffey et al., 1998). A European consortium of investigators published findings of 11.7 per 100,000 for focal dystonia and 3.5 per 100,000 for segmental and generalized primary dystonias (Warner et al., 2000). A survey of primary blepharospasm in the Puglia region of southern Italy found a prevalence of 13.3 per 100,000 (Defazio et al., 2001). The incidence rate of primary blepharospasm was found to be only 1.2 per 100,000 population per year in Olmstead County, Minnesota (Bradley et al., 2003).

In Belgrade, the prevalence rate for focal, segmental, and multifocal dystonia was 13.6 per 100,000 population (Pekmezovic et al., 2003). It was almost twice as common (25.4 per 100,000 population) in Oslo (Le et al., 2003). Gender appears to play a role in both the prevalence and the age at onset of focal dystonia, women being more at risk and having an earlier age at onset for writer's cramp but men having an earlier age at onset for cervical dystonia, blepharospasm, and laryngeal dystonia (Epidemiologic Study of Dystonia in Europe (ESDE) Collaborative Group, 1999).

Table 13-1 lists epidemiologic studies of PTD.

## CLASSIFICATION OF TORSION DYSTONIA

Box 13-2 presents the three ways to classify patients with torsion dystonia: by age at onset, by body distribution of abnormal movements, and by etiology. This method allows physicians and health-care providers some understanding of the nature of the dystonia, including prognosis.

Table 13-1 Prevalence of primary torsion dystonia

| Authors | | Population | Prevalence | Remarks |
|---|---|---|---|---|
| Zeman and Dyken | (1967) | Indiana | 1/200,000 | Essentially a white, non-Jewish population Generalized dystonia only |
| Zilber et al | (1984) | Israel: Jews of Eastern Europe | 1/15,000 | Generalized dystonia only |
| | | Afro-Asian Jews | 1/117,000 | Generalized dystonia only |
| Nutt et al. | (1988) | General dystonia(2) | 1/29,400 | Olmstead County |
| | | Focal dystonia | 1/3400 | From Mayo clinic records |
| Risch et al. | (1995) | New York area | Disease: 1/6000 | Based on cases seen at Columbia |
| | | Ashkenazi Jewish | Gene: 1/2000 | University Medical Center |
| Nakashima et al. | (1995) | Focal dystonia | 1/16,129 | Japan |
| Duffey et al. | (1998) | General dystonia | 1/62,000 | North of England survey |
| | | Focal dystonia | 1/8000 | |
| Warner et al. | (2000) | General and segmental dystonia | 1/28,500 | European consortium survey |
| | | Focal dystonia | 1/8500 | |
| Defazio et al. | (2001) | Blepharospasm | 1/7519 | Puglia region, Southern Italy |
| Pekmezovic et al. | (2003) | Focal dystonia, cervical dystonia | 1/8929 | Belgrade, Serbia |
| Le et al. | (2003) | Focal and segmental dystonia | 1/3534 | Europeans in Oslo, Norway |
| Matsumoto et al. | (2003) | Focal dystonia | 1/9900 | Kyoto, Japan |
| Bradley et al. | (2003) | Blepharospasm | Incidence rate: 1.2/100,000/year | Rochester, Minnesota |

**Box 13-2** Three ways to classify torsion dystonia

**By Age at Onset**
Early-onset: ≤26 years
Late-onset: >26 years

**By Distribution**
Focal
Segmental
Multifocal
Generalized
Hemidystonia

**By Etiology**
Primary (also known as idiopathic) dystonia
Dystonia-plus
Secondary dystonia
Heredodegenerative dystonia (usually presents as
   dystonia-plus)
A feature of another neurologic disease (e.g., dystonic
   tics, paroxysmal dyskinesias, PD, PSP)

**Table 13-2** Distribution of dystonia by body parts

| Type of Dystonia | n | Percentage |
|---|---|---|
| Focal | 1230 | 50% |
| Segmental | 837 | 34% |
| Generalized | 383 | 16% |
| | 2450 | 100% |

Data from the Center for Parkinson's Disease and Other Movement Disorders, Columbia University Medical Center, New York City.

## Classification by Age at Onset

Classification by age at onset is useful because this is the most important single factor related to prognosis of primary dystonia (Marsden et al., 1976; Fahn, 1986; Greene et al., 1995). Even for secondary dystonias, such as tardive dystonia, age is commonly a factor in the location of the dystonia. As a general rule, the younger the age at onset, the more likely it is that the dystonia will become severe and will spread to involve multiple parts of the body. In contrast, the older the age at onset, the more likely it is that the dystonia will remain focal. Onset of dystonia in a leg is the second most important predictive factor (Greene et al., 1995) (Video 13-11). Because a bimodal age distribution is seen with primary dystonia, the age classification consists of two categories: (1) age 26 years or below and (2) above age 26 (Bressman, 2004).

## Classification by Distribution

Since dystonia usually begins by affecting a single part of the body (focal dystonia) and since dystonia can either remain focal or spread to involve other body parts, it is useful to classify dystonia according to its distribution of involvement of the body. Body distribution is one method of defining the severity of dystonia, and knowing the body distribution of dystonia is very important in planning a therapeutic strategy (Fahn, 1995).

Focal dystonia indicates that only a single area of the body is affected. Frequently seen types of focal dystonia tend to have specific labels, such as blepharospasm (see Videos 1-42 and 13-1), torticollis (see Videos 1-45 and 13-2), oromandibular dystonia, spastic dysphonia (see Video 1-44), writer's cramp (see Videos 1-46 and 13-4), and occupational cramp (see Video 13-5). Adult-onset focal dystonias are much more common than are generalized dystonias (Fahn, 1986; Marsden, 1986) (Table 13-2). If dystonia spreads, it most commonly does so by next affecting a contiguous body part. When dystonia affects two or more contiguous parts of the body, it is referred to as segmental dystonia (see Video 1-43). Some of

the primary focal dystonias, such as blepharospasm and cervical dystonia, affect females more than males, while the reverse is seen for writer's cramp (Soland et al., 1996a).

*Generalized dystonia* is defined as representing a combination of segmental crural dystonia (i.e., both legs or legs plus trunk) plus involvement of any other area of the body (Videos 13-12, 13-13, 13-14, and 13-15). The term *multifocal dystonia* fills a gap in these designations. It applies to the involvement of two or more noncontiguous parts of the body. Dystonia affecting one half of the body is called hemidystonia. Almost always, hemidystonia indicates that the dystonia is symptomatic rather than primary (Narbona et al., 1984; Marsden et al., 1985; Pettigrew and Jankovic, 1985). A review of hemidystonia (Chuang et al., 2002) found that the most common etiologies were stroke, trauma, and perinatal injury; the mean age of onset was between 20 and 26 years; the mean latency from insult to dystonia was between 2.8 and 4.1 years, the longest latencies occurring after perinatal injury; and basal ganglia lesions were identified in 48% to 60% of the cases, most commonly involving the putamen.

Detailed clinical descriptions of how dystonia manifests itself in the different regions of the body have been summarized by Fahn (1984a). The most common primary focal dystonia seen in a movement disorder clinic is cervical dystonia (torticollis), followed by dystonias affecting cranial musculature, such as blepharospasm and spasmodic dysphonia (Table 13-3). The most common primary segmental dystonia involves the cranial structures, and these are commonly referred to as cranial-cervical dystonia and sometimes as

**Table 13-3** Distribution of focal dystonias

| Type of Dystonia | n | Percentage |
|---|---|---|
| Blepharospasm | 140 | 13.9 |
| Oromandibular | 31 | 3.1 |
| Spasmodic dysphonia | 257 | 25.5 |
| Torticollis | 447 | 44.4 |
| Right arm | 96 | 9.5 |
| Left arm | 20 | 2.0 |
| Trunk | 5 | 0.5 |
| Right leg | 4 | 0.4 |
| Left leg | 6 | 0.6 |
| | 1006 | 100 |

Data from the Center for Parkinson's Disease and Other Movement Disorders, Columbia University Medical Center, New York City.

**Table 13-4** Distribution of segmental dystonias

| Type of Dystonia | n | Percentage |
|---|---|---|
| Segmental cranial | 167 | 42.8 |
| Cranial + brachial | 56 | 14.4 |
| Cranial + axial | 14 | 3.6 |
| Segmental brachial | 83 | 21.3 |
| Segmental axial | 31 | 7.9 |
| Segmental crural | 13 | 3.3 |
| Multifocal | 26 | 6.7 |
| | 390 | 100 |

Data from the Center for Parkinson's Disease and Other Movement Disorders, Columbia University Medical Center, New York City.

Meige syndrome (Tolosa and Klawans, 1979; Tolosa et al., 1988a) (Table 13-4). Details of cervical dystonia have been reviewed (Dauer et al., 1998). Primary axial dystonia that presents in adulthood is much less common than the cranial-cervical dystonias. In 9 of the 18 patients collected by Bhatia and colleagues (1997), onset was in the back, with the other half spreading to the back from the cranial-cervical region. Probably because of the age at onset, it does not spread to the legs. About one third of their patients improved with high-dose anticholinergics with or without antidopaminergics.

## Classification by Etiology

Awareness of etiology is an ultimate aim in the clinical evaluation of dystonia, not only for treatment and genetic counseling but also because it should lead to understanding the pathophysiology of the illness and how to prevent dystonia. The etiologic classification (Fahn, Bressman, et al., 1998) divides the causes of dystonia into four major categories: primary (or idiopathic), secondary (environmental causes or symptomatic), dystonia-plus syndromes, and heredodegenerative diseases in which dystonia is a prominent feature (Box 13-3).

Primary dystonia is characterized as a pure dystonia (with the exception that tremor can be present) and excludes a symptomatic cause. Dystonia-plus syndromes, such as DRD and myoclonus-dystonia, were previously considered to be variants of primary dystonia (Fahn, 1989c). But because symptoms and signs other than dystonia (namely, parkinson-

**Box 13-3** Five categories of the etiologic classification of dystonia

Primary (also known as idiopathic) dystonia
Dystonia-plus
Secondary dystonia
Heredodegenerative diseases (usually present as dystonia-plus)
A feature of another neurologic disease (e.g., tics, paroxysmal dyskinesias, Parkinson disease, progressive supranuclear palsy)

ism and myoclonus, respectively) are present, these entities are placed in the dystonia-plus category. Another concept is that dystonia-plus syndromes, like the primary dystonias, are not neurodegenerative disorders but neurochemical ones (Fahn, Bressman, et al., 1998). Secondary dystonias are those due to environmental insult, while heredodegenerative dystonias are due to neurodegenerative diseases that are usually inherited.

### PRIMARY DYSTONIA

Primary dystonia consists of familial and nonfamilial (sporadic) types. Although most patients with torsion dystonia have a negative family history for this disorder, the presence of other affected family members allows the family to be investigated in terms of localizing the abnormal gene(s) for dystonia. In primary dystonia, the only neurologic abnormality is the presence of dystonic postures and movements, with the exception of tremor that can resemble essential tremor and can even be essential tremor in some individuals. There is no associated loss of postural reflexes, amyotrophy, weakness, spasticity, ataxia, reflex change, abnormality of eye movements, disorder of retina, dementia, or seizures except when they may be the result of a concomitant problem such as a complication from a neurosurgical procedure undertaken to correct the dystonia or the presence of some other incidental neurologic disease. Since many of the secondary dystonias have these neurologic findings, the presence of any of these findings in a patient with dystonia immediately suggests that one is dealing with a secondary dystonia, a dystonia-plus syndrome, or a heredodegenerative disorder (see Box 13-3). However, the absence of such neurologic findings does not necessarily exclude the possibility of a secondary dystonia, which may rarely present as a pure dystonia.

Tremor in the primary dystonias may be due to a dystonic tremor (Fahn, 1984b) that results from rhythmic group action potentials that occur in dystonia (Yanagisawa and Goto, 1971). It remains to be elucidated whether tremor that mimics essential tremor (see Video 13-10) and enhanced physiologic tremor that is seen in many patients with dystonia as well as in members of their families (Zeman et al., 1960; Yanagisawa et al., 1972; Couch, 1976; Deuschl et al., 1997) is actually a component of idiopathic dystonia (i.e., dystonic tremor). Hand tremor in patients with cervical dystonia more closely resembles enhanced physiologic tremor than dystonic tremor or essential tremor (Deuschl et al., 1997).

Within the primary dystonias are a variety of genetic disorders, some of which have had their genes already mapped to *DYT1, DYT2, DYT4, DYT6, DYT7,* and *DYT13*. Other familial primary dystonias have not yet been mapped. But most primary dystonias are sporadic and with an onset during adulthood, usually presenting as one of a variety of focal and segmental dystonias (see Tables 13-3 and 13-4). *DYT1* (Oppenheim dystonia) is discussed in more detail later in the chapter. Here, some of the other primary familial dystonias listed in Box 13-4 are discussed.

In the Mennonite and Amish populations, a mixed type of autosomal-dominant dystonia has been seen in which onset can be either in childhood or adulthood, with involvement of limbs and the cervical and cranial regions. Dysphonia and dysarthria are often the most disabling features. The abnormal

Box 13-4  Detailed etiologic classification of the dystonias

### A. Primary (also Known as Idiopathic) Dystonia

1. Oppenheim dystonia (originally called dystonia musculorum deformans)

   *Genetics*
   a. Autosomal-dominant
   b. Penetrance rate between 30% and 40%
   c. Deletion of one of a pair of GAG triplets (codes for glutamic acid) in the *DYT1* gene located on chromosome 9q34.1
   d. *DYT1* codes for the heat-shock, ATP-binding protein, torsinA, an AAA+ protein
   e. In the Ashkenazi Jewish population, there is a characteristic extended haplotype due to a founder's effect in which the mutation entered this population approximately 350 years ago.
   f. Gene prevalence is 1/2000 in the Ashkenazi Jewish population
   g. Commercial gene testing is available

   *Clinical Phenotype*
   a. Early onset (> age 40)
   b. Limbs usually affected first
   c. Spread to other sites is related to age at onset and site of onset
   d. Pure dystonia (no other neurologic feature except action tremor may be present)
   e. No known consistent pathology
   f. MRI normal
   g. FDG PET: increased lenticular and decreased thalamic metabolic activity consistent with increased direct striatopallidal activity

2. Childhood and adult onset, familial cranial and limb (*DYT6*)

   *Genetics*
   a. Autosomal-dominant
   b. Gene mapped to 8p21–q22

   *Clinical Phenotype*
   a. Childhood and adult onset
   b. Site of onset in arm or cranial, occasionally leg or neck
   c. Usually remains as upper body involvement
   d. Affects the Mennonite and Amish populations

3. Adult-onset familial torticollis

   *Genetics*
   a. Autosomal-dominant
      1) *DYT7* = a north German family: 18p (Leube et al., 1996). Platelet complex 1 activity may be decreased
      2) Gene specificity is uncertain in other torticollis patients in Northern Germany (Leube and Auburger, 1998; Klein, Ozelius, et al., 1998), and findings appear to be limited to one family.
      3) Other families with autosomal-dominant torticollis that are not *DYT1*, *DYT7*, or *DYT13*, and their gene mappings have not yet been published.

   *Clinical Phenotype*
   a. Mostly adult-onset, occasionally in adolescence
   b. Limited to neck in 85%
   c. Occasional involvement of arm

4. Adult-onset familial cervical-cranial predominant

   *Genetics*
   a. Autosomal-dominant
   b. Not *DYT1*
   c. One family has been mapped to chromosome 1p36.13–p36.32 (*DYT13*)

   *Clinical Phenotype*
   a. Mostly adult-onset, occasionally in childhood
   b. Site of onset usually in neck, which predominates
   c. Usually remains segmental as cranial-cervical
   d. Occasional involvement of arm

5. Other familial types to be identified as distinct entities

6. Sporadic, usually adult-onset
   a. Could be genetic, but uncertain
      1) In patients with cervical dystonia, a search of polymorphisms in the dopamine receptor (D1 to D5) and dopamine transporter genes found an increased number of polymorphisms in allele 2 of the D5 receptor gene and a decrease in allele 6 of this gene compared to controls (Placzek et al., 2001). Adult-onset dystonia typically is not associated with the *DYT1* gene, whereas almost all young-onset, limb-onset individuals have the *DYT1* mutation.
   b. Classify by age at onset:
      1) childhood-onset (<13)
      2) adolescent-onset (13 to 20)
      3) adult-onset (>20)
   c. No known pathology

### B. Dystonia-Plus Syndromes

1. Dystonia with parkinsonism
   a. Dopa-responsive dystonia (DRD)
      1) GTP cyclohydrolase I deficiency (*DYT5*). First step in tetrahydrobiopterin (BH4) synthesis

   *Genetics*
      a) Autosomal-dominant with different mutations of the gene for GTP cyclohydrolase I (GCH) located at 14q22.1

   *Clinical Phenotype*
      a) Childhood onset (<16) with leg and gait disorder

Adapted from Fahn S, Bressman SB, Marsden CD: Classification of dystonia. In Fahn S, Marsden CD, DeLong MR (eds): Dystonia 3: Advances in Neurology, vol 78. Philadelphia, Lippincott-Raven, 1998, pp 1–10, with more recent additions.

*Continued*

Box 13-4 Detailed etiologic classification of the dystonias—cont'd

b) Girls > boys
c) May be diurnal (no symptoms in morning, worse at night)
d) Parkinsonian signs present (bradykinesia, loss of postural reflexes, rigidity)
e) Markedly improves with low dose levodopa
f) Must differentiate from juvenile Parkinson disease
g) Adult onset with parkinsonism or a focal dystonia of neck, cranial, or arm involvement
h) No pathologic neurodegeneration
i) Normal fluorodopa PET and β-CIT single photon emission computed tomography
j) Abnormal phenylalanine loading test in GCH defect

2) Autosomal-recessive with mutation of tyrosine hydroxylase gene on chromosome 21; infantile onset
3) Other biopterin-deficient diseases; infantile or adult onset
   a) 6-pyruvoyltetrahydropterin synthase deficiency (second step in BH4 synthesis); autosomal-recessive
   b) pterin-4a-carbinolamine dehydratase deficiency (AR) (required for BH4 regeneration after oxidation); AR
   c) dihydropteridine reductase deficiency (required for BH4 regeneration after oxidation); AR
   d) Sepiapterin reductase deficiency; autosomal-recessive

b. Dopamine agonist–responsive dystonia
   1) Aromatic amino acid decarboxylase deficiency
   2) Autosomal-recessive
c. Rapid-onset dystonia-parkinsonism (RDP)

*Genetics*
1) Autosomal-dominant
2) Mutation found in the α3 subunit of the gene for the Na+/K+-ATPase (*ATP1A3*)

*Clinical Phenotype*
1) Adolescent and adult onset
2) Progresses to generalized over hours to a few weeks
3) Parkinsonian signs present
4) Tends to plateau
5) No known pathology

2. Dystonia with myoclonic jerks that respond to alcohol
a. Myoclonus-dystonia

*Genetics*
1) Autosomal-dominant
2) Gene mapped to chromosome 7q21
3) Mutations in the ε-sarcoglycan gene
4) Another locus on 18p11, gene not identified

*Clinical Phenotype*
1) Alcohol-responsive, lightning-like jerks present
2) Upper body affected, legs usually spared
3) Childhood, adolescent, and adult onset
4) Slowly progressive
5) Tends to plateau
6) Pathology unknown
7) May be same disorder as hereditary essential myoclonus

**C. Secondary Dystonia**

1. Perinatal cerebral injury
   a. Athetoid cerebral palsy
   b. Delayed onset dystonia
   c. Pachygyria

2. Encephalitis, infectious and postinfectious
   a. Reye syndrome
   b. Subacute sclerosing leukoencephalopathy
   c. Creutzfeldt-Jakob disease
   d. HIV infection

3. Head trauma

4. Thalamotomy and thalamic lesions

5. Lenticular nucleus lesions

6. Primary antiphospholipid syndrome

7. Focal cerebral vascular injury

8. Arteriovenous malformation

9. Hypoxia

10. Brain tumor

11. Multiple sclerosis

12. Brainstem lesion, including pontine myelinolysis

13. Posterior fossa tumors

14. Cervical cord injury or lesion, including syringomyelia

15. Lumbar canal stenosis

16. Peripheral injury

17. Electrical injury

18. Drug-induced
    a. Levodopa
    b. Dopamine D2 receptor blocking agents
       1) Acute dystonic reaction
       2) Tardive dystonia
    c. Ergotism
    d. Anticonvulsants

19. Toxins: Mn, CO, carbon disulfide, cyanide, methanol, disulfiram, 3-nitropropionic acid, wasp sting (Leopold et al., 1999)

20. Metabolic: hypoparathyroidism

Box 13-4  Detailed etiologic classification of the dystonias—cont'd

21. Immune encephalopathy: Sjögren syndrome, multiple myeloma, Rasmussen syndrome

22. Psychogenic

### D. Heredodegenerative Diseases (Typically Not Pure Dystonia)

1. X-linked recessive
   a. Lubag (X-linked dystonia-parkinsonism) (*DYT3*)

   *Genetics*
   1) X-linked autosomal-recessive
   2) *DYT3* gene mapped to centromere; Xq13, multiple transcript gene
   3) Extended haplotype

   *Clinical Phenotype*
   1) Filipino males
   2) Occasional Filipino female carriers affected; manifesting chorea or dystonia
   3) Young adult onset
   4) Cranial (oromandibular and lingual) dystonia or generalized dystonia
   5) Parkinsonism can appear at onset and be only feature or develop after and replace dystonia
   6) Steadily progressive → disabling
   7) Pathology: mosaic gliosis in striatum
   8) PET: normal fluorodopa; hypometabolic in striatum

   b. Deafness-dystonia syndrome (Mohr-Tranebjaerg syndrome) (Tranebjaerg et al., 2000; Ujike et al., 2001)

   *Genetics*
   a. X-linked recessive
   b. Mutations in DDP1 (deafness-dystonia peptide 1)
   c. DDP1 acts with human Tim13 in a complex in the intermembrane space of mitochondria (Rothbauer et al., 2001)

   *Clinical Phenotype*
   a. Deafness and dystonia in males
   b. Torticollis and writer's cramp also seen in female carriers (Swerdlow and Wooten, 2001)
   c. Pelizaeus-Merzbacher disease
   d. Mental retardation, seizures, and infantile spasms
   1) Mutations in Aristaless related homeobox gene, ARX. (Stromme et al., 2002)

2. X-linked-dominant
   a. Rett syndrome

3. Autosomal-dominant
   a. Juvenile parkinsonism (presenting with dystonia)
   b. Huntington disease (usually presents as chorea)
   1) Gene: IT15 located at 4p16.3 for protein named huntingtin
   c. Neuroferritinopathy
   d. Machado-Joseph disease (SCA3)
   e. Dentatorubro-pallidoluysian atrophy
   f. Other spinocerebellar degenerations
   g. Creutzfeldt-Jakob disease (Hellmann and Melamed, 2002)

4. Autosomal-recessive
   a. Wilson disease (can also present with tremor or parkinsonism)
   1) Gene: Cu-ATPase located at 13q14.3
   b. Niemann-Pick type C (dystonic lipidosis) (sea-blue histiocytosis) defect in cholesterol esterification; gene mapped to chromosome 18
   c. Juvenile neuronal ceroid-lipofuscinosis (Batten disease)
   d. GM1 gangliosidosis (Campdelacreu et al., 2002)
   e. GM2 gangliosidosis
   f. Metachromatic leukodystrophy
   g. Lesch-Nyhan syndrome
   h. Homocystinuria
   i. Glutaric acidemia
   j. Triosephosphate isomerase deficiency
   k. Methylmalonic aciduria
   l. Hartnup disease
   m. Ataxia telangiectasia
   n. Friedreich ataxia (Hou and Jankovic, 2003)
   o. Neurodegeneration with brain iron accumulation Type 1 (formerly called Hallervorden-Spatz syndrome), recently renamed pantothenate kinase–associated neurodegeneration (PKAN) (Hayflick et al., 2003)
   p. Neuroacanthocytosis
   q. Neuronal intranuclear hyaline inclusion disease
   r. Hereditary spastic paraplegia with dystonia
   s. Sjögren-Larsson syndrome (ichthyosis, spasticity, mental retardation) (Cubo and Goetz, 2000)
   t. Ataxia-amyotrophy-mental retardation-dystonia syndrome (Wilmshurst et al., 2000)

5. Probable autosomal-recessive
   a. Familial basal ganglia calcifications
   b. Progressive pallidal degeneration

6. Mitochondrial
   a. Leigh disease
   1) Genes: nuclear and mitochondrial DNA
   b. Leber disease
   1) Gene: mitochondrial DNA
   c. Other mitochondrial encephalopathies (Sudarsky et al., 1999)

7. Associated with parkinsonian syndromes
   a. Parkinson disease
   b. Progressive supranuclear palsy
   c. Multiple-system atrophy
   d. Cortical-basal ganglionic degeneration

gene has been mapped to 8p21–q22 and designated *DYT6* (Almasy et al., 1997).

Several families with adult-onset familial torticollis have been reported, with one of them (Family K in Northwest Germany) mapped to chromosome 18p, this locus being designated *DYT7* (Leube et al., 1996). Investigation of more families and of apparently sporadic cases of torticollis from this region showed that most have inherited the same mutation as Family K from a common ancestor and, in fact, owe their disease to autosomal-dominant inheritance at low penetrance (Leube et al., 1997a, 1997b). However, subsequent information from these authors now question whether their findings are incorrect (Klein, Ozelius, et al., 1998; Leube and Auburger, 1998). Other families with torticollis have been excluded from the chromosome 18p region and from *DYT1* (Bressman et al., 1996; Cassetta et al., 1999; Jarman et al., 1999).

Cervical-cranial-predominant dystonia is another form of autosomal-dominant primary dystonia; it has been seen in non-Jewish families that do not link to *DYT1* (Bressman, Heiman, et al., 1994; Bressman et al., 1996; Bentivoglio et al., 1997). The site of onset is usually in the neck, which continues to dominate, but dystonia often spreads to involve the cranial structures as well and occasionally the arm. Onset may be in childhood (Bentivoglio et al., 1997) or adulthood (Bressman, Heiman, et al., 1994). An autosomal-dominant Italian family described by Bentivoglio and colleagues (1997, 2004) with onset predominantly with cervical-cranial or brachial dystonia has been mapped to chromosome 1p36.13–p36.32 and has been categorized as *DYT13* (Valente et al., 2001).

## DYSTONIA-PLUS SYNDROMES

Dystonia-plus syndromes represent a group of dystonias that are associated with parkinsonism or myoclonus without known degeneration or loss of neurons; these include dopa-responsive dystonia, dopamine agonist–responsive dystonia, and myoclonus-dystonia. These are therefore considered neurochemical disorders instead of neurodegenerative ones. A neurodegenerative disease is a neurologic disorder due to progressive dying and loss of neurons in the central nervous system, visible by light microscopy, and often accompanied by gliosis and by intracellular inclusions. Many neurodegenerative diseases are inherited, and some are known to have specific metabolic causes, but all produce visible pathologic changes in the brain. A neurochemical disease is a neurologic disorder due to a primary biochemical defect that alters central nervous system function and is not associated with a loss of neurons.

Details of DRD (including GTP cyclohydrolase-1 deficiency, tyrosine hydroxylase (TH) deficiency, and pterin synthesis deficiencies), RDP, and myoclonus-dystonia are presented in their own sections later in the chapter.

A disorder that is analogous to DRD is dopamine agonist–responsive dystonia, which is considered here briefly. It was first described by Hyland and colleagues (1992) (Video 13-16), and a second family was described by Maller and colleagues (1997). It is due to an autosomal-recessive disorder beginning in the first few months of life with hypotonia, hypokinesia, and developmental delay. Eventually, the patient experiences autonomic dysfunction (hyperhidrosis, miosis, and ptosis), dystonia-parkinsonism, episodes of oculogyria and other paroxysmal movements, and bouts of deep sleep (Hyland et al., 1992; Pons et al., 2004). It is the result of reduced activity of aromatic L-amino acid decarboxylase, so there is reduced metabolism of dopa to dopamine and 5-hydroxytryptophan to serotonin (Hyland et al., 1992). There is reduced concentration of the metabolites of dopamine and serotonin in urine, namely, homovanillic acid and 5-hydroxyindoleacetic acid, respectively. The symptoms respond partially to dopamine agonists plus a monoamine oxidase inhibitor. No autopsy was performed on the two affected twin boys and their older sibling who died. The incomplete response to a dopamine agonist and a monoamine oxidase inhibitor makes it uncertain whether this is a neurochemical rather than a neurodegenerative disease; but without an autopsy to determine this, it is placed now in the dystonia-plus category. A report on six cases plus a review of the seven cases in the literature was recently published (Pons et al., 2004).

A similar clinical presentation occurs with several pterin disorders (Hyland et al., 1998). The autosomal-recessive biopterin deficiency states that are listed with the dopa-responsive dystonias in Box 13-4 should be mentioned here because they also manifest features of decreased norepinephrine and serotonin in addition to dystonia and parkinsonism. In this way, they more closely resemble the phenotype of aromatic amino acid decarboxylase deficiency. Their clinical features include miosis, oculogyria, rigidity, hypokinesia, chorea, myoclonus, seizures, temperature disturbance, and hypersalivation. The clinical syndrome can present at any age with generalized dystonia-parkinsonism and with marked diurnal fluctuation (Hanihara et al., 1997). These pterin enzyme deficiencies cause hyperphenylalaninemia, and they may respond partially to levodopa. There are no neuropathologic observations, and they have arbitrarily been listed in the dystonia-plus syndrome category rather than as a neurodegeneration.

## SECONDARY DYSTONIA AND HEREDODEGENERATIVE DISEASES

The secondary dystonias are subdivided into several categories. Those that are due to environmental causes are mainly due to lesions causing structural brain damage, but the secondary dystonias also include psychogenic dystonia (Fahn et al., 1987; Calne and Lang, 1988; Fahn and Williams, 1988) (see Box 13-4). The heredodegenerative disorders are the conditions that are associated with various hereditary neurologic disorders and those in which neuronal degeneration is present.

A major portion of the clinical investigation of dystonia (Fahn et al., 1987) concerns the tests that are required to uncover the etiology of secondary and heredodegenerative dystonias. Almost yearly, new etiologies of these types of dystonia are reported. These include the ingestion of mildewed sugar cane containing the mitochondrial toxin 3-nitropropionic acid (Ludolph et al., 1992), toxoplasmosis in AIDS (Tolge and Factor, 1991), disulfiram intoxication (Krauss et al., 1991), Creutzfeldt-Jakob disease (Sethi and Hess, 1991; Hellmann and Melamed, 2002), primary antiphospholipid syndrome (Angelini et al., 1993), spinal cord lesions (Uncini et al., 1994; Madhusudanan et al., 1995), lumbar canal stenosis resulting in foot dystonia on standing or walking (Blunt et al., 1996), ataxia-telangiectasia (Koepp et al.,1994), alternating hemiplegia of childhood (Andermann et al., 1994), organophosphorus insecticide poisoning (Senanayake and Sanmuganathan, 1995), pure thalamic degeneration (Yamamoto and Yamashita, 1995), midbrain hemorrhage (Munoz et al., 1996), bilateral lesions of the mesencephalon and vermis (Rousseaux et al., 1996), posterior fossa tumors (Krauss et al., 1997), electrical injury (Adler and Caviness, 1997), intracerebral arteritis from herpes zoster ophthalmicus (Burbaud et al., 1997), childhood-onset (Uc et al., 2000) or adult-onset Niemann-Pick type C disease (Lossos et al., 1997), adult GM1 gangliosidosis (Hirayama et al., 1997; Campdelacreu et al., 2002), optic glioma (Vandertop et al., 1997), neuroferritinopathy (Curtis et al., 2001; Mir et al., 2005), dystonia in spinocerebellar ataxia type 1 (Wu et al., 2004) and in type 6 (Sethi and Jankovic, 2002), hand dystonia due to neurofibromatosis type 1 (Di Capua et al., 2001), and striatal necrosis–induced dystonia with acidosis from 3-oxothiolase deficiency (Yalcinkaya et al., 2001). From HIV, there can be dystonia from striatal necrosis (Abbruzzese et al., 1990) or from secondary infections, such as toxoplasmosis (Tolge and Factor, 1991). See the discussion of hemidystonia (almost always secondary dystonia) in the section entitled "Classification by Distribution."

Dystonia can present in patients who have pyruvate dehydrogenase deficiency (Head et al., 2004). The main clue to the biochemical diagnosis is a raised concentration of lactate in the cerebrospinal fluid. These patients can respond to levodopa.

If dystonia occurs in the first year of life, the leading cause is cerebral palsy or a metabolic error, such as glutaric aciduria (Kyllerman et al., 1994). A number of cases of symptomatic dystonias, so-called delayed-onset dystonia, appear months to years after the cerebral insult. Often, such a delayed onset is seen with perinatal or early childhood asphyxia (Saint-Hilaire et al., 1991). Delayed onset of dystonia can also be seen with central pontine myelinolysis (Tison et al., 1991; Maraganore et al., 1992), cyanide intoxication (Valenzuela et al., 1992), head trauma (Lee et al., 1994), and a variety of other static brain lesions (Scott and Jankovic, 1996). Ingestion causes striatal necrosis and coma, and the dystonia evolves as the patient comes out of the coma (He et al., 1995). Dystonia from severe head trauma is usually delayed. Of 221 patients who survived severe head trauma with a Glasgow Coma Score of 8 or less, 4% later developed dystonia (Krauss et al., 1996). The dystonia appeared with a latency of 2 months to 2 years. Delayed-onset generalized dystonia due to cerebral anoxia can worsen over time and show a delay in magnetic resonance imaging (MRI) changes in the globus pallidi (Kuoppamaki et al., 2002). The delayed-onset dystonia from the ingestion of mildewed sugar cane containing the Arthrinium-produced mycotoxin 3-nitropropionic acid is not the same phenomenon. 3-Nitropropionic acid is a mitochondrial toxin that irreversibly inhibits complex II (Beal, 1995).

Clinicians have recognized that dystonia could become worse if an affected limb is casted and immobilized. Okun and colleagues (2002) reported on four patients who developed segmental dystonia following removal of a cast, which the authors attribute to the trauma of prolonged immobilization (Okun et al., 2002).

Dystonia is perhaps the most common movement disorder (often with hypokinesia seen with disorders causing striatal necrosis). Some of these causes are Wilson disease, toxins, metabolic acidosis (such as from 3-oxothiolase deficiency, propionic acidemia, methylmalonic acidemia, isovaleric acidemia, and glutaric aciduria type 1), HIV and other infections, Leigh disease and other mitochondrial encephalopathies, anoxia, wasp sting encephalopathy (Leopold et al., 1999), hemolytic uremia, vascular disease, and head trauma.

The gene for autosomal-recessive neurodegeneration with brain iron accumulation (NBIA) type 1 (formerly known as Hallervorden-Spatz syndrome) has been identified as pantothenate kinase (PANK2) (Zhou et al., 2001; Hartig et al, 2006; Valentino et al, 2006). In 49 families with typical phenotype and MRI for NBIA type 1, Hayflick and colleagues (2003) found that all had the PANK2 deficiency; in another 49 families with an atypical phenotype, only 17 had the enzyme deficiency. In another study, looking at 10 families with MRI positive for iron accumulation, only 4 were found to have a mutation on PANK2 (Thomas et al., 2004). The presence of a mutation in the PANK2 gene was associated with younger age at onset and a higher frequency of dystonia, dysarthria, intellectual impairment, and gait disturbance. Parkinsonism was seen predominantly in adult-onset patients, whereas dystonia seemed to be more frequent in the earlier-onset cases. In the most comprehensive study, involving 72 patients with NBIA, 48 (67%) were found to have a PANK2 mutation (Hartig et al, 2006). No strict correlation between the eye-of-the-tiger sign and PANK2 mutations was found. Not all patients with PANK2 deficiency have the eye-of-the-tiger sign on MRI; there is a report of one child whose eye-of-the-tiger sign disappeared on the MRI scan over time (Baumeister et al., 2005). Although the "eye-of-the-tiger" sign is very characteristic of PANK2 mutation, it may also be seen in patients with other NBIA syndromes, such as neuroferritinopathy and aceruloplasminemia, and in corticobasal degeneration progressive supranuclear palsy (Kumar et al, 2006).

## OTHER MOVEMENT DISORDERS IN WHICH DYSTONIA CAN BE PRESENT

There are some movement disorders, including Parkinson disease and Parkinson-plus syndromes (see Box 13-3) and dystonic tics and paroxysmal dyskinesias, listed in Box 13-5, in which dystonia is present but that are not typically classified as dystonia (see Box 13-5). Hypnogenic dystonia is commonly a manifestation of frontal lobe epilepsy (Sellal et al., 1991; Meierkord et al., 1992; Montagna, 1992) (see Chapter 23).

## PSEUDODYSTONIA

There are other neurologic syndromes in which sustained abnormal postures may be present but that are not considered true dystonias and hence are called pseudodystonias (Box 13-6). These include stiff-person syndrome, Isaacs syndrome, Satoyoshi syndrome (Merello et al., 1994), chronic inflammatory myopathy with involuntary complex repetitive discharges of muscle (Preston et al., 1996), and many others (see Box 13-6).

Box 13-5 Other movement disorders in which dystonia may be present

Tic disorders with dystonic tics
Paroxysmal dyskinesias with dystonia
   Paroxysmal kinesigenic dyskinesia
   Paroxysmal nonkinesigenic dyskinesia
   Paroxysmal exertional dyskinesia
   Benign infantile paroxysmal dyskinesias
Hypnogenic dystonia (sometimes these are seizures)

It has been found that congenital torticollis not only might be due to thickening and tightness of the sternomastoid muscle (labeled congenital muscular torticollis in Box 13-6) but is even more commonly associated with a palpable sternomastoid tumor (Cheng et al., 2001) and may also be due to other causes, including ocular problems. Most commonly, this is due to weakness of the superior oblique muscle, but it can also be due to paresis of the lateral rectus muscle or nystagmus (Williams et al., 1966). Nondystonic torticollis may be due to inflammation of joints (Uziel et al., 1998), soft tissue (Shale et al., 1988), and arteriovenous fistula at the craniocervical junction (Bayrakci et al., 1999). Treatment of congenital muscular torticollis by manual stretching is usually safe and effective; surgical treatment is necessary if this noninvasive treatment fails (Cheng et al., 2001).

Following are discussions of a few of the specific entities listed in Box 13-4.

Box 13-6 Pseudodystonias

These are not classified as dystonia but can be mistaken for dystonia because of sustained postures.
Sandifer syndrome
Stiff-person syndrome
Isaacs syndrome
Satoyoshi syndrome
Rotational atlantoaxial subluxation
Soft tissue nuchal mass
Bone disease
Ligamentous absence, laxity, or damage
Congenital muscular torticollis
Congenital postural torticollis
Juvenile rheumatoid arthritis
Ocular postural torticollis
Congenital Klippel-Feil syndrome
Posterior fossa tumor
Syringomyelia
Arnold Chiari malformation
Trochlear nerve palsy
Vestibular torticollis
Seizures manifesting as sustained twisting postures
Inflammatory myopathy
Torticollis from arteriovenous fistula at craniocervical junction

# OPPENHEIM DYSTONIA

## Clinical

The phenotype of Oppenheim dystonia (also known as *DYT1* dystonia) was characterized in the Ashkenazi Jewish population when detection of individuals with the *DYT1* mutation became possible because of the identification of the special genetic haplotype around the *DYT1* gene in this population (Bressman, de Leon, et al., 1994). The mean (± standard deviation) age at onset of symptoms is 12.5 ± 8.2 years. In 94% of patients, symptoms begin in a limb (arm or leg equally) (Videos 13-17 and 13-18); rarely, the disorder starts in the neck (3.3%) or larynx (2.2%). Even in the non-Jewish population, the same gene is responsible for most cases of early-onset and limb-onset PTD (Kramer et al., 1994). Over time, as diagnostic laboratory examinations for *DYT1* have become available, some variations of the phenotype have been observed (Edwards et al., 2003). The phenotype varies widely even in the same family, as has been reported in one large family with a proven *DYT1* gene mutation (Opal et al., 2002). The proband of this family died with a dystonic storm, while other family members carrying the same mutation either were asymptomatic or displayed dystonia that was focal, segmental, multifocal, or generalized in distribution. One family member had onset of her dystonia at age 64 years.

The phenotypes in families with non-*DYT1* dystonia overlap with each other but differ from those with *DYT1* dystonia. In the majority of non-*DYT1* families, the dystonia most commonly begins in the cranial-cervical region (Bentivoglio et al., 1997), whereas this site of onset is rare in *DYT1* dystonia (Bressman, de Leon, et al., 1994). Only in *DYT6* dystonia in the Mennonite population is there some clinical phenotypic overlap with Oppenheim dystonia (Almasy et al., 1997).

Sequence learning of motor tasks is reduced in manifesting and nonmanifesting gene carriers (Ghilardi et al., 2003). PET imaging obtained during motor task testing showed increased activation in the left premotor cortex and right supplementary motor area, with concomitant reduction in the posterior medial cerebellum. During sequence learning, activation responses in *DYT1* carriers were increased in the left ventral prefrontal cortex and lateral cerebellum. These findings suggest that abnormalities in motor behavior and brain function exist in clinically nonmanifesting *DYT1* carriers. Similarly, depression has been found in both manifesting and nonmanifesting *DYT1* carriers (Heiman et al., 2004).

## Genetics

In both Jewish (Bressman et al., 1989) and non-Jewish groups (Zeman and Dyken, 1967), Oppenheim dystonia is inherited as an autosomal-dominant disorder, and the gene has been localized to the long arm of chromosome 9 (9q34.1) (Ozelius et al., 1989; Kramer et al., 1990). This abnormal gene has been given the name *DYT1* but has been officially renamed TOR1A. The mutation that causes the disease has been identified as a deletion of one of a pair of GAG triplets (codes for glutamic acid) from the carboxy terminal in the previously unknown protein, designated, torsinA (Ozelius et al., 1997). The GAG deletion is the only sequence change that has been found thus far to be associated uniquely with the disease status, regardless of ethnic origin. Mutations causing this deletion are uncommon, but a few have been encountered (Klein, Brin, et al., 1998; Valente et al., 1999), and the unique haplotype found in North American and Russian Ashkenazi Jews with *DYT1* has also been seen in Great Britain (Valente et al., 1999).

Not every non-Jewish family with dystonia has the *DYT1* gene, so dystonia is genetically heterogeneous (Bressman, Heiman, et al., 1994; Bressman, Hunt, et al., 1994). But all Ashkenazi Jewish families with dystonia with limb onset and onset below the age of 49 in at least one member have so far been found to have the *DYT1* gene. Also most cases of non-Jewish individuals with limb-onset and childhood-onset have *DYT1* dystonia (Kramer et al., 1994). Intrafamilial correlation for age at onset of dystonia is low (Fletcher et al., 1991b). There is some evidence that dystonia in the Ashkenazi Jewish population tends to begin on the dominant side (Inzelberg et al., 1993). The penetrance rate of gene expression in the Ashkenazi Jewish population is approximately 30% (Bressman et al., 1989; Risch et al., 1990).

Previously, Eldridge (1970) proposed that dystonia in the Ashkenazi Jewish population was inherited as an autosomal–recessive disorder, whereas non-Jews inherited dystonia as an autosomal-dominant disorder. Reanalysis of Eldridge's data by segregation analysis has shown that dystonia in the Jewish population was also inherited as autosomal-dominant (Pauls and Korczyn, 1990). A detailed analysis of the clinical course of dystonia was compared in the Jewish and non-Jewish populations with inherited dystonia, and no major difference was found (Burke et al., 1986). The prevalence of dystonia among Jews of Eastern European ancestry has been estimated to be 1 per 15,000 (Zilber et al., 1984), while for non-Jews, the prevalence is 1 per 200,000 (Zeman and Dyken, 1967).

With the availability of direct testing for the *DYT1* mutation, Bressman and her colleagues (2000) have developed an algorithm as to which individuals who have the clinical diagnosis of PTD should be tested. They suggest testing in conjunction with genetic counseling for patients with PTD with onset before age 26 years, as this single criterion detected 100% of clinically ascertained carriers, with specificities of 43% to 63%. Testing patients with onset after age 26 years also may be warranted in those having an affected relative with early onset. The *DYT1* gene rarely is found in patients with musician's cramp (Friedman et al., 2000) or in patients with sporadic or familial writer's cramp (Kamm et al., 2000).

The relationship between essential tremor and dystonia has been debated (Lou and Jankovic, 1991; Lang et al., 1992). The finding that families with essential tremor do not have the *DYT1* gene by linkage analysis (Conway et al., 1993; Durr et al., 1993) indicates that the two disorders are not genetically identical.

## Molecular Biology

TorsinA is related to homologous proteins throughout the multicellular animal kingdom (Breakefield et al., 2001). It is a 332-amino acid protein and has a molecular weight of 37,813. The torsin family is a member of the AAA+ family of proteins. Their structures indicate that they are heat-shock and ATP-binding proteins. The impairment of torsinA could explain why stress has been able to induce the onset or the worsening of Oppenheim dystonia. Normal torsinA appears to protect against oxidative stress (Kuner et al., 2003), and torsinA is increased following exposure to the toxin MPTP (Kuner et al., 2004). A malfunctioning torsinA would have difficulty carrying out its chaperoning of damaged proteins that had been altered by a variety of stress factors.

TorsinA mRNA has been mapped in normal human brain and found to be localized in specific regions (Augood et al., 1998, 1999), which are listed in Box 13-7. A similar localization was found by using immunostaining for an antibody raised against torsinA (Augood et al., 2003). Although its location within dopamine neurons, among other types, have suggested to some investigators that dopamine is implicated in Oppenheim dystonia, clinical pharmacology has not yet seen a relationship, and biochemically, dopamine concentration is normal except for a 50% reduction in the rostral portions of the putamen and caudate nucleus in a single case (Furukawa et al., 2000) and a possible increase in striatal dopamine turnover in three cases (Augood et al., 2002). A morphometric analysis of the pigmented SNc neurons found no difference in neuron number, but the average size of neuronal cell bodies was increased, and dopaminergic SNc neurons were arranged in much closer apposition to each other than was observed in control tissue (Rostasy et al., 2003).

Antibodies to torsinA have been prepared in several laboratories. The normal protein is widely distributed in human, rat, and mouse brain (Shashidharan et al., 2000b; Konakova et al., 2001; Konakova and Pulst, 2001; Walker et al., 2001) and is found in endoplasmic reticulum (ER) (Hewett et al., 2000; Kustedjo et al., 2000). TorsinA immunohistochemistry investigation of a brain from a patient with Oppenheim dystonia failed to show any difference from control brains (Walker et al., 2002; Rostasy et al., 2003). The cholinergic neurons in rat striatum have a high content of torsinA during development, but then this concentration fades as the animal gets older (Oberlin et al., 2004). This temporal and anatomic pattern could fit with some clinical features of Oppenheim dystonia: young-onset with usual sparing after age 28 years and response to high-dose antimuscarinic agents.

---

**Box 13-7** Localization of torsinA

**Intense Expression**
Substantia nigra pars compacta dopamine neurons
Locus coeruleus
Cerebellar dentate nucleus
Purkinje cells
Basis pontis
Numerous thalamic nuclei
Pedunculopontine nucleus
Oculomotor nucleus
Hippocampal formation
Frontal cortex

**Moderate Expression**
Cholinergic neurons in the caudate-putamen
Numerous midbrain and hindbrain nuclei

**Weak Expression**
Noncholinergic striatal neurons
Globus pallidus
Subthalamic nucleus

Data from Augood SJ, Martin DM, Ozelius LJ, et al: Distribution of the mRNAs encoding torsinA and torsinB in the normal adult human brain. Ann Neurol 1999;46(5):761–769.

The AAA+ family of proteins is believed to serve as a chaperone in the processing and repair of damaged proteins. Six torsinA proteins are thought to join together to form a ring, with each of these six proteins bound to its neighbor by ATP. This structure is believed to function to repair other proteins that have been damaged. If the repair is unsuccessful, the damaged proteins can aggregate or die by apoptosis. In neural cultures (Hewett et al., 2000), the normal protein is found throughout the cytoplasm and neurites with a high degree of colocalization with the ER. In contrast, overexpression of the mutant protein in transgenic mice showed an accumulation of the protein in multiple, large inclusions in the cytoplasm around the nucleus. These inclusions were composed of membrane whorls, apparently derived from the ER. If disrupted processing of the mutant protein leads to its accumulation in multilayer membranous structures in vivo, these may interfere with membrane trafficking in neurons.

Immunohistochemical studies showed that torsinA is present in Lewy bodies (Shashidharan et al., 2000a; Sharma et al., 2001). A role of torsinA in α-synuclein, a major component of the Lewy body, was subsequently sought. Overexpression of wild-type torsinA dramatically reduced the number of transfected cells containing α-synuclein aggregates, whereas mutant torsinA failed to suppress α-synuclein aggregation (McLean et al., 2002)

TorsinA immunohistochemistry investigation of brains from patients with *DYT1* dystonia failed to show any difference from control brains (Walker et al., 2002; Rostasy et al., 2003). A morphometric analysis of the pigmented SNc neurons found no difference in neuron number, but the average size of neuronal cell bodies was increased, and dopaminergic SNc neurons were arranged in much closer apposition to each other than was observed in control tissue (Rostasy et al., 2003). Other evidence for a role in preventing protein aggregation comes from studies of the torsinA homologue in *Caenorhabditis elegans*, TOR-2 (Caldwell et al., 2003). TOR-2 also appears to be an ER protein, Overexpression of either TOR-2 or human wild-type torsinA significantly suppressed the aggregation of a polyglutamine repeat protein, whereas a mutant form of TOR-2 failed to reduce protein aggregation (Caldwell et al., 2003).

Wild-type torsinA is distributed throughout the cell and is particularly enriched in the lumen of the ER (Hewett et al., 2000; Kustedjo et al., 2000). Mutant torsinA concentrates in large clumps that are largely or completely segregated from the ER. The clumps of mutant torsinA immunostaining are not insoluble aggregates (Kustedjo et al., 2000), and they appear to be composed of whorled double-membrane structures, apparently derived from the ER (Hewett et al., 2000). This DeltaE302/303 mutation appears to be a stable protein and not toxic. The DeltaE302/3 mutation causes a striking redistribution of torsinA from the ER to the nuclear envelope (Gonzalez-Alegre and Paulson, 2004; Goodchild and Dauer, 2004; Hewett et al., 2004; Naismith et al., 2004). Oppenheim dystonia therefore appears to be a previously uncharacterized nuclear envelope disease and the first to selectively affect central nervous system function. Goodchild and Dauer (2005) found that normal torsinA binds a substrate in the lumen of the nuclear envelope, and the DeltaE mutation enhances this interaction. They identified lamina-associated polypeptide 1 (LAP1) as a torsinA-interacting protein. Goodchild and colleagues (2005) went on to show that genetic animal models without torsinA or with abnormal torsinA have severely abnormal nuclear membranes in neurons, whereas non-neuronal cell types appear normal. These observations demonstrate that neurons have a unique requirement for nuclear envelope localized torsinA function and suggest that loss of this activity is a key molecular event in the pathogenesis of *DYT1* dystonia. The mutant torsinA has also been shown to have a reduction of its normal ATPase activity (Konakova and Pulst, 2005). Membranous inclusions, which were found to occur in cells transfected with the mutant torsinA (Hewett et al., 2000), have now also been found in patients with Oppenheim dystonia (McNaught et al., 2004). They are present in the perinuclear region within brainstem cholinergic and other neurons in the pedunculopontine nucleus, cuneiform nucleus, and griseum centrale mesencephali. The inclusions stain positively for ubiquitin, torsinA, and the nuclear envelope protein lamin A/C. No inclusions were detected in the substantia nigra pars compacta, striatum, hippocampus, or selected regions of the cerebral cortex. McNaught and colleagues (2004) also noted tau/ubiquitin-immunoreactive aggregates in pigmented neurons of the substantia nigra pars compacta and locus coeruleus.

## DOPA-RESPONSIVE DYSTONIA

It should be mentioned that in addition to the genetic types described in this section, some patients with focal dystonias, including familial cases, might respond to levodopa therapy. A report of two families with a total of four members with childhood-onset cervical dystonia, all of whom had an excellent response to levodopa, illustrates this point (Schneider et al., 2006). Genetic testing on these patients showed that they did not have any of the genetic types discussed in this section. It is possible that these cases may represent new forms of dopa-responsive dystonia.

### Classic Dopa-Responsive Dystonia

Segawa and his colleagues (1976) described a syndrome of dystonia in children that has a diurnal pattern. The children may be relatively free of dystonic movements and postures in the morning and be severely afflicted in the late afternoon, evening, and night (Videos 13-19, 13-20, and 13-21). Segawa and colleagues (1976) called this disorder hereditary progressive dystonia with diurnal variation; they also mentioned that it responds to levodopa. Independently, Allen and Knopp (1976) described a form of childhood hereditary dystonia that had features of parkinsonism that showed sustained control by levodopa and anticholinergic medication. This was the same disorder.

Over time, several clinical features have been distinguished as highlighting this disorder: (1) Many patients with onset of dystonia in childhood have features of parkinsonism, including rigidity, bradykinesia, flexed posture, and loss of postural reflexes. (2) The disorder usually, but not exclusively, begins in childhood with a presentation of a peculiar gait, namely, a tendency to walk on the toes. (3) The disease can begin in infancy, thereby resembling cerebral palsy (Nygaard et al., 1994) (Videos 13-22 and 13-23), and there has now been a report of a neonatal onset of rigidity, tremor, and dystonia (Nardocci et al., 2003). (4) When the disorder begins in adulthood, it can present as a focal dystonia of the arm, neck, or cranium or present as parkinsonism, mimicking Parkinson disease (Nygaard et al.,

1992) (Video 13-24). (5) The patients respond remarkably well to low-dose levodopa. (6) Not all patients with childhood-onset dystonia have the diurnal fluctuation pattern. (7) Writer's cramp can be brought out with continued writing (Deonna et al., 1997). The term *dopa-responsive dystonia* (DRD) appears to be the preferred label for this disorder (Nygaard, 1989; Nygaard et al., 1990), because response to levodopa is the consistent finding, and the term also highlights the appropriate treatment. Moreover, the term *hereditary progressive dystonia* could apply to many genetic forms of dystonia and could certainly apply to the more virulent Oppenheim dystonia.

If levodopa therapy is delayed for a great many years, patients still respond to low doses of levodopa (Harwood et al., 1994) (Video 13-25). Even if the onset is in adulthood, presenting as parkinsonism and resembling Parkinson disease, it responds to low doses of levodopa and without adverse effects of response fluctuations (Nygaard et al., 1992; Harwood et al., 1994). Long-term treatment with levodopa does not cause the wearing-off phenomenon. Worsening of dystonia does not occur until 29 hours or more after levodopa withdrawal; the subjective feeling of wearing-off that is experienced by patients with DRD might be from one of the non-motor effects of levodopa, such as mood elevation (Dewey et al., 1998).

DRD is inherited in an autosomal-dominant pattern and needs to be recognized because it is so easily treated. The gene causing DRD has been mapped to chromosome 14q by Nygaard and colleagues (1993) and identified by Ichinose and colleagues (1994) as the gene for the enzyme GTP cyclohydrolase I (GCH), the rate-limiting enzyme in the biosynthesis of tetrahydrobiopterin (BH4), which is the cofactor of monoamine-synthesizing enzyme TH for dopamine and norepinephrine and tryptophan hydroxylase for serotonin. The genetic designation *DYT5* has been assigned to this form of dystonia (see Box 13-1). Clinically, only dystonia and parkinsonism are manifested. Approximately 40% to 50% of patients with DRD have no known mutations (Furukawa and Kish, 1999).

Different families have different mutations on the same GCH gene (Hirano et al., 1995; Ichinose et al., 1995; Bandmann et al., 1996; Furukawa et al., 1996, 1998b; Ichinose and Nagatsu, 1997; Jarman et al., 1997; Thony and Blau, 1997; Steinberger et al., 1998; Tamaru et al., 1998), and spontaneous mutations have been identified. The multiple mutations are scattered over the entire coding region for the six-exon-containing GCH gene.

Phenylalanine hydroxylase also requires the cofactor BH4 for its activity, and homozygous mutations and compound heterozygous mutations have been found in the GCH gene to cause the rare autosomal-recessively inherited form of hyperphenylalaninemia (Thony and Blau, 1997; Furukawa et al., 1998a). Such mutations are therefore clinically similar to the compound heterozygous or homozygous mutations spread over all six exons encoding 6-pyruvoyl-tetrahydropterin synthase, which manifests as an autosomal-recessively inherited variant of hyperphenylalaninemia, along with a deficiency of dopamine and serotonin. Hyperphenylalaninemia may be mild and go undetected neonatally; the child can develop dystonia later in childhood, along with developmental delay and seizures. The condition is treatable with levodopa, 5-hydroxytryptophan, and tetrahydrobiopterin (Demos et al., 2005). The other autosomal recessive pterin deficiency disorders also respond to levodopa, but they often have developmental delay, oculogyria, and dysautonomic features. Sepiapterin reductase deficiency appears to be fairly common in Malta (Neville et al., 2005). Although dystonia can respond to levodopa, cognitive impairment does not.

In some pedigrees with DRD, a mutation in the GCH gene has not been found. This fact, plus the multiple mutations in the GCH gene that have been discovered so far, indicated that genetic testing will not be an easy method to determine the presence of the molecular defect. Nagatsu and Ichinose (1997) found that GCH activity in lymphocytes is decreased to less that 20% of the mean value of healthy controls; that in unaffected carriers was 37%. The enzyme had normal activity in juvenile parkinsonism. These authors suggest that assay of GCH in blood cells might become a useful biochemical marker for the gene defect. A deficiency of neopterin is found in cerebrospinal fluid, but this is reduced in juvenile parkinsonism also.

PET scans for fluorodopa uptake and dopamine transport are normal, whereas those for the D2 receptor show increased binding, reflecting supersensitivity (Rinne et al., 2004). Network analysis, using FDG PET, shows that DRD has a unique metabolic architecture that differs from other inherited forms of dystonia (Asanuma et al., 2005a). The characteristic features are increases in metabolism in the dorsal midbrain, cerebellum, and supplementary motor area and reductions in motor and lateral premotor cortex and in the basal ganglia.

There has been a report of a patient with DRD who had a remission (Di Capua and Bertini, 1995), which perhaps should not come as a surprise because not every carrier of the mutation has symptoms. In fact, affected females outnumber affected males by a ratio of approximately 4:1 (Nagatsu and Ichinose 1997). This ratio has been explained by the observation that males have a higher GCH activity normally, so missing one of the two genes by a mutation may still leave sufficient enzyme intact to avoid symptoms. There is also a report that SSRI antidepressants reversed the benefit from levodopa therapy (Mathen et al., 1999).

The phenotype of DRD is not always easily distinguished from juvenile parkinsonism, but features that help in the differential diagnosis are presented in Table 13-5. Fluorodopa PET scanning reveals a normal or modest reduction of dopa uptake (Sawle et al., 1991; Nygaard et al., 1992; Snow et al., 1993; Turjanski et al., 1993), in contrast to the marked reduction in juvenile parkinsonism. A similar result is seen with β-CIT single photon emission computed tomography (Jeon, 1997; Naumann, Pirker, et al., 1997) or other dopamine transporter ligands (Huang et al., 2002). Another important difference is that long-term treatment with levodopa in DRD is not associated with the motor complications that are seen with levodopa therapy in juvenile (and adult) Parkinson disease (Nygaard et al., 1991; Nygaard et al., 1992; Harwood et al., 1994).

One unusual phenotypic expression is myoclonus, which occurred in one kindred and preceded the dystonia and bradykinesia (Leuzzi et al., 2002). Molecular genetics investigation found a missense mutation in exon 6 of the GCH gene. Another phenotype of DRD is adult-onset oromandibular dystonia and no obvious family history of dystonia, which was found in one individual who had a mutation of GCH and who responded positively to treatment with levodopa (Steinberger et al., 1999).

Table 13-5 Differential features between juvenile parkinsonism, dopa-responsive dystonia, and primary torsion dystonia

| Clinical Feature | Juvenile PD | DRD | Childhood PTD |
| --- | --- | --- | --- |
| Age Onset | Rare < 8 years | Infancy to 12 years | Uncommon below age 6 years |
| Gender | Predominantly male | Predominantly female | Equal |
| Initial Sign | Foot dystonia or PD | Foot, leg dystonia or gait disorder | Arm or leg dystonia |
| Dystonia | At onset | Throughout | Throughout |
| Diurnal | Perhaps | Sometimes | No |
| Sleep Benefit | Yes | Sometimes | No |
| Bradykinesia | Present | Present | No |
| Pull Test | Abnormal | Abnormal | Normal |
| Gait | Abnormal | Abnormal | Abnormal if leg or trunk is affected |
| Anticholinergic Response | Yes | Yes | Yes |
| Dopa Responsive | Yes | Yes | No, or mild |
| Dopa Dosage | Moderate to high | Very low | High |
| "Off" Episodes | Fluctuations | Stable | Unknown |
| Dyskinesias | Prominent | With high-dose dopa | Unknown |
| Fluorodopa PET | Decreased | Normal or borderline | Normal |
| ßCIT SPECT | Decreased | Normal | Normal |
| CSF HVA | Decreased | Decreased | Normal |
| CSF Neopterin | Moderately decreased | Marked decreased | Normal |
| Phenylalanine Test | Normal | Abnormal | Normal |
| Prognosis | Progressive | Plateaus | Usually worsens |

The first report of the pathology of a case of DRD-GCH type revealed decreased neuromelanin in the substantia nigra but otherwise normal nigral cell counts and morphology (Rajput et al., 1994). Biochemically, this patient had reduced concentrations of dopamine and its metabolite, homovanillic acid, in both the caudate and putamen. Furukawa and his colleagues (1999) carried out more extensive postmortem biochemistry in two patients with typical DRD. One had two GCH mutations, but the other had no mutation in the coding region of this gene. Striatal biopterin and neopterin levels were markedly reduced. Both had severely reduced (<3%) TH protein levels and normal concentrations of dopa decarboxylase protein, dopamine transporter, and vesicular monoamine transporters. The authors suggested that the reduction of TH protein might be explained by reduced enzyme stability/expression consequent to congenital BH4 deficiency.

A second autopsy report of DRD was on a patient with a different genetic locus, chromosome 14q13, and called *DYT14* by Grotzsch and colleagues (2002). This entity can be considered a third type of DRD, with TH deficiency, discussed in the next section, being the second type. The proband was an elderly, wheelchair-bound woman who had begun walking on her toes at age 3 years. Walking worsened gradually, and ankle release surgery was performed. Dystonia eventually spread to the upper body. At age 73, she was admitted for pneumonia, and rest tremor of one leg was recognized. She was treated with levodopa and improved dramatically, though she was still not able to walk. A diagnosis of DRD was made, and family members were found to be affected. An autopsy revealed a normal number of cells in the substantia nigra and locus coeruleus, which is typical of DRD and not Parkinson disease, but there was a decrease in neuromelanin. No Lewy bodies were seen. Genetic testing failed to find a mutation in the GCH gene. Linkage studies of family members found a >3 LOD score at 14q13.

## Tyrosine Hydroxylase Deficiency

TH deficiency is usually a more serious form of dopa-responsive dystonia and is transmitted as an autosomal-recessive disorder. The presence of dystonia and parkinsonism in infancy is the clinical clue that this disorder should be suspected. Biochemical analysis of cerebrospinal fluid will provide some evidence, but ultimately, testing for the gene mutation is required to establish the diagnosis.

At least eight different point mutations have now been discovered in the human TH gene, and more are reported regularly (Knappskog et al., 1995; Lüdecke et al., 1995, 1996; van den Heuvel et al., 1998; de Rijk-van Andel et al., 2000; Janssen et al., 2000; Swaans et al., 2000; Furukawa et al., 2001). Many of the reports are in Dutch families. The clinical features range from a mild syndrome of juvenile DRD to a more severe parkinsonism, dystonia, and oculogyric crises (all three representing dopamine deficiency) and also ptosis, miosis, oropharyngeal secretions, and postural hypotension (all representing norepinephrine deficiency). In the most severe form, the infant was virtually immobile, rigid, drooling saliva, with a tremor in tongue and hands. She responded dramatically to levodopa. The severity appears to be associated with the amount of loss of TH activity. Genetically, there can be homozygous mutations to heterozygous mutations. One compound heterozygote presented as spastic paraparesis, but a complete response to levodopa led to the correct diagnosis (Furukawa et al., 2001). Some patients with a mild form of the disorder live a normal life with a response to low-dose levodopa into adulthood. One reported problem is hypersensitivity to levodopa (Grattan-Smith et al., 2002). Hoffmann and colleagues (2003) reported four patients with TH deficiency and emphasized that most patients with this disorder have an encephalopathy that is not predominantly dystonia, but a progressive, often lethal encephalopathic disorder, which can be improved but not cured by levodopa. The DRD of TH deficiency can be as responsive to levodopa as is *DYT5* with GCH involvement. Schiller and colleagues (2004) report sustained benefit and excellent response to levodopa even when treatment was delayed for 20 years.

A phenylalanine-loading test has been recommended as a means to distinguish between DRD with GCH deficiency and that with TH deficiency (Hyland et al., 1997). In the former, phenylalanine is not metabolized rapidly, and the blood levels remain elevated for prolonged period. In TH deficiency, this test would be normal. One other potential method of differentiating GCH-deficient DRD from other DRDs or juvenile parkinsonism is the exquisite sensitivity to centrally acting anticholinergics. Some of the trihexyphenidyl responders reported by Fahn (1983) had responded to small doses, such as 6 mg per day. These patients were subsequently determined to have DRD. When trihexyphenidyl was first reported for the treatment of Parkinson disease, some papers pointed out that small doses could have a dramatic benefit in some children with dystonia (Corner, 1952; Burns, 1959). These children had diurnal fluctuations of their dystonia. Jarman and colleagues (1997) screened some of their patients with responsiveness to anticholinergics and found that some had a GCH mutation.

## RAPID-ONSET DYSTONIA-PARKINSONISM

RDP is an autosomal-dominant movement disorder characterized by sudden onset of persistent dystonia and parkinsonism, generally during adolescence or early adulthood (Dobyns and colleagues, 1993). Symptoms evolve over hours or days and generally stabilize within a few weeks, with slow or no progression. Members of a family who are wide apart in age may develop symptoms around the same time. Further follow-up of the original family revealed two members to have a more gradual progression of their disorder over 6 to 18 months. One of them experienced a rapid progression of symptoms 2 years after an initial stabilization of his condition. The phenotype therefore shows considerable variability. Two other, seemingly unrelated kindreds have now been reported (Brashear et al., 1997; Pittock et al., 2000).

Other features include little or no response to levodopa or dopamine agonists and low concentration of homovanillic acid in the cerebrospinal fluid in patients and in some asymptomatic suspected carriers (Brashear et al., 1998). PET studies indicate no loss of dopaminergic nerve terminals in RDP, suggesting that this disorder results from a functional deficit rather than being a neurodegenerative disease. An autopsied case revealed no neurodegeneration (Pittock et al., 2000).

The gene for RDP has been mapped to chromosome 19q13 (Kramer et al.., 1999) and has been identified as the gene for Na-K-ATPase (de Carvalho Aguiar et al., 2004). Six missense mutations in the $\alpha 3$ subunit (*ATP1A3*) were found in seven unrelated families with RDP. Functional studies and structural analysis of the protein suggest that these mutations impair enzyme activity or stability. This finding implicates the $Na^+/K^+$ pump, a crucial protein that is responsible for the electrochemical gradient across the cell membrane. The authors suggest that the rapid onset that is seen in the disorder is related to an inability to "keep up with a high demand for ion transport activity" in response to stressful situations. However, there is genetic hetereogeneity, because one large family with the RDP phenotype was found not to have a mutation in the *ATP1A3* gene (Kabakci et al., 2005).

Now that at least one gene for RDP has been found, genetic analysis can be carried out in dopa-nonresponsive parkinsonism. After being stable for 2.5 years, one patient thought to have Parkinson disease developed overnight oromandibular dystonia and more severe parkinsonian symptoms; he was found to have a missense mutation in the *ATP1A3* gene (Kamphuis et al., 2006).

## MYOCLONUS-DYSTONIA

Myoclonic movements were mentioned earlier in the chapter in the description of the phenomenology of dystonia. Although lightning-like movements can occur in Oppenheim dystonia, they can also be seen in a distinct autosomal-dominant disorder. Both conditions have unfortunately been called myoclonic dystonia, and in both, the myoclonic jerks can respond to alcohol. It has been recommended that when myoclonic jerks is part of Oppenheim dystonia, it should be referred to as dystonia with lightning-like jerks or as myoclonic dystonia (Quinn et al., 1988). The autosomal-dominant myoclonus-dystonia that is a distinct entity has been mapped to chromosome 7q21, and the mutated gene has been identified as the gene for $\varepsilon$-sarcoglycan (Zimprich et al., 2001; Asmus et al., 2002). The report of a mutation in the gene for the dopamine D2 receptor in a single family (Klein et al., 1999) has now been recognized to most likely represent a polymorphism (Klein, Gurvich, et al., 2000). This family has since been found to have genetic linkage to 7q21–q31 like the other families (Klein, Schilling, et al., 2000). Whether myoclonus-dystonia is an entity separate from hereditary essential myoclonus (Fahn and Sjaastad, 1991; Quinn, 1996) remains to be determined through genetic studies.

The onset can be in childhood or in adulthood. The myoclonus and dystonia are located predominantly in the arms and neck (Videos 13-26 and 13-27), and the symptoms  tend to plateau after a period of progression (Kyllerman et al., 1990). Obsessive-compulsive disorder and alcohol dependence are not uncommon in individuals who carry the gene (Saunders-Pullman et al., 2002). In an evaluation of the phenotype in three separate kindreds, other psychiatric problems were reported, including substance abuse, anxiety/panic/phobic disorders, and psychosis (Doheny et al., 2002). Cognitive testing showed impaired verbal learning and memory in one family, impaired memory in the second family, and no cognitive deficits in the third family.

In a family with myoclonus-dystonia containing a mutation in the $\varepsilon$-sarcoglycan gene, there was also another mutation (DeltaF323-Y328 mutation), this being in the *DYT1* gene in which a sequence of six amino acids was removed (Klein et al., 2002). This mutation in the *DYT1* gene does not appear to have produced any phenotypic alteration, and the localization of this mutant torsinA within the cell is similar to wild-type torsinA and unlike the DeltaE302/303 mutation (O'Farrell et al., 2002).

There is markedly reduced penetrance if the parent carrying the mutation is the mother (penetrance is about 5% to 10%, whereas if the father carries the mutation, the penetrance is about 90%). This pattern of phenotypic expression of myoclonus-dystonia is called maternal imprinting. As Asmus and Gasser (2004) explained, if the mutated allele is inherited from the father, inactivation of the maternal allele due to imprinting leads to complete ε-sarcoglycan deficiency and hence to the development of clinical symptoms. If, on the other hand, the mutated allele is inherited from the mother, the intact paternal allele is sufficient to sustain ε-sarcoglycan function. Making the inheritance pattern more complicated is one report of reduced penetrance in which the mutated gene was inherited from the father (Muller et al., 2002).

Another gene locus has recently been found for one family with myoclonus-dystonia on chromosome 18p11 (Grimes et al., 2002). In a study of Dutch families with myoclonus-dystonia, only 7 of 31 patients had carried a mutation in the ε-sarcoglycan gene (Gerrits et al., 2006).

## SECONDARY DYSTONIAS

In a movement disorders center, primary dystonias are much more common than are secondary dystonias. A screen for the *DYT1* gene in Ashkenazi Jewish patients with secondary dystonia failed to find any evidence that the *DYT1* mutation contributes to secondary dystonia (Bressman et al., 1997), including tardive dystonia and other environmental insults. The most common secondary dystonias seen at the Dystonia Clinical Research at Columbia University Medical Center are presented in Table 13-6.

### Tardive Dystonia

Tardive dystonia is the most common form of symptomatic dystonia seen at the Movement Disorders Center at Columbia University Medical Center (see Table 13-6). It can manifest itself exactly like PTD, but there is often accompanying classic tardive dyskinesia or tardive akathisia, which establishes the diagnosis. One form of clinical presentation seems more common in tardive dystonia: Many patients have retrocollis and extension of the elbows with internal rotation of the shoulders and flexion of the wrists. Tardive dystonia is a persistent dystonia as a result of a complication of drugs that block

Table 13-6 Common causes of torsion dystonia

| Cause | n |
| --- | --- |
| Primary | 1762 |
| Tardive dystonia | 184 |
| Birth injury | 83 |
| Psychogenic | 64 |
| Peripheral trauma | 51 |
| Head injury | 39 |
| Stroke | 27 |
| Encephalitis | 24 |
| Miscellaneous | 164 |
| Total | 2398 |

Data from the Center for Parkinson's Disease and Other Movement Disorders, Columbia University Medical Center, New York City.

dopamine receptors. Clinical features of tardive dystonia are discussed in detail in Chapter 20.

### Acute Dystonic Reactions

Acute dystonic reactions can occur from drugs that block dopamine receptors; these reactions are widely recognized and easily treated with antihistaminics and anticholinergics. Acute dystonia has also been reported with exposure to domperidone (Bonuccelli et al., 1991), amitriptyline (Ornadel et al., 1992), fluoxetine (Dave, 1994), clozapine (Kastrup et al., 1994; Thomas et al., 1994), and dextromethorphan (Graudins and Fern, 1996). Since domperidone is a peripherally acting dopamine receptor blocker, the acute dystonic reaction suggests that some of the drug entered the central nervous system, at least in the affected patient, who had polycystic ovary syndrome. Amitriptyline would ordinarily not be expected to produce such a reaction; the clinical description is that typical for acute dystonia after a neuroleptic, but no such drug was known to have been taken by the patient.

The so-called atypical antipsychotic drugs have been shown to have less risk for causing acute dystonic reactions. In one study evaluating a population of patients consecutively admitted to a psychiatric intensive-care unit, 1337 cases were treated with antipsychotics (Raja and Azzoni, 2001). The authors observed 41 cases (3.1%) of acute dystonic reactions. Four occurred with risperidone monotherapy, one with olanzapine, and one with quetiapine. The remaining cases were with medications labeled as typical antipsychotics.

Serotonergic agents have also been reported to induce acute dystonic reactions (Lopez-Alemany et al., 1997; Madhusoodanan and Brenner, 1997; Olivera, 1997). Serotonergic agents, such as fluoxetine, can inhibit dopaminergic neurons in the substantia nigra, worsening parkinsonism (Baldessarini and Marsh, 1992). This might somehow be related to the development of the dystonic reaction. How clozapine induces an acute dystonic reaction is unknown; it could relate to binding to the D2 receptor, the D4 receptor, or the 5-HT$_2$ receptor.

### Other Secondary Dystonias

A large number of injuries to the nervous system can result in secondary dystonia (see Box 13-4). Head trauma and peripheral trauma, including dental procedures (Schrag et al., 1999), can induce generalized and segmental dystonia and focal dystonia, respectively. Trauma may provoke the onset of PTD in an individual who carries the gene for this disorder (Fletcher et al., 1991c). Segmental axial dystonia was described with a closed head injury with small areas of encephalomalacia, including the caudate nucleus (Jabbari et al., 1992). Cervical dystonia can sometimes be secondary to lesions in the central nervous system, such as lacunar infarction in the putamen (Molho and Factor, 1993), and to lesions in the upper cervical spinal cord (Klostermann et al., 1993; Cammarota et al., 1995), including syringomyelia (Hill et al., 1999). Torticollis has also been reported to occur after electrocution (Colosimo et al., 1993) and in Moya-Moya disease (Yasutomo et al., 1993). Strokes can occasionally lead to delayed-onset hemidystonia. Perhaps in this category is the primary antiphospholipid syndrome, an immune-mediated vascular disorder that has been found to result in hemidystonia in children (Angelini et al., 1993). Sjögren syndrome, also considered an autoimmune disorder,

**Box 13-8** Clues that dystonia is symptomatic

History of possible etiologic factor (e.g., head trauma, peripheral trauma, encephalitis, toxin exposure, drug exposure, perinatal anoxia)

Presence of neurologic abnormality (e.g., dementia, seizures, ocular, ataxia, weakness, spasticity, amyotrophy)

Presence of false weakness on sensory examination or other clues of psychogenic etiology (see Box 13-9)

Onset of rest instead of action dystonia

Early onset of speech involvement

Hemidystonia

Abnormal brain imaging

Abnormal laboratory workup

---

has been associated with dystonia (van den Berg et al., 1999). Encephalitis, usually from severe equine encephalitis, results in permanent dystonia. The common Asian encephalitis known as Japanese encephalitis can cause severe dystonia (Kalita and Misra, 2000; Murgod et al., 2001). Occasionally, dystonia can be psychogenic in origin (see Chapter 26), and it is reasonable to consider psychogenic dystonia one of the many etiologies of secondary dystonia. Sometimes psychogenic dystonia occurs following trauma. When associated with pain, it may be diagnosed as reflex sympathetic dystrophy, but many of the patients have a psychogenic mechanism (Ochoa, 1999); this syndrome has also been called causalgia-dystonia (Bhatia et al., 1993b).

## Clues That Dystonia Might Be Secondary

In examining patients with dystonia, there are some clues in the history and neurologic examination that would suggest to the clinician that the patient's dystonia is secondary rather than primary (Box 13-8).

Perhaps the most difficult form of dystonia to diagnose is psychogenic dystonia, which can occur in up to 5% of children presenting with what otherwise appears to be primary dystonia. Clues suggesting a psychogenic etiology are false (give-way) weakness, false sensory findings, inconsistent movements with changing patterns of involvement, incongruent movements not fitting with typical organic dystonia, self-inflicting injuries, deliberate slowness of movement, and multiple types of abnormal dyskinesias that do not fit into a single organic etiology (Fahn and Williams, 1988). Box 13-9 lists the clinical situations that provide clues that the clinician might be encountering a psychogenic movement disorder. (Box 13-9 is from Chapter 26).

## LUBAG (X-LINKED DYSTONIA-PARKINSONISM)

While both DRD and classic PTD, as well as focal dystonias (Waddy et al., 1991), are inherited as autosomal-dominant disorders, there is a form of dystonia that is inherited as an X-linked recessive trait. This is present in males from the island of Panay in the Philippines (Lee et al., 1976; Fahn and Moskowitz, 1988). The disease can begin with either dystonia

---

**Box 13-9** Clues suggesting psychogenic dystonia

**Clues Relating to the Movements**

Abrupt onset

Inconsistent movements (changing characteristics over time)

Incongruous movements and postures (movements do not fit with recognized patterns or with normal physiologic patterns)

Presence of additional types of abnormal movements that are not consistent with the basic abnormal movement pattern or are not congruous with a known movement disorder, particularly rhythmic shaking, bizarre gait, deliberate slowness carrying out requested voluntary movement, bursts of verbal gibberish, excessive startle (bizarre movements in response to sudden, unexpected noise or threatening movement)

Spontaneous remissions

Movements decrease or disappear with distraction

Response to placebo, suggestion, or psychotherapy

Presence as a paroxysmal disorder

Dystonia beginning as a fixed posture

Twisting facial movements which move the mouth to one side or the other (note: organic dystonia of the facial muscles usually do not move the mouth sideways)

**Clues Relating to the Other Medical Observations**

False weakness

False sensory complaints

Multiple somatizations or undiagnosed conditions

Self-inflicted injuries

Obvious psychiatric disturbances

Employed in the health profession or in insurance claims

Presence of secondary gain, including continuing care by a "devoted" spouse

Litigation or compensation pending

Note: See also Chapter 26.

or parkinsonism; with progression, parkinsonism develops eventually, even in those who had dystonia earlier (Lee et al., 1991). Pure parkinsonism has been considered a more benign phenotype (Evidente et al., 2002). The symptoms may begin in the big toe with abnormal movements. Dystonia typically spreads from the limbs to axial musculature. Some patients with older onset may have focal dystonia involving the tongue and jaw (Videos 13-28 and 13-29). The families with this disorder refer to the condition as lubag ("shuffling"). Female heterozygotes have been discovered who manifest mild dystonia or chorea (Waters et al., 1993b). Evidente and colleagues (2004) reported eight more affected women. Six of the eight had parkinsonism, and only one had dystonia. The initial symptom was focal tremor or parkinsonism in four, chorea in three, and focal dystonia (cervical) in one. Seven of eight patients had slow or no progression of their symptoms and required no treatment. The patient with disabling parkinsonism was responsive to carbidopa/levodopa.

With the aid of molecular genetics for identification, the phenotype has been extended to also include tremor, myoclonus, chorea, and myorhythmia (Evidente et al., 2002). Deoxyglucose and fluorodopa PET scans show decreased metabolism in the striatum and no or little decrease of fluorodopa uptake (Eidelberg et al., 1992). Treatment is not satisfactory, but antimuscarinics and clonazepam appear to be somewhat helpful, as does zolpidem (Evidente, 2002).

The abnormal gene that causes lubag has been localized near the centromere of the X chromosome (Kupke et al., 1990, 1992; Wilhelmsen et al., 1991; Graeber et al., 1992; Haberhausen et al., 1995) and has been given the designation DYT3. The gene involves a multiple transcript system (Nolte et al., 2003). The mutation has been identified in the coding portion of DNA (i.e., an exon). However, this region of DNA is extremely complex, with genes being made from both strands, and multiple different RNAs (each encoding a different protein product) being made from each strand. Thus, while the investigators appear to have identified a specific mutation, they were not able to say which mutant protein (and there may be up to six from this mutation) is actually responsible for the disease. Subsequently, Makino and colleagues (2007) reported that it is the TAF1 gene in this region that is particularly affected, and its decreased function is likely the primary factor resulting in the disease.

The pathology of lubag has been reported (Altrocchi and Forno, 1983; Waters et al., 1993a). The neostriatum showed astrocytosis in a multifocal or mosaic pattern, due to islands of normal striatum sharply demarcated by gliotic tissue. The lateral part of the putamen was most severely gliotic, and the astrocytosis in this region was confluent rather than mosaic-like. The gliotic areas also exhibited neuronal loss involving both large and small populations in the putamen. In the body and head of the caudate nucleus, the gliosis was less extensive, and neuronal loss was equivocal. The tail of the caudate was also affected, showing a mild diffuse astrocytosis and loss of nerve cells. No areas of striatum seemed to be spared. The myelinated fiber bundles in caudate and putamen were thinned in affected foci. The brainstem was normal. In particular, there were no Lewy bodies or neurofibrillary tangles. In addition to the pathologic observations in the two Filipino men, a very similar pathologic finding was reported in a non-Filipino youth with progressive generalized dystonia with marked orolingual and pharyngeal involvement (Gibb et al., 1992) and in a non-Filipino man with a combination of

psychiatric symptoms, craniocervical dystonia, bulbar dysfunction, and parkinsonism (Factor and Barron, 1997). The similar pathology and clinical features of dystonia suggest that lubag might be present in other populations beside Filipinos. An Italian family with a mutation on the DYT3 gene could be another case (Fabbrini et al., 2005). Lubag is now a confirmed neurodegenerative disorder and deserves much more intensive study. The mechanism of its pathogenesis might shed light on normal basal ganglia function, in addition to leading to a better understanding of the pathophysiologic mechanisms underlying dystonia and parkinsonism.

Toward that end, Goto and colleagues (2005) found that with the dystonia phenotype, the striosomes in the striatum are severely depleted, while the matrix compartment of the striatum is relatively spared. But as the disease progresses, and the striosomes become involved, the clinical features become parkinsonian. This suggests that dystonia may result from an imbalance in the activity between the striosomal and matrix-based pathways.

# PATHOPHYSIOLOGY AND PATHOANATOMY OF PRIMARY DYSTONIA

## Pathophysiology

A major characteristic of dystonic movements is the presence of sustained simultaneous contractions of agonists and antagonists (Yanagisawa and Goto, 1971; Rothwell et al., 1983; Rothwell and Obeso, 1987). There are also contractions of adjoining and distant muscles, so-called overflow, particularly during a voluntary movement. Also, rhythmic contractions frequently occur on voluntary movement. None of these physiologic features is specific for dystonia. Increasing muscle spindle activity by the tonic vibration reflex maneuver induced dystonic postures or movements typical of those seen during writing in 11 out of 15 patients with writer's cramp but not in normal individuals (Kaji et al., 1995). The cutaneous electromyographic silent period during isometric contraction was studied in primary brachial dystonia. The duration of the silent period was significantly prolonged in dystonia and in Parkinson disease in both affected and unaffected arms compared with controls (Pullman et al., 1996).

Some physiologic reflexes, such as blink reflexes, have been found to be abnormal in primary cranial and cervical dystonias (Berardelli et al., 1985; Tolosa et al., 1988b). The R1 and R2 blink responses have increased amplitude and duration. This finding implies excess physiologic excitatory drive to the midbrain region. In a physiologic study, a sensory trick that reduced blepharospasm was found to decrease the R2 blink response (Gomez-Wong et al., 1998).

In limb dystonia, there is an abnormality of the normal reciprocal inhibition between agonist and antagonist. The second, longer phase of reciprocal inhibition is much reduced or even absent in affected limbs in dystonia (Nakashima et al., 1989). This has been interpreted as evidence for reduced presynaptic inhibition of muscle afferent input to the inhibitory interneurons as a result of defective descending motor control. Reduced reciprocal inhibition is a feature that is seen with other types of dystonia (Valls-Sole and Hallett, 1995). The early and late long-latency reflex responses are often abnormal in primary focal dystonia (Naumann and Reiners, 1997), and this can be influenced by botulinum toxin injections, indicating their influence by peripheral afferents. Cooling the affected limb in writer's cramp has been shown to reduce the dystonia and improve writing performance (Pohl et al., 2002).

There is a report of decreased N30 amplitude in somatosensory evoked potentials in patients with cervical dystonia (Mazzini et al., 1994). The excitability of the motor cortex was studied in 11 patients with task-specific dystonia and 11 age-matched controls by delivering transcranial magnetic stimuli at different stimulus intensities (Ikoma et al., 1996). With increasing stimulus intensity, the increase in the motor-evoked potentials in the flexor carpi radialis muscles was greater in patients than in normal subjects, suggesting that cortical motor excitability is increased in dystonia.

Blepharospasm has been studied in some detail, recording electromyographs simultaneously from both orbicularis oculi (OO) and levator palpebrae superioris (LPS) (Aramideh et al., 1994). Some patients had contractions only of the OO and simultaneous reciprocal inhibition of LPS; others had combined simultaneous contractions of both OO and LPS; and others had gradual cessation of LPS inhibition along with OO contraction (combination of blepharospasm, LP motor impersistence); a fourth group had a combination of blepharospasm and involuntary LP inhibition; a fifth group had involuntary inhibition of LPS activity, without any dystonic discharges in OO (apraxia of eyelid opening). Krack and Marion (1994) suggest that this so-called apraxia of lid opening is actually a dystonic phenomenon.

The cerebral cortex appears to play a physiologic role in dystonia. An animal model of producing focal dystonia by training overusage of a limb resulted in receptive fields in the sensorimotor cortex that were 10 to 20 times larger than normal (Byl et al., 1996) without local signs of tendon or nerve inflammation (Topp and Byl, 1999). A current concept is that in dystonia, there is a loss of surround inhibition in the cerebral cortex (Hallett, 2004; Sohn and Hallett, 2004). In writer's cramp, abnormal sensorimotor integration was found by studying contingent negative variation (Ikeda et al., 1996), and premotor cortex and supplementary motor area have increased blood flow as determined with PET blood flow scans (Playford et al., 1998). These results might represent a release of the thalamus from the normal inhibitory influence of the globus pallidus interna. Both the internal and external segments of the globus pallidus show a reduced neuronal firing pattern in dystonia, including "off" period dystonia in Parkinson disease (Hashimoto, 2000).

The interstitial nucleus of Cajal in the midbrain has been reported to function as a neural integrator for head posture (Klier et al., 2002). A bilateral imbalance in this structure, through either direct damage or inappropriate input, could be one of the mechanisms underlying torticollis.

New insights about occupational cramps, such as musician's cramp, which are associated with repetitive movements, have emerged. Studies in primates support the notion that repetitive motions of the hand can induce plasticity changes in the sensory cortex, leading to degradation of topographic representations of the hand (Chen and Hallett, 1998). Hand dystonia is represented by an abnormality of the normal homuncular organization of the finger representations in the primary somatosensory cortex (Bara-Jimenez et al., 1998).

Patients with focal hand dystonia have a decreased performance in sensory detection, suggesting a role for sensory dysfunction in the pathophysiology of dystonia (Bara-Jimenez et al., 2000). Functional MRI was utilized to study tactile stimulation in patients with focal hand dystonia. These patients, compared to normal controls, have a nonlinear interaction between the sensory cortical response to individual finger stimulation (Sanger et al., 2002). Levy and Hallett (2002) used two-dimensional J-resolved magnetic resonance spectroscopy to reveal GABA levels and found them decreased in sensorimotor cortex and lentiform nuclei contralateral to the affected hand in patients with writer's cramp. This finding correlates with physiologic studies showing reduced intracortical inhibition.

In addition to focal hand dystonia, focal facial dystonia (blepharospasm) has been studied physiologically. Suprathreshold transcranial magnetic stimuli were applied over the optimal representation of the relaxed abductor digiti minimi muscle of the dominant hand in both groups of subjects following conditioning stimuli (Sommer et al., 2002). Intracortical inhibition was reduced in both patient groups. Physiologic markers of primary dystonia, including cortical inhibition and cutaneous silent period, although abnormal when compared to healthy controls, however, were not different when patients with psychogenic and organic dystonia were compared. This suggests either that these abnormal findings represent a consequence rather than a cause of dystonia or that they are endophenotypic abnormalities that predispose to both types of dystonia (Espay et al., 2006).

A brief summary of the pathophysiology of dystonia is presented in Box 13-10, taken in part from Berardelli and colleagues (1998).

## Pathoanatomy

A number of pathologic studies have been carried out on patients who died with PTD. When these were reviewed by Zeman (1970), who also added his own cases, he concluded that whereas environmental etiologies leave their mark with

---

**Box 13-10** Highlights of pathophysiology of torsion dystonia

Reduced and irregular neuronal firing rate in the internal and external segments of the globus pallidus

Reduced pallidal inhibition of the thalamus with consequent overactivity of medial and prefrontal cortical areas and underactivity of the primary motor cortex during movements

Cortical abnormalities:
  Reduced preparatory activity in the EEG before the onset of voluntary movements
  Enhanced premotor and supplementary motor cortical excitability
  Reduced primary motor cortex activity

Reduced spinal cord and brainstem inhibition is seen in many reflex studies (long-latency reflexes, cranial reflexes, and reciprocal inhibition)

Cocontraction and overflow of electromyographic activity of inappropriate muscles is characteristic

alterations in the basal ganglia, the hereditary forms are without tangible pathologic abnormalities detectable by light microscopy. He felt that the earlier reports of positive findings could be explained as nonspecific alterations or as artifacts due to the agonal state prior to death. There have been few reports since then. Zweig and colleagues (1988) described the histology of the brainstem in four patients with PTD (Table 13-7). Two of them started in childhood or adolescence (Cases 1 and 2); Case 1 was Jewish, and Case 2 was non-Jewish. Case 1 had numerous neurofibrillary tangles in the locus coeruleus, along with mild neuronal loss and extracellular neuromelanin in this nucleus. There were rare neurofibrillary tangles in the substantia nigra pars compacta, pedunculopontine nucleus, and dorsal raphe.

The inconsistency of the histology in patients with primary dystonia makes it difficult to interpret the significance of the observations by Zweig and his colleagues (1988). Clearly, there is a large need to have many more cases studied pathologically. Bhatia and colleagues (1993a) found no abnormalities in a patient with orofacial dystonia and rest tremor.

Although primary dystonia is not associated with any known histopathologic lesion, the volume of the putamen is increased about 10% (Black et al., 1998). In secondary dystonia, however, the basal ganglia, particularly the putamen, is involved (Burton et al., 1984). Lesions in the pallidum also can result in dystonia, often with parkinsonism (Munchau et al., 2000). Actually, lesions can involve not only the basal ganglia but also connections to and from these nuclei, such as the thalamus and the cortex (Marsden et al., 1985). In primary cervical dystonia, an increase in gray matter density bilaterally in the motor cortex and in the cerebellar flocculus and unilat-

**Table 13-7** Description of brainstem pathology in four patients with primary torsion dystonia

| Case | Ethnicity | Age at Onset | Age at Death | Site at Onset | Final Classification | Clinical Remarks | Pathology of Interest |
|---|---|---|---|---|---|---|---|
| 1 | Jewish | 14 | 29 | Right foot | Generalized | Bilateral thalamotomies, head injury at age 23, seizures | Numerous NFTs, mild neuronal loss, and extracellular neuromelanin in locus coeruleus. Rare NFT in substantia nigra pars compacta, dorsal raphe, and pedunculopontine nucleus |
| 2* | Non-Jewish | 4 | 10 | Feet | Segmental crural (trunk and both legs) | Initially improved with anticholinergics | No notable abnormality found. |
| 3†‡ | Not stated | 33 | 68 | Eyelids | Cranial and cervical (face, jaw, tongue, and neck) | Initial diagnosis was postencephalitic, but no history of encephalitis. Marked improvement with baclofen and valproate. | Depigmentation of substantia nigra and locus coeruleus. Occasional NFT in nucleus basalis. Moderate to marked neuronal loss in substantia nigra pars compacta, dorsal raphe, pedunculopontine nucleus, and locus coeruleus. Extracellular pigment in substantia nigra and locus coeruleus. |
| 4*† | Not stated | 47 | 50 | Neck | Cervical | Intention tremor developed in right arm. Clonazepam was beneficial. Developed status epilepticus. | No notable abnormality found. |

*Cases 2 and 4 had no notable abnormality.
†Cases 3 and 4 had adult-onset cranial-cervical dystonia and cervical dystonia, respectively.
‡Case 3 had remarkable neuronal loss in the substantia nigra pars compacta, dorsal raphe, pedunculopontine nucleus, and locus coeruleus. The pigmented nuclei had extracellular pigment. There was occasional NFT in the nucleus basalis and infrequent NFT in the substantia nigra.
NFT, neurofibrillary tangles.

Data from Zweig RM, Hedreen JC, Jankel WR, et al: Pathology in brainstem regions of individuals with primary dystonia. Neurology 1988;38:702–706.

erally in the right globus pallidus internus was found by using voxel-based morphometry (Draganski et al., 2003). A survey of secondary cervical dystonia found that structural lesions were most commonly localized to the brainstem and cerebellum, and fewer cases were in the cervical spinal cord and basal ganglia (LeDoux and Brady, 2003).

Although no consistent cerebral anatomic abnormality has ever been reported in primary focal hand dystonia, a voxel-based morphometry study showed a significant bilateral increase in gray matter in the hand representation area of primary somatosensory and, to a lesser extent, primary motor cortices in 36 patients with unilateral focal hand dystonia compared with 36 controls (Garraux et al., 2004). The presence of anatomic changes in the perirolandic cortex for the unaffected hand as well as that for the affected hand suggested to the investigators that these disturbances might be, at least in part, primary.

In an MRI study of eight patients with secondary unilateral dystonia, lesions associated with dystonic spasms were located in the putamen posterior to the anterior commissure in all patients and extended variably into the dorsolateral part of the caudate nucleus, the posterior limb of the internal capsule, or the lateral segment of the globus pallidus (Lehericy et al., 1996). In imaging studies of dystonia developing after a stroke, focal lesions were seen in the striatopallidum and in different parts of the thalamus (Karsidag et al., 1998; Krystkowiak et al., 1998). A characteristic dystonic tremor following a stroke is commonly localized to the thalamus by imaging studies (Cho and Samkoff, 2000).

However, one should not assume that the basal ganglia are always the site of physiologic pathology in primary dystonia. It has been shown, for example, that the rostral brainstem (Jankovic and Patel, 1983; Kulisevsky et al., 1993), pontine tegmentum (Aramideh et al., 1996), and thalamus (Miranda and Millar, 1998) can be pathologically damaged in some cases of secondary blepharospasm. Lesions from stroke, multiple sclerosis, and encephalitis have all been seen.

An abnormality in the striatum in PTD is suggested by finding prolonged MRI T2 times in the lentiform nucleus in patients with primary cervical dystonia (Schneider et al., 1994). Findings on fluorodeoxyglucose and spiperone PET studies (discussed later) also support this implication. Intraoperative recordings for stereotaxic surgery for dystonia show an abnormal firing pattern in the internal segment of the globus pallidus (Lenz et al., 1998).

## BIOCHEMISTRY

Although no consistent morphologic abnormalities in PTD are seen on brain imaging (Rutledge et al., 1987) or histologic examination (Zeman, 1976; Zweig et al., 1988), some changes have been reported on postmortem biochemical analysis. Hornykiewicz and colleagues (1986) examined the biochemistry of the brain in two patients with childhood-onset generalized primary dystonia, and Jankovic and colleagues (1987) studied a single case of adult-onset primary cranial segmental dystonia. There were changes in norepinephrine, serotonin, and dopamine levels in various regions of brain. It is not clear which, if any, of these alterations is related to the pathophysiology of dystonia. In a patient with symptomatic dystonia due

to neuroacanthocytosis, de Yebenes and colleagues (1988) found large increases in norepinephrine in caudate, putamen, globus pallidus, and dentate nucleus. Again, it is not clear whether norepinephrine is related to dystonia. Many more biochemical studies need to be carried out.

Eidelberg and colleagues (1995) evaluated FDG PET in 11 patients with predominantly right-sided Oppenheim dystonia and 11 age-matched controls. They found that global and regional metabolic rates were normal in PTD. But the Scaled Subprofile Model analysis of the combined groups of PTD patients and controls revealed a significant topographic profile characterized by relative bilateral increases in the metabolic activity of the lateral frontal and paracentral cortices, associated with relative covariate hypermetabolism of the contralateral lentiform nucleus, pons, and midbrain. Subject scores for this profile correlated significantly with Fahn-Marsden disease severity ratings ($r = 0.67$, $P < .02$). Thalamic metabolism was decreased. Thus, in contrast to parkinsonism, lentiform and thalamic metabolism were dissociated in dystonia. In Parkinson disease, both regions show increased metabolism; in dystonia, the lentiform is increased while the thalamus is decreased. These authors concluded that PTD is characterized by relative metabolic overactivity of the lentiform nucleus and premotor cortices. The presence of lentiform-thalamic metabolic dissociation suggests that in this disorder hyperkinetic movements may arise through excessive activity of the direct putaminopallidal inhibitory pathway, resulting in inhibition of the globus pallidus interna. In direct physiologic recordings during surgery, both the internal and external segments of the globus pallidus show a reduced neuronal firing pattern in dystonia, including "off" period dystonia in Parkinson disease (Hashimoto, 2000).

Eidelberg and colleagues utilized FDG PET in nonmanifesting *DYT1* carriers using a network analytic approach and identified a pattern of abnormal regional glucose utilization in two independent cohorts (Eidelberg et al., 1998; Trost et al., 2002). They found increased metabolism in the posterior putamen/globus pallidus, cerebellum, and supplementary motor area. This abnormal torsion dystonia–related pattern (TDRP) was also present in clinically affected patients, persisting even following the suppression of involuntary dystonic movements by sleep induction, and also in non-*DYT1* patients who had just essential blepharospasm (Hutchinson et al., 2000). This shows that TDRP expression is not specific for the *DYT1* genotype. In fact, these investigators found the same TDRP expression in the primary dystonia (*DYT6*) that has been reported in the Amish/Mennonite population (Trost et al., 2002). The investigators propose that the TDRP feature in the resting state represents a metabolic trait of primary dystonia.

In other FDG PET studies, Galardi and colleagues (1996) found hypermetabolism in the lentiform, thalamus, premotor and motor cortices, and cerebellum in patients with primary cervical dystonia; this did not reveal the lentiform-thalamic metabolic dissociation. Magyar-Lehmann and colleagues (1997) also found lentiform hypermetabolism bilaterally in cervical dystonia.

Carbon and colleagues (2004b) found bilateral hypermetabolism in the presupplementary motor area and parietal association cortices of affected carriers of both *DYT1* and *DYT6* dystonia, compared with their respective nonmanifesting counterparts. But differences were seen between manifesting

*DYT1* and *DYT6* carriers. Increases in metabolism were found in the putamen, anterior cingulate, and cerebellar hemispheres of *DYT1* carriers, while hypometabolism of the putamen and hypermetabolism in the temporal cortex occurred in *DYT6* affected patients.

Fluorodopa PET reveals mild reduction of uptake or normal uptake in familial PTD (Playford et al., 1993). PET scans using a ligand to bind to striatal dopamine D2 receptors showed a trend to higher uptake in the contralateral striatum in subjects showing lateralization of clinical signs (Leenders et al., 1993). Spiperone PET scans in primary focal dystonia revealed a 29% decrease in binding in the putamina (Perlmutter et al., 1997a) and suggest an involvement of the D2 receptor. Single photon emission computed tomography scans evaluating epidepride binding of the D2 receptors also showed decreased binding in both striata in patients with torticollis (Naumann et al., 1998). Eidelberg and colleagues (Carbon et al., 2004c; Asanuma et al., 2005b) used $^{11}$C-raclopride and PET in a cohort of nonmanifesting *DYT1* gene carriers and found significant reductions in binding in both the putamen and caudate (18% and 12% of control values, respectively). The reductions in D2 receptor sensitivity in the striatum in all these studies suggest that this might be a component in the pathophysiology of primary dystonias.

Tempel and Perlmutter (1993) measured blood flow with PET in patients with writer's cramp. Subjects had blood flow scans at rest and during vibration of either the affected or unaffected hand. Vibration produced a consistent peak response in primary sensorimotor area and supplementary motor area, both contralateral to the vibrated hand. Both responses were significantly reduced approximately 25% in patients with writer's cramp whether the affected or unaffected hand was vibrated. This indicates that patients with unilateral writer's cramp have bilateral brain dysfunction. These investigators performed an analogous study in patients with blepharospasm (Feiwell et al., 1999). They found decreased activation of blood flow in the primary sensorimotor cortical area, both ipsilateral and contralateral to the side of facial stimulation.

Following the injection of MPTP into baboons, the animals transiently developed ipsilateral turning and contralateral hemidystonia involving arm and leg. This transient dystonia preceded hemiparkinsonism and corresponded temporally with a decreased striatal dopamine content and a transient decrease in D2-like receptor number (Perlmutter et al., 1997b). Todd and Perlmutter (1998) suggest that the pathophysiology of dystonia involves decreased D2 receptor inhibition.

By the use of diffusion tensor MRI, the microstructure of white matter pathways was assessed in mutation carriers and control subjects. Axonal integrity was found to be reduced in the subgyral white matter of the sensorimotor cortex of *DYT1* carriers (Carbon et al., 2004a). Abnormal anatomic connectivity of the supplementary motor area might contribute to the susceptibility of *DYT1* carriers to develop clinical manifestations of dystonia.

A biochemical study investigating copper proteins in PTD found Wilson protein and ceruloplasmin were increased in the lentiform nuclei in two patients with focal dystonia and reduced in the patient with generalized dystonia, and Menkes protein was reduced in all three patients (Berg et al., 2000). In another biochemical study, plasma concentration of homocysteine was elevated in patients with PTD compared with age- and sex-matched controls (Muller et al., 2000). Naumann and colleagues (1996) studied transcranial sonography of the basal ganglia in 86 patients with dystonic disorders, including primary dystonia (generalized and focal). The majority of primary and secondary dystonias had a hyperechogenic lesion of the middle segment of the lenticular nucleus on the side opposite to the clinical dystonic symptoms. Becker and colleagues (1997) found a similar result in patients with idiopathic torticollis. These changes support the proposal of increased copper content in the lentiform nuclei in primary focal dystonia (Becker et al., 2001). Although this increase was suggested to be due to reduced levels of the Menkes protein, a membrane ATPase exporting copper out of the cells, genetic analysis has failed to find an alteration in the genes for this Menkes protein, the Wilson protein (another copper ATPase), or the intracellular copper chaperone, ATOX1, in patients with primary focal dystonia (Bandmann et al., 2002).

In a study of platelet mitochondria, Benecke and colleagues (1992) found a defect in complex I in patients with primary dystonia, most of whom had torticollis (*DYT7*). However, Reichmann and colleagues (1994) could not replicate this. Schapira and colleagues (1997) found that platelet complex I activity is normal in familial dystonia (including *DYT1* dystonia) but is decreased in sporadic torticollis.

## References

Abbruzzese G, Rizzo F, Dall'Agata D, et al: Generalized dystonia with bilateral striatal computed: Tomographic lucencies in a patient with human immunodeficiency virus infection. Eur Neurol 1990;30:271–273.

Adler CH, Caviness JN: Dystonia secondary to electrical injury: Surface electromyographic evaluation and implications for the organicity of the condition. J Neurol Sci 1997;148:187–192.

Allen N, Knopp W: Hereditary parkinsonism-dystonia with sustained control by L-dopa and anticholinergic medication. Adv Neurol 1976;14:201–213.

Almasy L, Bressman SB, Raymond D, et al: Idiopathic torsion dystonia linked to chromosome 8 in two Mennonite families. Ann Neurol 1997;42:670–673.

Altrocchi PH, Forno LS: Spontaneous oral-facial dyskinesia: Neuropathology of a case. Neurology 1983;33:802–805.

Andermann F, Ohtahara S, Andermann E, et al: Infantile hypotonia and paroxysmal dystonia: A variant of alternating hemiplegia of childhood. Mov Disord 1994;9:227–229.

Angelini L, Rumi V, Nardocci N, et al: Hemidystonia symptomatic of primary antiphospholipid syndrome in childhood. Mov Disord 1993;8:383–386.

Aramideh M, de Visser BWO, Devriese PP, et al: Electromyographic features of levator palpebrae superioris and orbicularis oculi muscles in blepharospasm. Brain 1994;117:27–38.

Aramideh M, de Visser BWO, Holstege G, et al: Blepharospasm in association with a lower pontine lesion. Neurology 1996;46:476–478.

Asanuma K, Ma Y, Huang C, et al: The metabolic pathology of dopa-responsive dystonia. Ann Neurol 2005a;57(4):596–600.

Asanuma K, Ma Y, Okulski J, et al: Decreased striatal D2 receptor binding in non-manifesting carriers of the DYT1 dystonia mutation. Neurology 2005b;64(2):347–349.

Ashour R, Jankovic J: Joint and skeletal deformities in Parkinson's disease, multiple system atrophy, and progressive supranuclear palsy. Mov Disord 2006;21(11)1856–1863.

Asmus F, Gasser T: Inherited myoclonus-dystonia. In Fahn S, Hallett M, DeLong M (eds): Dystonia 4: Advances in Neurology, vol 94. Philadelphia, Lippincott Williams & Wilkins, 2004, pp 113–119.

Asmus F, Zimprich A, duMontcel ST, et al: Myoclonus-dystonia syndrome: Epsilon-sarcoglycan mutations and phenotype. Ann Neurol 2002;52(4):489–492.

Auburger G, Ratzlaff T, Lunkes A, et al: A gene for autosomal dominant paroxysmal choreoathetosis spasticity (CSE) maps to the vicinity of a potassium channel gene cluster on chromosome 1p, probably within 2 cM between D1S443 and D1S197. Genomics 1996;31:90–94.

Augood SJ, Hollingsworth Z, Albers DS, et al: Dopamine transmission in DYT1 dystonia: A biochemical and autoradiographical study. Neurology 2002;59(3):445–448.

Augood SJ, Keller-McGandy CE, Siriani A, et al: Distribution and ultrastructural localization of torsinA immunoreactivity in the human brain. Brain Res 2003;986(1–2):12–21.

Augood SJ, Martin DM, Ozelius LJ, et al: Distribution of the mRNAs encoding torsinA and torsinB in the normal adult human brain. Ann Neurol 1999;46(5):761–769.

Augood SJ, Penney JB, Friberg IK, et al: Expression of the early-onset torsion dystonia gene (DYT1) in human brain. Ann Neurol 1998; 43:669–673.

Baldessarini RJ, Marsh E: Fluoxetine and side effects. Arch Gen Psychiatry 1992;47:191–192.

Bandmann O, Asmus F, Sibbing D, et al: Copper genes are not implicated in the pathogenesis of focal dystonia. Neurology 2002;59(5): 782–783.

Bandmann O, Nygaard TG, Surtees R, et al: Dopa-responsive dystonia in British patients: New mutations of the GTP-cyclohydrolase I gene and evidence for genetic heterogeneity. Hum Mol Genet 1996;5:403–406.

Bara-Jimenez W, Catalan MJ, Hallett M, Gerloff C: Abnormal somatosensory homunculus in dystonia of the hand. Ann Neurol 1998;44:828–831.

Bara-Jimenez W, Shelton P, Hallett M: Spatial discrimination is abnormal in focal hand dystonia. Neurology 2000;55:1869–1873.

Baumeister FA, Auer DP, Hortnagel K, et al: The eye-of-the-tiger sign is not a reliable disease marker for Hallervorden-Spatz syndrome. Neuropediatrics 2005;36(3):221–222.

Bayrakci B, Aysun S, Firat M: Arteriovenous fistula: A cause of torticollis. Pediatr Neurol 1999;20:146–147.

Beal MF: Aging, energy, and oxidative stress in neurodegenerative diseases. Ann Neurol 1995;38:357–366.

Becker G, Berg D, Francis M, Naumann M: Evidence for disturbances of copper metabolism in dystonia: From the image towards a new concept. Neurology 2001;57(12):2290–2294.

Becker G, Naumann M, Scheubeck M, et al: Comparison of transcranial sonography, magnetic resonance imaging, and single photon emission computed tomography findings in idiopathic spasmodic torticollis. Mov Disord 1997;12:79–88.

Benecke R, Strumper P, Weiss H: Electron transfer complex-I defect in idiopathic dystonia. Ann Neurol 1992;32:683–686.

Bentivoglio AR, Del Grosso N, Albanese A, et al: Non-DYT1 dystonia in a large Italian family. J Neurol Neurosurg Psychiatry 1997;62: 357–360.

Bentivoglio AR, Ialongo T, Contarino MF, et al: Phenotypic characterization of DYT13 primary torsion dystonia. Mov Disord 2004; 19(2):200–206.

Berardelli A, Rothwell JC, Day BL, Marsden CD: Pathophysiology of blepharospasm and oromandibular dystonia. Brain 1985;108:593–609.

Berardelli A, Rothwell JC, Hallett M, et al: The pathophysiology of primary dystonia. Brain 1998;121:1195–1212.

Berg D, Weishaupt A, Francis MJ, et al: Changes of copper-transporting proteins and ceruloplasmin in the lentiform nuclei in primary adult-onset dystonia. Ann Neurol 2000;47:827–830.

Bhatia K, Daniel SE, Marsden CD: Orofacial dystonia and rest tremor in a patient with normal brain pathology. Mov Disord 1993a;8: 361–362.

Bhatia KP, Bhatt MH, Marsden CD: The causalgia-dystonia syndrome. Brain 1993b;116:843–851.

Bhatia KP, Quinn NP, Marsden CD: Clinical features and natural history of axial predominant adult onset primary dystonia. J Neurol Neurosurg Psychiatry 1997;63:788–791.

Black KJ, Ongur D, Perlmutter JS: Putamen volume in idiopathic focal dystonia. Neurology 1998;51:819–824.

Blau N, Bonafe L, Thony B: Tetrahydrobiopterin deficiencies without hyperphenylalaninemia: Diagnosis and genetics of DOPA-responsive dystonia and sepiapterin reductase deficiency. Mol Genet Metab 2001;74:172–185.

Blunt SB, Fuller G, Kennard C, Brooks D: Orolingual dystonia with tip of the tongue geste. Mov Disord 1994;9:466.

Blunt SB, Richards PG, Khalil N: Foot dystonia and lumbar canal stenosis. Mov Disord 1996;11:723–725.

Bonuccelli U, Nocchiero A, Napolitano A, et al: Domperidone-induced acute dystonia and polycystic ovary syndrome. Mov Disord 1991;6:79–81.

Bradley EA, Hodge DO, Bartley GB: Benign essential blepharospasm among residents of Olmsted County, Minnesota, 1976 to 1995: An epidemiologic study. Ophthal Plast Reconstr Surg 2003;19(3): 177–181.

Brancati F, Valente EM, Castori M, et al: Role of the dopamine D5 receptor (DRD5) as a susceptibility gene for cervical dystonia. J Neurol Neurosurg Psychiatry. 2003;74(5):665–666.

Brandfonbrener AG, Robson C: Review of 113 musicians with focal dystonia seen between 1985 and 2002 at a clinic for performing artists. In Fahn S, Hallett M, DeLong M (eds): Dystonia 4: Advances in Neurology, vol 94. Philadelphia, Lippincott Williams & Wilkins, 2004, pp 255–256.

Brashear A, Butler IJ, Hyland K, et al: Cerebrospinal fluid homovanillic acid levels in rapid-onset dystonia-parkinsonism. Ann Neurol 1998;43:521–526.

Brashear A, De Leon D, Bressman SB, et al: Rapid-onset dystonia-parkinsonism in a second family. Neurology 1997;48:1066–1069.

Breakefield XO, Kamm C, Hanson PI: TorsinA: Movement at many levels. Neuron 2001;31(1):9–12.

Bressman SB: Dystonia genotypes, phenotypes, and classification. In Fahn S, Hallett M, DeLong M (eds): Dystonia 4: Advances in Neurology, vol 94. Philadelphia, Lippincott Williams & Wilkins, 2004, pp 101–107.

Bressman SB, de Leon D, Brin MF, et al: Idiopathic torsion dystonia among Ashkenazi Jews: Evidence for autosomal dominant inheritance. Ann Neurol 1989;26:612–620.

Bressman SB, de Leon D, Kramer PL, et al: Dystonia in Ashkenazi Jews: Clinical characterization of a founder mutation. Ann Neurol 1994;36:771–777.

Bressman SB, de Leon D, Raymond D, et al: Secondary dystonia and the DYT1 gene. Neurology 1997;48:1571–1577.

Bressman SB, Heiman GA, Nygaard TG, et al: A study of idiopathic torsion dystonia in a non-Jewish family: Evidence for genetic heterogeneity. Neurology 1994;44:283–287.

Bressman SB, Hunt AL, Heiman GA, et al: Exclusion of the DYT1 locus in a non-Jewish family with early-onset dystonia. Mov Disord 1994;9:626–632.

Bressman SB, Sabatti C, Raymond D, et al: The DYT1 phenotype and guidelines for diagnostic testing. Neurology 2000;54:1746–1752.

Bressman SB, Warner TT, Almasy L, et al: Exclusion of the DYT1 locus in familial torticollis. Ann Neurol 1996;40:681–684.

Burbaud P, Berge J, Lagueny A, et al: Delayed-onset hemidystonia secondary to herpes zoster ophthalmicus-related intracerebral arteritis in an adolescent. J Neurol 1997;244:470–472.

Burke RE, Brin MF, Fahn S, et al: Analysis of the clinical course of non-Jewish, autosomal dominant torsion dystonia. Mov Disord 1986;1:163–178.

Burke RE, Fahn S, Marsden CD, et al: Validity and reliability of a rating scale for the primary torsion dystonias. Neurology 1985; 35:73–77.

Burns CLC: The treatment of torsion spasm in children with trihexyphenidyl (Artane). The Medical Press 1959;241:148–149.

Burton K, Farrell K, Li D, Calne DB: Lesions of the putamen and dystonia: CT and magnetic resonance imaging. Neurology 1984; 34:962–965.

Byl NN, Merzenich MM, Jenkins WM: A primate genesis model of focal dystonia and repetitive strain injury: 1. Learning-induced dedifferentiation of the representation of the hand in the primary somatosensory cortex in adult monkeys. Neurology 1996;47: 508–520.

Caldwell GA, Cao S, Sexton EG, et al: Suppression of polyglutamine-induced protein aggregation in *Caenorhabditis elegans* by torsin proteins. Hum Mol Genet 2003;12(3):307–319.

Calne DB, Lang AE: Secondary dystonia. Adv Neurol 1988;50:9–33.

Camfield L, Ben-Shlomo Y, Warner TT: Impact of cervical dystonia on quality of life. Mov Disord 2002;17(4):838–841.

Cammarota A, Gershanik OS, Garcia S, Lera G: Cervical dystonia due to spinal cord ependymoma: Involvement of cervical cord segments in the pathogenesis of dystonia. Mov Disord 1995; 10:500–503.

Campdelacreu J, Munoz E, Gomez B, et al: Generalised dystonia with an abnormal magnetic resonance imaging signal in the basal ganglia: A case of adult-onset GM1 gangliosidosis. Mov Disord 2002; 17(5):1095–1097.

Carbon M, Kingsley PB, Su S, et al: Microstructural white matter changes in carriers of the DYT1 gene mutation. Ann Neurol 2004a;56(2):283–286.

Carbon M, Su S, Dhawan V, et al: Regional metabolism in primary torsion dystonia: Effects of penetrance and genotype. Neurology 2004b;62(8):1384–1390.

Carbon M, Trost M, Ghilardi MF, Eidelberg D: Abnormal brain networks in primary torsion dystonia. In Fahn S, Hallett M, DeLong M (eds): Dystonia 4: Advances in Neurology, vol 94. Philadelphia, Lippincott Williams & Wilkins, 2004c, pp 155–161.

Cassetta E, Del Grosso N, Bentivoglio AR, et al: Italian family with cranial cervical dystonia: Clinical and genetic study. Mov Disord 1999;14:820–825.

Cavallaro R, Galardi G, Cavallini MC, et al: Obsessive compulsive disorder among idiopathic focal dystonia patients: An epidemiological and family study. Biol Psychiat 2002;52(4):356–361.

Chan J, Brin MF, Fahn S: Idiopathic cervical dystonia: Clinical characteristics. Mov Disord 1991;6:119–126.

Charness ME, Schlaug G: Brain mapping in musicians with focal task-specific dystonia. In Fahn S, Hallett M, DeLong M (eds): Dystonia 4: Advances in Neurology, vol 94. Philadelphia, Lippincott Williams & Wilkins, 2004, pp 231–238.

Chen R, Hallett M: Focal dystonia and repetitive motion disorders. Clin Orthop 1998;102–106.

Cheng JCY, Wong MWN, Tang SP, et al: Clinical determinants of the outcome of manual stretching in the treatment of congenital muscular torticollis in infants: A prospective study of eight hundred and twenty-one cases. J Bone Joint Surg Am 2001;83A:679– 687.

Cho C, Samkoff LM: A lesion of the anterior thalamus producing dystonic tremor of the hand. Arch Neurol 2000;57:1353–1355.

Chuang C, Fahn S, Frucht SJ: The natural history and treatment of acquired hemidystonia: Report of 33 cases and review of the literature. J Neurol Neurosurg Psychiat 2002;72:59–67.

Cohen LG, Hallett M, Sudarsky L: A single family with writer's cramp, essential tremor, and primary writing tremor. Mov Disord 1987;2:109–116.

Colosimo C, Kocen RS, Powell M, et al: Torticollis after electrocution. Mov Disord 1993;8:117–118.

Comella CL, Leurgans S, Wuu J, et al: Rating scales for dystonia: A multicenter assessment. Mov Disord 2003;18(3):303–312.

Comella CL, Stebbins GT, Goetz CG, et al: Teaching tape for the motor section of the Toronto Western Spasmodic Torticollis Scale. Mov Disord 1997;12:570–575.

Conway D, Bain PG, Warner TT, et al: Linkage analysis with chromosome-9 markers in hereditary essential tremor. Mov Disord 1993;8:374–376.

Cooper IS: The Victim Is Always the Same. New York, Norton, 1976.

Corner BD: Dystonia musculorum deformans in siblings; treated with Artane (trihexyphenidyl). Proc R Soc Med 1952;45:451–452.

Couch J: Dystonia and tremor in spasmodic torticollis. Adv Neurol 1976;14:245–258.

Cubo E, Goetz CG: Dystonia secondary to Sjögren-Larsson syndrome. Neurology 2000;55:1236–1237.

Curtis ARJ, Fey C, Morris CM, et al: Mutation in the gene encoding ferritin light polypeptide causes dominant adult-onset basal ganglia disease. Nat Genet 2001;28:345–349.

Dalvi A, Ford B, Fahn S: Dystonic storms. Mov Disord 1998;13: 611–612.

Dauer WT, Burke RE, Greene P, Fahn S: Current concepts on the clinical features, aetiology and management of idiopathic cervical dystonia. Brain 1998;121:547–560.

Dave M: Fluoxetine-associated dystonia. Am J Psychiatry 1994;151: 149.

Davidenkow S: Auf hereditar-abiotrophischer Grundlage akut auftretende, regressierende und episodische Erkrankungen des Nervensystems und Bemerkungen uber die familiare subakute, myoklonische Dystonie. Zeitschr ges Neurol Psychiat 1926;104:596–622.

de Carvalho Aguiar P, Sweadner KJ, et al: Mutations in the Na+/K+-ATPase alpha 3 gene ATP1A3 are associated with rapid-onset dystonia parkinsonism. Neuron 2004;43(2):169–175.

de Rijk-van Andel JF, Gabreels FJM, Geurtz B, et al: L-dopa-responsive infantile hypokinetic rigid parkinsonism due to tyrosine hydroxylase deficiency. Neurology 2000;55:1926–1928.

de Yebenes JG: Did Robert Schumann have dystonia? Mov Disord 1995;10:413–417.

de Yebenes JG, Vazquez A, Martinez A, et al: Biochemical findings in symptomatic dystonias. Adv Neurol 1988;50:167–175.

Defazio G, Livrea P, De Salvia R, et al: Prevalence of primary blepharospasm in a community of Puglia region, Southern Italy. Neurology 2001;56:1579–1581.

Demos MK, Waters PJ, Vallance HD, et al: 6-pyruvoyl-tetrahydropterin synthase deficiency with mild hyperphenylalaninemia. Ann Neurol 2005;58(1):164–167.

Deonna T, Roulet E, Ghika J, Zesiger P: Dope-responsive childhood dystonia: A forme fruste with writer's cramp, triggered by exercise. Dev Med Child Neurol 1997;39:49–53.

Deuschl G, Heinen F, Guschlbauer B, et al: Hand tremor in patients with spasmodic torticollis. Mov Disord 1997;12:547–552.

Dewey RB, Muenter MD, Kishore A, Snow BJ: Long-term follow-up of levodopa responsiveness in generalized dystonia. Arch Neurol 1998;55:1320–1323.

Di Capua M, Bertini E: Remission in dihydroxyphenylalanine-responsive dystonia. Mov Disord 1995;10:223.

Di Capua M, Lispi ML, Giannotti A, et al: Neurofibromatosis type 1 presenting with hand dystonia. J Child Neurol 2001;16:606–608.

Dobyns WB, Ozelius LJ, Kramer PL, et al: Rapid-onset dystonia-parkinsonism. Neurology 1993;43:2596–2602.

Doheny DO, Morrison CE, Smith CJ, et al: Phenotypic features of myoclonus-dystonia in three kindreds. Neurology 2002;59(8): 1187–1196.

Draganski B, Thun-Hohenstein C, Bogdahn U, et al: "Motor circuit" gray matter changes in idiopathic cervical dystonia. Neurology 2003;61(9):1228–1231.

Duffey POF, Butler AG, Hawthorne MR, Barnes MP: The epidemiology of the primary dystonias in the North of England. In Fahn S, Marsden CD, DeLong MR (eds): Dystonia 3: Advances in Neurology. Philadelphia, Lippincott-Raven, 1998, pp 121–125.

Durr A, Stevanin G, Jedynak CP, et al: Familial essential tremor and idiopathic torsion dystonia are different genetic entities. Neurology 1993;43:2212–2214.

Edwards M, Wood N, Bhatia K: Unusual phenotypes in DYT1 dystonia: A report of five cases and a review of the literature. Mov Disord 2003;18(6):706–711.

Eidelberg D, Dhawan V, Takikawa S, et al: Positron emission tomographic (PET) findings in Filipino X-linked dystonia-parkinsonism. Mov Disord 1992;7:298.

Eidelberg D, Moeller JR, Antonini A, et al: Functional brain networks in DYT1 dystonia. Ann Neurol 1998;44:303–312.

Eidelberg D, Moeller JR, Ishikawa T, et al: The metabolic topography of idiopathic torsion dystonia. Brain 1995;118:1473–1484.

Elble RJ, Moody C, Higgins C: Primary writing tremor: A form of focal dystonia. Mov Disord 1990;5:118–126.

Eldridge R: The torsion dystonias: Literature review and genetic and clinical studies. Neurology 1970;20(11: pt 2):1–78.

Eldridge R, Fahn S (eds): Dystonia: Advances in Neurology, vol 14, New York, Raven Press, 1976.

Epidemiologic Study of Dystonia in Europe (ESDE) Collaborative Group: Sex-related influences on the frequency and age of onset of primary dystonia. Neurology 1999;53:1871–1873.

Espay AJ, Morgante F, Purzner J, et al: Cortical and spinal abnormalities in psychogenic dystonia. Ann Neurol 2006;59:825–834.

Evidente VGH: Zolpidem improves dystonia in "Lubag" or X-linked dystonia-parkinsonism syndrome. Neurology 2002;58(4):662–663.

Evidente VGH, Gwinn-Hardy K, Hardy J, et al: X-linked dystonia ("Lubag") presenting predominantly with parkinsonism: A more benign phenotype? Mov Disord 2002;17:200–202.

Evidente VGH, Nolte D, Niemann S, et al: Phenotypic and molecular analyses of X-linked dystonia-parkinsonism ("Lubag") in women. Arch Neurol 2004;61(12):1956–1959.

Fabbrini G, Brancati F, Vacca L, et al: A novel family with an unusual early-onset generalized dystonia. Mov Disord 2005;20(1):81–86.

Factor SA, Barron KD: Mosaic pattern of gliosis in the neostriatum of a North American man with craniocervical dystonia and parkinsonism. Mov Disord 1997;12:783–789.

Fahn S: High dosage anticholinergic therapy in dystonia. Neurology 1983;33:1255–1261.

Fahn S: Atypical tremors, rare tremors, and unclassified tremors. In Findley LJ, Capildeo R (eds): Movement Disorders: Tremor. New York, Oxford University Press, 1984a, pp 431–443.

Fahn S: The varied clinical expressions of dystonia. Neurol Clin 1984b;2:541–554.

Fahn S: Generalized dystonia: Concept and treatment. Clin Neuropharmacol 1986;9(suppl 2):S37–S48.

Fahn S: Concept and classification of dystonia. Adv Neurol 1988; 50:1–8.

Fahn S: Assessment of the primary dystonias. In Munsat TL (ed): Quantification of Neurologic Deficit. Boston, Butterworths, 1989a, pp 241–270.

Fahn S: Clinical variants of idiopathic torsion dystonia. J Neurol Neurosurg Psychiatry 1989b;(suppl):96–100.

Fahn S: Dystonia: Where next? In Quinn NP, Jenner PG (eds): Disorders of Movement: Clinical, Pharmacological and Physiological Aspects. London, Academic Press, 1989c, pp 349–359.

Fahn S: Recent concepts in the diagnosis and treatment of dystonias. In Chokroverty S (ed): Movement Disorders. Costa Mesa, Calif, PMA Publishing Corp, 1990, pp 237–258.

Fahn S: Medical treatment of dystonia. In Tsui JJCT, Calne DB (eds): Handbook of Dystonia. New York, Marcel Dekker, 1995, pp 317–328.

Fahn S: Hypokinesia and hyperkinesia. In Goetz CG, Pappert EJ (eds): Textbook of Clinical Neurology. Philadelphia, WB Saunders, 1999, pp 267–284.

Fahn S, Bressman SB, Marsden CD: Classification of dystonia. In Fahn S, Marsden CD, DeLong MR (eds): Dystonia 3: Advances in Neurology, vol. 78. Philadelphia, Lippincott-Raven, 1998, pp. 1–10.

Fahn S, Hallett M, DeLong MR, eds: Dystonia: Advances in Neurology, vol. 4. Lippincott, Williams & Wilkins, Philadelphia, 2004.

Fahn S, Hening WA, Bressman S, et al: Long-term usefulness of baclofen in the treatment of essential blepharospasm. Adv Ophthalmic Plast Reconstr Surg 1985;4:219–226.

Fahn S, Marsden CD: The treatment of dystonia. In Marsden CD, Fahn S (eds): Movement Disorders, vol 2. London, Butterworths, 1987, pp 359–382.

Fahn S, Marsden CD, Calne DB: Classification and investigation of dystonia. In Marsden CD, Fahn S (eds): Movement Disorders, vol 2. London, Butterworths, 1987, pp 332–358.

Fahn S, Marsden CD, Calne DB (eds): Dystonia, 2: Advances in Neurology, vol 50. New York, Raven Press, 1988.

Fahn S, Marsden CD, DeLong MR (eds): Dystonia, 3: Advances in Neurology, vol 78. Philadelphia, Lippincott-Raven, 1998.

Fahn S, Moskowitz C: X-Linked recessive dystonia and parkinsonism in Filipino males. Ann Neurol 1988;24:179.

Fahn S, Sjaastad O: Hereditary essential myoclonus in a large Norwegian family. Mov Disord 1991;6:237–247.

Fahn S, Williams DT: Psychogenic dystonia. Adv Neurol 1988; 50:431–455.

Feiwell RJ, Black KJ, McGee-Minnich LA, et al: Diminished regional cerebral blood flow response to vibration in patients with blepharospasm. Neurology 1999;52:291–297.

Fink JK, Rainier S, Wilkowski J, et al: Paroxysmal dystonic choreoathetosis: Tight linkage to chromosome 2q. Am J Hum Genet 1996;59:140–145.

Fish DR, Sawyers D, Allen PJ, et al: The effect of sleep on the dyskinetic movements of Parkinson's disease, Gilles de La Tourette syndrome, Huntington's disease, and torsion dystonia. Arch Neurol 1991;48:210–214.

Flatau F, Sterling W: Progressiver Torsionspasms bie Kindern. Z Gesamte Neurol Psychiatr 1911;7:586–612.

Fletcher NA, Harding AE, Marsden CD: A case-control study of idiopathic torsion dystonia. Mov Disord 1991a;6:304–309.

Fletcher NA, Harding AE, Marsden CD: Intrafamilial correlation in idiopathic torsion dystonia. Mov Disord 1991b;6:310–314.

Fletcher NA, Harding AE, Marsden CD: The relationship between trauma and idiopathic torsion dystonia. J Neurol Neurosurg Psychiatry 1991c;54:713–717.

Fouad GT, Servidei S, Durcan S, et al: A gene for familial paroxysmal dyskinesia (FPD1) maps to chromosome 2q. Am J Hum Genet 1996;59:135–139.

Friedman JRL, Klein C, Leung J, et al: The GAG deletion of the DYT1 gene is infrequent in musicians with focal dystonia. Neurology 2000;55:1417–1418.

Frucht SJ: Focal task-specific dystonia in musicians. In Fahn S, Hallett M, DeLong M (eds): Dystonia 4: Advances in Neurology, vol 94. Philadelphia, Lippincott Williams & Wilkins, 2004, pp 225–230.

Frucht SJ, Fahn S, Greene PE, et al: The natural history of embouchure dystonia. Mov Disord 2001;16:899–906.

Furukawa Y, Graf WD, Wong H, et al: Dopa-responsive dystonia simulating spastic paraplegia due to tyrosine hydroxylase (TH) mutations. Neurology 2001;56:260–263.

Furukawa Y, Hornykiewicz O, Fahn S, Kish SJ: Striatal dopamine in early-onset primary torsion dystonia with the DYT1 mutation. Neurology 2000;54:1193–1195.

Furukawa Y, Kish SJ: Dopa-responsive dystonia: Recent advances and remaining issues to be addressed. Mov Disord 1999;14: 709–715.

Furukawa Y, Kish SJ, Bebin EM, et al: Dystonia with motor delay in compound heterozygotes for GTP-cyclohydrolase I gene mutations. Ann Neurol 1998a;44:10–16.

Furukawa Y, Lang AE, Trugman JM, et al: Gender-related penetrance and de novo GTP-cyclohydrolase I gene mutations in dopa-responsive dystonia. Neurology 1998b;50:1015–1020.

Furukawa Y, Nygaard TG, Gutlich M, et al: Striatal biopterin and tyrosine hydroxylase protein reduction in dopa-responsive dystonia. Neurology 1999;53:1032–1041.

Furukawa Y, Shimadzu M, Rajput AH, et al: GTP-cyclohydrolase I gene mutations in hereditary progressive and dopa-responsive dystonia. Ann Neurol 1996;39:609–617.

Galardi G, Perani D, Grassi F, et al: Basal ganglia and thalamo-cortical hypermetabolism in patients with spasmodic torticollis. Acta Neurol Scand 1996;94:172–176.

Garraux G, Bauer A, Hanakawa T, et al: Changes in brain anatomy in focal hand dystonia. Ann Neurol 2004;55(5):736–739.

Gerrits MC, Foncke EM, de Haan R, et al: Phenotype-genotype correlation in Dutch patients with myoclonus-dystonia. Neurology 2006;66(5):759–761.

Ghilardi MF, Carbon M, Silvestri G, et al: Impaired sequence learning in carriers of the DYT1 dystonia mutation. Ann Neurol 2003; 54(1):102–109.

Gibb WRG, Kilford L, Marsden CD: Severe generalised dystonia associated with a mosaic pattern of striatal gliosis. Mov Disord 1992; 7:217–223.

Gimenez-Roldan S, Delgado G, Marin M, et al: Hereditary torsion dystonia in gypsies. Adv Neurol 1988;50:73–81.

Goetz CG, Chmura TA, Lanska DJ: History of dystonia: Part 4 of the MDS-sponsored history of movement disorders exhibit, Barcelona, June, 2000. Mov Disord 2001;16:339–345.

Gomez-Wong E, Marti MJ, Cossu G, et al: The "geste antagonistique" induces transient modulation of the blink reflex in human patients with blepharospasm. Neurosci Lett 1998;251:125–128.

Gonzalez-Alegre P, Paulson HL: Aberrant cellular behavior of mutant torsinA implicates nuclear envelope dysfunction in DYT1 dystonia. J Neurosci 2004;24(11):2593–2601.

Goodchild RE, Dauer WT: Mislocalization to the nuclear envelope: An effect of the dystonia-causing torsinA mutation. Proc Nat Acad Sci U S A 2004;101(3):847–852.

Goodchild RE, Dauer WT: The AAA+ protein torsinA interacts with a conserved domain present in LAP1 and a novel ER protein. J Cell Biol 2005;168(6):855–862.

Goodchild RE, Kim CE, Dauer WT: Loss of the dystonia-associated protein torsinA selectively disrupts the neuronal nuclear envelope. Neuron 2005;48(6):923–932.

Goto S, Lee LV, Munoz EL, et al: Functional anatomy of the basal ganglia in X-linked recessive dystonia-parkinsonism. Ann Neurol 2005;58(1):7–17.

Graeber MB, Kupke KG, Muller U: Delineation of the dystonia-parkinsonism syndrome locus in Xq13. Proc Natl Acad Sci U S A 1992;89:8245–8248.

Grattan-Smith PJ, Wevers RA, Steenbergen-Spanjers GC, et al: Tyrosine hydroxylase deficiency: Clinical manifestations of catecholamine insufficiency in infancy. Mov Disord 2002;17(2): 354–359.

Graudins A, Fern RP: Acute dystonia in a child associated with therapeutic ingestion of a dextromethorphan containing cough and cold syrup. J Toxicol-Clin Toxicol 1996;34:351–352.

Greene P, Kang U, Fahn S, et al: Double-blind, placebo controlled trial of botulinum toxin injection for the treatment of spasmodic torticollis. Neurology 1990;40:1213–1218.

Greene P, Kang UJ, Fahn S: Spread of symptoms in idiopathic torsion dystonia. Mov Disord 1995;10:143–152.

Greene PE, Bressman S: Exteroceptive and interoceptive stimuli in dystonia. Mov Disord 1998;13:549–551.

Grimes DA, Han F, Lang AE, et al: A novel locus for inherited myoclonus-dystonia on 18p11. Neurology 2002;59:1183–1186.

Grotzsch H, Pizzolato GP, Ghika J, et al: Neuropathology of a case of dopa-responsive dystonia associated with new genetic locus, DYT14. Neurology 2002;58:1839–1842.

Haberhausen G, Schmitt I, Kohler A, et al: Assignment of the dystonia-parkinsonism syndrome locus, DYT3, to a small region within a 1.8-Mb YAC contig of Xq13.1. Am J Hum Genet 1995; 57:644–650.

Hallett M: Dystonia: Abnormal movements result from loss of inhibition. In Fahn S, Hallett M, DeLong M (eds): Dystonia 4: Advances in Neurology, vol 94. Philadelphia, Lippincott Williams & Wilkins, 2004, pp 1–9.

Han F, Lang AE, Racacho L, et al: Mutations in the epsilon-sarcoglycan gene found to be uncommon in seven myoclonus-dystonia families. Neurology 2003;61(2):244–246.

Hanihara T, Inoue K, Kawanishi C, et al: 6-Pyruvoyl-tetrahydropterin synthase deficiency with generalized dystonia and diurnal fluctuation of symptoms: A clinical and molecular study. Mov Disord 1997;12:408–411.

Hartig MB, Hortnagel K, Garavaglia B, et al: Genotypic and phenotypic spectrum of PANK2 mutations in patients with neurodegeneration with brain iron accumulation. Ann Neurol 2006; 59:248–256.

Harwood G, Hierons R, Fletcher NA, Marsden CD: Lessons from a remarkable family with DOPA-responsive dystonia. J Neurol Neurosurg Psychiatry 1994;57:460–463.

Hashimoto T: Neuronal activity in the globus pallidus in primary dystonia and off-period dystonia. J Neurol 2000;247:49–52.

Hayes MW, Ouvrier RA, Evans W, et al: X-linked dystonia-deafness syndrome. Mov Disord 1998;13:303–308.

Hayflick SJ, Westaway SK, Levinson B, et al: Genetic, clinical, and radiographic delineation of Hallervorden-Spatz syndrome. N Engl J Med 2003;348(1):33–40.

He FS, Zhang SL, Qian FY, Zhang CL: Delayed dystonia with striatal CT lucencies induced by a mycotoxin (3-nitropropionic acid). Neurology 1995;45:2178–2183.

Head RA, deGoede CGEL, Newton RWN, et al: Pyruvate dehydrogenase deficiency presenting as dystonia in childhood. Develop Med Child Neurol 2004;46(10):710–712.

Heiman GA, Ottman R, Saunders-Pullman RJ, et al: Increased risk for recurrent major depression in DYT1 dystonia mutation carriers. Neurology 2004;63(4):631–637.

Hellmann MA, Melamed E: Focal dystonia as the presenting sign in Creutzfeldt-Jakob disease. Mov Disord 2002;17(5):1097–1098.

Herz E: Dystonia. I. Historical review: Analysis of dystonic symptoms and physiologic mechanisms involved. Arch Neurol Psychiatr 1944a;51:305–318.

Herz E: Dystonia. II. Clinical classification. Arch Neurol Psychiatr 1944b;51:319–355.

Herz E: Dystonia. III. Pathology and conclusions. Arch Neurol Psychiatr 1944c;52:20–26.

Hewett J, Gonzalez-Agosti C, Slater D, et al: Mutant torsinA, responsible for early-onset torsion dystonia, forms membrane inclusions in cultured neural cells. Hum Mol Genet 2000;9:1403–1413.

Hewett JW, Kamm C, Boston H, et al: TorsinB: Perinuclear location and association with torsinA. J Neurochem 2004;89(5):1186–1194.

Hill MD, Kumar R, Lozano A, et al: Syringomyelic dystonia and athetosis. Mov Disord 1999;14:684–688.

Hirano M, Tamaru Y, Nagai Y, et al: Exon skipping caused by a base substitution at a splice site in the GTP cyclohydrolase I gene in a Japanese family with hereditary progressive dystonia/dopa-responsive dystonia. Biochem Biophys Res Commun 1995; 213:645–651.

Hirayama M, Kitagawa Y, Yamamoto S, et al: GM1 gangliosidosis type 3 with severe jaw-closing impairment. J Neurol Sci 1997; 152:99–101.

Hoffmann GF, Assmann B, Brautigam C, et al: Tyrosine hydroxylase deficiency causes progressive encephalopathy and dopa-nonresponsive dystonia. Ann Neurol 2003;54(suppl 6):S56–S65.

Hornykiewicz O, Kish SJ, Becker LE, et al: Brain neurotransmitters in dystonia musculorum deformans. N Engl J Med 1986;315:347–353.

Hou JGG, Jankovic J: Movement disorders in Friedreich's ataxia. J Neurol Sci 2003;206(1):59–64.

Huang CC, Yen TC, Weng YH, et al: Normal dopamine transporter binding in dopa responsive dystonia. J Neurol 2002;249(8): 1016–1020.

Hutchinson M, Nakamura T, Moeller JR, et al: The metabolic topography of essential blepharospasm: A focal dystonia with general implications. Neurology 2000;55(5):673–677.

Hyland K, Arnold LA, Trugman JM: Defects of biopterin metabolism and biogenic amine biosynthesis: Clinical, diagnostic, and therapeutic aspects. In Fahn S, Marsden CD, DeLong MR (eds): Dystonia 3: Advances in Neurology, vol. 78. Philadelphia, Lippincott-Raven, 1998, pp. 301–308.

Hyland K, Fryburg JS, Wilson WG, et al: Oral phenylalanine loading in dopa-responsive dystonia: A possible diagnostic test. Neurology 1997;48:1290–1297.

Hyland K, Surtees RAH, Rodeck C, Clayton PT: Aromatic L-amino acid decarboxylase deficiency: Clinical features, diagnosis, and treatment of a new inborn error of neurotransmitter amine synthesis. Neurology 1992;42:1980–1988.

Ichinose H, Nagatsu T: Molecular genetics of hereditary dystonia: Mutations in the GTP cyclohydrolase I gene. Brain Res Bull 1997;43:35–38.

Ichinose H, Ohye T, Segawa M, et al: GTP cyclohydrolase I gene in hereditary progressive dystonia with marked diurnal fluctuation. Neurosci Lett 1995;196:5–8.

Ichinose H, Ohye T, Takahashi E, et al: Hereditary progressive dystonia with marked diurnal fluctuation caused by mutations in the GTP cyclohydrolase I gene. Nat Genet 1994;8:236–242.

Ikeda A, Shibasaki H, Kaji R, et al: Abnormal sensorimotor integration in writer's cramp: Study of contingent negative variation. Mov Disord 1996;11:683–690.

Ikoma K, Samii A, Mercuri B, et al: Abnormal cortical motor excitability in dystonia. Neurology 1996;46:1371–1376.

Inzelberg R, Zilber N, Kahana E, Korczyn AD: Laterality of onset in idiopathic torsion dystonia. Mov Disord 1993;8:327–330.

Jabbari B, Paul J, Scherokman B, Vandam B: Posttraumatic segmental axial dystonia. Mov Disord 1992;7:78–81.

Jabusch HC, Altenmuller E: Three-dimensional movement analysis as a promising tool for treatment evaluation of musicians' dystonia. In Fahn S, Hallett M, DeLong M (eds): Dystonia 4: Advances in Neurology, vol 94. Philadelphia, Lippincott Williams & Wilkins, 2004, pp 239–245.

Jahanshahi M, Rowe J, Fuller R: Cognitive executive function in dystonia. Mov Disord 2003;18(12):1470–1481.

Jankovic J: Dystonia and other deformities in Parkinson's disease. J Neurol Sci 2005;239(1):1–3.

Jankovic J, Fahn S: Physiologic and pathologic tremors. Diagnosis, mechanism, and management. Ann Int Med 1980;93:460–465.

Jankovic J, Fahn S: Dystonic disorders. In Jankovic J, Tolosa E (eds): Parkinson's Disease and Movement Disorders, 3rd ed. Baltimore, Williams & Wilkins, 1998, pp 513–551.

Jankovic J, Patel SC: Blepharospasm associated with brainstem lesions. Neurology 1983;33:1237–1240.

Jankovic J, Penn AS: Severe dystonia and myoglobinuria. Neurology 1982;32:1195–1197.

Jankovic J, Svendsen CN, Bird ED: Brain neurotransmitters in dystonia. N Engl J Med 1987;316:278–279.

Janssen RJ, Wevers RA, Haussler M, et al: A branch site mutation leading to aberrant splicing of the human tyrosine hydroxylase gene in a child with a severe extrapyramidal movement disorder. Ann Hum Genet 2000;64(pt 5):375–382.

Jarman PR, Bandmann O, Marsden CD, Wood NW: GTP cyclohydrolase I mutations in patients with dystonia responsive to anticholinergic drugs. J Neurol Neurosurg Psychiatry 1997;63: 304–308.

Jarman PR, Del Grosso N, Valente EM, et al: Primary torsion dystonia: The search for genes is not over. J Neurol Neurosurg Psychiat 1999;67:395–397.

Jedynak CP, Bonnet AM, Agid Y: Tremor and idiopathic dystonia. Mov Disord 1991;6:230–236.

Jeon BS: Dopa-responsive dystonia: A syndrome of selective nigrostriatal dopaminergic deficiency. J Korean Med Sci 1997;12:269–279.

Jin H, Kendall E, Freeman TC, et al: The human family of deafness/dystonia peptide (DDP) related mitochondrial import proteins. Genomics 1999;61:259–267.

Jin H, May M, Tranebjaerg L, et al: A novel X-linked gene, DDP, shows mutations in families with deafness (DFN-1), dystonia, mental deficiency and blindness. Nat Genet 1996;14:177–180.

Kabakci K, Isbruch K, Schilling K, et al: Genetic heterogeneity in rapid onset dystonia-parkinsonism: Description of a new family. J Neurol Neurosurg Psychiatry 2005;76(6):860–862.

Kaji R, Rothwell JC, Katayama M, et al: Tonic vibration reflex and muscle afferent block in writer's cramp. Ann Neurol 1995;38: 155–162.

Kalita J, Misra UK: Markedly severe dystonia in Japanese encephalitis. Mov Disord 2000;15:1168–1172.

Kamm C, Naumann M, Mueller J, et al: The DYT1 GAG deletion is infrequent in sporadic and familial writer's cramp. Mov Disord 2000;15:1238–1241.

Kamphuis DJ, Koelman H, Lees AJ, Tijssen MA: Sporadic rapid-onset dystonia-parkinsonism presenting as Parkinson's disease. Mov Disord 2006;21(1):118–119.

Karsidag S, Ozer F, Sen A, Arpaci B: Lesion localization in developing poststroke hand dystonia. Eur Neurol 1998;40:99–104.

Kastrup O, Gastpar M, Schwarz M: Acute dystonia due to clozapine. J Neurol Neurosurg Psychiatry 1994;57:119.

Khan NL, Wood NW, Bhatia KP: Autosomal recessive, DYT2-like primary torsion dystonia: A new family. Neurology 2003;61(12): 1801–1803.

Klein C, Brin MF, de Leon D, et al: De novo mutations (GAG deletion) in the DYT1 gene in two non-Jewish patients with early-onset dystonia. Hum Mol Genet 1998;7:1133–1136.

Klein C, Brin MF, Kramer P, et al: Association of a missense change in the D2 dopamine receptor with myoclonus dystonia. Proc Nat Acad Sci U S A 1999;96:5173–5176.

Klein C, Gurvich N, Sena-Esteves M, et al: Evaluation of the role of the D2 dopamine receptor in myoclonus dystonia. Ann Neurol 2000;47:369–373.

Klein C, Liu L, Doheny D, et al: Epsilon-sarcoglycan mutations found in combination with other dystonia gene mutations. Ann Neurol 2002;52(5):675–679.

Klein C, Ozelius LJ, Hagenah J, et al: Search for a founder mutation in idiopathic focal dystonia from northern Germany. Amer J Hum Genet 1998;63:1777–1782.

Klein C, Schilling K, Saunders-Pullman RJ, et al: A major locus for myoclonus-dystonia maps to chromosome 7q in eight families. Amer J Hum Genet 2000;67:1314–1319.

Klier EM, Wang HY, Constantin AG, Crawford JD: Midbrain control of three-dimensional head orientation. Science 2002;295:1314–1316.

Klostermann W, Vieregge P, Kompf D: Spasmodic torticollis in multiple sclerosis: Significance of an upper cervical spinal cord lesion. Mov Disord 1993;8:234–236.

Knappskog PM, Flatmark T, Mallet J, et al: Recessively inherited L-DOPA-responsive dystonia caused by a point mutation (Q381K) in the tyrosine hydroxylase gene. Hum Mol Genet 1995;4:1209–1212.

Koehler CM, Leuenberger D, Merchant S, et al: Human deafness dystonia syndrome is a mitochondrial disease. Proc Nat Acad Sci U S A 1999;96:2141–2146.

Koepp M, Schelosky L, Cordes I, et al: Dystonia in ataxia telangiectasia: Report of a case with putaminal lesions and decreased striatal [I-123]iodobenzamide binding. Mov Disord 1994;9:455–459.

Konakova M, Huynh DP, Yong W, Pulst SM: Cellular distribution of torsin A and torsin B in normal human brain. Arch Neurol 2001;58:921–927.

Konakova M, Pulst SM: Immunocytochemical characterization of torsin proteins in mouse brain. Brain Res 2001;922(1):1–8.

Konakova M, Pulst SM: Dystonia-associated forms of torsinA are deficient in ATPase activity. J Mol Neurosci 2005;25(1):105–111.

Krack P, Marion MH: "Apraxia of lid opening," a focal eyelid dystonia: Clinical study of 32 patients. Mov Disord 1994;9:610–615.

Krack P, Schneider S, Deuschl G: Geste device in tardive dystonia with retrocollis and opisthotonic posturing. Mov Disord 1998;13:155–157.

Kramer PL, Heiman GA, Gasser T, et al: The DYTI gene on 9q34 is responsible for most cases of early limb-onset idiopathic torsion dystonia in non-Jews. Am J Hum Genet 1994;55:468–475.

Kramer PL, Mineta M, Klein C, et al: Rapid-onset dystonia-parkinsonism: Linkage to chromosome 19q13. Ann Neurol 1999;46:176–182.

Kramer PL, Ozelius L, de Leon D, et al: Dystonia gene in Ashkenazi Jewish population located on chromosome 9q32-34. Ann Neurol 1990;27:114–120.

Krauss JK, Mohadjer M, Wakhloo AK, Mundinger F: Dystonia and akinesia due to pallidoputaminal lesions after disulfiram intoxication. Mov Disord 1991;6:166–170.

Krauss JK, Seeger W, Jankovic J: Cervical dystonia associated with tumors of the posterior fossa. Mov Disord 1997;12:443–447.

Krauss JK, Trankle R, Kopp KH: Post-traumatic movement disorders in survivors of severe head injury. Neurology 1996;47:1488–1492.

Krystkowiak P, Martinat P, Defebvre L, et al: Dystonia after striatopallidal and thalamic stroke: Clinicoradiological correlations and pathophysiological mechanisms. J Neurol Neurosurg Psychiatry 1998;65:703–708.

Kulisevsky J, Avila A, Roig C, Escartin A: Unilateral blepharospasm stemming from a thalamomesencephalic lesion. Mov Disord 1993;8:239–240.

Kumar N, Boes CJ, Babovic-Vuksanovic D, Boeve BF: The "eye-of-the-tiger" sign is not pathognomonic of the PANK2 mutation. Arch Neurol 2006;63:292–293.

Kuner R, Teismann P, Trutzel A, et al: TorsinA protects against oxidative stress in COS-1 and PC12 cells. Neurosci Lett 2003;350(3):153–156.

Kuner R, Teismann P, Trutzel A, et al: TorsinA, the gene linked to early-onset dystonia, is upregulated by the dopaminergic toxin MPTP in mice. Neurosci Lett 2004;355(1–2):126–130.

Kuoppamaki M, Bhatia KP, Quinn N: Progressive delayed-onset dystonia after cerebral anoxic insult in adults. Mov Disord 2002;17(6):1345–1349.

Kupke KG, Graeber MB, Muller U: Dystonia-parkinsonism syndrome (XDP) locus: Flanking markers in Xq12-q21.1. Am J Hum Genet 1992;50:808–815.

Kupke KG, Lee LV, Muller U: Assignment of the X-linked torsion dystonia gene to Xq21 by linkage analysis. Neurology 1990;40:1438–1442.

Kurlan R, Behr J, Medved L, Shoulson I: Myoclonus and dystonia: A family study. Adv Neurol 1988;50:385–389.

Kustedjo K, Bracey MH, Cravatt BF: Torsin A and its torsion dystonia-associated mutant forms are lumenal glycoproteins that exhibit distinct subcellular localizations. J Biol Chem 2000;275:27933–27939.

Kutvonen O, Dastidar P, Nurmikko T: Pain in spasmodic torticollis. Pain 1997;69:279–286.

Kyllerman M, Forsgren L, Sanner G, et al: Alcohol responsive myoclonic dystonia in a large family. Dominant inheritance and phenotypic variation. Mov Disord 1990;5:270–279.

Kyllerman M, Skjeldal OH, Lundberg MA-H, et al: Dystonia and dyskinesia in glutaric aciduria type-I: Clinical heterogeneity and therapeutic considerations. Mov Disord 1994;9:22–30.

Lang A, Quinn N, Marsden CD, et al: Essential tremor. Neurology 1992;42:1432–1433.

Le KD, Nilsen B, Dietrichs E: Prevalence of primary focal and segmental dystonia in Oslo. Neurology 2003;61(9):1294–1296.

LeDoux MS, Brady KA: Secondary cervical dystonia associated with structural lesions of the central nervous system. Mov Disord 2003;18(1):60–69.

Lee LV, Kupke KG, Caballargonzaga F, et al: The phenotype of the X-linked dystonia-parkinsonism syndrome: An assessment of 42 cases in the Philippines. Medicine (Baltimore) 1991;70:179–187.

Lee LV, Pascasio FM, Fuentes FD, Viterbo GH: Torsion dystonia in Panay, Philippines. Adv Neurol 1976;14:137–152.

Lee MS, Rinne JO, Ceballos-Baumann A, et al: Dystonia after head trauma. Neurology 1994;44:1374–1378.

Leenders K, Hartvig P, Forsgren L, et al: Striatal [C-11]-N-methyl-spiperone binding in patients with focal dystonia (torticollis) using positron emission tomography. J Neural Transm Park Dis Dement Sect 1993;5:79–87.

Lehericy S, Vidailhet M, Dormont D, et al: Striatopallidal and thalamic dystonia: A magnetic resonance imaging anatomoclinical study. Arch Neurol 1996;53:241–250.

Lenz FA, Suarez JI, Metman LV, et al: Pallidal activity during dystonia: Somatosensory reorganisation and changes with severity. J Neurol Neurosurg Psychiatry 1998;65:767–770.

Leopold NA, Bara-Jimenez W, Hallett M: Parkinsonism after a wasp sting. Mov Disord 1999;14(1):122–127.

Lesser RP, Fahn S: Dystonia: A disorder often misdiagnosed as a conversion reaction. Am J Psychiatry 1978;153:349–452.

Leube B, Auburger G: Questionable role of adult-onset focal dystonia among sporadic dystonia patients. Ann Neurol 1998;44:984–985.

Leube B, Hendgen T, Kessler KR, et al: Evidence for DYT7 being a common cause of cervical dystonia (torticollis) in Central Europe. Am J Med Genet 1997a;74:529–532.

Leube B, Hendgen T, Kessler KR, et al: Sporadic focal dystonia in Northwest Germany: Molecular basis on chromosome 18p. Ann Neurol 1997b;42:111–114.

Leube B, Rudnicki D, Ratzlaff T, et al: Idiopathic torsion dystonia: Assignment of a gene to chromosome 18p in a German family with adult onset, autosomal dominant inheritance and purely focal distribution. Hum Mol Genet 1996;5:1673–1677.

Leuzzi V, Carducci C, Carducci C, et al: Autosomal dominant GTP-CH deficiency presenting as a dopa-responsive myoclonus-dystonia syndrome. Neurology 2002;59(8):1241–1243.

Levy LM, Hallett M: Impaired brain GABA in focal dystonia. Ann Neurol 2002;51:93–101.

Lim EC, Seet RC, Wilder-Smith EP, Ong BK: Dystonia gravidarum: A new entity? Mov Disord 2006;21:69–70.

Lobbezoo F, Tanguay R, Thon MT, Lavigne GJ: Pain perception in idiopathic cervical dystonia (spasmodic torticollis). Pain 1996;67:483–491.

Lopez-Alemany M, Ferrer-Tuset C, Bernacer-Alpera B: Akathisia and acute dystonia induced by sumatriptan. J Neurol 1997;244:131–132.

Lossos A, Schlesinger I, Okon E, et al: Adult-onset Niemann-pick type C disease: Clinical, biochemical, and genetic study. Arch Neurol 1997;54:1536–1541.

Lou JS, Jankovic J: Essential tremor: Clinical correlates in 350 patients. Neurology 1991;41:234–238.

Lüdecke B, Dworniczak B, Bartholomé K: A point mutation in the tyrosine hydroxylase gene associated with Segawa's syndrome. Hum Genet 1995;95:123–125.

Lüdecke B, Knappskog PM, Clayton PT, et al: Recessively inherited L-DOPA-responsive parkinsonism in infancy caused by a point mutation (L205P) in the tyrosine hydroxylase gene. Hum Mol Genet 1996;5:1023–1028.

Ludolph AC, Seelig M, Ludolph A, et al: 3-Nitropropionic acid decreases cellular energy levels and causes neuronal degeneration in cortical explants. Neurodegeneration 1992;1:155–161.

Madhusoodanan S, Brenner R: Reversible choreiform dyskinesia and extrapyramidal symptoms associated with sertraline therapy. J Clin Psychopharmacol 1997;17:138–139.

Madhusudanan M, Gracykutty M, Cherian M: Athetosis-dystonia in intramedullary lesions of spinal cord. Acta Neurol Scand 1995; 92:308–312.

Magyar-Lehmann S, Antonini A, Roelcke U, et al: Cerebral glucose metabolism in patients with spasmodic torticollis. Mov Disord 1997;12:704–708.

Makino S, Kaji R, Ando S, et al: Reduced neuron-specific expression of the TAF1 gene is associated with X-linked dystonia-parkinsonism. Am J Hum Genet 2007;80(3):393–406.

Maller R, Hyland K, Milstien S, et al: Aromatic L-amino acid decarboxylase deficiency: Clinical features, diagnosis, and treatment of a second family. J Child Neurol 1997;12:349–354.

Manji H, Howard RS, Miller DH, et al: Status dystonicus: The syndrome and its management. Brain 1998;121:243–252.

Maraganore DM, Folger WN, Swanson JW, Ahlskog JE: Movement disorders as sequelae of central pontine myelinolysis: Report of three cases. Mov Disord 1992;7:142–148.

Marsden CD: The focal dystonias. Clin Neuropharmacol 1986; 9(suppl 2):S49–S60.

Marsden CD, Harrison MJG, Bundey S: Natural history of idiopathic torsion dystonia. Adv Neurol 1976;14:177–187.

Marsden CD, Obeso JA, Zarranz JJ, Lang AE: The anatomical basis of symptomatic hemidystonia. Brain 1985;108:463–483.

Mathen D, Marsden CD, Bhatia KP: SSRI-induced reversal of levodopa benefit in two patients with dopa-responsive dystonia. Mov Disord 1999;14:874–876.

Matsumoto S, Nishimura M, Kaji R, et al: DYT1 mutation in Japanese patients with primary torsion dystonia. Neuroreport 2001;12: 793–795.

Matsumoto S, Nishimura M, Shibasaki H, Kaji R: Epidemiology of primary dystonias in Japan: Comparison with Western countries. Mov Disord 2003;18(10):1196–1198.

Mazzini L, Zaccala M, Balzarini C: Abnormalities of somatosensory evoked potentials in spasmodic torticollis. Mov Disord 1994; 9:426–430.

McLean PJ, Kawamata H, Shariff S, et al: TorsinA and heat shock proteins act as molecular chaperones: Suppression of alpha-synuclein aggregation. J Neurochem 2002;83(4):846–854.

McNaught KS, Kapustin A, Jackson T, et al: Brainstem pathology in DYT1 primary torsion dystonia. Ann Neurol 2004;56(4):540–547.

Meierkord H, Fish DR, Smith SJM, et al: Is nocturnal paroxysmal dystonia a form of frontal lobe epilepsy? Mov Disord 1992;7:38–42.

Merello M, Garcia H, Nogues M, Leiguarda R: Masticatory muscle spasm in a non-Japanese patient with Satoyoshi syndrome successfully treated with botulinum toxin. Mov Disord 1994;9:104–105.

Mir P, Edwards MJ, Curtis ARJ, et al: Adult-onset generalized dystonia due to a mutation in the neuroferritinopathy gene. Mov Disord 2005;20(2):243–245.

Miranda M, Millar A: Blepharospasm associated with bilateral infarcts confined to the thalamus: Case report. Mov Disord 1998; 13:616–617.

Misbahuddin A, Placzek MR, Chaudhuri KR, et al: A polymorphism in the dopamine receptor DRD5 is associated with blepharospasm. Neurology 2002;58:124–126.

Molho ES, Factor SA: Basal ganglia infarction as a possible cause of cervical dystonia. Mov Disord 1993;8:213–216.

Montagna P: Nocturnal paroxysmal dystonia and nocturnal wandering. Neurology 1992;42:61–67.

Moretti P, Hedera P, Wald J, Fink J: Autosomal recessive primary generalized dystonia in two siblings from a consanguineous family. Mov Disord 2005;20(2):245–247.

Muller B, Hedrich K, Kock N, et al: Evidence that paternal expression of the epsilon-sarcoglycan gene accounts for reduced penetrance in myoclonus-dystonia. Am J Hum Genet 2002;71(6):1303–1311.

Muller J, Wissel T, Masuhr F, et al: Clinical characteristics of the geste antagoniste in cervical dystonia. J Neurol 2001;248:478–482.

Muller T, Woitalla D, Hunsdiek A, Kuhn W: Elevated plasma levels of homocysteine in dystonia. Acta Neurol Scand 2000;101:388–390.

Müller U, Haberhausen G, Wagner T, et al: DXS106 and DXS559 flank the X-linked dystonia-parkinsonism syndrome locus (DYT3). Genomics 1994;23:114–117.

Munchau A, Filipovic SR, Oester-Barkey A, et al: Spontaneously changing muscular activation pattern in patients with cervical dystonia. Mov Disord 2001;16:1091–1097.

Munchau A, Mathen D, Cox T, et al: Unilateral lesions of the globus pallidus: Report of four patients presenting with focal or segmental dystonia. J Neurol Neurosurg Psychiat 2000;69:494–498.

Munchau A, Schrag A, Chuang C, et al: Arm tremor in cervical dystonia differs from essential tremor and can be classified by onset age and spread of symptoms. Brain 2001;124:1765–1776.

Munhoz RP, Lang AE: Gestes antagonistes in psychogenic dystonia. Mov Disord 2004;19(3):331–332.

Munoz JE, Tolosa E, Saiz A, et al: Upper-limb dystonia secondary to a midbrain hemorrhage. Mov Disord 1996;11:96–99.

Murgod UA, Muthane UB, Ravi V, et al: Persistent movement disorders following Japanese encephalitis. Neurology 2001;57(12): 2313–2315.

Naismith TV, Heuser JE, Breakefield XO, Hanson PI: TorsinA in the nuclear envelope. Proc Nat Acad Sci U S A 2004;101(20):7612–7617.

Nakashima K, Kusumi M, Inoue Y, Takahashi K: Prevalence of focal dystonias in the western area of Tottori Prefecture in Japan. Mov Disord 1995;10:440–443.

Nakashima K, Rothwell JC, Day BL, et al: Reciprocal inhibition between forearm muscles in patients with writer's cramp and other occupational cramps, symptomatic hemidystonia and hemiparesis due to stroke. Brain 1989;112:681–697.

Narbona J, Obeso JA, Tunon T, et al: Hemi-dystonia secondary to localised basal ganglia tumour. J Neurol Neurosurg Psychiatry 1984;47:704–709.

Nardocci N, Zorzi G, Blau N, et al: Neonatal dopa-responsive extrapyramidal syndrome in twins with recessive GTPCH deficiency. Neurology 2003;60(2):335–337.

Naumann M, Becker G, Toyka KV, et al: Lenticular nucleus lesion in idiopathic dystonia detected by transcranial sonography. Neurology 1996;47:1284–1290.

Naumann M, Magyar-Lehmann S, Reiners K, et al: Sensory tricks in cervical dystonia: Perceptual dysbalance of parietal cortex modulates frontal motor programming. Ann Neurol 2000;47:322–328.

Naumann M, Pirker W, Reiners K, et al: [I-123]beta-CIT single-photon emission tomography in DOPA-responsive dystonia. Mov Disord 1997;12:448–451.

Naumann M, Pirker W, Reiners K, et al: Imaging the pre- and postsynaptic side of striatal dopaminergic synapses in idiopathic cervical dystonia: A SPECT study using [I-123] epidepride and [I-123] beta-CIT. Mov Disord 1998;13:319–323.

Naumann M, Reiners K: Long-latency reflexes of hand muscles in idiopathic focal dystonia and their modification by botulinum toxin. Brain 1997;120:409–416.

Neville BG, Parascandalo R, Farrugia R, Felice A: Sepiapterin reductase deficiency: A congenital dopa-responsive motor and cognitive disorder. Brain 2005;128(pt 10):2291–2296.

Nolte D, Niemann S, Muller U: Specific sequence changes in multiple transcript system DYT3 are associated with X-linked dystonia parkinsonism. Proc Natl Acad Sci U S A 2003;100(18):10347–10352.

Nutt JG, Muenter MD, Aronson A, et al: Epidemiology of focal and generalized dystonia in Rochester, Minnesota. Mov Disord 1988;3:188–194.

Nygaard TG: Dopa-responsive dystonia: 20 years into the L-dopa era. In Quinn NP, Jenner PG (eds): Disorders of Movement: Clinical Pharmacological and Physiological Aspects. London, Academic Press Limited, 1989, pp 323–337.

Nygaard TG, Marsden CD, Fahn S: Dopa-responsive dystonia: Long-term treatment response and prognosis. Neurology 1991;41:174–181.

Nygaard TG, Raymond D, Chen CP, et al: Localization of a gene for myoclonus-dystonia to chromosome 7q21-q31. Ann Neurol 1999;46:794–798.

Nygaard TG, Takahashi H, Heiman GA, et al: Long-term treatment response and fluorodopa positron emission tomographic scanning of parkinsonism in a family with dopa-responsive dystonia. Ann Neurol 1992;32:603–608.

Nygaard TG, Trugman JM, de Yebenes JG, Fahn S: Dopa-responsive dystonia: The spectrum of clinical manifestations in a large North American family. Neurology 1990;40:66–69.

Nygaard TG, Waran SP, Levine RA, et al: Dopa-responsive dystonia simulating cerebral palsy. Pediatr Neurol 1994;11:236–240.

Nygaard TG, Wilhelmsen KC, Risch NJ, et al: Linkage mapping of dopa-responsive dystonia (DRD) to chromosome 14q. Nat Genet 1993;5:386–391.

Oberlin SR, Konakova M, Pulst S, Chesselet MF: Development and anatomic localization of torsinA. In Fahn S, Hallett M, DeLong M (eds): Dystonia 4: Advances in Neurology, vol 94. Philadelphia, Lippincott Williams & Wilkins, 2004, pp 61–65.

Obeso JA, Rothwell JC, Lang AE, Marsden CD: Myoclonic dystonia. Neurology 1983;33:825–830.

Ochoa JL: Truths, errors, and lies around "reflex sympathetic dystrophy" and "complex regional pain syndrome." J Neurol 1999;246:875–879.

O'Farrell C, Hernandez DG, Evey C, et al: Normal localization of Delta F323-Y328 mutant torsinA in transfected human cells. Neurosci Lett 2002;327(2):75–78.

Okun MS, Nadeau SE, Rossi F, Triggs WJ: Immobilization dystonia. J Neurol Sci 2002;201(1–2):79–83.

Olivera AA: Sertraline and akathisia: Spontaneous resolution. Biol Psychiatry 1997;41:241–242.

Opal P, Tintner R, Jankovic J, et al: Intrafamilial phenotypic variability of the DYT1 dystonia: From asymptomatic TOR1A gene carrier status to dystonic storm. Mov Disord 2002;17(2):339–345.

Oppenheim H: Uber eine eigenartige Krampfkrankheit des kindlichen und jugendlichen Alters (Dysbasia lordotica progressiva, Dystonia musculorum deformans). Neurol Centrabl 1911;30:1090–1107.

O'Riordan S, Raymond D, Lynch T, et al: Age at onset as a factor in determining the phenotype of primary torsion dystonia. Neurology 2004;63(8):1423–1426.

Ornadel D, Barnes EA, Dick DJ: Acute dystonia due to amitriptyline. J Neurol Neurosurg Psychiatry 1992;55:414.

Ozelius L, Kramer PL, Moskowitz CB, et al: Human gene for torsion dystonia located on chromosome 9q32-34. Neuron 1989;2:1427–1434.

Ozelius LJ, Hewett JW, Page CE, et al: The early-onset torsion dystonia gene (DYT1) encodes an ATP binding protein. Nat Genet 1997;17:40–48.

Pal PK, Samii A, Schulzer M, et al: Head tremor in cervical dystonia. Can J Neurol Sci 2000;27:137–142.

Paret G, Tirosh R, Benzeev B, et al: Rhabdomyolysis due to hereditary torsion dystonia. Pediatr Neurol 1995;13:83–84.

Parker N: Hereditary whispering dysphonia. J Neurol Neurosurg Psychiatry 1985;48:218–224.

Pauls DL, Korczyn AD: Complex segregation analysis of dystonia pedigrees suggests autosomal dominant inheritance. Neurology 1990;40:1107–1110.

Pekmezovic T, Ivanovic N, Svetel M, et al: Prevalence of primary late-onset focal dystonia in the Belgrade population. Mov Disord 2003;18(11):1389–1392.

Perlmutter JS, Stambuk MK, Markham J, et al: Decreased [F-18] spiperone binding in putamen in idiopathic focal dystonia. J Neurosci 1997a;17:843–850.

Perlmutter JS, Tempel LW, Black KJ, et al: MPTP induces dystonia and parkinsonism: Clues to the pathophysiology of dystonia. Neurology 1997b;1432–1438.

Pesenti A, Barbieri S, Priori A: Limb immobilization for occupational dystonia: A possible alternative treatment for selected patients. Adv Neurol 2004;94:247–254.

Pettigrew LC, Jankovic J: Hemidystonia: A report of 22 patients and a review of the literature. J Neurol Neurosurg Psychiatry 1985;48:650–657.

Pittock SJ, Joyce C, O'Keane V, et al: Rapid-onset dystonia-parkinsonism: A clinical and genetic analysis of a new kindred. Neurology 2000;55:991–995.

Placzek MR, Misbahuddin A, Chaudhuri KR, et al: Cervical dystonia is associated with a polymorphism in the dopamine (D5) receptor gene. J Neurol Neurosurg Psychiatry 2001;71:262–264.

Playford ED, Fletcher NA, Sawle GV, et al: Striatal [F-18]dopa uptake in familial idiopathic dystonia. Brain 1993;116:1191–1199.

Playford ED, Passingham RE, Marsden CD, Brooks DJ: Increased activation of frontal areas during arm movement in idiopathic torsion dystonia. Mov Disord 1998;13:309–318.

Pohl C, Happe J, Klockgether T: Cooling improves the writing performance of patients with writer's cramp. Mov Disord 2002;17(6):1341–1344.

Pons R, Ford B, Chiriboga CA, et al: Aromatic L-amino acid decarboxylase deficiency: Clinical features, treatment, and prognosis. Neurology 2004;62(7):1058–1065.

Preston DC, Finkleman RS, Munsat TL: Dystonic postures generated from complex repetitive discharges. Neurology 1996;46:257–258.

Pullman SL, Ford B, Elibol B, et al: Cutaneous electromyographic silent period findings in brachial dystonia. Neurology 1996;46:503–508.

Quinn NP: Essential myoclonus and myoclonic dystonia. Mov Disord 1996;11:119–124.

Quinn NP, Rothwell JC, Thompson PD, Marsden CD: Hereditary myoclonic dystonia, hereditary torsion dystonia and hereditary essential myoclonus: An area of confusion. Adv Neurol 1988;50:391–401.

Raja M, Azzoni A: Novel antipsychotics and acute dystonic reactions. Int J Neuropsychopharmacol 2001;4(4):393–397.

Rajput AH, Gibb WRG, Zhong XH, et al: DOPA-responsive dystonia: Pathological and biochemical observations in a case. Ann Neurol 1994;35:396–402.

Reichmann H, Naumann M, Hauck S, Janetzky B: Respiratory chain and mitochondrial deoxyribonucleic acid in blood cells from patients with focal and generalized dystonia. Mov Disord 1994;9:597–600.

Rinne JO, Iivanainen M, Metsahonkala L, et al: Striatal dopaminergic system in dopa-responsive dystonia: A multi-tracer PET study shows increased D2 receptors. J Neural Transm 2004;111(1):59–67.

Risch N, Bressman SB, deLeon D, et al: Segregation analysis of idiopathic torsion dystonia in Ashkenazi Jews suggests autosomal dominant inheritance. Am J Hum Genet 1990;46:533–538.

Risch N, De Leon D, Ozelius L, et al: Genetic analysis of idiopathic torsion dystonia in Ashkenazi Jews and their recent descent from a small founder population. Nat Genet 1995;9:152–159.

Roesch K, Curran SP, Tranebjaerg L, Koehler CM: Human deafness dystonia syndrome is caused by a defect in assembly of the DDP1/TIMM8a-TIMM13 complex. Hum Mol Genet 2002;11(5):477–486.

Rosenbaum F, Jankovic J: Focal task-specific tremor and dystonia: Categorization of occupational movement disorders. Neurology 1988;38:522–527.

Rostasy K, Augood SJ, Hewett JW, et al: TorsinA protein and neuropathology in early onset generalized dystonia with GAG deletion. Neurobiol Dis 2003;12:11–24.

Rothbauer U, Hofmann S, Muhlenbein N, et al: Role of the deafness dystonia peptide 1 (DDP1) in import of human Tim23 into the inner membrane of mitochondria. J Biol Chem 2001;276:37327–37334.

Rothwell JC, Obeso JA: The anatomical and physiological basis of torsion dystonia. In Marsden CD, Fahn S (eds): Movement Disorders 2. London, Butterworths, 1987, pp 313–331.

Rothwell JC, Obeso JA, Day BL, Marsden CD: The pathophysiology of dystonias. Adv Neurol 1983;39:851–863.

Rousseaux M, Cassim F, Benaim C, et al: Dystonia and tremor in a bilateral lesion of the posterior mesencephalon and vermis. Rev Neurol 1996;152:732–737.

Rutledge JN, Hilal SK, Silver AJ, et al: Study of movement disorders and brain iron by MR. Am J Neuroradiol 1987;8:397–411.

Sa DS, Mailis-Gagnon A, Nicholson K, Lang AE: Posttraumatic painful torticollis. Mov Disord 2003;18(12):1482–1491.

Saint-Hilaire M-H, Burke RE, Bressman SB, et al: Delayed-onset dystonia due to perinatal or early childhood asphyxia. Neurology 1991;41:216–222.

Sanger TD, Pascual-Leone A, Tarsy D, Schlaug G: Nonlinear sensory cortex response to simultaneous tactile stimuli in writer's cramp. Mov Disord 2002;17(1):105–111.

Saunders-Pullman R, Shriberg J, Heiman G, et al: Myoclonus dystonia: Possible association with obsessive-compulsive disorder and alcohol dependence. Neurology 2002;58:242–245.

Sawle GV, Leenders KL, Brooks DJ, et al: Dopa-responsive dystonia: [F-18]dopa positron emission tomography. Ann Neurol 1991; 30:24–30.

Schapira AHV, Warner T, Gash MT, et al: Complex I function in familial and sporadic dystonia. Ann Neurol 1997;41:556–559.

Scheidt CE, Schuller B, Rayki O, et al: Relative absence of psychopathology in benign essential blepharospasm and hemifacial spasm. Neurology 1996;47:43–45.

Schiller A, Wevers RA, Steenbergen GCH, et al: Long-term course of L-dopa-responsive dystonia caused by tyrosine hydroxylase deficiency. Neurology 2004;63(8):1524–1526.

Schneider S, Feifel E, Ott D, et al: Prolonged MRI T-2 times of the lentiform nucleus in idiopathic spasmodic torticollis. Neurology 1994;44:846–850.

Schneider SA, Mohire MD, Trender-Gerhard I, et al: Familial dopa-responsive cervical dystonia. Neurology 2006;66(4):599–601.

Schrag A, Bhatia KP, Quinn NP, Marsden CD: Atypical and typical cranial dystonia following dental procedures. Mov Disord 1999;14:492–496.

Schrag A, Trimble M, Quinn N, Bhatia K: The syndrome of fixed dystonia: An evaluation of 103 patients. Brain 2004;127:2360–2372.

Schramm A, Reiners K, Naumann M: Complex mechanisms of sensory tricks in cervical dystonia. Mov Disord 2004;19(4):452–458.

Schwalbe W: Eine eigentumliche tonische Krampfform mit hysterischen Symptomen. Inaug Diss, Berlin, G. Schade, 1908.

Scolding NJ, Smith SM, Sturman S, et al: Auctioneer's jaw: A case of occupational oromandibular hemidystonia. Mov Disord 1995; 10:508–509.

Scott BL, Jankovic J: Delayed-onset progressive movement disorders after static brain lesions. Neurology 1996;46:68–74.

Scott RB, Gregory R, Wilson J, et al: Executive cognitive deficits in primary dystonia. Mov Disord 2003;18(5):539–550.

Segawa M, Hosaka A, Miyagawa F, et al: Hereditary progressive dystonia with marked diurnal fluctuation. Adv Neurol 1976;14: 215–233.

Sekijima Y, Hashimoto T, Onodera O, et al: Severe generalized dystonia as a presentation of a patient with aprataxin gene mutation. Mov Disord 2003;18(10):1198–1200.

Sellal F, Hirsch E, Maquet P, et al: Postures et mouvements anormaux paroxystiques au cours du sommeil: Dystonie paroxystique hypnogenique ou epilepsie partielle? [Abnormal paroxysmal movements during sleep: Hypnogenic paroxysmal dystonia or focal epilepsy?] Rev Neurol 1991;147:121–128.

Senanayake N, Sanmuganathan PS: Extrapyramidal manifestations complicating organophosphorus insecticide poisoning. Hum Exp Toxicol 1995;14:600–604.

Sethi KD, Hess DC: Creutzfeldt-Jakob's disease presenting with ataxia and a movement disorder. Mov Disord 1991;6:157–162.

Sethi KD, Jankovic J: Dystonia in spinocerebellar ataxia type 6. Mov Disord 2002;17:150–153.

Sethi KD, Lee KH, Deuskar V, Hess DC: Orthostatic paroxysmal dystonia. Mov Disord 2002;17(4):841–845.

Shale H, Fahn S, Calne DB: What is it? Case 1, 1988: Head tilt in a young girl associated with neck pain and limitation of neck movement. Mov Disord 1988;3:347–351.

Shale HM, Truong DD, Fahn S: Tics in patients with other movement disorders. Neurology 1986;36(suppl 1):118.

Sharma N, Hewett J, Ozelius LJ, et al: A close association of torsinA and alpha-synuclein in Lewy bodies: A fluorescence resonance energy transfer study. Am J Pathol 2001;159(1):339–344.

Shashidharan P, Good PF, Hsu A, et al: TorsinA accumulation in Lewy bodies in sporadic Parkinson's disease. Brain Res 2000a;877:379–381.

Shashidharan P, Kramer BC, Walker RH, et al: Immunohistochemical localization and distribution of torsinA in normal human and rat brain. Brain Res 2000b; 853:197–206.

Sheehy MP, Marsden CD: Writer's cramp: A focal dystonia. Brain 1982;105:461–480.

Sibbing D, Asmus F, Konig IR, et al: Candidate gene studies in focal dystonia. Neurology 2003;61(8):1097–1101.

Simon DK, Friedman J, Breakefield XO, et al: A heteroplasmic mitochondrial complex I gene mutation in adult-onset dystonia. Neurogenetics 2003;4(4):199–205.

Snow BJ, Nygaard TG, Takahashi H, Calne DB: Positron emission tomographic studies of DOPA-responsive dystonia and early-onset idiopathic parkinsonism. Ann Neurol 1993;34:733–738.

Sohn YH, Hallett M: Disturbed surround inhibition in focal hand dystonia. Ann Neurol 2004;56(4):595–599.

Soland VL, Bhatia KP, Marsden CD: Sex prevalence of focal dystonias. J Neurol Neurosurg Psychiatry 1996a;60:204–205.

Soland VL, Bhatia KP, Volonte MA, Marsden CD: Focal task-specific tremors. Mov Disord 1996b;11:665–670.

Sommer M, Ruge D, Tergau F, et al: Intracortical excitability in the hand motor representation in hand dystonia and blepharospasm. Mov Disord 2002;17(5):1017–1025.

Steinberger D, Topka H, Fischer D, Muller U: GCH1 mutation in a patient with adult-onset oromandibular dystonia. Neurology 1999;52:877–879.

Steinberger D, Weber Y, Korinthenberg R, et al: High penetrance and pronounced variation in expressivity of GCH1 mutations in five families with dopa-responsive dystonia. Ann Neurol 1998;43: 634–639.

Stone LA, Jankovic J: The coexistence of tics and dystonia. Arch Neurol 1991;48:862–865.

Stromme P, Mangelsdorf ME, Scheffer IE, Geecz J: Infantile spasms, dystonia, and other X-linked phenotypes caused by mutations in Aristaless related homeobox gene, ARX. Brain Develop 2002; 24(5):266–268.

Sudarsky L, Plotkin GM, Logigian EL, Johns DR: Dystonia as a presenting feature of the 3243 mitochondrial DNA mutation. Mov Disord 1999;14:488–491.

Svetel M, Ivanovic N, Marinkovic J, et al: Characteristics of dystonic movements in primary and symptomatic dystonias. J Neurol Neurosurg Psychiatry 2004;75(2):329–330.

Swaans RJM, Rondot P, Renier WO, et al: Four novel mutations in the tyrosine hydroxylase gene in patients with infantile parkinsonism. Ann Hum Genet 2000;64:25–31.

Swerdlow RH, Wooten GF: A novel deafness/dystonia peptide gene mutation that causes dystonia in female carriers of Mohr-Tranebjaerg syndrome. Ann Neurol 2001;50:537–540.

Swoboda KJ, Saul JP, McKenna CE, et al: Aromatic L-amino acid decarboxylase deficiency: Overview of clinical features and outcomes. Ann Neurol 2003;54(suppl 6):S49–S55.

Szepetowski P, Rochette J, Berquin P, et al: Familial infantile convulsions and paroxysmal choreoathetosis: A new neurological syndrome linked to the pericentromeric region of human chromosome 16. Am J Hum Genet 1997;61:889–898.

Tamaru Y, Hirano M, Ito H, et al: Clinical similarities of hereditary progressive/dopa responsive dystonia caused by different types of mutations in the GTP cyclohydrolase I gene. J Neurol Neurosurg Psychiatry 1998;64:469–473.

Taylor TD, Litt M, Kramer P, et al: Homozygosity mapping of Hallervorden-Spatz syndrome to chromosome 20p12.3-p13. Nat Genet 1996;14:479–481.

Tempel LW, Perlmutter JS: Abnormal cortical responses in patients with writer's cramp. Neurology 1993;43:2252–2257.

Thomas M, Hayflick SJ, Jankovic J: Clinical heterogeneity of neurodegeneration with brain iron accumulation (Hallervorden-Spatz syndrome) and pantothenate kinase-associated neurodegeneration. Mov Disord 2004;19(1):36–42.

Thomas P, Lalaux N, Vaiva G, Goudemand M: Dose-dependent stuttering and dystonia in a patient taking clozapine. Am J Psychiatry 1994;151:1096.

Thony B, Blau N: Mutations in the GTP cyclohydrolase I and 6-pyruvoyl-tetrahydropterin synthase genes. Hum Mutat 1997;10:11–20.

Tison FX, Ferrer X, Julien J: Delayed onset movement disorders as a complication of central pontine myelinolysis. Mov Disord 1991; 6:171–173.

Todd RD, Perlmutter JS: Mutational and biochemical analysis of dopamine in dystonia: Evidence for decreased dopamine D-2 receptor inhibition. Mol Neurobiol 1998;16:135–147.

Tolge CF, Factor SA: Focal dystonia secondary to cerebral toxoplasmosis in a patient with acquired immune deficiency syndrome. Mov Disord 1991;6:69–72.

Tolosa E, Kulisevsky J, Fahn S: Meige syndrome: Primary and secondary forms. Adv Neurol 1988a;50:509–515.

Tolosa E, Montserrat L, Bayes A: Blink reflex studies in focal dystonias: Enhanced excitability of brainstem interneurons in cranial dystonia and spasmodic torticollis. Mov Disord 1988b;3:61–69.

Tolosa ES, Klawans HL: Meige's disease: A clinical form of facial convulsion, bilateral and medial. Arch Neurol 1979;36:635–637.

Tomita H, Nagamitsu S, Wakui K, et al: Paroxysmal kinesigenic choreoathetosis locus maps to chromosome 16p11.2-q12.1. Am J Hum Genet 1999;65:1688–1697.

Topp KS, Byl NN: Movement dysfunction following repetitive hand opening and closing: Anatomical analysis in owl monkeys. Mov Disord 1999;14:295–306.

Tranebjaerg L, Hamel BCJ, Gabreels FJM, et al: A de novo missense mutation in a critical domain of the X-linked DDP gene causes the typical deafness-dystonia-optic atrophy syndrome. Eur J Human Genet 2000;8:464–467.

Trost M, Carbon M, Edwards C, et al: Primary dystonia: Is abnormal functional brain architecture linked to genotype? Ann Neurol 2002;52(6):853–856.

Truong DD, Fahn S: An early description of dystonia: Translation of Schwalbe's thesis and information on his life. Adv Neurol 1988;50:651–664.

Tsui JJCT, Calne DB (eds): Handbook of Dystonia. New York, Marcel Dekker, 1995.

Turjanski N, Bhatia K, Burn DJ, et al: Comparison of striatal F-18-dopa uptake in adult-onset dystonia-parkinsonism, Parkinson's disease, and dopa-responsive dystonia. Neurology 1993;43:1563–1568.

Uc EY, Wenger DA, Jankovic J: Niemann-Pick disease type C: Two cases and an update. Mov Disord 2000;15:1199–1203.

Ujike H, Tanabe Y, Takehisa Y, et al: A family with X-linked dystonia-deafness syndrome with a novel mutation of the DDP gene. Arch Neurol 2001;58:1004–1007.

Uncini A, Dimuzio A, Thomas A, et al: Hand dystonia secondary to cervical demyelinating lesion. Acta Neurol Scand 1994;90:51–55.

Uziel Y, Rathaus V, Pomeranz A, et al: Torticollis as the sole initial presenting sign of systemic onset juvenile rheumatoid arthritis. J Rheumatol 1998;25:166–168.

Valente EM, Bentivoglio AR, Cassetta E, et al: DYT13, a novel primary torsion dystonia locus, maps to chromosome 1p36.13–36.32 in an Italian family with cranial-cervical or upper limb onset. Ann Neurol 2001;49:362–366.

Valente EM, Misbahuddin A, Brancati F, et al: Analysis of the epsilon-sarcoglycan gene in familial and sporadic myoclonus-dystonia: Evidence for genetic heterogeneity. Mov Disord 2003;18(9): 1047–1051.

Valente EM, Povey S, Warner TT, et al: Detailed haplotype analysis in Ashkenazi Jewish and non-Jewish British dystonic patients carrying the GAG deletion in the DYT1 gene: Evidence for a limited number of founder mutations. Ann Hum Genet 1999;63:1–8.

Valente EM, Spacey SD, Wali GM, et al: A second paroxysmal kinesigenic choreoathetosis locus (EKD2) mapping on 16q13-q22.1 indicates a family of genes which give rise to paroxysmal disorders on human chromosome 16. Brain 2000;123:2040–2045.

Valentino P, Annesi G, Ciro Candiano IC, et al: Genetic heterogeneity in patients with pantothenate kinase-associated neurodegeneration and classic magnetic resonance imaging eye-of-the-tiger pattern. Mov Disord 2006;21:252–254.

Valenzuela R, Court J, Godoy J: Delayed cyanide induced dystonia. J Neurol Neurosurg Psychiatry 1992;55:198–199.

Valls-Sole J, Hallett M: Modulation of electromyographic activity of wrist flexor and extensor muscles in patients with writer's cramp. Mov Disord 1995;10:741–748.

van den Berg JSP, Horstink MWIM, van den Hoogen FHJ, Oyen WJG: Dystonia: A central nervous system presentation of Sjogren's syndrome. Mov Disord 1999;14:374–375.

van den Heuvel LPWJ, Luiten B, Smeitink JAM, et al: A common point mutation in the tyrosine hydroxylase gene in autosomal recessive L-DOPA-responsive dystonia in the Dutch population. Hum Genet 1998;102:644–646.

Vandertop WP, Kamphuis DJ, Witkamp TD: Hemidystonia as presenting symptom of an optic glioma. Child Nerv Syst 1997;13:289–292.

Waddy HM, Fletcher NA, Harding AE, Marsden CD: A genetic study of idiopathic focal dystonias. Ann Neurol 1991;29:320–324.

Wahlström J, Ozelius L, Kramer P, et al: The gene for familial dystonia with myoclonic jerks responsive to alcohol is not located on the distal end of 9q. Clin Genet 1994;45:88–92.

Walker RH, Brin MF, Sandu D, et al: Distribution and immunohistochemical characterization of torsinA immunoreactivity in rat brain. Brain Res 2001;900:348–354.

Walker RH, Brin MF, Sandu D, et al: TorsinA immunoreactivity in brains of patients with DYT1 and non-DYT1 dystonia. Neurology 2002;58(1):120–124.

Warner T, Camfield L, Marsden CD, et al: A prevalence study of primary dystonia in eight European countries. J Neurol 2000;247:787–792.

Waters CH, Faust PL, Powers J, et al: Neuropathology of Lubag (X-linked dystonia-parkinsonism). Mov Disord 1993a;8:387–390.

Waters CH, Takahashi H, Wilhelmsen KC, et al: Phenotypic expression of X-linked dystonia-parkinsonism (lubag) in two women. Neurology 1993b;43:1555–1558.

Wilhelmsen KC, Weeks DE, Nygaard TG, et al: Genetic mapping of "lubag" (X-linked dystonia-parkinsonism) in a Filipino kindred to the pericentromeric region of the X chromosome. Ann Neurol 1991;29:124–131.

Williams CRP, O'Flynn E, Clarke NMP, Morris RJ: Torticollis secondary to ocular pathology. J Bone Joint Surg [Br] 1996;78:620–624.

Wilmshurst JM, Surtees R, Cox T, Robinson RO: Cerebellar ataxia, anterior horn cell disease, learning difficulties, and dystonia: A new syndrome. Develop Med Child Neurol 2000;42:775–779.

Wu YR, Lee-Chen GJ, Lang AE, et al: Dystonia as a presenting sign of spinocerebellar ataxia type 1. Mov Disord 2004;19(5):586–587.

Yalcinkaya C, Apaydin H, Ozekmekci S, Gibson KM: Delayed-onset dystonia associated with 3-oxothiolase deficiency. Mov Disord 2001;16:372–375.

Yamamoto T, Yamashita M: Thalamo-olivary degeneration in a patient with laryngopharyngeal dystonia. J Neurol Neurosurg Psychiatry 1995;59:438–441.

Yanagisawa N, Goto A: Dystonia musculorum deformans: Analysis with electromyography. J Neurol Sci 1971;13:39–65.

Yanagisawa N, Goto A, Narabayashi H: Familial dystonia musculorum deformans and tremor. J Neurol Sci 1972;16:125–136.

Yasutomo K, Hashimoto T, Miyazaki M, Kuroda Y: Recurrent torticollis as a presentation of Moya-Moya disease. J Child Neurol 1993;8:187–188.

Zabani I, Vaghadia H: Refractory dystonia during propofol anaesthesia in a patient with torticollis-dystonia disorder. Can J Anaesth 1996;43:1062–1064.

Zeman W: Pathology of the torsion dystonias (dystonia musculorum deformans). Neurology 1970;20(no. 11, pt 2):79–88.

Zeman W: Dystonia: An overview. Adv Neurol 1976;14:91–103.

Zeman W, Dyken P: Dystonia musculorum deformans; clinical, genetic and pathoanatomical studies. Psychiatr Neurol Neurochir 1967;70:77–121.

Zeman W, Kaelbling R, Pasamanick B: Idiopathic dystonia musculorum deformans: I. The hereditary pattern. Am J Hum Genet 1959;11:188–202.

Zeman W, Kaelbling R, Pasamanick B: Idiopathic dystonia musculorum deformans: II. The formes frustes. Neurology 1960;10:1068–1075.

Zhou B, Westaway SK, Levinson B, et al: A novel pantothenate kinase (PANK2) is defective in Hallervorden-Spatz syndrome. Nat Genet 2001; 28:350–354.

Zilber N, Korczyn AD, Kahana E, et al: Inheritance of idiopathic torsion dystonia among Jews. J Med Genet 1984;21:13–20.

Zimprich A, Grabowski M, Asmus F, et al: Mutations in the gene encoding epsilon-sarcoglycan cause myoclonus-dystonia syndrome. Nat Genet 2001;29:66–69.

Zweig RM, Hedreen JC, Jankel WR, et al: Pathology in brainstem regions of individuals with primary dystonia. Neurology 1988;38: 702–706.

# Chapter 14

# Treatment of Dystonia

Despite the paucity of knowledge about the cause and pathogenesis of dystonic disorders, the symptomatic treatment of dystonia has markedly improved, particularly since the introduction of botulinum toxin. In most cases of dystonia, the treatment is merely symptomatic, designed to improve posture and function and to relieve associated pain. In rare patients, however, dystonia can be so severe that it can produce not only abnormal postures and disabling dystonic movements, sometimes compromising respiration, but also muscle breakdown and life-threatening hyperthermia, rhabdomyolysis, and myoglobinuria. In such cases of dystonic storm or status dystonicus, proper therapeutic intervention can be life-saving (Jankovic and Penn, 1982; Vaamonde et al., 1994; Dalvi et al., 1998; Manji et al., 1998; Jankovic, 2006).

The assessment of various therapeutic interventions in dystonia is problematic for the following reasons: (1) Dystonia and its effects on function are difficult to quantitate; therefore, most trials utilize crude clinical rating scales, many of which have not been properly evaluated or validated; (2) dystonia is a syndrome with different etiologies, anatomic distributions, and heterogeneous clinical manifestations producing variable disability; (3) some patients, perhaps up to 15%, may have spontaneous, albeit transient, remissions; (4) many studies have used dosages that may have been insufficient or too short in duration to provide benefit; (5) the vast majority of therapeutic trials in dystonia are not double-blind, placebo-controlled; and (6) most studies, even those that have been otherwise well designed and controlled, have utilized small sample sizes, which makes the results difficult to interpret, particularly in view of a large placebo effect demonstrated in dystonia (Lindeboom et al., 1996). A variety of instruments have been used to assess the response in patients with cervical dystonia; the most frequently used is the Toronto Western Spasmodic Torticollis Rating Scale (TWSTRS) (Consky and Lang, 1994; Comella et al., 1997). TWSTRS (range: 0 to 87) consists of three subscales: severity (range: 0 to 35), disability (range: 0 to 23), and pain (range: 0 to 20). In addition, visual analog scale, global assessment of change, and pain analog assessments have been used in various clinical trials. Various scales, such as the Fahn-Marsden scale and the Unified Dystonia Rating Scale have also been used to assess patients with generalized dystonia (Burke et al., 1985a; Ondo et al., 1998; Comella et al., 2003). Another scale designed to capture the burden of dystonia on patients is the Cervical Dystonia Impact Profile scale (Cano et al., 2004). The Jankovic Rating Scale was initially used in the original study of BTX in patients with cranial dystonia, which led to the approval of BTX by the Food and Drug Administration (Jankovic and Orman, 1987), and in subsequent studies (Roggenkamper et al., 2006) to assess the severity and frequency of involuntary eyelid contractions in patients with blepharospasm. Subsequent studies have refined the clinical rating scales and included quality-of-life scales (Lindeboom et al., 1996). Health-related quality-of-life instruments, such as the craniocervical dystonia questionnaire (CDQ-24), are increasingly used to assess the function and the impact of treatment in patients with cranial, cervical, and other dystonias on activities of daily living and other measures of quality of life (Muller et al., 2004; Reimer et al., 2005; Hall et al., 2006). The selection of a particular choice of therapy is guided largely by personal clinical experience and by empirical trials (Greene et al., 1988; Greene, 1995; Jankovic, 1997; Brin, 1998; Jankovic, 2007; Jankovic, 2004a; Albanese et al., 2006; Jankovic, 2006) (Box 14-1). An evidence-based review concluded that except for botulinum toxin (BTX) in cervical dystonia and high-dose trihexyphenidyl in young patients with segmental and generalized dystonia (level A, class I-II), none of the methods of pharmacologic intervention have been confirmed as being effective according to evidence-based criteria (Balash and Giladi, 2004). The patient's age, the anatomic distribution of dystonia, and the potential risk of adverse effects are also important determinants of choice of therapy. The identification of a specific cause of dystonia, such as drug-induced dystonias or Wilson disease (Svetel et al., 2001), may lead to a treatment that is targeted to the particular etiology. It is therefore prudent to search for identifiable causes of dystonia, particularly when some atypical features are present. The diagnostic approach to patients with dystonia is based on being aware of the multiple causes of torsion dystonia, which is covered in Chapter 13 and in other reviews (Jankovic, 2007).

## PHYSICAL AND SUPPORTIVE THERAPY

Before reviewing pharmacologic and surgical therapy of dystonia, it is important to emphasize the role of patient education and supportive care, which are integral components of a comprehensive approach to patients with dystonia. Physical therapy and well-fitted braces are designed primarily to improve posture and to prevent contractures. Although braces are often poorly tolerated, particularly by children, they may be used in some cases as a substitute for a sensory trick. For example, some patients with cervical dystonia are able to construct neck-head braces that seem to provide sensory input by touching certain portions of the neck or head in a fashion similar to the patient's own sensory trick, thus enabling the patient to maintain a desirable head position. Various hand devices have been developed in an attempt to help patients with writer's cramp to use their hands more effectively and comfortably (Ranawaya and Lang, 1991; Tas et al., 2001). In one small study of five professional musicians with focal

Box 14-1    Treatment of dystonia

**Focal Dystonias**
*Blepharospasm*
Clonazepam, lorazepam
Botulinum toxin injections
Trihexyphenidyl
Orbicularis oculi myectomy

*Oromandibular Dystonia*
Baclofen
Trihexyphenidyl
Botulinum toxin injections

*Spasmodic Dysphonia*
Botulinum toxin injections
Voice and supportive therapy

*Cervical Dystonia*
Trihexyphenidyl
Diazepam, lorazepam, clonazepam
Botulinum toxin injections
Tetrabenazine
Cyclobenzaprine

Carbamazepine
Baclofen (oral)
Peripheral surgical denervation

**Task-Specific Dystonias (e.g., Writer's Cramp)**
Benztropine, trihexyphenidyl
Botulinum toxin injections
Occupational therapy

**Segmental and Generalized Dystonias**
Levodopa (in children to young adults)
Trihexyphenidyl, benztropine
Diazepam, lorazepam, clonazepam
Baclofen (oral, intrathecal)
Carbamazepine
Tetrabenazine
Triple therapy: tetrabenazine, fluphenazine,
    trihexyphenidyl
Intrathecal baclofen (ITB) infusion (axial dystonia)
Deep brain stimulation of GPi (in distal dystonia or
    hemidystonia)

dystonia, Candia and colleagues (1999) reported success with immobilization by splints of one or more of the digits other than the dystonic finger followed by intensive repetitive exercises of the dystonic finger. It is not clear, however, whether this therapy provides lasting benefits. In one study of eight patients with idiopathic occupational focal dystonia of the upper limb, immobilization with a splint for 4 to 5 weeks resulted in a significant improvement at a 24-week follow-up visit, based on Arm Dystonia Disability Scale (0 = normal; 3 = marked difficulty in playing) and the Tubiana and Champagne Score (0 = unable to play; 5 = returns to concert performances) and was considered marked in four and moderate in three, and the initial improvement disappeared in one (Priori et al., 2001). The splint was applied for 24 hours every day except for 10 minutes once a week when it was removed for brief local hygiene. Immediately on full removal of the splint, all patients reported marked clumsiness and weakness, which resolved in 4 weeks. There were also some local subcutaneous and joint edema and pain in the immobilized joint, and nail growth stopped; none of the patients developed contractures. While the mechanisms of action of immobilization is unknown, the authors have postulated that removing all motor and sensory input to a limb might allow the cortical map to "reset" to the previous normal topography. One major concern about immobilization of a limb, particularly dystonic limb, is that such immobilization can actually increase the risk of exacerbating or even precipitating dystonia, as has been well demonstrated in dystonia following casting or other peripheral causes of dystonia (Jankovic, 2001a). A variation of the immobilization therapy, constraint-induced movement therapy, has been used successfully in rehabilitation of patients after stroke and other brain insults, and the observed benefit has been attributed to cortical reorganization (Taub et al., 1999; Levy et al., 2001; Taub and Morris, 2001; Taub et al., 2002; Wolf et al., 2002).

Another technique, using a repetitive task during regional anesthesia of a weak arm in patients following stroke, was

also associated with improved hand function (Muellbacher et al., 2002). Some patients find various muscle relaxation techniques and sensory feedback therapy useful adjuncts to medical or surgical treatments. Since some patients with dystonia have impaired sensory perception, it has been postulated that sensory training may relieve dystonia. In a study of 10 patients with focal hand dystonia, Zeuner and colleagues (2002) showed that reading Braille for 30 to 60 minutes daily for 8 weeks improved spatial acuity and dystonia that was sustained for up to 1 year in some patients (Zeuner and Hallett, 2003). Sensory training to restore sensory representation of the hand along with mirror imagery and mental practice techniques has also been reported to be useful in the treatment of focal hand dystonia (Byl and McKenzie, 2000; Byl et al., 2003).

Siebner and colleagues (1999) showed that using repetitive transcranial magnetic stimulation delivered at low frequencies ($\leq 1$ Hz) for 20 minutes can temporarily (8 of 16 patients reported improvement that lasted longer than 3 hours) improve handwriting impaired by dystonic writer's cramp, presumably by increasing inhibition (and thus reducing excitability) of the underlying cortex. Finally, long-term neck muscle vibration of the contracting muscle might have a therapeutic value in patients with cervical dystonia. This is suggested by transient (minutes) improvement in head position in one patient who was treated for 15 minutes with muscle vibration (Karnath et al., 2000). Transcutaneous electrical stimulation has been found to improve dystonic writer's cramp for at least 3 weeks in a double-blind, placebo-controlled trial (Tinazzi et al., 2005). Such observation is consistent with the notion that proprioceptive sensory input affects cervical dystonia.

## DOPAMINERGIC THERAPY

Pharmacologic treatment of dystonia is based largely on an empirical rationale rather than a scientific one. Unlike

Parkinson disease, in which therapy with levodopa replacement is based on the finding of depletion of dopamine in the brains of parkinsonian animals and humans, the knowledge of biochemical alterations in idiopathic dystonia is very limited. One exception is dopa-responsive dystonia (DRD), in which the biochemical and genetic mechanisms have been elucidated by molecular DNA and biochemical studies in patients (Ichinose et al., 1994) and by studies of postmortem brains (Furukawa et al., 1999). Decreased neuromelanin in the substantia nigra with otherwise normal nigral cell count and morphology and normal tyrosine hydroxylase immunoreactivity were found in the brain of one patient with classic DRD (Rajput et al., 1994). There was a marked reduction in dopamine in the substantia nigra and the striatum. These findings suggested that in DRD, the primary abnormality was a defect in dopamine synthesis. This proposal is supported by the finding of a mutation in the GTP cyclohydrolase I gene on chromosome 14q that indirectly regulates the production of tetrahydrobiopterin, a cofactor for tyrosine hydroxylase, the rate-limiting enzyme in the synthesis of dopamine (Ichinose et al., 1994; Tanaka et al., 1995; Steinberger et al., 2000). Another form of DRD has been described in four cases belonging to two unrelated families of dopa-responsive cervical dystonia, presenting between 9 and 15 years of age and similar to classic DRD manifesting diurnal variation but no levodopa-induced dyskinesia (Schneider et al., 2006).

DRD usually presents in childhood with dystonia, mild parkinsonian features, and pseudopyramidal signs (hypertonicity and hyperreflexia) predominantly involving the legs. Many patients have a family history of dystonia or Parkinson disease. At least half of the patients have diurnal fluctuations, with marked progression of their symptoms toward the end of the day and a relief after sleep. Many patients with this form of dystonia are initially misdiagnosed as having cerebral palsy. Some patients with DRD are not diagnosed until adulthood, and family members of patients with typical DRD may present with adult-onset levodopa-responsive parkinsonism (Harwood et al., 1994). The take-home message from these reports is that a therapeutic trial of levodopa should be considered in all patients with childhood-onset dystonia, whether they have classic features of DRD or not.

Most patients with DRD improve dramatically even with small doses of levodopa (100 mg of levodopa with 25 mg of decarboxylase inhibitor), but some might require doses of levodopa as high as 1000 mg per day. In contrast to patients with juvenile Parkinson disease (Ishikawa and Miyatake, 1995), DRD patients usually do not develop levodopa-induced fluctuations or dyskinesias. If no clinically evident improvement is noted after 3 months of therapy, the diagnosis of DRD is probably in error, and levodopa can be discontinued. In addition to levodopa, patients with DRD also improve with dopamine agonists, anticholinergic drugs, and carbamazepine (Nygaard et al., 1991). In contrast to patients with DRD, patients with idiopathic or other types of dystonia rarely improve with dopaminergic therapy (Lang, 1988). While dopaminergic therapy is remarkably effective in treating DRD, this strategy is not useful in the treatment of primary dystonia. Apomorphine, however, may ameliorate dystonia, perhaps by decreasing dopamine as well as serotonin release (Zuddas and Cianchetti, 1996).

## ANTIDOPAMINERGIC THERAPY

Although dopamine receptor–blocking drugs were used extensively in the past, most clinical trials have produced mixed results with these drugs. Because of the poor response and the possibility of undesirable side effects, particularly sedation, parkinsonism, and tardive dyskinesia, the use of these drugs in the treatment of dystonia should be discouraged (Jankovic, 1995b). Clozapine, an atypical neuroleptic, has been reported in a small open trial to be moderately effective in the treatment of segmental and generalized dystonia, but its usefulness was limited by potential side effects (Karp et al., 1999). Although antidopaminergic drugs have been reported to be beneficial in the treatment of dystonia, the potential clinical benefit is usually limited by the development of side effects. Dopamine depleting drugs, however, such as tetrabenazine, have been found useful in some patients with dystonia, particularly those with tardive dystonia (Jankovic and Orman, 1988; Jankovic and Beach, 1997). Tetrabenazine, a vesicular monoamine transporter 2 (VMAT2) inhibitor, has the advantage over other antidopaminergic drugs in that it does not cause tardive dyskinesia, although it may cause transient acute dystonic reaction (Burke et al., 1985b; Jankovic and Beach, 1997; Kenney and Jankovic, 2006). Tetrabenazine is not readily available in the United States, but it is dispensed by prescription under the trade name "Nitoman" or "Xenazine 25" in other countries, including the United Kingdom. It is possible that some of the new atypical neuroleptic drugs will be useful not only as antipsychotics but also in the treatment of hyperkinetic movement disorders. Risperidone, a D2 dopamine receptor–blocking drug with a high affinity for 5-HT$_2$ receptors, has been reported to be useful in a 4-week trial of five patients with various forms of dystonia (Zuddas and Cianchetti, 1996). Clozapine, a D4 dopamine receptor blocker with relatively low affinity for the D2 receptors and high affinity for the 5-HT$_{2A}$ receptors, has been reported to ameliorate the symptoms of tardive dystonia (Trugman et al., 1994). The treatment of tardive dystonia and other tardive syndromes is discussed in Chapter 20 and in other reviews (Jankovic, 1995b).

## ANTICHOLINERGIC THERAPY

High-dosage anticholinergic medications, such as trihexyphenidyl, for dystonia were introduced by Fahn (1983) and confirmed in studies by several groups (Marsden et al., 1984; Greene et al., 1988; Jabbari et al., 1989; Hoon et al., 2001), including a double-blind study (Burke et al., 1986). Although anticholinergic therapy is helpful in all types of dystonias, the supremacy of botulinum toxin therapy for focal dystonias has relegated anticholinergic therapy to use largely in the treatment of generalized and segmental dystonia. In the experience of Greene and colleagues (1988), patients with blepharospasm, generalized dystonia, tonic (in contrast to clonic) dystonia, and onset of dystonia at age younger than 19 years seemed to respond better to anticholinergic drugs than did other subgroups, but this difference did not reach statistical significance. Except for short duration of symptoms before onset of therapy, there was no other variable, such as gender or severity, that reliably predicted a favorable response.

Treating patients within the first 5 years of disease onset was statistically significantly more successful than delaying treatment in both children (Table 14-1) and adults (Table 14-2) regardless of severity (Greene et al., 1988). Thus, early initiation of treatment is important. This therapy is generally well tolerated when the dose is increased slowly. It is recommended that therapy begin with a 5-mg preparation, a half-tablet at bedtime, with a half-tablet added each week, advancing up to 10 mg in four divided doses by the end of 4 weeks. Because there is a lag between reaching a dose and seeing a benefit, it is recommended that this dose be held for a month and that the dose then continue to be increased at the same rate over the next 4 weeks until the dose is 20 mg in four divided doses. It is recommended that the dose continue to be increased in this manner until there is adequate benefit or adverse effects that limit higher doses. Some patients require up to 60 to 140 mg per day, but may experience dose-related drowsiness, confusion, or memory difficulty that limit the dose. Children usually tolerate the very high dosages, whereas adults do not. In one study of 20 cognitively intact patients with dystonia,

Table 14-1 Treatment of dystonia with high-dosage anticholinergics in children

**A. Quality of Results of Treatment as a Function of Duration of Disease ($N = 67$)**

| Duration of Symptoms before Initiating Therapy | Good | Poor | Mean Age at Onset |
|---|---|---|---|
| 0–5 years | 17 | 6 | 8.8 years |
| > 5 years | 17 | 27 | 9.8 years |

**B. Onset of Treatment at Different Severities of Disease ($N = 62$)**

| Duration of Symptoms before Initiating Therapy | Mild | Moderate | Severe |
|---|---|---|---|
| 0–5 years | 7 | 6 | 8 |
| > 5 years | 7 | 25 | 9 |

**C. Treatment Outcome as a Function of Family History and Severity of Disease**

| Clinical Category | N | Good Response |
|---|---|---|
| All patients | 67 | 51% |
| Familal | 27 | 52% |
| Nonfamilial | 47 | 50% |
| Severity | | |
|    Mild | 14 | 50% |
|    Moderate | 31 | 48% |
|    Severe | 17 | 47% |

Age at onset in all subjects was less than 20 years. **A,** Results: $P < .01$ by chi-square; age at onset, NS by t-test. Results indicate that starting anticholinergic medication early in the course is more likely to provide a better outcome than delaying treatment beyond 5 years duration of symptoms. **B,** Results: $P < .025$ by chi-square. Severity of dystonia tends to be milder in those with a short duration. **C,** Patients with even more severe symptoms at the time therapy is started can have a beneficial outcome.

Data from Greene P, Shale H, Fahn S: Analysis of open-label trials in torsion dystonia using high dosage of anticholinergics and other drugs. Mov Disord 1988;3:46–60.

Table 14-2 Duration of disease at onset of high-dosage anticholinergic therapy has an impact on outcome regardless of age at onset of dystonia

**A. All Subjects with Focal, Segmental, or Generalized Dystonia**

| Duration of Symptoms before Initiating Therapy | Good | Poor |
|---|---|---|
| 0–5 years | 63 | 61 |
| > 5 years | 36 | 60 |

**B. Subjects with Cervical Dystonia**

| Duration of Symptoms before Initiating Therapy | Good | Poor |
|---|---|---|
| 0–5 years | 23 | 23 |
| > 5 years | 5 | 2 |

**A,** Results: $P < .025$ by chi-square. **B,** Results: $P < .05$ by chi-square.

Data from Greene P, Shale H, Fahn S: Analysis of open-label trials in torsion dystonia using high dosage of anticholinergics and other drugs. Mov Disord 1988;3:46–60.

only 12 of whom could tolerate 15 to 74 mg of daily trihexyphenidyl, drug-induced impairments of recall and slowing of mentation were noted, particularly in the older patients (Taylor et al., 1991). Diphenhydramine, a histamine $H_1$ antagonist with anticholinergic properties, has been reported to have an antidystonic effect in three of five patients (Truong et al., 1995). However, the drug was not effective in 10 other patients with cervical dystonia, and it was associated with sedation and other anticholinergic side effects in most patients. Pyridostigmine, a peripherally acting anticholinesterase, and eye drops of pilocarpine (a muscarinic agonist) often ameliorate many of the peripheral side effects, such as urinary retention and blurred vision. Pilocarpine (Salagen) 5 mg four times per day, Cevimeline (Evoxac) 30 mg three times per day, and synthetic saliva (Glandosane, Salagen, Salivart, Salix) have been found effective in the treatment of dry mouth.

## OTHER PHARMACOLOGIC THERAPIES

Many patients with dystonia require a combination of several medications and treatments (Jankovic, 2004b; Jankovic, 2006). High-dosage oral baclofen appears to be the next most effective agent for dystonia, particularly in combination with high-dosage anticholinergic treatment. Baclofen is a $GABA_b$ autoreceptor agonist that is used to treat spasticity. It has been found to produce substantial and sustained improvement in 29% of children at a mean dose of 92 mg per day (range: 40 to 180 mg per day) (Greene, 1992; Greene and Fahn, 1992a). Although baclofen was initially effective in 28 of 60 (47%) of adults with cranial dystonia, only 18% continued baclofen at a mean dose of 105 mg per day after a mean of 30.6 months (Fahn et al., 1985a).

Benzodiazepines (diazepam, lorazepam, or clonazepam) may provide additional benefit for patients whose response to anticholinergic drugs is unsatisfactory (Tables 14-3 and 14-4).

Table 14-3 Effectiveness of baclofen and clonazepam in torsion dystonia

| Category | Baclofen | | Clonazepam | |
|---|---|---|---|---|
| | N | Good | N | Good |
| All patients | 108 | 20% | 115 | 16% |
| Blepharospasm | 38 | 30% | 23 | 23% |
| Meige syndrome | 17 | 24% | 16 | 19% |
| Torticollis | 27 | 11% | 33 | 21% |
| Segmental dystonia | 14 | 24% | 35 | 17% |
| Generalized dystonia | 8 | 13% | 17 | 6% |
| Secondary dystonia | 19 | 16% | 22 | 27% |

Data from Greene P, Shale H, Fahn S: Analysis of open-label trials in torsion dystonia using high dosage of anticholinergics and other drugs. Mov Disord 1988;3:46–60.

Clonazepam might be particularly useful in patients with myoclonic dystonia. Muscle relaxants that are useful in the treatment of dystonia include cyclobenzaprine (Flexeril, 30 to 40 mg per day), metaxalone (Skelaxin, 800 mg two to three times per day), carisoprodol (Soma), methocarbamol (Robaxin oral and patch), orphenadrine (Norflex), and chlorzoxazone (Parafonforte). Structurally and pharmacologically similar to amitriptyline, cyclobenzaprine at doses of 30 to 40 mg per day has been found to be superior to placebo but equal to diazepam.

Narayan and colleagues (1991) first suggested that intrathecal baclofen (ITB) might be effective in the treatment of dystonia in 1991 in a report of an 18-year-old man with severe cervical and truncal dystonic spasms who was refractory to all forms of oral therapy and to large doses of paraspinal BTX injections. Muscle-paralyzing agents were necessary to relieve these spasms, which compromised his respiration. Within a few hours after the institution of ITB infusion, the patient's dystonia markedly improved, and he was able to be discharged from the intensive-care unit within 1 to 2 days. The subsequent experience with intrathecal infusions has been quite encouraging, and studies are currently in progress to further evaluate this form of therapy in patients with dystonia and other motor disorders (Penn et al., 1995; Dressler et al., 1997; van Hilten et al., 1999). In some patients who were treated with intrathecal baclofen for spasticity, the benefits persisted even after the infusion was stopped (Dressnandt and Conrad, 1996). Ford and colleagues (1996) reviewed the experience with ITB in 25 patients and concluded that this form of therapy may be "more effective when dystonia is associated with spasticity or pain." ITB could have a role in selected patients with dystonic storm (Dalvi et al., 1998) and in secondary dystonias associated with pain and spasticity (Ford et al., 1998a).

Table 14-4 Comparison of anticholinergics, baclofen, and clonazepam in the treatment of blepharospasm

| Medication | N | Good response |
|---|---|---|
| Anticholinergics | 22 | 55% |
| Baclofen | 38 | 29% |
| Clonazepam | 23 | 22% |

For example, Albright and colleagues (1998) found improvement in dystonia scores in 10 of 12 patients with cerebral palsy using an average daily dose of ITB of 575 µg; the improvement was sustained in 6 patients. In a subsequent study involving 86 patients ages 3 to 42 years (mean: 13 years) with generalized dystonia (secondary to cerebral palsy in 71% of patients), external infusion or bolus-dose screening was positive in approximately 90% of patients (Albright et al., 2001). Programmable pumps were implanted in 77 patients. Infusion began at 200 µg per day and increased by 10% to 20% per day until the best dose was achieved. The median duration of ITB therapy was 26 months. The mean dose increased over time, from 395 µg at 3 months to 610 µg at 24 months to 960 µg at 36 months. Patients and caregivers rated quality of life and ease of care as having improved in approximately 85% of patients. Seven patients, including four with cerebral palsy, lost their response to ITB during the study, usually during the first year. The most common side effects were increased constipation (19%), decreased neck and trunk control, and drowsiness. Surgical and device complications occurred in 38% of patients, including infections and catheter breakage and disconnection. Complication rates decreased over time. The authors conclude, "In our opinion, ITB is the treatment of choice for severe, generalized secondary dystonia after oral medications have been shown to be ineffective." One potentially serious complication of ITB is life-threatening intermittent catheter leakage, which might not be detectable by standard noninvasive methods (Bardutzky et al., 2003).

In a long-term (6 years) follow-up of ITB in 14 patients, 5 patients were found to have improvement in their rating scale scores, although only 2 patients had sustained "clear clinical benefit" (Walker et al., 2000). Hou and colleagues (2001) provided a follow-up on long-term effects of ITB in 10 patients (2 males and 8 females; mean age: 43.2 years; range: 21 to 66 years) with severe segmental or generalized dystonia who responded unsatisfactorily to oral medications and BTX injections. Three patients had peripherally induced dystonia, all with reflex sympathetic dystrophy, two were idiopathic (one with reflex sympathetic dystrophy), two suffered brain injury, two had static encephalopathy, and one had an unknown neurodegenerative disorder. Anatomically, three patients suffered segmental dystonia involving the neck, arms, or abdominal muscles. Seven others had generalized dystonia. The average duration of dystonia prior to implantation was 11 years (range: 1.7 to 35 years). All patients received test doses of bolus ITB before implantations. Two had relatively poor initial response to the test dose, but still received implantations for continuous infusion. Neurologic assessments were conducted immediately after the implantations, 1 month later, and every 3 months thereafter. The average duration of follow-up was 4.7 years (range: 0.7 to 11.1 years). Only one patient abandoned the pump after 22 months. Initially, five improved markedly, two improved moderately, two improved mildly, and one had no improvement. Both patients who failed to respond to the initial test of ITB improved on continuous infusion with pump. In four patients, the improvement lessened over time, although the patients were still better than they had been preoperatively. All 10 patients needed to continue oral medications, and 8 continued BTX injections at similar doses. Hou and colleagues (2001) concluded that patients with secondary (spastic) dystonia involving primarily legs and trunk appeared to be the best candidates for continuous ITB infusion. Continuous ITB has been found to be safe and effective in other series of patients with reflex sympathetic dystrophy and dystonia (van Hilten et al., 2000). It is not yet clear whether ITB can induce lasting remissions in patients with dystonia. The American Academy for Cerebral Palsy and Developmental Medicine has published a systematic review of the use of ITB for spastic and dystonic cerebral palsy (Butler et al., 2000). The limited published data show that ITB reduced spasticity and dystonia, particularly in the lower extremities.

There are other medications that are used in the treatment of dystonia. For example, slow-release morphine sulfate has been shown to improve not only pain but also dystonic movement in some patients with primary and tardive dystonia (Berg et al., 2001). Besides clonazepam, gamma-hydroxybutyrate, used in the treatment of alcohol abuse, has been found to be beneficial in the treatment of myoclonus-dystonia syndrome (Priori et al., 2000). It is not known whether acamprosate, another drug that is used in the treatment of alcohol abuse, is useful in the treatment of myoclonus-dystonia. Anticonvulsants, such as levetiracetam (Keppra) and zonisamide (Zonegran), have been reported to be effective in the treatment of cortical myoclonus, but it is not clear whether these drugs play a role in the treatment of dystonia.

Peripheral deafferentiation with anesthetic was previously reported to improve tremor (Pozos and Iaizo, 1992), but this approach might also be useful in the treatment of focal dystonia, such as writer's cramp (Kaji et al., 1995a) or oromandibular dystonia (Yoshida et al., 1998) that is unresponsive to other pharmacologic therapy. An injection of 5 to 10 mL of 0.5% lidocaine into the target muscle improved focal dystonia for up to 24 hours. This short effect can be extended for up to several weeks if ethanol is injected simultaneously. The observation that blocking muscle spindle afferents reduces dystonia suggests that somatosensory input is important in the pathogenesis of dystonia (Hallett, 1995; Kaji et al., 1995b). Mexiletine, an oral derivative of lidocaine, has been found to be effective in the treatment of cervical dystonia at doses ranging from 450 to 1200 mg per day (Ohara et al., 1998). Two thirds of the patients, however, experienced adverse effects, including heartburn, drowsiness, ataxia, and tremor. On the basis of a review and a rating of videotapes by a "blind" rater, Lucetti and colleagues (2000) reported a significant improvement in six patients with cervical dystonia who had been treated with mexiletine.

Local electromyograph (EMG) -guided injection of phenol is currently being investigated as a potential treatment of cervical dystonia, but the results have not been very encouraging because of pain associated with the procedure and unpredictable response (Ruiz and Bernardos, 2000; Massey, 2002). Chemomyectomy with muscle-necrotizing drugs, such as doxorubicin, has been tried in some patients with blepharospasm and hemifacial spasm (Wirtschafter, 1991), but because of severe local irritation, it is doubtful that this approach will be adopted into clinical practice.

Attacks of kinesigenic paroxysmal dystonia may be controlled with anticonvulsants (e.g., carbamazepine, phenytoin). The nonkinesigenic forms of paroxysmal dystonia are less responsive to pharmacologic therapy, although clonazepam and acetazolamide may be beneficial. Treatment of paroxysmal dyskinesias is covered in Chapter 23 and in other reviews (Fahn, 1994; Demirkiran and Jankovic, 1995). Table 14-5 lists the common medications and procedures utilized for dystonia.

Table 14-5 Therapeutic options for patients with dystonia

| Generic Name | Trade Name | Daily Dosage* | Mechanism of Action |
|---|---|---|---|
| Trihexyphenidyl | Artane | 6–100 | Anticholinergic |
| Benztropine | Cogentin | 4–15 | Anticholinergic |
| Orphenadrine | Norflex | 200–800 | Anticholinergic |
| Clonazepam | Klonopin | 1–12 | Serotonergic, relaxant |
| Lorazepam | Ativan | 1–16 | Relaxant |
| Diazepam | Valium | 10–100 | Relaxant |
| Cyclobenzaprine | Flexeril | 20–60 | Relaxant |
| Chlordiazepoxide | Librium | 10–100 | Relaxant |
| Baclofen | Lioresal | 40–120 | Antispastic, GABA agonist, substance P antagonist |
| Baclofen intrathecal infusion | Lioresal | 200–1500 µg/day | |
| Primidone | Mysoline | 50–800 | Antiepileptic, antitremor |
| Valproate | Depakote | 500–1500 | Antiepileptic, GABA-T inhibitor |
| Carbamazepine | Tegretol | 1600–1600 | Antiepileptic |
| Levodopa/carbidopa | Sinemet(CR) | 75/300 | Dopamine precursor 200/2000 |
| Lithium | Lithobid | 600–1800 | Antidopaminergic |
| Tetrabenazine | Xenazine 25 | 50–300 | Monoamine depleter and blocker |
| Botulinum toxin-A | BOTOX | 5–400 mouse units | Blocks acetylcholine release at the neuromuscular junction by cleaving SNAP-25 |
| Botulinum toxin-B | MYOBLOC | 100–15,000 mouse units | Blocks acetylcholine release at the neuromuscular junction by cleaving synaptobrevin (VAMP) |
| Surgery: peripheral denervation, myectomy, thalamotomy, pallidotomy, pallidal deep brain stimulation | | | |

*The dose is in milligrams unless otherwise specified.

In addition to conventional forms of therapy described previously, many patients with dystonia seek complementary or alternative forms of therapy. In one survey of 180 members of the German Dystonia Group, 131 (73%) patients used some form of alternative treatments, such as acupuncture (56%), relaxation techniques (44%), homeopathy (27%), and massages (26%) (Junker et al., 2004).

## BOTULINUM TOXIN

The introduction of BTX into clinical practice in the late 1980s revolutionized treatment of dystonia. The most potent biologic toxin, BTX has become a powerful therapeutic tool in the treatment of a variety of neurologic, ophthalmic, and other disorders that are manifested by abnormal, excessive, or inappropriate muscle contractions (Jankovic and Brin, 1991; Jankovic and Hallett, 1994; Brin et al., 2002; Thant and Tan, 2003; Jankovic, 2004a). In December 1989, after extensive laboratory and clinical testing, the Food and Drug Administration approved this biologic (BTX-A or BOTOX) as a therapeutic agent in patients with strabismus, blepharospasm, and other facial nerve disorders, including hemifacial spasm. In December 2000, the Food and Drug Administration approved BOTOX and BTX-B (MYOBLOC) as treatments for cervical dystonia. Although its widest application is still in the treatment of disorders manifested by abnormal, excessive, or inappropriate muscle contractions, the use of BTX is rapidly expanding to include treatment of a variety of ophthalmologic, gastrointestinal, urologic, orthopedic, dermatologic, painful, and cosmetic disorders (Tintner and Jankovic, 2001b; Jankovic and Brin, 2002; Thant and Tan, 2003; Jankovic, 2004a) (Box 14-2).

Few therapeutic agents have been better understood in terms of their mechanism of action before their clinical application or have had greater impact on patients' functioning than BTX. The therapeutic value of BTX is due to its ability to cause chemodenervation and to produce local paralysis when injected into a muscle. There are seven immunologically distinct toxins that share structurally homologous subunits. Synthesized as single-chain polypeptides (molecular weight of 150 kDa), these toxin molecules have relatively little potency until they are cleaved by trypsin or bacterial enzymes into a heavy chain (100 kDa) and a light chain (50 kDa). The 150-kDa protein, the active portion of the molecule, complexes with one or more nontoxin proteins that support its structure and protect it from degradation. Type A is the only serotype that forms the 900-kDa complex. Types A, B, C1, and hemagglutinin-positive D form the 500-kDa complex and 300-kDa complex; types E, F, and hemagglutinin-negative D form only the 300-kDa complex (Melling et al., 1998). The three-dimensional structure of the BTX complex is known (Hanson and Stevens, 2002). When linked by a disulfide bond, these dichains exert their paralytic action by preventing the release of acetylcholine. BTX therefore does not affect the synthesis or storage of acetylcholine, but it interferes with the release of acetylcholine from the presynaptic terminal. This is a three-step process that involves binding to the acceptors on presynaptic membrane (heavy chain), internalization (endocytosis), and an enzymatic action (light chain). BTX serotypes bind to different acceptors, which contain both protein components and gangliosides with more than one neuraminic acid residue. BTX-A has been found to enter neurons by binding to the synaptic vesicle protein SV2 (isoform C), which acts as the BTX-A receptor (Dong et al., 2006; Mahrhold et al., 2006). The neural membrane proteins Synaptotagmin-I and -II act as receptors for BTX-B and for BTX-G (Mahrhold et al., 2006). While the heavy chain of the toxin binds to the presynaptic cholinergic terminal, the light chain acts as a zinc-dependent protease that selectively cleaves proteins that are critical for fusion of the presynaptic vesicle with the presynaptic membrane. Thus, the light chains of BTX-A and BTX-E cleave SNAP-25 (synaptosome-associated protein), a protein that is needed for synaptic vesicle targeting and fusion with the presynaptic membrane. The light chains of BTX-B, BTX-D, and BTX-F prevent the quantal release of acetylcholine by proteolytically cleaving synaptobrevin-2, also known as VAMP (vesicle-associated membrane protein), an integral protein of the synaptic vesicle membrane. BTX-C cleaves syntaxin,

---

**Box 14-2** Clinical applications of botulinum toxin

**Focal Dystonia**
Blepharospasm
Lid apraxia
Oromandibular-facial-lingual dystonia
Cervical dystonia (torticollis)
Laryngeal dystonia (spasmodic dysphonia)
Task-specific dystonia (occupational cramps)
Other focal dystonias (idiopathic, secondary)

**Other Involuntary Movements**
Voice, head, and limb tremor
Palatal myoclonus
Hemifacial spasmatics

**Inappropriate Contractions**
Strabismus
Nystagmus
Myokymia

Bruxism
Stuttering
Painful rigidity
Muscle contraction headaches
Lumbosacral strain and back spasms
Radiculopathy with secondary muscle spasm
Spasticity
Spastic bladder
Achalasia (esophageal, pelvirectal)
Other spasmic disorders

**Other Potential Applications**
Protective ptosis
Cosmetic (wrinkles, facial asymmetry)
Debarking dogs
Other

Table 14-6 Botulinum neurotoxins

| Neurotoxin | Substrate | Localization |
|---|---|---|
| BTX-A, BTX-E | SNAP-25 | Presynaptic plasma membrane |
| BTX-B, BTX-D, BTX-F | VAMP/ synaptobrevin | Synaptic vesicle membrane |
| BTX-C | Syntaxin | Presynaptic plasma membrane |

another plasma membrane–associated protein (Table 14-6). A three-dimensional study showed that syntaxin 1a forms a complex with neuronal-Sec1, forming a recognition site for the arriving vesicle through a Rab protein and the subsequent formation of the syntaxin-VAMP-SNAP-25 complex promotes membrane fusion (Misura et al., 2000). Figure 14-1 illustrates the mechanisms of action of the different types of BTX.

The BTX-A has been studied most intensely and used most widely, but the clinical applications of other types of toxins, including BTX-B and BTX-F, are also expanding (Greene and Fahn, 1992b; Mezaki et al., 1995; Sheean and Lees, 1995; Figgit and Noble, 2002; Jankovic, 2004a). BTX-A is harvested from a culture medium after fermentation of a high-toxin-producing strain of *Clostridium botulinum* that lyses and liberates the toxin into the culture (Schantz and Johnson, 1992). The toxin is then extracted, precipitated, purified, and finally crystallized with ammonium sulfate. The crystalline toxin is diluted from milligram to nanogram concentrations, freeze-dried, and dispensed as a white powder in small vials containing 100 mouse units (U) of the toxin. When isolated from bacterial cultures, BTX is noncovalently associated with nontoxic macromolecules, such as hemagglutinin. These nontoxic proteins enhance toxicity by protecting the neurotoxin from proteolytic enzymes in the gut, but they apparently have no effect on the potency of the toxin if injected parenterally. Although the efficacy and duration of benefits of BTX-B or MYOBLOC, formerly NeuroBloc (Elan), are thought to be generally

comparable to those of BTX-A (BOTOX and Dysport), no head-to-head comparisons between the various products have been performed. An in vivo study using injections into the extensor digitorum brevis in healthy volunteers suggested that the muscle paralysis from BTX-B was not as complete or long-lasting as that from BTX-A (Sloop et al., 1997). Whether M-wave amplitude is a reliable measure of clinical response and whether the doses of BTX-A (7.5 to 10 U) and BTX-B (320 to 480 U), with a B/A ratio of about 45:1, are comparable are debatable. The apparently longer duration of action of BTX-A compared to that of BTX-B could possibly be explained by the observation that VAMP that is cleaved by BTX-B cannot form stable SNARE complex and it turns over to form new VAMP, whereas SNAP-25, the substrate for BTX-A, forms a truncated SNAP-25$_A$, which prevents degradation of SNARE, as a result of which the inhibition of exocytosis persists for 40 to 60 days. This correlates well with the reappearance of the original terminals (de Paiva et al., 1999). De Paiva and colleagues (1999) noted that a single intramuscular injection of BTX-A into the sternomastoid muscles of mice caused the formation of functional neuronal sprouts that connected with the muscle fiber. The primary BTX-A–intoxicated nerve terminal was incapable of neurotransmitter exocytosis; it produced new sprouts that were capable of exocytosis with subsequent upregulation of adjacent nicotinic receptors on the muscle fiber, thus forming a functional synapse. After a certain period of time, such as 3 months, consistent with return of clinical function of the muscle and wearing-off response from the previous injection, the original BTX-A–intoxicated terminal resumed exocytosis, and the sprouts regressed to return the neuromuscular junction to its original state. Other studies have also shown that the prolonged duration of action BTX-A is due to persistence of catalytically active enzyme in the muscle cell (Adler et al., 2001). A physiologic study in monkeys showed that BTX-B diffuses less extensively than BTX-A into adjacent and remote muscles (Arezzo et al., 2002). In contrast to BOTOX, MYOBLOC is a solution that does not require reconstitution, and it may be

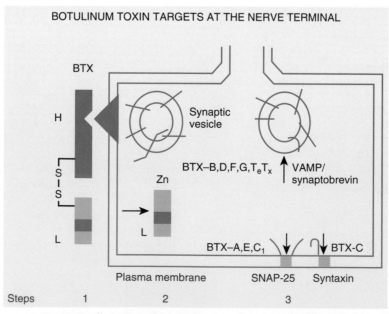

Figure 14-1 Diagram illustrating the mechanism of action of different types of BTX.

stored in a refrigerator rather than a freezer. The commercial preparations are complex proteins that must be dissociated from the active neurotoxin molecule to exert the paralytic effect. This dissociation, which is pH dependent, unmasks the binding site on the heavy chain.

In addition to BOTOX, MYOBLOC, and Dysport (Truong et al., 2005) (Tables 14-7 and 14-8), a new formulation of BTX Type A, NT 201, has been recently introduced (Benecke et al., 2005). This formulation of BTX type A, which is free of complexing proteins, has been reported to be equivalent, in terms of efficacy and safety, to BOTOX in healthy volunteers and in patients with blepharospasm (Roggenkamper et al., 2006) and cervical dystonia (Benecke et al., 2005). While low antigenicity has been predicted with this new formulation of BTX, no long-term data exist, and in view of the low frequency of blocking antibodies reported with the new formulation of BOTOX (see later) (Jankovic et al., 2003), it is not clear what role the new NT 201 BTX will play in the future treatment of dystonia.

The primary effect of BTX is to induce paralysis of injected skeletal muscles, especially the most actively contracting muscles. BTX paralyzes not only the extrafusal fibers but also the intrafusal fibers, thus decreasing the activity of Ib muscle afferents (Filippi et al., 1993). This might explain the effect of BTX on reciprocal inhibition. In untreated patients with dystonia, the second phase of reciprocal inhibition is usually decreased. BTX "corrects" the abnormal reciprocal inhibition by increasing the second phase, possibly through its effect on the muscle afferents (Priori et al., 1995). While the effect on intrafusal fibers might contribute in part to the beneficial action of BTX in patients with dystonia, this is not its main action because BTX is effective in facial dystonia, even though the facial muscles do not have spindles.

Measuring variations in fiber diameter and using acetylcholine-esterase staining as indexes of denervation, Borodic and colleagues (1994) showed that BTX diffuses up to 4.5 cm from the site of a single injection (10 U injected in the rabbit longissimus dorsi). Since the size of the denervation field is determined largely by the dose (and volume), multiple injections along the affected muscle rather than a single injection should therefore contain the biologic effects of the toxin in the targeted muscle (Borodic et al., 1992). Blackie and Lees (1990) also showed that frequency of dysphagia could be reduced by 50% when multiple rather than single injections are used.

A small percentage of patients receiving repeated injections develop antibodies against BTX, causing them to be com-

Table 14-7 Comparison of product characteristics

| | Botox | Dysport | Myobloc |
|---|---|---|---|
| Serotype | A | A | B |
| Complex MW | 900 kDa | 900 kDa | 700 kDa |
| Package (units) | 100 | 500 | 2500/5000/10000 |
| Neurotoxin Protein per Vial (ng) | 5 | 12.5 | 25/50/100 |
| Form | Vacuum Dried | Lyophilized | Solution |
| Storage | Freezer | – | Refrigerator |
| pH | 7 | 7 | 5.6 |

Table 14-8 Summary of labeling

| | Botox (N = 170) | Myobloc (N = 109) |
|---|---|---|
| Maximal efficacy | CDSS -20% | TWSTRS 20% -5,000 25% -10,000 |
| Duration | 3 months | 12–16 weeks |
| Adverse effects | Dysphagia Rhinitis | Dysphagia Dry mouth |
| Immunogenicity by MPA | 17% at entry 2% additional | 18% at 18 months |

pletely resistant to the effects of subsequent BTX injections (Greene et al., 1994; Jankovic and Schwartz, 1995; Jankovic, 2002). In one study, 24 of 559 (4.3%) patients treated for cervical dystonia developed BTX antibodies (Greene et al., 1994). The authors suggested that the true prevalence of antibodies might be more than 7%. In addition to patients with BTX antibodies, they studied eight patients from a cohort of 76 (10.5%) who stopped responding to BTX treatments. These BTX-resistant patients had a shorter interval between injections, more booster injections, and a higher dose at the non-booster injection compared to nonresistant patients treated during the same period. As a result of this experience, clinicians are warned against using booster injections and are encouraged to extend the interval between treatments as long as possible, certainly at least 1 month, and to use the smallest possible dose. In addition to high dosages, young age is a potential risk factor for the development of immunoresistance to BTX-A (Jankovic and Schwartz, 1995; Hanna and Jankovic, 1998; Hanna et al., 1999). Some of the patients who developed BTX-A antibodies have benefited from injections by immunologically distinct preparations, such as BTX-F and BTX-B (Greene and Fahn, 1992b; Mezaki et al., 1994). After 1 to 3 years, some patients become antibody negative, and when reinjected with the same type of toxin, they may again experience transient benefit (Sankhla et al., 1998). The original preparation of BOTOX contained 25 ng of neurotoxin complex protein per 100 units, but in 1997, the Food and Drug Administration approved a new preparation that contains only 5 ng per 100 units, which should have lower antigenicity (Aoki et al., 1999). In fact, in a 3-year follow-up of patients treated with the current BOTOX, no evidence of blocking antibodies was found, compared to a 9.4% frequency of blocking antibodies in patients treated with the original BOTOX for the same period of time (Jankovic et al., 2003) (Fig. 14-2). The preliminary data suggest that BTX-B provides clinical effects similar to those of BTX-A, but the duration of benefits is shorter (Comella et al., 2005) and MYOBLOC appears to have greater antigenicity than BOTOX, particularly in patients with prior resistance to BTX-A (Jankovic et al., 2006). To compare autonomic effects of BTX, Tintner and colleagues (2005) randomized patients with cervical dystonia to receive either BTX-A or BTX-B in a double-blind manner. Efficacy and physiologic questionnaire measures of autonomic function were assessed at baseline and 2 weeks after injection. Patients who were treated with BTX-B had significantly less saliva production (P < .01) and greater severity of constipation (P = .037) than did those treated with BTX-A but did not differ with respect to other tests of autonomic function, including changes in blood pressure, heart rate, and ocular

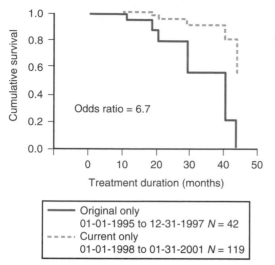

**ORIGINAL VS. CURRENT BOTOX IN CERVICAL DYSTONIA SURVIVAL WITHOUT EVIDENCE OF IMMUNORESISTANCE**

Odds ratio = 6.7

Original only
01-01-1995 to 12-31-1997 *N* = 42
Current only
01-01-1998 to 01-31-2001 *N* = 119

**Figure 14-2** Survival of patients before the development of antibodies after the use of original or current BTX. (Reprinted with permission from Jankovic J, Vuong KD, Ahsan J: Comparison of efficacy and immunogenicity of original versus current botulinum toxin in cervical dystonia. Neurology 2003;60:1186–1188.)

function. The autonomic effects of BTX-B were reviewed in several additional reports (Wan et al., 2005).

Many clinical studies have provided evidence not only that BTX is safe and effective but also that this therapy leads to meaningful improvements in quality of life (Naumann and Jankovic, 2004; Jankovic et al., 2004), and the benefits are long-lasting (Mejia et al., 2005) (Video 14-1). Despite its proven therapeutic value, there are still many unresolved issues and concerns about BTX. These include lack of standardization of biologic activity of the different preparations of BTX, poor understanding of toxin antigenicity, variations in the methods of injection, and inadequate assays for BTX antibodies. Training guidelines for the use of botulinum toxin have been established (American Academy of Neurology, 1994). Clinicians who are interested in utilizing BTX chemodenervation in their practice must be aware of these concerns and must exercise proper precautions to minimize the potential risks associated with BTX. Most important, they should become thoroughly familiar with the movement disorders that they intend to treat and with the anatomy at the injection site. Possible contraindications to the use of BTX include the presence of myasthenia gravis (Emerson, 1994), Eaton-Lambert syndrome, motor neuron disease, aminoglycoside antibiotics, and pregnancy. Besides occasional complications, usually related to local weakness, a major limitation of BTX therapy is its high cost. Several studies analyzing the cost-effectiveness of BTX treatment, however, have demonstrated that the loss of productivity as a result of untreated dystonia and the cost of medications or surgery more than justify the financial expense of BTX treatments. It is likely that future research will result in the development of new, more effective neuromuscular blocking agents that provide therapeutic chemodenervation with long-term benefits and at lower cost.

## Blepharospasm

The effectiveness of BTX in blepharospasm was first demonstrated in double-blind, placebo-controlled trials (Fahn et al., 1985b; Jankovic and Orman, 1987). In a subsequent report of experience with BTX in 477 patients with various dystonias and hemifacial spasm, Jankovic and colleagues (1990) reviewed the results in 90 patients who had been injected with BTX for blepharospasm. Moderate or marked improvement was noted in 94% of the patients. The average latency from the time of the injection to the onset of improvement was 4.2 days; the average duration of maximum benefit was 12.4 weeks, but the total benefit lasted considerably longer: an average of 15.7 weeks. While 41% of all treatment sessions were followed by some side effects (ptosis, blurring of vision or diplopia, tearing, and local hematoma), only 2% of these affected patient's functioning. Complications usually improved spontaneously in less than 2 weeks. These results are consistent with those of other studies (Elston, 1994). There is no apparent decline in benefit, and the frequency of complications actually decreases after repeat BTX treatments (Jankovic and Schwartz, 1993a).

Reasons for the gradual enhancement in efficacy and reduction in the frequency of complications with repeat treatments include greater experience and improvements in the injection technique. For example, one controlled study showed that an injection into the pretarsal rather than preseptal portion of the orbicularis oculi is associated with significantly lower frequency of ptosis (Jankovic, 1996). Ptosis can be prevented also by injecting initially only the lateral and medial portions of the upper lid, thus avoiding the midline levator muscle. Usually an initial injection of 5 U is made in each site in the upper lid and 5 U in the lower lid laterally only. This finding has been confirmed by others (Cakmur et al., 2002).

The functional improvement, experienced by the vast majority of patients after BTX injection, is difficult to express numerically. Many patients could not work, drive, watch television, or read prior to the injections. As a result of reduced eyelid and eyebrow spasms, most can now function normally. In addition to the observed functional improvement, there is usually a meaningful amelioration of discomfort, and because of less embarrassment, the patients' self-esteem also frequently improves. BTX injections are now considered by many to be the treatment of choice for blepharospasm (American Academy of Ophthalmology, 1989; American Academy of Neurology, 1990). In addition to idiopathic blepharospasm, BTX injections have been used effectively in the treatment of blepharospasm induced by drugs (e.g., levodopa in parkinsonian patients or neuroleptics in patients with tardive dystonia), dystonic eyelid and facial tics in patients with Tourette syndrome, and blepharospasm associated with apraxia of eyelid opening (Jankovic, 1994; Aramideh et al., 1995; Lepore et al., 1995; Jankovic, 1996; Forget et al., 2002).

## Oromandibular Dystonia

Oromandibular dystonia is among the most challenging forms of focal dystonia to treat with BTX (Blitzer et al., 1989); it rarely improves with medications, there are no surgical treatments, and BTX therapy can be complicated by swallowing problems. The masseter muscles are usually injected in patients with jaw-closure dystonia; in patients with jaw-opening dystonia, either the submental muscle complex or the lateral pterygoid muscles are injected. In a total of 91 patients treated in 271 visits, the overall improvement was rated as 2.6 (0 = no response to 4 = marked improvement in spasms and function) (Jankovic and Schwartz, 1991b). A meaningful reduction in the oromandibular-lingual spasms and an improvement in chewing and speech were achieved in more than 70% of patients. The improvement was noted within an average of 5.5 days after injection and lasted an average of 11.5 weeks. Patients with dystonic jaw closure responded better than those with jaw-opening dystonia. Temporary swallowing problem, noted in fewer than one third of patients and in only 17% of all treatment sessions, was the most frequent complication. Early treatment with BTX may prevent dental and other complications, including temporomandibular joint syndrome and other oral and dental problems (Blitzer and Brin, 1991). BTX can provide lasting improvement not only in patients with primary (idiopathic) dystonia but also in orolingual-mandibular tardive dystonia. Clenching and bruxism are frequent manifestations of oromandibular dystonia, although nocturnal and diurnal bruxism can occur even without evident dystonia (Tan and Jankovic, 1999, 2000). Oromandibular involuntary movements caused by hemimasticatory spasms and other disorders such as Satoyoshi syndrome have also been successfully treated with BTX (Merello et al., 1994).

## Laryngeal Dystonia (Spasmodic Dysphonia)

Until the introduction of BTX, the therapy of spasmodic dysphonia was disappointing. The anticholinergic and benzodiazepine drugs only rarely provide meaningful improvement in voice quality. Unilateral transection of the recurrent laryngeal nerve, although effective in most patients, frequently causes unacceptable complications, and the voice symptoms often recur (Dedo and Izdebski, 1983). A surgical procedure that involves denervation of the adductor branch of the recurrent laryngeal nerve with reinnervation of the distal sumps with branches of the ansa cervicalis nerve was reported to produce marked improvement in patients with adductor spasmodic dysphonia (Berke et al., 1999), but further studies are need to confirm this initial observation.

Several studies have established the efficacy and safety of BTX in the treatment of laryngeal dystonia, and this approach is considered by most to be the treatment of choice for spasmodic dysphonia (Brin et al., 1987; Blitzer et al., 1988; Jankovic et al., 1990; Brin et al., 1992; Ludlow, 1990; Brin et al., 1998; Blitzer et al., 2002). Before a patient can be considered a potential candidate for BTX injections, the diagnosis of spasmodic dysphonia must be confirmed by detailed neurologic, otolaryngologic, and voice assessment and documented by video and voice recordings.

Three approaches are currently used in the BTX treatment of spasmodic dysphonia: (1) unilateral EMG-guided injection of 5 to 30 U (Jankovic et al., 1990), (2) bilateral approach, injecting with EMG-guidance 1.25 to 4 U in each vocal fold (Brin et al., 1992), and (3) an injection via indirect laryngoscopy without EMG (Ford et al., 1990). Irrespective of the technique, most investigators report about 75% to 95% improvement in voice symptoms. One controlled study, however, concluded that unilateral injections "may provide both superior and longer lasting benefits" than bilateral injections (Adams et al., 1993). The dosage can be adjusted depending on the severity of glottal spasms and the response to previous injections. Adverse experiences include transient breathy hypophonia, hoarseness, and rare dysphagia with aspiration.

Although more complicated and less effective, BTX injections into the posterior cricoarytenoid muscle with the EMG needle placed posterior to the thyroid lamina may be used in the treatment of the abductor form of spasmodic dysphonia (Brin et al., 1989; Brin et al., 1992). Using a multidisciplinary team approach, consisting of an otolaryngologist who is experienced in laryngeal injections and a neurologist who is knowledgeable about motor disorders of speech and voice, BTX injections can provide effective relief for most patients with spasmodic dysphonia (American Academy of Neurology, 1990; American Academy of Otolaryngology, 1990). Outcome assessments clearly show that BTX injections for spasmodic dysphonia produce measurable improvements in the quality of life of patients with this disorder (Courey et al., 2000). BTX may be useful in the treatment of voice tremor and stuttering, but the results are less predictable (Ludlow, 1990; Brin et al., 1994; Warrick et al., 2000).

## Cervical Dystonia

The goal of therapy of cervical dystonia is not only to improve abnormal posture of the head and associated neck pain but also to prevent the development of secondary complications such as contractures, cervical radiculopathy, and cervical myelopathy (Treves and Korczyn, 1986; Waterston et al., 1989).

With the use of TWSTRS and other scales, the efficacy and safety of BTX in the treatment of cervical dystonia have been demonstrated in several controlled and open trials (Greene et al., 1990; Jankovic and Schwartz, 1990; Poewe et al., 1992; Jankovic et al., 1994; Tintner and Jankovic, 2001b; Jankovic, 2002, 2004c; Truong et al., 2005) (Videos 14-2 and 14-3). In one double-blind, placebo-controlled study of 55 patients with cervical dystonia, 61% improved after BTX-A injection (Greene et al., 1990). BTX has been found to be superior not only to placebo but also to trihexyphenidyl (Brans et al., 1996). In a study of 66 consecutive patients with idiopathic cervical dystonia, Brans and colleagues (1996) compared the effectiveness of BTX-A (Dysport) with that of trihexyphenidyl in a prospective, randomized, double-blind design. Dysport or saline was injected under EMG guidance at study entry and again after 8 weeks. Patients were assessed for efficacy at baseline and after 12 weeks by different clinical rating scales. Sixty-four patients completed the study, 32 in each group. The mean dose of BTX-A was 292 U (first session) and 262 U (second session). The mean dose of trihexyphenidyl was 16.25 mg. TWSTRS (primary outcome) and other scales showed a significant improvement in favor of BTX-A, and adverse effects were significantly less frequent than in the group of patients randomized to trihexyphenidyl. In a multicenter, double-blind, randomized, controlled trial assessing the safety and efficacy of Dysport in cervical dystonia patients, 80 patients were randomly assigned to receive one treatment with Dysport (500 units) or placebo (Truong et al., 2005). Dysport was significantly more efficacious than placebo at weeks 4, 8, and 12 as assessed by TWSTRS (10 point versus 3.8 point reduction in total score, respectively, at week 4; $P \leq .013$). Of participants in the Dysport group, 38% showed positive treatment response, compared to 16% in the placebo group (95% confidence interval 0.02 to 0.41). The median duration of response to Dysport was 18.5 weeks. Side effects were generally similar in the two treatment groups; only blurred vision and weakness occurred significantly more often with Dysport. No participants in the Dysport group converted from negative to positive antibodies after treatment. These results confirm previous reports that Dysport (500 units) is safe, effective, and well tolerated in patients with cervical dystonia.

Open-label studies generally report a more dramatic improvement, partly because of a placebo effect and, more important, because of greater flexibility in selecting the proper dosage and site of injection. Most trials report that about 90% of patients experience improvement in function and control of the head and neck and in pain. The average latency between injection and the onset of improvement (and muscle atrophy) is 1 week, and the average duration of maximum improvement is 3 to 4 months. On the average, the injections are repeated every 4 to 6 months. Patients with long-duration dystonia have been found to respond less well than those who were treated relatively early, possibly because prolonged dystonia produced contractures (Jankovic and Schwartz, 1991b). In one study, 28% of patients experienced some complication, such as swallowing difficulties, neck weakness, and nausea, sometime during the course of their treatment (some patients had up to 12 visits in 5 years). Dysphagia, the most common complication, was encountered in 14% of all 659 visits, but in only five instances was this problem severe enough to require changing to a soft or liquid diet. Complications are usually related to focal weakness, although distant and systemic subclinical and clinical effects, such as generalized weakness and malaise, rarely occur, possibly as a result of blood distribution or retrograde axonal transport to the spinal motor neurons (Garner et al., 1993). Most complications resolve spontaneously, usually within 2 weeks. An injection into one or both sternocleidomastoid muscles was most frequently associated with dysphagia (Jankovic and Schwartz, 1991b; Comella, Tanner, et al., 1992). One study showed that dosages as small as 20 units administered as a single injection into the sternocleidomastoid muscle completely eliminated muscle activity and could produce neck weakness and dysphagia (Buchman et al., 1994). In an analysis of patients who received five or more injections, the beneficial response was maintained and the frequency of complications with repeat injections actually declined, presumably as a result of improving skills (Jankovic and Schwartz, 1993a). Lindeboom and colleagues (1998), found that neurologic impairment and pain usually improve following BTX injections, but only functional status measures differentiate between patients who improve and those who have an insufficient response. There have been only a few long-term studies of BTX treatment in cervical dystonia. Brashear and colleagues (2000) showed that two thirds of patients who received BTX reported the injections always helped. Another long-term study showed that 75% of patients continued to benefit for at least 5 years, only 7.5% developed secondary unresponsiveness, and only 1.3% discontinued BTX therapy because of intolerable side effects (Hsiung et al., 2002).

Results similar to those obtained with BTX-A have been obtained in patients treated for cervical dystonia with BTX-B

(Tsui et al., 1995; Lew et al., 1997; Figgitt and Noble, 2002). In a double-blind, controlled trial of 122 patients with cervical dystonia treated with BTX-B, there was a dose response effect, particularly at doses of 10,000 units (Lew et al., 1997). Using TWSTRS, 77% of the patients were found to respond at week 4. Other studies have subsequently confirmed the efficacy of BTX-B (Brashear et al., 1999), even in patients who are resistant to BTX-A (Brin et al., 1999). In a 16-week, randomized, multicenter, double-blind, placebo-controlled trial of BTX-B, 109 patients, who previously responded well to BTX-A, were randomized into one of the treatment groups: placebo, 5,000 U, and 10,000 U administered into two to four cervical muscles (Brashear et al., 1999). At week 4, the total TWSTRS score improved by 4.3, 9.3 ($P = .01$), and 11.7 ($P = .0004$), respectively, when compared to baseline, and this was accompanied by significant improvements in pain, disability, and severity. The estimated median time until the total TWSTRS score returned to baseline was 63, 114, and 111 days, respectively. The most frequent side effects associated with BTX-B included dysphagia and dry mouth. An identical design was used in another study of BTX-B in cervical dystonia with one exception: The patients were resistant to BTX-A as determined by the F-TAT (Brin et al., 1999). A total of 77 patients were randomized to receive placebo or 10,000 U of BTX-B. At week 4, the total TWSTRS scores improved by 2 (placebo) and 11 (10,000 U) ($P = .0001$). There was also significant improvement in secondary and tertiary outcome measures, including global assessments and pain visual analog scores, as well as other measures of pain, disability, and severity. The estimated duration of effect, based on a Kaplan-Meier survival analysis, was 112 days (12 to 16 weeks). Subsequent studies have suggested that dosages as high as 45,000 U of BTX-B (MYOBLOC) per session may be effective and safe in patients with cervical dystonia.

The most important determinants of a favorable response to BTX treatments are a proper selection of the involved muscles and an appropriate dosage (Box 14-3). EMG may be helpful in some patients with obese necks or in whom the involved

---

**Box 14-3** Examination of patients with cervical dystonia

1. Find the most uncompensated position
   The patient is instructed to allow the head to "draw" into the maximal abnormal posture without resisting the dystonic "pulling" (with eyes open and closed)
   Examine while standing, walking, sitting, and writing
2. Passively move the head
   To define the dystonic posture
   To localize the contracting muscles
   To determine the full range of motion
   To determine whether there are contractures
3. Palpate contracting muscles
   To localize the involved muscles
   To estimate the muscle mass
   To find points of tenderness
4. EMG (needed rarely)
   To localize involved muscles that cannot be palpated
   To guide the injection into the muscles that are difficult to access

muscles are difficult to identify by palpation (Dubinsky et al., 1991; Gelb et al., 1991). One study attempted to determine the usefulness of EMG-assisted BTX injections and found that the percentage of patients who showed any improvement after BTX was similar whether the injections were assisted by EMG or not (Comella, Buchman, et al., 1992). They also noted that "a significantly greater magnitude of improvement" was present in patients treated with EMG-assisted method and that there was "a significantly greater number of patients with marked benefit" in the group that was randomly assigned to the EMG-assisted method of treatment. Since the majority (70% to 79%) of patients had previously been treated with BTX, some might have been experiencing residual effects from previous injections, making the interpretation of the results difficult. Furthermore, the patients who were treated without EMG assistance received a higher dose, indicating more severe dystonia, thus possibly explaining the lesser degree of observed improvement. The general consensus among most BTX users is that EMG is not needed in the vast majority of patients, except in rare instances when the muscles cannot be adequately palpated or the patient does not obtain adequate relief of symptoms with the conventional approach (Jankovic, 2001b). Not only does BTX treatment provide effective symptomatic relief in patients with cervical dystonia; it has also dramatically changed the natural history of the disease, as it also prevents contractures. Early introduction of BTX has been shown to prevent contractures even in patients with congenital torticollis (Collins and Jankovic, 2006).

## Writer's Cramp and Other Limb Dystonias

Treatments of writer's cramp with muscle relaxation techniques, physical and occupational therapy, and medical and surgical therapies have been disappointing. Several open (Rivest et al., 1990; Jankovic and Schwartz, 1993b; Karp et al., 1994; Priori et al., 1995; Pullman et al., 1996; Quirk et al., 1996; Wissel et al., 1996) and double-blind controlled (Yoshimura et al., 1992; Tsui et al., 1993; Cole et al., 1995) trials have concluded that BTX injections into selected hand and forearm muscles probably provide the most effective relief in patients with these task-specific occupational dystonias. In some studies, fine wire electrodes were used to localize bursts of muscle activation during the task, and the toxin was injected through a hollow EMG needle into the belly of the most active muscle (Cole et al., 1995). Similar beneficial results, however, were obtained in other studies without complex EMG studies (Rivest et al., 1990). Several lines of evidence support the notion that an intramuscular injection of BTX into the forearm muscles corrects the abnormal reciprocal inhibition (Priori et al., 1995).

Jankovic and Schwartz (1993b) studied the effects of BTX in 46 patients with hand dystonia who had injections into their forearm muscles in 130 treatment sessions. The average age was 49.4 years, and the dystonic symptoms had been present for an average of 8.6 years. After careful examination and palpation of the forearm muscles during writing, the toxin was injected into either the wrist flexors (116 injections) or the wrist extensors (52 injections). The average baseline severity of dystonia was 3.5 on a 0 to 4 rating scale. The average peak effect response for all treatment sessions was 2.3 (0 = no response to 4 = maximum benefit). The latency from injection to onset of effect averaged 5.6 days, and the benefit lasted an average of 9.2 weeks. Temporary hand weakness, the chief complication of this treatment, occurred in 54% of patients and in 34% of all treatment sessions. However, nearly all patients preferred the temporary weakness, which was usually mild, to the disabling writer's cramps. Although one study showed that only 14 of 38 (37%) of needle placement attempts reached the proper hand muscles in the absence of EMG guidance, this does not mean that placement with EMG guidance correlates with better results, since the selection of the muscle involved in the hand dystonia is based on clinical examination, not on EMG (Molloy et al., 2002). One study showed that voluntary activity of the hand immediately after the treatment for 30 minutes enhanced the weakness produced by the injection (Chen et al., 1999).

In addition to improving writer's cramp, BTX might provide relief in other task-specific disorders affecting typists, draftsmen, musicians, athletes, and other people who depend on skilled movements of their hands (Schuele et al., 2005). Other focal distal dystonias, besides those involving the hands, might be amenable to treatment with BTX. Patients with Parkinson disease, progressive supranuclear palsy, corticobasal degeneration, and other forms of parkinsonism or stroke-related hemiplegia occasionally develop secondary fixed dystonia of the hand (dystonic clenched fist), which might benefit in terms of pain and hygiene from local BTX injections (Cordivari et al., 2001). Patients with foot dystonia as a manifestation of primary (idiopathic) dystonia and patients with parkinsonism who experience foot dystonia as an early symptom of their disease or, more commonly, as a complication of levodopa therapy might benefit from local BTX infections (Pacchetti et al., 1995). BTX injections into the foot-toe flexors or extensors not only might alleviate the disability, pain, and discomfort that are often associated with such dystonia but also might improve gait. Whether BTX injections will play an important role in the treatment of recurrent painful physiologic foot and calf cramps has yet to be determined.

## Other Indications for Botulinum Toxin

It is beyond the scope of this chapter to review the rapidly broadening indications for BTX therapy (see Box 14-2). The reader is referred to some recent reviews on this topic (Brin et al., 2002; Jankovic and Brin, 2002; Jankovic 2004a).

## SURGICAL TREATMENT OF DYSTONIA

Although surgery has been used in the treatment of dystonia for long time (Cooper 1965), there has been a recent resurgence in this approach, largely because of improvements in surgical and imaging techniques and as a result of surgical benefits observed in patients with tremor and Parkinson disease (Jankovic, 1998; Lang, 1998; Ondo et al., 2001).

### Central Ablative Procedures and Deep Brain Stimulation

Improved understanding of the functional anatomy of the basal ganglia and physiologic mechanisms underlying movement disorders, coupled with refinements in imaging and surgical techniques, has led to a resurgence of interest in thalamotomy in patients with disabling tremors, dystonia, and other hyperkinetic movement disorders (Grossman and Hamilton, 1993; Jankovic et al., 1996; Ondo et al., 2001). The observation, supported by both physiologic and positron emission tomographic studies, that there is a disruption of pallidothalamic-cortical projections in dystonia provides some rationale for treating dystonia by interrupting the abnormal outflow from the thalamus to the overactive prefrontal motor cortex (Lenz et al., 1990; Mitchel et al., 1990; Ceballos-Baumann et al., 1995) (Fig. 14-3).

In a longitudinal study of 17 patients with severe dystonia, 8 (47%) had a moderate to marked improvement in their abnormal postures and functional disability following thalamotomy (Cardoso et al., 1995). Patients with primary and secondary dystonia had similar responses, but 43% of the patients with primary dystonia deteriorated during a mean follow-up of 32.9 months, whereas only 30% of patients with secondary dystonia deteriorated during a mean follow-up of 41.0 months. Neurologic complications were observed in 6 of 17 patients (35%) immediately after surgery, but deficits (contralateral weakness, dysarthria, pseudobulbar palsy) persisted in only one subject. Mild weakness contralateral to the surgery was the most common complication, noted in 3 patients immediately following the procedure. The one patient who underwent bilateral procedures had no detectable dysarthria. These results are consistent with other studies that have reported improvement in 34% to 70% of patients with dystonia following thalamotomy (Cooper, 1976; Andrew et al., 1983; Tasker et al., 1988). While most studies concluded that distal dystonia responded more favorably to thalamotomy than does axial dystonia, Andrew and colleagues (1983) felt that their patients with axial dystonia, including torticollis, also improved after thalamotomy. Most investigators, however, feel that the best candidates for thalamotomy are patients who have disabling, particularly unilateral, dystonia (hemidystonia) that is unresponsive to medical therapy.

Patients with pre-existing dysarthria are also good candidates because they have less to lose from thalamotomy-related speech disturbance. Patients with secondary (symptomatic) dystonia seem to respond better than do those with idiopathic dystonia. Thalamotomy should not be recommended for patients with facial, laryngeal, and cervical or truncal dystonia.

The role of pallidotomy in the treatment of dystonia is currently being reevaluated in view of emerging use of deep brain stimulation (Jankovic et al., 1997; Eltahawy et al., 2004). In one study of eight patients with severe generalized dystonia, there was 59% and 62.5% improvement in the Fahn-Marsden Dystonia Scale and in the Unified Dystonia Rating Scale, respectively, following pallidotomy (Ondo et al., 1998). The experience with pallidotomy continues to show favorable long-term effects, particularly in patients with primary dystonia (Ondo et al., 2001; Yoshor et al., 2001). Although the surgery does not slow or halt the progression of the underlying disease, most patients continue to benefit. The procedure is usually well tolerated, and the benefits have persisted during for more than 10 years in most patients with primary dystonia. Pallidotomy has also been reported to be effective in a 47-year-old woman with paroxysmal dystonia induced by exercise (Bhatia et al., 1998).

Although there are no data from normal humans, microelectrode recordings from patients with generalized dystonia indicate that the mean discharge rates (about 50 Hz) in the globus pallidus internum (GPi) are lower than those in patients with Parkinson disease (80 to 85 Hz) (Lozano et al., 1997) or parkinsonian primates (70 to 75 Hz) (Filion and Tremblay, 1991) but higher than those in hemiballism (Vitek et al., 1998, 1999) and that the proportion of GPi cells that respond to stimulation is higher in patients with dystonia than in those with hemiballism (Lenz et al., 1998). In comparison to normal or parkinsonian primates, the GPi discharges in patients with dystonia seem to be more irregular, with more bursting and pauses, and the receptive fields to passive and active movements seem to be widened (Kumar et al.,

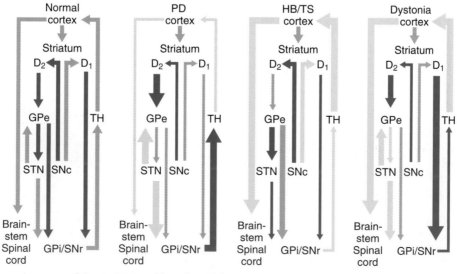

**MODELS OF BASAL GANGLIA DYSFUNCTION**

Figure 14-3 Schematic diagram of connections of basal ganglia in normal subjects and patients with Parkinson disease, hemiballism (HB) or Tourette syndrome (TS), and dystonia. *Light arrows,* inhibitory pathways; *dark arrows,* excitatory pathways.

1999). The intraoperative neurophysiologic recordings in 15 patients with dystonia were compared with those of 78 patients with Parkinson disease undergoing pallidotomy; the discharge rates were lower in frequency and more irregular in the GPi and GPe of patients with dystonia (Fig. 14-4) (Sanghera et al., 2003).

Although the physiologic studies, based on lower mean discharge rates in GPe and GPi (Vitek et al., 1998, 1999), suggest overactivity of both direct (striatum-GPi) and indirect (striatum-GPe-GPi) pathways, the dopamine receptor ligand PET studies (Perlmutter et al., 1997; Asanuma et al., 2005) suggest increased activity in the direct and decreased activity in the indirect pathway. This is compatible with FDG PET studies supportive of excessive activity in the direct pathway (Eidelberg et al., 1995). In multiple reports, pallidotomy (Lozano et al., 1997; Ondo et al., 1998; Vitek et al., 1999) and GPi DBS (Coubes et al., 2000; Tronnier and Fogel, 2000; Vercueil et al., 2001; Bereznai et al., 2002; Vidailhet et al., 2005; Diamond et al., 2006) appear to be effective procedures for patients with dystonia (Videos 14-4, 14-5, and 14-6). Both procedures may provide benefit by disrupting the abnormal GPi pattern and thus reduce cortical overactivation, characteristic of dystonia (Eidelberg et al., 1995). Primary dystonia clearly responds better than secondary dystonia to either pallidotomy or GPi DBS, although patients with pantothenate kinase–associated neurodegeneration also experience marked improvement (Coubes et al., 2000; Eltahawy et al., 2004).

In a prospective, multicenter study of 22 patients with generalized dystonia, seven of whom had a *DYT1* mutation, the Fahn-Marsden Dystonia Scale score improved after bilateral GPi DBS from a mean of 46.3 ± 21.3 to 21.0 ± 14.1 at 12 months (*P* < .001) (Vidailhet et al., 2005). A "blinded" review of the videos at 3 months showed improvement with stimulation from a mean of 34.63 ± 12.3 to 24.6 ± 17.7. The improvement in mean dystonia motor scores was 51%, and one third of the patients improved more than 75% compared to preoperative scores. In addition, there was a significant improvement in health-related quality of life as measured by the SF-36, but there was no change in cognition or mood. Although the sample was rather small, the authors were not able to find any predictors of response such as *DYT1* gene status, anatomic distribution of the dystonia, or location of the electrodes. Patients with the phasic form of dystonia improved more than those with tonic contractions and posturing. The maximum benefit was not achieved in some patients until 3 to 6 months after surgery. Vercueil and colleagues (2001) described 10 patients with bilateral GPi DBS; 5 had a major improvement, 2 had a moderated improvement, and 1 had a minor improvement after 14 months. They concluded that GPi DBS is much more effective than thalamic DBS for the treatment of dystonia. In a 2-year follow-up of 31 patients with primary generalized dystonia, Coubes and colleagues (2004), noted a mean improvement in clinical and functional Fahn-Marsden Dystonia Rating Scale of 79% and 65%, respectively. There was no difference in response between DYT1-positive and DYT1-negative patients, but the magnitude of improvement was greater in children than in adults. Since an ablative lesion or high-frequency stimulation of the GPi can both produce and improve dystonia, this suggests it is the pattern of discharge in the basal ganglia rather than the actual location or frequency of discharge that is pathophysiologically relevant to dystonia (Münchau et al., 2000). In addition to primary dystonia, GPi DBS has been reported to be effective in patients with tardive dystonia (Trottenberg et al., 2005), cranial-cervical

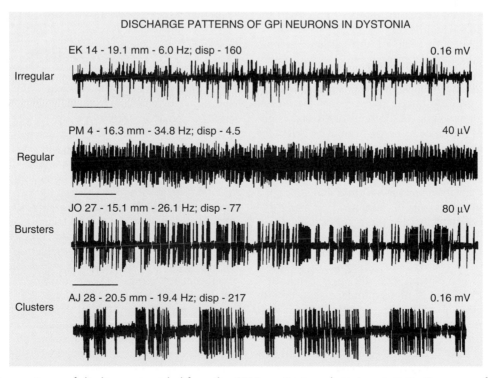

**Figure 14-4** Various patterns of discharge recorded from the GPi in patients undergoing stereotactic surgery for dystonia. (Reprinted with permission from Sanghera M, Grossman RG, Kalhorn CG, et al: Basal ganglia neuronal discharge in primary and secondary dystonia in patients undergoing pallidotomy. Neurosurgery 2003;52:1358–1373.)

dystonia (Foote et al., 2005), and other forms of segmental dystonia (Krauss et al., 2002).

## Peripheral Surgery

Peripheral denervation procedures were used extensively for cervical dystonia prior to the advent of BTX therapy. In one series of patients with cervical dystonia seen before 1990, 40 of 300 (13%) patients elected to have this type of surgery (Jankovic et al., 1991). While 10% of the patients noted worsening after the surgery, 38% experienced a noticeable improvement in the ability to control their head position or in reduction of the neck pain.

Three procedures have been used in the treatment of cervical dystonia: (1) extradural selective sectioning of posterior (dorsal) rami (posterior ramisectomy) with or without myotomy, (2) intradural sectioning of anterior cervical roots (anterior cervical rhizotomy), and (3) microvascular decompression of the spinal accessory nerve. Although the first procedure, championed by Bertrand (Bertrand and Molina-Negro, 1988), is considered by many clinicians to be the procedure of choice, no study has compared the different surgical approaches. Bertrand and Molina-Negro (1988) reported that 97 of 111 (87%) patients had "excellent" or "very good" results. In a smaller series, five of nine (56%) patients had moderate benefit that was sustained during up to 21 months of follow-up (Davis et al., 1991). The procedure is performed under general anesthesia without a paralyzing agent so that intraoperative nerve root stimulation can be used to identify the innervation to the dystonic muscles. This information, coupled with preoperative EMG, is used to avulse selected nerve roots, usually the branches of the spinal accessory nerve and the posterior rami of C1 through C6. Thorough avulsion of the peripheral branches is believed to be essential in preventing recurrences. Pain seems to improve more than the abnormal posture following the cervical muscle denervation, although some patients complain of stiff neck, sometimes lasting several months after the surgery. Other complications may include local numbness, neck weakness, and rarely dysphagia. The chief disadvantage of anterior rhizotomy compared to posterior primary ramisectomy is that the former procedure causes denervation of both involved and uninvolved muscles, and it cannot be carried out at or below the C4 level because of the potential for involvement of the roots to the phrenic nerve, leading to paralysis of the diaphragm. The posterior ramisectomy (C2 to C6) allows more selective denervation of the involved muscles. Krauss and colleagues (1997) reported the effects of 70 intradural or extradural approaches in 46 patients with severe cervical dystonia. During a mean duration of follow-up of 6.5 years, 21 (46%) of the patients reported excellent or marked improvement on a global outcome scale. There was no difference in the distribution of outcome when patients who still responded to BTX were compared with the BTX nonresponders. According to a modified TWSTRS scale, there was statistically significant improvement not only in the severity of dystonia but also in the ability to perform occupational and domestic tasks and various activities of daily living. The results of this study are comparable to those of Ford and colleagues (1998b) who reported a retrospective study of an open-label selective denervation for severe cervical dystonia (torticollis) in 16 patients who were refractory to injections with BTX-A. The surgery

was performed elsewhere, and the patients were followed by these authors. Using functional capacity scales, they concluded that 6 (37.5%) patients had "a moderate or complete return of normal neck function." Despite some improvement in 12 of 14 (85.7%) patients on the TWSTRS dystonia rating scale applied to "blinded" ratings of videotaped examinations, the surgery failed to return patients to their occupations. On the basis of the reported experience, one can conclude that surgical treatment tailored to the specific pattern of dystonic activity in the individual patient is a valuable alternative in the long-term management of cervical dystonia, particularly for patients who are anxious to avoid the intracranial surgical procedure of DBS targeting the GPi.

Surgical treatments, such as facial nerve lysis and orbicularis oculi myectomy, once used extensively in the treatment of blepharospasm, have been essentially abolished because BTX treatment is usually very effective and because postoperative complications, such as ectropion, exposure keratitis, facial droop, and postoperative swelling and scarring, are common (Chapman et al., 1999). Similarly, recurrent laryngeal nerve section, once used in the treatment of spasmodic dysphonia (Dedo et al., 1983), is used rarely and only when BTX fails to provide a satisfactory relief. Another once popular procedure, spinal cord stimulation for cervical dystonia, has been shown to be ineffective by a controlled trial (Goetz et al., 1988).

## OTHER THERAPIES

Inhibiting expression of mutant torsinA could be potentially a powerful therapeutic strategy in DYT1 dystonia. Using small interfering RNA (siRNA) to silence the expression of mutant torsinA, Gonzalez-Alegre and colleagues (2003) successfully suppressed expression of this abnormal protein in transfected cells that was allele-specific.

## THERAPEUTIC GUIDELINES

In summary, patients with segmental or generalized dystonia beginning in childhood or adolescence should be initially tried on levodopa/carbidopa up to 1000 mg of levodopa per day (Fig. 14-5). If this therapy is successful, it should be maintained at a lowest possible dose. If it is ineffective after 3 months, then high-dose anticholinergic (e.g., trihexyphenidyl) therapy should be instituted, and the dosage should be increased to the highest tolerated level. If the results are poor, then baclofen, benzodiazepines, carbamazepine, and tetrabenazine should be tried. Some patients may require triple therapy consisting of an anticholinergic agent (e.g., trihexyphenidyl), a monoamine-depleting drug (e.g., tetrabenazine), and a dopamine receptor–blocking drug (e.g., fluphenazine, pimozide, risperidol, or clozapine) (Marsden et al., 1984). Tetrabenazine alone or with anticholinergic drugs is particularly useful in the treatment of tardive dystonia. In some patients, BTX injections may be helpful to control the most disabling symptom of the segmental or generalized dystonia. In most patients with adult-onset dystonia, the distribution is usually focal; therefore, BTX injections are usually considered the treatment of choice. In addition to the abnormal movement and posture, pain, associated depression, anxiety, and other psychological comorbidities can have

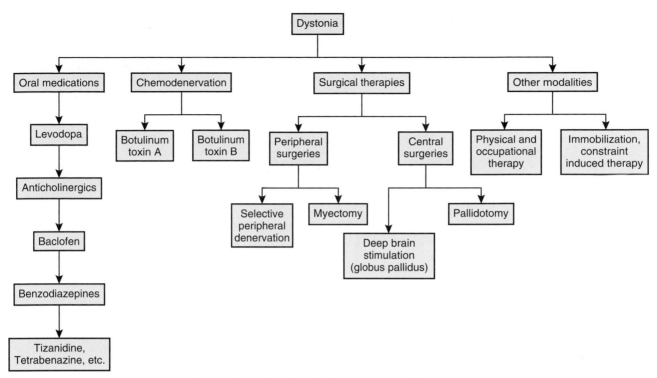

**Figure 14-5** Algorithm for the treatment of dystonia.

an important impact on the quality of life of patients with cervical dystonia and must be treated appropriately (Ben-Shlomo et al., 2002). In some patients, this treatment might need to be supplemented by other drugs noted previously or by surgical peripheral denervation. DBS should be reserved only for patients whose symptoms continue to be disabling despite optimal medical therapy. Any form of therapy should, of course, be preceded by a thorough evaluation designed to rule out secondary causes of dystonia. Finally, it is important to emphasize that patient education and counseling are essential components of a comprehensive therapeutic approach to all patients with dystonia (see Appendix 14-1).

# References

Adams SG, Hunt EJ, Charles DA, Lang AE: Unilateral versus bilateral botulinum toxin injections in spasmodic dysphonia: Acoustic and perceptual results. J Otolaryngol 1993;22:171–175.

Adler M, Keller JE, Sheridan RE, Deshpande SS: Persistence of botulinum neurotoxin A demonstrated by sequential administration of serotypes A and E in rat EDL muscle. Toxicon 2001;39:233–243.

Albanese A, Barnes MP, Bhatia KP, et al: A systematic review on the diagnosis and treatment of primary (idiopathic) dystonia and dystonia plus syndromes: Report of an EFNS/MDS-ES Task Force. Eur J Neurol 2006;13:433–444.

Albright AL, Barry MJ, Painter MJ, Shultz B: Infusion of intrathecal baclofen for generalized dystonia in cerebral palsy. J Neurosurg 1998;88:73–76.

Albright AL, Barry MJ, Shafron DH, Ferson SF: Intrathecal baclofen for generalized dystonia. Dev Med Child Neurol 2001;43:652–657.

American Academy of Neurology: Assessment: The clinical usefulness of botulinum toxin-A in treating neurologic disorders: Report of the Therapeutics and Technology Assessment Subcommittee of the American Academy of Neurology. Neurology 1990;40:1332–1336.

American Academy of Neurology: Training guidelines for the use of botulinum toxin for the treatment of neurologic disorders: Report of the Therapeutics and Technology Assessment Subcommittee of the American Academy of Neurology. Neurology 1994;44(12):2401–2403.

American Academy of Ophthalmology: Botulinum toxin therapy of eye muscle disorders: Safety and effectiveness. Ophthalmology 1989;96(2):37–41.

American Academy of Otolaryngology: Position statement on the clinical usefulness of botulinum toxin in the treatment of spasmodic dysphonia. Arch Otolaryngol Head Neck Surg Bull 1990;9:8.

Andrew J, Fowler CJ, Harrison MJG: Stereotaxic thalamotomy in 55 cases of dystonia. Brain 1983;106:981–1000.

Aoki KR, Merlino G, Spanoyannis AF, Wheeler LA: BOTOX (Botulinum Toxin Type A) Purified Neurotoxin Complex prepared from the new bulk toxin retains the same preclinical efficacy as the original but with reduced antigenicity. Neurology 1999;52(suppl 2):A521–522.

Aramideh M, Ongerboer de Visser BW, Koelman JHTM, Speelman JD: Motor persistence of orbicularis oculi muscle in eyelid-opening disorders. Neurology 1995;45:897–902.

Arezzo JC, Litwak MS, Caputo FA, et al: Spread of paralysis to nearby and distant noninjected muscles in a monkey hand model: Comparison of BoNT-B and BoNT-A. In Brin MF, Hallett M, Jankovic J (eds): Scientific and Therapeutic Aspects of Botulinum Toxin. Philadelphia, Lippincott Williams & Wilkins, 2002, pp 123–134.

Asanuma K, Ma Y, Okulski J, et al: Decreased striatal D2 receptor binding in non-manifesting carriers of the DYT1 dystonia mutation. Neurology 2005;64(2):347–349.

Balash Y, Giladi N: Efficacy of pharmacological treatment of dystonia: Evidence-based review including meta-analysis of the effect of botulinum toxin and other cure options. Eur J Neurol 2004;11:361–370.

Bardutzky J, Tronnier V, Schwab S, Meinck HM: Intrathecal baclofen for stiff-person syndrome: Life-threatening intermittent catheter leakage. Neurology 2003;60:1976–1978.

Benecke R, Jost WH, Kanovsky P, et al: A new botulinum toxin type A free of complexing proteins for treatment of cervical dystonia. Neurology 2005;64:1949–1951.

Ben-Shlomo Y, Camfield L, Warner T: What are the determinants of quality of life in people with cervical dystonia? J Neurol Neurosurg Psychiatry 2002;72:608–614.

Bereznai B, Steude U, Seelos K, Botzel K: Chronic high-frequency globus pallidus internus stimulation in different types of dystonia: A clinical, video, and MRI report of six patients presenting with segmental, cervical, and generalized dystonia. Mov Disord 2002;17:138–144.

Berg D, Becker G, Naumann M, Reiners K: Morphine in tardive and idiopathic dystonia. J Neural Transm 2001;108:1035–1041.

Berke GS, Blackwell KE, Gerratt BR, et al: Selective laryngeal adductor denervation-reinnervation: A new surgical treatment for adductor spasmodic dysphonia. Ann Otol Rhinol Laryngology 1999;108:227–237.

Bertrand CM, Molina-Negro P: Selective peripheral denervation in 111 cases of spasmodic torticollis: Rationale and results. In Fahn S, Marsden CD, Calne DB (eds): Dystonia: Advances in Neurology, vol 50. New York, Raven Press, 1988, pp 637–643.

Bhatia KP, Marsden CD, Thomas DGT: Posteroventral pallidotomy can ameliorate attacks of paroxysmal dystonia induced by exercise. J Neurol Neurosurgy Psychiatry 1998;65:604–615.

Blackie JD, Lees AJ: Botulinum toxin treatment in spasmodic torticollis. J Neurol Neurosurg Psychiatry 1990;53:640–643.

Blitzer A, Brin MF, Fahn S, Lovelace RE: The use of botulinum toxin for the treatment of focal laryngeal dystonia (spastic dysphonia). Laryngoscope 1988;98:193–197.

Blitzer A, Brin MF: Laryngeal dystonia: A series with botulinum toxin therapy. Ann Otol Rhinol Laryngol 1991;100:85–90.

Blitzer A, Brin MF, Greene PE, Fahn S: Botulinum toxin injection for the treatment of oromandibular dystonia. Ann Otol Rhinol Laryngol 1989;98:93–97.

Blitzer A, Zalvan C, Gonzalez-Yanez O, Brin MF: Botulinum toxin type A injections for the management of the hyperfunctional larynx. In Brin MF, Hallett M, Jankovic J (eds):. Scientific and Therapeutic Aspects of Botulinum Toxin. Philadelphia, Lippincott Williams & Wilkins, 2002, pp 207–216.

Borodic GE, Ferrante R, Pearce LB, Smith K: Histologic assessment of dose-related diffusion and muscle fiber response after therapeutic botulinum A toxin injections. Mov Disord 1994;9:31–39.

Borodic GE, Pearce LB, Smith K, Joseph M: Botulinum A toxin for spasmodic torticollis: Multiple vs single injection points per muscle. Head Neck 1992;14:33–37.

Brans JWM, Lindeboom R, Snoek JW, et al: Botulinum toxin versus trihexyphenidyl in cervical dystonia: A prospective, randomized, double-blind controlled trial. Neurology 1996;46:1066–1072.

Brashear A, Bergan K, Wojcieszek J, et al: Patients' perception of stopping or continuing treatment of cervical dystonia with botulinum toxin type A. Mov Disord 2000;15:150–153.

Brashear A, Lew MF, Dykstra DD, et al: Safety and efficacy of NeuroBloc (botulinum toxin type B) in type A-responsive cervical dystonia. Neurology 1999;53:1439–1446.

Brin MF: Treatment of Dystonia. In Jankovic J, Tolosa E (eds): Parkinson's Disease and Movement Disorders, 3rd ed. Baltimore, Williams & Wilkins, 1998, pp 553–578.

Brin MF, Blitzer A, Fahn S, Gould W, Lovelace RE. Adductor laryngeal dystonia (spastic dysphonia): Treatment with local injections of Botulinum toxin (Botox). Mov Disord 1989;4:287-296.

Brin MF, Blitzer A, Stewart C: Laryngeal dystonia (spasmodic dysphonia) observations of 901 patients and treatment with botulinum toxin. Adv Neurol 1998;78:1–10.

Brin MF, Blitzer A, Stewart C, Fahn S: Treatment of spasmodic dysphonia (laryngeal dystonia) with local injections of botulinum toxin: Review and technical aspects. In Blitzer A, Brin MF, Sasaki CT, et al. (eds): Neurologic Disorders of the Larynx. New York, Thieme Medical Publishers, 1992, pp 214–228.

Brin MF, Fahn S, Moskowitz C, et al: Localized injections of botulinum toxin for the treatment of focal dystonia and hemifacial spasm. Mov Disord 1987:2:237–254.

Brin MF, Hallett M, Jankovic J (eds): Scientific and Therapeutic Aspects of Botulinum Toxin. Philadelphia, Lippincott Williams & Wilkins, 2002.

Brin MF, Lew MF, Adler CH, et al: Safety and efficacy of NeuroBloc (botulinum toxin type B) in type A-resistant cervical dystonia. Neurology 1999;53:1431–1438.

Brin MF, Stewart C, Blitzer A, et al: Laryngeal botulinum toxin injections for disabling stuttering in adults. Neurology 1994;44:2262–2266.

Buchman AS, Comella CL, Stebbins GT, et al: Determining a dose-effect curve for botulinum toxin in the sternocleidomastoid muscle in cervical dystonia. Clin Neuropharmacol 1994;17:188–193.

Burke RE, Fahn S, Marsden CD: Torsion dystonia: A double-blind, prospective trial of high-dosage trihexyphenidyl. Neurology 1986;36:160–164.

Burke RE, Fahn S, Marsden CD, et al: Validity and reliability of a rating scale for the primary torsion dystonias. Neurology 1985a; 35:73–77.

Burke RE, Reches A, Traub MM, et al: Tetrabenazine induces acute dystonic reactions. Ann Neurol 1985b;17:200–202.

Butler C, Campbell S, AACPDM Treatment Outcomes Committee Review Panel: Evidence of the effects of intrathecal baclofen for spastic and dystonic cerebral palsy. Dev Med Child Neurol 2000;42:634–645.

Byl NN, McKenzie A: Treatment effectiveness for patients with a history of repetitive hand use and focal hand dystonia: A planned, prospective follow-up study. J Hand Ther 2000;13:289–301.

Byl NN, Nagajaran S, McKenzie AL: Effect of sensory discrimination training on structure and function in patients with focal hand dystonia: A case series. Arch Phys Med Rehab 2003;84:1505–1514.

Cakmur R, Ozturk V, Uzunel F, et al: Comparison of preseptal and pretarsal injections of botulinum toxin in the treatment of blepharospasm and hemifacial spasm. J Neurol 2002;249:64–68.

Candia V, Elbert T, Altenmüller E, et al: Constraint-induced movement therapy for focal hand dystonia in musicians. Lancet 1999;53:42.

Cano SJ, Warner TT, Linacre JM, et al: Capturing the true burden of dystonia on patients: The Cervical Dystonia Impact Profile (CDIP-58). Neurology 2004;63:1629–1633.

Cardoso F, Jankovic J, Grossman R, Hamilton W: Outcome after stereotactic thalamotomy for dystonia and hemiballismus. Neurosurgery 1995;36:501–508.

Ceballos-Baumann AO, Passingham RE, Warner T, et al: Overactive prefrontal and underactive motor cortical areas in idiopathic dystonia. Ann Neurol 1995;37:363–372.

Chapman KL, Bartley GB, Waller RR, Hodge DO: Follow-up of patients with essential blepharospasm who underwent eyelid protractor myectomy at the Mayo Clinic from 1980 through 1995. Ophthal Plast Reconstr Surg 1999;15:106–110.

Chen R, Karp BI, Goldstein SR, et al: Effect of muscle activity immediately after botulinum toxin injection for writer's cramp. Mov Disord 1999;14:307–312.

Cole R, Hallett M, Cohen LG: Double-blind trial of botulinum toxin for treatment of focal hand dystonia. Mov Disord 1995;10:466–471.

Collins A, Jankovic J: Botulinum toxin injection for congenital muscular torticollis presenting in children and adults. Neurology 2006;67:1083–1085.

Comella CL, Buchman AS, Tanner CM, et al: Botulinum toxin injection for spasmodic torticollis: Increased magnitude of benefit with electromyographic asssistance. Neurology 1992;42:878–882.

Comella CL, Jankovic J, Shannon KM, et al: Comparison of botulinum toxin serotypes A and B for the treatment of cervical dystonia. Neurology 2005;65:1423–1429.

Comella CL, Leurgans S, Wuu J, et al: Rating scales for dystonia: A multicenter assessment. Mov Disord 2003;18:303–312.

Comella CL, Stebbins GT, Goetz CG, et al: Teaching tape for the motor section of the Toronto Western Spasmodic Torticollis Scale. Mov Disord 1997;12:570–575.

Comella Cl, Tanner CM, DeFoor-Hill L, Smith C: Dysphagia after botulinum toxin injections for spasmodic torticollis. Clinical and radiologic findings. Neurology 1992;42:1307–1310.

Consky ES, Lang AE: Clinical assessments of patients with cervical dystonia. In Jankovic J, Hallett M (eds): Therapy with botulinum toxin. New York, Marcel Dekker, 1994, pp 211–237.

Cooper IS: Clinical and physiologic implications of thalamic surgery for disorders of sensory communication. II: Intention tremor, dystonia, Wilson's disease and torticollis. J Neurol Sci 1965; 2:520–533.

Cooper IS: 20-year followup study of the neurosurgical treatment of dystonia musculorum deformans. In Eldridge R., Fahn S (eds): Dystonia. Advances in Neurology, vol 14. New York, Raven Press, 1976, pp 423–452.

Cordivari C, Misra P, Catania S, Lees AJ: Treatment of dystonic clenched fist with botulinum toxin. Mov Disord 2001;16:907–913.

Coubes P, Cif L, El Fertit H, et al: Electrical stimulation of the globus pallidus internus in patients with primary generalized dystonia: Long-term results. J Neurosurg 2004;101:189–194.

Coubes P, Roubertie A, Vayssiere N, et al: Treatment of DYT1-generalised dystonia by stimulation of the internal globus pallidus. Lancet 2000;355:2220–2221.

Courey MS, Garrett CG, Billante CR, et al: Outcomes assessment following treatment of spasmodic dysphonia with botulinum toxin. Ann Otol Rhinol Laryngol 2000;109:819–822.

Dalvi A, Fahn S, Ford B: Intrathecal baclofen in the treatment of dystonic storm. Mov Disord 1998;13:611–612.

Davis DH, Ahlskog JE, Litchy WJ, Root LM: Selective peripheral denervation for torticollis: Preliminary results. Mayo Clin Proc 1991;66:365–371.

de Paiva A, Meunier FA, Molgó J, et al: Functional repair of motor endplates after botulinum neurotoxin A poisoning: Bi-phasic switch of synaptic activity between nerve sprouts and their parent terminals. Proc Natl Acad Sci U S A 1999;96:3200–3205.

Dedo HH, Izdebski K: Intermediate results of 306 recurrent laryngeal nerve sections for spastic dysphonia. Laryngoscope 1983; 93:9–15.

Demirkiran M, Jankovic J: Paroxysmal dyskinesias: Clinical features and classification. Ann Neurol 1995;38:571–579.

Diamond A, Shahed J, Azher S, et al: Globus pallidus deep brain stimulation in dystonia. Mov Disord 2006;21:692–695.

Dong M, Yeh F, Tepp WH, et al: SV2 is the protein receptor for botulinum neurotoxin A. Science 2006;312:592–596.

Dressler D, Oeljeschlager R-O, Ruther E: Severe tardive dystonia: Treatment with continuous intrathecal baclofen administration. Mov Disord 1997;12:585–587.

Dressnandt J, Conrad B: Lasting reduction of severe spasticity after ending chronic treatment with intrathecal baclofen. J Neurol Neurosurg Psychiatry 1996;60:168–173.

Dubinsky RM, Gray CS, Vetere-Overfield B, Koller WC: Electromyographic guidance of botulinum toxin treatment in cervical dystonia. Clin Neuropharmacol 1991;14:262–267.

Eidelberg D, Moeller JR, Ishikawa T, et al: The metabolic topography of idiopathic torsion dystonia. Brain 1995;118:1473–1484.

Elston JS: Botulinum toxin for blepharospasm. In Jankovic J, Hallett M (eds): Therapy with Botulinum Toxin. New York, Marcel Dekker, 1994, pp 191–198.

Eltahawy HA, Saint-Cyr J, Giladi N, et al: Primary dystonia is more responsive than secondary dystonia to pallidal interventions: Outcome after pallidotomy or pallidal deep brain stimulation. Neurosurgery 2004;54:613–619.

Emerson J: Botulinum toxin for spasmodic torticollis in a patient with myasthenia gravis. Mov Disord 1994;9:367.

Fahn S: High dosage anticholinergic therapy in dystonia. Neurology 1983;33:1255–1261.

Fahn S: Paroxysmal dyskinesias. In Marsden CD, Fahn S (eds): Movement Disorders 3. Oxford, Butterworth-Heinemann, 1994, pp 310–345.

Fahn S, Henning WA, Bressman S, et al: Long-term usefulness of baclofen in the treatment of essential blepharospasm. Adv Ophthalm Plast Reconstr Surg 1985a;4:219–226.

Fahn S, List T, Moskowitz C, et al: Double-blind controlled study of botulinum toxin for blepharospasm. Neurology 1985b;35(suppl 1): 271–272.

Figgitt DP, Noble S: Botulinum toxin B: A review of its therapeutic potential in the management of cervical dystonia. Drugs 2002; 62:705–755.

Filion M, Tremblay L: Abnormal spontaneous activity of globus pallidus neurons in monkeys with MPTP-induced parkinsonism. Brain Res 1991;547:142–151.

Filippi GM, Errico P, Samtarelli R, et al: Botulinum A toxin effects on rat jaw muscle spindles. Acta Otolaryngol (Stockh) 1993;113:400–404.

Foote KD, Sanchez JC, Okun MS: Staged deep brain stimulation for refractory craniofacial dystonia with blepharospasm: Case report and physiology. Neurosurgery 2005;56(2):E415.

Ford B, Greene P, Louis ED, et al: Use of intrathecal balcofen in the treatment of patients with dystonia. Arch Neurol 1996;53:1241–1246.

Ford B, Greene PE, Louis ED, et al: Intrathecal baclofen in the treatment of dystonia. Adv Neurol 1998a;78:199–210.

Ford B, Louis ED, Greene P, Fahn S: Outcome of selective ramisectomy for botulinum toxin resistant torticollis. J Neurol Neurosurg Psychiatry 1998b;65:472–478.

Ford CN, Bless DM, Lowery JD: Indirect laryngoscopic approach for injection of botulinum toxin in spasmodic dysphonia. Otolaryngol Head Neck Surg 1990;103:752–758.

Forget R, Tozlovanu V, Iancu A, Boghen D: Botulinum toxin improves lid opening in blepharospasm-associated apraxia of lid opening. Neurology 2002;58:1843–1846.

Furukawa Y, Nygaard TG, Gutlich M, et al: Striatal biopterin and tyrosine hydroxylase protein reduction in dopa-responsive dystonia. Neurology 1999;53:1032–1041.

Garner CG, Straube A, Witt TN, et al: Time course effects of local injections of botulinum toxin. Mov Disord 1993;8:33–37.

Gelb DJ, Yoshimura DM, Olney RK, et al: Change in pattern of muscle activity following botulinum toxin injections for torticollis. Ann Neurol 1991;29:370–376.

Goetz CG, Penn RD, Tanner CM: Efficacy of cervical cord stimulation in dystonia. In Fahn S, Marsden CD, Calne DB (eds): Dystonia: Advances in Neurology, vol 50. New York, Raven Press, 1988, pp 645–649.

Gonzalez-Alegre P, Miller VM, Davidson BL, Paulson HL: Toward therapy for DYT1 dystonia: Allele-specific silencing of mutant TorsinA. Ann Neurol 2003;53:781–787.

Greene P: Baclofen in the treatment of dystonia. Clin Neuropharmacol 1992;15:276–288.

Greene P: Medical and surgical therapy of idiopathic torsion dystonia. In Kurlan R (ed): Treatment of Movement Disorders. Philadelphia, J B Lippincott, 1995, pp 153–181.

Greene PE, Fahn S: Baclofen in the treatment of idiopathic dystonia in children. Mov Disord 1992a;7:48–52.

Greene P, Fahn S: Treatment of torticollis with injections of botulinum toxin type F in patients with antibodies to botulinum toxin type A. Mov Disord 1992b;7(suppl 1):134.

Greene P, Fahn S, Diamond B: Development of resistance to botulinum toxin type A in patients with torticollis. Mov Disord 1994;9:213–217.

Greene P, Kang U, Fahn S, et al: Double-blind, placebo controlled trial of botulinum toxin injection for the treatment of spasmodic torticollis. Neurology 1990;40:1213–1218.

Greene P, Shale H, Fahn S: Analysis of open-label trials in torsion dystonia using high dosage of anticholinergics and other drugs. Mov Disord 1988;3:46–60.

Grossman RG, Hamilton WJ: Surgery for movement disorders. In Jankovic J, Tolosa E (eds): Parkinson's Disease and Movement Disorders, 2nd ed. Baltimore, Williams & Wilkins, 1993, pp 531–548.

Hall TA, McGwin G Jr, Searcey K, et al: Health-related quality of life and psychosocial characteristics of patients with benign essential blepharospasm. Arch Ophthalmol 2006;124:116–119.

Hallett M: Is dystonia a sensory disorder? Ann Neurol 1995;38:139–140.

Hanna PA, Jankovic J: Mouse bioassay versus Western blot assay for botulinum toxin antibodies: Correlation with clinical response. Neurology 1998;50:1624–1629.

Hanna PA, Jankovic J, Vincent A: Comparison of mouse bioassay and immunoprecipitation assay for botulinum toxin antibodies. J Neurol Neurosurg Psychiatry 1999;66:612–616.

Hanson MA, Stevens RC: Structural view of botulinum neurotoxin in numerous functional states. In Brin MF, Hallett M, Jankovic J (eds): Scientific and Therapeutic Aspects of Botulinum Toxin. Philadelphia, Lippincott Williams & Wilkins, 2002, pp 11–28.

Harwood G, Hierons R, Fletcher NA, Marsden CD: Lessons from a remarkable family with dopa-responsive dystonia. J Neurol Neurosurg Psychiatry 1994;57:460–463.

Hoon AH Jr, Freese PO, Reinhardt EM, et al: Age-dependent effects of trihexyphenidyl in extrapyramidal cerebral palsy. Pediatr Neurol 2001;25:55–58.

Hou JG, Ondo W, Jankovic J: Intrathecal baclofen for dystonia. Mov Disord 2001;16:1201–1202.

Hsiung GY, Das SK, Ranawaya R, et al: Long-term efficacy of botulinum toxin A in treatment of various movement disorders over a 10-year period. Mov Disord 2002;17(9):1288–1293.

Ichinose H, Ohye T, Takahi E, et al: Hereditary progressive dystonia with marked diurnal fluctuation caused by mutations in the GTP cyclohydrolase I gene. Nat Genet 1994;8:236–242.

Ishikawa A, Miyatake T: A family with hereditary juvenile dystonia-parkinsonism. Mov Disord 1995;10:482–488.

Jabbari B, Scherokman B, Gunderson CH, et al: Treatment of movement disorders with trihexyphenidyl. Mov Disord 1989;4:202–212.

Jankovic J: Botulinum toxin in the treatment of dystonic tics. Mov Disord 1994;9:347–349.

Jankovic J: Apraxia of eyelid opening [Letter to the editor]. Mov Disord 1995a;10:686–687.

Jankovic J: Tardive syndromes and other drug-induced movement disorders. Clin Neuropharmacol 1995b;18:197–214.

Jankovic J: Pretarsal injection of botulinum toxin for blepharospasm and apraxia of eyelid opening. J Neurol Neurosurg Psychiatry 1996;60:704.

Jankovic J: Treatment of dystonia. In Watts RL, Koller WC (eds): Movement Disorders: Neurologic Principles and Practice. New York, McGraw Hill, 1997, pp 443–454.

Jankovic J: Re-emergence of surgery for dystonia [Editorial Commentary]. J Neurol Neurosurg Psychiatry 1998;65:434.

Jankovic J: Can peripheral trauma induce dystonia and other movement disorders? Yes! Mov Disord 2001a;16:7–12.

Jankovic J: Needle EMG guidance is rarely required. Muscle Nerve 2001b;24:1568–1570.

Jankovic J: Botulinum toxin: Clinical implications of antigenicity and immunoresistance. In Brin MF, Hallett M, Jankovic J (eds): Scientific and Therapeutic Aspects of Botulinum Toxin. Philadelphia, Lippincott Williams & Wilkins, 2002, pp 409–416.

Jankovic J: Botulinum toxin in clinical practice. J Neurol Neurosurg Psychiatry 2004a;75:951–957.

Jankovic J: Dystonia: Medical therapy and botulinum toxin. In Fahn S, Hallett M, DeLong DR (eds): Dystonia 4. Advances in Neurology, vol 94. Philadelphia, Lippincott Williams & Wilkins, 2004b, pp 275–286.

Jankovic J: Treatment of cervical dystonia with botulinum toxin. Mov Disord 2004c;19(suppl 8):S109–S115.

Jankovic J: Treatment of dystonia. Lancet Neurol 2006;5:864–872.

Jankovic J: Dystonic disorders. In Jankovic J, Tolosa E (eds): Parkinson's Disease and Movement Disorders, 5th ed. Philadelphia, Lippincott Williams & Wilkins, 2007, pp 321–347.

Jankovic J, Beach J: Long-term effects of tetrabenazine in hyperkinetic movement disorders. Neurology 1997;48:358–362.

Jankovic J, Brin MF: Therapeutic uses of botulinum toxin. N Engl J Med 1991;324:1186–1194.

Jankovic J, Brin M: Botulinum toxin: Historical perspective and potential new indications. In Mayer NH, Simpson DM (eds): Spasticity: Etiology, Evaluation, Management and the Role of Botulinum Toxin. New York, WEMOVE, 2002, pp 100–109.

Jankovic J, Brin MF, Comella C: Handbook of botulinum toxin treatment for cervical dystonia. New York, Churchill Livingstone, 1994.

Jankovic J, Esquenazi A, Fehling D, et al: Evidence-based review of patient reported outcomes with botulinum toxin type A. Clin Neuropharmacol 2004;27:234–244.

Jankovic J, Hallett M (eds): Therapy with botulinum toxin. New York, Marcel Dekker, 1994.

Jankovic J, Hamilton W, Grossman RG: Thalamic surgery for movement disorders. In Obeso JA, DeLong M, Ohye C, Marsden CD (eds): Advances in Understanding the Basal Ganglia and New Surgical Approaches for Parkinson's Disease. Advances in Neurology, vol 74. New York, Raven Press, 1997, pp 221–233.

Jankovic J, Hunter C, Atassi MZ: Botulinum toxin type B observational study (BOS). Mov Disord 2005;20(suppl 10):S31.

Jankovic J, Hunter C, Dolimbek BZ, et al: Clinico-immunologic aspects of botulinum toxin type B treatment of cervical dystonia. Neurology 2006;67(12):2233–2235.

Jankovic J, Leder S, Warner D, Schwartz K: Cervical dystonia: Clinical findings and associated movement disorders. Neurology 1991;41:1088–1091.

Jankovic J, Orman J: Botulinum A toxin for cranial-cervical dystonia: A double-blind, placebo-controlled study. Neurology 1987;37:616–623.

Jankovic J, Orman J: Tetrabenazine treatment in dystonia, chorea, tics and other dyskinesias. Neurology 1988;38:391–394.

Jankovic J, Penn A: Severe dystonia and myoglobinuria. Neurology 1982;32:1195–1197.

Jankovic J, Schwartz K: Botulinum toxin injections for cervical dystonia. Neurology 1990;41:277–280.

Jankovic J, Schwartz K: Botulinum toxin treatment of tremors. Neurology 1991a;41:1185–1188.

Jankovic J, Schwartz K: Clinical correlates of response to botulinum toxin injections. Arch Neurol 1991b;48:1253–1256.

Jankovic J, Schwartz K: Longitudinal follow-up of botulinum toxin injections for treatment of blepharospasm and cervical dystonia. Neurology 1993a;43:834–836.

Jankovic J, Schwartz K: The use of botulinum toxin in the treatment of hand dystonias. J Hand Surg 1993b;18A:883–887.

Jankovic J, Schwartz K: Response and immunoresistance to botulinum toxin injections. Neurology 1995;45:1743–1746.

Jankovic J, Schwartz K, Clemence W, et al: A randomized, double-blind, placebo-controlled study to evaluate botulinum toxin type A in essential hand tremor. Mov Disord 1996;11:250–256.

Jankovic J, Schwartz K, Donovan DT: Botulinum toxin treatment of cranial-cervical dystonia, spasmodic dysphonia, other focal dystonias and hemifacial spasm. J Neurol Neurosurg Psychiatry 1990;53:633–639.

Jankovic J, Vuong KD, Ahsan J: Comparison of efficacy and immunogenicity of original versus current botulinum toxin in cervical dystonia. Neurology 2003;60:1186–1188.

Junker J, Oberwittler C, Jackson D, Berger K: Utilization and perceived effectiveness of complementary and alternative medicine in patients with dystonia. Mov Disord 2004;19:158–161.

Kaji R, Kohara N, Katayama M, et al: Muscle afferent block by intramuscular injection of lidocaine for the treatment of writer's cramp. Muscle Nerve 1995a;18:234–235.

Kaji R, Rothwell JC, Katayama M, et al: Tonic vibration reflex and muscle afferent block in writer's cramp. Ann Neurol 1995b;38:155–162.

Karnath H-O, Konczak J, Dichgans J: Effect of prolonged neck muscle vibration on lateral head tilt in severe spasmodic torticollis. J Neurol Neurosurg Psychiatry 2000;69:658–660.

Karp BI, Cole RA, Cohen LG, et al: Long-term botulinum toxin treatment of focal hand dystonia. Neurology 1994;44:70–76.

Karp BI, Goldstein SR, Chen R, et al: An open trial of clozapine for dystonia. Mov Disord 1999;14:652–657.

Kenney C, Jankovic J: Tetrabenazine in the treatment of hyperkinetic movement disorders. Expert Rev Neurotherapeutics 2006;6:7–17.

Krauss JK, Loher TJ, Pohle T, et al: Pallidal deep brain stimulation in patients with cervical dystonia and severe cervical dyskinesias with cervical myelopathy. J Neurol Neurosurg Psychiatry 2002; 72:249–256.

Krauss JK, Toops EG, Jankovic J, Grossman RG: Symptomatic and functional outcome of surgical treatment of cervical dystonia. J Neurol Neurosurg Psychiatry 1997;63:642–648.

Kumar R, Dagher A, Hutchison WD, et al: Globus pallidus deep brain stimulation (DBS) for generalized dystonia: Clinical efficacy and reversal of the abnormal PET activation pattern. Neurology 1999;53:871–874.

Lang AE: Dopamine agonists and antagonists in the treatment of idiopathic dystonia. In Fahn S, Marsden CD, Calne DB (eds): Dystonia: Advances in Neurology, vol 50. New York, Raven Press, 1988, pp 561–570.

Lang AE: Surgical treatment of dystonia. Adv Neurol 1998;78:185–198.

Lenz FA, Martin R, Kwan HC, et al: Thalamic single-unit activity occurring in patients with hemidystonia. Stereotact Funct Neurosurg 1990;55:159–162.

Lenz FA, Suarez JI, Verhagen Metman L, et al: Pallidal activity during dystonia: Somatosensory reorganization and changes with severity. J Neurol Neurosurg Psychiatry 1998;65:767–770.

Lepore V, Defazio G, Acquistapance D, et al: Botulinum A toxin for the so-called apraxia of lid opening. Mov Disord 1995;10:525–526.

Levy CE, Nichols DS, Schmalbrock PM, et al: Functional MRI evidence of cortical reorganization in upper-limb stroke hemiplegia treated with constraint-induced movement therapy. Am J Phys Med Rehabil 2001;80:4–12.

Lew MF, Adomato BT, Duane DD, et al: Botulinum toxin type B: A double-blind, placebo-controlled, safety and efficacy study in cervical dystonia. Neurology 1997;49:701–707.

Lindeboom R, Brans JWM, Aramindeh M, et al: Treatment of cervical dystonia: A comparison of measures for outcome assessment. Mov Disord 1998;13:706–712.

Lindeboom R, de Haan RJ, Brans JWM, Speelman JD: Treatment outcomes in cervical dystonia: A clinimetric study. Mov Disord 1996;11:371–376.

Lozano AM, Kumar R, Gross RE, et al: Globus pallidus internus pallidotomy for generalized dystonia. Mov Disord 1997;12:865–870.

Lucetti C, Nuti A, Gambaccini G, et al: Mexiletine in the treatment of torticollis and generalized dystonia. Clin Neuropharmacol 2000;23:186–189.

Ludlow CL: Treatment of speech and voice disorders with botulinum toxin. JAMA 1990;264:2671–2675.

Mahrhold S, Rummel A, Bigalke H, et al: The synaptic vesicle protein 2C mediates the uptake of botulinum neurotoxin A into phrenic nerves. FEBS Lett 2006;580:2011–2014.

Manji H, Howard RS, Miller DH, et al: Status dystonicus: The syndrome and its management. Brain 1998;121:243–252.

Marsden CD, Marion M-H, Quinn N: The treatment of severe dystonia in children and adults. J Neurol Neurosurg Psychiatry 1984; 47:1166-1173.

Massey JM: EMG-Guided chemodenervation with phenol in cervical dystonia (spasmodic torticollis). In Brin MF, Hallett M, Jankovic J (eds): Scientific and Therapeutic Aspects of Botulinum Toxin. Philadelphia, Lippincott Williams & Wilkins, 2002, pp 459–462.

Mejia NI, Vuong KD, Jankovic J: Long-term botulinum toxin efficacy, safety and immunogenicity. Mov Disord 2005;20:592–597.

Melling J, Hambleton P, Shone CC: Clostridium botulinum toxins: Nature and preparation for clinical use. Eye 1998;2:16–23.

Merello M, Garcia H, Nogues M, Leiguarda R: Masticatory muscle spasm in a non-Japanese patient with Satoyoshi syndrome successfully treated with botulinum toxin. Mov Disord 1994;9:104–105.

Mezaki T, Kaji R, Hamano T, et al: Optimisation of botulinum treatment for cervical and axial dystonias: Experience with Japanese type A toxin. J Neurol Neurosurg Psychiatry 1994;57:1535–1537.

Mezaki T, Kaji R, Kohara N, et al: Comparison of therapeutic efficacies of type A and F botulinum toxins for blepharospasm: A double-blind, controlled study. Neurology 1995;45:506–508.

Misura KMS, Scheller RH, Weis WI: Three-dimensional structure of the neuronal-Sec1-syntaxin 1a complex. Nature 2000;404:355–362.

Mitchel IJ, Luquin R, Boyce S: Neural mechanisms of dystonia: Evidence from a 2-deoxyglucose uptake study in a primate model of dopamine agonist-induced dystonia. Mov Disorder 1990;5:49–54.

Molloy FM, Shill HA, Kaelin-Lang A, Karp BI: Accuracy of muscle localization without EMG: Implications of limb dystonia. Neurology 2002;58:805–807.

Muellbacher W, Richards C, Ziemann U, et al: Improving hand function in chronic stroke. Arch Neurol 2002;59:1278–1282.

Muller J, Wissel J, Kemmler G, et al: Craniocervical dystonia questionnaire (CDQ-24): Development and validation of a disease-specific quality of life instrument. J Neurol Neurosurg Psychiatry 2004;75:749–753.

Münchau A, Mathen D, Cox T, et al: Unilateral lesions of the globus pallidus: Report of four patients presenting with focal or segmental dystonia. J Neurol Neurosurg Psychiatry 2000;69:494–498.

Narayan RK, Loubser PG, Jankovic J, et al: Intrathecal baclofen for intractable axial dystonia. Neurology 1991;41:1141–1142.

Naumann M, Jankovic J: Safety of botulinum toxin type A: A systematic review and meta-analysis. Curr Med Res Opin 2004;20:981–990.

Nygaard TG, Marsden CD, Fahn S: Dopa-responsive dystonia: Long-term treatment response and prognosis. Neurology 1991;41:174–181.

Ohara S, Hayashi R, Momoi H, et al: Mexiletine in the treatment of spasmodic torticollis. Mov Disord 1998;13:934–940.

Ondo WG, Desaloms JM, Jankovic J, Grossman R: Surgical pallidotomy for the treatment of generalized dystonia. Mov Disord 1998;13:693–698.

Ondo WG, Desaloms JM, Jankovic J, Grossman RG: Pallidotomy and thalamotomy for dystonia. In Krauss JK, Jankovic J, Grossman RG (eds): Surgery for Parkinson's Disease and Movement Disorders. Philadelphia, Lippincott Williams & Wilkins, 2001, pp 299–306.

Pacchetti C, Albani G, Martignoni E, et al: "Off" painful dystonia in Parkinson's disease treated with botulinum toxin. Mov Disord 1995;10:333–336.

Penn RD, Gianino JM, York MM: Intrathecal baclofen for motor disorders. Mov Disord 1995;10:675–677.

Perlmutter JS, Stambuk MK, Markham J, et al: Decreased [$^{18}$F]spiperone binding in putamen in idiopathic focal dystonia. J Neurosci 1997;17:843–850.

Poewe W, Schlosky L, Kleedorfer B, et al: Treatment of spasmodic torticollis with local injections of botulinum toxin. J Neurol 1992;239:21–25.

Pozos RS, Iaizo PA: Effects of topical anesthesia on essential tremor. Electromyogr Clin Neurophysiol 1992;32:369–372.

Priori A, Berardelli A, Mercuri B, Mafredi M: Physiological effects produced by botulinum toxin treatment of upper limb dystonia: Changes in reciprocal inhibition between forearm muscles. Brain 1995;118:801–807.

Priori A, Bertolasi L, Pesenti A, et al: Gamma-hydroxyburinic acid for alcohol-sensitive myoclonus in dystonia. Neurology 2000;54:1706.

Priori A, Pesenti A, Cappellari A, et al: Limb immobilization for the treatment of focal occupational dystonia. Neurology 2001;57:405–409.

Pullman SL, Greene P, Fahn S, Pederson SF: Approach to the treatment of limb disorders with botulinum toxin. Arch Neurol 1996;53:617–624.

Quirk JA, Sheean GL, Marsden CD, Lees AJ: Treatment of nonoccupational limb and trunk dystonia with botulinum toxin. Mov Disord 1996;11:377–383.

Rajput AH, Gibb WRG, Zhong XH, et al: DOPA-responsive dystonia: Pathological and biochemical observations in a case. Ann Neurol 1994;35:396–402.

Ranawaya R, Lang A: Usefulness of a writing device in writer's cramp. Neurology 1991;41:1136–1138.

Reimer J, Gilg K, Karow A, et al: Health-related quality of life in blepharospasm or hemifacial spasm. Acta Neurol Scand 2005;111:64–70.

Rivest J, Lees AJ, Marsden CD: Writer's cramp: Treatment with botulinum toxin injections. Mov Disord 1990;6:55–59.

Roggenkamper P, Jost WH, Bihari K, et al for the NT 201 Blepharospasm Study Team: Efficacy and safety of a new Botulinum Toxin Type A free of complexing proteins in the treatment of blepharospasm. J Neural Transm 2006;113:303–312.

Ruiz PJG, Bernardos VS: Intramuscular phenol injection for severe cervical dystonia. J Neurol 2000;247146–147.

Sanghera M, Grossman RG, Kalhorn CG, et al: Basal ganglia neuronal discharge in primary and secondary dystonia in patients undergoing pallidotomy. Neurosurgery 2003;52:1358–1373.

Sankhla C, Jankovic J, Duane D: Variability of the immunologic and clinical response in dystonic patients immunoresistant to botulinum toxin injections. Mov Disord 1998;13:150–154.

Schantz EJ, Johnson EA: Properties and use of botulinum toxin and other microbial neurotoxins in medicine. Microbiol Rev 1992;56:80–99.

Schneider SA, Mohire MD, Trender-Gerhard I, et al: Familial dopa-responsive cervical dystonia. Neurology 2006;66:599–601.

Schuele S, Jabusch HC, Lederman RJ, Altenmuller E: Botulinum toxin injections in the treatment of musician's dystonia. Neurology 2005;64:341–343.

Sheean GL, Lees AJ: Botulinum toxin F in the treatment of torticollis clinically resistant to botulinum toxin A. J Neurol Neurosurg Psychiatry 1995;59:601–607.

Siebner HR, Tormos JM, Ceballos-Baumann AO, et al: Low-frequency repetitive transcranial magnetic stimulation of the motor cortex in writer's cramp. Neurology 1999;52:529–537.

Sloop RR, Cole BA, Escutin RO: Human response to botulinum toxin injection: Type B compared with type A. Neurology 1997;49:189–194.

Steinberger D, Korinthenber R, Topka H, et al: Dopa-responsive dystonia: Mutation analysis of GCH1 and analysis of therapeutic doses of L-dopa. Neurology 2000;55:1735–1737.

Svetel M, Kozic D, Stefanoval E, et al: Dystonia in Wilson's disease. Mov Disord 2001;16:719–723.

Tan E-K, Jankovic J: Botulinum toxin A in patients with oromandibular dystonia: Long-term follow-up. Neurology 1999;53:2102–2105.

Tan E-K, Jankovic J: Treating severe bruxism with botulinum toxin. J Am Dent Assoc 2000;131:211–216.

Tanaka H, Endo K, Tsuji S, et al: The gene for hereditary progressive dystonia with marked diurnal fluctuation maps to chromosome 14q. Ann Neurol 1995;37:405–408.

Tas N, Karatas K, Sepici V: Hand orthosis as a writing aid in writer's cramp. Mov Disord 2001;16:1185–1189.

Tasker RR, Doorly T, Yamashiro K: Thalamotomy in generalized dystonia. In Fahn S, Marsden CD, Calne DB (eds): Dystonia 2: Advances in Neurology, vol 50. New York, Raven Press, 1988, pp 615–631.

Taub E, Morris DM: Constraint-induced movement therapy to enhance recovery after stroke. Curr Atheroscler Rep 2001;3:279–286.

Taub E, Uswatte G, Elbert T: New treatments in neurorehabilitation founded on basic research. Nat Rev Neurosci 2002;3:226–236.

Taub E, Uswatte G, Pidikiti R: Constraint-induced movement therapy: A new family of techniques with broad application to physical rehabilitation—A clinical review. J Rehabil Res Dev 1999;36:237–251.

Taylor AE, Lang AE, Saint-Cyr JA, et al: Cognitive processes in idiopathic dystonia treated with high-dose anticholinergic therapy: Implications for treatment strategies. Clin Neuropharmacol 1991;14:62–77.

Thant ZS, Tan EK: Emerging therapeutic applications of botulinum toxin. Med Sci Monit 2003;9:40–48.

Tinazzi M, Farina S, Bhatia K, et al: TENS for the treatment of writer's cramp dystonia: A randomized, placebo-controlled study. Neurology 2005;64:1946–1948.

Tintner R, Gross R, Winzer UF, et al: Autonomic function after botulinum toxin type A or B: A double-blind, randomized trial. Neurology 2005;65:765–767.

Tintner R, Jankovic J: Botulinum toxin for the treatment of cervical dystonia. Expert Opin Pharmacother 2001a;2:1985–1994.

Tintner R, Jankovic J: Focal dystonia: The role of botulinum toxin. Curr Neurol Neurosci 2001b;1:337–345.

Treves T, Korczyn AD: Progressive dystonia and paraparesis in cerebral palsy. Eur Neurol 1986;25:148–153.

Tronnier VM, Fogel W: Pallidal stimulation for generalized dystonia: Report of three cases. J Neurosurg 2000;92:453–456.

Trottenberg T, Volkmann J, Deuschl G, et al: Treatment of severe tardive dystonia with pallidal deep brain stimulation. Neurology 2005;64:344–346.

Trugman JM, Leadbetter R, Zalis M, et al: Treatment of severe axial tardive dystonia with clozapine: Case report and hypothesis. Mov Disord 1994;9:441–446.

Truong D, Duane DD, Jankovic J, et al: Efficacy and safety of botulinum type A toxin (Dysport) in cervical dystonia: Results of the first US randomized, double-blind, placebo-controlled study. Mov Disord 2005;20:783–791.

Truong DD, Sandromi P, van der Noort S, Matsumoto RR: Diphenhydramine is effective in the treatment of idiopathic dystonia. Arch Neurol 1995;52:405–407.

Tsui JKC, Bhatt M, Calne S, Calne DB: Botulinum toxin in treatment of writer's cramp: A double-blind study. Neurology 1993;43:183–185.

Tsui JKC, Hayward M, Mak EKM, Schulzer M: Botulinum toxin type B in the treatment of cervical dystonia: A pilot study. Neurology 1995;45:2109–2110.

Vaamonde J, Narbona J, Weiser R, et al: Dystonic storms: A practical management problem. Clin Neuropharmacol 1994;17:344–347.

van Hilten BJ, van de Beek WJ, Hoff JI, et al: Intrathecal baclofen for the treatment of dystonia in patients with reflex sympathetic dystrophy. N Engl J Med 2000;343:625–630.

van Hilten JJ, Hoff JI, Thang MC, et al: Clinimetric issues of screening for responsiveness to intrathecal baclofen in dystonia. J Neural Transm 1999;106931–106941.

Vercueil L, Pollak P, Fraix V, et al: Deep brain stimulation in the treatment of severe dystonia. J Neurol 2001;248:695–700.

Vidailhet M, Vercueil L, Houeto JL, et al: French Stimulation du Pallidum Interne dans la Dystonie (SPIDY) Study Group. Bilateral deep-brain stimulation of the globus pallidus in primary generalized dystonia. N Engl J Med 2005;352:459–467.

Vitek JL, Chockkan V, Zhang J-Y, et al: Neuronal activity in the basal ganglia in patients with generalized dystonia and hemiballism. Ann Neurol 1999;46:22–35.

Vitek JL, Zhang J, Evatt M, et al: GPi pallidotomy for dystonia: Clinical outcome and neuronal activity. In Fahn S, Marsden CD, DeLong DR (eds): Dystonia 3: Advances in Neurology, vol 78. Philadelphia, Lippincott-Raven, 1998, pp 211–219.

Walker RH, Danisi FO, Swope DM, et al: Intrathecal baclofen for dystonia: Benefits and complications during six years of experience. Mov Disord 2000;15:1242–1247.

Wan XH, Vuong KD, Jankovic J: Clinical application of botulinum toxin type B in autonomic symptoms. Chin Med Sci J 2005;20:44–47.

Warrick P, Dromey C, Irish JC, et al: Botulinum toxin for essential tremor of the voice with multiple anatomical sites of tremor: A crossover design study of unilateral versus bilateral injection. Laryngoscope 2000;110:1366–1374.

Waterston JA, Swash M, Watkins ES: Idiopathic dystonia and cervical spondylotic myelopathy. J Neurol Neurosurg Psychiatry 1989;52:1424–1426.

Wirtschafter JD: Clinical doxorubicin chemomyectomy: An experimental treatment for benign essential blepharospasm and hemifacial spasm. Ophthalmology1991;98:357–366.

Wissel J, Kabus C, Wenzel R: Botulinum toxin in writer's cramp: Objective response evaluation in 31 patients. J Neurol Neurosurg Psychiatry 1996;61:172–175.

Wolf SL, Blanton S, Baer H, et al: Repetitive task practice: A critical review of constraint-induced movement therapy in stroke. Neurology 2002;8:325–338.

Yoshida K, Kaji R, Kubori T, et al: Muscle afferent block for the treatment of oromandibular dystonia. Mov Disord 1998;13:699–705.

Yoshimura DM, Aminoff MJ, Olney RK: Botulinum toxin therapy for limb dystonias. Neurology 1992;42:627–630.

Yoshor D, Hamilton WJ, Ondo W, et al: Comparison of thalamotomy and pallidotomy for the treatment of dystonia. Neurosurgery 2001;48:818–824.

Zeuner KE, Bara-Jimenez W, Noguchi PS, et al: Sensory training for patients with focal hand dystonia. Ann Neurol 2002;51:593–598.

Zeuner KE, Hallett M: Sensory training as treatment for focal hand dystonia: A 1-year follow-up. Mov Disord 2003;18:1044–1047.

Zuddas A, Cianchetti C: Efficacy of risperidone in idiopathic segmental dystonia. Lancet 1996;347:127–128.

## APPENDIX 14-1

## Patient Organizations

Several organizations, some listed here, are dedicated to educating patients and their families about dystonia. These organizations provide guidance to local support groups, and they are instrumental in increasing public awareness about dystonia. Another major aim is to raise funds to support research dedicated to finding the cause, cure, and new symptomatic treatments for this disorder.

### Dystonia Medical Research Foundation
One East Wacker Drive, Suite 2430
Chicago, IL 60601-1905
Telephone: (312) 755-0198 in Canada (800) 361-8061
Fax: (312) 803-0138
E-mail: dystonia@dystonia-foundation.org
Website: http://www.dystonia-foundation.org/

### National Spasmodic Torticollis Association
9920 Talbert Avenue #233
Fountain Valley, CA 92708
Telephone: 800-HURTFUL
E-mail: nstamail@aol.com
Website: http://www.torticollis.org

### Bachmann-Strauss Dystonia and Parkinson Foundation
One Gustave L. Levy Place, Box 1490
New York, NY 10029
Telephone: (212) 241-5614
Fax: (212) 987-0662
E-mail: Bachmann.Strauss@mssm.edu
Website: http://www.dystonia-parkinsons.org

### Spasmodic Torticollis/Dystonia
P.O. Box 28
Mukwonago, WI 53149
Telephone: 1-888-445-4598
E-mail: info@spasmodictorticollis.org
Website: http://www.spasmodictorticollis.org

### Care4Dystonia
440 East 78th Street
New York, NY 10021
Telephone: 212-249-2808
E-mail: bekadys@aol.com
Website: http://www.care4dystonia.org/

### Benign Essential Blepharospasm Research Foundation
P.O. Box 12468
Beaumont, TX 77726-2468
Telephone: 409-832-0788
Fax: 409-832-0890
E-mail: bebrf@ih2000.net

For further information about movement disorders, contact

### WE MOVE: Worldwide Education and Awareness for Movement Disorders
204 West 84th Street
New York, NY 10024
Telephone: 800-437-6682 (MOV2)
Fax: 212-875-8389
E-mail: jblazer@wemove.org
Website: www.wemove.org

# Chapter 15

# Huntington Disease

George Huntington published his essay "On Chorea" in 1872 (Huntington, 1872). Soon afterward, the eponym *Huntington's chorea* was adapted in the literature to draw attention to chorea (derived from the Latin *choreus*, meaning "dance" and Greek *choros*, meaning "chorus") as the clinical hallmark of this neurodegenerative disorder. However, since many other manifestations of the disease exist and since chorea might not even be present, the term *Huntington disease* (HD) is more appropriate (Penney and Young, 1998; Jankovic and Ashizawa, 2003). Although chorea (known as the dancing mania) has been recognized since the Middle Ages, the origin of the affected families described by Huntington was traced to the early seventeenth century in the village of Bures in southeast England. The inhabitants of this area later migrated to various parts of the world, accounting for the marked variation in the regional prevalence of HD. While the estimated prevalence of HD in the United States is 2 to 10 per 100,000 population (Kokmen et al., 1994), the prevalence in certain regions of the world is as high as 52 per 100,000 (Lake Maracaibo, Venezuela) and 560 per 100,000 (Moray Firth, Scotland) (Harper, 1992). Americo Negrette, a Venezuelan physician, first observed the dancing mania of Maracaibo in the 1950s, and his findings later led to the discovery of the gene locus and gene mutation for HD (Okun and Thommi, 2004). Because many epidemiologic studies were done before the advent of genetic testing, the true prevalence of the HD gene is not known. DNA testing has largely replaced other tests, such as magnetic resonance imaging (MRI) of the brain, in the evaluation of patients with HD.

## CLINICAL ASPECTS

In a study involving 1901 patients with HD, the following were considered the most frequent presenting symptoms, in descending order: chorea, trouble walking, unsteadiness, irritability, depression, clumsiness, speech difficulty, memory loss, dropping of objects, lack of motivation, paranoia, intellectual decline, sleep disturbance, hallucination, weight loss, and sexual problems (Foroud et al., 1999). While hyperkinesia, usually in the form of chorea, is typically present in adult-onset HD, parkinsonism (an akinetic-rigid syndrome) is characteristic of juvenile HD. Besides chorea, other motor symptoms that typically affect patients with HD include dysarthria, dysphagia, aerophagia, postural instability, ataxia, dystonia, bruxism, myoclonus, tics, and tourettism (Vogel et al., 1991; Carella et al., 1993; Thompson et al., 1994; Ashizawa and Jankovic, 1996; Hu and Chaudhuri, 1998; Louis et al., 1999; Tan and Jankovic, 2000; Jankovic and Ashizawa, 2003) (Videos 15-1, 15-2, 15-3, and 15-4). A very characteristic feature of HD is the inability to maintain tongue protru-

sion (Videos 15-5 and 15-6), representing motor impersistence or negative chorea. Hung-up and pendular reflexes are also typically present in patients with HD (see Video 15-6). Some patients can "camouflage" their chorea by incorporating the involuntary movements into semipurposeful activities, so-called parakinesia (Video 15-7). Myoclonus is particularly common in patients with juvenile HD (Video 15-8). and progressive myoclonic epilepsy has been reported as the initial presentation of juvenile HD (Gambardella et al., 2001). Rarely, patients with HD present with tics and other features suggestive of adult-onset Tourette syndrome (Jankovic and Ashizawa, 1995) (Video 15-9).

It is beyond the scope of this chapter to review the differential diagnosis of chorea and HD (which is covered, instead, in Chapter 16), but in addition to HD-like diseases (HDL1, HDL2, and HDL3) and dentatorubral-pallidoluysian atrophy, SCA17 may present as HD-like phenotype (Toyoshima et al., 2004).

The Unified Huntington's Disease Rating Scale (UHDRS) was developed to assess and quantify various clinical features of HD, specifically motor function, cognitive function, behavioral abnormalities, and functional capacity (Huntington Study Group, 1996; Siesling et al., 1998). A shortened version of the UHDRS has been validated (Siesling et al., 1997). In addition, assessment protocol has been developed to evaluate various neurologic and behavioral features in HD patients who are undergoing striatal grafting (CAPIT-HD Committee, 1996). Variability in isometric grip forces while grasping an object has been found to correlate well with UHDRS and progressive motor deficits associated with HD (Reilmann et al., 2001).

In a study of 593 members of a large kindred in Venezuela, generation of fine motor movements and of rapid eye saccades was found to be impaired in about 50% of at-risk individuals (Penney et al., 1990). Since at-risk individuals with these findings were more likely than those without them to develop overt HD within several years, these abnormalities were thought to represent the earliest clinical manifestations of the disease. If the first examination was normal, there was only a 3% risk of developing symptomatic HD within 3 years. HD patients seem to have greater defects in initiating internally than externally generated saccades (Tian et al., 1991). In 215 individuals at risk for HD or recently diagnosed with HD, a high resolution, video-based eye tracking system demonstrated three types of significant abnormalities while performing memory guided and antisaccade tasks: increased error rate, increased saccade latency, and increased variability of saccade latency (Blekher et al., 2006). In another study, initiation deficits of voluntary-guided but not reflexive saccades were found in individuals with preclinical HD (Golding et al., 2006). Using quantitative assessments, Siemers and colleagues (1996) found subtle but significant abnormalities in simple and choice movement time and reaction time in 103 truly presymptomatic carriers of the HD gene. These deficits correlated well with the number of cytosine-adenine-guanine (CAG) trinucleotide repeats (see later). In a follow-up longitudinal study of 43 at-risk individuals, Kirkwood and colleagues (1999) found that the following variables declined more rapidly among the presymptomatic gene carriers ($n = 12$) than among the noncarriers ($n = 31$): psychomotor speed (digit symbol subscale of the Wechsler Adult Intelligence Scale), optokinetic nystagmus, and rapid alternating movements. In the Predict-HD study, 505 at-risk individuals—452 of whom had more than 39 CAG repeats but have not yet met clinical criteria for the diagnosis of HD—the triatum MRI volume decreased from 17.06 cm³ at diagnostic confidence level of 0 (no signs, mean CAG repeat 42.23, mean motor score 1.20) to 14.89 cm³ at diagnostic confidence level of 3 (probable HD, mean CAG repeat number 44.33, mean motor score 16.92), and higher diagnostic confidence rating was associated with poorer cognitive performance (Paulsen et al., 2006).

Besides chorea, the other two components of the HD triad include cognitive decline and various psychiatric symptoms, particularly depression (Litvan et al., 1998; Paulsen et al., 2001a). While some studies (Foroud et al., 1995) showed that cognitive deficits correlated with the number of CAG repeats in asymptomatic carriers of the HD gene, other studies found no correlation between cognitive decline and CAG repeats in symptomatic patients with HD (Zappacosta et al., 1996). The neurobehavioral symptoms typically consist of personality changes, agitation, irritability, anxiety, apathy, social withdrawal, impulsiveness, depression, mania, paranoia, delusions, hostility, hallucinations, psychosis, and various sexual disorders (Fedoroff et al., 1994; Litvan et al., 1998). In a study of 52 patients with HD, Paulsen and colleagues (2001a) found the following neuropsychiatric symptoms in descending order of frequency: dysphoria, agitation, irritability, apathy, anxiety, disinhibition, euphoria, delusions, and hallucinations (Video 15-10).  Behaviors such as agitation, anxiety, and irritability have been related to hyperactivity of the medial and orbitofrontal cortical circuitry (Litvan et al., 1998). This is in contrast to the apathy and hypoactive behaviors that are seen in progressive supranuclear palsy, attributed to a dysfunction in the frontal cortex and associated circuitry. Progressive decline in attention and executive function, consistent with frontostriatal pathology, has been found in early HD (Ho et al., 2003). Criminal behavior, closely linked to the personality changes, depression, and alcohol abuse, has been reported to be more frequent in patients with HD than in nonaffected first-degree relatives (Jensen et al., 1998). Such behavior might be a manifestation of an impulsive disorder as part of disinhibition, seen not only in HD but also in other frontal lobe-basal ganglia disorders, particularly Tourette syndrome (Brower et al., 2001).

Cognitive changes, manifested chiefly by loss of recent memory, poor judgment, and impaired concentration and acquisition, occur in nearly all patients with HD; but some patients with late-onset chorea never develop dementia (Britton et al., 1995). In one study, dementia was found in 66% of 35 HD patients (Pillon et al., 1991). Tasks requiring psychomotor or visuospatial processing, such as skills required by Trail Making B and Stroop Interference Test, are impaired early in the course of the disease and deteriorate at a more rapid rate than memory impairment (Bamford et al., 1995). In addition to deficits in visual and auditory perception,

patients with HD have impaired recognition of emotional facial expression (Sprengelmeyer et al., 1996). The presence of apraxia and other "cortical" features has cast doubt on this classification (Shelton and Knopman, 1991). In one study, ideomotor apraxia was found in three of nine HD patients, and seven of nine made some apraxic errors. It could not be determined whether the apraxia was due to involvement of frontal cortex or to involvement of subcortical structures (Shelton and Knopman, 1991).

Although neurobehavioral symptoms precede motor disturbances in some cases, de Boo and colleagues (1997) showed that motor symptoms are more evident than cognitive symptoms in early stages of HD. Asymptomatic at-risk individuals who are positive for the HD gene or the marker do seem to differ in their cognitive performance from asymptomatic at-risk individuals who are negative for the HD gene or marker (Foroud et al., 1995; Giordani et al., 1995; Lawrence et al., 1998). Most studies have found that neuropsychological tests do not differentiate between presymptomatic individuals who are positive for the HD gene and those who are negative (Strauss and Brandt, 1990; de Boo et al., 1997), but some studies have found that cognitive changes might be the first symptoms of HD (Hahn-Barma et al., 1998). In a longitudinal study by the Huntington Study Group of 260 individuals who were considered to be at risk for HD, Paulsen and colleagues (2001b) found that this group had worse scores on the cognitive section of the UHDRS at baseline, an average of 2 years before the development of motor manifestations of the disease.

About 10% of HD cases have their onset before age 20, but the typical peak age at onset is in the fourth and fifth decades. Young-onset patients usually inherit the disease from their father; older-onset patients are more likely to inherit the gene from their mother. Juvenile HD (onset of symptoms before age 20 years) typically presents with the combination of progressive parkinsonism, dementia, ataxia, and seizures (Table 15-1 and Videos 15-11 and 15-12; see also Video 15-8). In contrast,  adult HD usually presents with the insidious onset of clumsiness and adventitious movements, which might be wrongly attributed to simple nervousness. Bradykinesia is usually evident in patients with the rigid form of HD, but when it coexists with chorea, it might not be fully appreciated on a routine examination (van Vugt et al., 1996; Sanchez-Pernaute et al., 2000). Fast simple wrist flexion movements were found to be

Table 15-1 Huntington disease

| Features | Adult Onset | Juvenile Onset |
|---|---|---|
| Age at onset | 35–40 | <15 |
| Inheritance | AD | AD (usually from the father) |
| Initial features | Personality changes, chorea | Personality changes, rigidity, bradykinesia, dystonia |
| Late features | Dementia, dysarthria, abnormal eye movements, dystonia, rigidity | Dementia, dysarthria, abnormal eye movements, tremor, seizures, ataxia, myoclonus |
| Duration | 15–30 years | 5–20 years |

significantly slower in 17 patients with HD compared to controls (Thompson et al., 1988). While bradykinesia was most pronounced in the rigid-akinetic patients, it was also evident in patients with the typical choreic variety of HD. When bradykinesia predominates, the patients exhibit parkinsonian findings, some of which can be subtle. Using a continuous wrist-worn monitor of motor activity, van Vugt and colleagues (1996) also provided evidence of hypokinesia in patients with HD, particularly when they were treated with neuroleptics. Micrographia may be one manifestation of underlying parkinsonism; when chorea predominates, the handwriting is characterized by macrographia (Phillips et al., 1994). Bradykinesia in HD may be an expression of postsynaptic parkinsonism as a result of involvement of both direct and indirect pathways. This might explain why a reduction in chorea with antidopaminergic drugs rarely improves overall motor functioning and indeed can cause an exacerbation of the motor impairment. In their excellent review, Berardelli and colleagues (1999) argue that "bradykinesia results from degeneration of the basal ganglia output to the supplementary motor areas concerned with the initiation and maintenance of sequential movements" and "may reflect failure of thalamocortical relay of sensory information." Although bradykinesia associated with HD usually does not respond to dopaminergic therapy, late-onset levodopa-responsive HD presenting as parkinsonism has been well documented (Reuter et al., 2000).

In addition to motor, cognitive, and behavioral abnormalities, most patients with HD lose weight during the course of their disease, despite increased appetite. Weight loss is not unique for HD among the neurodegenerative disorders; for example, it is typically seen in patients with Parkinson disease (Jankovic et al., 1992). The pathogenesis of weight loss in HD is unknown, but one study showed that patients with HD have a 14% higher sedentary energy expenditure than that of controls and that this appears to be correlated with the severity of the movement disorder (Pratley et al., 2000). The lower body mass index in HD parallels the weight loss in transgenic mice, suggesting that it represents a clinical expression of the gene abnormality associated with HD (Djousse et al., 2002).

The natural course of HD varies; on the average, duration of illness from onset to death is about 15 years for adult HD, but it is about 4 to 5 years shorter for the juvenile variant. Patients with juvenile onset (<20 years) and with late onset (>50 years) of symptoms have the shortest duration of the disease (Foroud et al., 1999) (Fig. 15-1; see also Videos 15-11 and 15-12). Using the Total Functional Capacity Scale, longitudinal follow-up of patients with HD showed a 0.72 unit/year rate of decline (Marder et al., 2000). Clinical-pathologic studies have demonstrated a strong inverse correlation between the age at onset and the severity of striatal degeneration (Myers et al., 1988). A review of clinical and pathologic data in 163 HD patients showed that patients with juvenile or adolescent onset had much more aggressive progression of the disease than did patients with onset in middle and late life. Analysis of data collected by the Huntington Study Group on 1026 patients with HD, followed for a median of 2.7 years, concluded that the rate of progression was significantly more rapid with a younger age at onset and longer CAG repeats (Mahant et al., 2003). Although chorea and dystonia were not major determinants of disability, chorea was associated with weight loss.

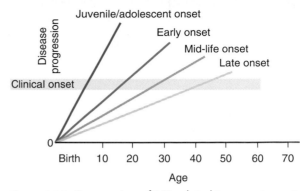

**Figure 15-1** Progression of HD related to age at onset.

Progressive motor dysfunction, dementia, dysphagia, and incontinence eventually lead to institutionalization and death from aspiration, infection, and poor nutrition (Leopold and Kagel, 1985). Among 4809 HD subjects, 3070 of whom had a definite diagnosis of HD, 228 (7.4%) resided in a skilled nursing facility, and these residents had worse chorea, bradykinesia, gait abnormality, and imbalance, as well as more obsessions, compulsions, delusions, and auditory hallucinations, and they were more aggressive and disruptive than their counterparts living at home (Wheelock et al., 2003). Quality of life is markedly affected by HD; the "work" and "alertness behavior" domains of the Sickness Impact Profile are affected the most (Helder et al., 2001).

## NEUROIMAGING

Caudate atrophy, as measured by the ratio of intercaudate to outer-table distances, has traditionally been used as an index of striatal atrophy in HD, and it has been demonstrated to correlate well with the degree of cognitive impairment in early HD (Bamford et al., 1995). Except for atrophy, MRI is unremarkable, although patients with the akinetic-rigid form of HD are more likely to show striatal hyperintensity on T2-weighted MRI than are patients with the choreic form of HD (Oliva et al., 1993). Subsequent studies, however, showed that a reduction in the volume of putamen measured by MRI was a more sensitive index of neurologic dysfunction than was caudate atrophy (Harris et al., 1992; Rosas et al., 2001). This suggests that the putamen is underdeveloped in HD or that it is one of the earliest structures to atrophy. Striatal volume loss correlates with length of CAG repeats (Rosas et al., 2001). Several MRI volumetric and single photon emission computed tomography blood flow studies have shown that basal ganglia volume and blood flow are reduced even before individuals become symptomatic with HD (Harris et al., 1999; Aylward et al., 2004) and that widespread degeneration occurs in early and middle stages of HD (Rosas et al., 2003). Other techniques, such as real-time sonography, showed abnormalities not only in the caudate but also in the substantia nigra of patients with HD (Postert et al., 1999).

In addition to striatal atrophy shown by neuroimaging studies, a variety of techniques, such as positron emission tomography (PET) scans of $^{18}$F-2-fluoro-2-deoxyglucose uptake and single photon emission computerized tomography, have been used to demonstrate hypometabolism and reduced regional cerebral blood flow in the basal ganglia and the cortex (Kuwert et al., 1990; Hasselbach et al., 1992; Harris et al., 1999). Abnormalities in striatal metabolism measured by PET scans may precede caudate atrophy (Grafton et al., 1990). Regional cerebral metabolic rate of glucose consumption has been found to be decreased by 62% in the caudate, 56% in the lenticular nucleus, and 17% in the frontal cortex (Kuwert et al., 1990). Bilateral reduction in the uptake of technetium 99m HM-PAO and iodine 123 IMP in the caudate and putamen has been demonstrated by single photon emission computed tomography in patients with HD (Nagel et al., 1991). Using PET and [$^{11}$C]Flumazenil binding to GABA receptors in the striatum, Künig and colleagues (2000) found marked reduction in the caudate (but not in the putamen) of HD patients compared to normal controls. The authors interpreted these findings as indicative of compensatory GABA receptor upregulation in the striatal (putamen) GABAergic medium spiny neurons projecting to the pallidum. Using voxel-based MRI morphometry to identify differences between presymptomatic carriers and gene-negative controls, Thieben and colleagues (2002) found significant reductions in the gray matter volume in the left striatum, bilateral insula, dorsal midbrain, and bilateral intraparietal sulcus in the gene carriers. None of the imaging studies, however, including PET scans, are sensitive enough to reliably detect evidence of disease in truly presymptomatic individuals. Using a novel statistical method called tensor-based morphometry, Kipps and colleagues (2005) were able to demonstrate progression of gray matter atrophy in presymptomatic HD mutation carriers compared to controls. This suggests that neuroimaging could be used as a surrogate marker in future trials of putative neuroprotective agents.

## NEUROPATHOLOGY AND NEUROCHEMISTRY

Postmortem changes in HD brains include neuronal loss and gliosis in the cortex and the striatum, particularly the caudate nucleus (Box 15-1). Morphometric analysis of the prefrontal cortex in HD patients reveals loss of cortical pyramidal cells, particularly in layers III, V, and VI (Sotrel et al., 1991). Both neuroimaging and postmortem studies indicate that regional thinning of the cortical ribbon, particularly involving the sensorimotor region, is affected in early HD and "might provide a sensitive prospective surrogate marker for clinical trials of neuroprotective medications" (Rosas et al., 2002). Chorea seems to be related to the loss of medium spiny striatal neurons projecting to the lateral pallidum (GPe), whereas rigid-akinetic symptoms correlate with the additional loss of striatal neurons projecting to the substantia nigra compacta (SNc) and medial pallidum (GPi) (Albin, Young, et al., 1990; Albin, 1995). Pathologic studies have suggested that the earliest changes associated with HD consist of degeneration of the striato-SNc neurons followed by striato-GPe and striato-SNr neurons and finally striato-GPi neurons (Hedreen and Folstein, 1995; Albin, 1995) (Fig. 15-2). There appears to be a correlation between the number of CAG repeats and the severity of pathology; longer trinucleotide repeat length is associated with greater neuronal loss in the caudate and puta-

Neuronal loss and gliosis in the cortex and striatum (caudate and putamen)
Early loss of medium-sized, spiny striatal neurons: SNc, GPe, SNr, GPi
Loss of large (17 to 44 μm) striatal interneurons
Loss (<40%) of neurons in SN
Intranuclear inclusions and dystrophic neurons in cortex and striatum

men (Furtado et al., 1996). Increased density of oligodendrogliocytes and intranuclear inclusions were found in the tail of the caudate nucleus among presymptomatic HD gene carriers, suggesting that pathologic changes occur long before the onset of symptoms (Gómez-Tortosa et al., 2001). In addition to neuronal loss in the basal ganglia, there is evidence of increased iron in this brain area as measured by MRI, which in part might contribute to the regional neurotoxicity (Bartzokis et al., 1999).

Using specific monoclonal antibodies against phosphorylated and nonphosphorylated neurofilaments and neuronal cell adhesion molecules, Nihei and Kowall (1992) found marked abnormalities in these cytoskeletal components in the striatal neurons of HD brains. The earliest degenerative changes, the loss of medium-sized spiny neurons containing calbindin, enkephalin, and substance P immunoreactivity, occur in the dorsomedial aspect of the caudate and putamen (Ferrante et al., 1991). The enkephalin neurons appear to die before the substance P neurons. In contrast, the spiny striatal cholinergic and somatostatin-containing interneurons are spared. As a result of these degenerative changes, the matrix zone of the striatum is reduced in size, while the patches (striosomes) remain unaltered. In one postmortem study, however, calbindin D28k mRNA in the striata of HD brains was normal, while the preproenkephalin neurons were markedly reduced in the HD caudate nucleus (Richfield et al., 1995). Another class of medium-sized (8 to 18 μm) striatal

PATHOLOGY OF HD

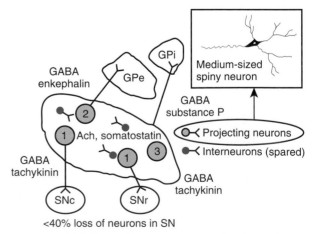

Figure 15-2 Pathologic changes associated with HD from the earliest stages (1) to more advanced stages (3). Ach, acetylcholine; GABA, gamma-aminobutyric acid.

interneurons, characterized by intense immunostaining against calcium-binding protein calretinin, was found to be markedly increased in the striatum of brains of patients with HD compared to controls (Cicchetti and Parent, 1997). In contrast, the density of the larger, 17- to 44-µm, interneurons was markedly decreased. Since both populations of interneurons express calretinin, the implication of the findings of the study is that calretinin, for some yet unknown reason, protects the medium-sized neurons but not the large neurons against HD-related degeneration. The basal ganglia–thalamocortical circuitry, particularly the associative striatum, and its relevance to HD have been reviewed by Joel (2001). Curtis and colleagues (2003) observed an interesting phenomenon in the brains of patients with HD. When they were compared to non-HD control brains, there was marked increase in cell proliferation in the subependymal layer, and the degree of cell proliferation increased with pathologic severity and increasing CAG repeats in the HD gene. These results suggest that progenitor cell proliferation and neurogenesis occur in the diseased adult human brain, providing further evidence for regeneration.

Huntingtin, the product of the HD gene, is expressed throughout the brain in both affected and unaffected regions; therefore, its contribution to neurodegeneration in HD is unclear. Since the mutated huntingtin is not limited to vulnerable neurons, other factors besides mutated huntingtin must play a role in the neuronal degeneration associated with HD (Gourfinkel-An et al., 1997). An immunohistochemical study showed that neuronal staining for huntingtin is reduced in the striatal medium-sized spiny neurons, but the large striatal neurons that are spared in HD retain normal levels of huntingtin (Sapp et al., 1997). Surprisingly, however, huntingtin staining was markedly reduced in both segments of the globus pallidus. This suggests a postsynaptic response to a reduction in striatal inputs; or it might indicate that the globus pallidus is for some yet unknown reason preferentially involved in HD.

The finding of neuronal intranuclear inclusions and dystrophic neurites in the two regions that are most affected in HD, the cortex and striatum, has revolutionized our understanding of the genetic-pathologic mechanisms of this heredodegenerative disorder (DiFiglia et al., 1997). Using an antiserum against the NH$_2$-terminal of huntingtin, DiFiglia and colleagues (1997) found intense labeling localized to neuronal intranuclear inclusions in brains of three juvenile and six adult cases of HD. These inclusions had an average diameter of 7.1 µ and were almost twice as large as the nucleolus. The neurons with these inclusions were found in all cortical layers and the medium-sized neurons of the striatum but not in the globus pallidus or the cerebellum. They were more frequent in juvenile HD, and in these cases, the inclusions were found not only in the nuclei but also in the cytoplasm. The inclusions were not found in the cortex of one subject who had the HD gene but was still asymptomatic but were found in his striatum, thus providing evidence that these changes preceded clinical onset and might be critical in the pathogenesis of the disease. In addition, the investigators found spherical and slightly ovoid dystrophic neurites in cortical layers 5 and 6. None of the control brains demonstrated this finding, and antibodies raised against the internal site of huntingtin failed to differentiate the HD brains from those of controls. Subsequent studies showed that the NH$_2$-terminus

of mutant huntingtin is cleaved by apopain and is ubiquitinated. Thus, ubiquitin staining can also be used to localize these inclusions. These inclusions are composed of granules, straight and tortuous filaments, and fibrils, and they are not membrane bound. Similar inclusions have been demonstrated in the HD transgenic mouse (Davies et al., 1997). Since the aggregates in the nucleus consist mostly of N-terminal fragments of the whole huntingtin protein, it has been postulated that the protein has to be cleaved before it enters the nucleus. Mutant huntingtin fragments accumulate in axon terminals and interfere with glutamate uptake (Li et al., 2000) and, as occurs in other polyglutamine disease, impair axonal transport (Szebenyi et al., 2003; Gunawardena and Goldstein, 2005). The authors suggest that "given the susceptibility of medium spiny striatal neurons to glutamate excitotoxic lesions, the inhibitory effect of mutant huntingtin on vesicular glutamate uptake may contribute to endogenous excitotoxicity in HD." Using a yeast artificial chromosome transgenic mouse model of HD, Tang and colleagues (2005) found that repetitive application of glutamate elevates cytosolic Ca$^{2+}$ levels in medium spiny neurons from the HD mouse but not from the wild-type or control mouse. They further found that the FDA-approved anticoagulant enoxaparin (Lovenox), a calcium blocker, and the mitochondrial Ca$^{2+}$ uniporter blocker Ruthenium 360, are neuroprotective. Thus, abnormal Ca$^{2+}$ signaling seems to be directly linked with the degeneration of medium spiny neurons in the caudate nucleus in HD; therefore, calcium channel blockers could have a therapeutic potential for treatment of HD.

While some studies have shown a moderate (40%) degree of neuronal degeneration in the substantia nigra, particularly noticeable in the medial and lateral thirds (Oyanagi et al., 1989), this is probably not sufficient to cause bradykinesia either in choreic or rigid-akinetic HD patients (Albin, Reiner et al., 1990). Measurements of brain dopamine concentrations and cerebrospinal fluid (CSF) homovanillic acid levels have yielded conflicting results (Box 15-2). In one study, CSF homovanillic acid was normal in 51 patients with early HD, and there was no correlation between homovanillic acid levels and degree of parkinsonism (Kurlan et al., 1988). Dopamine, acetylcholine, and serotonin receptors are decreased in the striatum. Using PET imaging of dihydrotetrabenazine as a marker of striatal vesicular monoamine transporter (VMAT)

**Box 15-2** Huntington disease: Neurotransmitters, peptides, and receptors

↓↓ CAT
↓↓ GABA, GAD
↓↓ enkephalin, substance-P, cholecystokinin, angiotensin, and met-enkephalin
↑ somatostatin, TRH, neurotensin, neuropeptide-Y
↓ Glutamate (↑ CSF glutamate)
   ↑↑ 3-hydroxyanthranilic acid oxidase
DA, GABA, cholinergic-muscarinic, and benzodiazepine receptors
↓↓ NMDA, ↓ phenyclidine and quisqualate receptors

CAT, choline acetyl transferase; DA, dopamine; GABA, gamma-aminobutyric acid; GAD, glutamic acid decarboxylase; NMDA, N-methyl-D-aspartate receptors; TRH, thyroid releasing hormone.

type-2, Bohnen and colleagues (2000) found reduced binding especially in the posterior putamen, similar to Parkinson disease, particularly in patients with akinetic-rigid HD.

Postsynaptic loss of dopamine receptors might be responsible for the parkinsonian findings in some HD patients (Sánchez-Pernaute et al., 2000). Dopamine D2 receptors, imaged with iodobenzamide–single photon emission computed tomography, have provided evidence of D2 receptor loss in HD (Brucke et al., 1991). Using PET to measure binding of specific D1 and D2 receptor ligands in the striatum, Weeks and colleagues (1996) found that these two receptors are markedly decreased in individuals who have the HD mutation but who are still presymptomatic. In another study, Andrews and colleagues (1999) showed that loss of striatal D1 and D2 binding as determined by PET was significantly greater in the known mutation carriers than in the combined at-risk and gene-negative patients. Although some studies found that the loss of D2 receptors correlates significantly with motor and cognitive slowing (Sánchez-Pernaute et al., 2000), other studies failed to show any correlation between clinical and psychological assessments and the loss of striatal D2 receptors (Pavese et al., 2003). Turjanski and colleagues (1995) showed that HD patients with rigidity had more pronounced reduction of these receptors (also measured by PET) compared with HD patients without rigidity. Since D2 binding was normal in a patient with chorea associated with systemic lupus erythematosus, the authors concluded that the presence of chorea is not determined by alterations in striatal dopamine receptor binding.

Loss of the medium-sized spiny neurons, which normally constitute 80% of all striatal neurons, is associated with a marked decrease in GABA and enkephalin levels. After examining two brains of presymptomatic individuals carrying the HD gene, Albin and colleagues (1992) concluded that striatal neurons projecting to the GPe and SN, but not those that project to the GPi, are preferentially involved in early stages of HD and even in the presymptomatic phase. Similarly, cannabinoid receptors are preferentially lost in the GPe (Richfield and Herkenham, 1994). In contrast, the cholinergic and somato-statin striatal interneurons seem to be relatively spared in HD. Other neuropeptide alterations in HD include a decrease in substance-P, cholecystokinin, and met-enkephalin and an increase in somatostatin, thyrotropin-releasing hormone, neurotensin, and neuropeptide Y (see Box 15-2).

## GENETICS AND PATHOGENESIS

For some time, HD has been regarded as truly an autosomal-dominant disease in that homozygotes were thought to be no different from heterozygotes. However, subsequent studies have provided evidence that homozygotes ($n = 8$) have a more severe clinical course than that of heterozygotes ($n = 75$), even though the age at onset is similar (Squitieri et al., 2003). This suggests that the more rapid progression is a consequence of greater toxic effects because of doubling of mutated proteins and aggregate formation (see later). Linkage studies in HD families from various ethnic origins and countries have found that, despite the marked variability in phenotypic expression, genetic heterogeneity is unlikely. Localization of a gene marker near the tip of the short arm of chromosome 4 in 1983 by Gusella and colleagues (1983) initiated an intensive search for the abnormal gene, which was finally cloned 10 years later (Bates et al., 1991; Pritchard et al., 1991; Wexler et al., 1991; Huntington's Disease Collaborative Research Group, 1993). The mutation that is responsible for the disease consists of an unstable enlargement of the CAG repeat sequence (codes for glutamine) in the 5′ end of a large (210 kb) gene called *IT15* (Huntington's Disease Collaborative Research Group, 1993). This gene, located at 4p16.3, contains 67 exons and encodes a previously unknown 348-kDa protein, named huntingtin, without homology to known protein sequences (Fig. 15-3). The expanded CAG repeat, located in exon 1, alters huntingtin by elongating a polyglutamine segment near the $NH_2$-terminus.

The study of HD, the prototype of trinucleotide repeat neurodegenerative diseases, has provided important insights into

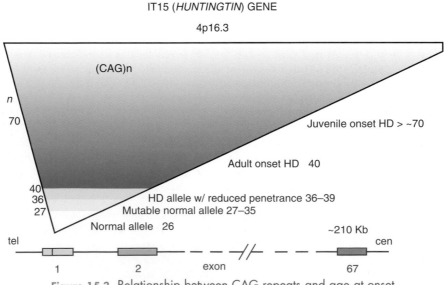

Figure 15-3 Relationship between CAG repeats and age at onset.

the pathogenesis of a growing number of disorders caused by accumulation of misfolded proteins (Everett and Wood, 2004). Whereas the number of repeats varies between 10 and 29 copies in unaffected individuals, the HD gene contains 36 to 121 of such repeats (Kremer et al., 1994). The intermediate-sized CAG repeats range from 30 to 35. Only 1% of patients diagnosed as having HD had a normal CAG repeat length. In the case of a 50-year-old man with typical symptoms of HD since age 43 but without a family history of HD, his maternally derived allele had 17 CAG repeats, but his paternally derived allele had 45 CAG expands. His completely asymptomatic 80-year-old father and 76-year-old paternal uncle had 30 CAG repeats each. This patient indicates that a relatively short expansion (of 30 CAG repeats) might be unstable, particularly if it is of paternal origin, and might spontaneously expand in successive generations resulting in so-called sporadic HD (Alford et al., 1996). Approximately 11% of patients with clinically suspected HD exhibit no family history of HD, and some of these patients might have "new" mutations (Goldberg et al., 1993; Davis et al.,1994). In a study of 28 patients with clinically probable HD, but without a family history of HD, 25 (89%) patients were confirmed by DNA testing to have HD, and 5 of 16 (31%) patients with clinically doubtful HD had expanded triplet repeats, confirming the diagnosis of HD (Davis et al., 1994). There are some alleles that do not cause HD in individuals carrying the allele but become unstable in the next generation. These alleles are termed *intermediate*, and their lower limit of CAG repeats might be as low as 27 (Nance, 1996). Of the 11 cases that lacked the triplet expansion, 5 had a prior history of Sydenham chorea during childhood, indicating the possibility of recurrence of autoimmune chorea.

Several studies have demonstrated that the number of repeats inversely correlates with the age at onset (anticipation) (Duyao et al., 1993; Snell et al., 1993; Ashizawa et al., 1994; Gusella and MacDonald, 1995; Furtado et al., 1996; Brinkman et al., 1997; Nance and the U.S. Huntington Disease Genetic Testing Group, 1997; Maat-Kievit et al., 2002; Marder et al., 2002). Brinkman and colleagues (1997) retrospectively examined the relationship between CAG length and age at onset and found a 50% probability of developing HD symptoms by age 65 when the CAG repeat length is 39 and by age 30 when the CAG repeat length is 50. The inverse relationship between age of onset and number of CAG repeats was confirmed in a Dutch cohort of 755 affected patients (Maat-Kievit et al., 2002). The correlation was stronger for paternal inheritance than for maternal inheritance. CAG repeat length also inversely correlates with late-stage outcomes, such as nursing home admission and placement of percutaneous endoscopic gastrostomy (Marder et al., 2002).

The Huntington Study Group is conducting the Pilot Huntington At Risk Observational Study to prospectively characterize the transition from health to illness (phenoconversion). Although some studies suggest a possible correlation between the length of CAG repeats and the rate of progression (Illarioshkin et al., 1994; Brandt et al., 1996; Antonini et al., 1998), other studies have found no correlation between the CAG repeats and progression (Ashizawa et al., 1994; Kieburtz et al., 1994; Claes et al., 1995) or between age at onset and progression of disease (Feigin et al., 1995). The rate of disease progression is generally faster in paternally transmitted HD independent of the CAG repeat length (Ashizawa et al., 1994). Because of the poor correlation between the number of CAG

repeats and the rate of progression, some investigators have argued that the number of CAG repeats should not be disclosed to the patient or even to the physician. Some practical guidelines follow: (1) The CAG repeat size should be disclosed to appropriately informed physicians and counselors who take care of the patient, (2) appropriate training should be provided to inform physicians and counselors about the implications of the CAG repeat size in HD, and (3) information regarding the CAG repeat size should be disclosed to patients on the patient's request, given that appropriate counseling is made available to the patient (Jankovic et al., 1995). When appropriate genetic counseling and a multidisciplinary approach are used in presymptomatic testing, the risk of adverse events such as psychological distress and depression requiring hospitalization or leading to attempted suicide may be as low as 2% (no difference between carriers and noncarriers) (Goizet et al., 2002).

There is no difference in the mean number of repeats between patients presenting with psychiatric symptoms and those with chorea and other motor disorders, although, as expected, the rigid juvenile patients have the largest number of repeats (MacMillan et al., 1993; Nance and the U.S. Huntington Disease Genetic Testing Group, 1997). The trinucleotide repeat is relatively stable over time in lymphocyte DNA but may be unstable in sperm DNA. This appears to account for the marked increase in the number of trinucleotide repeats to offspring by affected fathers, leading to a 10:1 ratio of juvenile HD when the affected parent is the father. However, after isolating X- and Y-bearing sperm of HD transgenic mice, Kovtun and colleagues (2004) found that the CAG distribution is the same as that in the founding fathers, suggesting that the "gender-dependent changes in CAG repeat length arise in the embryo." Using quantitative in situ hybridization methods, Landwehrmeyer and colleagues (1995) showed that the expression of huntingtin mRNA was not selectively increased in the neurons that were particularly susceptible to degeneration in HD. The authors suggested that this lack of correlation indicates that the gene mutation is not sufficient to produce the disease and that other factors probably also play a role in its pathogenesis.

N-terminal mutant huntingtin also binds to synaptic vesicles and inhibits their glutamate uptake in vitro (Li et al., 2000). Using a transgenic mouse model generated by introducing mutant polyQ tract into one of the mouse genes, Li and colleagues (2000) found aggregated huntingtin only in medium striatal neurons, neurons that are most susceptible to degeneration in HD. These investigators identified a protein, called huntingtin-associated protein (HAP1), that specifically binds to huntingtin. Subsequent studies have demonstrated that HAP1 and huntingtin are anterogradely transported in axons. HAP1 normally interacts with kinesin light chain, a subunit of the kinesin motor complex that drives anterograde transport along microtubules, and it links to transport proteins such as growth factor receptor tyrosine kinase (TrkA) (Rong et al., 2006). However, when mutant huntingtin is present, HAP1 is unable to carry out its trafficking function, leading to degeneration of nerve terminals. Other huntingtin-interacting proteins have been identified, such as glyceraldehyde-3-phosphate dehydrogenase (GAPDH), HAP1, HIP14, apopain, α-adaptin, ubiquitin, calmodulin, and PSD95 (Reddy et al., 1999; Young, 2003; Yanai et al., 2006). The huntingtin protein might also interact with clathrin and adaptor protein-2, which are involved in endocytosis and other proteins (Li and Li, 2004). The long tract of glutamines in mutant HD protein weakens the interaction with huntingtin-associated protein, which is then free to bind the protein Hippi and activate apoptosis through caspase-8 and caspase-3. The latter also cleaves Htt, producing fragments that eventually form intraneuronal inclusions (Gervais et al., 2002). It has been found that wild-type huntingtin partially protects cells against noxious stimuli, and removal of the caspase sites is beneficial for the cells (Young, 2003). Huntingtin has been found to be normally palmitoylated at cysteine 214, which is essential for its trafficking and function, and this process is regulated by the palmitoyl transferase huntingtin interacting protein 14 (HIP14). Expansion of the polyglutamine tract of htt results in reduced interaction between mutant htt and HIP14 and, consequently, in a marked reduction in palmitoylation and increased formation of inclusions and neuronal toxicity (Yanai et al., 2006). These pathologic changes may be partly corrected by overexpression of HIP14.

The aggregated huntingtin was first found in neuronal nucleus and later in synaptic terminals. Scherzinger and colleagues (1999) found that the aggregation of huntingtin protein is time- and concentration-dependent, suggesting "a nucleation-dependent polymerization." Aggregation was proportional to repeat length, and no aggregation could be induced for a repeat length of 27 or fewer glutamines. This might in part explain the inverse correlation of repeat length and age at onset. Since the probability of neural death in HD with time is constant and since the age at onset is inversely dependent on the length of repeats, it has been suggested that the polyglutamine aggregates are toxic when directed to the nucleus and cause the cell death in HD (Yang et al., 2002) (Fig. 15-4). This is supported by the physics of protein aggregation as a result of transition to a new intramolecular configuration (Perutz and Windle, 2001).

Analyzing DNA for the expansion of respective trinucleotide repeats utilizing polymerase chain reaction and Southern blotting has provided means for a reliable diagnostic test that does not require participation of other family members. Such a test is helpful not only in confirming the diagnosis in index cases but also in clarifying the diagnosis in atypical cases and asymptomatic at-risk individuals. In one study, 4 of 15 tests on presymptomatic individuals using linkage analysis were positive for the HD gene (Meissen et al., 1988). While all the individuals with positive results experienced transient symptoms of depression, none reported suicidal ideation. One year after the results of gene testing were disclosed, both increased-risk and the decreased-risk individuals had overall no increase in depression or deterioration in psychological well-being (Wiggins et al., 1992). A high rate of suicidal ideation, however, was found in a Swedish study of 13 HD carriers and 21 noncarriers (Robins Wahlin et al., 2000). In another study of 171 presymptomatic gene carriers compared to 414 noncarriers, Kirkwood and colleagues (2000) found that the carriers performed significantly worse on the digit symbol, picture arrangement, and arithmetic subscales of the Weschler Adult Intelligence Scale–Revised and various movement and choice time measures.

Other studies have addressed the natural history and progression of HD in the early and middle stages (Kirkwood et al., 2001). An adjustment to results of testing appears to depend more on the individual's psychological makeup before the testing than on the testing itself (Meiser and Dunn, 2000). Because of potential psychological and legal implications of positive identification of an HD gene mutation in an asymptomatic, at-risk individual, predictive testing must be performed by a team of clinicians and geneticists who are not only knowledgeable about the disease and the genetic techniques but also sensitive to the psychosocial and ethical issues associated with such testing. Although, as a result of the discovery of the HD gene, the cost of presymptomatic testing has been substantially reduced, the currently recommended extensive pretesting and posttesting counseling is still quite costly. An assessment of the cost-benefit ratio should be carried out. When the DNA test for HD became available, it was thought that demand for testing for HD in asymptomatic at-risk individuals would be high (Tyler et al., 1992), but recent studies have demonstrated a decline in the number of applicants (Maat-Kievit et al., 2000). In one study only 3% to 4% of at-risk individuals have requested a presymptomatic test, and requests for prenatal diagnosis are rare (Lacone et al., 1999).

## HD CELLULAR MECHANISM

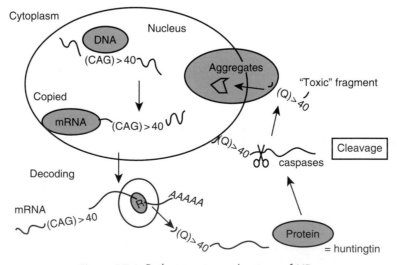

**Figure 15-4** Pathogenetic mechanisms of HD.

Important insights into the potential function of huntingtin have been gained by the study of various mouse models in which the HD homolog gene was inactivated (knockout models) (Duyao et al., 1995) or expanded CAG repeats are introduced into the mouse hypoxanthine phosphoribosyltransferase gene (knock-in models) (Reddy et al., 1999). Homozygous inactivation resulted in embryonic death, suggesting that huntingtin is critical for early embryonic development. Since this model does not mimic adult HD and homozygote individuals apparently are indistinguishable from heterozygotes, it suggests that the HD gene mutation involves "gain" rather than "loss" in function. This hypothesis, however, has been challenged because the earlier studies suggesting no phenotypic difference between heterozygous and homozygous HD were based on linkage studies and focused predominantly on the age at onset (Cattaneo et al., 2001). Furthermore, homozygous transgenic mice expressing mutant huntingtin cDNA have a shorter life span than that of heterozygous mice. This suggests that either a double-dose of mutant huntingtin or loss of the normal allele (loss of function) contributes to the disease. Either wild-type or mutant huntingtin is needed for normal brain development. Huntingtin is associated with vesicle membranes and microtubules and as such probably has a role in endocytosis, intracellular trafficking, and membrane recycling. Thus, HD appears to result from new toxic property of the mutant protein (gain of function) and loss of neuroprotective activity of the normal huntingtin (loss of function) (Cattaneo et al., 2001).

There are currently three types of HD transgenic models: (1) mice expressing fragments, usually one or two exons of the human *huntingtin* gene that contain the polyglutamine expansion (R6/2 and N-171-82Q mice); (2) transgenic mice expressing the full-length human *huntingtin* gene with expanded polyglutamine tract (YAC128 mice); and (3) knock-in mice with pathogenic CAG repeats inserted into the existing CAG expansion (*HdhQIII*) (Hersch and Ferrante, 2004). Interestingly, the more genetically accurate the model, the more variable and subtle is the phenotype. Thus, the fragment models are used more frequently for therapeutic research, and these studies are then confirmed in the full-length models. Full-length huntingtin, when expressed in transgenic mice, does not appear to produce neurologic disease, but only the shortened or truncated form of the protein appears to be toxic to neuronal cells. Except for the mouse model that expresses the full-length huntingtin gene with 72 CAG repeats and that displays selective striatal pathology at 12 months of age (Hodgson et al., 1999), all transgenic-mouse cell lines develop intranuclear inclusions and neurodegeneration in widespread areas of the brain. Using viral-vector mediated expression, several investigators have been able to produce aggregates starting within 5 days after transduction and associated with striatal degeneration in rats and even in primates (Kirik and Bjorklund, 2003). Formation of inclusions correlated with longer CAG expansions and shorter protein fragments. Overexpression of a short fragment of huntingtin, carrying 82 glutamine repeats, in the putamen produced progressive dyskinesia and putaminal intranuclear aggregates and striatal degeneration (Regulier et al., 2003). Although intranuclear inclusions in HD are traditionally thought to be neurotoxic, recent studies provide evidence that they are actually neuroprotective (Arrasate et al., 2004). Using a robotic microscope imaging system that can follow the survival of individual neurons over several days, the authors found that neuronal death was related to the length of polyglutamine expansions in the huntingtin protein, not to the increase in size or number of inclusion bodies. Therefore, this study suggests that the inclusions protect neurons by reducing the levels of toxic diffuse forms of mutant huntingtin. Furthermore, compounds that promote the formation of inclusions lessen the pathology of HD (Bodner et al., 2006).

Although multiple processes have been postulated to relate CAG expansion to neurodegeneration, a growing body of evidence suggests that the expansion leads to dysregulation of the transcription factor cAMP-response element binding protein (CREB)-binding protein (CBP)-mediated gene expression (Nucifora et al., 2001).

Mutant huntingtin has been postulated to cause cell toxicity through various mechanisms, including the formation of inclusions and aggregates and by decreasing transcriptional activation by CBP, a mediator of cell survival signals containing a short polyglutamine stretch (Nucifora et al., 2001; Mantamadiotis et al., 2002). CBP is a coactivator for the transcription factor CREB linking DNA-binding proteins to RNA polymerase II transcription complex and functioning in histone acetyltransferase complex. By recruiting CREB into cellular aggregates, the mutant huntingtin prevents it from participating as a coactivator in CREB-mediated transcription, supporting the toxic gain-of-function mechanism of cell death in HD. The polyglutamine-containing domain of abnormal huntingtin protein directly binds the acetyltransferase domains of CBP and p300/CBP-associated factor (P/CAF) (Steffan et al., 2001). This reduces acetyltransferase activity and decreases acetylation of histones, proteins that package DNA. This in turn results in a decrease in gene transcription. Therefore, histone-deacetylase inhibitors could prevent HD-related neurodegeneration. Indeed, inhibition of histone deacetylase by sodium butyrate has been shown to partially protect HD R6/2 mice from neurodegeneration and against 3-nitropropionic acid neurotoxicity (Ferrante et al., 2003). Transcriptional dysregulation as a pathogenic mechanism of neurodegeneration in HD has also been suggested by the study by Dunah and colleagues (2002), which showed that huntingtin interacts with the transcriptional activator Sp1 and coactivator TAFII130. Sp1, the first of many transcriptional activators isolated from human cells, binds to GC-box on the promoter region of DNA. It contains glutamine-rich activation domains that selectively bind to core components of the transcriptional machinery, such as TAFII13 subunit of TFIID, which contains TATA-box-binding protein and multiple TATA-box-binding protein–associated factors. Therefore, one of the earliest steps in the development of HD may involve deregulation of specific transcriptional programs as suggested by Dunah and colleagues (2002), who demonstrated that mutant huntingtin inhibited Sp1 binding to DNA in postmortem brain tissues of both presymptomatic and affected HD patients. As a result, the RNA polymerase II is not able to locate the dopamine D2 receptor promoter region, and the gene cannot be transcribed (Freiman and Tjian, 2002).

Several transgenic murine models of HD have been developed (Mangiarini et al., 1999). The R6/2 transgenic mouse line has been best studied most extensively (Mangiarini et al., 1999; Ona et al., 1999). These mice develop normally until 5 to 7 weeks of age, when they start manifesting irregular gait, abrupt shuddering movements, and resting tremors, followed by epileptic seizures, muscle wasting, and premature death at 14 to 16 weeks. Striatal neurons show ubiquitinated neuronal inclusions, similar to those seen in the brains of patients with HD. Analysis of glutamate receptors in symptomatic 12-week-old R6/2 mice revealed decreases compared with age-matched littermate controls (Cha et al., 1998). Other neurotransmitter receptors that are known to be affected in HD were also decreased in R6/2 mice, including dopamine and muscarinic cholinergic, but not gamma-aminobutyric acid (GABA) receptors. D1-like and D2-like dopamine receptor binding was drastically reduced to one third of control in the brains of 8- and 12-week-old R6/2 mice. Altered expression of neurotransmitter receptors precedes clinical symptoms in R6/2 mice and may contribute to subsequent pathology. Biochemical analysis at 12 weeks shows a marked reduction in striatal aconitase (Tabrizi et al., 2000), indicative of damage by superoxide ($O_2^{\cdot}$) and peroxynitrite ($ONOO^-$), similar to human HD (Tabrizi et al., 1999). In addition, the R6/2 transgenic mouse has a marked reduction in striatal and cortical mitochondrial complex IV activity and increased immunostaining for inducible nitric oxide synthase and nitrotyrosine (Tabrizi et al., 2000). Since these changes occur before evidence of neuronal death, the described findings suggest that mitochondrial dysfunction and free radical damage play an important role in the pathogenesis of HD. Indeed, mutant huntingtin has been found to attach to the outer mitochondrial membrane, causing the mitochondria permeability transition pores to open, allowing an influx of calcium and releasing cytochrome c (Choo et al., 2004). N171 mice, in which the transgene is driven by the prion promoter, have been used also as models of HD, but they have not been subjected to as rigorous examination as have the R6/2 mice. In another study, mice in which the PGC-1a gene had been knocked out developed brain lesions in the striatum, and PGC-1a levels in those particular neurons were much lower among mice with the HD mutation than in normal mice (Cui et al., 2006). Since PGC1a is involved in energy metabolism, this study shows that transcriptional repression of PGC-1a leads to mitochondrial dysfunction and supports other studies that suggest that energy deficits contribute to neurodegeneration in HD. In addition to the mouse models, there are several Drosophila models (Zoghbi and Botas, 2002). These are now being utilized for testing drugs that might have a potential for favorably modifying the disease (Agrawal et al., 2005).

It has been postulated that the common theme linking all the diseases pathogenetically with polyglutamine-tract expansion is that the various proteins (e.g., huntingtin, atrophin, androgen receptor, and ataxins), as a result of an increase in size of their intrinsic polyglutamine sequences, accumulate in the nucleus, forming insoluble amyloid-like fibrils and then somehow interfere with normal cellular metabolism (Davies et al., 1998). Proteolytic cleavage of a glutathione-S-transferase-huntingtin fusion protein results in spontaneous formation of insoluble aggregates. The aggregate formation is directly related to huntingtin and polyglutamine length; a polyglutamine tract of 51 glutamines or longer result in these aggregates (Scherzinger et al., 1997; Martindale et al., 1998). It has been hypothesized that after the expanded CAG repeat in the HD gene is transcribed in the huntingtin mRNA and then translated as an expanded polyglutamine tract in huntingtin, the mutated protein is cleaved (e.g., by caspase,

apopain). This, the earliest step in the pathogenesis of HD, is followed by the liberation of polyglutamine-containing fragments, which are linked by transglutaminase to other proteins containing lysine residues, resulting in formation of perinuclear aggregates, eventually leading to neuronal apoptosis (Bates, 2003). The formation of inclusions, however, is not required for the initiation of cell death; in fact, neuronal intranuclear inclusions might have a protective role (Saudou et al., 1998). Kuemmerle and colleagues (1999) found that aggregate formation occurs predominantly in spared striatal interneurons rather than in the spiny neurons that are typically affected in HD. Thus, huntingtin aggregates do not predict neuronal death and might actually protect against polyglutamine-induced neurotoxicity. Several lines of evidence suggest that the expanded polyglutamine fragment of mutant huntingtin decreases protein degradation by the proteasome (Martin, 1999; Bence et al., 2001). The protein aggregates appear to be simultaneously inhibitors of the ubiquitin-proteasome system and the products that result from its inhibition. Arfaptin 2 has been shown to promote huntingtin protein aggregation, possibly by impairing proteasome function (Peters et al., 2002). Aggregating proteins besides huntingtin, including α-synuclein, tau, mutant SOD1, and mutant ubiquitin, inhibit proteasome function (Cookson, 2004). In addition to the brain, proteasomal dysfunction has been demonstrated in the skin fibroblasts of patients with HD (Seo et al., 2004). In the striatum, however, dysfunction of the proteasomal system correlated with neuronal pathology and decreased levels of brain-derived neurotrophic factor (BDNF), which is normally upregulated by wild-type huntingtin; decreased mitochondrial complex II/III activity; and increased levels of ubiquitin (Seo et al., 2004).

The impairment of proteasomal degradation of mutant huntingtin leads to caspase-mediated apoptosis (Jana et al., 2001). Jana and colleagues (2001), for example, found "massive accumulation" of polyubiquitinated mutant, but not normal, huntingtin after 2 days of expression in mouse neural cells, indicating lack of proteasomal processing of the mutant protein. Decline of proteasomal activity with time in the soluble fraction of the cell and an increase in the insoluble portion correlated with increased accumulation of proteasomal components in cell aggregates. The expression of mutant huntingtin (or inhibition of proteasomes with lactacystin) was associated with activation of caspases and release of mitochondrial cytochrome c, indicators of apoptosis. Studies have demonstrated that wild-type huntingtin upregulates transcription of cortically derived BDNF (Zuccato et al., 2001). Thus, a decrease in BDNF appears to play an important role in the pathology in HD by causing dysfunction of striatal enkephalinergic neurons (Canals et al., 2004). Furthermore, since wild-type huntingtin has been found to transport BDNF, it is not surprising that mutated huntingtin interferes with intracellular transport of this trophic factor (Gauthier et al., 2004). This suggests that as a result of mutated huntingtin in HD, there is insufficient neurotrophic support for striatal neurons and that treatment with BDNF might possibly restore or rescue the damaged striatal neurons. Rapamycin, an antibiotic that acts as a specific inhibitor of mTOR, a kinase that regulates important cellular processes, has been found to attenuate huntingtin accumulation and cell death in cell models of HD, possibly by enhancing the clearance of proteins that abnormally accumulate and aggregate in the cytoplasm (Ravikumar et al., 2004). Therefore, drugs such as rapamycin might play a role also in other neurodegenerative diseases that result from accumulation of unwanted protein aggregates.

Huntingtin also interacts with chaperone proteins that unfold the expanded mutant huntingtin protein, preventing the aggregate formation in a cell culture model (Jana et al., 2001). Studies have shown that processing of polyglutamine-containing proteins by proteases (e.g., caspases) liberates truncated fragments with expanded polyglutamine tracts that can form aggregates through hydrogen bonding or transglutaminase activity and may be toxic to the cell. Abnormalities in proteasome function are associated with altered expression of stress-response proteins or heat shock proteins that function as chaperones. The chaperones normally maintain proteins in an appropriate conformation and denature misfolded proteins (aggregates) (Kobayashi and Sobue, 2001). Overexpression of these chaperone proteins protects cells from toxicity induced by huntingtin with expanded polyglutamines (Jana et al., 2001; Kobayashi and Sobue, 2001). It has been postulated that the mutant huntingtin with an expanded polyglutamine tract, which is resistant to proteasome-mediated protein processing, overloads the proteasome machinery, enhancing the pathogenic effects of mutant huntingtin. Since truncated proteins that contain the expanded polyglutamine tract appear to be more toxic than the full-length protein, blocking proteolytic processing, aggregation, and nuclear uptake might be reasonable therapeutic strategies.

To examine the possible role of caspase-1, a cysteine protease that is important in regulating apoptosis, in the pathogenesis of cell death associated with HD, Ona and colleagues (1999) crossbred R6/2 with a transgenic mouse expressing dominant-negative mutant of caspase-1 in the brain. The inhibition of caspase-1 delayed the disease onset by 7.3 days and prolonged survival by 20.4 days. Furthermore, it significantly delayed the appearance of neuronal inclusions and neurotransmitter alterations. Although abnormal protein aggregation has been postulated to play an important role in the pathogenesis of HD, DiFiglia and colleagues (Kim et al., 1999) showed that aggregation was not intimately involved in cell death. While general inhibitors of caspases prolonged cell life, they did not alter aggregation, whereas specific caspase 3 inhibitors inhibited aggregation but had no effect on survival. Thus, continuous influx of the mutant protein is required to maintain inclusions. To determine whether caspase cleavage of huntingtin is a key event in the selective neurodegeneration in HD, Graham and colleagues (2006) found that mice expressing mutant huntingtin, resistant to cleavage by caspase-6 but not caspase-3, maintained normal neuronal function, did not develop striatal neurodegeneration, and were protected against neurotoxicity induced by multiple stressors, including NMDA, quinolinic acid, and staurosporine. These findings suggest that proteolysis of huntingtin at the caspase-6 cleavage site is critical for neurodegeneration in HD, which is enhanced by excitotoxicity. This and other studies provide strong evidence that caspases are important in the pathogenesis of cell death in HD and other neurodegenerative diseases.

The finding that N-methyl-D-aspartate (NMDA) receptors are markedly reduced in the putamen and cerebral cortex was the first clue that suggested an NMDA-mediated excitotoxicity as a mechanism of neuronal degeneration in HD (Young et al., 1988; Tabrizi et al., 1999). In addition to the 92% reduction in

NMDA binding, phencyclidine binding was reduced by 67% and quisqualate by 55% in the same HD brains. The NMDA receptor density was decreased by 50% in the brain of a presymptomatic HD gene carrier, suggesting that the loss of the excitatory receptors occurred early in the course of the disease (Albin, Young, et al., 1990). In contrast to the study by Young and colleagues (1988), no single excitatory amino acid receptor was selectively affected. Using quantitative in vitro autoradiography, Dure and colleagues (1991) found a 50% to 60% reduction in binding sites of all the major excitatory receptors (NMDA, MK-801, glycine, kainate, and AMPA) in the caudate nucleus of HD brains. Furthermore, as was noted earlier, mutated huntingtin protein might interfere with vesicular glutamate uptake and thus contribute to excitotoxicity (Li et al., 2000).

In support of the excitotoxic theory is the observation that certain excitatory neurotoxins produce useful animal models of HD. Although the activity of 3-hydroxyanthranilic acid oxidase, the synthesizing enzyme for quinolinic acid, is markedly increased in the striatum of HD brains (Schwarcz et al., 1988), the concentration of quinolinic acid, an NMDA agonist, in the CSF and brains of patients with HD is normal (Heyes et al., 1991). Nevertheless, intrastriatal injections of quinolinic acid preferentially damage the medium-sized spiny neurons containing calbindin Dk28, enkephalin, and substance P, the very same neurons that degenerate in HD (Beal, Ferrante, et al., 1991; Ferrante et al., 1993). The striatal patch-matrix pattern closely resembles that seen in HD. Pretreatment with MK-801, a noncompetitive NMDA antagonist, protects the striatum from the quinolinic acid neurotoxicity. Despite neuronal loss and astrogliosis, the axons are spared, which might account for relatively normal dopamine, norepinephrine, and serotonin levels. GABA levels are markedly decreased in the GPe of these animals, similar to HD, indicating early loss of GABA afferents from the striatum to the GPe in both HD and the experimental model. In addition to pathologic and biochemical similarities between this animal model and HD, the animals exhibit choreic movements. In addition to quinolinic acid, another excitotoxin that has been implicated in the pathogenesis of HD is glutamate. The observation that glutamate levels are decreased in the striatum of HD brains has been interpreted to be a result of chronic failure of the normal reuptake mechanism for glutamate released from the corticostriatal afferent terminals (Perry and Hansen, 1990). The resulting increase in concentration of glutamate at synapses might cause damage to the striatal neurons. The increased extracellular glutamate might also explain the finding of increased CSF glutamate in some patients with HD. Additional support for the excitotoxic theory of HD is provided by the observation that a lesion with the excitotoxin ibotenic acid, a glutaric acid agonist, in a striatum of the baboon produces behavioral and neuropathologic changes similar to those seen in patients with HD (Hantraye et al., 1990).

One hypothesis of mechanisms of cell death in HD is that a defect in mitochondrial energy metabolism makes certain neurons more vulnerable to the excitotoxic effects of endogenous glutamate (Beal, 1992). Panov and colleagues (2002) showed that lymphoblast mitochondria from patients with HD and brain mitochondria from transgenic HD mice have a lower membrane potential and depolarize at lower calcium loads than do mitochondria from controls. Since this defect preceded the onset of pathologic or behavioral abnormalities by months, the authors concluded that "mitochondrial calcium abnormalities occur early in HD pathogenesis and may be a direct effect of mutant huntingtin on the organelle." Intrastriatal injections of inhibitors of oxidative phosphorylation, such as aminooxyacetic acid or MPP[+], or a systemic administration of 3-nitropropionic acid (3-NP), a mitochondrial poison, into animals produce even more striking resemblance to HD than when "pure" excitotoxins are used (Beal, Swartz, et al., 1991; Storey et al., 1992; Brouillet et al., 1993; Beal et al., 1993). Studies have shown that 3-NP induces striatal neurodegeneration via c-Jun N-terminal kinase/c-Jun module (Garcia et al., 2002). Accidental ingestion of 3-NP has resulted in putaminal necrosis and delayed onset of dystonia and chorea in humans (Ludolph et al., 1991). The age-dependent neurotoxicity of 3-NP, demonstrated by increased striatal lactate levels in the older animals, appears to be related to the effect of 3-NP on energy metabolism. Severe defects have been demonstrated in the activities particularly of complexes II and III in the caudate nuclei of HD patients (Gu et al., 1996; Tabrizi et al., 1999). Using spectrophotometric techniques, Browne and colleagues (1997) found 29% and 67% reductions in the activity of the complex II to III in the caudate and putamen of HD brains, respectively. In addition, there was a 62% reduction in the complex IV activity. This finding provides further support for the potential role of oxidative damage in the pathogenesis of HD. The possibility that mitochondrial function is impaired in HD is supported by the observation of 5-fold to 11-fold increase in cortical mitochondrial DNA deletion in the brains of HD patients (Horton et al., 1995). Dichloroacetate, which stimulates pyruvate dehydrogenase complex, has been found to increase survival and improve motor function and prevent striatal atrophy in R6/2 and N171-82Q transgenic mouse models of HD (Andreassen et al., 2001).

Defects in mitochondrial oxidative phosphorylation have been postulated to decrease cellular ATP production, resulting in a concomitant decrease in sodium-potassium ATPase activity and partial membrane depolarization. Under normal circumstances, the NMDA receptor-associated channels are blocked by a voltage-dependent $Mg^{2+}$ system that pumps $Mg^{2+}$ out of the cell. As a result of decreased APTase activity, caused by the inhibition of oxidative phosphorylation, the normal resting potential cannot be maintained, resulting in the opening of the channel and influx of calcium. This triggers a cascade of events leading to a production of free radicals and associated oxidative damage to various cellular elements. Thus, as a result of inhibition of oxidative phosphorylation, even low levels of excitatory amino acids become toxic, a process that is referred to as slow excitotoxicity.

It has been suggested that in HD, as a result of prolonged excitatory neurotransmission, certain neurons become "exhausted" and switch from aerobic to anaerobic glycolytic metabolism, leading to the production and accumulation of lactate. Increased lactate concentration in the cerebral cortex of patients and animal models of HD, postulated to be due to global cerebral energy failure, has been demonstrated by proton magnetic resonance spectroscopy (Jenkins et al., 1998). Subsequently 1H magnetic resonance spectroscopy was used to measure N-acetylaspartate, creatine, and choline, and a reduction in these markers correlated well with the progression of the disease and with striatal atrophy (Sánchez-Pernaute et al.,

1999). Administration of agents that improve energy metabolism, such as coenzyme Q10 and nicotinamide, might protect animals against toxicity produced by malonate, a complex II inhibitor (Beal et al., 1994). Using 31P magnetic resonance spectroscopy to measure lactate in the muscle and 1H magnetic resonance spectroscopy to measure lactate in the basal ganglia and the cortex, Koroshetz and colleagues (1997) showed that treatment with coenzyme Q10 was associated with a significant decrease in cortical lactate concentrations in patients with HD. There is, however, no evidence that this biochemical change is in any way associated with clinical improvement or slowing of disease progression. Furthermore, increased lactate could not be confirmed by other studies (Hoang et al., 1998). A National Institutes of Health–sponsored multicenter study designed to evaluate the efficacy of coenzyme Q10 and remacemide, an NMDA antagonist, is currently being conducted by the Huntington Study Group (see later).

The obvious question still to be answered is how the mutation in the HD gene leads to selective damage of certain neuronal populations. One of the most provocative clues to the selective vulnerability of neuronal damage in HD was provided initially by Li and colleagues (1995). These investigators identified a protein, called huntingtin-associated protein, that specifically bound to huntingtin. Huntingtin-associated protein binding is enhanced by expansion of the polyglutamine tract in huntingtin. Other huntingtin-interacting proteins have been identified, such as glyceraldehyde-3-phosphate dehydrogenase, huntingtin-interacting protein, apopain, α-adaptin, ubiquitin, calmodulin, and PSD95 (Reddy et al., 1999; Young, 2003). The huntingtin protein might also interact with clathrin and adaptor protein-2, which are involved in endocytosis and other proteins (Li and Li, 2004). The long tract of glutamines in mutant HD protein weakens the interaction with huntingtin-associated protein, which is then free to bind the protein Hippi and activate apoptosis through caspase-8 and caspase-3. The latter also cleaves Htt, producing fragments that eventually form intraneuronal inclusions (Gervais et al., 2002). Wild-type huntingtin has been found to partially protect cells against noxious stimuli, and removal of the caspase sites is beneficial for the cells (Young, 2003).

The relationship of these proteins to the pathogenesis of HD, however, is still unclear (Paulson and Fischbeck, 1996; Roses, 1996). It is possible that as the huntingtin polyglutamine tract expands and changes its tertiary configuration, it blocks the ATP-dependent import mechanisms for succinate dehydrogenase entry into the mitochondria in the striatum. This might lead to selective, localized energy depletion and pathologic changes that are typically associated with HD. As the expansion increases, the impairment of import mechanism becomes less selective, and the pathology becomes more widespread. Thus, in HD, in addition to the typical involvement of the striatum, the GPe and GPi, SNc, and cerebellum become involved, and the patient manifests additional features, such as rigidity, bradykinesia, and ataxia (Furtado et al., 1996). Morphometric analyses of structural MRI demonstrated marked cerebellar atrophy and white matter loss in patients with HD (Fennema-Notestine et al., 2004). Although activity of glyceraldehyde-3-phosphate dehydrogenase, a huntingtin-binding protein, is normal in the brains of patients with HD, the activity of aconitase, an Fe-S-containing tricarboxylic acid cycle enzyme, is reduced to 8% in the caudate, 27% in the putamen, and 52% in the cerebral cortex

POSSIBLE PATHOGENESIS OF HD

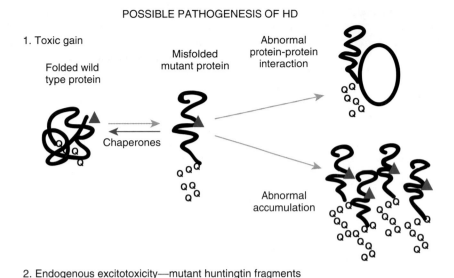

**Figure 15-5** Mechanisms of neurodegeneration in HD.

of HD brains (Tabrizi et al., 1999). Since this enzyme is particularly sensitive to inhibition by peroxynitrite ($ONOO^-$) and superoxide ($O_2^-$), it is considered be a good marker of excitotoxic cell damage.

Huntingtin may also contribute to the apoptotic cell death in HD; it has been found to be cleaved by apopain, an apoptosis-specific cystein protease (Goldberg et al., 1996). It has been postulated that the aggregates of mutant huntingtin (DiFiglia et al., 1997) cannot be properly removed from the cell and therefore might interfere with the metabolic activities of the affected neurons. Since ubiquitin is important in protein degradation and this process requires energy, the cells that are most vulnerable to the accumulation of the ubiquitin-huntingtin aggregates are those whose metabolic function has been already compromised, possibly as a result of toxins that interfere with oxidative phosphorylation. This concept then might link this new finding of region-selective accumulation of huntingtin aggregates and inclusions (DiFiglia et al., 1997) with the theories of regional impairment of energy metabolism (Beal et al., 1994) (Figs. 15-5 and 15-6). More recently, the molecular pathogenesis of HD has been considered to result from a decrease in specific chaperone proteins, such as Hdj1, Hsp70, $\alpha$SGT, and $\beta$SGT, as demonstrated in R6/2 mice (Hay et al., 2004). Antigliadin antibodies have been demonstrated in 44% of patients with HD, but this probably represents an epiphenomenon and a nonspecific finding, as it has also been demonstrated in ataxia and other neurodegenerative disorders (Bushara et al., 2004).

## TREATMENT

HD is one of few neurodegenerative diseases in which the diagnosis can be made long before the onset of clinical symptoms. This offers an opportunity to intervene in the earliest stages of the neurodegenerative cascade, perhaps even before the disease-related cell loss is initiated (Yamamoto et al., 2000). Thus, HD is an excellent model for testing early neuroprotective treatments (Beal and Ferrante, 2004; Leegwater-

Kim and Cha, 2004; Ryu and Ferrante, 2005; Bodner et al., 2006). There is currently no treatment to stop or slow the progression of HD, but experimental therapeutics in transgenic mouse models promise to translate some of the pathogenesis-targeted strategies into clinical trials (Beal and Ferrante, 2004). These models, for example, have been used to demonstrate potential disease-modifying effects of caspase inhibitors (Ona et al., 1999; Chen et al., 2000; Yamamoto et al., 2000). In another study, 2% creatine has been found to increase survival from 97.7 days to 114.6 days, and this was associated with a reduction in the number of huntingtin-positive aggregates in the striatum of transgenic HD mice (Ferrante et al., 2000). In a pilot study, 10 g per day of creatine was well tolerated for 12 months by 13 patients with HD, except for transient nausea and diarrhea in 2 patients (Tabrizi et al., 2003). In a randomized, double-blind, placebo-controlled study of 64 patients with HD, 8 g per day of creatine administered for 16 weeks was well tolerated and was associated with an increase in serum and brain creatine and a reduction in serum 8-hydroxy-2'-deoxyguanosine, an indicator of oxidative injury to DNA (Hersch et al., 2006). In a placebo-controlled trial, using 5 g per day of creatine, Verbessem and colleagues (2003) showed no improvement in functional, neuromuscular, or cognitive status in patients with early to moderate HD. Although weight loss is very common in HD, paradoxically, food restriction (fasting) slows disease progression in transgenic mice (Duan et al., 2004). The same group also showed that paroxetine, a serotonin-uptake inhibitor, improves survival in transgenic mice while preventing weight loss (Duan et al., 2004). Using the R6/1 HD mice, van Dellen and colleagues (2000) showed that the onset of neurologic deficit was significantly delayed if the mice were raised in an enriched and stimulating environment. Furthermore, environmental enrichment delayed the degenerative loss of peristriatal cerebral volume and rescued protein deficits, possibly through rescuing transcription or protein transport problems (Spires et al., 2004). Similarly, environmental stimulation was found to enhance the health and life expectancy in R6/2 mice that were transgenic for exon 1 (Carter et al., 2000). It is therefore possible that occupational

HD PATHOGENESIS

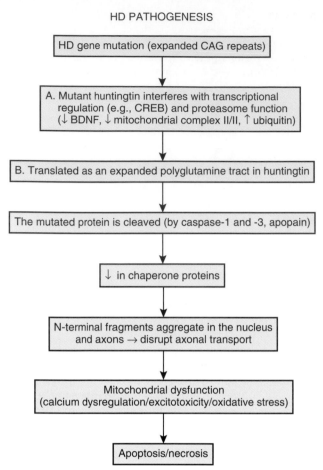

**Figure 15-6** Possible sequence of mechanisms and pathways leading to cell death in HD.

therapy, based on the principle of environmental enrichment, could delay the onset of HD. These findings showing that environmental enrichment slows disease progression in HD mouse models have been confirmed by other studies (Hockly et al., 2002). In support of the role of environment in expression of HD symptoms is the observation of discordance after 7 years in monozygotic twins with HD (Friedman et al., 2005).

Although several agents, such as coenzyme Q10 (CoQ10) and nicotinamide, are being tested in clinical trials to determine whether they exert a neuroprotective effect in humans, only symptomatic treatments have been found to be useful in HD patients at this time. CoQ10 (ubiquinone) carries electrons from complexes I and II to complex II of the mitochondrial electron transport chain (Jankovic and Ashizawa, 2003; Ryu and Ferrante, 2005). As such, it can act as an antioxidant or as a pro-oxidant, depending on the cell's redox potential (Shults and Schapira, 2001). In the pilot study, CoQ10, at doses of 600 and 1200 mg per day, has been found to be well tolerated, although some patients may experience adverse effects, such as headache, heartburn, fatigue, and increased involuntary movements (Feigin et al., 1996). In a multicenter clinical trial conducted by the Huntington Study Group that compared CoQ10 and remacemide, an NMDA ion channel blocker, 347 patients with documented HD were randomized to receive CoQ10 300 mg twice daily, remacemide hydrochloride

200 three times daily, both, or placebo (Huntington Study Group, 2001). The patients were evaluated every 4 to 5 months for 30 months. Although patients who were treated with CoQ10 showed a trend toward slowing in total functional capacity decline (13%), this difference failed to reach statistical significance. Furthermore, CoQ10 was associated with higher frequency of stomach upset, and remacemide treatment was associated with higher frequency of nausea, vomiting, and dizziness. Because of these rather disappointing results, routine use of CoQ10 in patients with HD is not warranted. Similarly, remacemide, although relatively well tolerated at 200 and 600 mg per day (Kieburtz et al., 1996), cannot be recommended for the treatment of HD. In a 6-week open-label trial, another antiglutamatergic drug, riluzole (100 mg per day), was found to be well tolerated and to be associated with a 35% reduction in the chorea rating score (Rosas et al., 1999). The Huntington Study Group (2003) also found that riluzole at 200 mg per day significantly improved chorea scores but without improving functional capacity, and because of abnormalities in liver transaminase, this drug could not be recommended for routine use in HD. The potentially useful role of riluzole in favorably modifying the progression of HD is also supported by studies in animal models of HD (Schiefer et al., 2002). Schiefer and colleagues (2002) were able to significantly increase survival time of R6/2 HD transgenic mice treated with riluzole. Furthermore, they showed that striatal neuronal intranuclear inclusions were less ubiquitinated and were surrounded by ubiquitinated microaggregates in riluzole-treated animals compared to controls. Staining with antibodies directed against the mutated huntingtin revealed no significant difference in this component of neuronal intranuclear inclusions. Minocycline has been shown to delay disease progression in animal models of HD by reducing the production of caspase-1 and caspase-3 and by decreasing inducible nitric oxide synthetase activity (Chen et al., 2000). Minocycline, a second-generation antibiotic with high levels of blood-brain barrier permeability, has been shown to delay disease progression in the mouse model R6/2 of HD, possibly by inhibiting caspase-1 and caspase-3 mRNA upregulation and decreasing inducible nitric oxide synthase. Thirty patients (19 women and 11 men) between the ages of 21 and 66 years with symptomatic and genetically confirmed HD were treated with minocycline at the Baylor College of Medicine Huntington Disease Center for at least 6 months (Thomas et al., 2003). Assessments included the Abnormal Involuntary Movements Scale, the UHDRS, and the Mini-Mental State Examination, performed at baseline and every 2 months throughout the study period. Laboratory studies at baseline and at 2-month intervals included complete blood and platelet counts and renal and liver function tests. In this pilot study, we showed that minocycline was well tolerated over the 6-month observation period, although no significant improvement was observed on any clinical assessment. No changes were noted in any of the laboratory tests. There was no evidence of any adverse interaction between minocycline and any of the concomitant medications. Our findings are similar to those reported by others (Bonelli et al., 2003). Future multicenter trials should focus not only on the long-term tolerability of minocycline but also, more importantly, on its potential disease-modifying effects. Interestingly, paroxetine, a commonly used serotonin reuptake inhibitor, has been found to slow the progression in huntingtin mutant mice (Duan et al., 2004). Ethyl eicosapentaenoate (LAX-101),

another caspase inhibitor, has also been shown to have potential neuroprotective effects in animals and is currently being tested in clinical trials. Early and sustained treatment with essential fatty acids has been demonstrated to protect against motor deficits in R6/1 transgenic mice expressing exon 1 and a portion of intron 2 of the *huntingtin* gene (Clifford et al., 2002).

A growing body of evidence supports the notion that preformed polyglutamine aggregates are highly toxic when directed to the cell nucleus; therefore, recent research has focused on pharmacologic intervention aimed at inhibiting aggregate formation (Bates et al., 2003; Sanchez et al., 2003; Bossy-Wetzel et al., 2004; Hay et al., 2004). One such strategy is to use histone deacetylase inhibitors, such as phenylbutyrate, suberoylanilide hydroxamic acid, and pyroxamide, to arrest polyglutamine-dependent neurodegeneration (Marks et al., 2001; Steffan et al., 2001). In *Drosophila* flies expressing 93Q huntingtin, the histone deacetylase inhibitors suberoylamide hydroxamic acid and sodium butyrate suppressed neuronal degeneration (Steffan et al., 2001; Kazantsev et al., 2002; Agrawal et al., 2005). Suberoylamide hydroxamic acid also ameliorates motor deficits in the R6/2 mouse model of HD (Hockly et al., 2003). Geldanamycin, a benzoquinone ansamycin antibiotic that binds to Hsp90 and activates the stress response, has been found in some in vitro cell culture models of HD to prevent polyQ aggregation, presumably by activating a heat shock response (Sittler et al., 2001). Geldanamycin and radicicol have been found to delay aggregate formation in cell cultures and to increase soluble exon 1 huntingtin at concentrations that are capable of inducing Hsp40 and Hsp70 expression, indicating that chaperone induction favorably changes the biophysical properties of the aggregates (Hay et al., 2004). These drugs do not cross the blood-brain barrier, however, and therefore might not be clinically useful. Intraperitoneal injections of cystamine, an amino acid derivative that competitively inhibits transglutaminase, into transgenic HD mice ameliorated tremor and gait abnormalities and prolonged survival from 92 to 103 days (Karpuj et al., 2002). Keene and colleagues (2002) reported that treatment with tauroursodeoxycholic acid, a hydrophilic bile acid, prevented neuropathology and associated behavioral deficits in the 3-nitropropionic acid rat model of HD and reduced striatal neuropathology in the R6/2 transgenic HD mouse. Inhibition of polyglutamine oligomerization by the azo dye Congo red interferes with the ability of expanded polyglutamine to induce cytotoxic events, thus facilitating the degradation of expanded polyglutamine by making it more accessible to proteasome (Sanchez et al., 2003). Congo red has also been found to inhibit the assembly of protofibrils into fibrils, thus preventing toxicity from mature fibrils (Poirier et al., 2002). Trehalose, a disaccharide composed of two glucose molecules, has been found to alleviate polyglutamine-mediated pathology in the R6/2 transgenic model of HD, including a 30% reduction in brain aggregates (Tanaka et al., 2004). Trehalose, which appears to bind directly to proteins with expanded polyglutamines, is highly soluble and therefore can be administered orally. Since it appears to have no toxicity, the drug is a promising therapeutic agent for various polyglutamine diseases, not just HD. Another strategy to reduce the toxic effects of pathogenic fragment of huntingtin by small ubiquitin-like modifier (SUMO)-1, which at least partially prevents aggregation of huntingtin in vitro (Steffan et al., 2004). However, in a Drosophila model of HD, SUMOylation of huntingtin fragment exacerbates neurode-generation, whereas ubiquitination reduces HD pathology. These findings suggest that SUMO-1 blockers might delay the progression of HD. Some unorthodox attempts are under way to test various putative neuroprotective agents, such as CoQ10, creatine, cystamine, omega-3 fatty acids, trehalose, and blueberry extract (Couzin, 2004).

Transglutaminase inhibitors, such as cystamine and monodansyl cadaverine, reduce aggregate formation and, as such, might be potential therapeutic agents in diseases caused by CAG-repeat expansion (Igarashi et al., 1998). By inhibiting the HD mutant transgene with tetracycline, Yamamoto and colleagues (2000) were able to show that the neurodegeneration can be not only prevented but also reversed. In another report, Chen and colleagues (2000) found that minocycline delays disease progression, possibly by reducing the production of caspase-1 and caspase-3 and by decreasing inducible nitric oxide synthetase activity in R6/2 mice. Preliminary data based on pilot clinical trials suggest that minocycline is well tolerated and that it is not associated with serious adverse events or laboratory test abnormalities (Bonelli et al., 2003; Thomas et al., 2004). In a pilot safety and tolerability study of 30 patients with HD who were given minocycline over a 6-month period, minocycline was found to be well tolerated during this study period, and no serious adverse events were noted (Thomas et al., 2004). Minocycline was also found to be well tolerated in a larger, double-blind, placebo-controlled study of 60 HD patients (Huntington Study Group, 2004). It has also been found to have a potential neuroprotective role in other neurodegenerative disorders (Zemke and Majid, 2004). Smith and colleagues (2003), however, found no effect of minocycline or doxycycline on behavioral abnormalities or huntingtin aggregates in R6/2 mice. Another caspase inhibitor with potential neuroprotective effects, currently being tested in patients with HD, is ethyl eicosapentaenoate (LAX-101 or Miraxion). This pure, highly unsaturated fatty acid, concentrated chiefly in fish oil, has been found to be effective in some pilot trials in HD and schizophrenia. In a small ($n = 24$) double-blind, placebo-controlled study of LAX-101, Vaddadi and colleagues (2002) showed possible improvement in both the orofacial and total components of the UHDRS after 6 months of treatment. LAX-101 is currently undergoing phase 3 clinical trials in the United States and Europe. These important observations, of course, have obvious therapeutic implications and suggest that caspase inhibitors might play a role in the treatment of HD and related neurodegenerative disorders (Friedlander, 2000; Sanchez Mejia and Friedlander, 2001) (Fig.15-7).

Until effective neuroprotective therapy is found, the management of patients with HD will focus primarily on relief of symptoms designed to improve their quality of life. Psychosis, one of the most troublesome symptoms, usually improves with neuroleptics, such as haloperidol, pimozide, fluphenazine, and thioridazine. These drugs, however, can induce tardive dyskinesia and other adverse effects; therefore, they should be used only if absolutely needed to control symptoms. Clozapine (Clozaril), an atypical antipsychotic drug that does not cause tardive dyskinesia, might be a useful alternative to the typical neuroleptics, but its high cost, risk of agranulocytosis, and other potential side effects might limit its use (Bonuccelli et al., 1994). It is likely that the other atypical antipsychotics, such as olanzapine (Zyprexa) (Paleacu et al., 2002) and quetiapine fumarate (Seroquel), will also provide a beneficial effect. Anxiolytics and antidepressants also might be useful in some patients with psychiatric problems. Donepezil,

PATHOGENESIS → THERAPEUTICS

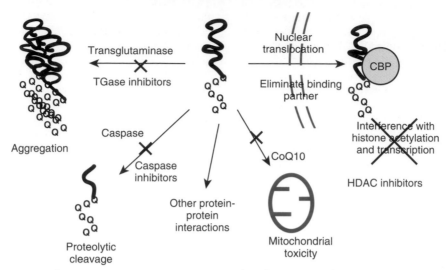

Figure 15-7 Therapeutic strategies in HD targeted to the suspected pathogenic mechanisms.

a procholinergic drug that is used in the treatment of Alzheimer disease, was found to be ineffective in the treatment of cognitive impairment or chorea associated with HD (Fernandez et al., 2000).

One of the most effective drugs in the treatment of hyperkinetic movement disorders, including chorea, is tetrabenazine (TBZ) (Jankovic and Beach, 1997). This drug, currently marketed in several European countries and Canada as either Xenazine 25 or Nitoman, is a potent and selective depletor of dopamine and, to a lesser degree, norepinephrine and serotonin from nerve terminals. The effects of TBZ are largely restricted to the CNS, which differentiates it from another monoamine depletor, reserpine, an old antihypertensive drug that produces both central and peripheral depletion. By inhibiting the brain synaptic VMAT, TBZ impairs uptake of monoamines and serotonin into synaptic vesicles, causing them to remain in the cytoplasm, where they are rapidly degraded by monoamine oxidases. There are two types of VMAT: type 1 (VMAT1) and type 2 (VMAT2), which are coded by two distinct genes, 8p21.3 and 10q25, respectively. In humans, VMAT2 is nearly exclusively expressed in the CNS neurons, whereas VMAT1 is present in the peripheral nerve terminals. TBZ exhibits a 10,000-fold higher affinity for human VMAT2 than for human VMAT1, reversibly binding to the intravesicular part of VMAT2. Reserpine, on the other hand, binds irreversibly to the cytoplasmic site of both VMAT1 (peripheral) and VMAT2 (central). These pharmacologic differences probably account for the absence of hypotension and gastrointestinal side effects with TBZ compared to reserpine. Also, the duration of action is much shorter with TBZ, about 12 hours versus several days. In contrast to reserpine, which depletes all the monoamines and serotonin equally, TBZ preferentially depletes dopamine. Finally, despite early reports of dopamine receptor inhibition, more recent studies suggest that since the affinity of TBZ for the dopamine $D_2$ receptor is 1000-fold lower than its affinity for VMAT2, it is unlikely that the weak DA $D_2$ receptor antagonism is involved in the therapeutic effects of TBZ. This might be one reason why tardive dyskinesia has never been reported to

occur with TBZ, one of the chief advantages of this drug over the neuroleptic, dopamine receptor–blocking, drugs.

Although TBZ can cause or exacerbate depression, sedation, akathisia, and parkinsonism, in our experience it is clearly the most effective and safest antichorea drug (Jankovic and Beach, 1997; Ondo et al., 2002; Kenney et al., 2007a) (Video 15-13). The intermediate-sized CAG repeats range from 29 to 35, but rare cases with CAG repeats in this range develop the full symptomatology of HD. An autopsy-proven case of HD with only 29 CAG repeats has been reported (Kenney et al., 2007b). In one study of 15 patients who were treated for an average of 7 months at a mean dose of TBZ of $68 \pm 27.1$ mg per day (range: 25 to 150 mg per day), a "blinded" rating of videotapes showed improvement in motor scores in 12 (80%), and the mean score improved from $16 \pm 3.6$ to $13 \pm 3.8$ (Ondo et al., 2002). Adverse events included akathisia, insomnia, constipation, depression, drooling, and subjective weakness. Paradoxically, some patients with HD benefit from dopaminergic drugs, particularly when the disease is associated with parkinsonism (Racette and Perlmutter, 1998). In a multicenter, double-blind, placebo-controlled trial of TBZ involving 84 ambulatory patients with HD, TBZ treatment resulted in a reduction of 5.0 units in chorea severity compared with a reduction of 1.5 units on placebo treatment (adjusted mean effect size = $-3.5 \pm 0.8$ UHDRS units [mean ± standard error]; 95% confidence interval: $-5.2, -1.9$; $P < .0001$) (Huntington Study Group, 2006). There was also a significant benefit on ratings of clinical global improvement. There were five study withdrawals in the TBZ group and five serious adverse events in four subjects (drowning suicide, complicated fall, restlessness/suicidal ideation, and breast cancer), compared with one withdrawal and no serious adverse events in the placebo group. This study concluded that TBZ, at adjusted dosages of up to 100 mg per day, was effective for the treatment of chorea in HD and was generally safe and well tolerated.

A novel dopaminergic modulator, OSU6162, has been reported to improve chorea in a patient with HD (Tedroff et al., 1999), but further studies on the pharmacology and clinical efficacy of the drug are needed. Baclofen, a putative GABA agonist, provides neither symptomatic nor protective effects in HD (Shoulson et al., 1989). Whether blocking glutamate release from the presynaptic terminals by drugs such as riluzole or lamotrigine (Brodie, 1992) or whether other antiglutamatergic drugs will be effective in slowing down the otherwise inexorable progression of the disease awaits further studies. In a double-blind, placebo-controlled trial, lamotrigine failed to slow HD progression but was found to improve symptoms and lessen chorea; 54% of patients on lamotrigine reported symptomatic improvement versus 15% of those on placebo, and the chorea subscale measure showed less deterioration for lamotrigine than for placebo (Kremer et al., 1999). Dystonia and bruxism, occasionally present in patients with HD, can be effectively treated with local injections of botulinum toxin (Tan and Jankovic, 2000). Pallidotomy, known to be effective in the treatment of levodopa-induced dyskinesias in patients with Parkinson disease, has been found also useful in the treatment of dystonia associated with HD (Cubo et al., 2000). Bilateral pallidal stimulation at 40 and 130 Hz improved chorea in one patient with HD (Moro et al., 2004).

Since NMDA supersensitivity might be responsible in part for chorea in patients with HD, selective NMDA antagonists might ameliorate this symptom. In a double-blind, controlled trial of 22 patients with HD, amantadine (400 mg per day) reduced extremity chorea by 36% (Verhagen Metman et al., 2002). In addition to symptomatic effect, amantadine might confer a neuroprotective effect. In another randomized placebo-controlled trial, amantadine at 300 mg per day had no effect on HD-associated chorea (O'Suilleabhain and Dewey, 2003). A 2-hour intravenous infusion of amantadine in a double-blind, randomized crossover study showed reduction in dyskinesias scores after both intravenous and oral administration (Lucetti et al., 2003).

Following up on some encouraging results from animal studies, the delivery of trophic factors, such as nerve growth factor and ciliary neutrophic factor by genetically modified cells, into the striatum of patients with HD has become a reachable goal (Kordower et al., 1999; Mittoux et al., 2000; McBride et al., 2004). Implantation of nerve growth factor–producing fibroblasts into the rat striatum appeared to protect these animals against neurotoxic effects of the excitatory amino acids quinolate and quisqualate (Schumacher et al., 1991). Whether intrastriatal implantations of genetically engineered cells designed to produce trophic factors, such as ciliary neutrophic factor (Emerich et al., 1997; Kordower et al., 1999), or fetal cells will be useful in the treatment of HD awaits the results of further animal and clinical studies (Freeman et al., 2000; Bachoud-Levi et al., 2002; Peschanski et al., 2004). The observation that implanted fetal neuronal cells survive in the HD brain and reconstitute damaged neuronal connections suggests that the host HD disease process does not affect the grafted tissue. No change in functional status or hyperkinetic movements was observed in 12 HD patients who were treated with transplantation of fetal porcine striatal cells (St. Hillaire et al., 1998), but in another study (Bachoud-Levi et al., 2000), motor and cognitive improvement was noted in three of five patients after staged grafting of both striatal areas with human fetal neuroblasts. In their subsequent study, the investigators showed that the three patients who received fetal striatal allografts and demonstrated clinical improvement had a reduction of striatal and cortical hypometabolism as measured by F-deoxyglucose PET, whereas

in the two patients who did not show clinical improvement, the striatal and cortical metabolism progressed (Gaura et al., 2004). Hauser and colleagues (2002) reported the results of an uncontrolled pilot study of transplantation of fetal striatal cells into the postcommissural putamen of seven patients with HD. There was no change in the primary outcome variable, the motor component of UHDRS, and three subjects suffered four subdural hemorrhages. Furthermore, the placebo effect, which was the same as the treatment effect (>20% improvement), lasted 18 months. Although the authors conclude that transplantation of human fetal striatal cells is feasible and that "a lack of significant worsening might reflect clinical benefit in a progressive neurodegenerative disease," this study should be viewed as a negative study. It should, however, provide a stimulus for future randomized, blind, and adequately controlled studies (Greenamyre and Shoulson, 2002). Five patients with HD who were followed for up to 6 years were found to improve during the first 2 years, and then their function again deteriorated (Bachoud-Levi et al., 2006). These studies are currently in progress in multiple, chiefly European, countries (Peschanski et al., 2004). In addition, a new initiative, Systemic Evaluation of Treatment for Huntington's Disease, has been developed to systematically evaluate various strategies as potential treatments for HD (http://www.huntingtonproject.org; Walker and Raymond, 2004).

Finally, RNA interference (RNAi) has been suggested as a promising therapeutic strategy, but further work is needed to determine whether this method can suppresses the expression of only the mutated, but not the normal, *huntingtin* (*HTT*) gene (Harper et al., 2005). A listing of available and experimental therapies for HD is provided in Box 15-3.

**Box 15-3** Treatment of Huntington disease

Adequate nutrition
Physical, speech, and occupational therapy
Treat/prevent aspiration, fecal impaction, incontinence
Support: life-planning, disability benefits, household
  help, home equipment, supervised smoking, child
  care, day care, institutional care, hospice
Caregiver support
Anxiolytics: benzodiazepines, propranolol, clonidine
Antidepressants: tricyclics (nortriptyline, amitriptyline,
  imipramine);
SSRIs (fluoxetine, sertraline, fluvoxamine, paroxetine,
  venlafaxine, citalopram)
DA receptor–blocking drugs or DA-depleting drugs for
  severe chorea, psychosis:
    quetiapine, olanzapine, ziprasidone, clozapine,
    fluphenazine, risperidone, haloperidol, tetrabena-
    zine (TBZ)
Glutamate release inhibitors and receptor blockers
  (remacemide, riluzole)
Mitochondrial electron transport enhancers and free
  radical scavengers
(CoQ10, nicotinamide, creatine)
Caspase and iNOS inhibitors (minocycline, ethyl eico-
  sapentaenoate or ethyl-EPA, LAX-101)
Histone deacetylase inhibitors
Trophic factors
Fetal transplants

# References

Agrawal N, Pallos J, Slepko N, et al: Identification of combinatorial drug regimens for treatment of Huntington's disease using Drosophila. Proc Natl Acad Sci U S A 2005;102:3777–3781.

Albin RL: Selective neurodegeneration in Huntington's disease. Ann Neurol 1995;38:835–836.

Albin RL, Reiner A, Anderson KD, et al: Striatal and nigral neuron subpopulations in rigid Huntington's disease: Implications for the functional anatomy of chorea and rigidity-akinesia. Ann Neurol 1990;27:357–365.

Albin RL, Reiner A, Anderson KD, et al: Preferential loss of striato-external pallidal projection neurons in presymptomatic Huntington's disease. Ann Neurol 1992;31:425–430.

Albin RL, Young AB, Penney JB, et al: Abnormalities of striatal projection neurons and N-methyl-D-aspartate receptors in presymptomatic Huntington's disease. N Engl J Med 1990;332:1293–1298.

Alford RL, Ashizawa T, Jankovic J, et al: Molecular detection of new mutations, resolution of ambiguous results and complex genetic counseling issues in Huntington's disease. Am J Med Genet 1996;66:281–286.

Andreassen OA, Ferrante RJ, Huang H-M, et al: Dichloroacetate exerts therapeutic effects in transgenic models of Huntington disease. Ann Neurol 2001;50:112–117.

Andrews TC, Weeks RA, Turjanski N, et al: Huntington's disease progression. PET and clinical observations. Brain 1999;122:2353–2363.

Antonini A, Leenders KL, Eidelberg D: [11C] Raclopride-PET studies of the Huntington's disease rate of progression: Relevance of the trinucleotide repeat length. Ann Neurol 1998;43:253–255.

Arrasate M, Mitra S, Schweitzer ES, et al: Inclusion body formation reduces levels of mutant huntingtin and the risk of neuronal death. Nature 2004;431:805–810.

Ashizawa T, Jankovic J: Cervical dystonia as the initial presentation of Huntington's disease. Mov Disord 1996;11:457–459.

Ashizawa T, Wong L-JC, Richards CS, et al: CAG repeat size and clinical presentation in Huntington's disease. Neurology 1994;44:1137–1143.

Aylward EH, Sparks BF, Field KM, et al: Onset and rate of striatal atrophy in preclinical Huntington disease. Neurology 2004;63:66–72.

Bachoud-Levi A-C, Gaura V, Brugieres P, et al: Effect of fetal neural transplants in patients with Huntington's disease 6 years after surgery: A long-term follow-up study. Lancet Neurol 2006;5:303–309.

Bachoud-Levi A-C, Hantraye P, Peschanski M: Fetal neural grafts for Huntington's disease: A prospective view. Mov Disord 2002;17:439–444.

Bachoud-Levi A-C, Remy P, Nguyen J-P, et al: Motor and cognitive improvements in patients with Huntington's disease after neural transplantation. Lancet 2000;356:1975–1979.

Bamford KA, Caine ED, Kido DK, et al: A prospective evaluation of cognitive decline in early Huntington's disease. Neurology 1995;45:1867–1873.

Bartzokis G, Cummings J, Perlman S, et al: Increased basal ganglia iron levels in Huntington disease. Arch Neurol 1999;56:569–574.

Bates G: Huntingtin aggregation and toxicity in Huntington's disease. Lancet 2003;361:1642–1644.

Bates GP, MacDonald ME, Baxendale S, et al: Defined physical limits of the Huntington disease gene candidate region. Am J Hum Genet 1991;49:7–16.

Beal MF: Does impairment of energy metabolism result in excitotoxic neuronal degeneration in neurodegenerative diseases? Ann Neurol 1992;31:119–130.

Beal MF, Brouillet E, Jenkins BG, et al: Neurochemical and histologic characterization of striatal excitotoxic lesions produced by the mitochondrial toxin 3-nitropropionic acid. J Neurosci 1993;13:4181–4192.

Beal MF, Ferrante RJ: Experimental therapeutics in transgenic mouse models of Huntington's disease. Nat Rev Neurosci 2004;5:373–384.

Beal MF, Ferrante RJ, Swartz KJ, Kowall NW: Chronic quinolinic acid lesions in rats closely resemble Huntington's disease. J Neurosci 1991;11:1649–1659.

Beal MF, Henshaw DR, Jenkins BG, et al: Coenzyme Q10 and nicotinamide block striatal lesions produced by the mitochondrial toxin malonate. Ann Neurol 1994;36:882–888.

Beal MF, Swartz KJ, Hyman BT, et al: Aminooxyacetic acid results in excitotoxin lesions by a novel indirect mechanism. J Neurochemistry 1991;57:1068–1073.

Bence NF, Sampat RM, Kopito RR: Impairment of the ubiquitin-proteasome system by protein aggregation. Science 2001;292:1552–1555.

Berardelli A, Noth J, Thompson PD, et al: Pathophysiology of chorea and bradykinesia in Huntington's disease. Mov Disord 1999;14:398–403.

Blekher T, Johnson SA, Marshall J, et al: Saccades in presymptomatic and early stages of Huntington disease. Neurology 2006;67:394–399.

Bodner RA, Outeiro TF, Altmann S, et al: Pharmacological promotion of inclusion formation: A therapeutic approach for Huntington's and Parkinson's diseases. Proc Natl Acad Sci U S A 2006; 103:4246–4251.

Bohnen NI, Koeppe RA, Meyer P, et al: Decreased striatal monoaminergic terminals in Huntington disease. Neurology 2000;54:1753–1759.

Bonelli RM, Heuberger C, Reisecker F: Minocycline for Huntington's disease: An open label study. Neurology 2003;60:883–884.

Bonuccelli U, Ceravolo R, Maremmani C, et al: Clozapine in Huntington's chorea. Neurology 1994;44:821–823.

Bossy-Wetzel E, Schwarzenbacher R, Lipton SA: Molecular pathways to neurodegeneration. Nat Med 2004;10(suppl 7):S2–S9.

Brandt J, Bylsma FW, Gross H, et al: Trinucleotide repeat length and clinical progression in Huntington's disease. Neurology 1996;46:526–531.

Brinkman RR, Mezei MM, Theilmann J, et al: The likelihood of being affected with Huntington disease by a particular age, for a specific CAG size. Am J Hum Genet 1997;60:1201–1210.

Britton JW, Uiti RJ, Ahlskog JE, et al: Hereditary late-onset chorea without significant dementia: Genetic evidence for substantial phenotypic variation in Huntington's disease. Neurology 1995;45:443–447.

Brodie MJ: Lamotrigine. Lancet 1992;339:1397–1400.

Brouillet E, Jenkins BG, Hyman BT, et al: Age-dependent vulnerability of the striatum to the mitochondrial toxin 3-nitropropionic acid. J Neurochemistry 1993;60:356–359.

Brower M, Price B: Neuropsychiatry of frontal lobe dysfunction in violent and criminal behavior: A critical review. J Neurol Neurosurg Psychiatry 2001;71:720–726.

Browne SE, Bowling AC, MacGarvey U, et al: Oxidative damage and metabolic dysfunction in Huntington's disease: Selective vulnerability of the basal ganglia. Ann Neurol 1997;41:646–653.

Brucke T, Podreka I, Wenger S, et al: Dopamine D2 receptor imaging with SPECT: Studies in different neuropsychiatric disorders. J Cereb Blood Flow Metab 1991;11:220–228.

Bushara KO, Nance M, Gomez CM: Antigliadin antibodies in Huntington's disease. Neurology 2004;62:132–133.

Canals JM, Pineda JR, Torres-Peraza JF, et al: Brain-derived neurotrophic factor regulates the onset and severity of motor dysfunction associated with enkephalinergic neuronal degeneration in Huntington's disease. J Neurosci 2004;24:7727–7739.

CAPIT-HD Committee: Core assessment program for intracerebral transplantation in Huntington's disease (CAPIT-HD). Mov Disord 1996;11:143–150.

Carella F, Scaioli V, Ciano C, et al: Adult onset myoclonic Huntington's disease. Mov Disord 1993;8:201–205.

Carter RJ, Hunt MJ, Morton AJ: Environmental stimulation increases survival in mice transgenic for Exon 1 of the Huntington's disease gene. Mov Disord 2000;15:925–937.

Cattaneo E, Rigamonti D, Coffredo D, et al: Loss of normal huntingtin function: New developments in Huntington's disease research. Trends Neurosci 2001;24:182–188.

Cha JH, Kosinski CM, Kerner JA, et al: Altered brain neurotransmitter receptors in transgenic mice expressing a portion of an abnormal human huntington disease gene. Proc Natl Acad Sci U S A 1998;95:6480–6485.

Chen M, Ona VO, Li M, et al: Minocycline inhibits caspase-1 and caspase-3 expression and delays mortality in a transgenic mouse model of huntington disease. Nat Med 2000;6:797–801.

Choo YS, Johnson GV, MacDonald M, et al: Mutant huntingtin directly increases susceptibility of mitochondria to the calcium-induced permeability transition and cytochrome c release. Hum Mol Genet 2004;13:1407–1420.

Cicchetti F, Parent A: Striatal interneurons in Huntington's disease: Selective increase in the density of calretinin-immunoreactive medium-sized neurons. Mov Disord 1997;11:619–626.

Claes S, Zand KV, Legius E, et al: Correlations between triplet repeat expansion and clinical features in Huntigton's disease. Arch Neurol 1995;113:749–753.

Clifford JJ, Drago J, Natoli AL, et al: Essential fatty acids given from conception prevent topographies of motor deficit in a transgenic model of Huntington's disease. Neuroscience 2002;109:81–88.

Cookson MR: Roles of the proteasome in neurodegenerative disease: Refining the hypothesis. Ann Neurol 2004;56:315–316.

Couzin J: Unorthodox clinical trials meld science care. Science 2004;304:816–817.

Cubo E, Shannon KM, Penn RD, Kroin JS: Internal globus pallidotomy in dystonia secondary to Huntington's disease. Mov Disord 2000;15:1248–1251.

Cui L, Jeong H, Borovecki F, et al: Transcriptional repression of PGC-1alpha by mutant huntingtin leads to mitochondrial dysfunction and neurodegeneration. Cell 2006;127:59–69.

Curtis MA, Penney EB, Pearson AG, et al: Increased cell proliferation and neurogenesis in the adult human Huntington's disease brain. Proc Natl Acad Sci U S A 2003;100(15):9023–9027.

Davies SW, Beardsall K, Turmaine M, et al: Are neuronal intranuclear inclusions the common neuropathology of triplet-repeat disorders with polyglutamine-repeat expansions? Lancet 1998;351:131–133.

Davies SW, Turmaine M, Cozens BA, et al: Formation of neuronal intranuclear inclusions underlies the neurological dysfunction in mice transgenic for the HD mutation. Cell 1997;90:537–548.

Davis MB, Bateman D, Quinn NP, et al: Mutation analysis in patients with possible but apparently sporadic Huntington's disease. Lancet 1994;344:714–717.

de Boo GM, Tibben A, Lanser JB, et al: Early cognitive and motor symptoms in identified carriers of the gene for Huntington's disease. Arch Neurol 1997;54:1353–1357.

DiFiglia M, Sapp E, Chase KO, et al: Aggregation of Huntingtin in neuronal intranuclear inclusions and dystrophic neurites in brain. Science 1997;277:1990–1993.

Djousse L, Knowlton B, Cupples LA, et al: Weight loss in early stage of Huntington's disease. Neurology 2002;59:1325–1330.

Duan W, Guo Z, Jiang H, et al: Paroxetine retards disease onset and progression in Huntingtin mutant mice. Ann Neurol 2004;55:590–594.

Dunah AW, Jeong H, Griffin A, et al: Sp1 and TAFII130 transcriptional activity disrupted in early Huntington's disease. Science 2002;296:2238–2243.

Dure LS, Young AB, Penney JB: Excitatory amino acid binding sites in the caudate nucleus and frontal cortex of Huntington's disease. Ann Neurol 1991;30:785–793.

Duyao M, Ambrose C, Myers R, et al: Trinucleotide repeat length instability and age of onset in Huntington's disease. Nat Genet 1993;4:387–392.

Duyao MP, Auerbach AB, Ryan A, et al: Inactivation of the mouse Huntington's disease gene homolog Hdh. Science 1995;269:407–410.

Emerich DF, Winn SR, Hantraye PM, et al: Protective effect of encapsulated cells producing neurotrophic factor CNTF in a monkey model of Huntington's diseease. Nature 1997;386:395–399.

Everett CM, Wood NW: Trinucleotide repeats and neurodegenerative disease. Brain 2004;127:2385–2405.

Fedoroff JP, Peyser C, Franz ML, Folstein SE: Sexual disorders in Huntington's disease. J Neuropsychiatry Clin Neurosci 1994;6:147–153.

Feigin A, Kieburtz K, Bordwell K, et al: Functional decline in Huntington's disease. Mov Disord 1995;10:211–214.

Feigin A, Kieburtz K, Como P, et al: Assessment of coenzyme Q10 tolerability in Huntington's disease. Mov Disord 1996;11:321–323.

Fennema-Notestine C, Archibald SL, Jacobson MW, et al: In vivo evidence of cerebellar atrophy and cerebral white matter loss in Huntington disease. Neurology 2004;63:989–995.

Fernandez HH, Friedman JH, Grace J, Beason-Hazen S: Donepezil for Huntington's disease. Mov Disord 2000;15:173–176.

Ferrante RJ, Andreassen OA, Jenkins BG, et al: Neuroprotective effects of creatine in a transgenic mouse model of Huntington's disease. J Neuroscience 2000;204:389–397.

Ferrante RJ, Kowall NW, Cipolloni PB, et al: Excitotoxin lesions in primates as a model for Huntington's disease: Histopathological and neurochemical characterization. Exp Neurology 1993;119:46–71.

Ferrante RJ, Kowall NW, Richardson EP: Proliferative and degenerative changes in striatal spiny neurons in Huntington's disease: A combined study using the section-Golgi method and calbindin D28k immunocytochemistry. J Neurosci 1991;11:3877–3887.

Ferrante RJ, Kubilus JK, Lee J, et al: Histone deacetylase inhibition by sodium butyrate chemotherapy ameliorates the neurodegenerative phenotype in Huntington's disease mice. J Neurosci 2003;23:9418–9427.

Foroud T, Gray J, Ivashina J, Conneally PM: Differences in duration of Huntington's disease based on age at onset. J Neurol Neurosurg Psychiatry 1999;66:52–56.

Foroud T, Siemers E, Kleindorfer D, et al: Cognitive scores in carriers of Huntington's disease gene compared to noncarriers. Ann Neurol 1995;37:657–664.

Freeman TB, Cicchetti F, Hauser RA, et al: Transplanted fetal striatum in Huntington's disease: Phenotypic development and lack of pathology. Proc Natl Acad Sci U S A 2000;97:13877–13882.

Freiman RN, Tjian R: A glutamine-rich trail leads to transcription factors. Science 2002;296:2149–2150.

Friedlander RM: Role of caspase 1 in neurologic disease. Arch Neurol 2000;57:1273–1276.

Friedman JH, Trieschmann ME, Myers RH, Fernandez HH: Monozygotic twins discordant for Huntington disease after 7 years. Arch Neurol 2005;62:995–997.

Furtado S, Suchowersky O, Rewcastle NB, et al: Relationship between trinucleotide repeats and neuropathological changes in Huntington's disease. Ann Neurol 1996;39:132–136.

Gambardella A, Muglia M, Labate A, et al: Juvenile Huntington's disease presenting as progressive myoclonic epilepsy. Neurology 2001;57:708–711.

Garcia M, Vanhoutte P, Pages C, et al: The mitochondrial toxin 3-nitropropionic acid induces striatal neurodegeneration via c-Jun N-terminal kinase/c-Jun module. J Neurosci 2002;22:2174–2184.

Gaura V, Bachoud-Levi AC, Ribeiro MJ, et al: Striatal neural grafting improves cortical metabolism in Huntington's disease patients. Brain 2004;127:65–72.

Gauthier LR, Charrin BC, Borrell-Pages M, et al: Huntingtin controls neurotrophic support and survival of neurons by enhancing BDNF vesicular transport along microtubules. Cell 2004;118:127–138.

Gervais FG, Singaraja R, Xanthoudakis S, et al: Recruitment and activation of caspase-8 by the Huntingtin-interacting protein Hip-1 and a novel partner Hippi. Nat Cell Biol 2002;4:95–105.

Giordani B, Berent S, Boivin MJ, et al: Longitudinal neuropsychological and genetic linkage analysis of persons at risk for Huntington's disease. Arch Neurol 1995;52:59–64.

Goizet C, Lesca G, Durr A: Presymptomatic testing in Huntington's disease and autosomal dominant cerebellar ataxias. Neurology 2002;59:1330–1336.

Goldberg YP, Kremer B, Andrew SE, et al: Molecular analysis of new mutations for Huntington's disease: Intermediate alleles and sex of origin effects. Nat Genet 1993;5:174–179.

Goldberg YP, Nicholson DW, Rasper DM, et al: Cleavage of huntingtin by apopain, a proapoptotic cystein protease, is modulated by the polyglutamine tract. Nat Genet 1996;13:442–449.

Golding CV, Danchaivijitr C, Hodgson TL, et al: Identification of an oculomotor biomarker of preclinical Huntington disease. Neurology 2006;67:485–487.

Gómez-Tortosa E, MacDonald M, Friend JC, et al: Quantitative neuropathological changes in presymptomatic Huntington's disease. Ann Neurol 2001;49:29–34.

Gourfinkel-An I, Cancel G, Trottier Y, et al: Differential distribution of the normal and mutated forms of huntingtin in the human brain. Ann Neurol 1997;42:712–719.

Grafton ST, Mazziotta JC, Pahl JJ, et al: A comparison of neurological, metabolic, structural, and genetic evaluations in persons at risk for Huntington's disease. Ann Neurol 1990;28:614–621.

Graham RK, Deng Y, Slow EJ, et al: Cleavage at the caspase-6 site is required for neuronal dysfunction and degeneration due to mutant huntingtin. Cell 2006;125:1179–1191.

Greenamyre JT, Shoulson I: We need something better, and we need it now: Fetal striatal transplantation in Huntington's disease? Neurology 2002;58:675–676.

Gu M, Gash MT, Mann VM, et al: Mitochondrial defect in Huntington's disease caudate nucleus. Ann Neurol 1996;39:385–389.

Gunawardena S, Goldstein LS: Polyglutamine diseases and transport problems: Deadly traffic jams on neuronal highways. Arch Neurol 2005;62:46–51.

Gusella JF, MacDonald ME: Huntington's disease: CAG genetics expands neurobiology. Curr Opin Neurobiol 1995;5:656–662.

Gusella JF, Wexler NS, Conneally PM, et al: A polymorphic DNA marker genetically linked to Huntington's disease. Nature 1983;306:234–238.

Hahn-Barma V, Deweer B, Dürr A, et al: Are cognitive changes the first symptoms of Huntington's disease? A study of gene carriers. J Neurol Neurosurg Psychiatry 1998;64:172–177.

Hantraye P, Riche D, Maziere M, Isacson O: A primate model of Huntington's disease: Behavioral and anatomical studies of unilateral excitotoxic lesions of the caudate putamen in the baboon. Exp Neurol 1990;106:91–104.

Harper PS: The epidemiology of Huntington's disease. Hum Genet 1992;89:365–376.

Harper SQ, Staber PD, He X, et al: RNA interference improves motor and neuropathological abnormalities in a Huntington's disease mouse model. Proc Natl Acad Sci U S A 2005;102:5820–5825.

Harris GJ, Codori AM, Lewis RF, et al: Reduced basal ganglia blood flow and volume in pre-symptomatic, gene-tested persons at-risk for Huntington's disease. Brain 1999;122:1667–1678.

Harris GJ, Pearlson GD, Peyser CE, et al: Putamen volume reduction on magnetic resonance imaging exceeds caudate changes in mild Huntington's disease. Ann Neurol 1992;31:69–75.

Hasselbach SG, Oberg G, Sorensen SA, et al: Reduced regional cerebral blood flow in Huntington's disease studied by SPECT. J Neurol Neurosurg Psychiatry 1992;55:1018–1023.

Hauser RA, Furtado S, Cimino CR, et al: Bilateral human fetal striatal transplantation in Huntington's disease. Neurology 2002;58:687–695.

Hay DG, Sathasivam K, Tobaben S, et al: Progressive decrease in chaperone protein levels in a mouse model of Huntington's disease and induction of stress proteins as a therapeutic approach. Hum Mol Genet 2004;13:1389–1405.

Hedreen JC, Folstein SE: Early loss of striosome neurons in Huntington's disease. J Neuropathol Exp Neurol 1995;54:105–120.

Helder DI, Kaptein AA, van Kempen GMJ, et al: Impact of Huntington's disease on quality of life. Mov Disord 2001;16:325–330.

Hersch SM, Ferrante RJ: Translating therapies for Huntington's disease from genetic animal models to clinical trials. NeuroRx 2004;1:298–306.

Hersch SM, Gevorkian S, Marder K, et al: Creatine in Huntington disease is safe, tolerable, bioavailable in brain and reduces serum 8OH2'dG. Neurology 2006;66:250–252.

Heyes MP, Swartz KJ, Markey SP, Beal MF: Regional brain and cerebrospinal fluid quinolinic acid concentrations in Huntington's disease. Neurosci Lett 1991;122:265–269.

Ho AK, Sahakian BJ, Brown RG, et al: Profile of cognitive progression in early Huntington's disease. Neurology 2003;61:1702–1706.

Hoang TQ, Bluml S, Dubowitz DJ, et al: Quantitative proton-decoupled $^{31}$P MRS and $^{1}$H MRS in the evaluation of Huntington's and Parkinson's disease. Neurology 1998;50:1033–1040.

Hockly E, Cordery PM, Woodman B, et al: Environmental enrichment slows disease progression in R6/2 Huntington's disease mice. Ann Neurol 2002;51:235–242.

Hockly E, Richon VM, Woodman B, et al: Suberoylanilide hydroxamic acid, a histone deacetylase inhibitor, ameliorates motor deficits in a mouse model of Huntington's disease. Proc Natl Acad Sci U S A 2003;100:2041–2046.

Hodgson JG, Agopyan N, Gutekunst CA, et al: A YAC mouse model for Huntington's disease with full-length mutant huntingtin, cytoplasmic toxicity, and selective striatal neurodegeneration. Neuron 1999;23:181–192.

Horton TM, Graham BH, Corral-Debrinski M, et al: Marked increase in mitochondrial DNA deletion levels in the cerebral cortex of Huntington's disease patients. Neurology 1995;45:1879–1883.

Hu MTM, Chaudhuri KR: Repetitive belching, aerophagia, and torticollis in Huntington's disease: A case report. Mov Disord 1998;13:363–365.

Huntington G: On chorea. Medical and Surgical Reporter 1872;26:320–321.

Huntington Study Group: Unified Huntington's Disease Rating Scale: Reliability and consistency. Mov Disord 1996;11:136–142.

Huntington Study Group: A randomized, placebo-controlled trial of coenzyme Q10 and remacemide in Huntington's disease. Neurology 2001;57:397–404.

Huntington Study Group: Dosage effects of riluzole in Huntington's disease: A multicenter placebo-controlled study. Neurology 2003;61:1551–1556.

Huntington Study Group: Minocycline safety and tolerability in Huntington disease. Neurology 2004;63:547–549.

Huntington Study Group: A randomized, double-blind, placebo-controlled trial of tetrabenazine as antichorea therapy in Huntington disease. Neurology 2006;66:366–372.

Huntington's Disease Collaborative Research Group: A novel gene containing a trinucleotide repeat that is expanded and unstable on Huntington's disease chromosomes. Cell 1993;72:971–983.

Igarashi S, Koide R, Shimohata T, et al: Suppression of aggregate formation and apoptosis by transglutaminase inhibitors in cells expressing truncated DRPLA proteins with an expanded polyglutamine stretch. Nat Genet 1998;18:111–117.

Illarioshkin SN, Igarashi S, Onodera O, et al: Trinucleotide repeat length and rate of progression of Huntington's disease. Ann Neurol 1994;36:630–635.

Jana NR, Zemskov EA, Wang G-H, Nukina N: Altered proteasomal function due to the expression of polyglutamine-expanded truncated N-terminal huntingtin induces apoptosis by caspase activation through mitochondrial cytochrome c release. Hum Mol Genet 2001;10:1049–1059.

Jankovic J, Ashizawa T: Tourettism associated with Huntington's disease. Mov Disord 1995;10:103–105.

Jankovic J, Ashizawa T: Huntington's disease. In Noseworthy J (ed): Neurological Therapeutics: Principles and Practice. London, Martin Dunitz, 2003, pp 2550–2561.

Jankovic J, Beach J: Long-term effects of tetrabenazine in hyperkinetic movement disorders. Neurology 1997;48:358–362.

Jankovic J, Beach J, Ashizawa T: Emotional and functional impact of DNA testing on patients with symptoms of Huntington's disease. J Med Genet 1995;32:516–518.

Jankovic J, Wooten M, Van der Linden C, Jansson B: Weight loss in Parkinson's disease. South Med J 1992;85:351–354.

Jenkins BG, Rosas HD, Chen YCI, et al: $^1$H NMR spectroscopy studies of Huntington's disease: Correlations with CAG repeat numbers. Neurology 1998;50:1357–1365.

Jensen P, Fenger K, Bowling TG, Sorensen SA: Crime in Huntington's disease: A study of registered offences among patients, relatives, and controls. J Neurol Neurosurg Psychiatry 1998;65:467–471.

Joel D: Open interconnected model of basal ganglia-thalamocortical circuitry and its relevance to the clinical syndrome of Huntington's disease. Mov Disord 2001;16:407–423.

Karpuj MV, Becher MW, Springer JE, et al: Prolonged survival and decreased abnormal movements in transgenic model of Huntington disease, with administration of the transglutaminase inhibitor cystamine. Nat Med 2002;8:143–149.

Kazantsev A, Walker HA, Slepko N, et al: A bivalent Huntingtin binding peptide suppresses polyglutamine aggregation and pathogenesis in Drosophila. Nat Genet 2002;30:367–376.

Keene CD, Rodrigues CM, Eich T, et al: Tauroursodeoxycholic acid, a bile acid, is neuroprotective in a transgenic animal model of Huntington's disease. Proc Natl Acad Sci U S A 2002;99:10671–10676.

Kenney C, Hunter C, Davidson A, Jankovic J: Short-term effects of tetrabenazine on chorea associated with Huntington's disease. Mov Disord 2007a;22(1)10–13.

Kenney C, Powell S, Jankovic J: Autopsy-proven Huntington's disease with 29 trinucleotide repeats. Mov Disord 2007b;22:127–130.

Kieburtz K, Feigin A, McDermott M, et al: A controlled trial of remacemide hydrochoride in Huntington's disease. Mov Disord 1996;11:273–277.

Kieburtz K, MacDonald M, Shih C, et al: Trinucleotide repeat length and progression of illness in Huntington's disease. J Med Genet 1994;31:872–874.

Kim M, Lee HS, LaForet G, et al: Mutant huntingtin expression in clonal striatal cells: Dissociation of inclusion formation and neuronal survival by caspase inhibition. J Neurosci 1999;19:964–973.

Kipps CM, Duggins AJ, Mahant N, et al: Progression of structural neuropathology in preclinical Huntington's disease: A tensor based morphometry study. J Neurol Neurosurg Psychiatry 2005;76:650–655.

Kirik D, Bjorklund A: Modeling CNS neurodegeneration by overexpression of disease-causing proteins using viral vectors. Trends Neurosci 2003;26:386–392.

Kirkwood SC, Siemers E, Hodes ME, et al: Subtle changes among presymptomatic carriers of the Huntington's disease gene. J Neurol Neurosurg Psychiatry 2000;69:773–779.

Kirkwood SC, Siemers E, Stout JC, et al: Longitudinal cognitive and motor changes among presymptomatic Huntington disease gene carriers. Arch Neurol 1999;56:563–568.

Kirkwood SC, Su JL, Conneally P, Foroud T: Progression of symptoms in the early and middle stages of Huntington disease. Arch Neurol 2001;58:273–278.

Kobayashi Y, Sobue G: Protective effects of chaperons on polyglutamine diseases. Brain Res Bull 2001;56:165–168.

Kokmen E, Özekmekci S, Beard CM, et al: Incidence and prevalence of Huntington's disease in Olmsted county, Minnesota (1950–1989). Arch Neurol 1994;51:696–698.

Kordower JH, Isacson O, Emerich DF: Cellular delivery of trophic factors for the treatment of Huntington's disease: Is neuroprotection possible? Exp Neurol 1999;159:4–20.

Koroshetz WJ, Jenkins BG, Rosen BR, Beal MF: Energy metabolism defects in Huntington's disease and effects of coenzyme Q10. Ann Neurol 1997;41:160–165.

Kovtun IV, Spiro C, McMurray CT: Triplet repeats and DNA repair: Germ cell and somatic cell instability in transgenic mice. Methods Mol Biol 2004;277:309–320.

Kremer B, Clark CM, Almqvist EW, et al: Influence of lamotrigine on progression of early Huntington disease. Neurology 1999;53:1000–1011.

Kremer B, Goldberg P, Andrew SE, et al: A worldwide study of the Huntington's disease mutation: The sensitivity and specificity of measuring CAG repeats. N Engl J Med 1994;330:1401–1406.

Kuemmerle S, Gutekunst C-A, Klein AM, et al: Huntingtin aggregates may not predict neuronal death in Huntington's disease. Ann Neurol 1999;46:842–849.

Künig G, Leenders KL, Sanchez-Pernaute R, et al: Benzodiazepine receptor binding in Huntington's disease: [$^{11}$C]Flumazenil uptake measured using positron emission tomography. Ann Neurol 2000;47:644–648.

Kurlan R, Goldblatt D, Zaczek R, et al: Cerebrospinal fluid homovanillic acid and parkinsonism in Huntington's disease. Ann Neurol 1988;24:282–284.

Kuwert T, Lange HW, Langen K-J, et al: Cortical and subcortical glucose consumption measured by PET in patients with Huntington's disease. Brain 1990;113:1405–1423.

Lacone F, Engel U, Holinski-Feder E, et al: DNA analysis of Huntington's disease: Five years of experience in Germany, Austria, and Switzerland. Neurology 1999;53:801–806.

Landwehrmeyer GB, McNeil SM, Dure LS, et al: Huntington's disease gene: Regional and cellular expression in brain of normal and affected individuals. Ann Neurol 1995;37:218–230.

Lawrence ADM, Godges JR, Rosser AE, et al: Evidence for specific cognitive deficits in preclinical Huntington's disease. Brain 1998; 121:1329–1341.

Leegwater-Kim J, Cha J-HJ: The paradigm of Huntington's disease: Therapeutic opportunities in neurodegeneration. NeuroRx 2004;1:128–138.

Leopold NA, Kagel MC: Dysphagia in Huntington's disease. Arch Neurol 1985;42:57–60.

Li H, Li SH, Johnston H, et al: Amino-terminal fragments of mutant huntingtin show selective accumulation in striatal neurons and synaptic toxicity. Nat Genet 2000;25:385–389.

Li SH, Li XJ: Huntingtin-protein interactions and the pathogenesis of Huntington's disease. Trends Genet 2004;20:146–154.

Li XJ, Li SH, Sharp AH, et al: A huntingtin-associated protein enriched in brain with implications for pathology. Nature 1995; 378:398–402.

Litvan I, Paulsen JS, Mega MS, Cummings JL: Neuropsychiatric assessment of patients with hyperkinetic and hypokinetic movement disorders. Arch Neurol 1998;55:1313–1319.

Louis ED, Lee P, Quinn L, Marder K: Dystonia in Huntington's disease: Prevalence and clinical characteristics. Mov Disord 1999; 14:95–101.

Lucetti C, Del Dotto P, Gambaccini G, et al: IV amantadine improves chorea in Huntington's disease. An acute randomized, controlled study. Neurology 2003;60:1995–1997.

Ludolph AC, He F, Spencer PS, et al: 3-Nitropropionic acid: Exogenous animal neurotoxin and possible human striatal toxin. Can J Neurol Sci 1991;18:492–498.

Maat-Kievit, A, Losekoot, M, Zwinderman, K, et al: Predictability of age of onset in Huntington disease in the Dutch population. Medicine 2002;81:251–259.

Maat-Kievit A, Vegter-van der Vlis M, Zoeteweij M, et al: Paradox of a better test for Huntington's disease. J Neurol Neurosurg Psychiatry 2000;69:579–583.

MacMillan JC, Snell RG, Tyler A, et al: Molecular analysis and clinical correlations of the Huntington's disease mutation. Lancet 1993;342:954–958.

Mahant N, McCusker EA, Byth K, Graham S: Huntington's disease: Clinical correlates of disability and progression. Neurology 2003;61:1085–1092.

Mangiarini L, Sathasivam K, Bates GP: Molecular pathology of Huntington's disease: Animal models and nuclear mechanisms. Neuroscientist 1999;5:383–391.

Mantamadiotis T, Lemberger T, Bleckmann SC, et al: Disruption of CREB function in brain leads to neurodegeneration. Nat Genet 2002;31:47–54.

Marder K, Sandler S, Lechich A, et al: Relationship between CAG repeat length and late-stage outcomes in Huntington's disease. Neurology 2002;59:1622–1624.

Marder K, Zhao H, Myers RH, et al: Rate of functional decline in Huntington's disease. Neurology 2000;54:452–458.

Marks PA, Richon Vam, Breslow R, Rifkind RA: Histone deactylase inhibitors as new cancer drugs. Curr Opin Oncol 2001;13:377–483.

Martin JB: Molecular basis of the neurodegenerative disorders. N Engl J Med 1999;340:1970–1980.

Martindale D, Hackman A, Wieczorek A, et al: Length of huntingtin and its polyglutamine tract influences localization and frequency of intracellular aggregates. Nat Genet 1998;18:150–154.

McBride JL, Behrstock SP, Chen EY, et al: Human neural stem cell transplants improve motor function in a rat model of Huntington's disease. J Comp Neurol 2004;475:211–219.

Meiser B, Dunn S: Psychological impact of genetic testing for Huntington's disease: An update of the literature. J Neurol Neurosurg Psychiatry 2000;69:574–578.

Meissen GJ, Myers RH, Mastromauro CA, et al: Predictive testing for Huntington's disease with use of linked DNA marker. N Engl J Med 1988;318:535–542.

Mittoux V, Joseph JM, Conde F, et al: Restoration of cognitive and motor functions by ciliary neurotrophic factor in a primate model of Huntington's disease. Hum Gene Ther 2000;11:1177–1187.

Moro E, Lang AE, Strafella AP, et al: Bilateral globus pallidus stimulation for Huntington's disease. Ann Neurol 2004;56:290–294.

Myers RH, Vonsattel JP, Stevens TJ, et al: Clinical and neuropathologic assessment of severity in Huntington's disease. Neurology 1988;38:341–347.

Nagel JS, Ichise M, Holman BL: The scintigraphic evaluation of Huntington's disease and other movement disorders using single photon emission computed tomography perfusion brain scans. Sem Nucl Med 1991;21:11–23.

Nance MA: Huntington's disease: Another chapter rewritten. Am J Hum Genet 1996;59:1–6.

Nance MA, US Huntington Disease Genetic Testing Group: Genetic testing of children at risk for Huntington's disease. Neurology 1997;49:1048–1053.

Nihei K, Kowall NW: Neurofilament and neural cell adhesion molecule immunocytochemistry of Huntington's disease striatum. Ann Neurol 1992;31:59–63.

Nucifora FC, Sasaki M, Peters MF, et al: Interference by huntingtin and atrophin-1 with CBP-mediated transcription leading to cellular toxicity. Science 2001;291:2423–2428.

Okun MS, Thommi N: Americo Negrette (1924 to 2003): Diagnosing Huntington disease in Venezuela. Neurology 2004;63:340–343.

Oliva D, Carella F, Savoiardo M, et al: Clinical and magnetic resonance features of the classic and akinetic-rigid variants of Huntington's disease. Arch Neurol 1993;50:17–19.

Ona VO, Li M, Vonsattel JPG, et al: Inhibition of caspase-1 slows disease progression in a mouse model of Huntington's disease. Nature 1999;399:263–267.

Ondo WG, Tintner R, Thomas M, Jankovic J: Tetrabenazine treatment for Huntington's disease-associated chorea. Clin Neuropharmacol 2002;25:300–302.

O'Suilleabhain P, Dewey RB Jr: A randomized trial of amantadine in Huntington disease. Arch Neurol 2003;60:996–998.

Oyanagi K, Takeda S, Takashi H, et al: A quantitative investigation of the substantia nigra in Huntington's disease. Ann Neurol 1989; 26:13–19.

Paleacu D, Anca M, Giladi N: Olanzapine in Huntington's disease. Acta Neurol Scand 2002;105:441–444.

Panov AV, Gutekunst CA, Leavitt BR, et al: Early mitochondrial calcium defects in Huntington's disease are a direct effect of polyglutamines. Nat Neurosci 2002;5:731–736.

Paulsen JS, Hayden M, Stout JC, et al: Preparing for preventive clinical trials: The Predict-HD study. Arch Neurol 2006;63:883–890.

Paulsen JS, Ready RE, Hamilton JM, et al: Neuropsychiatric aspects of Huntington's disease. J Neurol Neurosurg Psychiatry 2001a;71:310–314.

Paulsen JS, Zhao H, Stout JC, et al: Clinical markers of early disease in persons near onset of Huntington's disease. Neurology 2001b;57:658–662.

Paulson HL, Fischbeck KH: Trinucleotide repeats in neurogenetic disorders. Annu Rev Neurosci 1996;19:79–107.

Pavese N, Andrews TC, Brooks DJ, et al: Progressive striatal and cortical dopamine receptor dysfunction in Huntington's disease: A PET study. Brain 2003;126:1127–1135.

Penney JB, Young AB: Huntington's disease. In Jankovic J, Tolosa E (eds): Parkinson's Disease and Movement Disorders, 3rd ed. Baltimore, Williams & Wilkins, 1998, pp 341–356.

Penney JB, Young AB, Snodgrass SR, et al: Huntington's disease in Venezuela: 7 years of follow-up on symptomatic and asymptomatic individuals. Mov Disord 1990;5:93–99.

Perry TL, Hansen S: What excitotoxin kills striatal neurons in Huntington's disease? Clues from neurochemical studies. Neurology 1990;40:20–24.

Perutz MF, Windle AH: Cause of neural death in neurodegenerative diseases attributable to expansion of glutamine repeats. Nature 2001;412:143–144.

Peschanski M, Bachoud-Levi AC, Hantraye P: Integrating fetal neural transplants into a therapeutic strategy: The example of Huntington's disease. Brain 2004;127:1219–1228.

Peters PJ, Ning K, Palacios F, et al: Arfaptin 2 regulates the aggregation of mutant huntingtin protein. Nat Cell Biol 2002; 4:240–245.

Phillips JG, Bradshaw JL, Chiu E, Bradshaw JA: Characteristics of handwriting of patients with Huntington's disease. Mov Disord 1994;9:521–530.

Pillon B, Dubois B, Ploska A, Agid Y: Severity and specificity of cognitive impairment in Alzheimer's, Huntington's, and Parkinson's diseases and progressive supranuclear palsy. Neurology 1991;41:634–643.

Poirier MA, Li H, Macosko J, et al: Huntingtin spheroids and protofibrils as precursors in polyglutamine fibrilization. J Biol Chem 2002;277:41032–41037.

Postert T, Lack B, Kuhn W, et al: Basal ganglia alterations and brain atrophy in Huntington's disease depicted by transcranial real time sonography. J Neurol Neurosurg Psychiatry 1999;67:457–462.

Pratley RE, Salbe AD, Ravussin E, Caviness JN: Higher sedentary energy expenditure in patients with Huntington's disease. Ann Neurol 2000;47:64–70.

Pritchard C, Cox DR, Myers RM: Invited editorial: The end in sight for Huntington disease? Am J Hum Genet 1991;49:1–6.

Racette BA, Perlmutter JS: Levodopa responsive parkinsonism in an adult with Huntington's disease. J Neurol Neurosurg Psychiatry 1998;65:577–579.

Ravikumar B, Vacher C, Berger Z, et al: Inhibition of mTOR induces autophagy and reduces toxicity of polyglutamine expansions in fly and mouse models of Huntington disease. Nat Genet 2004;36:585–595.

Reddy PH, Williams M, Tagle DA: Recent advances in understanding the pathogenesis of Huntington's disease. Trends Neurosci 1999;22:248–255.

Regulier E, Trottier Y, Perrin V, et al: Early and reversible neuropathology induced by tetracycline-regulated lentiviral overexpression of mutant huntingtin in rat striatum. Hum Mol Genet 2003;12:2827–2836.

Reilmann R, Kirsten F, Quinn L, et al: Objective assessment of progression in Huntington's disease: A 3-year follow-up study. Neurology 2001;57:920–924.

Reuter I, Hu MTM, Andrews TC, et al: Late onset levodopa responsive Huntington's disease with minimal chorea masquerading as Parkinson plus syndrome. J Neurol Neurosurg Psychiatry 2000;68:238–241.

Richfield EK, Herkenham M: Selective vulnerability in Huntington's disease: Preferential loss of cannabinoid receptors in lateral globus pallidus. Ann Neurol 1994;36:577–584.

Richfield EK, Maguire-Zeiss KA, Vonkeman HE, Voorn P: Preferential loss of preproenkephalin versus preprotachykinin neurons from the striatum of Huntington's disease patients. Ann Neurol 1995;38:852–861.

Robins Wahlin T-B, Bäckman L, Haegermark A, et al: High suicidal ideation in persons testing for Huntington's disease. Acta Neurol Scand 2000;102:150–161.

Rong J, McGuire JR, Fang ZH, et al: Regulation of intracellular trafficking of huntingtin-associated protein-1 is critical for TrkA protein levels and neurite outgrowth. J Neurosci 2006;26:6019–6030.

Rosas HD, Goodman J, Chen YI, et al: Striatal volume loss in HD as measured by MRI and the influence of CAG repeat. Neurology 2001;57:1025–1028.

Rosas HD, Koroshetz WJ, Chen YI, et al: Evidence for more widespread cerebral pathology in early HD: An MRI-based morphometric analysis. Neurology 2003;60:1615–1620.

Rosas HD, Koroshetz WJ, Jenkins BG, et al: Riluzole therapy in Huntington's disease (HD). Mov Disord 1999;14:326–330.

Rosas HD, Liu AK, Hersch S, et al: Regional and progressive thinning of the cortical ribbon in Huntington's disease. Neurology 2002;58:695–701.

Roses AD: From genes to mechanisms to therapies: Lessons to be learned from neurological disorders. Nat Med 1996;2:267–269.

Ryu H, Ferrante RJ: Emerging chemotherapeutic strategies for Huntington's disease. Expert Opin Emerg Drugs 2005;10:345–363.

Sanchez I, Mahlke C, Yuan J: Pivotal role of oligomerization in expanded polyglutamine neurodegenerative disorders. Nature 2003;421:373–379.

Sanchez Mejia RO, Friedlander RM: Caspases in Huntington's disease. Neuroscientist 2001;7:480–489.

Sánchez-Pernaute R, Garcia-Segura JM, Alba AB, et al: Clinical correlation of striatal $^1$H MRS changed in Huntington's disease. Neurology 1999;53:806–812.

Sánchez-Pernaute R, Künig G, del Barrio Albe A, et al: Bradykinesia in early Huntington's disease. Neurology 2000;54:119–125.

Sapp E, Schwartz C, Chase K, et al: Huntingtin localization in brains of normal and Huntington's disease patients. Ann Neurol 1997;42:604–612.

Saudou F, Finkbeiner S, Devys D, Greenberg ME: Huntingtin acts in the nucleus to induce apoptosis but death does not correlate with the formation of intranuclear inclusions. Cell 1998;95:55–66.

Scherzinger E, Lurz R, Turmaine M, et al: Huntingtin-encoded polyglutamine expansions for amyloid-like protein aggregates in vitro and in vivo. Cell 1997;90:537–548.

Scherzinger E, Sittler A, Schweiger K, et al: Self-assembly of polyglutamine-containing huntingtin fragments into amyloid-like fibrils. Implications for Huntington's disease pathology. Proc Natl Acad Sci U S A 1999;96:4604–4609.

Schiefer J, Landwehrmeyer GB, Luesse HG, et al: Riluzole prolongs survival time and alters nuclear inclusion formation in a transgenic mouse model of Huntington's disease. Mov Disord 2002;17:748–757.

Schumacher JM, Short MP, Hyman BT, et al: Intracerebral implantation of nerve growth factor-producing fibroblasts protects striatum against neurotoxic levels of excitatory amino acids. Neuroscience 1991;45:561–570.

Schwarcz R, Okuno E, White RJ, et al: 3-hydroxyanthranilate oxygenase activity is increased in the brains of Huntington disease victims. Proc Natl Acad Sci U S A 1988;85:4079–4081.

Seo H, Sonntag KC, Isacson O: Generalized brain and skin proteasome inhibition in Huntington's disease. Ann Neurol 2004;56:319–328.

Shelton PA, Knopman DS: Ideomotor apraxia in Huntington's disease. Arch Neurol 1991;48:35–41.

Shoulson I, Odoroff C, Oakes D, et al: A controlled trial of baclofen as protective therapy in early Huntington's disease. Ann Neurol 1989;25:252–259.

Shults CW, Schapira AHV: A cue to queue for CoQ? Neurology 2001;57:375–376.

Siemers E, Foroud T, Bill DJ, et al: Motor changes in presymptomatic Huntington disease gene carriers. Arch Neurol 1996;53:487–492.

Siesling S, van Vugt JPP, Zwinderman KAH, et al: Unified Huntington's Disease Rating Scale: A follow up. Mov Disord 1998;13:915–919.

Siesling S, Zwinderman AH, van Vugt JPP, et al: Shortened version of the motor section of the Unified Huntington's Disease Rating Scale. Mov Disord 1997;229–234.

Sittler A, Lurz R, Lueder G, et al: Geldanamycin activates a heat shock response and inhibits huntingtin aggregation in a cell culture model of Huntington's disease. Hum Mol Genet 2001;10:1307–1315.

Smith DL, Woodman B, Mahal A, et al: Minocycline and doxycycline are not beneficial in a model of Huntington's disease. Ann Neurol 2003;54:186–196.

Snell RG, MacMillan JC, Cheadle JP, et al: Relationship between trinucleotide repeat expansion and phenotypic variation in Huntington's disease. Nat Genet 1993;4:393–397.

Sotrel A, Paskevich PA, Kiely DK, et al: Morphometric analysis of the prefrontal cortex in Huntington's disease. Neurology 1991;41:1117–1123.

Spires TL, Grote HE, Varshney NK, et al: Environmental enrichment rescues protein deficits in a mouse model of Huntington's disease, indicating a possible disease mechanism. J Neurosci 2004;24:2270–2276.

Sprengelmeyer R, Young AW, Calder AJ, et al: Loss of disgust. Perception of faces and emotions in Huntington's disease. Brain 1996;119:1647–1665.

Squitieri F, Gellera C, Cannella M, et al: Homozygosity for CAG mutation in Huntington disease is associated with a more severe clinical course. Brain 2003;126:946–955.

St. Hillaire M, Shannon K, Schumacher J, et al: Transplantation of fetal porcine striatal cells in Huntington's disease: Preliminary safety and efficacy results [abstract]. Neurology 1998;50:A80–A81.

Steffan JS, Agrawal N, Pallos J, et al: SUMO modification of Huntingtin and Huntington's disease pathology. Science 2004;304:100–104.

Steffan JS, Bodai L, Pallos J, et al: Histone deacetylase inhibitors arrest polyglutamine dependent neurodegeneration in Drosophila. Nature 2001;413:739–743.

Storey E, Hyman BT, Jenkins B, et al: 1-methy-4-phenylpyridinium produces excitotoxic lesions in rat striatum as a result of impairment of oxidative metabolism. J Neurochem 1992;58:1975–1978.

Strauss ME, Brandt J: Are there neuropsychologic manifestations of the gene for Huntington's disease in asymptomatic, at-risk individuals? Arch Neurol 1990;47:905–908.

Szebenyi G, Morfini GA, Babcock A, et al: Neuropathogenic forms of huntingtin and androgen receptor inhibit fast axonal transport. Neuron 2003;40:41–52.

Tabrizi SJ, Blamire AM, Manners DN, et al: Creatine therapy for Huntington's disease: Clinical and MRS findings in a 1-year pilot study. Neurology 2003;61:141–142.

Tabrizi SJ, Cleeter MWJ, Xuereb J, et al: Biochemical abnormalities and excitotoxicity in Huntington's disease brain. Ann Neurol 1999;45:25–32.

Tabrizi SJ, Workman J, Hart PE, et al: Mitochondrial dysfunction and free radical damage in the Huntington R6/2 transgenic mouse. Ann Neurol 2000;47:80–86.

Tan E-K, Jankovic J: Bruxism in Huntington's disease. Mov Disord 2000;15:171–173.

Tanaka M, Machida Y, Niu S, et al: Trehalose alleviates polyglutamine-mediated pathology in a mouse model of Huntington disease. Nat Med 2004;10:148–154.

Tang TS, Slow E, Lupu V, et al: Disturbed Ca2+ signaling and apoptosis of medium spiny neurons in Huntington's disease. Proc Natl Acad Sci U S A 2005;102:2602–2607.

Tedroff J, Ekesob A, Sonesson C, et al: Long-lasting improvement following (-)-OSU6162 in a patient with Huntington's disease. Neurology 1999;53:1605–1606.

Thieben MJ, Duggins AJ, Good CD, et al: The distribution of structural neuropathology in pre-clinical Huntington's disease. Brain 2002;125:1815–1828.

Thomas M, Ashizawa T, Jankovic J: Minocycline in Huntington's disease: A pilot study. Mov Disord 2004;19:692–695.

Thomas M, Le W, Jankovic J: Minocycline and other tetracycline derivatives: A neuroprotective strategy in Parkinson's disease and Huntington's disease. Clin Neuropharmacol 2003;26:18–23.

Thompson PD, Berardelli A, Rothwell JC, et al: The coexistence of bradykinesia and chorea in Huntington's disease and its implications for theories of basal ganglia control of movement. Brain 1988;111:223–244.

Thompson PD, Bhatia KP, Brown P, et al: Cortical myoclonus in Huntington's disease. Mov Disord 1994;9:633–641.

Tian JR, Zee DS, Lasker AG, Folstein SE: Saccades in Huntington's disease: Predictive tracking and interaction between release of fixation and initiation of saccades. Neurology 1991;41:875–881.

Toyoshima Y, Yamada M, Onodera O, et al: SCA17 homozygote showing Huntington's disease-like phenotype. Ann Neurol 2004;55:281–286.

Turjanski N, Weeks R, Dolan R, et al: Striatal D1 and D2 receptor binding in patients with Huntington's disease and other choreas. A PET study. Brain 1995;118:689–696.

Tyler A, Ball D, Craufurd D, et al: Presymptomatic testing for Huntington's disease in the United Kingdom. BMJ 1992;304:1593–1596.

Vaddadi KS, Soosai E, Chiu E, Dingjan P: A randomized, placebo-controlled, double blind study of treatment of Huntington's disease with unsaturated fatty acids. Neuroreport 2002;13:29–33.

van Dellen A, Blakemore C, Deacon R, et al: Delaying the onset of Huntington's in mice. Nature 2000;404:721–722.

Van Vugt JPP, van Hilten BJ, Roos RAC: Hypokinesia in Huntington's disease. Mov Disord 1996;11:384–388.

Verbessem P, Lemiere J, Eijnde BO, et al: Creatine supplementation in Huntington's disease: A placebo-controlled pilot trial. Neurology 2003;61:925–930.

Verhagen Metman L, Morris MJ, Farmer C, et al: Huntington's disease: A randomized, controlled trial using the NMDA-antagonist amantadine. Neurology 2002;59:694–699.

Vogel CM, Drury I, Terry LC, Young AB: Myoclonus in adult Huntington's disease. Ann Neurol 1991;29:213–215.

Walker FO, Raymond LA: Targeting energy metabolism in Huntington's disease. Lancet 2004;364:312–313.

Weeks RA, Piccini P, Harding AE, Brooks DJ: Striatal D1 and D2 dopamine receptor loss in asymptomatic mutation carriers of Huntington's disease. Ann Neurol 1996;40:49–54.

Wexler NS, Rose EA, Housman DE: Molecular approaches to hereditary diseases of the nervous system: Huntington's disease as a paradigm. Ann Rev Neurosci 1991;14:503–529.

Wheelock VL, Tempkin T, Marder K, et al: Predictors of nursing home placement in Huntington disease. Neurology 2003;60:998–1001

Wiggins S, Whyte P, Huggins M, et al: The psychological consequences of predictive testing for Huntington's disease. N Engl J Med 1992;327:1401–1405.

Yamamoto A, Lucas JJ, Hen R: Reversal of neuropathology and motor dysfunction in a conditional model of Huntington's disease. Cell 2000;101:57–66.

Yanai A, Huang K, Kang R, et al: Palmitoylation of huntingtin by HIP14 is essential for its trafficking and function. Nat Neurosci 2006;9:824–831.

Yang W, Dunlap JR, Andrews RB, Wetzel R: Aggregated polyglutamine peptides delivered to nuclei are toxic to mammalian cells. Hum Mol Genet 2002;11:2905–2917.

Young AB: Huntingtin in health and disease. J Clin Invest 2003;111:299–302.

Young AB, Greenamyre JT, Hollingsworth Z, et al: NMDA receptor losses in putamen from patients with Huntington's disease. Science 1988;241:981–983.

Zappacosta B, Monza D, Meoni C, et al: Psychiatric symptoms do not correlate with cognitive decline, motor symptoms, or CAG repeat length in Huntington's disease. Arch Neurol 1996;53:493–497.

Zemke D, Majid A: The potential of minocycline for neuroprotection in human neurologic disease. Clin Neuropharmacol 2004;27:293–298.

Zoghbi HY, Botas J: Mouse and fly models of neurodegeneration. Trends Genet 2002;18:463–471.

Zuccato C, Ciammola A, Rigamonti D, et al: Loss of huntingtin-mediated BDNF gene transcription in Huntington's disease. Science 2001;293:493–498.

## APPENDIX 15-1

### Patient Organizations

Several organizations, some listed here, are dedicated to educating patients and their families about Huntington disease. These organization provide guidance to local support groups, and they are instrumental in increasing public awareness about Huntington disease. Another major aim is to raise funds to support research dedicated to finding the cause, cure, and new symptomatic treatments for this disorder.

### Huntington's Disease Society of America

158 West 29th Street, 7th Floor
New York, New York 10001-5300
Telephone: (800) 345-HDSA/ (212) 242-1968
Fax: (212) 239-3430
Website: http://www.hdsa.org

### Huntington Study Group

Telephone: 800-942-0424
Website: www.huntington-study-group.org

### International Huntington Association

Gerrit Dommerholt
Callunahof 8, 7217 ST Harfsen
The Netherlands
Telephone: 31-573311595
Fax: 31-703500050
Website: http://www.hdlighthouse.org

*Other Related Websites*
http://clix.to/HDSupportInfo
http://www.wemove.org

## Chapter 16

# Chorea, Ballism, Athetosis
## Phenomenology and Etiology

Chorea consists of involuntary, continual, abrupt, rapid, brief, unsustained, irregular movements that flow randomly from one body part to another. Patients can partially and temporarily suppress the chorea and frequently camouflage some of the movements by incorporating them into semipurposeful activities (parakinesia). The inability to maintain voluntary contraction (motor impersistence), such as manual grip (milkmaid grip) or tongue protrusion, is a characteristic feature of chorea and results in dropping of objects and clumsiness. Chorea should be differentiated from pseudochoreoathetosis, a movement disorder that is phenomenologically similar to chorea or athetosis (slow chorea) due to loss of proprioception (Sharp et al., 1994). Muscle stretch reflexes are often "hung-up" and "pendular." Affected patients typically have a peculiar, irregular, and dance-like gait. The pathophysiology of chorea is poorly understood, but in contrast to parkinsonism, dystonia, and other movement disorders, intracortical inhibition of the motor cortex is normal in chorea (Hanajima et al., 1999). In addition, semiquantitative analysis of single photon emission computed tomography in patients with hemichorea due to various causes suggests that there is an increase in activity in the contralateral thalamus, possibly due to disinhibition as a result of loss of normal pallidal inhibitory input (Kim et al., 2002).

Chorea may be a manifestation of a primary neurologic disorder, such as Huntington disease (HD), or it may occur as a neurologic complication of systemic, toxic, or other disorders (Rosenblatt et al., 1998; Cardoso, 2004) (Box 16-1). Chorea may be seen in normal infants, but these movements usually disappear by age 8 months (Shoulson, 1986), and some of the movements may be purposeful (Van der Meer et al., 1995).

Before the discussion of non-HD causes of chorea, it is important to point out that HD-like phenotypes without the HD genotype are increasingly being described. Several neurodegenerative disorders, some with expanded trinucleotide repeats, have been reported as phenocopies of HD, including spinocerebellar atrophy, particularly SCA2 and SCA3 (Kawaguchi et al., 1994), pure cerebello-olivary degeneration (Fox et al., 2003), and dentatorubral-pallidoluysian atrophy (DRPLA) (see later) (La Spada et al., 1994; Ikeuchi et al., 1995; Komure et al., 1995; Warner et al., 1995; Ross et al., 1997; Rosenblatt et al., 1998).

## DENTATORUBRAL-PALLIDOLUYSIAN ATROPHY AND HUNTINGTON DISEASE–LIKE DISORDERS

DRPLA is an autosomal-dominant neurodegenerative disorder that is particularly prevalent in Japan, but it has also been identified in Europe and in African-American families (Haw River syndrome) (Burke et al., 1994; Thomas and Jankovic, 2001) (Fig. 16-1). Usually beginning in the fourth decade, the disorder may occur as an early-onset DRPLA (before 20 years of age), manifested by a variable combination of myoclonus, epilepsy, mental retardation, or late-onset DRPLA (after 20 years of age), manifested by cerebellar ataxia, choreoathetosis, dystonia, rest and postural tremor, parkinsonism, and dementia (Video 16-1).

Neuroimaging studies often show evidence of cortical, brainstem, and cerebellar atrophy and widespread white matter changes (Koide et al., 1997; Muñoz et al., 1999, 2004). Neuropathologic findings consist chiefly of degeneration of dentatorubral system, globus pallidum externa (GPe), subthalamic nucleus, and—to a lesser extent—striatum, substantia nigra, inferior olive, and thalamus (Warner et al., 1994), as well as demyelination and reactive astrogliosis in the cerebral white matter (Muñoz et al., 2004). Involvement of oligodendrocytes in autopsied brains and an increased number of affected glia, as well as larger expansions in CAG in these glia, in transgenic mice might explain the widespread demyelination (Yamada et al., 2002). Several pathologic reports have noted widespread deposition of lipofuscin. As with HD and other diseases associated with CAG repeat expansions, DRPLA has been associated with the formation of perinuclear aggregates that can be prevented by the use of transglutaminase inhibitors, such as cystamine and monodansyl cadaverine (Igarashi et al., 1998). These intranuclear inclusions stain intensely with ubiquitin (Becher and Ross, 1998). Subsequent studies have demonstrated accumulation of mutant atrophin-1 in the neuronal nuclei, rather than neuronal intranuclear inclusions, as the predominant pathologic feature in this neurodegenerative disorder (Yamada et al., 2001).

Unstable CAG expansion has been identified as the mutation in a gene on chromosome 12 (Koide et al., 1994; Komure et al., 1995; Warner et al., 1995; Becher et al., 1997; Ross et al., 1997). As with HD, there is an inverse correlation between the age at onset and the number of CAG repeats (Ikeuchi et al., 1995). The early onset of DRPLA is associated with greater number of CAG repeats (62 to 79) as compared with the late-onset type (54 to 67 repeats) (Ikeuchi et al., 1995). Testing for the various gene mutations will undoubtedly lead to better recognition and appreciation of the spectrum of clinical and pathologic changes associated with these disorders. For example, a family with spastic paraplegia, truncal ataxia, and dysarthria but without other clinical features of DRPLA has been found to show homozygosity for an allele that carries intermediate CAG repeats in the DRPLA gene (Kuroharas et al., 1997). The DRPLA gene is expressed predominantly in neurons, but neurons that are vulnerable to degeneration in DRPLA do not selectively express the gene (Nishiyama et al., 1997). DRPLA protein has been identified as a phosphoprotein, c-Jun NH(2)-terminal kinase, one of the major factors involved in its phosphorylation. In DRPLA, this protein

Box 16-1  Differential diagnosis of chorea

**Developmental/Aging Choreas**
Physiologic chorea of infancy
Kernicterus
Cerebral palsy
Minimal cerebral dysfunction (choreiform syndrome)
Buccal-oral-lingual dyskinesias of aging
Senile (essential) chorea

**Hereditary Choreas**

*Onset Usually in Infancy, Childhood, or Adolescence*
Benign hereditary chorea
Amino acid disorders: glutaric acidemia, cystinuria,
    homocystinuria, phenylketonuria, Hartnup disease,
    argininosuccinic acidemia
Carbohydrate disorders: mucopolysaccharidoses,
    mucolipidoses, galactosemia, pyruvate dehydrogenase
    deficiency
Lipid disorders: sphingolipidosis (Krabbe), globoid cell
    leukodystrophy, metachromatic leukodystrophy,
    Gaucher disease, GM1 and GM2 gangliosidosis,
    ceroid lipofuscinosis
Lesch-Nyhan syndrome
Hallervorden-Spatz syndrome
Ataxia-telangiectasia
Tuberous sclerosis
Sturge-Weber syndrome
Wilson disease
Ataxia-myoclonus syndrome
Hemoglobin SC disease
Xeroderma pigmentosum
Leigh disease and other mitochondrial cytopathies
Pelizaeus-Merzbacher
Sulfite-oxidase deficiency
Familial striatal necrosis
Early-onset ataxia with hypoalbuminemia
Paroxysmal nonkinesigenic choreoathetosis

*Onset Usually in Adolescence or Adulthood*
Wilson disease
Huntington disease
Huntington disease-like 1 (HDL1): AD, seizures, linked
    to 20p
Huntington disease–like 2 (HDL2)
Huntington disease–like 3 (HDL3): AR, onset first
    decade, linked to 4p15.3
Benign familial chorea (hereditary chorea without
    dementia)
Neuroacanthocytosis with normal or abnormal lipids
    (see Box 16-2)
Dentatorubropallidoluysian atrophy (DRPLA)
Porphyria
Paroxysmal kinesigenic choreoathetosis
Paroxysmal dystonic choreoathetosis (Mount-Reback)
Familial calcification of basal ganglia
Joseph disease
Olivopontocerebellar atrophies (hereditary ataxias)
Associated with peroneal atrophy, epilepsy, and
    cerebellar ataxia

**Drug-Induced and Toxic Choreas**
Dopamine receptor blocking (neuroleptic) drugs:
    tardive dyskinesia
Antiparkinsonian drugs
Dopaminergic (e.g., levodopa, bromocriptine,
    pergolide)

*Anticonvulsants*
Phenytoin
Carbamazepine
Valproate

*Noradrenergic Stimulants*
Amphetamines
Methylphenidate, pemoline
Aminophyline, theophyline

*Steroids*
Oral contraceptives
Anabolic steroids

*Opiates*
Methadone

*Miscellaneous Drugs*
Amoxapine
Antihistamines
Cimetidine
Cyclizine
Diazoxide
Digoxin
Isoniazid
Lithium
Methyldopa
Metoclopramide
Reserpine
Triazolam
Tricyclic antidepressants

*Toxins*
Alcohol intoxication and withdrawal
Carbon monoxide
Manganese
Mercury
Thallium
Toluene (glue sniffing)

**Metabolic/Endocrine/Nutritional Choreas**

*Metabolic*
Hyponatremia and hypernatremia
Hypocalcemia
Hypoglycemia and hyperglycemia
Hypomagnesemia
Propionic acidemia
Glutaric aciduria
GM1 gangliosidosis
Hepatic encephalopathy (acquired hepatocerebral
    degeneration)
Renal encephalopathy
Cardiac surgery

**Box 16-1** Differential diagnosis of chorea—cont'd

*Endocrine*
Hyperthyroidism
Hypoparathyroidism
Psudohypoparathyroidism
Hyperparathyroidism
Chorea gravidarum (pregnancy)
Addison disease

*Nutritional*
Beriberi
Pellagra
Vitamin deficiency (B12, D)

**Infectious/Immunologic Choreas**
*Infectious*
Scarlet fever (streptococcal erythrogenic toxin)
Diphtheria
Pertussis
Typhoid fever
Viral encephalitis (mumps, measles, varicella, ECHO,
    influenza)
Neurosyphilis
Mononucleosis
Legionnaire disease
Lyme disease
Toxoplasmosis
Bacterial endocarditis
Sarcoidosis
Tuberculosis
Herpes zoster ophthalmicus

*Postinfectious*
Sydenham disease (poststreptococcal)
Postinfectious encephalitis (chickenpox, measles,
    mumps, rubella)

*Immunologically Mediated*
Systemic lupus erythematosus (SLE)
Periarteritis nodosa
Behcet syndrome
Henoch-Schonlein purpura
Multiple sclerosis
Antiphospholipid antibody syndrome
Postvaccinial meningoencephalitis
Acquired immune deficiency syndrome (AIDS)

**Cerebrovascular Choreas**
Basal ganglia infarction/hemorrhage
Arteriovenous malformation
Polycythemia vera
Migraine
Transient cerebral ischemia

**Miscellaneous Choreas**
Posttraumatic
Epidural hematoma
Subdural hematoma
Electrical injury to the nervous system
Brain tumors
Pick disease
Degeneration of nucleus centrum medianum of thalamus
Post cardiac surgery

---

appears to be slowly phosphorylated; thus, it may delay a process that is essential in keeping neurons alive (Okamura-Oho et al., 2003).

An autosomal-dominant HD-like neurodegenerative disorder, now classified as Huntington disease-like 1 (HDL1), was mapped to chromosome 20p (Xiang et al., 1998). A 192-nucleotide insertion in the region of the prion protein gene (*PRNP*) encoding an octapeptide repeat in the prion protein

was found in a single family with HD phenotype, suggesting that *PRNP* mutations can result in HD phenocopies (Moore et al., 2001). Another disorder, termed *HD-like 2* or *HDL2*, is characterized by onset in the fourth decade, involuntary movements such as chorea and dystonia as well as other movement disorders (bradykinesia, rigidity, tremor), dysarthria, hyperreflexia, gait abnormality, psychiatric symptoms, weight loss, and dementia with progression from onset

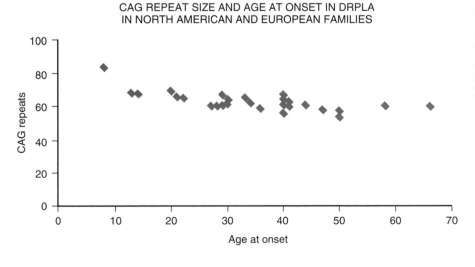

CAG REPEAT SIZE AND AGE AT ONSET IN DRPLA
IN NORTH AMERICAN AND EUROPEAN FAMILIES

**Figure 16-1** Inverse correlation between CAG repeats and age at onset of DRPLA. (Reprinted with permission from Thomas M, Jankovic J: Dentatorubropallidoluysian atrophy in North American families. Ann Neurol 2001;50[suppl 1]:S65.)

to death in about 20 years (Margolis et al., 2001, 2004; Walker, Jankovic, et al., 2003). The disorder appears to be present exclusively or predominantly in individuals of African origin. The neuroimaging and neuropathologic findings are very similar to those in HD, but the intranuclear inclusions stain with 1C2 but not antihuntingtin antibodies. Unlike the family linked to chromosome 20p, seizures are not present in this latter family. All 10 affected family members had a CAG repeat expansion of 50 to 60 triplets. The gene was later mapped to chromosome 16q24.3 and was found to encode junctophilin-3, a protein of the junctional complex linking the plasma membrane and the endoplasmic reticulum (Holmes et al., 2001). The mutation associated with HDL2 has been identified as a CTG/CAG trinucleotide repeat expansion within the junctophilin-3 (*JPH3/HDL2*) gene. In the normal population, the repeat length ranges from 6 to 27 CTG triplets, whereas affected individuals have 41 to 58 triplets. One family, previously described as "autosomal dominant chorea-acanthocytosis with polyglutamine-containing neuronal inclusions" (see later) (Walker et al., 2002), was subsequently found to have the triple nucleotide expansion of HDL2 (Stevanin et al., 2003; Walker, Rasmussen, et al., 2003).The CTG repeat expansion at the HDL2 locus has been found to be responsible for 2% of patients with typical features of HD but without expanded CAG repeats in the *IT15* gene and 0.2% of all HD families, again providing evidence that HD is clinically and genetically heterogeneous (Stevanin et al., 2002). This group later analyzed 252 patients with a HDL phenotype, including 60 with typical HD, who had tested negative for pathologic expansion in the *IT15* gene and found two patients that had an abnormal CTG expansion in the *JPH3* gene and two other patients with abnormal CAG expansion in the gene coding for TATA-binding protein (TBP/SCA17) (Stevanin et al., 2003; Toyoshima et al., 2004). Thus, the frequency of mutation in either *JPH3* gene or *TBP* gene among patients with HDL phenotype is about 3%. Initially, the TBP expansion was found in the family with SCA17, characterized clinically by intellectual deterioration, cerebellar ataxia, epilepsy, and chorea. Although acanthocytosis was emphasized by Walker and colleagues (2002; Walker, Rasmussen, et al., 2003) in their initial report and in one of three patients reported subsequently (Walker, Rasmussen, et al., 2003), we have not been able to confirm the presence of acanthocytes in one member of the original family or in the other members when we carefully examined the peripheral smear.

While the majority of genetic forms of chorea are inherited in an autosomal-dominant pattern, a novel autosomal-recessive neurodegenerative Huntington-like disorder has been described (Kambouris et al., 2000). Beginning at 3 to 4 years of age and manifested by chorea, dystonia, ataxia, gait disorder, spasticity, seizures, mutism, intellectual impairment, and bilateral frontal and caudate atrophy, this neurodegenerative disorder has been linked to 4p15.3, different from the 4p16.3 HD locus. This disorder has now been classified as HDL3.

Some cases of neuronal intranuclear inclusion disease, caused by expanded CAG repeats and characterized by the combination of extrapyramidal signs, lower motor neuron signs, and cognitive and behavioral abnormalities resulting in death by the third decade, also show intranuclear aggregates, similar to the other CAG disorders (Lieberman et al., 1998).

# NEUROACANTHOCYTOSIS

After HD, neuroacanthocytosis is perhaps the most common form of hereditary chorea. Previously also referred to as chorea-acanthocytosis, it is now recognized that this multisystem, neurodegenerative disorder can be expressed by a wide variety of clinical and laboratory abnormalities, hence the term *neuroacanthocytosis* (Spitz et al., 1985; Danek et al., 2005) (Box 16-2). Symptoms usually first begin in the third and fourth decades of life (range: 8 to 62 years) with lip and tongue biting followed by orolingual (eating) dystonia, motor and phonic tics, generalized chorea, and stereotypies (Video 16-2). Other features include cognitive and personality changes, seizures, dysphagia, dysarthria, vertical ophthalmoparesis, parkinsonism, amyotrophy, areflexia, evidence of axonal neuropathy, and elevated serum creatine kinase without evidence of myopathy. Hardie and colleagues (1991) reviewed the clinical, hematologic, and pathologic findings in 19 patients (10 males and 9 females) with a mean age of 32 years (range: 8 to 62 years) with more than 3% acanthocytes on peripheral blood smear. Twelve of these patients with neuroacanthocytosis were familial, and seven were sporadic; two had the McLeod phenotype (see later). In their series, Hardie and colleagues (1991) found a variety of movement disorders, including chorea (58%), orofacial dyskinesia (53%), dystonia (47%), vocalizations (47%), tics (42%), and parkinsonism (34%). Although lip and tongue biting was observed in only 16% of the patients, this feature and tongue protrusion when eating (eating dystonia) are characteristic of neuroacanthocytosis and when present strongly suggest the diagnosis. Besides movement disorders other associated features included dysarthria (74%); absent or reduced reflexes (68%); dementia (63%); psychiatric problems such as depression, anxiety, and obsessive-compulsive disorder (58%); dysphagia (47%); seizures (42%);

Box 16-2 Classification of neuroacanthocytosis

**A. Normal Lipids**
  1. Autosomal-dominant
     a. Without inclusions
     b. With polyglutamine-containing neuronal inclusions (Walker et al., 2002)
  2. Autosomal–recessive: 9q21 (73 exons)
     a. Multiple mutations in the chorea acanthocytosis gene coding for chorein (Rampoldi et al., 2001; Ueno et al., 2001)
  3. Sporadic
**B. Hypobetalipoproteinemia (Mars et al., 1969)**
**C. Abetalipoproteinemia (Bassen and Kornzweig, 1950)**
**D. Aprebetalipoproteinemia (Bohlega et al., 1998)**
**E. Hypoprebetalipoproteinemia**
  1. HARP syndrome: Hypoprebetalipoproteinemia, acanthocytosis, retinitis pigmentosa, and pallidal degeneration: similar to NBIA-1 (HSD)
**F. X-linked (McLeod syndrome) (Allen et al., 1961) Xp21**
  1. Neuroacanthocytosis: http://www.geocities.com/nanews2003/

muscle weakness and wasting (16%); and elevated creatine phosphokinase (CK) in 58%. Magnetic resonance volumetry and fluorodeoxyglucose positron emission tomography (PET) show striatal atrophy in patients with neuroacanthocytosis (Jung et al., 2001).

Although autosomal-dominant, X-linked recessive, and sporadic forms of neuroacanthocytosis have been reported, the majority of the reported families indicate autosomal recessive inheritance. Genomewide scan for linkage in 11 families with autosomal-recessive inheritance showed a linkage to a marker on chromosome 9q21, indicating a single locus for the disease (Rubio et al., 1997). Ueno and colleagues (2001) carried out a linkage-free analysis in the region of chromosome 9q21 in the Japanese population and identified a 260-bp deletion in the EST (expressed sequence tags) region K1AA0986 in exon 60, 61 that was homozygous in patients with neuroacanthocytosis and heterozygous in their parents. Further sequencing has identified a polyadenylation site with a protein with 3096 amino acid residues that has been named "Chorein" by the authors. This deletion is not found in normal Japanese and European populations (Ueno et al., 2001). In another study by Rampoldi and colleagues (2001) in European patients, a novel gene encoding a 3174-amino-acid protein on chromosome 9q21 with 73 exons was identified. They identified 16 mutations in the chorea acanthocytosis (CHAC) gene, now renamed *VPS13A* gene. These mutations were identified in various exons. They suggested that chorea acanthocytosis encodes an evolutionarily conserved protein that is involved in protein sorting (Rampoldi et al., 2002). Other single heterozygous mutations have been identified in this gene (Saiki et al., 2003). Molecular analysis by screening all 73 exons of the *VPS13A* gene shows marked genotype-phenotype heterogeneity (Lossos et al., 2005). Walker and colleagues (2002) described a family with chorea or parkinsonism as well as cognitive changes, inherited in an autosomal-dominant pattern. At autopsy, there was marked degeneration of the striatum and intranuclear inclusion bodies immunoreactive for ubiquitin, expanded polyglutamine CGG repeats, and torsinA. Interestingly, one of the patients had fragile X syndrome, and two had expanded trinucleotide repeats at permutation range, previously associated with postural/kinetic tremor, parkinsonism, ataxia, and cognitive decline (Hagerman et al., 2001). The family reported by Walker and colleagues (2002) turned out to have the trinucleotide repeat expansion associated with HDL2, but subsequent analysis of the family shed doubt on the presence of acanthocytes as a feature of the HDL2 syndrome (Walker, Jankovic, et al., 2003).

Two patients from the original study by Rubio and colleagues (1997) were found to have the McLeod phenotype, an X-linked (Xp21) recessive form of acanthocytosis associated with depression, bipolar and personality disorder, and neurologic manifestations, including chorea, involuntary vocalizations, seizures, motor axonopathy, hemolysis, liver disease, and high creatine kinase levels (Witt et al., 1992; Danek et al., 2001a, 2001b). Neuroimaging usually reveals caudate and occasionally cerebellar atrophy with a rim of increased T2-intensity in the lateral putamen. Functional neuroimaging studies show evidence of downregulation of D2 dopamine receptors. In contrast to the autosomal-recessive form of neuroacanthocytosis linked to chromosome 9, patients with McLeod syndrome usually do not exhibit lip-biting or dysphagia. This multisystem disorder is associated with low reactivity of Kell erythrocyte antigens (weak antigenicity of red cells) due to absence of KX 37 kDa, 444 AA, membrane protein that forms a complex with the Kell protein. The disorder is caused by different mutations in the *XK* gene encoding for the KX protein (Ho et al., 1996; Danek et al., 2001a; Jung et al., 2001). Mutations identified by various authors include frame shift mutations in exon 2 at codon 151, deletion at codon 90 in exon 2 and at codon 408 in exon 3, and splicing mutations in intron 2 of the *XK* gene (Dotti et al., 2000; Ueyama et al., 2000; Danek et al., 2001a; Jung et al., 2001). Rarely, neuroacanthocytosis may be associated with abetaliproteinemia due to mutations in the microsomal triglyceride transfer protein (Sharp et al., 1993). In addition to acanthocytosis, the patients exhibit retinopathy; malabsorption, including that of vitamin E; low serum cholesterol levels; and abnormal serum lipoprotein electrophoresis. Aprebetalipoproteinemia can also cause movement disorders and acanthocytosis (Bohlega et al., 1998). Another syndrome that is associated with acanthocytosis is the hypoprebetalipoproteinemia, acanthocytosis, retinitis pigmentosa, and pallidal degeneration (HARP syndrome) (Orrell et al., 1995). This disorder is associated with dystonia, particularly involving the oromandibular region, rather than chorea and self-mutilation, and it is clinically and neuroradiologically similar to pantothenate kinase-associated neurodegeneration (PKAN), formerly known as Hallervorden-Spatz disease (see later). Indeed, a homozygous nonsense mutation in exon 5 of the *PANK2* gene that creates a stop codon at amino acid 371, found in the original HARP patient, establishes that HARP is part of the pantothenate kinase-associated neurodegeneration disease spectrum (Ching et al., 2002; Houlden et al., 2003). Because of Hallervorden's terrible past and his shameless involvement in active euthanasia (Shevell, 2003), the disorder has been renamed neurodegeneration with brain iron accumulation type 1 (NBIA-1). NBIA-1, an autosomal-recessive disorder characterized by childhood-onset progressive rigidity, dystonia, choreoathetosis, spasticity, optic nerve atrophy, and dementia, has been associated with acanthocytosis (Malandrini et al., 1996; Racette et al., 2001; Thomas et al., 2004). Although chorea is not a typical feature of NBIA-1, "senile chorea" has been described in a patient with pathologically proven NBIA-1 (Grimes et al., 2000).

Linkage analyses initially localized the NBIA-1 gene on 20p12.3–p13; subsequently, 7-bp deletion and various missense mutations were identified in the coding sequence of the *PANK2* gene, which codes for pantothenate kinase (Zhou et al., 2001; Hayflick et al., 2003). Pantothenate kinase is an essential regulatory enzyme in coenzyme A biosynthesis. It has been postulated that as a result of phosphopantothenate deficiency, cysteine accumulates in the globus pallidus of brains of patients with NBIA-1. It undergoes rapid autooxidation in the presence of nonheme iron that normally accumulates in globus pallidus internus and substantia nigra, generating free radicals that are locally neurotoxic. Interestingly, atypical subjects were found to be compound heterozygotes for certain mutations for which classic subjects were homozygous. The disorder with the clinical phenotype of NBIA associated with mutations in the *PANK2* gene is now referred to as pantothenate kinase–associated neurodegeneration (Thomas et al., 2004). On the basis of an analysis of 123 patients from 98 families with NBIA-1, Hayflick and colleagues (2003) found that "classic Hallervorden-Spatz syndrome" was associated with *PANK2* mutation in all cases and that one third of "atypical" cases had the mutations within the *PANK2* gene. Those who had the *PANK2* mutation were more likely to have dysarthria and psychiatric symptoms, and all had the typical "eye of a tiger" abnormality on magnetic resonance imaging (MRI) with a specific pattern of hyperintensity within the hypointense globus pallidum interna (GPi).

An examination of wet blood or Wright-stained, fast dry, blood smear usually reveals over 15% of red blood cells as acanthocytes. In mild forms of acanthocytosis, scanning electron microscopy might be required to demonstrate the red blood cell abnormalities (Feinberg et al., 1991). In a recent study of two patients with pathologically proven neuroacanthocytosis, Feinberg and colleagues (1991) noted that the yield in demonstrating acanthocytosis may be increased by using a coverslip because the contact with glass causes the fragile cells to undergo morphologic changes. Diluting the blood with normal saline, incubating the Wright-stained smear with EDTA, using a scanning electron microscope, and other techniques designed to increase "echinocytotic stress" are also helpful (Feinberg et al., 1991; Orrell et al., 1995). The characteristic acanthocytic appearance of red blood cells has been attributed to abnormalities in transmembrane glycoprotein band 3 that can be demonstrated on gel electrophoresis. It is not yet clear how the gene mutation leads to the abnormal morphology of the red cells.

By using high-performance liquid chromatography, fatty acids of erythrocyte membrane proteins were analyzed in six patients with neuroacanthocytosis (Sakai et al., 1991). In comparison with normal controls and patients with HD, erythrocytes of patients with neuroacanthocytosis showed a marked abnormality in the composition of covalently bound fatty acids: an increase in palmitic acid (C16:0) and a decrease in stearic acid (C18:0).

Brain MRI in patients with neuroacanthocytosis usually shows caudate and more generalized brain atrophy, but some cases also show extensive white matter abnormalities (Nicholl et al., 2004). Caudate hypometabolism and atrophy have been demonstrated by PET studies and by neuroimaging. Similar to the findings in Parkinson disease, PET scans findings in six patients with neuroacanthocytosis showed a reduction to 42% of normal in [$^{18}$F]dopa uptake in the posterior putamen; in contrast to Parkinson disease, however, there was a marked reduction in the striatal [$^{11}$C]raclopride (D2) receptor binding (Brooks et al., 1991).

Neuronal loss and gliosis were particularly prominent in the striatum and pallidum but may also affect the thalamus, substantia nigra, and anterior horns of the spinal cord (Rinne et al., 1994b). The neuronal loss in the substantia nigra is most evident in the ventrolateral region, similar to Parkinson disease, but the nigral neuronal loss is more widespread in neuroacanthocytosis (Rinne et al., 1994a). The preservation of the cerebral cortex, cerebellum, subthalamic nucleus, pons, and medulla may serve to differentiate pathologically between neuroacanthocytosis, HD, and DRPLA. Brain biochemical analyses showed low substance P in the substantia nigra and striatum and increased levels of norepinephrine in the putamen and pallidum (DeYebenes et al., 1988).

Unfortunately, there is no effective treatment for patients with neuroacanthocytosis. The associated parkinsonism rarely improves with dopaminergic therapy, probably because there is loss of postsynaptic dopamine receptors. We have seen some patients whose condition remained static for several years, followed by further progression and an eventual demise as a result of aspiration pneumonia or other complications of chronic illness.

## OTHER FAMILIAL CHOREAS

Besides HD and neuroacanthocytosis, genetically transmitted choreas include benign hereditary chorea, a nonprogressive chorea of childhood onset (Wheeler et al., 1993). The patients may have a slight motor delay because of chorea, slight gait ataxia, and their handwriting may be impaired, but the disorder is self-limiting after adolescence in most cases, although it may persist as a mild chorea beyond age 60 years. Inherited as an autosomal-dominant disorder, benign hereditary chorea has been linked to a marker on chromosome 14q13.1–q21.1 (de Vries et al., 2000; Fernandez et al., 2001; Breedveld et al., 2002) and a novel single nucleotide substitution in the *TITF-1* gene (also referred to as *TTF, Nkx2.1*, and *T/ebp*), coding for a transcription essential for the organogenesis of the lung, thyroid, and basal ganglia, has been identified in one Canadian family (Kleiner-Fisman et al., 2003). The *TITF-1* gene mutation should be considered in children and adults with chorea, mental retardation, congenital hypothyroidism, and chronic lung disease (hence, the term *brain-thyroid-lung syndrome*, proposed for this disease [Willemsen et al., 2005]). Benign hereditary chorea has been associated with congenital hypothyroidism and, surprisingly, marked improvement with levodopa (Asmus et al., 2005). The existence of this entity has been questioned, however, since many patients who were initially diagnosed with benign hereditary chorea were later found to have some other diagnosis, such as myoclonic dystonia, hereditary essential myoclonus, tics, and HD (Schrag et al., 2000). Essential chorea is a form of adult-onset, nonprogressive chorea without family history of chorea or other symptoms suggestive of HD and without evidence of striatal atrophy on neuroimaging studies. Sometimes referred to as senile chorea, essential chorea usually has its onset after age 60, and in contrast to HD, it is not associated with dementia or positive family history. Some cases of senile chorea, however, have been reported to have pathologic changes identical to HD; others have had predominant degeneration of the putamen rather than the caudate (Friedman and Ambler, 1990). The CAG repeat length should, by definition, be normal, but Ruiz and colleagues (1997) found abnormal CAG expansion in three of six clinically diagnosed cases of senile chorea. Although the authors suggest that some patients with senile chorea have a sporadic form of HD, the term *essential* (or *senile*) *chorea* should be reserved for those patients with late-onset chorea without family history, without dementia, without psychiatric problems, and without CAG expansion. These criteria are necessary in order to separate senile or essential chorea from HD. Hereditary chorea without dementia and with a benign course has also been described (Behan and Bone, 1977). This benign hereditary chorea usually starts in early childhood and progresses until the second decade, after which time it remains static or even spontaneously improves. It appears to be inherited in an autosomal-dominant pattern and has been linked to the 6.93-KcM region on chromosome 14q (Fernandez et al., 2001).

Choreathetosis, along with developmental arrest, pendular nystagmus, optic atrophy, dysphagia, and severe bilateral striatal atrophy with response to biotin, is a feature of familial infantile bilateral necrosis, an autosomal-recessive disorder that has been mapped to 19q13.32–13.41 (Straussberg et al., 2002; Basel-Vanagaite et al., 2004).

## INFECTIOUS CHOREA

A variety of infections that affect the central nervous system have been associated with chorea. Acute manifestations of bacterial meningitis, encephalitis, tuberculous meningitis, and aseptic meningitis include movement disorders such as chorea, athetosis, dystonia, or hemiballismus (Alarcon et al., 2000). Human immunodeficiency virus (HIV) has also been reported to cause chorea and other features of HD, either as the result of human immunodeficiency virus encephalitis (Sevigny et al., 2005) or as the result of focal opportunistic infections such as toxoplasmosis (Nath et al., 1987; Gallo et al., 1996; Pardo et al., 1998; Piccolo et al., 1999).

## POSTINFECTIOUS AND AUTOIMMUNE CHOREAS

Occasionally still referred to as St. Vitus chorea or St. Vitus dance (Krack, 1999), Sydenham disease, an autoimmune chorea that was described originally by Thomas Sydenham, an English physician, is considered a consequence of infection with group A streptococcus (Swedo, 1994; Cardoso et al., 1997; Cardoso, 2004) (Videos 16-3 and 16-4). Osler, in his seminal paper "On Chorea and Choreiform Affections," published in 1894, drew attention to the distinction between Sydenham disease and HD (Goetz, 2000). Since chorea is only one of many manifestations, the term *Sydenham disease* is preferred, rather than *Sydenham chorea*, but the latter is used so frequently in the literature that its usage will be difficult to change. Some features of Sydenham disease overlap with those of Tourette syndrome. There is controversy as to whether pediatric autoimmune neuropsychiatric disorders associated with streptococcal infections, which may be associated with motor and phonic tics, is a variant of Sydenham disease or a separate entity (Kurlan, 2004). Although tics are often differentiated from chorea by the presence of premonitory sensation, reported by more than 90% of patients with Tourette syndrome (Kwak et al., 2003a), some patients with chorea also report sensory symptoms (Rodopman-Arman et al., 2004). Other features of Sydenham disease include dysarthria and decreased verbal output, hypometric saccades, oculogyric crisis, papilledema, central retinal artery occlusion, and seizures. Like Tourette syndrome (Kwak et al., 2003b), migraine is more common in children with Sydenham disease than in controls (Teixeira et al., 2005). Unlike arthritis and carditis, which occur soon after streptococcal infection, chorea and various neurobehavioral symptoms may be delayed for 6 months or longer and may be the sole manifestation of rheumatic fever (Stollerman, 1997). In 50 consecutive patients with rheumatic fever, 26% developed chorea, but arthritis was more frequent in patients without chorea (84%) than in those with chorea (31%) (Cardoso et al., 1997). Although the majority of the patients have bilateral involvement, the distribution of chorea is usually asymmetric, and pure hemichorea can be seen in 20% of all Sydenham disease patients. The individual contractions are slightly longer in Sydenham disease (>100 msec) compared to those in HD (50 to 100 msec) (Hallett and Kaufman, 1981). Behavioral problems associated with Sydenham disease include irritability, emotional lability, obsessive-compulsive disorder, hyperactivity, learning disorders, and other behavioral problems that are typically observed in patients with Tourette syndrome. One study compared 56 patients with Sydenham disease with 50 rheumatic fever patients and 50 healthy subjects and found that obsessive-compulsive behavior was present in 19%, obsessive-compulsive disorder in 23.2%, and attention deficit-hyperactivity disorder in 30.4%, all significantly more frequently than in the diseased or healthy controls (Maia et al., 2005). The neurobehavioral symptoms usually begin within 2 to 4 weeks after the onset of the choreic movements. The disorder tends to resolve spontaneously in 3 to 4 months but may persist in half of the patients during a 3-year follow-up (Cardoso et al., 1999). Female gender and the presence of carditis might be risk factors for persistent disease. In some cases of Sydenham disease, the chorea recurs during pregnancy (chorea gravidarum) or when the patient is exposed to estrogen. Sydenham disease, once relatively common, is now encountered relatively rarely in developed countries (Eshel et al., 1993). Recurrences of Sydenham disease are not associated with anti–basal ganglia antibodies (Harrison et al., 2004).

In addition to elevated titers of antistreptolysin, the majority of patients have been found to have IgG antibodies reacting with neurons in the caudate and subthalamic nuclei (Kiessling et al., 1993; Swedo et al., 1993). High antistreptolysin titer is not specific for group A streptococcal infection; it can also reflect group G. These antineuronal antibodies are found in nearly all patients with Sydenham disease (Swedo, 1994; Abraham et al., 1997; Mittleman, 1997). The rheumatic B-cell alloantigen D8/17 is also frequently found in patients with rheumatic chorea, but it is not clear whether this could be used as a diagnostic test (Feldman et al., 1993). Anti–basal ganglia antibodies have been identified in patients with acute and persistent Sydenham disease, providing further evidence that the disease is an antibody-mediated disorder (Church et al., 2002).

Although cephalosporins are equally effective, 500 to 1000 mg of penicillin G four times per day or one intramuscular injection of 600,000 to 1.2 million U of benzathine penicillin is considered the drug of choice for pharyngitis caused by beta-hemolytic streptococcal infection (Garvey and Swedo, 1997). Despite an adequate (10-day) course, the bacteriologic failure rate is as high as 15%, and some patients develop rheumatic fever. Therefore, oral rifampin 20 mg/kg every 24 hours for four doses is recommended during the last 4 days of the 10-day course of penicillin therapy. Alternatively, oral rifampin 10 mg/kg can be given every 12 hours for eight doses with one dose of intramuscular benzathine penicillin G. Another alternative is oral clindamycin 20 mg/kg per day in three doses for 10 days. The best prevention of rheumatic fever is accurate diagnosis and adequate treatment of the initial acute pharyngitis. Penicillin prophylaxis is advisable in all patients for at least 10 years after rheumatic fever. Symptomatic treatment usually consists of antidopaminergic drugs, valproic acid, and carbamazepine until the condition resolves spontaneously. A double-blind placebo controlled study of prednisone showed beneficial effects on Sydenham disease (Paz et al., 2006).

Besides Sydenham disease associated with rheumatic fever, chorea has been recognized in a variety of other autoimmune processes, such as systemic lupus erythematosus (SLE). Choreic movements associated with pregnancy (chorea gravidarum) and with birth control pills probably result from common pathogenesis, and chorea gravidarum may be the first manifestation of SLE or may represent a variant of Sydenham disease. Chorea in SLE has been associated with the presence of antiphospholipid antibodies, a heterogeneous group of antibodies that produce platelet endothelial dysfunction and promote thrombogenesis. The primary antiphospholipid syndrome is characterized by the presence of antiphospholipid antibodies in patients who have autoimmune phenomena but insufficient clinical or serologic features to be classified as having SLE. This syndrome is associated with migraine, chorea, and venous or arterial thrombosis (Gutrecht et al., 1991; Cervera et al., 1997). Other clinical features include spontaneous abortions, arthralgias, Raynaud phenomenon, digital infarctions, transient ischemic attacks, and stroke (Lang et al., 1991). Anticardiolipin antibodies, frequently found in SLE, are absent in patients with Sydenham disease. Chorea occurs in 2% of patients with SLE, and choreic movements precede the diagnosis of SLE in 22% of these cases.

MRI is usually normal in patients with Sydenham disease except for selective enlargement of the caudate, putamen, and globus pallidus (Giedd et al., 1995). In contrast to other choreic disorders, PET scans in patients with Sydenham disease indicate increased rather than decreased striatal glucose consumption (Weindl et al., 1993). Contralateral striatal hypermetabolism was documented by a $^{18}$F-fluorodeoxyglucose PET scan in a 23-year-old woman with alternating hemichorea and antiphospholipid syndrome (Furie et al., 1994). The striatal D1 and D2 receptor binding, measured by PET scans, was normal in one patient with SLE (Turjanski et al., 1995).

## OTHER CHOREAS

One of the most common forms of chorea encountered in a movement disorder clinic is drug-induced chorea associated with the use of dopaminergic or antidopaminergic drugs, anticonvulsants, and other drugs (Hyde et al., 1991; Jankovic, 1995). Levodopa-induced dyskinesia is often manifested by stereotypies, dystonia, and myclonus, as well as by chorea (Jankovic, 2005) (Video 16-5). Although the dominant hyperkinetic movement disorder that is seen in patients with tardive dyskinesia is stereotypy, some patients have associated chorea, and chorea is the chief manifestation in children with withdrawal emergent syndrome (see Chapter 20). Chorea, often accompanied by ataxia and deafness, has also been associated with mitochondrial DNA mutations (Nelson et al., 1995) and other evidence of mitochondrial cytopathy (Caer et al., 2005). The disorder of early-onset ataxia with oculomotor apraxia and hypoalbuminemia due to mutations in the *aprataxin* gene on chromosome 19p13 has also been associated with chorea (Shimazaki et al., 2002).

Besides vasculitis, chorea has been associated with a variety of other vascular etiologies, but few have been documented pathologically. The topic of vascular chorea has been reviewed in a report of an 85-year-old woman who developed progressive dementia and chorea at age 70 (Bhatia et al., 1994). At autopsy, her brain showed neostriatal neuronal loss and gliosis associated with congophilic angiopathy and atherosclerosis.

During the 1980s, there was an increase in the number of children with chorea as sequelae to cardiac surgery, but with modification of treatment strategies during the perioperative period, the incidence of this complication has subsequently decreased (Robinson et al., 1988). This postpump chorea appears to be associated with prolonged time on pump, deep hypothermia, and circulatory arrest (Medlock et al., 1993; Newburger et al., 1993; du Plessis et al., 2002) (Videos 16-6 and 16-7). Others have suggested that hypoxia rather than hypothermia is critical in the development of CHAP syndrome (choreathetosis and orofacial dyskinesia, hypotonia, and pseudobulbar signs) after surgery for congenital heart disease. In most patients, the chorea persists, and fewer than 25% improve with antidopaminergic therapy such as haloperidol. Steroid-responsive chorea was described in a patient after heart transplant (Blunt et al., 1994). Although the chorea may improve, long-term studies have shown that these children have persistent deficits in memory, attention, and language (du Plessis et al., 2002).

A variety of systemic (Janavs and Aminoff, 1998), metabolic, and neurodegenerative disorders can be associated with chorea, such as hypocalcemia or hypercalcemia, hyperglycemia (Ahlskog et al., 2001; Chu et al., 2002; Oh et al., 2002), hyperthyroidism (Pozzan et al., 1992), B12 deficiency (Pacchetti et al., 2002), Lesch-Nyhan syndrome (Jankovic et al., 1988; Jinnah et al., 1994; Ernst et al., 1996), propionic acidemia (Nyhan et al., 1999), and other metabolic disorders such as glutaric aciduria and GM1 gangliosidosis (Shulman et al., 1995; Stacy and Jankovic, 1995). Chorea (with or without associated ballism) has been reported as the presenting feature of renal chorea (Kujawa et al., 2001) and paraneoplastic striatal encephalitis (Tani et al., 2000; Vernino et al., 2002; Kinirons et al., 2003). In a series of 16 patients with paraneoplastic chorea, 11 had small-cell carcinoma, all had CRMP-5 IgGG, and 6 had ANNA-1 (anti-Hu) antibodies (Vernino et al., 2002). Another metabolic cause of chorea is liver disease, particularly chronic acquired hepatocerebral degeneration (Thobois et al., 2002) (Video 16-8). Many of the metabolic choreas are associated with abnormalities on MRI scans. For example, hepatocerebral degeneration and hyperglycemic chorea are often associated with high signal intensity on T1-weighted MRI, involving the striatum and pallidum (Ahlskog et al., 2001; Thobois et al., 2002). In a report of two patients with hyperglycemic hemichorea-hemiballism, Chu and colleagues (2002) found high signal intensities on T1- and T2-weighted images as well as on diffusion-weighted MRI accompanied by a reduction in diffusion coefficient, suggestive of suggesting hyperviscosity, rather than petechial hemorrhages, as the mechanism of edema in the striatum. Other disorders frequently associated with this MRI abnormality include manganese toxicity, Wilson disease, abnormal calcium metabolism, neurofibromatosis, hypoxia, and hemorrhage.

## TREATMENT OF CHOREA

The first step in the treatment of chorea is the identification of a specific etiology. Chorea has been treated successfully with drugs that interfere with central dopaminergic function, such as the dopamine receptor–blocking drugs (neuroleptics), reserpine, and tetrabenazine (Jankovic and Beach, 1997; Chatterjee and Frucht, 2003; Kenney and Jankovic, 2006).

Indeed, tetrabenazine provides the most effective relief of chorea with only minimal, dose-related side effects, such as drowsiness, insomnia, depression, and parkinsonism. Tetrabenazine is effective not only for the treatment of chorea associated with HD (Ondo et al., 2002; Huntington Study Group, 2006) but also for choreatic disorders associated with tardive dyskinesia (Ondo et al., 1999), cerebral palsy, and post-pump encephalopathy (Chatterjee and Frucht, 2003) (see Video 16-6). While some studies have suggested that sodium valproate may be effective in the treatment of chorea (Daoud, 1990; Hoffman and Feinberg, 1990), other reports have been less conclusive (Sethi and Patel, 1990). Levetiracetam has been reported to markedly improve a patient with cerebral palsy and postinfectious chorea (Recio et al., 2005). Clonazepam can sometimes suppress chorea (Peiris et al., 1976).

There is no consensus as to the optimal management of autoimmune chorea. Patients with Sydenham disease should be treated with penicillin prophylactically to prevent rheumatic fever. Symptomatic suppression of chorea with dopamine antagonists may lessen disability. Anticoagulation, immuno-suppressants, and plasmapheresis have been utilized with variable success, and the frequent occurrence of spontaneous remissions makes the results of treatment difficult to interpret. Until prospective therapeutic trials can be designed, careful selection of treatment that best seems to suit the severity of the patient's illness might be indicated. The presence of true vasculitis might require more aggressive management. Steroids are sometimes recommended for the treatment of autoimmune chorea, and this treatment was found effective also in chorea associated with heart transplant (Blunt et al., 1994). Stereotactic surgery is occasionally needed in very severe and disabling cases of hemichorea/hemiballism (Krauss and Mundinger, 2000).

## BALLISM

Chorea, athetosis, and ballism represent a continuum of involuntary, hyperkinetic movement disorders. Ballism is a form of forceful, flinging, high-amplitude, coarse, chorea (Videos 16-9 and 16-10). Ballism and chorea are often inter-related and may occur in the same patient (Harbord and Kobayashi, 1991). The involuntary movement usually affects only one side of the body; the term *hemiballism* is used to describe unilateral ballism. Although various structural lesions have been associated with ballism (Rossetti et al., 2003), damage to the subthalamic nucleus and the pallidosub-thalamic pathways appears to play a critical role in the expression of this hyperkinetic movement disorder (Guridi and Obeso, 2001). Subthalamotomy has been found to ameliorate the motor disturbances in human and experimental parkin-sonism, but the procedure can produce transient or perma-nent hemiballism (Bergman et al., 1990; Aziz et al., 1991; Guridi and Obeso, 2001; Chen et al., 2002).

When caused by a hemorrhagic or ischemic stroke, the movement disorder is often preceded by hemiparesis. Anterior parietal artery stroke, without any evidence of involvement of the basal ganglia, thalamus, or subthalamic nucleus, has been associated with contralateral hemiballism and neurogenic pain (Rossetti et al., 2003). This and other similar cases sug-gest that the lesion associated with hemiballism may extend beyond the contralateral subthalamic nucleus and connecting structures into the adjacent internal capsule. Less common

causes of hemiballism include abscess, arteriovenous mal-formation, cerebral trauma, hyperosmotic hyperglycemia (Ahlskog et al., 2001), multiple sclerosis, and tumor (Glass et al., 1984). Rarely, ballism occurs bilaterally (paraballism), usually due to bilateral basal ganglia strokes or calcification (Inbody and Jankovic, 1986; Vidakovic et al., 1994). In a series of 21 patients with hemiballism, hemichorea, or both, an iden-tifiable cause was found in all (Dewey and Jankovic, 1989). Stroke was the most common cause, followed by tumors, abscesses, encephalitis, vasculitis, and other causes. In a series of 23 patients with hemiballism and 2 with biballism, Vidakovic and colleagues (1994) found ischemic and hemor-rhagic strokes to be the most common causes of hemiballism. Other causes included encephalitis, Sydenham disease, SLE, basal ganglia calcifications, nonketotic hyperglycemia, tuber-ous sclerosis, and overlap between Fisher syndrome and Guillain-Barré syndrome (Odaka et al., 1999). Only two patients had "pure" hemiballism, and only six showed a lesion in the subthalamic nucleus on neuroimaging studies. The prognosis for spontaneous remission was good; nine patients completely recovered, and in seven additional patients, there was complete recovery of the ballism, but mild chorea had per-sisted. While hemichorea-hemiballism is usually contralateral to a basal ganglia lesion, ipsilateral hemichorea-hemiballism has been described in patients with contralateral hemiparesis (Krauss et al., 1999). The mechanism of this peculiar phenom-enon is unknown. Survival rates following vascular hemiballis-mus are similar to those of vascular disease, with only 32% survival and 27% stroke-free survival 150 months following the onset of the movement disorder (Ristic et al., 2002).

## TREATMENT OF BALLISM

The frequent occurrence of spontaneous remission makes the assessment of therapy difficult. Dopamine receptor–blocking drugs such as perphenazine, haloperidol, chlorpromazine, pimozide, and atypical neuroleptics have been used most fre-quently (Dewey and Jankovic, 1989; Shannon, 1990; Bashir and Manyam, 1994). Dopamine-depleting drugs, such as reserpine and tetrabenazine, have also been used successfully (Jankovic and Beach, 1997). Some clinicians consider tetra-benazine the preferred drug for its rapid onset of action and its effectiveness, without the danger of inducing tardive dysk-inesia if chronic antidopaminergic treatment is needed. Other drugs that are sometimes beneficial in the treatment of bal-lism include sodium valproate and clonazepam. Finally, ven-trolateral thalamotomy and other stereotactic surgeries may be needed to control violent and disabling contralateral hemiballism (Cardoso et al., 1995; Krauss and Mundinger, 2000). Although effective and relatively safe, this procedure should be used only as a last resort in patients with disabling and medically intractable movement disorder.

## ATHETOSIS

Athetosis is a slow form of chorea that consists of writhing movements resembling dystonia, but in contrast to dystonia, these movements are not sustained, patterned, repetitive, or painful. Originally described by Hammond in acquired hemidystonia and by Shaw in cerebral palsy, athetosis should be viewed as a movement disorder separate from dystonia (Morris et al., 2002a). The relationship of athetosis to chorea is highlighted not only by the continuously changing direction of movement, but also by the observation that chorea often evolves into athetosis or vice versa. In some patients, particularly children, chorea and athetosis often coexist, hence the term *choreoathetosis*. Dystonia, particularly involving the trunk causing opisthotonic posturing, also frequently accompanies athetosis, particularly in children with cerebral palsy (Video 16-11). In contrast to idiopathic dystonia, athetosis associated with perinatal brain injury often causes facial grimacing and spasms, particularly during speaking and eating and the bulbar function is usually impaired.

Athetosis most often accompanies cerebral palsy, an umbrella term for a group of motor-sensory cerebral disorders manifested since early childhood and attributed to various etiologies (Kyllerman, 1982; Foley, 1983; Murphy et al., 1995; Goddard-Finegold, 1998; Morris et al., 2002b; Cowan et al., 2003; Ashwal et al., 2004; Koman et al., 2004; Keogh and Badawi, 2006). In addition to motor disorders manifested chiefly by weakness and hypertonia (i.e., spasticity, rigidity, athetosis, dystonia), patients with cerebral palsy may have cognitive impairment, mental retardation, epilepsy, visual and hearing problems, and other neurologic deficits. As a result of hypertonia, many patients with untreated cerebral palsy develop fixed contractures. With the advent of botulinum toxin treatment, intrathecal baclofen infusion, and selective dorsal rhizotomy, coupled with aggressive physical therapy and antispastic drugs, these sequelae can be largely prevented.

Although there has been a steady decline in infant mortality, the incidence of cerebral palsy has remained unchanged. Because of the higher frequency of premature births, the frequency of certain types of cerebral palsy, such as spastic diplegia, has been increasing. In one study of children born at 25 or fewer completed weeks of gestation, half of the patients at 30 months of age were considered disabled, 18% were diagnosed with cerebral palsy, and 24% had gait difficulties (Wood et al., 2000). Kernicterus, once a common cause of cerebral palsy, is now rare. Besides delayed developmental milestones and athetotic or dystonic movements, patients with kernicterus often exhibit vertical ophthalmoparesis, deafness, and dysplasia of the dental enamel. Although improved perinatal care has reduced the frequency of birth-related injuries, birth asphyxia with anoxia is still a relatively common cause of cerebral palsy (Kuban and Leviton, 1994; Cowan et al., 2003). Intrauterine insults, particularly chorioamnionitis and prolonged rupture of membranes (Murphy et al., 1995), might be responsible for many of the cases of cerebral palsy. In one study of 351 full-term infants with neonatal encephalopathy, early seizures, or both, excluding infants with congenital malformations and obvious chromosomal disorders, MRI showed evidence of an acute insult in 69% to 80% (Cowan et al., 2003). The higher figure correlated with evidence of perinatal asphyxia. Both above-normal and below-normal weight at birth are also significant risk factors for cerebral palsy (Jarvis et al., 2003). These data strongly suggest that events in the immediate perinatal period are most important in the neonatal brain injury. An analysis of 58 brains of patients with clinical diagnosis of cerebral palsy showed wide morphologic variation, but the authors were able to classify the brains into three major categories: thinned cerebral mantle ($n = 10$), hydrocephalus ($n = 3$), and microgyria-pachygyria ($n = 45$)

(Tsusi et al., 1999). Of the 19 brains that were examined microscopically, four showed heterotopic gray matter, three showed cortical folding (cortical dysplasia), and three showed neuronal cytomegaly. The majority of the examined brains showed a variable degree of laminal disorganization in the cortex and disorientation of neurons, suggesting impaired neuronal migration during cortical development. Because of 5% to 10% of family history of athetoid cerebral palsy, genetic factors are considered important in the pathogenesis of this disorder (Fletcher and Foley, 1993). In a study based on the Swedish registry, 40% of cases of cerebral palsy were thought to have a genetic basis (Costeff, 2004). A growing number of studies also draw attention to inflammation and coagulation abnormalities in children with cerebral palsy. The increased concentrations of interleukins, tumor necrosis factor, reactive antibodies to lupus anticoagulant, anticardiolipin, antiphospholipid, antithrombin III, epidermal growth factor, and other abnormal cytokine patterns may play an important role in the etiology of cerebral palsy (Nelson et al., 1998; Kaukola et al., 2004). Kadhim and colleagues (2001) suggest that an early macrophage reaction and associated cytokine production and coagulation necrosis, coupled with intrinsic vulnerability of the immature oligodendrocyte, lead to periventricular leukomalacia, the most common neuropathologic changes found in premature infants who develop cerebral palsy. Although infection and inflammation, along with free radicals, can activate the process that leads to periventricular leukomalacia and even to delayed progression (Scott and Jankovic, 1996), the cause or pathogenesis of cerebral palsy is still not well understood.

Often referred to as static encephalopathy, the neurologic deficit associated with cerebral palsy may progress with time. Motor development curves derived by assessing patients with the Gross Motor Function Measure, used to prognosticate gross motor function in patients with cerebral palsy, indicate that, depending on their level of impairment (levels I to V) 3 to 10 years after birth, the natural course becomes static (Rosenbaum et al., 2002). We and others, however, found that some patients continue to progress, and others may progress after a period of static course. In about half of the patients with cerebral palsy, the abnormal movements become apparent within the first year of life, but in some cases, they might not appear until the fifth decade or even later. The mechanism by which such "delayed-onset" movement disorder becomes progressive after decades of a static course is unknown (Scott and Jankovic, 1996), but aberrant regeneration and sprouting of nerve fibers has been considered. In contrast to the other forms of cerebral palsy (e.g., diplegic or spastic and hemiplegic), the athetoid variety, which constitutes only about a quarter of all cases, is usually not associated with significant cognitive impairment or epilepsy. Although here athetosis is emphasized, the most common movement disorder in patients with cerebral palsy is spasticity (Albright, 1995).

Many other disorders associated with developmental delay and mental retardation can cause athetosis. Some are due to errors in metabolism and include acidurias, lipidoses, and Lesch-Nyhan syndrome (Jankovic et al., 1988; Stacy and Jankovic, 1995; see Box 16-1). Although athetosis is usually associated with perinatal brain injury, the neuroimaging studies often fail to show basal ganglia pathology. Finally, athetotic movements, or "pseudoathetosis," can be seen in patients with severe proprioceptive deficit (Sharp et al., 1994).

## TREATMENT OF ATHETOSIS

Athetosis usually does not respond well to pharmacologic therapy. Because dopa-responsive dystonia is sometimes confused with athetoid cerebral palsy, it is prudent to treat all these patients with levodopa. If levodopa fails to provide any meaningful benefit, then anticholinergic drugs should be tried in the same manner as is done in treating dystonia. Although generally recommended, physical therapy might or might not prevent contractures, and its role in altering the eventual outcome is uncertain (Palmer et al., 1988). Other complications of cerebral palsy, such as carpal tunnel syndrome, cervical spondylosis with radiculopathy, and myelopathy, require independent assessment and treatment (Hirose and Kadoya, 1984; Treves and Korczyn, 1986).

## References

Abraham S, O'Gorman M, Shulman ST: Anti-nuclear antibodies in Sydenham's chorea. Adv Exp Med Biol 1997;418:153–156.

Ahlskog JE, Nishimo H, Evidente VGH, et al : Persistent chorea triggered by hyperglycemic crisis in diabetics. Mov Disord 2001; 16:890–898.

Alarcon F, Duenas G, Cevallos N, et al: Movement disorders in 30 patients with tuberculous meningitis. Mov Disord 2000;15: 561–569.

Albright AL : Spastic cerebral palsy. Approaches to drug treatment. CNS Drugs 1995;4:17–27.

Allen FH Jr, Krabbe SM, Corcoran PA: A new phenotype (McLeod) in the Kell blood-group system.Vox Sang 1961;6:555–560.

Ashwal S, Russman BS, Blasco PA, et al: Practice parameter: Diagnostic assessment of the child with cerebral palsy: Report of the Quality Standards Subcommittee of the American Academy of Neurology and the Practice Committee of the Child Neurology Society. Neurology 2004;62:851–863.

Asmus F, Horber V, Pohlenz J, et al: A novel TITF-1 mutation causes benign hereditary chorea with response to levodopa. Neurology 2005;64:1952–1954.

Aziz TZ, Peggs D, Sambrook MA, Crossman AR: Lesion of the sub-thalamic nucleus for the alleviation of 1-methyl-4-phenyl-1,2,3,6-tetrahydropyridine (MPTP)-induced parkinsonism in the primate. Mov Disord 1991;6:288–292.

Basel-Vanagaite L, Straussberg R, Ovadia H, et al: Infantile bilateral striatal necrosis maps to chromosome 19q. Neurology 2004;62: 87–90.

Bashir K, Manyam BV: Clozapine for the control of hemiballism. Clin Neuropharmacol 1994;17:477–480.

Bassen FA, Kornzweig AL: Malformation of the erythrocytes in a case of atypical retinitis pigmentosa. Blood 1950;5:381–387.

Becher MW, Ross CA: Intranuclear neuronal inclusions in DRPLA. Mov Disord 1998;13:852–953.

Becher MW, Rubinsztein DC, Leggo J, et al: Dentatorubral and pallidoluysian atrophy (DRPLA): Clinical and neuropathological findings in genetically confirmed North American and European pedigrees. Mov Disord 1997;12:519–530.

Behan PO, Bone A: Hereditary chorea without dementia. J Neurol Neurosurg Psychiatry 1977;40:687–691.

Bergman H, Wichmann T, Delong MR: Reversal of experimental parkinsonism by lesions of the subthalamic nucleus. Science 1990;249:1436–1438.

Bhatia KP, Lera G, Luthert PJ, Marsden CD: Vascular chorea: Case report with pathology. Mov Disord 1994;9:447–450.

Blunt SB, Brooks DJ, Kennard C: Steroid-responsive chorea in childhood following cardiac transplantation. Mov Disord 1994; 9:112–113.

Bohlega S, Riley W, Powe J, et al: Neuroacanthocytosis and aprebetalipoproteinemia. Neurology 1998;50:1912–1914.

Breedveld GJ, Percy AK, MacDonald ME, et al: Clinical and genetic heterogeneity in benign hereditary chorea. Neurology 2002;59: 579–584.

Brooks DJ, Ibanez V, Playford ED, et al: Presynaptic and postsynaptic striatal dopaminergic function in neuroacanthocytosis: A positron emission tomographic study. Ann Neurol 1991;30: 166–171.

Burke JR, Wingfield MS, Lewis KE, et al: The Haw River syndrome: Entatorubropallidoluysian atrophy in an African-American family. Nat Genet 1994;7:521–524.

Caer M, Viala K, Levy R, et al: Adult-onset chorea and mitochondrial cytopathy. Mov Disord 2005;20:490–492.

Cardoso F: Chorea: Non-genetic causes. Curr Opin Neurol 2004; 17:433–436.

Cardoso F, Eduardo C, Silva AP, Mota CC: Chorea in 50 consecutive patients with rheumatic fever. Mov Disord 1997;12:701–703.

Cardoso F, Jankovic J, Grossman RG, Hamilton WJ: Outcome following stereotactic thalamotomy for dystonia and hemiballism. Neurosurgery 1995;36:501–508.

Cardoso F, Vargas AP, Oliveira LD, et al: Persistent Sydenham's chorea. Mov Disord 1999;14:805–807.

Cervera R, Asherson RA, Font J, et al: Chorea in the antiphospholipid syndrome: Clinical, radiologic, and immunologic characteristics of 50 patients from our clinics and the recent literature. Medicine 1997;76:203–212.

Chatterjee A, Frucht SJ: Tetrabenazine in the treatment of severe pediatric chorea. Mov Disord 2003;18:703–706.

Chen CC, Lee ST, Wu T, et al: Hemiballism after subthalamotomy in patients with Parkinson's disease: Report of 2 cases. Mov Disord 2002;17:1367–1371.

Ching KHL, Westway SK, Gitschier J, et al: HARP syndrome is allelic with pantothenate-kinase-associated neurodegeneration. Neurology 2002;58:1673–1674.

Chu K, Kang DW, Kim DE, et al: Diffusion-weighted and gradient echo magnetic resonance findings of hemichorea-hemiballismus associated with diabetic hyperglycemia: A hyperviscosity syndrome? Arch Neurol 2002;59:448–452.

Church AJ, Cardoso F, Dale RC, et al: Anti-basal ganglia antibodies in acute and persistent Sydenham's chorea. Neurology 2002;59: 227–231.

Costeff H: Estimated frequency of genetic and nongenetic causes of congenital idiopathic cerebral palsy in west Sweden. Ann Hum Genet 2004;68:515–520.

Cowan F, Rutherford M, Groenendaal F, et al: Origin and timing of brain lesions in term infants with neonatal encephalopathy. Lancet 2003;361:736–742.

Danek A, Jung HH, Melone MA, et al: Neuroacanthocytosis: New developments in a neglected group of dementing disorders. J Neurol Sci 2005;229–230:171–186.

Danek A, Rubio JP, Rampoldi L, et al: McLeod neuroacanthocytosis: Genotype and phenotype. Ann Neurol 2001a;50:755–764.

Danek A, Tison F, Rubio J, et al: The chorea of McLeod syndrome. Mov Disord 2001b;16:882–889.

Daoud AS, Zaki M, Shakir R, Al-Saleh Q: Effectiveness of sodium valproate in the treatment of Sydenham's chorea. Neurology 1990; 40:1140–1141.

de Vries BB, Arts WF, Breedveld GJ, et al: Benign hereditary chorea of early onset maps to chromosome 14q. Am J Hum Genet 2000; 66:136–142.

Dewey RB, Jankovic J: Hemiballism-hemichorea: Clinical and pharmacologic findings in 21 patients. Arch Neurol 1989;46:862–867.

DeYebenes JG, Brin MF, Mena MA, et al: Neurochemical findings in neuroacanthocytosis. Mov Disord 1988;3:300–312.

Dotti MT, Battisti C, Malandrini A, et al: McLeod syndrome and neuroacanthocytosis with a novel mutation in the XK gene. Mov Disord 2000;15 (6):1282–1284.

du Plessis AJ, Bellinger DC, Gauvreau K, et al: Neurologic outcome of choreoathetoid encephalopathy after cardiac surgery. Pediatr Neurol 2002;27:9–17.

Ernst M, Zametkin AJ, Matochik JA, et al: Presynaptic dopaminergic deficits in Lesch-Nyhan disease. N Engl J Med 1996;334:1568–1572.

Eshel G, Lahat E, Azizi E, et al: Chorea as a manifestation of rheumatic fever: A 30-year survey (1960–1990). Eur J Pediatr 1993; 152:645–646.

Feinberg TE, Cianci CD, Morrow JS, et al: Diagnostic tests for choreoacanthocytosis. Neurology 1991;41:1000–1006.

Feldman BM, Zabriskie JB, Silverman ED, Laxer RM: Diagnostic use of B-cell alloantigen D8/17 in rheumatic chorea. J Pediatr 1993;123:84–86.

Fernandez M, Raskind W, Matsushita M, et al: Hereditary benign chorea: Clinical and genetic features of a distinct disease. Neurology 2001;57:106–110.

Fletcher NA, Foley J: Parental age, genetic mutation, and cerebral palsy. J Med Genet 1993;30:44–46.

Foley J: The athetoid syndrome: A review of a personal series. J Neurol Neurosurg Psychiatry 1983;46:289–298.

Fox SH, Nieves A, Bergeron C, Lang AE: Pure cerebello-olivary degeneration of Marie, Foix, and Alajouanine presenting with progressive cerebellar ataxia, cognitive decline, and chorea. Mov Disord 2003;18:1550–1554.

Friedman JH, Ambler M: A case of senile chorea. Mov Disord 1990; 5:251–253.

Furie R, Ishikawa T, Dhawan V, Eidelberg D: Alternating hemichorea in primary antiphospholipid syndrome: Evidence for contralateral striatal hypermetabolism. Neurology 1994;44:2197–2199.

Gallo BV, Shulman LM, Weiner WJ, et al: HIV encephalitis presenting with severe generalized chorea. Neurology 1996;46:1163–1165.

Garvey MA, Swedo SE: Sydenham's chorea. Clinical and therapeutic update. Adv Exp Med Biol 1997;418:115–120.

Giedd JN, Rapoport JL, Kruesi MJP, et al: Sydenham's chorea: Magnetic resonance imaging of the basal ganglia. Neurology 1995;45:2199–2202.

Glass JP, Jankovic J, Borit A: Hemiballismus and metastatic brain tumor. Neurology 1984;34:204–207.

Goddard-Finegold J: Perinatal aspects of cerebral palsy. In Miller G, Clark GD (eds): The Cerebral Palsies. Boston, Butterworth-Heinemann, 1998, pp 151–173.

Goetz CG: William Osler: On Chorea: On Charcot. Ann Neurol 2000;47:404–407.

Grimes DA, Lang AE, Bergeron C: Late adult onset chorea with typical pathology of Hallervorden-Spatz syndrome. J Neurol Neurosurg Psychiatry 2000;69:392–395.

Guridi J, Obeso JA: The subthalamic nucleus, hemiballismus and Parkinson's disease: Reappraisal of a neurosurgical dogma. Brain 2001;124:5–19.

Gutrecht JA, Kattwinkel N, Stillman MJ: Retinal migraine, chorea, and retinal artery thrombosis in a patient with primary antiphospholipid antibody syndrome. J Neurol 1991;238:55–56.

Hagerman RJ, Leehey M, Heinrichs W, et al: Intention tremor, parkinsonism, and generalized brain atrophy in male carriers of fragile X. Neurology 2001;57:127–130.

Hallett M, Kaufman C: Physiological observations in Sydenham's chorea. J Neurol Neurosurg Psychiatry 1981;44:829–832.

Hanajima R, Ugawa Y, Terao Y, et al: Intracortical inhibition of the motor cortex is normal in chorea. J Neurol Neurosurg Psychiatry 1999;66:783–786.

Harbord MG, Kobayashi JS: Fever producing ballismus in patients with choreoathetosis. J Child Neurol 1991;6:49–52.

Hardie RJ, Pullon HWH, Harding AE, et al: Neuroacanthocytosis: A clinical, haematological and pathological study of 19 cases. Brain 1991;114:13–49.

Harrison NA, Church A, Nisbet A, et al: Late recurrences of Sydenham's chorea are not associated with anti-basal ganglia antibodies. J Neurol Neurosurg Psychiatry 2004;75:1478–1479.

Hayflick SJ, Westaway SK, Levinson B, et al: Genetic, clinical, and radiographic delineation of Hallervorden-Spatz syndrome. N Engl J Med 2003;348:33–40.

Hirose G, Kadoya S: Cervical spondylotic radiculo-myelopathy in patients with athetoid-dystonic cerebral palsy: Clinical evaluation and surgical treatment. J Neurol Neurosurg Psychiatry 1984;47:775–780.

Ho MF, Chalmers RM, Davis MB, et al: A novel point mutation in the McLeod syndrome gene in neuroacanthocytosis. Ann Neurol 1996;39:672–675.

Hoffman AS, Feinberg TE: Successful treatment of age-related chorea with sodium valproate. J Am Geriatr Soc 1990;38:56–58.

Holmes SE, O'Hearn E, Rosenblatt A, et al: A repeat expansion in the gene encoding junctophilin-3 is associated with Huntington disease-like 2. Nat Genet 2001;29:377–378.

Houlden H, Lincoln S, Farrer M, et al: Compound heterozygous PANK2 mutations confirm HARP and Hallervorden-Spatz syndromes are allelic. Neurology 2003;61:1423–1426.

Huntington Study Group: Tetrabenazine as antichorea therapy in Huntington disease: A randomized controlled trial. Neurology 2006;66:366–372.

Hyde TM, Hotson JR, Kleinman JE: Differential diagnosis of choreiform tardive dyskinesia. J Neuropsychiatry 1991;3:255–268.

Igarashi S, Koide R, Shimohata T, et al: Suppression of aggregate formation and apoptosis by transglutaminase inhibitors in cells expressing truncated DRPLA proteins with an expanded polyglutamine stretch. Nat Genet 1998;18:111–117.

Ikeuchi T, Koide R, Tanaka H, et al: Dentatorubral-pallidoluysian atrophy: Clinical features are closely related to unstable expansions of trinucleotide (CAG) repeat. Ann Neurol 1995;37:769–775.

Inbody S, Jankovic J: Hyperkinetic mutism: Bilateral ballism and basal ganglia calcification. Neurology 1986;36:825–827.

Janavs J, Aminoff MJ: Dystonia and chorea in acquired systemic disorders. J Neurol Neurosurg Psychiatry 1998;65:436–445.

Jankovic J: Tardive syndromes and other drug-induced movement disorders. Clin Neuropharmacol 1995;18:197–214.

Jankovic J: Motor fluctuations and dyskinesias in Parkinson's disease: Clinical manifestations. Mov Disord 2005;20(suppl 11):S11–S6.

Jankovic J, Beach J: Long-term effects of tetrabenazine in hyperkinetic movement disorders. Neurology 1997;48:358–362.

Jankovic J, Caskey TC, Stout JT, Butler I: Lesch-Nyhan syndrome: A study of motor behavior and CSF monoamine turnover. Ann Neurol 1988;23:466–469.

Jarvis S, Glinianaia SV, Torrioli MG, et al: Surveillance of Cerebral Palsy in Europe (SCPE) collaboration of European Cerebral Palsy Registers. Cerebral palsy and intrauterine growth in single births: European collaborative study. Lancet 2003;362:1106–1111.

Jinnah HA, Wojcik BE, Hunt M, et al: Dopamine deficiency in a genetic mouse model of Lesch-Nyhan disease. J Neurosci 1994; 14:1164–1175.

Jung HH, Hergerberg M, Kneifel S, et al: McLeod syndrome: A novel mutation, predominant psychiatric manifestations, and distinct striatal imaging findings. Ann Neurol 2001;49:384–392.

Kadhim H, Tabarki B, Verellen G, et al: Inflammatory cytokines in the pathogenesis of periventricular leukomalacia. Neurology 2001;56:1278–1284.

Kambouris M, Bohlega S, Al-Tahan A, Meyer BF: Localization of the gene for a novel autosomal recessive neurodegenerative Huntington-like disorder to 4p15.3. Am J Hum Genet 2000;66: 445–452.

Kaukola T, Satyaraj E, Patel DD, et al: Cerebral palsy is characterized by protein mediators in cord serum. Ann Neurol 2004;55:186–194.

Kawaguchi Y, Okamoto T, Taniwaki M, et al: CAG expansions in a novel gene from Machado-Joseph's disease at chromosome 14q32.1. Nat Genet 1994;8:221–228.

Kenney C, Jankovic J: Tetrabenazine in the treatment of hyperkinetic movement disorders. Expert Rev Neurotherapeutics 2006;6:7–17.

Keogh JM, Badawi N: The origins of cerebral palsy. Curr Opin Neurol 2006;19:129–134.

Kiessling LS, Marcotte AC, Culpepper L: Antineuronal antibodies in movement disorders. Pediatrics 1993;92:39–43.

Kim J-S, Lee K-S, Le K-H, et al: Evidence of thalamic disinhibition in patients with hemichorea: Semiquantitative analysis using SPECT. J Neurol Neurosurg Psychiatry 2002;72:329–333.

Kinirons P, Fulton A, Keoghan M, et al: Paraneoplastic limbic encephalitis (PLE) and chorea associated with CRMP-5 neuronal antibody. Neurology 2003;61:1623–1624.

Kleiner-Fisman G, Rogaeva E, Halliday W, et al: Benign hereditary chorea: Clinical, genetic, and pathological findings. Ann Neurol 2003;54:244–247.

Koide R, Ikeuchi T, Onodera O, et al: Unstable expansion of CAG repeat in hereditary dentatorubral-pallidoluysian atrophy (DRPLA). Nat Genet 1994;6:9–13.

Koide R, Onodera O, Ikeuchi T, et al: Atrophy of the cerebellum and brainstem in dentatorubral pallidoluysian atrophy: Influence of CAG repeat size on MRI findings. Neurology 1997;49:1605–1612.

Koman LA, Smith BP, Shilt JS: Cerebral palsy. Lancet 2004; 363:1619–1631.

Komure O, Sano A, Nishino N, et al: DNA analysis in hereditary dentatorubral-pallidolusian atrophy: Correlation between CAG repeat length and phenotypic variation and the molecular basis anticipation. Neurology 1995;45:143–149.

Krack P: Relicts of dancing mania: The dancing procession of Echternach. Neurology 1999;55:2169–2172.

Krauss JK, Mundinger F: Surgical treatment of hemiballism and hemichorea. In Krauss JK, Jankovic J, Grossman RG (eds): Surgery for Movement Disorders. Philadelphia, Lippincott Williams & Wilkins, 2000, pp 397–403.

Krauss JK, Pohle T, Borremans JJ: Hemichorea and hemiballism associated with contralateral hemiparesis and ipsilateral basal ganglia lesions. Mov Disord 1999;14:497–501.

Kuban KCK, Leviton A: Cerebral palsy. N Engl J Med 1994; 330: 188–195.

Kujawa KA, Niemi V, Tomasi MA, et al: Ballistic-choreic movement as the presenting feature of renal cancer. Arch Neurol 2001; 58:1133–1135.

Kurlan R: The PANDAS hypothesis: Losing its bite? Mov Disord 2004;19:371–374.

Kuroharas K, Kuroda Y, Maruyama H, et al: Homozygosity for an allele carrying intermediate CAG repeats in the dentatorubral-pallidoluysian atrophy (DRPLA) gene results in spastic paraplegia. Neurology 1997;48:1087–1090.

Kwak C, Dat Vuong K, Jankovic J: Premonitory sensory phenomenon in Tourette's syndrome. Mov Disord 2003a;18:1530–1533.

Kwak C, Vuong KD, Jankovic J: Migraine headache in patients with Tourette syndrome. Arch Neurol 2003b;60:1595–1598.

Kyllerman M: Dyskinetic cerebral palsy: II. Pathogenetic risk factors and intrauterine growth. Acta Paediatr Scand 1982;71:551–558.

La Spada AR, Paulson HL, Fischbeck KH: Trinucleotide repeat expansion in neurological disease. Ann Neurol 1994;36:814–822.

Lang AE, Sethi KD, Provias JP, Deck JH: What is it? Case 1,1991: A severe and fatal systemic illness first presenting with a movement disorder. Mov Disord 1991;6:362–370.

Lieberman AP, Robitaille Y, Trojanowski JQ, et al: Polyglutamine-containing aggregates in neuronal intranuclear inclusion disease. Lancet 1998;351:884.

Lossos A, Dobson-Stone C, Monaco AP, et al: Early clinical heterogeneity in choreoacanthocytosis. Arch Neurol 2005;62:611–614.

Maia DP, Teixeira AL Jr, Quintao Cunningham MC, Cardoso F: Obsessive compulsive behavior, hyperactivity, and attention deficit disorder in Sydenham chorea. Neurology 2005;64:1799–1801.

Malandrini A, Fabrizi GM, Bartalucci P, et al: Clinicopathological study of familial late infantile Hallervorden-Spatz disease: A particular form of neuroacanthocytosis. Childs Nerv Syst 1996;12:155–160.

Margolis RL, Holmes SE, Rosenblatt A, et al: Huntington's disease-like 2 (HDL2) in North America and Japan. Ann Neurol 2004; 56:670–674.

Margolis RL, O'Hearn E, Rosenblatt A, et al: A disorder similar to Huntington's disease is associated with a novel CAG repeat expansion. Ann Neurol 2001;50:373–380.

Mars H, Lewis LA, Robertson AL Jr, et al: Familial hypo-beta-lipoproteinemia: A genetic disorder of lipid metabolism with nervous system involvement. Am J Med 1969;46(6):886–900.

Medlock MD, Cruse RS, Winek SJ, et al: A 10-year experience with postpump chorea. Ann Neurol 1993;34:820–826.

Mittleman BB: Cytokine networks in Sydenham's chorea and PANDAS. Adv Exp Med Biol 1997;418:933–935.

Moore RC, Xiang F, Monaghan J, et al: Huntington disease phenocopy is a familial prion disease. Am J Hum Genet 2001;69:1385–1388.

Morris JGL, Jankelowitz SK, Fung VSC, et al: Athetosis: I. Historical considerations. Mov Disord 2002a;17:1278–1280.

Morris JGL, Grattan-Smith P, Jankelowitz SK, et al: Athetosis: II. The syndrome of mild athetoid cerebral palsy. Mov Disord 2002b; 17:1281–1287.

Muñoz E, Campdelacreu J, Ferrer I, et al: Severe cerebral white matter involvement in a case of dentatorubropallidoluysian atrophy studied at autopsy. Arch Neurol 2004;61:946–949.

Muñoz E, Mila M, Sanchez A, et al: Dentatorubropallidoluysian atrophy in a Spanish family: A clinical, radiological, pathological, and genetic study. J Neurol Neurosurg Psychiatry 1999;67:811–814.

Murphy DJ, Sellers S, MacKenzie IZ, et al: Case-control study of antenatal and intrapartum risk factors for cerebral palsy in very preterm singleton babies. Lancet 1995;346:1449–1454.

Nath A, Jankovic J, Pettigrew LC: Movement disorders and AIDS. Neurology 1987;37:36–41.

Nelson I, Hanna MG, Alsanjari N, et al: A new mitochondrial DNA mutation associated with progressive dementia and chorea: A clinical, pathological, and molecular genetic study. Ann Neurol 1995;37:400–403.

Nelson KB, Dambrosia JM, Grether JK, Phillips TM: Neonatal cytokines and coagulation factors in children with cerebral palsy. Ann Neurol 1998;44:665–675.

Newburger JW, Jonas RA, Wernovsky G, et al: A comparison of the perioperative neurologic effects of hypothermic circulatory arrest versus low-flow cardiopulmonary bypass in infant heart surgery. N Engl J Med 1993;329:1057–1064.

Nicholl DJ, Sutton I, Dotti MT, et al: White matter abnormalities on MRI in neuroacanthocytosis. J Neurol Neurosurg Psychiatry 2004;75:1200–1201.

Nishiyama K, Nakamura K, Murayama S, et al: Regional and cellular expression of the dentatorubral-pallidoluysian atrophy gene in brains of normal and affected individuals. Ann Neurol 1997; 41:599–605.

Nyhan WL, Bay C, Beyer EW, Mazi M: Neurologic nonmetabolic presentation of propionic acidemia. Arch Neurol 1999;56:1143–1147.

Odaka M, Yuki N, Hirata K: Bilateral ballism in a patient with overlapping Fisher's and Guillain-Barré syndromes. J Neurol Neurosurg Psychiatry 1999;67:206–208.

Oh S-H, Lee K-Y, Im J-H, Lee M-S: Chorea associated with nonketotic hyperglycemia and hyperintensity basal ganglia lesion on T1-weighted brain MRI study: A meta-analysis of 53 cases including four present cases. J Neurol Sci 2002;200:57–62.

Okamura-Oho Y, Miyashita T, Nagao K, et al: Dentatorubral-pallidoluysian atrophy protein is phosphorylated by c-Jun NH(2)-terminal kinase. Hum Mol Genet 2003;12:1535–1542.

Ondo WG, Hanna PA, Jankovic J: Tetrabenazine treatment for tardive dyskinesia: Assessment by randomized videotape protocol. Am J Psychiatry 1999;156:1279–1281.

Ondo WG, Tintner R, Thomas M, Jankovic J: Tetrabenazine treatment for Huntington's disease-associated chorea. Clin Neuropharmacol 2002;25:300–302.

Orrell RW, Amrolia PJ, Heald A, et al: Acanthocytosis, retinitis pigmentosa, and pallidal degeneration: A report of three patients, including the second reported case with hypoprebetalipoproteinemia (HARP) syndrome. Neurology 1995;45:487–492.

Pacchetti C, Cristina S, Nappi G, et al: Reversible chorea and focal dystonia in vitamin $B_{12}$ deficiency. N Engl J Med 2002;347:295.

Palmer FB, Shapiro BK, Wachtel RC, et al: The effects of physical therapy on cerebral palsy: A controlled trial in infants with spastic diplegia. N Engl J Med 1988;318:803–808.

Pardo J, Marcos A, Bhathal H, et al: Chorea as a form of presentation of human immunodeficiency virus-associated dementia complex. Neurology 1998;50:568–569.

Paz JA, Silva CA, Marques-Dias MJ: Randomized double-blind study with prednisone in Sydenham's chorea. Pediatr Neurol 2006; 34:264–269.

Peiris JB, Boralessa H, Lionel ND: Clonazepam in the treatment of choreiform activity. Med J Aust 1976;1(8):225–227.

Piccolo I, Causarano R, Sterzi R, et al: Chorea in patients with AIDS. Acta Neurol Scand 1999;100:332–336.

Pozzan GB, Battistella PA, Rigon F, et al: Hyperthyroid-induced chorea in an adolescent girl. Brain Dev 1992;14:126–127.

Racette BA, Perry A, D'Avossa G, Perlmutter JS: Late-onset neurodegeneration with brain iron accumulation type 1: Expanding the clinical spectrum. Mov Disord 2001;16:1148–1152.

Rampoldi L, Danek A, Monaco AP: Clinical features and molecular basis of neuroacanthocytosis. J Mol Med 2002;80:475–491.

Rampoldi L, Dobson-Stone C, Rubio JP, et al: A conserved sorting-associated protein is mutant in chorea-acanthocytosis. Nat Genet 2001;28:119–120.

Recio MV, Hauser RA, Louis ED, et al: Chorea in a patient with cerebral palsy: Treatment with levetiracetam. Mov Disord 2005;20:762–764.

Rinne JO, Daniel SE, Scaravilli F, et al: Nigral degeneration in neuroacanthocytosis. Neurology 1994a;44:1629–1632.

Rinne JO, Daniel SE, Scaravilli F, et al: The neuropathological features of neuroacanthocytosis. Mov Disord 1994b;9:297–304.

Ristic A, Marinkovic J, Dragasevic N, et al: Long-term prognosis of vascular hemiballismus. Stroke 2002;33:2109–2111.

Robinson RO, Samuels M, Pohls KRE: Choreic syndrome after cardiac surgery. Arch Dis Child 1988;63:1466–1469.

Rodopman-Arman A, Yazgan Y, Berkem M, Eraksoy M: Are sensory phenomena present in Sydenham's chorea? Evaluation of 13 cases. Neuropediatrics 2004;35:242–245.

Rosenbaum PL, Walter SD, Hanna SE, et al: Prognosis for gross motor function in cerebral palsy: Creation of motor development curves. JAMA 2002;288:1357–1363.

Rosenblatt A, Ranen NG, Rubinsztein DC, et al: Patients with features similar to Huntington's disease, without CAG expansion in huntingtin. Neurology 1998;51:215–220.

Ross CA, Margolis RL, Rosenblatt A, et al: Huntington disease and the related disorder, dentatorubral-pallidoluysian atrophy (DRPLA). Medicine (Baltimore) 1997;76:305–308.

Rossetti AO, Ghika JA, Vingerhoets F, et al: Neurogenic pain and abnormal movements contralateral to an anterior parietal artery stroke. Arch Neurol 2003;60:1004–1006.

Rubio JP, Danek A, Stone C, et al: Chorea-acanthocytosis: Genetic linkage to chromosome 9q21. Am J Hum Genet 1997;61:899–908.

Ruiz G, Gomez-Tortosa E, del Barrio A, et al: Senile chorea: A multicenter prospective study. Acta Neurol Scand 1997;95:180–183.

Saiki S, Sakai K, Kitagawa Y, et al: Mutation in the CHAC gene in a family of autosomal dominant chorea-acanthocytosis. Neurology 2003;61:1614–1616.

Sakai T, Antoku Y, Iwashita H, et al: Chorea-acanthocytosis: Abnormal composition of covalently bound fatty acids of erythrocyte membrane proteins. Ann Neurol 1991;29:664–669.

Schrag A, Quinn NP, Bhatia KP, et al: Benign hereditary chorea: Entity or syndrome? Mov Disord 2000;15:280–288.

Scott B, Jankovic J: Delayed-onset progressive movement disorders. Neurology 1996;46:68–74.

Sethi KD, Patel BP: Inconsistent response to divalproex sodium in hemichorea/hemiballism. Neurology 1990,40:1630–1631.

Sevigny JJ, Chin SS, Milewski Y, et al: HIV encephalitis simulating Huntington's disease. Mov Disord 2005;20:610–613.

Shannon KM: Hemiballismus. Clin Neuropharm 1990;13:413–425.

Sharp D, Blinderman L, Combs KA, et al: Cloning and gene defects in microsomal triglyceride transfer protein associated with abeta-lipoproteinemia. Nature 1993;365(6441):65–69.

Sharp FR, Rando TA, Greenberg SA, et al: Pseudochoreoathetosis: Movements associated with loss of proprioception. Arch Neurol 1994;51:1103–1109.

Shevell M: Hallervorden and history. N Engl J Med 2003;348:3–4.

Shimazaki H, Takiyama Y, Sakoe K, et al: Early-onset ataxia with ocular motor apraxia and hypoalbuminemia: The aprataxin gene mutations. Neurology 2002;59:590–595.

Shoulson I: On chorea. Clin Neuropharmacol 1986;9(suppl 2):S85–S99.

Shulman LM, Lang AE, Jankovic J, et al: What is it? Case 1, 1995: Psychosis, dementia, chorea, ataxia, and supranuclear gaze dysfunction. Mov Disord 1995;10:257–262.

Spitz MC, Jankovic J, Killian JM: Familial tic disorder, parkinsonism, motor neuron disease, and acanthocytosis: A new syndrome. Neurology 1985;35:366–377.

Stacy M, Jankovic J: Rare childhood movement disorders associated with metabolic and neurodegenerative disorders. In Roberts MM, Eapen V (eds): Movement and Allied Disorders in Childhood. Chichester, England, John Wiley & Sons, 1995, pp 177–197.

Stevanin G, Camuzat A, Holmes SE, et al: CAG/CTG repeat expansions at the Huntington's disease-like 2 locus are rare in Huntington's disease patients. Neurology 2002;58:965–967.

Stevanin G, Fujigasaki H, Lebre AS, et al: Huntington's disease-like phenotype due to trinucleotide repeat expansions in the TBP and JPH3 genes. Brain 2003;126:1599–1603.

Stollerman GH: Rheumatic fever. Lancet 1997;349:935–942.

Straussberg R, Shorer Z, Weitz R, et al: Familial infantile bilateral striatal necrosis: Clinical features and response to biotin treatment. Neurology 2002;59:983–989.

Swedo SE: Sydenham's chorea. A model for childhood autoimmune neuropsychiatric disorders. JAMA 1994;272:1788–1791.

Swedo SE, Leonard HL, Schapiro MB, et al: Sydenham's chorea: Physical and psychological symptoms of St Vitus dance. Pediatrics 1993;91:706–713.

Tani T, Piao Y-S, Mori S, et al: Chorea resulting from paraneoplastic striatal encephalitis. J Neurol Neurosurg Psychiatry 2000;69:512–515.

Teixeira AL Jr, Meira FCA, Maia DP, et al: Migraine headache in patients with Sydenham's chorea. Cephalalgia 2005;25:542-4.

Thobois S, Giraud P, Debat P, et al: Orofacial dyskinesias in a patient with primary biliary cirrhosis: A clinicopathological case report and review. Mov Disord 2002;17:415–419.

Thomas M, Hayflick SJ, Jankovic J: Clinical heterogeneity of neurodegeneration with iron accumulation–1 (Hallervorden-Spatz syndrome) and pantothenate kinase associated neurodegeneration (PKAN). Mov Disord 2004;19:36–42.

Thomas M, Jankovic J: Dentatorubropallidoluysian atrophy in North American families. Ann Neurol 2001;50(suppl 1):S65.

Toyoshima Y, Yamada M, Onodera O, et al: SCA17 homozygote showing Huntington's disease-like phenotype. Ann Neurol 2004;55:281–286.

Treves T, Korczyn AD: Progressive dystonia and paraparesis in cerebral palsy. Eur Neurol 1986;25:148–153.

Tsusi Y, Nagahama M, Mizutani A: Neuronal migration disorders in cerebral palsy. Neuropathology 1999;19:14–27.

Turjanski N, Weeks R, Dolan R, et al: Striatal D1 and D2 receptor binding in patients with Huntington's disease and other choreas. A PET study. Brain 1995;118:689–696.

Ueno S, Maruki Y, Nakamura M, et al: The gene encoding a newly discovered protein, chorein, is mutated in chorea-acanthocytosis. Nat Genet 2001;28:121–122.

Ueyama H, Kumamoto T, Nagao S, et al: A novel mutation of the McLeod syndrome gene in a Japanese family. J Neurol Sci 2000; 176(2):151–154.

Van der Meer, van der Weel, Lee DN: The functional significance of arm movements in neonates. Science 1995;267:693–695.

Vernino S, Tuite P, Adler CH, et al: Paraneoplastic chorea associated with CRMP-5 neuronal antibody and lung carcinoma. Ann Neurol 2002;51:625–630.

Vidakovic A, Dragasevic N, Kostic VS: Hemiballism: Report of 25 cases. J Neurol Neurosurg Psychiatry 1994;57:945–949.

Walker RH, Jankovic J, O'Hearn E, Margolis RL: Phenotypic features of Huntington disease-like 2. Mov Disord 2003;18:1527–1530.

Walker RH, Morgello S, Davidoff-Feldman B, et al: Autosomal dominant chorea-acanthocytosis with polyglutamine-containing neuronal inclusions. Neurology 2002;58:1031–1037.

Walker RH, Rasmussen A, Rudnicki D, et al. Huntington's disease-like 2 can present as chorea-acanthocytosis. Neurology 2003; 61:1002–1004.

Warner TT, Lennox GG, Janota I, Harding AE: Autosomal-dominant dentatorubropallidoluysian atrophy in the United Kingdom. Mov Disord 1994;9:289–296.

Warner TT, Williams LD, Walker RWH, et al: A clinical and molecular genetic study of dentatorubropallidoluysian atrophy in four European families. Ann Neurol 1995;37:452–459.

Weindl A, Kuwert T, Leenders KL, et al: Increased striatal glucose consumption in Sydenham's chorea. Mov Disord 1993;8:437–444.

Wheeler PG, Weaver DD, Dobyns WB: Benign hereditary chorea. Pediatr Neurol 1993;9:337–340.

Willemsen MA, Breedveld GJ, Wouda S, et al: Brain-thyroid-lung syndrome: A patient with a severe multi-system disorder due to a de novo mutation in the thyroid transcription factor 1 gene. Eur J Pediatr 2005;164:28–30.

Witt TN, Danek A. Hein MU, et al: McLeod syndrome: A distinct form of neuroacanthocytosis. J Neurol 1992;239:302–306.

Wood NS, Marlow N, Costeloe K, et al: Neurologic and developmental disability after extremely preterm birth. N Engl J Med 2000; 343:378–384.

Xiang F, Almqvist EW, Huq M, et al: A Huntington disease-like neurodegenerative disorder maps to chromosome 20p. Am J Hum Genet 1998;63:1431–1438.

Yamada M, Sato T, Tsuji S, Takahashi H: Oligodendrocytic polyglutamine pathology in dentatorubral-pallidoluysian atrophy. Ann Neurol 2002;52:670–674.

Yamada M, Wood JD, Shimohata T, et al: Widespread occurrence of intranuclear atrophin-1 accumulation in the central nervous system neurons of patients with dentatorubral-pallidoluysian atrophy. Ann Neurol 2001;49:14–23.

Zhou B, Westaway SK, Levinson B, et al: A novel pantothenate kinase gene (PANK2) is defective in Hallervorden-Spatz syndrome. Nat Genet 2001; 28:345–349.

# Chapter 17

# Tics and Tourette Syndrome

Tourette syndrome (TS) is a neurologic disorder manifested by motor and vocal or phonic tics usually starting during childhood and often accompanied by obsessive-compulsive disorder (OCD), attention-deficit hyperactivity disorder (ADHD), poor impulse control, and other comorbid behavioral problems (Shapiro and Shapiro, 1992; Cohen and Leckman, 1994; Hyde and Weinberger, 1995; Feigin and Clarke, 1998; Leckman and Cohen, 1999; Freeman et al., 2000; Robertson, 2000; Jankovic, 2001b; Leckman et al., 2001; Leckman, 2002; Stein, 2002; Singer, 2005; Albin and Mink, 2006). Once considered a rare psychiatric curiosity, TS is now recognized as a relatively common and complex neurobehavioral disorder. There has been speculation that many notable historical figures, including Dr. Samuel Johnson and possibly Wolfgang Amadeus Mozart (Simkin, 1992), were afflicted with TS.

One of the earliest reports of TS dates to 1825, when Itard (1825) described a French noblewoman with body tics, barking sounds, and uncontrollable utterances of obscenities. Sixty years later, the French neurologist and a student of Charcot, Georges Gilles de la Tourette (1885) reviewed Itard's original case and added eight more patients. He noted that all nine patients shared one feature: They all exhibited brief involuntary movements or tics; additionally, six made noises, five shouted obscenities (coprolalia), five repeated the words of others (echolalia), and two mimicked others' gestures (echopraxia) (Goetz and Klawans, 1982; Kushner, 1999). Although Tourette considered the disorder he described to be hereditary, the etiology was ascribed to psychogenic causes for nearly a century following the original report. The perception of TS began to change in the 1960s, when the beneficial effects of neuroleptic drugs on the symptoms of TS began to be recognized (Shapiro and Shapiro, 1968). This observation helped to refocus attention from psychogenic etiology to central nervous system (CNS) etiology.

The cause of TS is yet unknown, but the disorder appears to be inherited in the majority of patients (Pauls et al., 1988, 1991; Tolosa and Jankovic, 1998; Jankovic, 2001b; Leckman, 2002; Paschou et al., 2004; Singer, 2005). The clinical expression of this genetic defect varies from one individual to another, fluctuations in symptoms are seen within the same individual, and different manifestations occur in various family members (Kurlan, 1994). This variable expression from one individual to another, even within members of the same family, contributes to diagnostic confusion. Without a specific biologic marker, the diagnosis depends on a careful evaluation of the patient's symptoms and signs by an experienced clinician. Educational efforts directed to physicians, educators, and the general public have increased awareness about TS. In addition, the media have drawn increasing public attention to this condition. As a result of this improved awareness, the self-referral rate of patients has increased, and the correct diagnosis is made earlier than was the case in the past. Many patients, however, still remain undiagnosed, or their symptoms are wrongly attributed to habits, allergies, asthma, dermatitis, hyperactivity, nervousness, and many other conditions (Jankovic et al., 1998; Hogan and Wilson, 1999).

## PHENOMENOLOGY OF TICS

Tics, the clinical hallmark of TS, are relatively brief and intermittent movements (motor tics) or sounds (vocal or phonic tics). Motor tics typically consist of sudden, abrupt, transient, often repetitive and coordinated (stereotypic) movements that may resemble gestures and mimic fragments of normal behavior, vary in intensity, and are repeated at irregular intervals (Videos 17-1 to 17-8). Currently accepted criteria for the diagnosis of TS require both types of tics to be present (Robertson, 1989; Golden, 1990; Tourette Syndrome Classification Study Group, 1993; Singer, 2000). This division into motor and vocal/phonic tics, however, is artificial, because vocal/phonic tics are actually motor tics that involve respiratory, laryngeal, pharyngeal, oral, and nasal musculature. Contractions of these muscles may produce sounds by moving air through the nose, mouth, or throat. The term *phonic tic* is preferable, since not all sounds produced by TS patients involve the vocal cords.

To better understand the categorization of tics and how they fit in the general schema of movement disorders, it might be helpful to provide a simple classification of movements (Jankovic, 1992) (see Chapter 1). All movements can be categorized into one of four classes:

1. Voluntary
   a. Intentional (planned, self-initiated, internally generated)
   b. Externally triggered in response to some stimulus (e.g., turning the head toward a loud noise or withdrawing the hand from a hot plate)
2. Semivoluntary (unvoluntary)
   a. Induced by an inner sensory stimulus (e.g., the need to "stretch" a body part)
   b. Induced by an unwanted feeling or compulsion (e.g., compulsive touching or smelling)
3. Involuntary
   a. Nonsuppressible (e.g., reflexes. seizures, myoclonus)
   b. Suppressible (e.g., tics, tremor, dystonia, chorea, stereotypy)
4. Automatic
   a. Learned motor behaviors performed without conscious effort (e.g., the act of walking or speaking)

Recent studies have shown that automatic, learned behaviors appear to be encoded in the sensorimotor portion of the striatum (Jog et al., 1999). Some support for the proposed classification is provided by the findings of Papa and colleagues (1991). They recorded normal premovement (readiness) electroencephalographic, slow, negative potential (the Bereitschaftspotential) 1 to 1.5 seconds prior to self-induced, internally generated (voluntary) movement in normal individuals but not before externally triggered movement induced by electrical stimulation. Most tics can be categorized as either semivoluntary (unvoluntary) or involuntary (suppressible). In some cases, learned voluntary motor skills are incorporated into the tic repertoire. This is exemplified by a case of a woman with TS who incorporated sign language into her tic behavior, suggesting that semantics is more important than phonology in the generation of tics (Lang et al., 1993).

Tics may be simple or complex. Simple motor tics involve only one group of muscles, causing a brief, jerk-like movement. They are usually abrupt in onset and rapid (clonic tics), but they may be slower, causing a briefly sustained abnormal posture (dystonic tics) or an isometric contraction (tonic tics) (Jankovic and Fahn, 1986; Jankovic, 1992). Examples of simple clonic motor tics include blinking, nose twitching, and head jerking. Simple dystonic tics include blepharospasm, oculogyric movements, bruxism, sustained mouth opening,  torticollis, and shoulder rotation (Video 17-9; see also Videos  17-1 to 17-3). Tensing of abdominal or limb muscles is an example of a tonic tic (Video 17-10). To characterize clonic and dystonic tics further, 156 patients with TS were studied; 89 (57%) exhibited dystonic tics, including oculogyric deviations (28%), blepharospasm (15%), and dystonic neck movements (7%) (Jankovic and Stone, 1991). Since patients with dystonic tics did not differ significantly on any clinical variables from those with only clonic tics, we concluded that despite previous reports (Feinberg et al., 1986), the presence of dystonic tics should not be considered atypical or unusual. In fact, subsequent observation of the patient in the Feinberg and colleagues (1986) case report was actually a case of TS with typical dystonic tics (Fahn, 1987). Dystonic tics should be distinguished from persistent dystonia, which is typically seen in patients with primary dystonia (Jankovic and Fahn, 2002). Dystonic (and tonic) muscle contraction might be  responsible for so-called blocking tics (Video 17-11). These blocking tics are due to either prolonged tonic or dystonic tics that interrupt ongoing motor activity such as speech (intrusions) or a sudden inhibition of ongoing motor activity (negative tic). Clonic and dystonic tics may occasionally occur in patients with primary dystonia more frequently than in the general population. In nine patients with coexistent TS and persistent primary dystonia, the onset of tics was at a mean age of 9 years, while dystonia followed the onset of tics by a mean of 22 (10 to 38) years (Stone and Jankovic, 1991). Other reports have drawn attention to the possible association of tics and dystonia in the same family, providing additional evidence for a possible etiologic relationship between TS and primary dystonia (Németh et al., 1999). Dopa-responsive dystonia with mutations in the GCH1 gene and TS was found in various members of a large Danish family (Romstad et al., 2003).

Motor (particularly dystonic) and phonic tics are preceded by premonitory sensations in over 80% of patients (Cohen and Leckman, 1992; Banaschewski et al., 2003; Kwak et al., 2003b). This premonitory phenomenon consists of localizable sensations or discomforts, such as a burning feeling in the eye

before an eye blink, tension or a crick in the neck that is relieved by stretching of the neck or jerking of the head, a feeling of tightness or constriction that is relieved by arm or leg extension, nasal stuffiness before a sniff, a dry or sore throat before throat clearing or grunting, and itching before a rotatory movement of the scapula. Rarely, these premonitory sensations, termed in one report *extracorporeal phantom tics*, involve sensations in other people and objects and are temporarily relieved by touching or scratching them (Karp and Hallett, 1996). In one study, premonitory sensations were experienced by 92% of 135 patients with TS, and these were localized chiefly to the shoulder girdle, palms, midline abdominal region, posterior thighs, feet, and eyes (Cohen and Leckman, 1992). We administered a questionnaire regarding various aspects of premonitory sensations associated with their motor tics to 50 TS patients with a mean age of 23.6 ± 16.7 years (Kwak et al., 2003b). Forty-six of 50 (92%) subjects reported some premonitory sensations, the most common of which was an urge to move and an impulse to tic ("had to do it"). Other premonitory sensations included an itch, tingling/burning, numbness, and coldness. Thirty-seven (74%) also reported intensification of premonitory sensations if the patient was prevented from performing a motor tic; 36 (72%) reported relief of premonitory sensations after performing the tic; and 24 (48%) stated that their motor tic would not have occurred if they had had no premonitory sensation. Twenty-seven of 40 patients (68%) described a motor tic as a voluntary motor response to an involuntary sensation rather than as a completely involuntary movement. Besides the local or regional premonitory sensations, this premonitory phenomenon may be a nonlocalizable, less specific, and poorly described feeling, such as an urge, anxiety, anger, and other psychic sensations. The observed movement or sound sometimes occurs in response to these premonitory phenomena, and these movements or sounds have been previously referred to as sensory tics (Kurlan et al., 1989; Chee and Sachdev, 1997). In a study of 60 patients with tic disorders, 41 (68%) thought that all their tics were intentionally produced, and 15 (25%) additional patients had both voluntary and involuntary movements; thus, 93% of the tics were perceived to be "irresistibly but purposefully executed" (Lang, 1991). This "intentional" component of the movement may be a useful feature in differentiating tics from other hyperkinetic movement disorders, such as myoclonus and chorea. The sensations or feelings that often precede motor tics usually occur out of a background of relative normalcy and are clearly involuntary, even though the movements (motor tics) or noises (phonic tics) that occur in response to these premonitory symptoms may be regarded as semivoluntary or unvoluntary. Chee and Sachdev (1997) suggest that sensory tics, which we and others refer to as premonitory sensations, "represent the subjectively experienced component of neural dysfunction below the threshold for motor and phonic tic production." Many patients report that they have to repeat a particular movement to relieve the uncomfortable urge until "it feels good." The "just right" feeling has been associated with compulsive behavior, and as such, the "unvoluntary" movement may be regarded as a compulsive tic (Leckman et al., 1994).

Complex motor tics consist of coordinated, sequenced movements resembling normal motor acts or gestures that are  inappropriately intense and timed (Videos 17-12 and 17-13; see also Video 17-6). They may be seemingly nonpurposeful, such as head shaking or trunk bending, or they may seem purposeful, such as touching, throwing, hitting, jumping, and kicking. Additional examples of complex motor tics include gesturing "the finger" and grabbing or exposing one's genitalia (copropraxia) or imitating gestures (echopraxia). Burping, vomiting, and retching have been described as part of the clinical picture of TS, but it is not clear whether this phenomenon represents a complex tic or some other behavioral manifestation of TS (Rickards and Robertson, 1997). Another unusual tic is ear dyskinesia, which consists of anterior-posterior displacement of the external ear (Cardoso and Faleiro, 1999). Complex motor tics may be difficult to differentiate from compulsions, which frequently accompany tics, particularly in TS. A complex, repetitive movement may be considered a compulsion when it is preceded by, or associated with, a feeling of anxiety or panic, as well as an irresistible urge to perform the movement or sound because of fear that if it is not promptly or properly executed, "something bad" will happen. However, this distinction is not always possible, particularly when the patient is unable to verbalize such feelings. Some coordinated movements resemble complex motor tics but may actually represent pseudovoluntary movements (parakinesias) that are designed to camouflage the tics by incorporating them into seemingly purposeful acts, such as adjusting one's hair during a head jerk.

Simple phonic tics typically consist of sniffing, throat clearing, grunting, squeaking, screaming, coughing, blowing, and sucking sounds. Complex phonic tics include linguistically meaningful utterances and verbalizations, such as shouting of obscenities or profanities (coprolalia), repetition of someone else's words or phrases (echolalia), and repetition of one's own utterances, particularly the last syllable, word or phrase in a sentence (palilalia). Some TS patients also manifest sudden and transient cessation of all motor activity (blocking tics) without alteration of consciousness.

In contrast to other hyperkinetic movement disorders, tics are usually intermittent and may be repetitive and stereotypic (Table 17-1). Tics may occur as short-term bouts or bursting or long-term waxing and waning (Peterson and Leckman, 1998). They vary in frequency and intensity and often change distribution. Typically, tics can be volitionally suppressed, although this might require intense mental effort (Banaschewski et al., 2003). Suppressibility, although characteristic and common in tics, is not unique or specific for tics, and this phenomenon has been well documented in other hyperkinetic movement disorders (Koller and Biary, 1989; Walters et al., 1990). Using functional magnetic resonance imaging (MRI), Peterson and colleagues (1998a) showed decreased neuronal activity during periods of suppression in the ventral globus pallidus, putamen, and thalamus. There was increased activity in the right caudate nucleus, right frontal cortex, and other cortical areas that are normally involved in the inhibition of unwanted impulses (prefrontal, parietal, temporal, and cingulate cortices). Besides temporary suppressibility, tics are characterized by suggestibility and exacerbation with stress, excitement, boredom, fatigue, and exposure to heat (Lombroso et al., 1991). Tics may also increase during relaxation after a period of stress.

In contrast to other hyperkinetic movement disorders that are usually completely suppressed during sleep, motor and phonic tics may persist during all stages of sleep (Jankovic et al., 1984; Silvestri et al., 1990; Fish et al., 1991; Rothenberger et al., 2001; Hanna and Jankovic, 2003). In addition, patients

with TS often have disturbances of sleep, such as increased sleep fragmentation, higher frequency of arousals, decreased rapid eye movement (REM) sleep, and enuresis (Hanna and Jankovic, 2003). Many patients note a reduction in their tics when they are distracted while concentrating on mental or physical tasks (such as when playing a video game or during an orgasm). Other patients experience increased frequency and intensity of their tics when distracted, especially when they no longer have the need to suppress the tics. Tics are also typically exacerbated by dopaminergic drugs and by CNS stimulants, including methylphenidate and cocaine (Cardoso and Jankovic, 1993). Finally, it should be noted that there is a broad spectrum of movements that may be present in patients with TS that can be confused with tics, such as akathisia, chorea, dystonia, compulsive movements, and fidgeting as part of hyperactivity associated with ADHD (Jankovic, 1997; Kompoliti and Goetz, 1998; Wilens et al., 2004).

**Table 17-1** Differential diagnosis of tics

| Classification | Differential Diagnosis |
|---|---|
| **Simple Motor Tics** | |
| Clonic | Myoclonus |
| | Chorea |
| | Seizures |
| Dystonic | Dystonia |
| | Athetosis |
| Tonic | Muscle spasms and cramps |
| **Complex Motor Tics** | |
| | Mannerisms |
| | Stereotypies |
| | Restless legs syndrome |
| | Seizures |
| Phenomenology | |
| Abrupt | Myoclonus |
| | Chorea |
| | Hyperekplexia |
| | Paroxysmal dyskinesia |
| | Seizures |
| Sensory phenomenon (urge relief) | Akathisia-stereotypy |
| | Restless legs syndrome |
| | Dystonia |
| Perceived as voluntary | Akathisia |
| Suppressibility | All hyperkinesias but less than tics |
| Decrease with distraction | Akathisia |
| | Psychogenic movements |
| Increase with stress | Most hyperkinesias |
| Increase with relaxation (after a period of stress) | Parkinsonian tremor |
| Multifocal, migrate | Chorea |
| | Myoclonus |
| Fluctuate spontaneously | Paroxysmal dyskinesias |
| | Seizures |
| Present during sleep | Myoclonus (segmental) |
| | Periodic movements |
| | Painful legs/moving toes |
| | Other hyperkinesias |
| | Seizures |

## CLINICAL FEATURES OF TOURETTE SYNDROME

### Motor Symptoms

TS, the most common cause of tics, is manifested by a broad spectrum of motor and behavioral disturbances. This clinical heterogeneity often causes diagnostic difficulties and presents a major challenge in genetic linkage studies. To aid in the diagnosis of TS, the Tourette Syndrome Classification Study Group (1993) formulated the following criteria for definite TS: (1) Both multiple motor and one or more phonic tics have to be present at some time during the illness, although not necessarily concurrently. (2) Tics must occur many times a day, nearly every day, or intermittently throughout a period of more than 1 year. (3) The anatomic location, number, frequency, type, complexity, or severity of tics must change over time. (4) Onset must be before age 21. (5) Involuntary movements and noises cannot be explained by other medical conditions. (6) Motor and/or phonic tics must be directly witnessed by a reliable examiner at some point during the illness or must be recorded by videotape or cinematography. Probable TS type 1 meets all the criteria except for number 3 and/or number 4, and probable TS type 2 meets all the criteria except for number 1; it includes either a single motor tic with phonic tics or multiple motor tics with possible phonic tics. In contrast to the criteria outlined by the Diagnostic and Statistical Manual of Mental Disorders, fourth edition (DSM-IV) (1994), the Tourette Syndrome Classification Study Group criteria do not include a statement about "impairment." There is considerable controversy about the DSM-IV criteria, which require that "marked distress or significant impairment in social, occupational or other important areas of functioning" be present. Therefore, patients with mild tics that do not produce an impairment would not satisfy the diagnostic criteria for TS, according to DMS-IV. This criterion will be deleted from the fifth edition of the DSM. Kurlan (1997) suggested another set of diagnostic criteria for genetic studies and introduced the term *Tourette disorder* for patients who have "functional impairment." This, however, does not take into account the marked fluctuation in symptoms and severity; some patients may be relatively asymptomatic at one time and clearly functionally impaired at another time. The TSA International Genetic Collaboration developed the Diagnostic Confidence Index, which consists of 26 confidence factors, with weightings given to each of them and a total maximum score of 100. The most highly weighted diagnostic confidence factors include history of coprolalia, complex motor or vocal tics, a waxing and waning course, echophenomenon, premonitory sensations, an orchestrated sequence, and age at onset. The Diagnostic Confidence Index was found to be a useful instrument in assessing the lifetime likelihood of TS (Robertson et al., 1999). Several instruments, some based on ratings of videotapes, have been developed to measure and quantitate tics, but they all have some limitations (Goetz and Kampoliti, 2001; Goetz et al., 2001).

The clinical criteria are designed to assist in accurate diagnosis, in genetic linkage studies, and in differentiating TS from other tic disorders (Box 17-1) (Jankovic, 1993b). There is a body of evidence to support the notion that many, if not all, patients with other forms of idiopathic tic disorders represent

---

**Box 17-1 Causes of tics**

**A. Primary**
1. Sporadic
   a. Transient motor or phonic tics (<1 year)
   b. Chronic motor or phonic tics (>1 year)
   c. Adult-onset (recurrent) tics
   d. TS
   e. Primary dystonia
2. Inherited
   a. TS
   b. Huntington disease
   c. Primary dystonia
   d. Neuroacanthocytosis
   e. Neurodegeneration with brain iron accumulation (Hallervorden-Spatz)
   f. Tuberous sclerosis
   g. Wilson disease
   h. Duchenne muscular dystrophy

**B. Secondary**
1. Infections: encephalitis, Creutzfeldt-Jakob disease, neurosyphilis, Sydenham disease
2. Drugs: amphetamines, methylphenidate, pemoline, levodopa, cocaine, carbamazepine, phenytoin, phenobarbital, lamotrigine, antipsychotics, and other dopamine receptor–blocking drugs (tardive tics, tardive tourettism)
3. Toxins: carbon monoxide
4. Developmental: static encephalopathy, mental retardation syndromes, chromosomal abnormalities, autistic spectrum disorders (Asperger syndrome)
5. Chromosomal disorders: Down syndrome, Kleinfelter syndrome, XYY karyotype, fragile-X, triple-X and 9p mosaicism, partial trisomy 16, 9p monosomy, citrullinemia, Beckwith-Wiedemann syndrome
6. Other: head trauma, stroke, neurocutaneous syndromes, schizophrenia, neurodegenerative diseases

**C. Related Manifestations and Disorders**
1. Stereotypies/habits/mannerisms
2. Self-injurious behaviors (SIBs)
3. Motor restlessness
4. Akathisia
5. Compulsions
6. Excessive startle
7. Jumping Frenchman

---

one end of the spectrum in a continuum of TS (Kurlan et al., 1988). The most common and mildest of the idiopathic tic disorders is the transient tic disorder (TTD) of childhood. This disorder is essentially identical to TS except the symptoms last less than 1 year and therefore the diagnosis can be made only in retrospect. Transient tic disorder has been estimated to occur in up to 24% of schoolchildren (Shapiro et al., 1988). Chronic multiple tic disorder is also similar to TS, but the patients have either only motor or, less commonly, only phonic tics lasting at least 1 year. Chronic single tic disorder is the same as chronic multiple tic disorder, but the patients have only a single motor or phonic tic. This separation into transient tic disorder, chronic multiple tic disorder, and chronic single tic disorder seems artificial because all can occur in the same family and probably represent a variable expression of the same genetic defect (Kurlan et al., 1988).

Although the diagnostic criteria require that the onset is present before the age of 21, in 96% of patients the disorder is manifested by age 11 (Robertson, 1989). In 36% to 48% of patients, the initial symptom is eye blinking, followed by tics involving the face and head. Blink rate in TS is about double of that of normal, age-matched controls (Tulen et al., 1999). During the course of the disease, nearly all patients exhibit tics involving the face or head, two thirds have tics in the arms, and half have tics involving the trunk or legs. According to one study, the average age at onset of tics is 5.6 years, and the tics usually become most severe at age 10; by 18 years of age, half of the patients are tic-free (Leckman et al., 1998). In a study of 58 adults who had been diagnosed with TS during childhood, Goetz and colleagues (1992) found that tics persisted in all patients but were moderate or severe in only 24%, although 60% had moderate or severe tics during the course of the disease. Tic severity during childhood had no predictive value for the future course, but patients with mild tics during the preadult period had mild tics during adulthood. In another study, the investigators reviewed videotapes of 31 patients, with an average age of 24.2 ± 3.5 years, approximately 12 years after their initial video and found that 90% of the adults still had tics, even though they often considered themselves tic-free (Pappert et al., 2003). There was, however, a significant improvement in tic disability and tic severity.

In another study designed to address the long-term prognosis of children with TS as they reach adulthood, 46 children with TS underwent a structured interview at a mean age of 11.4 years and again at 19.0 years (Bloch et al., 2006). The mean worst-ever tic severity score was 31.6 out of a possible 50 on the YGTSS and occurred at a mean age of 10.6 years. By the time of the second interview, the mean YGTSS score had decreased to 10. This first prospective longitudinal study also showed that only 22% continued to experience mild or greater tic symptoms (YGTSS scores ≥ 10) at follow-up, while nearly one third were in complete remission of tic symptoms at follow-up. In contrast to the study by Goetz and colleagues (1992), the severity of childhood tics was predictive of increased tic severity at follow-up. The peak OCD severity occurred 2 years after peak tic severity. Interestingly, a 10-point increase in baseline IQ increased the risk of OCD symptoms at follow-up by 2.8-fold. The authors point out that the later average onset of OCD symptoms indicates the importance of counseling parents about the possibility of OCD development in children who have recently been diagnosed with tics. Although the long-term prognosis for TS is generally favorable for most patients, a minority of cases may have persistent, severe tic symptoms that may be resistant to medications (Eapen et al., 2002).

Although the vast majority of tics in adults represent recurrences of childhood-onset tics, in rare cases patients may have their first tic occurrence during adulthood (Chouinard and Ford, 2000; Jankovic and Mejia, 2006). In adults with new onset tics, it is important to search for secondary causes, such  as infection, trauma, stroke, cocaine use, neuroleptic exposure, and peripheral injury (Video 17-14) (Chouinard and Ford, 2000; Jankovic, 2001a; Jankovic and Mejia, 2006). One study of eight patients with adult-onset tics (three of whom had childhood-onset OCD and three of whom had a family history of tics and OCD) found that in comparison to the

patients with more typical childhood-onset tics, the former group had more severe symptoms, greater social morbidity, and less favorable response to medications (Eapen et al., 2002). Poor motor control, which can lead to poor penmanship and, at times, almost illegible handwriting, can contribute to the academic difficulties faced by many patients with TS. Tics, although rarely disabling, can be quite troublesome for TS patients because they cause embarrassment, interfere with social interactions, and at times can be quite painful or uncomfortable. Rarely, cervical tics may be so forceful and violent, the so-called whiplash tics, that they might cause secondary neurologic deficits, such as compressive cervical myelopathy (Krauss and Jankovic, 1996) (see Video 17-2). The truncal bending tics, which resemble intermittent, repetitive camptocormis, may cause secondary degenerative changes in the thoracic spine (Azher and Jankovic, 2005) (see Video 17-5).

Vocalizations have been reported as the initial symptom in 12% to 37% of patients, throat clearing being the most common (Robertson, 1989). Phonic tics can be quite troublesome for patients and those around them. In addition to involuntary noises, some patients have speech dysfluencies that resemble developmental stuttering, and up to half of all patients with developmental stuttering have been thought to have undiagnosed TS (Abwender et al., 1998). Coprolalia, perhaps the most recognizable and certainly one of the most distressing symptoms of TS, is actually present in only half of patients (Video 17-15; see also Video 17-8). When describing the distress caused by his severe coprolalia, one of our patients remarked that immediately after shouting an obscenity, he reaches out with his hand in an attempt to "catch the word and bring it back before others can hear it." Coprolalia appears to be markedly influenced by cultural background. Although in one retrospective analysis of 112 children with TS, only 8% exhibited coprolalia (Goldenberg et al., 1994), the true prevalence of coprolalia in TS children and adults is about 50% in the U.S. population, when mental coprolalia (without actual utterance) is included. Coprolalia has been reported to occur in only 26% of Danish patients and 4% of Japanese patients (Robertson, 1989). Copropraxia has been found in about 20% of patients, echolalia in 30%, echopraxia in 25%, and palilalia in 15%.

Except tics, the neurologic examination in patients with TS is usually normal. In one case-control study, TS patients were found to have a shorter duration of saccades, but the saccades were performed with a greater mean velocity than in normal controls, and the TS patients had fewer correct antisaccade responses, suggesting a mild oculomotor disturbance in TS (Farber et al., 1999). Although the ability to inhibit reflexive saccades is normal, TS patients make more timing errors, indicating an inability to appropriately inhibit or delay planned motor programs (LeVasseur et al., 2001).

## Behavioral Symptoms

In addition to motor and phonic tics, patients with TS often exhibit a variety of behavioral symptoms, particularly ADHD and OCD (Fig. 17-1). In the Tourette International Consortium (TIC) database, which includes information on 3500 patients with TS evaluated by neurologists or psychiatrists, only 12% had tics only, without other comorbidities (Freeman et al., 2000). Kurlan and colleagues (2002) inter-

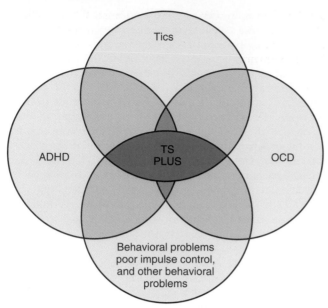

**Figure 17-1** An overlap of disorders typically coexisting in patients with TS. (Reprinted with permission from Jankovic J: Tourette's syndrome. N Engl J Med 2001;345:1184–1192.)

viewed 1596 children, ages 9 to 17, in schools in Rochester and Monroe Counties, New York, and identified tics in 339 children (21%) after 60 to 150 minutes of observation. They found the following behavioral problems more frequently ($P < .05$) in children with tics than in those without tics: OCD, ADHD, separation anxiety, overanxious disorder, simple phobia, social phobia, agoraphobia, mania, major depression, and oppositional defiant behavior. Also, children with tics were younger (mean age: 12.5 versus 13.3 years) and were more likely to require special education services (27% versus 19.8%). A thorough discussion of the pathogenesis of comorbid disorders and their relationship to TS is beyond the scope of this review, and the reader is referred to some recent reviews on these topics (Tannock, 1998; Stein, 2002). The diagnosis of ADHD and OCD is based on clinical history; there are no laboratory or other tests that reliably diagnose these neurobehavioral disorders (Dulcan and AACAP Works Group on Quality Issues, 1997; Goldman et al., 1998; Swanson et al., 1998) (Box 17-2). These comorbid behavioral conditions often interfere with learning and with academic and work performance (Singer, Schuerholz, et al., 1995). In contrast to tics, ADHD and obsessional symptom severity are significantly associated with impaired social and emotional adjustment (Carter et al., 2000). The clinician should be skilled not only in the recognition and treatment of ADHD but also in documenting the ADHD-related deficits (Richard et al., 1998). Such documentation is essential for the parents and educators in order to provide the optimal educational setting for the affected individual.

Since nearly all studies on the frequency of associated features have been based on a population of TS patients who have been referred to physicians, usually specialists, there is a certain selection bias; therefore, accurate figures on the prevalence of these behavioral disorders in TS patients are not available. It has been estimated, however, that 3% to 6% of

school-aged population suffers from ADHD (Goldman et al., 1998), and probably a majority of patients with TS have had symptoms of ADHD, OCD, or both at some time during the course of their illness (Coffey and Park, 1997). In a review of 1500 patients with TS, 48% were diagnosed as having ADHD, a figure that is consistent with the results of other studies (Comings and Comings, 1988b). The symptoms of ADHD may be the initial manifestations of TS and may precede the onset of motor and phonic tics by about 3 years. During this time, therapy with stimulant drugs may trigger the onset of tics and may precipitate the emergence of other TS symptoms (Price et al., 1986).

There are three types of ADHD: predominantly inattentive, predominantly hyperactive-impulsive, and combined (Dulcan et al., 1997) (see Box 17-2). ADHD is one of the most common neurobehavioral disorders, affecting 3% to 10% of children and 4% of adults (Wilens et al., 2004; Rappley, 2005). Adults with ADHD often have childhood histories of educational and discipline problems; and during adulthood, they usually have lower socioeconomic status,

**Box 17-2** Attention-Deficit Hyperactivity Disorder/ Hyperkinetic Disorder (ICD-10 and DSM-IV)

**Inattention (IN)**
Fails to attend to details
Difficulty sustaining attention
Does not seem to listen
Fails to finish
Difficulty organizing tasks
Avoids sustained effort
Loses things
Distracted by external stimuli
Forgetful

**Hyperactivity (H)**
Fidgets with hands or feet
Leaves seat in classroom
Runs about or climbs
Difficulty playing quietly
Motor excess ("on the go")
Talks excessively

**Impulsivity (IMP)**
Talks excessively
Blurts out answers
Difficulty waiting turn
Interrupts or intrudes on others

**Attention-Deficit Hyperactivity Disorder Diagnostic Subtypes (DSM-IV)**
Combined: six or more from the IN domain and six or more from the H/IMP domain
Inattentive: six or more from the IN domain and less than six from the H/IMP domain
Hyperactive/impulsive: six or more from the H/IMP domain and fewer than six from the IN domain

**HKD (ICD-10)**
Six or more from the IN domain, three or more from the H domain, and one or more from the IMP domain

lower rates of professional employment, and higher rates of marital problems, driving violations, and other life failures. In a genome scan of 106 families, including 128 affected sibpairs with estimated heritability of 60% to 80%, multipoint MLS values above 1 were evidence of a gene locus on chromosomes 4, 9, 10, 11, 12, 16, and 17 (Smalley et al., 2001). Although attention deficit is certainly one of the most common and disabling symptoms of TS, in many patients the inability to pay attention is due to not only a coexistent ADHD but also uncontrollable intrusions of thoughts. Some patients are unable to pay attention because of a compulsive fixation of gaze. For example, while they are sitting in a classroom or a theater or during a conversation, their gaze becomes fixated on a particular object, and despite concentrated effort, they are unable to break the fixation. As a result, they miss the teacher's lesson or a particular action in a play. Another reason for impaired attention in some TS patients is mental concentration exerted in an effort to suppress tics. Yet another cause for inattention is the sedative effect of anti-TS medications. It is therefore important to determine which mechanism or mechanisms are most likely to be responsible for the patient's attention deficit. This is particularly important in selecting the best therapeutic approach. Despite growing publicity about ADHD, there is little evidence of widespread overdiagnosis or overtreatment of ADHD (Goldman et al., 1998). One study showed that children and adolescents with ADHD as compared to those without ADHD are more likely to have major injuries and asthma, and their 9-year medical costs are double (Leibson et al., 2001). The mechanism of ADHD with or without TS is not well understood, and there are no specific pathologic abnormalities identified. However, by using high-resolution MRI, abnormal morphology was observed in the frontal cortices, reduction in the anterior temporal cortices, and increased gray matter in the posterior and inferior parietal cortices in children and adolescents with ADHD (Sowell et al., 2003).

That OCD is a part of the spectrum of neurobehavioral manifestations in TS is now well accepted (Rapoport, 1988; Towbin, 1988; Black, 1992; Stein, 2002). OCD, with an estimated lifetime prevalence of 2% to 3% (Sasson et al., 1997; Snider and Swedo, 2000) and an incidence of 0.55 per 1000 person-years (Nestadt et al., 1998) is one of the most frequent causes of disability (Jenike, 2004). It may occur alone without other features of TS (Micallef and Blin, 2001). The instrument used most frequently to measure the severity of OCD is the Yale-Brown Obsessive Compulsive Scale (Scahill et al., 1997). A distinction should be made between obsessive-compulsive symptoms or traits, obsessive-compulsive personality disorder, and OCD. Obsessions are characterized by intense, intrusive thoughts, such as concerns about bodily wastes and secretions; unfounded fears; need for exactness, symmetry, evenness, and neatness; excessive religious concerns; perverse sexual thoughts; and intrusions of words, phrases, or music. Compulsions consist of subjective urges to perform meaningless and irrational rituals, such as checking, counting, cleaning, washing, touching, smelling, hoarding, and rearranging. Leckman and colleagues (1994) have drawn attention to the frequent occurrence of the "just right" perception in patients with OCD and TS. While obsessional slowness accounts for some of the school problems experienced by TS patients, cognitive slowing (bradyphrenia) is also a contributing factor (Singer, Schuerholz, et al., 1995). Patients with OCD can usu-

ally be divided into those with a predominantly cognitive form (in which an idea is followed by a ritual) and those with a sensorimotor type (in which a physical sensation is followed by a movement). In contrast to primary OCD, in which the symptoms relate chiefly to hygiene and cleanliness, the obsessive symptoms that are associated with TS usually involve concerns with symmetry, violent aggressive thoughts, forced touching, fear of harming self or others, and need for saying or doing things "just right" (Eapen et al., 1997b). A principal-components factor analysis of 13 categories that are used to group types of obsessions and compulsions in the Yale-Brown Obsessive Compulsive Scale symptom checklist identified the obsessions and checking and the symmetry and ordering factors as particularly common in patients with tic disorders (Leckman, Grice, et al., 1997). Miguel and colleagues (2000) showed that patients who have OCD associated with TS tend to have more bodily sensations occurring either before or during the patient's performance of the repetitive behaviors as well as mental sensations including urge only, energy release (mental energy that builds up and needs to be discharged), and "just right" perceptions. In addition to an idiopathic sporadic or familial disorder and TS, OCD has been reported to occur as a result of a variety of lesions in the frontal-limbic-subcortical circuits (Berthier et al., 1996; Kwak and Jankovic, 2002; Voon, 2004). Although both ADHD and OCD are regarded as integral findings of the syndrome, only OCD has been shown to be genetically linked to TS (Alsobrook and Pauls, 1997). A pathogenic link between TS and OCD is also suggested by the finding in one study that 59% of 54 patients with OCD had a lifetime history of tics, and 14% fulfilled the criteria for TS during the 2- to 7-year follow-up (Leonard, 1992). Alsobrook and Pauls (2002) identified four significant factors: (1) aggressive phenomena (e.g., kicking, temper fits, argumentativeness), (2) purely motor and phonic tic symptoms, (3) compulsive phenomena (e.g., touching of others or objects, repetitive speech, throat clearing), and (4) tapping and absence of grunting, which accounted for 61% of the phenotypic symptom variance in TS probands and their first-degree relatives.

An important link between motor and behavioral manifestations of TS is the loss of impulse control. Many TS patients suffer from poor impulse control, disinhibition of aggression and emotions, and obsessive thoughts that may dictate their actions. Indeed, many behavioral symptoms of TS, including some complex tics, coprolalia, copropraxia, and many behavioral problems, can be explained by loss of normal inhibitory mechanisms (disinhibition) manifested by poor impulse control. It is as though the TS patients have lost their ability to suppress vestiges of primitive behavior. Poor impulse control might also explain the inability to control anger, as a result of which many patients have frequent and sometimes violent, temper outbursts, and rages. Rarely, TS patients exhibit inappropriate sexual aggressiveness and antisocial, oppositional, and even violent, unlawful, or criminal behavior. TS, indeed, serves as a model medical disorder that can predispose one to engage in uncontrollable and offensive behaviors that are misunderstood by the law-abiding community and the legal justice system (Jankovic et al., 2006). The social and legal aspects of TS patients have yet to be investigated, but there is growing concern regarding media misrepresentation that attributes violent criminal behavior in certain individuals to TS. Although TS should not be used as an excuse to justify unlawful or criminal behaviors, studies are needed to determine whether TS-related symptoms and neurobehavioral comorbidities predispose TS patients to engage in such behaviors. Often, the avolitional nature of behaviors in response to involuntary internal thought and emotional patterns is supported by the subsequent remorse and lack of secondary gain. This suggests that the preponderance of unlawful acts committed by TS patients are not premeditated but may result from a variety of TS-related mechanisms such as poor impulse control, OCD associated with addictive behavior (e.g., drugs, alcohol, gambling), attention-deficit disorder (ADD), and distractibility (e.g., motor vehicle accidents). A previous study (Comings and Comings, 1987) compared conduct in 246 TS patients to that of controls for behaviors such as lying, stealing, fighting or inability to stop fighting, violence against animals, physically attacking peers or parents, vandalism, running away from home, starting fires, poor temper control, alcohol and drug abuse, and other misdemeanors. Thirty-five percent of TS patients had a conduct score higher than 13, significantly greater than the 2.1% of controls with high scores ($P < .0005$). All behaviors with the exception of running away from home and trouble with the law occurred at a significantly greater rate in TS patients. Although no difference was found for the law variable, TS patients were significantly more likely to vandalize ($P < .0005$), fight ($P < .0005$), abuse drugs or alcohol ($P < .003$), and steal ($P < .015$). An interesting finding in this study was that certain behaviors, such as starting fires, shouting, and physically attacking, were significantly greater only in TS patients with comorbid ADD, supporting the well-established association of ADD in conduct disorder. It was estimated from this study that 10% to 30% of conduct disorder cases in non–economically disadvantaged children may be attributed to a possible TS gene. In a more recent study, however, TS accounted for only 2% of all cases that were referred for forensic psychiatric investigation in Stockholm, Sweden, between 1990 and 1995; 15% of the subjects had ADHD, 15% had PDD, and 3% had Asperger syndrome (Siponmaa et al., 2001).

Focal frontal lobe dysfunction, demonstrated in TS by various functional and imaging studies, has been associated with impulsive subtype of aggressive behavior (Brower and Price, 2001). It has been postulated that impulse disorders stem from exaggerated reward-, pleasure-, or arousal-seeking brain centers, resulting in failure of inhibition. Animal studies of rats with lesions of the nucleus accumbens core (AcbC), the brain region that is noted for reward and reinforcement, showed that the lesioned rats preferred small, immediate rewards over larger, delayed rewards (Cardinal et al., 2001). In addition to the ventromedial prefrontal cortices, lesions in the amygdala have also been known to result in altered decision-making processes and a disregard for future consequences (Bechara et al., 2000).

One of the most distressing symptoms of TS is a self-injurious behavior (SIB), which has been reported in up to 53% of all patients (Robertson, 1989; Robertson et al., 1990). A common form of SIB is damage of skin by biting, scratching, cutting, engraving, or hitting, particularly in the eye and throat (compulsions), often accompanied by an irresistible urge (obsession) (Jankovic et al., 1998) (Videos 17-16 and 17-17). Thus, SIB appears to be related to OCD, which has treatment implications. Besides OCD, SIB also correlates with impulsivity and impulse control (Mathews et al., 2004). Conduct dis-

orders and problems with discipline at home and in school are recurrent themes during discussions of behavioral problems with TS families. The inability to suppress or "edit" intentions due to a "dysfunctional intention editor" has been proposed as one of the chief reasons for poor impulse control in patients with TS (Baron-Cohen et al., 1994).

The TS gene(s) may, in addition to tics, ADHD, and OCD, express itself in a variety of behavioral manifestations, including learning and conduct disorders, schizoid and affective disorders, antisocial behaviors, oppositional defiant disorder, anxiety, depression, conduct disorder, severe temper outbursts, rage attacks, impulse control problems, inappropriate sexual behavior, and other psychiatric problems (Comings, 1987; Robertson, 2000). Personality disorder and depression have been reported in 64% of patients with TS (Robertson et al., 1997). Whether these behavioral problems indeed occur with higher frequency in TS patients and whether they are pathogenically linked to TS are debatable (Comings and Comings, 1988a; Pauls et al., 1988).

Besides comorbid behavioral conditions, TS has been reported to be frequently associated with migraine headaches. In one study, 26.6% of TS patients, with a mean age of 11.9 years, exhibited migraine headaches (Barabas et al., 1984). Kwak and colleagues (2003a) found migraine headaches in 25 carefully screened TS patients at a significantly greater rate than the estimated 11% to 13% in the general adult population ($P < .0001$) and the general pediatric population ($P < .04$). This compares to 4.0% to 7.4% in the general population of school-aged children. Tourette International Consortium Database (Freeman et al., 2000), which at the time of publication included information on 3500 patients with TS collected from 64 centers from around the world, showed that only 12% of patients with TS had no other disorders; ADHD was seen in 60%, symptoms of OCD in 59%, anger control problems in 37%, sleep disorder in 25%, learning disability in 23%, mood disorders in 20%, anxiety disorders in 18%, and SIB in 14%. The natural history of TS varies from one person to another, but patients typically start with attention deficit, followed by motor and then phonic tics, and then the development of OCD, which often persists until adulthood (Jankovic, 2001a) (Fig. 17-2).

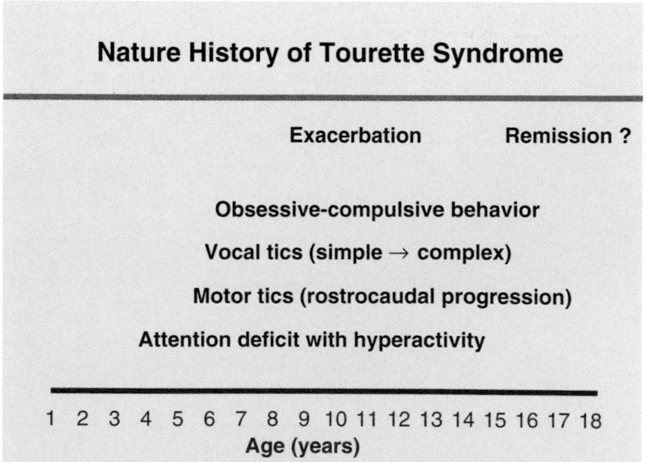

**Nature History of Tourette Syndrome**

Exacerbation        Remission ?

Obsessive-compulsive behavior

Vocal tics (simple → complex)

Motor tics (rostrocaudal progression)

Attention deficit with hyperactivity

1 2 3 4 5 6 7 8 9 10 11 12 13 14 15 16 17 18
**Age (years)**

**Figure 17-2** Typical progression of symptoms in patients with TS. (Reprinted with permission from Jankovic J: Tourette's syndrome. N Engl J Med 2001;345:1184–1192.)

# PATHOGENESIS

## Neurophysiology

Although the pathogenic mechanisms of TS are still unknown, the weight of evidence supports an organic rather than psychogenic origin (Leckman, Peterson, et al., 1997; Palumbo et al., 1997; Jankovic, 2001b; Leckman, 2002; Berardelli et al., 2003). Despite the observation that some tics may be voluntary, at least in part, physiologic studies suggest that tics are not mediated through normal motor pathways utilized for willed movements (Obeso et al., 1982). Using back-averaging techniques, Obeso and colleagues (1982) observed normal Bereitschaftspotential in six subjects who voluntarily simulated ticlike movements, but no such premovement potential was noted in association with an actual tic. The common absence of premotor potentials in simple motor tics suggests that tics are truly involuntary or that they occur in response to some external cue (Papa et al., 1991). Karp and colleagues (1996), however, documented premotor negativity in two of five patients with simple motor tics. Although the investigators could not correlate the presence of Bereitschaftspotential with the premonitory sensation, the physiology of the premovement phenomenon requires further studies.

Conventional neurophysiologic investigations have found that TS patients have defective inhibitory mechanisms, as is suggested by the increased duration of the late response of the blink reflex and reduced inhibition at paired pulse testing (Smith and Lees, 1989; Berardelli et al., 2003). TS patients also have exaggerated audiogenic startle response (Gironell et al., 2000). About 20% of patients with TS have exaggerated startle responses, which may fail to habituate with repetition (Stell et al., 1995).

As was noted before, functional MRI showed decreased neuronal activity during periods of suppression in the ventral globus pallidus, putamen, and thalamus and increased activity in the right caudate nucleus, right frontal cortex, and other cortical areas that are normally involved in the inhibition of unwanted impulses (prefrontal, parietal, temporal, and cingulate cortices) (Peterson et al., 1998a). In another study of three patients with TS, functional MRI showed marked reduction or absence of activity in secondary motor areas while the patient attempted to maintain a stable grip-load force control (Serrien et al., 2002). The authors interpreted the findings as an ongoing activation of the secondary motor reflecting patients' involuntary urges to move. In a study of children with ADHD, functional MRI showed increased frontal activation and reduced striatal activation on various tasks and an enhancement of striatal function after treatment with methylphenidate (Vaidya et al., 1998). Transcranial magnetic stimulation studies have demonstrated a shortened cortical silent period and defective intracortical inhibition (determined in a conditioning test paired-stimulus paradigm) in patients with TS (Ziemann et al., 1997; Orth et al., 2005) and OCD (Greenberg et al., 1998), thus providing a possible explanation for intrusive phenomena. Subsequent studies utilizing the same technique have demonstrated that patients with tic-related OCD have more abnormal motor cortex excitability than do OCD patients without tics (Greenberg et al., 2000). Transcranial magnetic stimulation studies have also demonstrated that TS children have a shorter cortical silent period but that their intracortical inhibition was not different from that of controls, although intracortical inhibition is reduced in children with ADHD (Moll et al., 2001). There is evidence of additive inhibitory deficits, as demonstrated by reduced intracortical inhibition and a shortened cortical silent period in children with TS and comorbid ADHD. In another study, ADHD more than tics were associated with short-interval intracortical inhibition (Gilbert et al., 2004). Both short-interval intracortical inhibition and short-interval afferent inhibition were reduced in eight patients with TS (ages 24 to 38 years) as compared to ten matched healthy controls (Orth et al., 2005). Comprehensive discussion of the neuroscience of ADHD is beyond the scope of this chapter, but the reader is referred to some recent reviews of this topic (Castellanos and Tannock, 2002).

Sleep studies have provided additional evidence that some tics are truly involuntary. Polysomnographic studies in 34 TS patients recorded motor tics in various stages of sleep in 23 patients and phonic tics in 4 patients (Glaze et al., 1983; Jankovic and Rohaidy, 1987). Additional sleep studies have suggested that some patients with TS have alterations of arousal, decreased percentage (up to 30%) of stage 3/4 (slow wave) sleep, decreased percentage of rapid eye movement sleep, paroxysmal events in stage 4 sleep with sudden intense arousal, disorientation and agitation, restless legs syndrome, and periodic leg movement in sleep (Voderholzer et al., 1997; Chokroverty and Jankovic, 1999; Picchietti et al., 1999). Restless legs syndrome has been reported to be present in about 10% of patients with TS and in 23% of parents (Lesperance et al., 2004). Other sleep-related disorders that are associated with TS include sleep apnea, enuresis, sleepwalking and sleep talking, nightmares, myoclonus, bruxism, and other disturbances (Rothenberger et al., 2001; Hanna and Jankovic, 2003).

## Neuroimaging

Although standard anatomic neuroimaging studies in TS are unremarkable, by using special volumetric, metabolic, blood flow, ligand, and functional imaging techniques, several interesting findings have been reported that have strong implications for the pathophysiology of TS (Peterson, 2001). Careful volumetric MRI studies have suggested that the normal asymmetry of the basal ganglia is lost in TS (Peterson et al., 1993; Singer et al., 1993; Peterson, 2001). In one study, the normal left > right asymmetry (Singer et al., 1993) in the volume in the right anterior brain, right caudate, and right pallidum was reversed in TS subjects (Castellanos et al., 1996). This finding, however, has not been consistently confirmed by other studies (Moriarty et al., 1997). In another volumetric MRI study, Frederickson and colleagues (2002) found evidence of smaller gray matter volumes in the left frontal lobes of patients with TS, further supporting the findings of loss of normal left > right asymmetry. Quantitative MRI studies have found a subtle, but possibly important, reduction in the volume of caudate nuclei in patients with TS. In 10 pairs of monozygotic twins, the right caudate was smaller in the more severely affected individuals, providing evidence for the role of environmental events in the pathogenesis of TS (Hyde et al., 1995). In contrast, the corpus callosum has been found to be larger in children with TS than in normal controls (Baumgardner et al., 1996). Subsequent study showed that this finding was gender-related and was present only in boys with TS (Mostofsky et al., 1999). Voxel-based morphometry and high-resolution MRI used in 31 TS patients showed increased gray matter in the left mesencephalon compared to 31 controls (Garraux et al., 2006). This finding, however, could not be replicated using the same technique in a smaller study of 14 boys with TS (Ludolph et al., 2006). This latter study found increased gray matter volumes in bilateral ventral putamen and regional decreases in gray matter volumes in the left hippocampus gyrus. The difference was attributed to younger mean age in the latter study compared with the previous study (12.5 versus 32 years). Dopaminergic hyperfunction (Albin et al., 2003), possibly as a result of overproduction of synapses in midchildhood (Giedd et al., 1999), might be associated with increased striatal volume in childhood, which may be lost in adulthood. Functional MRI studies show decreased neuronal activity during periods of suppression in the ventral globus pallidus, putamen, and thalamus and increased activity in the caudate, frontal cortex, and other cortical areas that are normally involved in the inhibition of unwanted impulses (prefrontal, parietal, temporal, and cingulated cortical areas) (Peterson, 2001).

Positron emission tomography (PET) scanning has shown variable rates of glucose utilization in basal ganglia as compared to controls. In one study, $[^{18}F]$fluorodeoxyglucose PET has shown evidence of increased metabolic activity in the lateral premotor and supplementary motor association cortices and in the midbrain (pattern 1), and decreased metabolic activity in the caudate and thalamic areas (limbic basal ganglia–thalamocortical projection system) (pattern 2) (Eidelberg et al., 1997). Pattern 1 is reportedly associated with tics, and pattern 2 correlates with the overall severity of TS. In contrast to dystonia, which is characterized by lentiform nucleus-thalamic metabolic dissociation, attributed to overactivity of the direct striatopallidal inhibitory pathway, the pattern of TS is characterized by concomitant metabolic reduction in striatal and thalamic function. The authors suggested that this pattern can be explained by a reduction in the indirect pathway resulting in reduction in subthalamic nucleus (STN) activity. Using event-related $[^{15}O]H_2O$ PET combined with time-synchronized audiotaping and videotaping of six patients with TS, Stern and colleagues (2000) found increased activity in the sensorimotor, language, executive, paralimbic, and frontal-subcortical areas that were temporarily related to the motor and phonic tics and the irresistible urge that precedes these behaviors. Rauch and colleagues (1997) showed bilateral medial temporal (hippocampal/parahippocampal) activation on PET in patients with OCD as compared to normal controls and absence of activation of inferior striatum, seen in normal controls. Various neuroimaging studies have also demonstrated moderate reduction in the size of the corpus callosum, basal ganglia (particularly caudate and globus pallidus), and frontal lobes (Filipek et al., 1997) and striatal hypoperfusion (Vaidya et al., 1998) in patients with ADHD.

## Neurochemistry

An alteration in the central neurotransmitters has been suggested chiefly because of relatively consistent responses to modulation of the dopaminergic system. Dopamine antagonists and depletors generally have an ameliorating effect on tics, whereas drugs that enhance central dopaminergic activity exacerbate tics (Jankovic and Rohaidy, 1987; Jankovic and

Orman, 1988). Low cerebrospinal fluid homovanillic acid, coupled with a favorable response to dopamine receptor–blocking drugs, has been interpreted as evidence in support of the notion that tics and TS are due to supersensitive dopamine receptors (Singer, 2000). Postmortem binding studies of dopamine receptors, however, have failed to provide support for this hypothesis (Singer, 2000).

Neurochemical studies of TS have been hampered by the lack of available postmortem brain tissue. Biochemical abnormalities in the few postmortem brains that have been studied include low serotonin, low glutamate in the medial globus pallidus, and low cyclic AMP in the cortex (Singer, 2000). Haber and Wolfer (1992) reported that in a blind rating of five TS brains, three had low dynorphin immunoreactivity in the ventral portion of the medial globus pallidus. A defect in tryptophan oxygenase in TS has been proposed by Comings (1990), who analyzed 1400 blood samples from patients with TS or ADHD and their relatives and controls; he found decreased platelet serotonin and low blood tryptophan levels in TS patients and their parents.

One intriguing hypothesis, supported partly by the increased $^3$H-mazindol binding to the presynaptic dopamine uptake carrier sites, suggests that TS represents a developmental disorder resulting in dopaminergic hyperinnervation of the ventral striatum and the associated limbic system (nucleus accumbens) (Singer et al., 1991). Using $[^{11}C]$Raclopride PET and amphetamine stimulation, Singer and colleagues (2002) found evidence for increased dopamine release in the putamen of patients with TS. They postulate that in TS, there is increased activity of the dopamine transporter leading to increased dopamine concentration in the dopamine terminals and stimulus-dependent increase in dopaminergic transmission. Support for this hypothesis has been provided by the imaging studies of Albin and colleagues (2003). The authors used PET with the vesicular monoamine transporter type 2 ligand $[(^{11})C]$dihydrotetrabenazine to quantify striatal monoaminergic innervation in patients with TS ($n = 19$) and control subjects ($n = 27$). With voxel-by-voxel analysis, the investigators found increased $[(^{11})C]$dihydrotetrabenazine binding in the ventral striatum (right > left) in patients with TS as compared to age-matched controls. A postmortem examination of two brains of patients with typical childhood-onset TD and one with adult-onset tics showed that the prefrontal cortex rather than the striatum showed most abnormalities, including increased D2 receptor protein, as well as increases in dopamine transporter, VAMP-2, and α-2A (Minzer et al., 2004).

Although this idea is highly speculative, it is possible that the genetic defect in TS somehow interferes with the normal regulation of the neuronal progenitor cells during development, thus resulting in the increased innervation of the ventral striatum (Ikonomidou et al., 1999; Itoh et al., 2001; Hanashima et al., 2004). This implies that the genetic defect somehow interferes with the programmed cell suicide that is needed to control cell proliferation in normal development and growth. The ventral striatum is the portion of the basal ganglia that is anatomically and functionally linked to the limbic system. The link between the basal ganglia and the limbic system might explain the frequent association of tics and complex behavioral problems, and a dysfunction in the basal ganglia and the limbic system seems to provide the best explanation for the most fundamental behavioral disturbance in TS, namely, loss of impulse control and a state of apparent "disinhibition." The notion that deficits in inhibitory functions are at the core of clinical phenotype associated with TS is supported by studies by Baron-Cohen and colleagues (1994) showing that patients with TS are not able to appropriately edit their intentions and by Swerdlow and colleagues (1996) showing that TS patients demonstrate deficits on the visuospatial priming tasks.

Functional neuroimaging studies have been used to aid in the understanding of neurotransmitter and receptor alterations in TS. Using [$^{123}$I]β-carboxymethoxy-3 β-(4-iodophenyl) tropane (CIT) single photon emission computed tomography scans, Malison and colleagues (1995) demonstrated a mean of 37% increase in binding of this dopamine transporter ligand in the striatum in five adult patients with TS as compared to age-matched controls. In contrast, Heinz and colleagues (1998) found no difference in [$^{123}$I]β-CIT binding in the midbrain, thalamus, or basal ganglia between 10 TS patients and normal control subjects. There was, however, a significant negative correlation between the severity of phonic tics and β-CIT binding in the midbrain and thalamus. In another study involving 12 TS adult patients, β-CIT scans showed evidence of increased dopamine transporter binding (Müller-Vahl et al., 2000). Combining single photon emission computed tomography and MRI, Wolf and colleagues (1996) found 17% greater binding of IBZM, a D2 receptor ligand, in the caudate (but not putamen) nucleus in five of the more affected monozygotic twins who were discordant for TS. It is important to note, however, that two of the five subjects were taking neuroleptics for up to 6 weeks prior to the single photon emission computed tomography studies. These findings, if confirmed by other studies of neuroleptic-naive patients, support the notion that the presynaptic dopamine function is enhanced in TS. This might, in turn, lead to a reduced inhibitory pallidal output to the mediodorsal thalamus. The observation that in patients with Parkinson disease the severity of childhood-onset tics was not influenced by the development of parkinsonism or by its treatment with levodopa, however, argues against the role of dopamine in the pathogenesis of TS symptoms (Kumar and Lang, 1997a). This is supported by the results of PET ligand studies showing normal D2 receptor density (Turjanski et al., 1994). Furthermore, Meyer and colleagues (1999) used PET imaging of (+)-α-[$^{11}$C]dihydrotetrabenazine to determine the density of vesicular monoamine transporter type 2, a cytoplasm-to-vesicle transporter that is linearly related to monoaminergic nerve terminal density unaffected by medications, in 8 TS patients and 22 controls. This study showed no significant difference in terminal density between patients and controls, thus failing to provide support for the concept of increased striatal innervation. However, these studies do not exclude the possibility of abnormal regulation of dopamine release and uptake. Subsequent study involving 19 adult patients with TS showed that the [($^{11}$C]dihydrotetrabenazine-binding potential is significantly increased, thus supporting the notion that striatal monoaminergic innervation is increased in the ventral striatum (right > left) of TS patients (Albin et al., 2003). The results of this study contrasted with previous findings of 30% to 40% increase in dopamine transporter (Müller-Vahl et al., 2000; Singer et al., 2001). Furthermore, in a small sample of TS patients, PET studies have demonstrated a 25% increase in accumulation of fluorodopa in the left caudate ($P = .03$) and

a 53% increase in the right midbrain ($P = .08$) (Ernst et al., 1999). These findings indicate possible dopaminergic dysfunction in the cells of origin and in the dopaminergic terminals, which suggests increased activity of DOPA decarboxylase.

Despite some limitations and inconsistencies, the imaging, ligand, and biochemical studies provide support for the hypothesis that the corticostriatal-thalamic-cortical circuit plays an important role in the pathogenesis of TS and related disorders (Witelson, 1993; Peterson, 2001). The dorsolateral prefrontal circuit, which links Brodmann area 9 and 10 with the dorsolateral head of the caudate, appears to be involved with executive functions (manipulation of previously learned knowledge, abstract reasoning, organization, verbal fluency, and problem solving; it is closely related to intelligence, education, and social exposure) and motor planning. An abnormality in this circuit has been implicated in ADHD. The lateral orbitofrontal circuit originates in the inferior lateral prefrontal cortex (area 10) and projects to the ventral medial caudate. An abnormality to this circuit is associated with personality changes, mania, disinhibition, and irritability. Last, the anterior cingulate circuit arises in the cingulate gyrus (area 24) and projects to the ventral striatum, which also receives input from the amygdala, hippocampus, medial orbitofrontal cortex, and entorhinal and perirhinal cortex. A variety of behavioral problems, including OCD, may be linked to an abnormality in this circuit.

Reduced metabolism or blood flow to the basal ganglia, particularly in the ventral striatum, most often in the left hemisphere, has been demonstrated in a majority of the studies involving TS subjects. These limbic areas are thought to be involved in impulse control, reward contingencies, and executive functions, and these behavioral functions appear to be abnormal in most patients with TS. The radioligand studies have been less consistent, but they provide some support for increased D2 receptor density in the caudate nucleus. Imaging studies of presynaptic markers such as dopa decarboxylase, dopamine, and dopamine transporter have produced results that are even less consistent. Future imaging and ligand studies should include children, since this population has been largely excluded because of ethical considerations. In addition, the studies should rigorously characterize comorbid disorders and should take into consideration potential confounding variables, such as the secondary effects of chronic illness and medications.

## Immunology

The potential role of immunologic mechanisms and specifically antineuronal antibodies is currently being explored in a variety of neurologic disorders, including TS (Allen, 1997; Hallett and Kiessling, 1997; Hallett et al., 2000; Morshed et al., 2001; Church et al., 2003). Several studies have suggested that exacerbations of TS symptoms correlated with an antecedent group A β-hemolytic streptococcus (GABHS) infection (demonstrated by elevated antistreptococcal titers) and the presence of serum antineuronal antibodies (Kiessling et al., 1993). Epitopes of streptococcal M proteins have been found to cross-react with the human brain, particularly the basal ganglia, and may be pathogenetically important in various neurologic disorders, such as Sydenham disease, TS-like syndrome, dystonia, and parkinsonism (Bronze and Dale, 1993;

Dale et al., 2001). In 10 patients with poststreptococcal acute disseminated encephalomyelitis (PSADEM) following exposure to GABHS, Dale and colleagues (2001) showed antibasal ganglia antibodies in all with three (60, 67, and 80 kDa) dominant bands. Furthermore, MRI showed hyperintense basal ganglia in 80% of the patients. The B lymphocyte antigen D8/17 is considered to be a marker for rheumatic fever but is also frequently overexpressed in patients with tics, OCD, and autism (Murphy et al., 1997; Swedo et al., 1997; Hoekstra et al., 2001). In one study, children and adults with TS had significantly higher serum levels of antineuronal antibodies against the putamen, but not the caudate or globus pallidus, as compared to controls (Singer et al., 1998). The potential relevance of this finding has been questioned, however, since there is no relationship between the presence of the antineuronal antibodies and age at onset, severity of tics, or the presence of comorbid disorders. Trifiletti and Packard (1999) have confirmed the presence of a specific brain protein at an apparent molecular weight of 83 kDa that is recognized by antibodies in the serum of 80% to 90% of patients with TS or OCD (Trifiletti and Packard 1999). They concluded that there may be a subset of patients with TS and OCD, perhaps up to 10% of all cases, in whom a streptococcal infection triggers the onset of symptoms. In a large case-control study of 150 patients with tics compared to 150 control subjects, Cardona and Orefici (2001) found a correlation between the occurrence of tics and prior exposure to streptococcal antigens and a correlation between the severity of tic disorder and the magnitude of the serologic response to streptococcal antigens measured by antistreptolysin O (ASO) titers (38% of the children with tics compared with 2% of the control subjects had ASO titers $\geq$ 500 IU, [$P < .001$]). In another study involving 25 adult patients with TS and 25 healthy controls, increased antibody titers against streptococcal M12 and M19 proteins were found in the TS group as compared to the healthy controls (Müller et al., 2001). In yet another study involving 81 patients with TS, 27 with Sydenham disease, 52 with autoimmune disorders, and 67 normal controls, Morshed and colleagues (2001) found elevated titers of IGG antineuronal antibodies in diseased individuals compared to controls, but there was no relationship between the antibody titers and the age, severity of TS, or comorbid disorders. Church and colleagues (2003) studied 100 patients with TS, 50 children with neurologic disease, 40 with recent uncomplicated streptococcal infection, and 50 healthy adults. They found elevated ASO titers in 64% of TS children compared with 15% of pediatric controls ($P < .0001$) and in 68% of adults with TS compared with 12% of adult neurologic controls and 8% of adult healthy controls ($P < .05$). Evidence of basal ganglia antibodies was found in 20% to 27% of TS patients, compared to 2% to 4% of controls. Similar to the proposed antigen in Sydenham disease, the most common antigen in TS was 60-kDa protein. Furthermore, 91% of patients with positive basal ganglia antibodies were found to have elevated ASO titers, whereas only 57% of those without such antibodies had high ASO titers. The authors concluded that these findings "suggest a pathogenic similarity between Sydenham disease and some patients with TS. In another study, 65% of 65 patients with atypical movement disorders, including dystonia and tics, had antibasal ganglia antibodies (Edwards et al., 2004b). Edwards and colleagues (2004a) also reported four adult cases of tic disorder and stereotypies associated with the presence of antibasal ganglia antibodies.

Development of dyskinesias (paw and floor licking, head and paw shaking) and phonic utterances has been reported in rodents after the microinfusion of dilute IgG from TS subjects into their striatum (Hallett et al., 2000). They extended their initial observations by demonstrating that intrastriatal microinfusion of TS sera or gamma immunoglobulins (IgG) in rats produced stereotypies and episodic utterances, analogous to involuntary movements seen in TS, and confirmed the presence of IgG selectively bound to striatal neurons (Hallett et al., 2000). Peterson and colleagues (2000) found that ADHD was associated significantly with titers of two distinct antistreptococcal antibodies, ASO and antideoxyribonuclease B, but no significant association was seen between antibody titers and a diagnosis of either chronic tic disorder or OCD. When basal ganglia volumes were included in these analyses, the relationships between antibody titers and basal ganglia volumes were significantly different in OCD and ADHD subjects compared with other diagnostic groups. Higher antibody titers in these subjects were associated with larger volumes of the putamen and globus pallidus nuclei.

Variably referred to as pediatric autoimmune neuropsychiatric disorders associated with streptococcal infections (PANDAS) or pediatric infection-triggered autoimmune neuropsychiatric disorders (PITANDS), this area is one of the most controversial topics in pediatric neurologic and psychiatric literature (Kurlan, 1998b; Trifiletti and Packard, 1999; Hoekstra et al., 2002; Murphy and Pichichero, 2002; Church et al., 2003; Snider and Swedo, 2003; Kurlan, 2004). The following are the diagnostic criteria for pediatric infection-triggered autoimmune neuropsychiatric disorders, which are similar to those for PANDAS except that they define an episode of illness more specifically:

1. The patient must have met diagnostic criteria for a tic disorder or OCD at some point in life,.
2. Symptom onset must have occurred between 3 years of age and puberty.
3. Symptom onset must be clinically sudden or demonstrate a pattern of sudden, recurrent clinically significant symptom exacerbations and remissions.
4. Increased symptoms must be pervasive and severe enough to warrant consideration of a treatment intervention or, if untreated, last for at least 4 weeks. Symptom exacerbations should not occur exclusively during a period of stress or illness.
5. There must be evidence of an antecedent or concomitant infection. This evidence might include a positive throat culture; positive GABHS serologic findings (antistreptolysin O antibodies with a peak at 3 to 6 weeks or anti-DNAase B antibodies with highest titers at 6 to 8 weeks); or a history of illness such as pharyngitis, sinusitis, or flu-like symptoms (Allen et al., 1997). Since GABHS infections are quite common (an average of three episodes during childhood), it is difficult to make the association between such infections and the subsequent development or exacerbation of tics or OCD.

The PANDAS concept has some other shortcomings: (1) The streptococcal infection may cause stress, which can exacerbate tics; (2) some patients with PANDAS may simply have a variant of Sydenham disease; and (3) there is no established temporal link between antecedent streptococcal infection and the exacerbation of tics. One piece of evidence supporting the notion that PANDAS simply represents one spectrum of Sydenham disease is the frequent occurrence of TS comorbidities in patients with Sydenham disease. One study compared 56 patients with Sydenham disease with 50 rheumatic fever patients and 50 healthy subjects; it found that obsessive-compulsive behavior (OCB) was present in 19%, OCD in 23.2%, and ADHD in 30.4% of Sydenham disease patients, all significantly more frequent than in the diseased or healthy controls (Maia et al., 2005). Nevertheless, the concept of postinfectious OCD is gradually seeping into the literature, even though definite proof is still lacking (Leonard et al., 1999). One observation, yet to be confirmed, that has been used in support of the autoimmune hypothesis of TS is that infusion of sera from patients with TS who have high titers of antibodies against nuclear or neural protein into ventrolateral striata of rats was associated with a higher rate of oral stereotypies as recorded by "blinded" raters (Taylor et al., 2002). This observation, however, could not be reproduced by other investigators who infused sera from patients with TS who had antiputaminal antibodies ($n = 9$) and from patients with PANDAS ($n = 8$) into the striatum of rats (Loiselle et al., 2004). No stereotypic behavior or abnormal movements were observed. Furthermore, there was no difference in anti–basal ganglia antibodies between patients with PANDAS and patients with TS as measured by enzyme-linked immunosorbent assay (Singer et al., 2004).

Untreated GABHS infection is often complicated by rheumatic fever within 10 to 14 weeks and by Sydenham disease within several months. Several studies have provided evidence for an overlap between TS and Sydenham disease, tics and OCD being manifested in both disorders (Church et al., 2003). It is therefore not clear whether TS and OCD are independent sequelae of GABHS or whether the observed symptoms of TS and OCD are manifestations of Sydenham disease. In a 3-year prospective study of 12 children, 5 to 11 years old, with documented acute GABHS tonsillopharyngitis, Murphy and Pichichero (2002) noted a sudden onset of OCD symptoms in all patients and tics in 3 patients concurrently with the acute infection or within 4 weeks. These symptoms resolved in all patients within 2 weeks of initiation of antibiotic therapy. Although this intriguing hypothesis requires further studies, plasmaphoresis, intravenous IGG, and immunosuppressant therapies are currently being investigated in the treatment of TS (Allen, 1997). In a study of 30 children in whom OCD or tics were presumably triggered or exacerbated by GABHS, there were striking improvements in various measures of OCD after intravenous immunoglobulin (IVIG) and in tics after plasma exchange (Perlmutter et al., 1999). Twenty-nine children with PANDAS were randomized in a partially double-blind fashion (no sham plasmapheresis) to an IVIG, IVIG placebo (saline), and plasmapheresis (PEX) group. One month after treatment, the severity of obsessive compulsive symptoms (OCS) were improved by 58% and 45% in the PEX and IVIG groups, respectively, compared to only 3% in the IVIG control group. In contrast, tic scores were improved only after PEX treatment (i.e., reductions of 49% [PEX], 19% [IVIG], and 12% [IVIG placebo]). Improvements in both tics and OCS were sustained for 1 year. However, there was no control PEX group, and the control comparisons were limited to the 1-month visit. Furthermore, there was no relationship between rate of antibody removal and therapeutic response.

Until the results of this study are confirmed, these treatment modalities are not justified in patients with TS. Furthermore, because of uncertainties about the possible cause-and-effect relationship between GABHS and tics and OCD, an antibiotic treatment for acute exacerbations of these symptoms is currently considered unwarranted (Kurlan, 1998b). Some studies have suggested that encephalitis lethargica is also part of the spectrum of poststreptococcal autoimmune diseases (Dale et al., 2004; Vincent, 2004).

## Other Hypotheses

Although direct evidence is still lacking, TS is currently viewed as a disorder of synaptic transmission involving disinhibition of the corticostriatal-thalamic-cortical circuitry. Several studies have provided evidence in support of the notion that the basal ganglia, particularly the caudate nucleus, and the inferior prefrontal cortex play an important role in the pathogenesis of not only TS but also comorbid disorders, particularly OCD (Baxter et al., 1992; McGuire, 1995; Swoboda and Jenike, 1995). For example, Laplane and colleagues (1989) described eight patients with bilateral basal ganglia lesions (anoxic or toxic encephalopathy) who showed stereotyped activities and OCB; extrapyramidal signs were mild or absent. Several imaging studies (reviewed earlier in the chapter) have implicated the ventral striatum-limbic system complex as playing an important role in the primitive reproductive behavior. A disturbance in sex hormones and certain excitatory neurotransmitters that normally influence the development of these structures may be ultimately expressed as TS (Kurlan, 1992). This hypothesis may explain the remarkable gender difference in TS, with males outnumbering females by 3 to 1; the exacerbation of symptoms at puberty and during the estrogenic phase of the menstrual cycle (Schwabe and Konkol, 1992); the characteristic occurrence of sexually related complex motor and phonic tics; and a variety of behavioral manifestations with sexual content. According to this hypothesis, the gene defect in TS results in an abnormal production of gonadal steroid hormones and increased trophic influence exerted by the excitatory amino acids, causing disordered development and increased innervation of the striatum and the limbic system. This is consistent with the finding of increased presynaptic dopamine uptake sites in brains of patients with TS (Singer et al., 1991).

Although there are no animal models, several families of horses with equine self-mutilation syndrome have been described with features that resemble human TS (Dodman et al., 1994). These horses exhibit a variety of stereotypic behaviors, such as glancing, biting at the flank or pectoral areas, bucking, kicking, rubbing, spinning, rolling, and vocalizing (squealing). Similar to TS, this condition is much more common in young males, is typically exacerbated by stress and during restful nonvigilance or boredom, and may be triggered by head trauma and relieved by castration. Genetic factors, however, seem to be most important.

## GENETICS

Finding a genetic marker and, ultimately, the gene has been the highest priority in TS research during the past decade. Unfortunately, despite concentrated effort by many investigators, the TS gene has thus far eluded this intensive search. A systematic genome scan using 76 affected sib-pair families with a total of 110 sib-pairs showed two regions, 4q and 8p, with an LOD score of 2.38 and 2.09, respectively; four additional regions, on chromosomes 1, 10, 13, and 19, had an LOD score over 1.0 (Tourette Syndrome Association International Consortium on Genetics, 1999). An analysis of 91 Afrikaner nuclear families with one or more affected children on chromosomes provided evidence of linkage to loci on chromosomes 2p11, 8q22, and 11q23–24, respectively (Simonic et al., 2001). This provides support for the finding in a previous study of a large French Canadian family of an LOD score of 3.24 for association with chromosome 11q23 (Merette et al., 2000). Other gene loci that are of interest in TS include 17q25 (Paschou et al., 2004) and 18q22 (Cuker et al., 2004). Assuming that genetic heterogeneity is not an important factor in TS, over 95% of the genome has been already excluded (Pakstis et al., 1991; Heutink et al., 1992). A linkage of TS with a known gene defect may help in the search for the TS gene. In this regard, a 16-year-old boy with typical TS was found to have a deletion of the terminal portion of the short arm of chromosome 9 (Taylor et al., 1991). A 7;18 translocation was identified in a patient with sporadic form of TS, and the relevant regions in chromosome 18q22.3 and 7q22–q31 will be searched for possible markers (Boghosian-Sell et al., 1996; Patel, 1996). The identification of balanced reciprocal translocation near 18q22.1 in families with TS and a deletion in the same locus in one patient with tics and OCD (and dysmorphic facial features) led to the tentative assignment of the TS gene in this region (Alsobrook and Pauls, 1997). Two families with translocations involving the 8q13 have been identified (Crawford et al., 2003). Linkage disequilibrium has been demonstrated between a D4 receptor locus (on chromosome 11) and TS (Grice et al., 1996). It is possible that the clue to the TS gene(s) will come from genetic studies of ADHD. In this regard, it is of interest that a genomewide scan in patients with ADHD identified five "hot spots": 17p11 (MLS = 2.98) and four nominal regions with MLS values greater than 1.0, including 5p13, 6q14, 11q25, and 20q13 (Ogdie et al., 2003). On the basis of analysis of several genomic regions, 17q25 appears to be of special interest, having the highest LOD score of 2.61 ($P = .002$) (Paschou et al., 2004).

A major advance in the search for the elusive TS gene or genes has been made by the discovery of a frameshift mutation in the Slit and Trk-like 1 (*SLITRK1*) gene on chromosome 13q31.1 (Abelson et al., 2005). These variants were absent in 172 other TS and 3600 control chromosomes. One parent of a TS patient carried the *SLITRK1* mutation but displayed only symptoms of trichotillomania. In a study of 44 families in which one or more members had trichotillomania, two mutations in the *SLITRK1* gene were found among some individuals with trichotillomania but not among their unaffected family members (Zuchner et al., 2006). *SLITRK1* mutations have been estimated to account for 5% of trichotillomania cases. The *SLITRK1* gene has been found to be expressed in brain regions previously implicated in TS—such as the cortex; the hippocampus; the thalamic, subthalamic, and globus pallidus nuclei; the striatum; and the cerebellum—and it appears to play a role in dendritic growth.

Current concepts of the genetics of TS support a sex-influenced autosomal-dominant mode of inheritance with a nearly complete penetrance for males and 56% penetrance for females when only tics are considered and 70% when OCD is included (Robertson, 1989; Pauls et al., 1991). Comings (1992), however, has proposed that TS is a semidominant, semirecessive disorder. This model takes into account the common observation that both parents of a TS child often exhibit TS or a forme fruste of TS and that the full and more severe motor-behavioral syndrome in the offspring represents a homozygous state (Fig. 17-3). Indeed, bilineal transmission was noted in 33% (considering tics) and 41% (considering tics or OCB) of TS families (Kurlan et al., 1994). In another study, McMahon and colleagues (1996) examined 175 members of a large, four-generation TS family as well as 16 spouses who married into this family. Interestingly, they found evidence of TS in 36% of the family members and in 31% of the married-in spouses (some form of a tic was found in 67% and 44%, respectively). Multivariate analysis showed that tics were more severe in the offspring of both parents with tics. This study raises the possibility of assortative mating (like marrying like) in TS, in contrast to random, nonassortative mating, which is presumed in the general population. Thus, bilineal transmission may lead to frequent homozygosity and high density of TS in some families. Walkup and colleagues (1996) failed to find TS in both parents, but when the broader definition was allowed, 19% of families had both parents affected. Using rigorous diagnostic criteria, we found that 25% of our TS cases had both parents with some features of TS: tics, 8%; OCB, 4%; and ADD, 12% (Fig. 17-4) (Hanna et al., 1999). The TS patients were compared with a control population of 1142 students who were observed in second-, fifth-, and eighth-grade classrooms. In contrast to the 5% frequency of ADD in one parent of controls, the occurrence of tics was 31% in at least one parent of TS cases, 45% in at least one parent of ADD cases, and 41% in at least one parent of OCB cases. Among all the parents of TS cases, tics were present in 24%, OCB in 25%, and ADD in 34%, whereas only 3% of parents of controls exhibited ADD. Bilineal transmission violates the standard principle of one-trait-one-locus, and it might explain why a gene marker has not yet been identified in TS despite intense collaborative research effort. These results are similar to those of Lichter and colleagues (1999), who found bilineal transmission in 6% of patients; tics or OCB were represented bilineally in 22% of patients. In a large family study and segregation analysis,

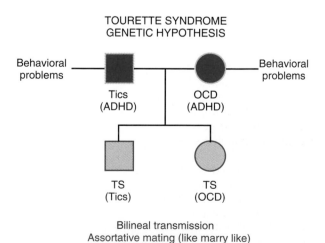

TOURETTE SYNDROME
GENETIC HYPOTHESIS

**Figure 17-3** Typical pattern of inheritance in patients with TS supporting bilineal transmission (both parents affected).

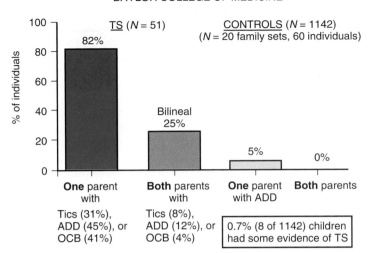

EPIDEMIOLOGIC GENETICS OF TOURETTE SYNDROME
BAYLOR COLLEGE OF MEDICINE

**Figure 17-4** Using rigid criteria for the diagnosis of tics, ADD, and OCB, this epidemiologic genetic study provided evidence of bilineal transmission in 25% of patients with TS. (Reprinted with permission from Hanna PA, Janjua FN, Contant CF, Jankovic J: Bilineal transmission in Tourette syndrome. Neurology 1999;53: 813–818.)

Walkup and colleagues (1996) provided evidence for a mixed model of inheritance rather than a simple autosomal mode of inheritance. This complex model of inheritance suggests that the majority of TS patients have two copies of the gene, one from each parent. This is consistent with the observation that many TS patients have both parents affected.

Twin studies, showing 89% concordance for TS and 100% concordance for either TS or chronic multiple tic disorder, provide strong support for the genetic etiology of TS (Alsobrook and Pauls, 1997; Singer, 2000). How much influence environmental factors have on the phenotypic expression of this disorder is not known. In searching for nongenetic factors in the pathogenesis of TS, Leckman and colleagues (1990) found that maternal life stress, nausea, and vomiting during first trimester of pregnancy were some of the perinatal factors that influenced the expression of the TS gene. In a study of 16 pairs of monozygotic twins, 94% of whom were concordant for tics, low birth weight was a strong predictor of tic severity, supporting a relationship between birth weight and phenotypic expression of TS (Hyde et al., 1992). Kurlan (1994) hypothesized that the clinical features associated with TS may occur to a variable degree in the course of normal childhood development and that genetic influences determine the severity of clinical symptoms in a given individual with TS. Eapen and colleagues (1997a) found evidence for earlier age at onset in maternally transmitted cases, suggesting genomic imprinting. The evidence for genomic imprinting in TS is, however, quite weak, and the genetic mechanism of TS remains elusive (Sadovnick and Kurlan, 1997). Because of phenotypic overlap between TS and Rett syndrome and myoclonus-dystonia, the genes for the latter disorders were examined, and no mutations in them were found in the TS population (De Carvalho et al., 2004).

One of the major concerns with the genetic linkage studies has been the lack of specificity of the current clinical criteria for diagnosis of TS. The boundaries of neurologic and behavioral manifestations of TS have not been clearly defined. While some investigators believe that the spectrum of behavioral expression of TS gene is quite broad, encompassing, in addition to ADHD and OCD, such diverse symptoms as conduct disorders, stuttering, dyslexia, panic attacks, phobias, depression, mania, and severe anxiety (Comings, 1987; Comings and Comings 1988a), others argue that more restrictive criteria for TS are needed, particularly for genetic linkage studies (Pauls et al., 1991). Pauls and colleagues (1991) studied 338 biological relatives of 86 TS probands and compared them to 21 biologically unrelated relatives of adopted TS probands. They confirmed their earlier observations and concluded that TS and OCD are etiologically related. The debate as to whether TS, OCD, and ADHD are genetically related or whether they merely represent comorbid neurobehavioral disorders will not be resolved until a TS-specific genetic marker is found.

Discovering the gene for OCD would have important implications for TS and would help to clarify the relationship between the two disorders. One study showed that men with OCD are significantly more likely to have both alleles of the gene for catechol-o-methyltransferase in a low activity form (L/L) than in the L/H form (Karayiorgou et al., 1997). As was noted earlier, the B lymphocyte antigen D8/17 has been suggested to be a possible peripheral marker for childhood-onset OCD and TS (Murphy et al., 1997).

## ETIOLOGY OF TICS (SECONDARY TOURETTISM)

While TS is probably the most common cause of tics, many other neurologic disorders are manifested by tics and other symptoms of TS (Fig. 17-5), supporting the notion of a multifactorial genesis of TS (see Box 17-1) (Jankovic, 2001b; Jankovic and Mejia, 2006). Of these, tics associated with static encephalopathy, autistic spectrum disorders, neuroacanthocytosis (Spitz et al., 1985; Saiki et al., 2004), Huntington disease (Jankovic and Ashizawa, 1995), pantothenate kinase–associated neurodegeneration (Pellecchia et al., 2005), beta-mannosidase deficiency (Sedel et al., 2006), and certain drugs (such as dopamine receptor–blocking drugs, cocaine, and antiepileptics [Cardoso and Jankovic, 1993; Bharucha and Sethi, 1995; Kumar and Lang, 1997b; Lombroso, 1999]) are particularly important to consider, especially in patients who do not fulfill the clinical criteria of TS. In one report, lamotrigine, a phenyltriazine drug that is structurally unrelated to other

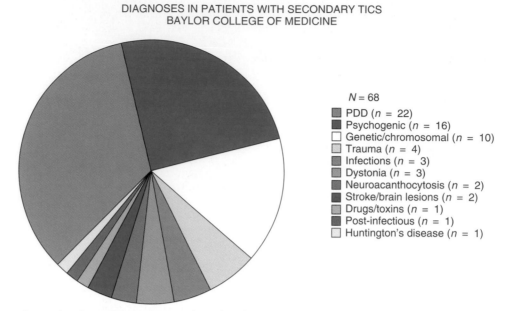

DIAGNOSES IN PATIENTS WITH SECONDARY TICS
BAYLOR COLLEGE OF MEDICINE

*N* = 68
- PDD (*n* = 22)
- Psychogenic (*n* = 16)
- Genetic/chromosomal (*n* = 10)
- Trauma (*n* = 4)
- Infections (*n* = 3)
- Dystonia (*n* = 3)
- Neuroacanthocytosis (*n* = 2)
- Stroke/brain lesions (*n* = 2)
- Drugs/toxins (*n* = 1)
- Post-infectious (*n* = 1)
- Huntington's disease (*n* = 1)

**Figure 17-5** Causes of tics other than TS in patients evaluated at the Baylor College of Medicine Movement Disorders Clinic. (Reprinted with permission from Jankovic J, Mejia NI: Tics associated with other disorders. In Walkup J, Mink J, Hollenbeck P [eds]: Tourette Syndrome. Advances in Neurology, vol 99. Philadelphia, Lippincott Williams & Wilkins, Philadelphia, 2006, pp 61–68.)

antiepileptic medications, was associated with dose-related motor and phonic tics in three children and features of OCD in one (Lombroso, 1999). The author speculated that in these rare cases, lamotrigine in high doses inhibited the presynaptic release of excitatory amino acids and resulted in an abnormal regulation of dopamine uptake in the striatum, leading to the production of tics and related TS symptoms. Rarely, "tourettism" can follow head trauma (Fahn, 1982; Krauss and Jankovic, 1997; Kumar and Lang, 1997b); nonspecific cerebral insults, such as ischemia, hypoxia, and hypothermia (Singer et al., 1997); or striatal encephalitis due to varicella zoster (Dale et al., 2003). The study of the mechanisms of the secondary tourettism could provide insights into the pathogenesis of TS. For example, while TS symptoms have been reported to be exacerbated by various structural lesions involving the basal ganglia and the limbic system (Jankovic, 2001b), one patient with TS had complete resolution of tics after an MRI-proven midbrain lesion due to Wernicke encephalopathy (Pantoni et al., 1997). This suggests that an intact midbrain tegmentum is required for the expression of motor tics.

Autistic spectrum disorders represent one of the largest groups of pediatric disorders in which features of TS, such as tics, ADHD, and OCD, may be present. Autism is a behaviorally defined syndrome manifested by poor social interaction; disordered language; and atypical responses to people, objects, and events (Volkmar and Pauls, 2003). The syndrome is typically associated with severe disturbances in cognition, language, and behavior that appear before the age of 30 months. Stereotypic movements include body rocking, repeated touching and sniffing of objects, ritualistic ordering, and insistence on precisely following routines. Similar to TS, there is about 3:1 male:female preponderance. A study of children 3 to 10 years old found a 0.34% prevalence of autism with cognitive impairment in 68% (Yeargin-Allsopp et al., 2003). A review of home videos during early development in 17 autistic children found evidence of abnormal movement at the age of 4 to 6 months and sometimes

even at birth, long before the diagnosis of autism (Teitelbaum et al., 1998). The authors suggest that their findings support the view that movement disturbances play an intrinsic part in the phenomenon of autism, that movement disturbances in autistic children are present at birth, and that such movement disturbances can be used to diagnose the presence of autism in the first few months of life. Other studies have suggested that TS symptoms are more common than expected in patients with autism, with an estimated frequency of 6.5% (Baron-Cohen et al., 1999). Asperger syndrome is a form of pervasive developmental disorder in which language and self-help skills are relatively intact. It is often considered a mild form of autism, but its relationship to other autistic disorders has not been well defined. Asperger syndrome patients frequently exhibit repetitive movements (stereotypies) and may have motor and phonic tics in addition to other behavioral abnormalities (Ringman and Jankovic, 2000). Other childhood behavioral disorders that may overlap in symptomatology with autism and TS include Williams syndrome, characterized by remarkable conversational skills and excessive empathy; Prader-Willi syndrome, associated with temper tantrums and obsessive-compulsive behavior; Angelman syndrome, characterized by hyperactivity and a constantly happy disposition (Cassidy and Morris, 2002); and Rett syndrome, an X-linked autistic disorder associated with stereotypies and other movement disorders. However, mutations in the *MECP2* gene on chromosome X28, responsible for Rett syndrome, were excluded (Rosa et al., 2003). Also excluded were mutations in the *SGCE* gene, responsible for the dystonia-myoclonus syndrome, which shares some clinical features with TS, in a population of well-defined TS (De Carvalho Aguiar et al., 2004).

Other related conditions that may have resemblance to tics and TS are the jumping Frenchmen of Maine, "ragin' Cajuns" of Louisiana, latah of the Malays, and myriachit of Siberia (Lees, 2001). First described in 1878, this culture-bound condition is characterized by an excessive startle response, sometimes with echolalia, echopraxia, or forced obedience.

It is considered by some as an operant conditioned behavior rather than a neurologic or even hysteric disorder (Saint-Hilaire et al., 1986). The rare late-onset startle-induced tics may resemble these culture-bound syndromes and other startle responses (Tijssen et al., 1999). Rarely, psychogenic tics are present in patients with TS, but this very rare occurrence is difficult to confirm clinically (Kurlan et al., 1992).

The discussion of the numerous causes of tics and other manifestation of TS is beyond the scope of this review, and the reader is referred to other reviews of secondary causes of tics (Kumar and Lang, 1997b; Jankovic 2001a; Jankovic and Mejia, 2006).

## EPIDEMIOLOGY

Discovery of a disease-specific marker will be helpful not only in improving current understanding of this complex neurobehavioral disorder but also in clarifying the epidemiology of TS (Scahill et al., 2001). The prevalence rates have varied markedly and have been estimated to be as high as 4.2% when all types of tic disorders are included (Costello et al., 1996) and 1/83 (1.2%) (Comings and Comings, 1988b) or as low as 28.7/100,000 (0.03%) (Caine et al., 1988) and 1/10,000 (0.01%) (Singer, 2000). There are many reasons for this wide variation, the most important of which are different ascertainment methods, different study populations, and different clinical criteria. Since about one third of patients with tics do not even recognize their presence, it is difficult to derive more accurate prevalence figures for TS without a well-designed door-to-door survey (Kurlan et al., 1987). In one study, 3034 students in three schools in Los Angeles were monitored over a 2-year period by a school psychologist; the frequency of definite TS was 1 in 95 males and 1 in 759 females (Comings et al., 1990). Because the observed population included special education children, the authors adjusted the final prevalence figure to 0.63%. This figure is similar to that derived from the observational study of 1142 children in second, fifth, and eighth grades of a general school population, among whom 8 children (0.7%) had some evidence of TS (Hanna et al., 1999). In another school-based study involving 167 randomly selected 13- and 14-year-olds in English high schools, the prevalence of TS based on DSM III-R was estimated at 3%, but 18% screened positive for tics (Mason et al., 1998). Snider and colleagues (2002) observed 553 schoolchildren (kindergarten to sixth grade) monthly over an 8-month period and found tics in 135 (24%); 34 children had persistent tics (6.1%). Those with persistent tics were more likely to be males and had more behavioral problems than those without persistent tics. Kurlan and colleagues (2001) found that 27% of 341 special education students had tics compared to 19.7% of 1255 students in regular classroom programs; the frequency of TS was 7% and 3.8%, respectively. In another study, based on an interview of 1596 children, Kurlan and colleagues (2002) found that 339 (21%) had tics. Children with tics were younger, were more likely to be male and attend special education classes, and had a lower mean IQ.

## TREATMENT

The first step in the management of patients with TS is proper education of the patient, relatives, teachers, and other individuals who frequently interact with the patient about the nature of the disorder (Scahill et al., 2006). School principals, teachers, and students can be helpful in implementing the therapeutic strategies. In addition, the parents and the physician should work as partners in advocating the best possible school environment for the child. This might include extra break periods and a refuge area to allow release of tics, waiving time limitations on tests or adjusting timing of tests to the morning, and other measures designed to relieve stress. National and local support groups can provide additional information and can serve as a valuable resource for the patient and his or her family (see Appendix 17-1).

Before deciding *how* to treat TS-related symptoms, it is important to decide *whether* to treat them. Even in our referrals, and presumably in more severely affected population of patients, about 20% do not need pharmacologic therapy. Counseling and behavioral modification might be sufficient for those with mild symptoms. Medications, however, may be considered when symptoms begin to interfere with peer relationships, social interactions, academic or job performance, or activities of daily living. Because of the broad range of neurologic and behavioral manifestation and varying severity, therapy of TS must be tailored specifically to the needs of the individual patient (Table 17-2 and Box 17-3) (Jimenez-Jimenez and Garcia-Ruiz, 2001; Lang, 2001; Silay and Jankovic, 2005). The most troublesome symptoms should be targeted first. Medications should be instituted at low doses, titrated gradually to the lowest effective dosage, and tapered during nonstressful periods (e.g., summer vacations). Another important principle of therapy in TS is to give each medication and dosage regimen an adequate trial. This approach will avoid needless changes made in response to variations in symptoms during the natural course of the disease.

Before discussing pharmacologic therapy of TS symptoms, it is appropriate to make a few remarks about behavioral therapy (Piacentini and Chang, 2001). Different forms of behavioral modification have been recommended since the disorder was first described, but until recently, very few studies of behavioral treatments have been subjected to rigorous scientific scrutiny. Most of the reported studies suffer from poor or unreliable assessments, small sample size, short follow-up, lack of controls, no validation of compliance, and other methodologic flaws. Given these limitations, the following behavioral techniques have been reported to provide at least some benefit: (1) massed (negative) practice (voluntary and effortful repetition of the tic leads to a build up of a state termed *reactive inhibition*, at which point the subject is forced to rest and not perform the tic due to a build-up of a negative habit), (2) operant techniques/contingency management (tic-free intervals are positively reinforced, and tic behaviors are punished), (3) anxiety management techniques (relaxation training), (4) exposure-based treatment (desensitization to address tic triggering phenomena such as premonitory sensory urges), (5) awareness training (direct visual feedback, self-monitoring, and awareness-enhancing techniques, such as saying the letter "T" after each tic), and (6) habit-reversal training (HRT), consisting of reenactment of tic movements while looking in a mirror, training to detect and increase awareness of one's tics, identification of high-risk situations, training to isometrically contract the tic-opposing muscles, and training to recognize and resist tic urges (Piacentini and Chang, 2001). Wilhelm and colleagues (2003) studied 32 patients with TS who were randomly assigned to 14 sessions

**Table 17-2 Pharmacology of Tourette syndrome**

| Drugs | Initial Dosage (mg/day) | Clinical Effect |
|---|---|---|
| **Dopamine Receptor Blockers** | | **Tics** |
| Fluphenazine | 1 | +++ |
| Pimozide | 2 | +++ |
| Haloperidol | 0.5 | +++ |
| Risperidone | 0.5 | ++ |
| Ziprasidone | 20 | ++ |
| Thiothixene | 1 | ++ |
| Trifluoperazine | 1 | ++ |
| Molindone | 5 | ++ |
| **Dopamine Depleters** | | **Tics** |
| Tetrabenazine | 25 | ++ |
| **CNS Stimulants** | | **ADHD** |
| Methylphenidate | 5 | +++ |
| Concerta | 18 | +++ |
| Metadate CD | 20 | +++ |
| Metadate ER | 20 | +++ |
| Ritalin SR | 20 | +++ |
| Adderall | 10 | +++ |
| Atomoxetine | 25 | +++ |
| Pemoline | 18.75 | ++ |
| Dextroamphetamine | 5 | ++ |
| Dexedrine Spansules | 20 | ++ |
| **Noradrenergic Drugs** | | **Impulse Control/ADHD** |
| Clonidine | 0.1 | ++ |
| Guanfacine | 1.0 | ++ |
| **Serotoninergic Drugs** | | **OCD** |
| Fluoxetine | 20 | +++ |
| Clomipramine | 25 | +++ |
| Sertraline | 50 | +++ |
| Paroxetine | 20 | +++ |
| Fluvoxamine | 50 | +++ |
| Venlafaxine | 25 | +++ |
| Citalopram | 40 | +++ |
| Escitalopram | 20 | +++ |
| Nefazodone | 300 | +++ |

+, minimal improvement; ++, moderate improvement; +++, marked improvement.

**Box 17-3 Treatment strategies in Tourette syndrome**

**TICS**
Clonazepam
Fluphenazine
Pimozide
Haloperidol
Thiothixene
Trifluoperazine
Molindone
Sulpiride
Tiapride
Flunarizine
Olanzapine
Risperidone
Quetiapine
Clozapine
Tetrabenazine
Pergolide
Topiramate
Nicotine
Naltrexone
Flutamide
Cannabinoid
Botulinum toxin

**Obsessive-Compulsive Disorder**
Imipramine
Clomipramine
Fluoxetine
Sertraline
Nefazodone
Fluvoxamine
Paroxetine
Venlafaxine
Citalopram
Lithium
Buspirone
Clonazepam
Trazodone
Clonazepam

**Attention-Deficit Disorder/Attention-Deficit Hyperactivity Disorder**
Clonidine
Imipramine
Nortriptyline
Desipramine
Deprenyl
Bupropion
Guanfacine
Carbamazepine
Dextroamphetamine
Methylphenidate
Adderal
Pemoline
Modafinil
Atomoxetine
Mecamylamine
Neurosurgery

of either HRT (awareness training, self-monitoring, relaxation training, competing response training, and contingency management) or supportive psychotherapy. The 16 patients who were assigned to the HRT group "improved significantly" and "remained significantly improved over pretreatment at 10-month follow-up." This approach has also been found useful in the management of phonic tics (Woods et al., 2003). It is not clear whether patients without premonitory urges would benefit from this form of therapy. There is also some concern as to whether the mental effort required to fully comply with HRT could actually interfere with patient's attention and learning. Given hype demands on time and effort on the part of the patient, the therapist, and parents, it is not surprising that even if HRT is effective, its benefits are usually only temporary. These therapies, however, may be useful ancillary techniques in patients whose response to other therapies, including pharmacotherapy, is not entirely satisfactory.

## Management of Tics

The goal of treatment should be not to completely eliminate all the tics but to achieve a tolerable suppression of the tics. Because of the variability of tics in terms of severity, frequency, and distribution, the assessment of efficacy of a therapeutic intervention on tics is often quite problematic. A number of tic-rating scales have been utilized, but none of them are ideal. Although at-home videotapes can be used to capture tics that are not appreciated by patients or when patients are examined in the clinic, video-based tic-rating scales have many shortcomings (Goetz et al., 1999, 2001).

Despite these limitations, controlled and open trials have found that of the pharmacologic agents that are used for tic suppression, the dopamine receptor–blocking drugs (neuroleptics) are clearly most effective (Robertson, 2000; Jimenez-Jimenez and Garcia-Ruiz, 2001) (see Table 17-2 and Box 17-3). Haloperidol (Haldol) and pimozide (Orap) are the only neuroleptics that have actually been approved by the Food and Drug Administration for the treatment of TS. In one randomized, double-blind, controlled study, pimozide was found to be superior to haloperidol with respect to efficacy and side effects (Sallee et al., 1997). However, instead of starting with a neuroleptic, which can cause sedation, bradykinesia, and even tardive dyskinesia, some clinicians (preferring to begin with agents without such risks) utilize clonazepam and clonidine, even though these drugs are not as effective as the neuroleptics. Clonazepam can be useful, particularly in the treatment of clonic tics. When neuroleptics are needed, some clinicians prefer fluphenazine (Prolixin) as the first of these agents, since it appears to have a lower incidence of sedation and other side effects. If fluphenazine fails to control tics adequately, risperidone (Risperdal) or pimozide can be substituted. Clinicians may start with fluphenazine, risperidone, and pimozide at 1 mg at bedtime and increase by 1 mg every 5 to 7 days. If these drugs fail to control tics adequately, then administration of haloperidol, thioridazine (Mellaril), trifluoperazine (Stelazine), molindone (Moban), or thiothixene (Navane) may be attempted. Risperidone, a neuroleptic with both dopamine- and serotonin-blocking properties, has been shown to be effective in reducing tic frequency and intensity in most (Bruun and Budman, 1996; Bruggeman et al., 2001), but not in all studies (Robertson et al., 1996). A double-blind, placebo-controlled, 8-week trial in which 24 patients were randomly assigned risperidone in doses of 0.5 to 6.0 mg per day (median dose of 2.5 mg per day) and 24 were assigned to placebo, risperidone was found to be significantly ($P < .05$) superior to placebo on the Global Severity Rating of the Tourette Syndrome Severity Scale (Dion et al., 2002). The proportion of patients who improved by at least one point on this seven-point scale was 60.8% in the risperidone group and 26.1% in the placebo group. Hypokinesia and tremor increased in the risperidone group, but there were no other extrapyramidal side effects. Fatigue and somnolence were the most common adverse events associated with risperidone. In another placebo-controlled study, 12 patients who were randomized to risperidone had a 36%

reduction in tic symptoms compared to 11% reduction in the 14 patients receiving placebo (Scahill et al., 2003). One randomized, double-blind study found risperidone to be more effective than clonidine in the treatment of TS-associated OCD (Gaffney et al., 2002). Risperidone has also been found to be effective in the treatment of tantrums, aggression, and SIB in children with autism (Research Units on Pediatric Psychopharmacology Autism Network, 2002). Some atypical, second-generation neuroleptics have been found to increase the risk of obesity and type 2 diabetes, but risperidone and ziprasidone appear to be associated with a lower risk of these complications (Gianfrancesco et al., 2002; Stahl and Shayegan, 2003). It is not clear whether the atypical neuroleptics, such as clozapine (Clozaril), olanzapine (Zyprexa), or quetiapine (Seroquel), will be effective in the treatment of tics and other manifestations of TS. Quetiapine (Seroquel), a dibenzothiazepine that blocks not only D1 and D2 receptors but also $5\text{-}HT_{1A}$ and $5\text{-}HT_2$ receptors, has been reported to provide beneficial effects in some patients with TS, but the clinical improvement might not be sustained. Ziprasidone (Geodon), one of the more recently introduced atypical neuroleptics and a potent blocker of $5\text{-}HT_{2A}$, $5\text{-}HT_{2C}$, $5\text{-}HT_{1A}$, $5\text{-}HT_{1D}$, and $\alpha_1$ receptors more than D2 or D3 receptors, was found to decrease tic severity by 35% compared to a 7% change in the placebo group (Sallee et al., 2000). Because of its relatively high D2 receptor occupancy, ziprasidone is pharmacologically more similar to risperidone and olanzapine than to clozapine and quetiapine (Mamo et al., 2004). Similar to pimozide, ziprasidone may prolong the QT interval (Blair et al., 2005) but has the advantage over other atypical neuroleptics that it is less likely to cause weight gain and sexual side effects. It also appears to have strong antiapathy, promotivational, and antidepressant effects. The clinical significance of a prolonged QT interval is controversial, but it may be associated with *torsades de pointe*s, which can potentially degenerate into ventricular fibrillation and sudden death. Besides pimozide and ziprasidone, other drugs that can prolong the QT interval include haloperidol, risperidone, thioridazine, and desipramine. However, according to experts, the low rate of QTc prolongation in *torsades de pointes* is not likely to be a serious problem (Glassman and Bigger, 2001).

Aripiprazole (Abilify) is the most recent addition to the new class of atypical antipsychotic medications (Goodnick and Jerry, 2002). Typical antagonist of D2 receptors in the mesolimbic pathway, aripiprazole is also a partial D2 agonist and displays strong $5\text{-}HT_{2A}$ receptor antagonism and is similar to ziprasidone in also having agonistic activity at the $5\text{-}HT_{1A}$ receptor. Among the atypical antipsychotics, aripiprazole displays the lowest affinity for α1-adrenergic (α1), histamine (H1), and muscarinic (M1) receptors and, as such, has a relatively low incidence of side effects, including orthostatic hypotension, weight gain, sedation, dry mouth, and constipation. This drug has not yet been studied in TS. Tetrabenazine, a monoamine-depleting and dopamine receptor–blocking drug, is a powerful anti-tic drug (Fig. 17-6), but it is not yet readily available in the United States (Jankovic and Beach, 1997; Kenney and Jankovic, 2006; Kenney et al., 2007). This drug has been found very effective in the treatment of TS, and it has the advantage over the conventional neuroleptics in that it does not cause tardive dyskinesias. Other drugs that are used in the treatment of tics include sulpiride, tiapride,

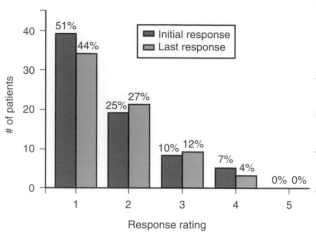

RESPONSE TO TETRABENAZINE IN PATIENTS WITH
TOURETTE SYNDROME (*N* = 77)

Duration of Rx = 23.7 ± 41.1 months
TBZ dose = 50.4 ± 27.0 mg

1. Marked reduction in abnormal movements, excellent improvement in function
2. Moderate reduction in abnormal movements, very good improvement in function
3. Moderate reduction in abnormal movements, only mild or no improvement in function
4. Poor or no response in abnormal movements or function
5. Worsening of the movement disorder and/or deterioration in function

**Figure 17-6** Tetrabenazine, a monoamine-depleting drug, provides marked to moderate improvement in most patients with TS.

metoclopramide, and piquindone (Jimenez-Jimenez and Garcia-Ruiz, 2001).

The side effects associated with neuroleptics, such as sedation, depression, weight gain, and school phobia, seem to be somewhat less frequent with fluphenazine than with haloperidol and the other neuroleptics (Bruun and Budman, 1996). The most feared side effects of chronic neuroleptic therapy include tardive dyskinesia and hepatotoxicity. In addition, pimozide may prolong the QT interval; therefore, patients who are treated with the drug must have an electrocardiogram before starting therapy. We repeat the electrocardiogram about 3 months later and once a year thereafter. It is important to note that certain antibiotics, such as clarithromycin, can raise the blood levels of pimozide and indirectly contribute to the drug's cardiotoxicity. Tardive dyskinesia, usually manifested by stereotypic involuntary movements, is only rarely persistent in children. However, tardive dystonia, a variant of tardive dyskinesias that is most frequently encountered in young adults, may persist and occasionally progresses to a generalized and disabling dystonic disorder (Singh and Jankovic, 1988; Silva et al., 1993) (Video 17-18). Other movement disorders that are associated with neuroleptics include bradykinesia, akathisia, and acute dystonic reactions (Jankovic, 1995). Therefore, careful monitoring of the patients is absolutely essential, and whenever possible, the dosage should be reduced or even discontinued during periods of remission or during vacations.

Several nonneuroleptic treatments have been reported to be effective in the treatment of tics. The dopamine agonist pergolide was found to be useful in an open-label trial in 32 patients with TS, particularly if the TS is associated with restless legs syndrome (Lipinski et al., 1997). In another study, 24 patients with TS (ages 7 to 17 years) who were medication-free for 4 weeks prior to treatment were randomized to receive either placebo or pergolide (150 to 300 mg daily) for 6 weeks, followed by a 2-week washout, and then crossed over to the other treatment arm (Gilbert et al., 2000). Nineteen patients completed the study. Tic severity, as determined by the main outcome measure, the Yale Global Tic Severity Scale, fell by 50% on pergolide versus 42% on placebo ($P < .0011$). There was no significant difference between the two treatments on the Clinical Global Impression-Severity scale or on the parent-rated Tic Severity Self Report. In a follow-up, randomized, placebo-controlled trial, the researchers concluded that "pergolide appeared to be an efficacious and safe medication for tic reduction in children, and may also improve attention deficit hyperactivity disorder symptoms" (Gilbert et al., 2003). Ropinirole, another dopamine agonist, has also been found to be effective in the treatment of TS (Anca et al., 2004). These findings seem paradoxical in view of the well-known beneficial effects of dopamine receptor blockers. It is possible, however, that the observed effects of dopamine agonists could be mediated by their action on dopamine D2 autoreceptors, thus reducing endogenous dopamine turnover. A single-blind levodopa challenge in six adult patients with TS resulted in a decrease in self-rated tic severity (Black and Mink, 2000), but this preliminary study needs to be confirmed by a larger and well-designed clinical trial.

Clonazepam is another drug that is sometimes useful in treating patients with TS, particularly in the treatment of clonic tics. Since some of the premonitory sensations resemble obsessions and the tics may be viewed as "compulsive" movements, anti-OCD medications can also be helpful. Treatment of the premonitory sensations may lead to improvement of these tics. Since sex steroids affect the expression of TS gene and also modulate multiple neurotransmitter systems, antiadrogens have been tried in the treatment of TS. Flutamide, an acetanilid nonsteroidal androgen antagonist, has been found in one double-blind, placebo-controlled study to modestly and transiently reduce motor, but not phonic, tics, with a mild improvement in associated symptoms of OCD (Peterson et al., 1998b). Because of potentially serious side effects, such as diarrhea and fulminant hepatic necrosis, this drug should be reserved only for those patients in whom tics remain a disabling problem despite optimal anti-tic therapy. Ondansetron, a selective 5-HT$_3$ antagonist at 8 to 16 mg per day for 3 weeks, has been associated with a decrease in severity of tics (Toren et al., 1999). Baclofen, a GABA$_B$ autoreceptor agonist, has been found to markedly decrease the severity of motor and phonic tics in 95% of 264 patients with TS (Awaad, 1999), but a double-blind, placebo-controlled, crossover trial of nine patients with TS showed that the beneficial response to baclofen was due to improvement in the overall impairment score rather than a reduction of tic activity (Singer et al., 2001). Donepezil, a noncompetitive inhibitor of acetylcholinesterase, has been reported anecdotally to suppress tics (Hoopes, 1999).

Ever since the discovery that cannabinoids markedly potentiate neuroleptic-induced hypokinesis in rats and that their effects on the extrapyramidal motor system may be mediated through nicotinic cholinergic receptors, there has been growing interest in nicotine as a treatment of various movement disorders, including TS (Sanberg et al., 1993). Nicotine gum (e.g., Nicorette, 2 mg) and transdermal nicotine patch (e.g., Nicoderm, 7 mg) have been reported to potentiate the anti-tic effects of neuroleptics, but this observation needs to be confirmed by a placebo-controlled study (Silver et al., 1996; Sanberg et al., 1998; Hughes et al., 1999). Open trials indicate that nicotine may suppress tics even in patients who have not been treated with D2 receptor–blocking drugs. The onset of anti-tic effect is quite rapid (0.5 to 3 hours) and the effects appear to persist for about 10 days after a 24-hour application of the patch (to the deltoid area). Side effects of the nicotine patch include local irritation and itching, nausea (in up to 70% lasting 4 to 6 hours), and transient headache with or without dizziness. There was apparently no evidence of nicotine dependence in these open trials. Although nicotine is a potent agonist of nicotinic acetylcholine receptors, when used chronically it causes desensitization of these receptors, thus exerting an antagonist effect. This is consistent with the observation that mecamylamine (Inversine, approved by the Food and Drug Administration as an antihypertensive and antismoking drug at 2.5 mg twice a day), an antihypertensive agent that acts as a peripheral ganglionic blocker with central antinicotinic, anticholinergic properties, improved tics as well as behavioral problems in 11 of 13 patients with TS at doses up to 5 mg per day (Sanberg et al., 1998). A subsequent double-blind, placebo-controlled study, however, failed to demonstrate a significant benefit on the symptoms associated with TS (Silver et al., 2001). Nicotine also causes the presynaptic release of acetylcholine, GABA, norepinephrine, dopamine, serotonin, vasopressin, and β-endorphins (Toth et al., 1992). Although the mechanism of action of nicotine in TS is unknown, it is interesting that nicotine initially activates midbrain dopamine neurons, but after longer exposure to nicotine, these neurons become desensitized, thus possibly accounting for the antidopaminergic (and anti-tic) effect of the drug (Pidoplichko et al., 1997). Recent studies suggest that nicotine inhibits some (e.g., α4β2), but not other (e.g., α3β4), striatal nicotinic receptors and that this inhibition could persist for several days (Lindstrom, 1997). Finally, there have been several anecdotal reports of marijuana helping various symptoms of TS. This is consistent with the finding that cannabinoid receptors are densely located in the output nuclei of the basal ganglia and that activation of these receptors increases GABAergic transmission and inhibition of glutamate release (Müller-Vahl et al., 1999). Some patients clearly benefit from taking the cannabinoid dronabinol (Marinol) at doses of 2.5 to 10 mg twice a day. Although levetiracetam has been found to be effective in the treatment of tics in an open-label trial involving 60 patients with TS (Awaad et al., 2005), it is not clear whether this or other anticonvulsants, such as topiramate

(Abuzzahab and Brown, 2001), which is currently undergoing clinical trials, will be useful in the treatment of TS.

Motor tics may be successfully treated with botulinum toxin (BTX) injections in the affected muscles (Video 17-19; see also Video 17-15).  Such focal chemodenervation ameliorates not only the involuntary movements but also the premonitory sensory component. Ten TS patients were treated with BTX injections into the involved muscles, and all experienced moderate to marked improvement in the intensity and frequency of their tics (Jankovic, 1994). Subsequent experience with a large number of patients has confirmed the beneficial effects of BTX injections in the treatment of motor and phonic tics, including severe coprolalia (Scott et al., 1996). Furthermore, those patients in whom premonitory sensations preceded the onset of tics noted lessening of these sensory symptoms. The benefits last 3 to 4 months, on the average, and there are usually no serious complications. In a follow-up study of 35 patients treated for troublesome or disabling tics in 115 sessions, the mean peak effect response was 2.8 (range: 0 to 4) (Kwak et al., 2000). The mean duration of benefit was 14.4 weeks (up to 45 weeks). The latency to onset of benefit was 3.8 days (up to 10 days). The mean duration of tics prior to initial injections was 15.3 years (range: 1 to 62 years), and the mean duration of follow-up was 21.2 months (range: 1.5 to 84 months). Twenty-one of 25 (84%) patients with notable premonitory sensory symptoms derived marked relief of these symptoms from BTX (mean benefit: 70.6%). Patients reported an overall global response of 62.7%. The total mean dose (units) was 502.1 (range: 15 to 3550), the number of visits was 3.3 (range: 1 to 16), and the mean dose per visit was 119.9 (range: 15 to 273). The sites of injections in descending order were as follows: cervical or upper thoracic (17), upper face (14), lower face (7), voice (4), upper back and shoulder (3), scalp (1), forearm (1), leg (1), and rectus abdominis (1). Complications included mild, transient neck weakness (4); mild, transient dysphagia (2); ptosis (2); nausea, 1 day (1); hypophonia (1); fatigue (1); and generalized weakness, 7 days (1). We concluded that BTX is effective and well tolerated in the treatment of tics. An additional and consistent finding was the relief of disturbing premonitory sensations. In a placebo-controlled study of 18 patients with simple motor tics, Marras and colleagues (2001) found a 39% reduction in the number of tics per minute within 2 weeks after injection with BTX compared to an 6% increase in the placebo group (P = .004). In addition, there was a 0.46 reduction in urge scores with BTX compared to a 0.49 increase in the placebo group (P = .02). This preliminary study, however, lacked the power to show significant differences in other measured variables, such as severity score, tic suppression, pain, and patient global impression. Furthermore, the full effect of BTX might not have been appreciated at only 2 weeks; a single treatment protocol does not reflect the clinical practice of evaluating patients after several adjustments in doses and sites of injections; and the patients' symptoms were relatively mild, since the patients "did not rate themselves as significantly compromised by their treated tics" at baseline (Kurlan, 2001). A larger sample and a longer follow-up will be needed to further evaluate the efficacy of BTX in the treatment of tics and to demonstrate that this treatment offers clinically meaningful benefit. A single-blind, placebo-controlled trial of two 20 minute applications of repetitive transcranial magnetic stimulation on two consecutive days provided no evidence that repetitive transcranial magnetic stimulation is of any benefit for patients with TS (Munchau et al., 2002).

Surgical treatment of TS is controversial, and the overall experience of stereotactic surgery in the treatment of tics has been rather disappointing (Temel and Visser-Vandewalle, 2004). Experience with 17 patients, with a median age of 23 years (range: 11 to 40 years), who were treated between 1970 and 1998 was reviewed by Babel and colleagues (2001). Unilateral zona incerta and VL/LM lesioning was used, and occasional second surgery on the contralateral side was performed. The authors concluded that the procedure(s) "sufficiently" reduced both motor and phonic tics. Transient complications were reported in 68% of patients; only one patient suffered permanent complication. Although stereotactic surgery has not been found generally useful in the treatment of tics (see the section entitled "Surgical Treatments" later in this chapter), a preliminary report of a 42-year-old man with severe motor and phonic tics controlled by high-frequency deep brain stimulation (DBS) of thalamus is quite encouraging (Vandewalle et al., 1999). In another report of a 36-year-old woman with a childhood history of tics, severe coprolalia, and SIB, stimulation of either the thalamus (centromedian-parafascicular complex) or the anteromedial part of the internal globus pallidus markedly improved the three components of her TS (Houeto et al., 2005). Globus pallidus has been increasingly used as the target in patients with disabling tics because of its extensive connections to the prefrontal cortex, an area that influences cognition and mood (Diederich et al., 2005; Shahed et al., 2007) (see Appendix 17-1). Finally, the observation that vagal nerve stimulation also favorably modifes the frequency and intensity of facial tics suggests that the brainstem plays a role in generation of modulation of tics (Diamond et al., 2006).

## Management of Behavioral Symptoms

### ATTENTION-DEFICIT HYPERACTIVITY DISORDER

Behavioral modification, school and classroom adjustments, and other techniques described previously may be useful in the management of behavioral problems associated with TS for some selected patients, but in our experience, these approaches are rarely effective and at best play an ancillary role. Such behavioral strategies, however, may provide important emotional support for the patient and the family members and may be helpful in raising self-esteem and improve motivation (Peterson and Cohen, 1998).

Pharmacologic therapy is usually required when behavioral measures do not allow for a satisfactory adaptation and the symptoms of ADHD impair interpersonal relationships and interfere with academic or occupational performance (Elia et al., 1999; Zametkin and Ernst, 1999; Riddle and Carlson, 2001; Silay and Jankovic, 2005). CNS stimulants, such as methylphenidate (Ritalin and Ritalin LA), controlled-release methylphenidate (Concerta), controlled-delivery methylphenidate (Metadate CD), dexmethylphenidate (Focalin), dextroamphetamine (Dexedrine), a mixture of amphetamine salts with a 75:25 ratio of dextroamphetamine and levoamphetamine (Adderall), and pemoline (Cylert) are clearly the most effective agents in the treatment of ADHD. The National Institute of Mental Health (NIMH) Collaborative Multimodal Treatment Study of Children with Attention Deficit Hyperactivity Disorder, the most comprehensive study of treatment strategies for ADHD, found medication to be superior to behavioral treatment (MTA Cooperative Group, 1999). The initial dose for methylphenidate is 5 mg in the morning, and the dose can be gradually advanced up to 20 to 60 mg per day (0.3 to 0.7 mg/kg per dose). Methylphenidate has been found useful not only in the treatment of attention deficit but also as a short-term therapy for conduct disorders (Klein et al., 1997). Dextroamphetamine doses are usually one half of those of methylphenidate. Pemoline should be given as a single morning dose that is approximately 6 times the daily dose of methylphenidate. These drugs usually have a rapid onset of action but also have a relatively short half-life. The long-acting preparations, such as Ritalin-SR (20 mg), are less reliable and less effective than two doses of standard preparation. Dexedrine Spansule has the advantage of greater range of available doses (5, 10, and 15 mg). Some studies (Manos et al., 1999; Pliszka et al., 2000), supported by our own experience, suggest that Adderall is better tolerated, produces less anorexia and sedation, and may be longer lasting than methylphenidate, and it can be used as a one-time morning dose. Only future studies will determine the utility of the new formulation of methylphenidate using a novel controlled-release delivery system designed for once-daily oral dosing (Concerta: 18 to 36 mg methylphenidate; Metadate CD: 20 mg methylphenidate; Adderall XR: 5 to 30 mg per day). Metadate CD is formulated to release 6 mg of methylphenidate from immediate-release and 14 mg from extended-release beads. Tolerance, while rare, is more likely to occur with the long-acting formulations, but this has not been demonstrated in patients with ADHD. Besides the possible development of tolerance, potential side effects of these stimulant drugs include nervousness, irritability, insomnia, anorexia, abdominal pain, and headaches. In one study, dextroamphetamine was found to cause more insomnia and negative emotional symptoms than does methylphenidate (Efron et al., 1997). Pemoline can rarely produce chemical hepatitis and even fulminant liver failure. Liver enzymes should be assessed before administration, but because the onset of hepatitis is unpredictable, routine laboratory studies are not useful. The parents should be instructed to notify the physician if nausea, vomiting, lethargy, malaise, or jaundice appears. Although some studies have suggested growth retardation, this effect, if present at all, is very minimal and probably clinically insignificant. Whether other CNS stimulants such as those used as appetite suppressants (e.g., sibutramine, Meridia, and Reductil) would be useful in the treatment of ADD or tics is not known (Arterburn et al., 2004).

CNS stimulants may exacerbate or precipitate tics in up to 25% of patients (Robertson and Eapen, 1992). If the symptoms of ADHD are troublesome and interfere with patient's functioning, however, it is reasonable to use these CNS stimulants and titrate the dosage to the lowest effective level (Wilens et al., 1995) (see Table 17-2 and Box 17-3). More recent studies suggest that while CNS stimulants may exacerbate tics when they are introduced into the anti-TS treatment regimen, with continued use these drugs can be well tolerated without tic exacerbation (Gadow et al., 1999; Law and Schachtar, 1999; Kurlan, 2002; Tourette Syndrome Study Group, 2002). The dopamine receptor–blocking drugs can be combined with the CNS stimulants if the latter produce unacceptable exacerbation of tics. If one stimulant is ineffective or poorly tolerated, another stimulant should be tried.

While methylphenidate was initially thought to work by raising brain levels of dopamine, more recent studies have suggested that its beneficial effects on ADHD are mediated via the serotonin system (Gainetdinov et al., 1999). A strain of mice with an inactivated gene for dopamine transporter has been described to have behavioral symptoms similar to those in children with ADHD. The hyperactivity of the mice was markedly ameliorated by methylphenidate, and this improvement correlated with an increase in brain serotonin. Other investigators have provided evidence that ADHD is a noradrenergic disorder (Biederman and Spencer, 1999). Although it has been suggested that long-term use of CNS stimulants might lead to substance abuse, some studies have demonstrated that untreated ADHD is a significant risk factor for substance abuse and that treatment of ADHD with CNS stimulants significantly reduces the risk for substance use disorder (Biederman et al., 1999).

$\alpha_2$-Adrenergic agonists and tricyclic antidepressants are also useful in the treatment of ADHD, particularly if CNS stimulants are not well tolerated or are contraindicated. Clonidine (Catapres), a presynaptic $\alpha_2$-adrenergic agonist that is used as an antihypertensive because it decreases plasma norepinephrine, improves symptoms of ADHD and of impulse control problems. Although initially found to be marginally effective in controlling motor tics (Leckman et al., 1991), clonidine has not been found to be an effective anti-tic agent in other studies. Singer, Brown, and colleagues (1995) reported a double-blind, placebo-controlled study involving children with ADHD ($n = 37$) randomized to 6-week medication cycles with clonidine (0.05 mg four times a day), desipramine (25 mg four times a day), or placebo. Desipramine, but not clonidine, was significantly more effective than placebo. The usual starting dose is 0.1 mg at bedtime, and the dosage is gradually increased up to 0.5 mg per day in three divided doses. Although a multicenter controlled clinical trial showed that clonidine alone or in combination with methylphenidate is an effective anti-tic drug (Tourette Syndrome Study Group, 2002), our experience has suggested that the perceived benefit might not be due to a specific anti-tic efficacy, but rather might be a nonspecific anxiolytic effect or due to its benefit for comorbid disorders (see later). The drug is also available as a transdermal patch (Catapres TTS-1, TTS-2, TTS-3, corresponding to 0.1, 0.2, and 0.3 mg, respectively) that should be changed once a week, using a different skin location. Side effects include sedation, lightheadedness, headache, dry mouth, and insomnia. Because of its sedative effects, some clinicians use clonidine as a nighttime soporific agent. Although the patch can cause local irritation, it seems to cause fewer side effects than oral clonidine.

Another drug that is increasingly used in the treatment of ADHD and impulse control problems is guanfacine (Tenex), which is available as 1-mg or 2-mg tablets. The initial dose is 0.5 mg at bedtime with gradual increases, as needed, to final doses up to 4 to 6 mg per day. Pharmacologically similar to clonidine, guanfacine may be effective in patients in whom clonidine failed to control the behavioral symptoms. Guanfacine may have some advantages over clonidine in that it has a longer half-life, it appears to be less sedating, and it produces less hypotension. It also seems to be a more selective $\alpha_2$-noradrenergic receptor agonist and binds more selectively to the postsynaptic $\alpha_{2A}$-adrenergic receptors located in the prefrontal cortex. While both clonidine and guanfacine appear to be effective in the treatment of attention deficit with and without hyperactivity, they appear to be particularly useful in the management of oppositional, argumentative, impulsive, and aggressive behavior. Although less effective than methylphenidate (Ritalin) (see later), the drugs have an advantage over methylphenidate in that they do not increase tics (Horrigan and Barnhill, 1995). The efficacy of this drug is supported by a pilot study of 13 patients with ADHD (but without TS) (Hunt et al., 1995). Another study, a 4-week, double-blind, placebo-controlled study of mild TS patients, however, failed to show significant neuropsychiatric or tic benefits (Cummings et al., 2002). The most frequently encountered side effects of the two drugs include sedation, dry mouth, itchy eyes, dizziness, headaches, fatigability, and postural hypotension. The beneficial effects might not be appreciated for several weeks after initiation of therapy, and the symptoms might markedly intensify if the medications are withdrawn abruptly. We have found deprenyl or selegiline (Eldepryl), an monoamine oxidate–B inhibitor, to be effective in controlling the symptoms of ADHD without exacerbating tics (Jankovic, 1993a). Using the DuPaul Attention Deficit Hyperactivity Scale, the efficacy of this drug in ADHD has been confirmed by a double-blind placebo-controlled study (Feigin et al., 1996). It is not clear how deprenyl improves symptoms of ADHD, but the drug is known to metabolize into amphetamines. Other drugs that are frequently used in relatively mild cases of ADHD include imipramine (Tofranil), nortriptyline (Pamelor), and desipramine (Norpramin). Because of potential cardiotoxicity, an electrocardiogram or cardiologic evaluation might be needed before initiation of desipramine therapy, and follow-up electrocardiograms should be performed every 3 to 6 months. Bupropion (Wellbutrin), an atypical antidepressant with stimulant properties, may also be useful in the management of ADHD, although like the other CNS stimulants, it may possibly exacerbate tics (Spencer et al., 1993). It is not yet known whether nonstimulant drugs such as modafinil or atomoxetine (inhibitor of presynaptic norepinephrine transporter) (Michelson et al., 2001; Kratochvil et al., 2002) will be useful in the treatment of ADHD associated with TS. Atomoxetine (Strattera), not a controlled substance, which was approved by the Food and Drug Administration in 2002, is the first anti-ADHD medication to be approved for adults as well as children. Metabolized primarily through the CYP2D6 enzymatic pathway and excreted in the urine, atomoxetine has a mean half-life of 5.2 hours. The usual starting dose is 0.5 mg/kg of body weight or 25 mg per day, and the dose can be gradually increased up to 40 to 50 mg twice a day. Anorexia, insomnia, sedation, tremor, and sexual dysfunction are the most frequent side effects. In one study (Kelsey et al., 2004), the efficacy of atomoxetine administered once daily among children with ADHD was assessed throughout the day, including the evening and early morning. This study was a randomized, multicenter, double-blind, placebo-controlled trial conducted at 12 outpatient sites in the United States. A total of 197 children, 6 to 12 years of age, who had been diagnosed as having ADHD on the basis of the criteria of the Diagnostic and Statistical Manual of Mental Disorders, fourth edition, were randomized to receive 8 weeks of treatment with atomoxetine or placebo, dosed once daily in the mornings. ADHD symptoms were assessed with parent and investigator rating scales. Among children 6 to 12 years of age who had been diagnosed as having ADHD, once-daily administration of atomoxetine in the morning provided safe, rapid, continuous symptom relief that lasted beyond the evening hours, into the morning hours. Overall, atomoxetine treatment was safe and well tolerated. Another prospective, multicenter open-label assessment of atomoxetine in non–North American children and adolescents with ADHD supported the efficacy and safety of atomoxetine (Buitelaar et al., 2004). Comparative studies assessing the relative efficacy and safety of atomoxetine versus CNS stimulants in patients with TS and comorbid ADHD are needed.

Modafinil, a nonscheduled stimulant, $\alpha_1$ receptor agonist that also acts on GABA and glutamate, has been found to be ineffective in a double-blind, placebo-controlled study of ADHD (Pliszka, 2003). Desmopressin, either as a nasal spray or in tablet form, with or without imipramine, can be used in the treatment of enuresis, which is frequently associated with ADHD.

## OBSESSIVE-COMPULSIVE DISORDER

The role of cognitive-behavioral therapy in the treatment of OCD has not been well defined, although some investigators argue that when used alone or in combination of pharmacotherapy, it is the psychotherapeutic treatment of choice (March et al., 2001; Micallef and Blin, 2001; Jenike, 2004). This therapy utilizes repeated exposure to provocative stimuli in an attempt to prevent the rituals and other compulsions. The Pediatric OCD Treatment Study showed that cognitive-behavioral therapy alone or in combination with a selective serotonin uptake inhibitor (SSRI) provides the best results in children and adolescents with OCD (Pediatric OCD Treatment Study Team, 2004).

Although imipramine and desipramine have been reported to be useful in the treatment of OCD, the most effective drugs are the SSRIs (Dolberg et al., 1996; Flament and Bisserbe, 1997; Grados and Riddle, 2001; Hensiek and Trimble, 2002; Silay and Jankovic, 2005). These include fluoxetine (Prozac), fluvoxamine (Luvox), clomipramine (Anafranil), paroxetine (Paxil), sertraline (Zoloft), venlafaxine (Effexor), citalopram (Celexa), and escitalopram (Lexapro), the S-enantiomer of citalopram. Controlled trials have found all these agents, except for escitalopram, to be effective in the treatment of OCD. Only a few comparative studies have been performed of the various agents in patients with TS and OCD, but clomipramine (Anafranil), fluvoxamine (Luvox), fluoxetine (Prozac), and sertraline (Zoloft) are particularly effective. The initial dosage of clomipramine is 25 mg at bedtime, and the dosage can be gradually increased up to 250 mg per day, using 25-, 50-, or 75-mg capsules after meals or at bedtime. Fluoxetine, paroxetine, and citalopram should be started at 20 mg after breakfast, and the dosage can be increased up to 80 mg per day. In contrast to clomipramine and fluvoxamine, the other SSRIs should be started as a morning, after-breakfast dose.

Although comparative trials have been lacking, meta-analyses have provided some useful information. In one such analysis, venlafaxine was found to be particularly effective in the treatment of depression and inducing remission compared to the other SSRIs, possibly because of its dual effect by inhibiting both serotonin and noradrenaline (Thase et al., 2001). Long-term clinical trials indicate that fluoxetine and sertraline are the best tolerated of the SSRIs (Flament and

Bisserbe, 1997). A double-blind comparison of fluvoxamine and clomipramine showed equal efficacy, although clomipramine had a more rapid onset of effect, but fluvoxamine was better tolerated (Milanfranchi et al., 1997). In addition to its antidepressant and anti-OCD effects, fluvoxamine has been found to be an effective treatment for children and adolescents with social phobia and anxiety (Research Unit on Pediatric Psychopharmacology Anxiety Study Group, 2001). There is some evidence that fluvoxamine sensitizes sigma receptors, which may lead to potentiation of dystonia in animals (Stahl, 1998). In a multicenter, randomized controlled study of 187 children and adolescents, sertraline was found to be safe and effective in the treatment of OCD (March et al., 1998). Up to 25% of patients with OCD show no meaningful improvement with the SSRIs and may therefore require polypharmacy (Laird, 1996). Certain drugs, such as lithium and buspirone, have been reported to augment the SSRIs. There is little information about the potential synergistic effects of different SSRIs, although some patients clearly feel that the combination of two SSRIs is more effective than when they are used as monotherapy. In some treatment-refractory cases, SSRIs might need to be combined with buspirone, clonazepam, lithium, and even neuroleptics (Goodman et al., 1998). When a combination or polypharmacy is used, it is prudent practice to discuss with the patients potential adverse reactions, including the serotonin syndrome (confusion, hypomania, agitation, myoclonus, hyperreflexia, sweating, tremor, diarrhea, and fever), withdrawal phenomenon, and possible extrapyramidal side effects. Acute parkinsonism was reported in adult patients with TS who were treated with the combination of serotonin reuptake inhibitors and neuroleptics (Kurlan, 1998a). Despite unsubstantiated evidence about an increased risk of suicide, some regulatory agencies, including the British Medicines and Health Care Products Regulatory Agency, found in December 2003 that the "balance of risks and benefits for the treatment of major depressive disorder in under 18s is judged to be unfavorable for sertraline, citalopram and escitalopram"; fluoxetine has been exempt because of its favorable "balance of risks and benefits" (see www.mhra.gov.uk). Systematic review of published and unpublished data on SSRIs in the treatment of childhood depression raised some questions about the safety and efficacy of these drugs in this population of depressed patients (Whittington et al., 2004). In addition to the SSRIs, anxiolytics, such as alprazolam and clonazepam, have been used with modest success. Similarly, monoamine oxidate (MAO) inhibitors, trazodone, and buspirone have limited efficacy in the treatment of OCD.

## OTHER BEHAVIORAL PROBLEMS

There are many other behavioral problems that may be even more troublesome for patients with TS than ADHD or OCD is. As was noted, treatment of ADHD often improves impulse control problems that are frequently associated with TS. Sudden, explosive attacks of rage, which occur in a considerable proportion of patients with TS, have been found to respond to SSRIs, such as paroxetine (Bruun and Budman, 1998).

It can be only speculated at this time whether antagonists of excitatory amino acids or antiadrenergic agents, such as flutamide, will exert a protective effect in TS. However, future therapeutic interventions should include strategies that are designed not only to control symptoms but also to alter the natural course of the disease.

## Surgical Treatments

Surgical treatment of TS is controversial. While the overall experience of stereotactic ablative surgery in the treatment of tics has been rather disappointing, an increasing number of reports have provided evidence that DBS involving the thalamus, globus pallidus, and other targets might be a very effective strategy for treating uncontrollable tics (Temel and Visser-Vandewalle, 2004; Diederich et al., 2005; Houeto et al., 2005; Ackermans et al., 2006; Shahed et al., 2007). Babel and colleagues (2001) reviewed experience with 17 patients with a median age of 23 years (range: 11 to 40 years) who were treated with ablative procedures between 1970 and 1998. Unilateral zona incerta and VL/LM lesioning was used, and occasionally second surgery on the contralateral side was performed. The authors concluded that the procedure(s) "sufficiently" reduced both motor and phonic tics. Transient complications were reported in 68% of patients; only one patient suffered any permanent complication. The medial thalamus has long been considered a target not only in ablative procedures but also in DBS treatment of tics and OCD (Nuttin et al., 1999; Vandewalle et al., 1999; Diederich et al., 2005). Nuttin and colleagues (2003) noted beneficial effects in OCD with bilateral anterior capsular stimulation after 1 year of stimulation, but all six patients remained defective in several domains of health-related quality of life. A report of a 42-year-old man with severe motor and phonic tics controlled by high-frequency DBS of the thalamus is quite encouraging (Vandewalle et al., 1999). In another report, in a 36-year-old woman with a childhood history of tics, severe coprolalia, and SIB, stimulation of either the thalamus (centromedian-parafascicular complex) or the anteromedial part of the internal globus pallidus markedly improved the three components of her TS (Houeto et al., 2005). This selection is supported by previous reports of successful treatment with bilateral GPi DBS in two TS patients. In one study, a comparison of bilateral GPi to bilateral medial thalamic stimulation in the same patient found greater tic reduction (95% versus 80%) at lower settings with GPi stimulation (Diederich et al., 2005), but another report described similar degrees of improvement using either site (Ackermans et al., 2006). In a 16-year-old boy with disabling, medically intractable TS, bilateral GPi DBS resulted in a 63% improvement in the Yale Global Tourette Syndrome Scale, an 85% improvement in the Tic Symptom Self Report, and a 51% improvement in SF-36, a quality-of-life measure (Shahed et al., 2007). Furthermore, the patient was able to return to school. Although these observations must be confirmed by a controlled trial before DBS can be recommended even for severely affected patients, they suggest that stimulation of certain targets involved in the limbic striatopallidal-thalamocortical system could be beneficial in the treatment of various aspects of TS. Although DBS may be associated with behavioral and cognitive complications, neuropsychological and psychiatric comorbidities in TS should not necessarily be a contraindication for DBS, as these conditions may in fact improve after GPi stimulation. Careful selection of patients, experience with DBS procedure, and comprehensive assessments at baseline and at follow-up visits are essential for successful outcome of DBS in TS (Mink et al., 2006).

## References

Abelson JF, Kwan KY, O'Roak BJ, et al: Sequence variants in SLITRK1 are associated with Tourette's syndrome. Science 2005;310:317–320.

Abuzzahab FS, Brown VL: Control of Tourette's syndrome with topiramate. Am J Psychiatry 2001;158:968.

Abwender DA, Trinidad K, Jones KR, et al: Features resembling Tourette's syndrome in developmental stutterers. Brain Lang 1998;62:455–464.

Ackermans L, Temel Y, Cath D, et al: Deep brain stimulation in Tourette's syndrome: Two targets? Mov Disord 2006;21:709–713.

Albin RL, Koeppe RA, Bohnen NI, et al: Increased ventral striatal monoaminergic innervation in Tourette syndrome. Neurology 2003;61:310–315.

Albin RL, Mink JW: Recent advances in Tourette syndrome research. Trends Neurosci 2006;29:175–182.

Allen AJ: Group A streptococcal infections and childhood neuropsychiatric disorders: Relationships and therapeutic implications. CNS Drugs 1997;8:267–275.

Alsobrook JP, Pauls DL: The genetics of Tourette syndrome. In Jankovic J (ed): Tourette Syndrome. Neurologic Clinics of North America, vol 15. Philadelphia, WB Saunders, 1997, pp 381–394.

Alsobrook JP II, Pauls DL: A factor analysis of tic symptoms in Gilles de le Tourette's syndrome. Am J Psychiatry 2002;159:291–296.

Anca MH, Giladi N, Korczyn AD: Ropinirole in Gilles de la Tourette syndrome. Neurology 2004;62:1626–1627.

Arterburn DE, Crane PK, Veenstra DL: The efficacy and safety of sibutramine for weight loss: A systematic review. Arch Intern Med 2004;164:994–1003.

Awaad Y: Tics in Tourette syndrome: New treatment options. J Child Neurol 1999;14:316–319.

Awaad Y, Michon AM, Minarik S: Use of levetiracetam to treat tics in children and adolescents with Tourette syndrome. Mov Disord 2005;20:714–718.

Azher SN, Jankovic J: Camptocormia: Pathogenesis, classification, and response to therapy. Neurology 2005;65:355–359.

Babel TB, Warnke PC, Ostertag CB: Immediate and long term outcome after infrathalamic and thalamic lesioning for intractable Tourette's syndrome. J Neurol Neurosurg Psychiatry 2001;70:666–671.

Banaschewski T, Woerner W, Rothenberger A: Premonitory sensory phenomena and suppressibility of tics in Tourette syndrome: Developmental aspects in children and adolescents. Dev Med Child Neurol 2003;45:700–703.

Barabas G, Matthews WS, Ferrari M: Tourette's syndrome and migraine. Arch Neurol 1984;41:871–872.

Baron-Cohen S, Cross P, Crowson M, Robertson M: Can children with Gilles de la Tourette syndrome edit their intentions? Psychol Med 1994;24:29–40.

Baron-Cohen S, Scahill VL, Izaguirre J, et al: The prevalence of Gilles de la Tourette syndrome in children and adolescents with autism: A large scale study. Psychol Med 1999;29:1151–1159.

Baumgardner TL, Singer HS, Denckla MB, et al: Corpus callosum morphology in children with Tourette syndrome and attention. Neurology 1996;47:477–482.

Baxter LR, Schwartz JM, Bergman KS, et al: Caudate glucose metabolic rate changes with both drug and behavioral therapy for obsessive-compulsive disorder. Arch Gen Psychiatry 1992;49:681–689.

Bechara A, Tranel D, Damasio H: Characterization of the decision-making deficit of patients with ventromedial prefrontal cortex lesions. Brain 2000;123:2189–2202.

Berardelli A, Curra A, Fabbrini G, et al: Pathophysiology of tics and Tourette syndrome. J Neurol 2003;250:781–787.

Berthier ML, Kulisevsky J, Gironell A, Heras JA: Obsessive-compulsive disorder associated with brain lesions: Clinical phenomenology, cognitive function, and anatomic correlates. Neurology 1996;47:353–361.

Bharucha KJ, Sethi KD: Tardive tourettism after exposure to neuroleptic therapy. Mov Disord 1995;10:791–793.

Biederman J, Spencer T: Attention-deficit/hyperactivity disorder (ADHD) as a noradrenergic disorder. Biol Psychiatry 1999;46:1234–1242.

Biederman J, Wilens T, Mick E, et al: Pharmacotherapy of attention-deficit/hyperactivity disorder reduces risk of substance abuse disorder. Pediatrics 1999;104:e20.

Black JL: Obsessive compulsive disorder: A clinical update. Mayo Clin Proc 1992;67:266–275.

Black KJ, Mink JW: Response to levodopa challenge in Tourette syndrome. Mov Disord 2000;15:1194–1198.

Blair J, Scahill L, State M, Martin A: Electrocardiographic changes in children and adolescents treated with ziprasidone: A prospective study. J Am Acad Child Adolesc Psychiatry 2005;44:73–79.

Bloch MH, Peterson BS, Scahill L, et al: Adulthood outcome of tic and obsessive-compulsive symptom severity in children with Tourette syndrome. Arch Pediatr Adolesc Med 2006;160:65–69.

Boghosian-Sell L, Comings DE, Overhauser J: Tourette syndrome in a pedigree with a 7;18 translocation: Identification of a YAC spanning the translocation breakpoint at 18q22.3 Am J Hum Genet 1996;59:999–1005.

Bronze MS, Dale JB: Epitopes of streptococcal M proteins that evoke antibodies that cross-react with human brain. J Immunol 1993; 151:2820–2828.

Brower M, Price B: Neuropsychiatry of frontal lobe dysfunction in violent and criminal behavior: A critical review. J Neurol Neurosurg Psychiatry 2001;71:720–726.

Bruggeman R, Van der Linden C, Buitellar JK, et al: Risperidone versus pimozide in Tourette's syndrome: A comparative double-blind parallel-group study. J Clin Psychiatry 2001;62:50–56.

Bruun RD, Budman CL: Risperidone as a treatment for Tourette's syndrome. J Clin Psychiatry 1996;57:29–31.

Bruun RD, Budman CL: Paroxetine treatment of episodic rages associated with Tourette's disorder. J Clin Psychiatry 1998;59:581–584.

Buitelaar JK, Danckaerts M, Gillberg C, et al: A prospective, multicenter, open-label assessment of atomoxetine in non–North American children and adolescents with ADHD. Eur Child Adolesc Psychiatry 2004;13:249–257.

Caine ED, McBride MC, Chiverton P, et al: Tourette's syndrome in Monroe County school children. Neurology 1988;38:472–475.

Cardinal R, Pennicott D, Sugathapala C, et al: Impulsive choice induced in rats by lesions of the nucleus accumbens core. Science 2001;292:2499–2501.

Cardona F, Orefici G: Group A streptococcal infections and tic disorders in an Italian pediatric population. J Pediatr 2001;138:71–75.

Cardoso F, Faleiro R: Tourette syndrome: Another cause of movement disorder of the ear. Mov Disord 1999;12:531–535.

Cardoso FEC, Jankovic J: Cocaine related movement disorders. Mov Disord 1993;8:175–178.

Carter AS, O'Donnell DA, Schultz RT, et al: Social and emotional adjustment in children affected with Gilles de la Tourette's syndrome associations with ADHD and family functioning. J Child Psychol Psychiatry 2000;41:215–223.

Cassidy SB, Morris CA: Behavioral phenotype in genetic syndromes: Genetic clues to human behavior. Adv Pediatr 2002;49: 59–86.

Castellanos FX, Giedd JN, Hamburger SD, et al: Brain morphometry in Tourette's syndrome: The influence of comorbid attention-deficit/hyperactivity disorder. Neurology 1996;47:1581–1583.

Castellanos FX, Tannock R: Neuroscience of attention-deficit/hyperactivity disorder: The search for endophenotypes. Nat Rev Neurosci 2002;3:617–628.

Chee K-Y, Sachdev P: A controlled study of sensory tics in Gilles de la Tourette syndrome and obsessive-compulsive disorder using a structured interview. J Neurol Neurosurg Psychiatry 1997;62:188–192.

Chokroverty S, Jankovic J: Restless legs syndrome: A disease in search of identity. Neurology 1999;52:907–910.

Chouinard S, Ford B: Adult onset tic disorders. J Neurol Neurosurg Psychiatry 2000;68:738–743.

Church AJ, Dale RC, Lees AJ, et al: Tourette's syndrome: A cross sectional study to examine the PANDAS hypothesis. J Neurol Neurosurg Psychiatry 2003;74:602–607.

Coffey BJ, Park KS: Behavioral and emotional aspects of Tourette syndrome. In Jankovic J, (ed): Tourette syndrome. Neurologic Clinics of North America, vol 15. Philadelphia, WB Saunders, 1997, pp 277–290.

Cohen DJ, Leckman JF: Sensory phenomena associated with Gilles de la Tourette's syndrome. J Clin Psychiatry 1992;53:319–323.

Cohen DJ, Leckman JF: Developmental psychopathology and neurobiology of Tourette's syndrome. J Am Acad Child Adolesc Psychiatry 1994;33:2–15.

Comings DE: A controlled study of Tourette syndrome, VII. Summary: A common genetic disorder causing disinhibition of the limbic system. Am J Hum Genet 1987;41:839–866.

Comings DE: Blood serotonin and tryptophan in Tourette syndrome. Am J Med Genet 1990;36:418–430.

Comings DE, Comings BG: A controlled study of Tourette syndrome: II. Conduct. Am J Hum Genet 1987;41:742–760.

Comings DE, Comings BG: A controlled study of Tourette syndrome: Revisited. Am J Hum Genet 1988a;43:209–217.

Comings DE, Comings BG: Tourette's syndrome and attention deficit disorder. In Cohen DJ, Bruun RD, Leckman JF (eds): Tourette's Syndrome and Tic Disorders. New York, John Wiley & Sons, 1988b, pp 119–135.

Comings DE, Comings BG: Alternative hypotheses on the inheritance of Tourette syndrome. In Chase T, Friedhoff A, Cohen DJ (eds): Tourette's Syndrome. Advances in Neurology, vol 58. New York, Raven Press, 1992, pp 189–200.

Comings DE, Himes JA, Comings BG: An epidemiologic study of Tourette's syndrome in a single school district. J Clin Psychiatry 1990;51:463–469.

Costello EJ, Angold A, Burns BJ, et al: The Great Smokey Mountains study of youth: Goals, design, methods, and the prevalence of DSM-III-R disorders. Arch Gen Psychiatry 1996;53:1129–1136.

Crawford FC, Ait-Ghezala G, Morris M, et al: Translocation breakpoint in two unrelated Tourette syndrome cases, within a region previously linked to the disorder. Hum Genet 2003;113:154–161.

Cuker A, State MW, King RA, et al: Candidate locus for Gilles de la Tourette syndrome/obsessive compulsive disorder/chronic tic disorder at 18q22. Am J Med Genet 2004;130A:37–39.

Cummings DD, Singer HS, Krieger M, et al: Neuropsychiatric effects of guanfacine in children with mild tourette syndrome: A pilot study. Clin Neuropharmacol 2002;25:325–332.

Dale R, Church AJ, Cardoso F, et al: Poststreptococcal acute disseminated encephalomyelitis with basal ganglia involvement and auto-reactive antibasal ganglia antibodies. Ann Neurol 2001;50:588–595.

Dale RC, Church AJ, Heyman I: Striatal encephalitis after varicella zoster infection complicated by tourettism. Mov Disord 2003;18: 1554–1556.

Dale RC, Church AJ, Surtees RA, et al: Encephalitis lethargica syndrome: 20 new cases and evidence of basal ganglia autoimmunity. Brain 2004;127:21–33.

De Carvalho Aguiar P, Fazzari M, Jankovic J, Ozelius LJ: Examination of the SGCE gene in Tourette syndrome patients with obsessive-compulsive disorder. Mov Disord 2004;19:1237–1238.

Diagnostic and Statistical Manual, 4th ed (DSM-IV). Washington, DC, American Psychiatric Association, 1994, pp 100–105.

Diamond A, Kenney C, Jankovic J: The effect of vagal nerve stimulation in a case of Tourette's syndrome and complex partial epilepsy. Mov Disord 2006;21:1273–1275.

Diederich NJ, Kalteis K, Stamenkovic M, et al: Efficient internal pallidal stimulation in Gilles de la Tourette syndrome: A case report. Mov Disord 2005;20:1496–1499.

Dion Y, Annable L, Sandor P, Chouinard G: Risperidone in the treatment of Tourette syndrome: A double-blind, placebo-controlled trial. J Clin Psychopharmacol 2002;22:31–39.

Dodman NH, Normile JA, Shuster L, Rand W: Equine self-mutilation syndrome (57 cases). J Am Vet Med Assoc 1994;204:1219–1223.

Dolberg OT, Iancu I, Sasson Y, Zohar J: The pathogenesis and treatment of obsessive-compulsive disorder. Clin Neuropharmacol 1996;19:129–147.

Dulcan M, AACAP Works Group on Quality Issues: Practice parameters for the assessment and treatment of children, adolescents, and adults with attention-deficit/hyperactivity disorder. J Am Acad Child Adolesc Psychiatry 1997;36:(suppl 10): 85S–121S.

Eapen V, Lees AJ, Lakke JPWF, et al: Adult-onset tic disorders. Mov Disord 2002;17:735–740.

Eapen V, O'Neill J, Hugh MD, et al: Sex of parent transmission effect in Tourette's syndrome: Evidence for earlier age at onset in maternally transmitted cases suggests a genomic imprinting effect. Neurology 1997a;48:934–937.

Eapen V, Robertson MM, Alsobrook JP, Pauls DL: Obsessive-compulsive symptoms in Gilles de la Tourette syndrome and obsessive compulsive disorder: Differences by diagnosis and family history. Am J Med Genet 1997b;74:432–438.

Edwards MJ, Dale RC, Church AJ, et al: Adult-onset tic disorder, motor stereotypes, and behavioural disturbance associated with antibasal ganglia antibodies. Mov Disord 2004a;19:1190–1196.

Edwards MJ, Trikouli E, Martino D, et al: Anti-basal ganglia antibodies in patients with atypical dystonia and tics: A prospective study. Neurology 2004b;63:156–158.

Efron D, Jarman F, Barker M, et al: Side effects of methylphenidate and dextroamphetamine in children with attention deficit hyperactivity disorder: A double-blind, crossover trial. Pediatrics 1997;100:662–666.

Eidelberg D, Moeller JR, Antonini A, et al: The metabolic anatomy of Tourette's syndrome. Neurology 1997;48:927–934.

Elia J, Ambrosini PJ, Rapoport JL: Treatment of attention-deficit-hyperactivity disorder. N Engl J Med 1999;340:780–788.

Ernst M, Zametkin AJ, Jons PH, et al: High presynaptic dopaminergic activity in children with Tourette's disorder. J Am Acad Child Adolesc Psychiatry 1999;38:86–94.

Fahn S: A case of post-traumatic tic syndrome. Adv Neurol 1982; 35:349–350.

Fahn S: Paroxysmal myoclonic dystonia with vocalisations. J Neurol Neurosurg Psychiatry 1987;50:117.

Farber RH, Swerdlow NR, Clementz BA: Saccadic performance characteristics and the behavioural neurology of Tourette's syndrome. J Neurol Neurosurg Psychiatry 1999;66:305–312.

Feigin A, Clarke H: Tourette syndrome: Update and review of the literature. Neurologist 1998;4:188–195.

Feigin A, Kurlan R, McDermott MP, et al: A controlled trial of deprenyl in children with Tourette's syndrome and attention deficit hyperactivity disorder. Neurology 1996;46:965–968.

Feinberg TE, Shapiro AK, Shapiro E: Paroxysmal myoclonic dystonia with vocalisations: New entity or variant of preexisting syndromes? J Neurol Neurosurg Psychiatry 1986;49:52–57.

Filipek P, Semrud-Clikeman M, Steinggard RJ, et al: Volumetric MRI analysis comparing subjects having attention deficit-hyperactivity disorder with normal controls. Neurology 1997;48:589–601.

Fish DR, Sawyers D, Allen PJ, et al: The effect of sleep on the dyskinetic movements of Parkinson's disease, Gilles de la Tourette syndrome, Huntington's disease, and torsion dystonia. Arch Neurol 1991;48:210–214.

Flament MF, Bisserbe J-C: Pharmacologic treatment of obsessive-compulsive disorder: Comparative studies. J Clin Psychiatry 1997;58(suppl 12):18–22.

Frederickson KA, Cutting LE, Kates WR, et al: Disproportionate increases of white matter in right frontal lobe in Tourette syndrome. Neurology 2002;58:85–89.

Freeman RD, Fast DK, Burd L, et al: Tourette Syndrome International Database Consortium: An international perspective on Tourette syndrome selected findings from 3500 individuals in 22 countries. Dev Med Child Neurol 2000;42:436–447.

Gadow KD, Sverd J, Sprafkin J, et al: Long-term methylphenidate therapy in children with comorbid attention-deficit hyperactivity and chronic multiple tic disorder. Arch Gen Psychiatry 1999;56: 330–336.

Gaffney GR, Perry PJ, Lund BC, et al: Risperidone versus clonidine in the treatment of children and adolescents with Tourette's syndrome. J Am Acad Child Adolesc Psychiatry 2002;41:330–336.

Gainetdinov RR, Wetsel WC, Jones SR, et al: Role of serotonin in the paradoxical calming effect of psychostimulants in hyperactivity. Science 1999;283:397–401.

Garraux G, Goldfine A, Bohlhalter S, et al: Increased midbrain gray matter in Tourette's syndrome. Ann Neurol 2006;59:381–385.

Gianfrancesco FD, Grogg AL, Mahmoud RA, et al: Differential effects of risperidone, olanzapine, clozapine, and conventional antipsychotics on type 2 diabetes: Findings from a large health plan database. J Clin Psychiatry 2002;63:920–930.

Giedd JN, Blumenthal J, Jeffries NO, et al: Brain development during childhood and adolescence: A longitudinal MRI study. Nat Neurosci 1999;2(10):861–863.

Gilbert DL, Bansal AS, Sethuraman G, et al: Association of cortical disinhibition with tic, ADHD, and OCD severity in Tourette syndrome. Mov Disord 2004;19:416–425.

Gilbert DL, Dure L, Sethuraman G, et al: Tic reduction with pergolide in a randomized controlled trial in children. Neurology 2003;60:606–611.

Gilbert DL, Sethuraman G, Sine L, et al: Tourette's syndrome improvement with pergolide in a randomized, double-blind crossover trial. Neurology 2000;54:1310–1315.

Gilles de la Tourette G: Étude sur une affection nerveuse caracterisée par de l'incoordination motrice accompagnée d'echolalie et de copralalie. Arch Neurol 1885;9:19–42, 158–200.

Gironell A, Rodriguez-Fornells A, Kulisevsky J, et al: Abnormalities of the acoustic startle reflex and reaction time in Gilles de la Tourette syndrome. Clin Neurophysiol 2000;111:1366–1371.

Glassman A, Bigger J: Antipsychotic drugs: Prolonged QTc, torsades de pointes, and sudden death. Am J Psychiatry 2001;158:1774–1782.

Glaze DG, Frost JD, Jankovic J: Sleep in Gilles de la Tourette syndrome: Disorder of arousal. Neurology 1983;33:586–592.

Goetz CG, Kompoliti K: Rating scales and quantitative asssement of tics. In Cohen DJ, Jankovic J, Goetz CG (eds): Tourette Syndrome. Advances in Neurology, vol 85. Philadelphia, Lippincott Williams & Wilkins, 2001, pp 31–42.

Goetz CG, Klawans HL: Gilles de la Tourette on Tourette syndrome. Adv Neurol 1982;35:1–16.

Goetz CG, Leurgans S, Chumara TA: Home alone: Methods to maximize tic expression for objective videotape assessments in Gilles de la Tourette syndrome. Mov Disord 2001;16:693–697.

Goetz CG, Pappert EJ, Louis ED, et al: Advantages of a modified scoring method for the Rush video-based tic rating scale. Mov Disord 1999;14:502–506.

Goetz CG, Tanner CM, Stebbins GT, et al: Adult tics in Gilles de la Tourette's syndrome: Description and risk factors. Neurology 1992;42:784–788.

Golden GS: Tourette syndrome: Recent advances. Neurol Clin 1990; 8:705–714.

Goldenberg JN, Brown SB, Weiner WJ: Coprolalia in younger patients with Gilles de la Tourette syndrome. Mov Disord 1994;9:622–625.

Goldman LS, Genel M, Bezman RJ, et al: Diagnosis and treatment of attention-deficit/hyperactivity disorder in children and adolescents. JAMA 1998;279:1100–1107.

Goodman WK, Ward HE, Murphy TK: Biologic approaches to treatment-refractory obsessive-compulsive disorder. Psychiatr Ann 1998;28:641–649.

Goodnick PJ, Jerry JM: Aripiprazole: Profile on efficacy and safety. Expert Opin Pharmacother 2002;3:1773–1781.

Grados MA, Riddle MA: Pharmacologic treatment of childhood obsessive-compulsive disorder: From theory to practice. J Child Psychol Psychiatry 2001;30:67–79.

Greenberg BD, Ziemann U, Cora-Locatelli G, et al: Altered cortical excitability in obsessive-compulsive disorder. Neurology 2000; 54:142–147.

Greenberg BD, Ziemann U, Harmon A, et al: Decreased neuronal inhibition in cerebral cortex in obsessive-compulsive disorder on transcranial magnetic stimulation. Lancet 1998;352:881–882.

Grice DE, Leckman JF, Pauls DL, et al: Linkage disequilibrium between an allele at the dopamine D4 receptor locus and Tourette syndrome, by the transmission-disequilibrium test. Am J Hum Genet 1996;59:644–652.

Haber S, Wolfer D: Basal ganglia peptidergic staining in Tourette syndrome: A follow-up study. In Chase T, Friedhoff A, Cohen DJ (eds): Tourette's Syndrome. Advances in Neurology, vol 58. New York, Raven Press, 1992, pp 145–150.

Hallett JJ, Harling-Berg CJ, Knopf PM, et al: Anti-striatal antibodies in Tourette syndrome cause neuronal dysfunction. J Neuroimmunol 2000;111:195–202.

Hallett JJ, Kiesling LS: Neuroimmnulogy of tics and other childhood hyperkinesias. In Jankovic J (ed): Tourette Syndrome, Neurologic Clinics. Philadelphia, WB Saunders, 1997, pp 333–344.

Hanashima C, Li SC, Shen L, et al: Foxg1 suppresses early cortical cell fate. Science 2004;303:56–59.

Hanna PA, Janjua FN, Contant CF, Jankovic J: Bilineal transmission in Tourette syndrome. Neurology 1999;53:813–818.

Hanna PA, Jankovic J: Sleep and tic disorders. In Chokroverty S, Hening W, Walters A (eds): Sleep and Movement Disorders. Woburn, MA, Butterworth-Heinemann, 2003, pp 464–471.

Heinz A, Knable MB, Wolf SS, et al: Tourette's syndrome. [I-123] β-CIT SPECT correlates of vocal tic severity. Neurology 1998;51:1069–1074.

Hensiek AE, Trimble MR: Relevance of new psychotropic drugs for the neurologist. J Neurol Neurosurg Psychiatry 2002;72:281–285.

Heutink P, Breedveld GJ, Niermeijer MF, et al: Progress in gene localization. In Kurlan R (ed): Handbook of Tourette's Syndrome and Related Tic and Behavioral Disorders. New York, Marcel Dekker, 1992, pp 317–335.

Hoekstra PJ, Bijzet J, Limburg PC, et al: Elevated D8/17 expression on B lymphocytes, a marker of rheumatic fever, measured with flow cytometry in tic disorder patients. Am J Psychiatry 2001;158: 605–610.

Hoekstra PJ, Kallenberg CG, Korf J, Minderaa RB: Is Tourette's syndrome an autoimmune disease? Mol Psychiatry 2002;7:437–445.

Hogan MB, Wilson NW: Tourette's syndrome mimicking asthma. J Asthma 1999;36:253–256.

Hoopes SP: Donezepil for Tourette's disorder and ADHD. J Clin Psychopharmacol 1999;19:381–382.

Horrigan JP, Barnhill LJ: Guanfacine for the treatment of attention deficit hyperactivity disorder in boys. J Child Adolesc Psychopharmacol 1995;5:215–223.

Houeto JL, Karachi C, Mallet L, et al: Tourette's syndrome and deep brain stimulation. J Neurol Neurosurg Psychiatry 2005;76:992–995.

Hughes JR, Goldstein MG, Hurt RD, Shiffman S: Recent advances in the pharmacotherapy of smoking. JAMA 1999;281:72–76.

Hunt RD, Arnsten AFT, Asbell MD: An open trial of guanfacine in the treatment of attention-deficit hyperactivity disorder. J Am Acad Child Adolesc Psychiatry 1995;34:50–54.

Hyde TM, Aaronson BA, Randolph C, et al: Relationship of birth weight to the phenotypic expression of Gilles de la Tourette's syndrome in monozygotic twins. Neurology 1992;42:652–658.

Hyde TM, Stacey ME, Copoola R, et al: Cerebral morphometric abnormalities in Tourette's syndrome: A quantitative MRI study of monozygotic twins. Neurology 1995;45:1176–1182.

Hyde TM, Weinberger DR: Tourette's syndrome: A model neuropsychiatric disorder. JAMA 1995;273:498–501.

Ikonomidou C, Bosch F, Miksa M et al: Blockade of NMDA receptors and apoptotic neurodegeneration in the developing brain. Science 1999;283:70–74.

Itard JMG: Mémoire sur quelques fonctions involuntaires des appareils de la locomotion de la préhension et de la voix. Arch Gen Med 1825;8:385–407.

Itoh K, Suzuki K, Bise K, et al: Apoptosis in the basal ganglia of the developing human nervous system. Acta Neuropath 2001;101:92–100.

Jankovic J: Diagnosis and classification of tics and Tourette's syndrome. In Chase T, Friedhoff A, Cohen DJ (eds): Tourette's Syndrome. Advances in Neurology, vol 58. New York, Raven Press, 1992, pp 7–14.

Jankovic J: Deprenyl in attention deficit associated with Tourette's syndrome. Arch Neurol 1993a;50:286–288.

Jankovic J: Tics in other neurologic disorders. In Kurlan R (ed): Handbook of Tourette's Syndrome and Related Tic and Behavioral Disorders. New York, Marcel Dekker, 1993b, pp 167–182.

Jankovic J: Botulinum toxin in the treatment of dystonic tics. Mov Disord 1994;9:347–349.

Jankovic J: Tardive syndromes and other drug-induced movement disorders. Clin Neuropharmacol 1995;18:197–214.

Jankovic J: Tourette's syndrome. N Engl J Med 2001a;345:1184–1192.

Jankovic J: Differential diagnosis and etiology of tics. In Cohen DJ, Jankovic J, Goetz CG (eds): Tourette Syndrome. Advances in Neurology, vol 85. Philadelphia, Lippincott Williams & Wilkins, 2001b, pp 15–29.

Jankovic J, Ashizawa T: Tourettism associated with Huntington's disease. Mov Disord 1995;10:103–105.

Jankovic J, Beach J: Long-term effects of tetrabenazine in hyperkinetic movement disorders. Neurology 1997;48:358–362.

Jankovic J, Fahn S: The phenomenology of tics. Mov Disord 1986;1:17–26.

Jankovic J, Fahn S: Dystonic disorders. In Jankovic J, Tolosa E (eds): Parkinson's Disease and Movement Disorders, 4th ed. Philadelphia, Lippincott Williams & Wilkins, 2002, pp 331–357.

Jankovic J, Glaze DG, Frost JD: Effect of tetrabenazine on tics and sleep of Gilles de la Tourette's syndrome. Neurology 1984;34:688–692.

Jankovic J, Kwak C, Frankoff R: Tourette syndrome and the law. J Neuropsychiatry Clin Neurosci 2006;18:86–95.

Jankovic J, Mejia NI: Tics associated with other disorders. In Walkup J, Mink J, Hollenbeck P (eds.): Tourette Syndrome. Advances in Neurology, vol 99. Philadelphia, Lippincott Williams & Wilkins, Philadelphia, 2006, pp 61–68.

Jankovic J, Orman J: Tetrabenazine therapy of dystonia, chorea, tics and other dyskinesias. Neurology 1988;38:391–394.

Jankovic J, Rohaidy H: Motor, behavioral and pharmacologic findings in Tourette's syndrome. Can J Neurol Sci 1987;14:541–546.

Jankovic J, Sekula SL, Milas D: Dermatological manifestations of Tourette's syndrome and obsessive-compulsive disorder. Arch Dermatol 1998;134:113–114.

Jankovic J, Stone L: Dystonic tics in patients with Tourette's syndrome. Mov Disord 1991;6:248–252.

Jenike MA: Obsessive-compulsive disorder. N Engl J Med 2004; 350:259–265.

Jimenez-Jimenez FJ, Garcia-Ruiz PJ: Pharmacological options for the treatment of Tourette's Disorder. Drugs 2001;61:2207–2220.

Jog MS, Kubota Y, Connolly CI, et al: Building neural representations of habits. Science 1999;286:1745–1749.

Karayiorgou M, Altemus M, Galke BL, et al: Genotype determining low catechol-o-methyltransferase activity as a risk factor for obsessive-compulsive disorder. Proc Natl Acad Sci U S A 1997;94:4572–4575.

Karp BI, Hallett M: Extracorporeal phantom tics in Tourette's syndrome. Neurology 1996;46:38–40.

Karp BI, Porter S, Toro C, Hallett M: Simple motor tics may be preceded by a premotor potential. J Neurol Neurosurg Psychiatry 1996;61:103–106.

Kelsey DK, Sumner CR, Casat CD, et al: Once-daily atomoxetine treatment for children with attention-deficit/hyperactivity disorder, including an assessment of evening and morning behavior: A double-blind, placebo-controlled trial. Pediatrics 2004;114:1–8.

Kenney C, Hunter C, Mejia N, Jankovic J: Tetrabenazine in the treatment of Tourette syndrome. J Ped Neurol 2007 (in press).

Kenney C, Jankovic J: Tetrabenazine in the treatment of hyperkinetic movement disorders. Expert Rev Neurotherapeutics 2006;6:7–17.

Kiessling LS, Marcotte AC, Culpepper L: Antineuronal antibodies in movement disorders. Pediatrics 1993;92:39–43.

Klein RG, Abikoff H, Klass E, et al: Clinical efficacy of methylphenidate in conduct disorder with and without attention deficit hyperactivity disorder. Arch Gen Psychiatry 1997;54:1073–1080.

Koller WC, Biary NM: Volitional control of involuntary movements. Mov Disord 1989;4:153–156.

Kompoliti K, Goetz CG: Hyperkinetic movement disorders misdiagnosed as tics in Gilles de la Tourette syndrome. Mov Disord 1998;13:477–480.

Kratochvil CJ, Heiligenstein JH, Dittmann R, et al: Atomoxetine and methylphenidate treatment in children with ADHD: A prospective, randomized, open-label trial. J Am Acad Child Adolesc Psychiatry 2002;41:776–784.

Krauss JK, Jankovic J: Severe motor tics causing cervical myelopathy in Tourette's syndrome. Mov Disord 1996;11:563–566.

Krauss JK, Jankovic J: Tics secondary to craniocerebral trauma. Mov Disord 1997;12:776–782.

Kumar R, Lang AE: Coexistence of tics and parkinsonism: Evidence for non-dopaminergic mechanisms in tic pathogenesis. Neurology 1997a;49:1699–1701.

Kumar R, Lang AE: Secondary tic disorders. In Jankovic J (ed): Tourette Syndrome. Neurologic Clinics of North America, vol 15. Philadelphia, WB Saunders, 1997b, pp 309–332.

Kurlan R: The pathogenesis of Tourette's syndrome: A possible role for hormonal and excitatory neurotransmitter influences in brain development. Arch Neurol 1992;49:874–876.

Kurlan R: Hypothesis II: Tourette's syndrome is part of a clinical spectrum that includes normal brain development. Arch Neurol 1994;51:1145–1150.

Kurlan R: Diagnostic criteria for genetic studies of Tourette syndrome. Arch Neurol 1997;54:517–518.

Kurlan R: Acute parkinsonism induced by the combination of a serotonin reuptake inhibitor and a neuroleptic in adults with Tourette's syndrome. Mov Disord 1998a;13:178–179.

Kurlan R: Tourette's syndrome and "PANDAS": Will the relation bear out? Neurology 1998b;50:1530–1534.

Kurlan R: New treatments for tics? Neurology 2001;56:580–581.

Kurlan R: Methylphenidate to treat ADHD is not contraindicated in children with tics. Mov Disord 2002;17:5–6.

Kurlan R: The PANDAS hypothesis: Losing its bite? Mov Disord 2004;19:371–374.

Kurlan R, Behr J, Medved L, Como P: Transient tic disorder and the clinical spectrum of Tourette's syndrome. Arch Neurol 1988;45:1200–1201.

Kurlan R, Behr J, Medved L, et al: Severity of Tourette's syndrome in one large kindred: Implication for determination of disease prevalence rate. Arch Neurol 1987;44:268–269.

Kurlan R, Como PG, Miller B, et al: The behavioral spectrum of tic disorders: A community-based study. Neurology 2002;59:414–420.

Kurlan R, Deeley C, Como P: Psychogenic movement disorder (pseudo-tics) in a patient with Tourette's syndrome. J Neuropsychiatry Clin Neurosci 1992;4:347–349.

Kurlan R, Eapen V, Stern J, et al: Bilineal transmission in Tourette's syndrome families. Neurology 1994;44:2336–2342.

Kurlan R, Lichter D, Hewitt D: Sensory tics in Tourette's syndrome. Neurology 1989;39:731–734.

Kurlan R, McDermott MP, Deeley C, et al: Prevalence of tics in schoolchildren and association with placement in special education. Neurology 2001;57:1383–1388.

Kushner HI: From Gilles de la Tourette's disease to Tourette syndrome: A history. CNS Spectr 1999;4:24–35.

Kwak C, Jankovic J: Tourettism and dystonia after subcortical stroke. Mov Disord 2002;17:821–825.

Kwak C, Vuong KD, Jankovic J: Migraine headache in patients with Tourette syndrome. Arch Neurol 2003a;60:1595–1598.

Kwak C, Vuong KD, Jankovic J: Premonitory sensory phenomenon in Tourette's syndrome. Mov Disord 2003b;18:1530–1533.

Kwak CH, Hanna PA, Jankovic J: Botulinum toxin in the treatment of tics. Arch Neurol 2000;57:1190–1193.

Laird LK: Issues in the monopharmacotherapy and polypharmacotherapy of obsessive-compulsive disorder. Psychopharmacol Bull 1996;32:569–576.

Lang A: Patient perception of tics and other movement disorders. Neurology 1991;41:223–228.

Lang AE: Update on the treatment of tics. In Cohen DJ, Jankovic J, Goetz CG (eds): Tourette Syndrome. Advances in Neurology, vol 85. Philadelphia, Lippincott Williams & Wilkins, 2001, pp 355–362.

Lang AE, Consky E, Sandor P: "Signing tics": Insights into the pathophysiology of symptoms in Tourette's syndrome. Ann Neurol 1993;33:212–215.

Laplane D, Levasseur M, Pillon B, et al: Obsessive-compulsive and other behavioural changes with bilateral basal ganglia lesions: A neuropsychological, magnetic resonance and positron tomography study. Brain 1989;112:699–726.

Law SF, Schachtar RT: Do typical clinical doses of methylphenidate cause tics in children treated for attention-deficit hyperactivity disorder? J Am Acad Child Adolesc Psychiatry 1999;38:944–951.

Leckman J, Cohen D, Goetz C, Jankovic J: Tourette syndrome: Pieces of the puzzle. In Cohen DJ, Jankovic J, Goetz CG (eds): Tourette Syndrome. Advances in Neurology, vol 85. Philadelphia, Lippincott Williams & Wilkins, 2001, pp 369–390.

Leckman JF: Tourette's syndrome. Lancet 2002;360:1577–1586.

Leckman JF, Cohen DJ: Tourette's Syndrome—Tics, Obsessions, Compulsions: Developmental Psychopathology and Clinical Care. New York, John Wiley, 1999.

Leckman JF, Dolnansky ES, Hardin MT, et al: Perinatal factors in the expression of Tourette's syndrome: An exploratory study. J Am Acad Child Adolesc Psychiatry 1990;29:220–226.

Leckman JF, Grice DE, Boardman J, et al: Symptoms of obsessive-compulsive disorder. Am J Psychiatry 1997;154:911–917.

Leckman JF, Hardin MT, Riddle MA, et al: Clonidine treatment of Gilles de la Tourette's Syndrome. Arch Gen Psychiatry 1991;48:324–328.

Leckman JF, Peterson BS, Anderson GM, et al: Pathogenesis of Tourette's syndrome. J Child Psychol Psychiatry 1997;38:119–142.

Leckman JF, Walker DE, Goodman WK, et al: "Just right" perceptions associated with compulsive behavior in Tourette's syndrome. Am J Psychiatry 1994;151:675–680.

Leckman JF, Zhang H, Vitale A, et al: Course of tic severity in Tourette syndrome: The first two decades. Pediatrics 1998;102:14–19.

Lees A: Jumpers. Mov Disord 2001;16:403–404.

Leibson CL, Katusic SK, Barbaresi WJ, et al: Use and costs of medical care for children and adolescents with and without attention-deficit/hyperactivity disorder. JAMA 2001;285:60–66.

Leonard H: Tourette syndrome and obsessive compulsive disorder. In Chase T, Friedhoff A, Cohen DJ (eds): Tourette's Syndrome. Advances in Neurology. New York, Raven Press, 1992, pp 83–94.

Leonard H, Swedo SE, Garvey M, et al: Postinfectious and other forms of obsessive-compulsive disorder. Child Adolesc Psychiatr Clin N Am 1999;8:497–511.

Lesperance P, Djerroud N, Diaz Anzaldua A, et al: Restless legs in Tourette syndrome. Mov Disord 2004;19:1084–1087.

LeVasseur AL, Flanagan JR, Riopelle RJ, Munoz DP: Control of volitional and reflexive in Tourette's syndrome. Brain 2001;124:2045–2058.

Lichter DG, Dmochowski J, Jackson LA, Trinidad KS: Influence of family history on clinical expression of Tourette's syndrome. Neurology 1999;52:308–316.

Lindstrom J: Nicotine acetylcholine receptors in health and disease. Mol Neurobiol 1997;15:193–222.

Lipinski JF, Sallee FR, Jackson C, Sethuraman G: Dopamine agonist treatment of Tourette disorder in children: Results of an open-label trial of pergolide. Mov Disord 1997;12:402–407.

Loiselle CR, Lee O, Moran TH, Singer HS: Striatal microinfusion of Tourette syndrome and PANDAS sera: Failure to induce behavioral changes. Mov Disord 2004;19:390–396.

Lombroso CT: Lamotrigine-induced tourettism. Neurology 1999;52:1191–1194.

Lombroso PJ, Mack G, Scahill L, et al: Exacerbation of Gilles de la Tourette's syndrome associated with thermal stress: A family study. Neurology 1991;41:1984–1987.

Ludolph AG, Juengling FD, Libal G, et al: Grey-matter abnormalities in boys with Tourette syndrome: Magnetic resonance imaging study using optimised voxel-based morphometry. Br J Psychiatry 2006;188:484–485.

Maia DP, Teixeira AL Jr, Quintao Cunningham MC, Cardoso F: Obsessive compulsive behavior, hyperactivity, and attention deficit disorder in Sydenham chorea. Neurology 2005;64:1799–1801.

Malison RT, McDougle CJ, van Dyck CH, et al: [$^{123}$I]β-CIT SPECT imaging of striatal dopamine transporter binding in Tourette's disorder. Am J Psychiatry 1995;152:1359–1361.

Mamo D, Kapur S, Shammi CM, et al: A PET study of dopamine D2 and serotonin 5-HT2 receptor occupancy in patients with schizophrenia treated with therapeutic doses of ziprasidone. Am J Psychiatry 2004;161:818–825.

Manos MJ, Short EJ, Findling RL: Differential effectiveness of methylphenidate and Adderall$^R$ in school-age youths with attention-deficit/hyperactivity disorder. J Am Acad Child Adolesc Psychiatry 1999;38:813–819.

March JS, Biederman J, Wolkow R, et al: Sertraline in children and adolescents with obsessive-compulsive disorder: A multicenter controlled trial. JAMA 1998;280:1752–1756.

March JS, Franklin M, Nelson A, Foa E: Cognitive-behavioral psychotherapy for pediatric obsessive-compulsive disorder. J Child Psychology 2001;30:8–18.

Marras C, Andrews D, Sime EA Lang AE: Botulinum toxin for simple motor tics: A randomized, double-blind, controlled clinical trial. Neurology 2001;56:605–610.

Mason A, Banerjee S, Zeitlin H, Robertson MM: The prevalence of Tourette syndrome in a mainstream school population. Dev Med Child Neurol 1998;40:292–296.

Mathews CA, Waller J, Glidden D, et al: Self injurious behaviour in Tourette syndrome: Correlates with impulsivity and impulse control. J Neurol Neurosurg Psychiatry 2004;75:1149–1155.

McGuire PK: The brain in obsessive-compulsive disorder. J Neurol Neurosurg Psychiatry 1995;59:457–459.

McMahon WM, van der Wetering BJ, Filoux F, et al: Bilineal transmission and phenotypic variations of Tourette's disorder in a large pedigree. J Am Acad Child Adolesc Psychiatry 1996;35:672–680.

Merette C, Brassard A, Potvin A, et al: Significant linkage for Tourette syndrome in a large French Canadian family. Am J Hum Genet 2000;67:1008–1013.

Meyer P, Bohnen NI, Minshima S, et al: Striatal presynaptic monoaminergic vesicles are not increased in Tourette's syndrome. Neurology 1999;53:371–374.

Micallef J, Blin O: Neurobiology and clinical pharmacology of obsessive-compulsive disorder. Clin Neuropharmacol 2001;24:191–207.

Michelson D, Faries D, Wernicke J, et al: Atomoxetine in the treatment of children and adolescents with attention-deficit/hyperactivity disorder: A randomized, placebo-controlled, dose-response study. Pediatrics 2001;108:1–9.

Miguel EC, do Rosario-Campos MC, Prado HS, et al: Sensory phenomena in obsessive-compulsive disorder and Tourette's disorder. J Clin Psychiatry 2000;61:150–156.

Milanfranchi A, Ravagli S, Lensi P, et al: A double-blind study of fluvoxamine and clomipramine in the treatment of obsessive-compulsive disorder. Int Clin Psychopharmacol 1997;12:131–136.

Mink JW, Walkup J, Frey KA, et al: Patient selection and assessment guidelines for deep brain stimulation in Tourette syndrome. Mov Disord 2006;21:1831–1838.

Minzer K, Lee O, Hong JJ, Singer HS: Increased prefrontal D2 protein in Tourette syndrome: A postmortem analysis of frontal cortex and striatum. J Neurol Sci 2004;219:55–61.

Moll GH, Heinrich H, Troo GE, et al: Children with comorbid attention-deficit-hyperactivity disorder and tic disorder: Evidence for additive inhibitory deficits with the motor systems. Ann Neurol 2001;49:393–396.

Moriarty J, Varma AR, Stevens J, et al: A volumetric MRI study of Gilles de la Tourette's syndrome. Neurology 1997;49:410–415.

Morshed SA, Parveen S, Leckman JF, et al: Antibodies against neural, nuclear, cytoskeletal, and streptococcal epitopes in children and adults with Tourette's syndrome, Sydenham's chorea, and autoimmune disorders. Biol Psychiatry 2001;50:566–577.

Mostofsky SH, Wendlandt J, Cutting L, et al: Corpus callosum measurement in girls with Tourette syndrome. Neurology 1999;53:1345–1347.

MTA Cooperative Group: A 14-month randomized clinical trial of treatment strategies for attention-deficit/hyperactivity disorder: The MTA Cooperative Group. Multimodal Treatment Study of Children with ADHD. Arch Gen Psychiatry 1999;56:1073–1086.

Müller N, Kroll B, Schwartz MJ, et al: Increased titers of antibodies against streptococcal M12 and M19 proteins in patients with Tourette's syndrome. Psychiatry Res 2001;101:187–193.

Müller-Vahl KR, Berding G, Brücke T, et al: Dopamine transporter binding in Gilles de la Tourette syndrome. J Neurol 2000;247:514–520.

Müller-Vahl KR, Kolbe H, Schneider U, Emrich HM: Cannabis in movement disorders. Forsch Komplementarmed 1999;6(suppl 3):23–27.

Munchau A, Bloem BR, Thilo KV, et al: Repetitive transcranial magnetic stimulation for Tourette syndrome. Neurology 2002;59:1789–1791.

Murphy ML, Pichichero ME: Prospective identification and treatment of children with pediatric autoimmune neuropsychiatric disorder associated with group A streptococcal infection (PANDAS). Arch Pediatr Adolesc Med 2002;156:356–361.

Murphy TK, Goodman WK, Fudge MW, et al: B lymphocyte antigen D8/17: A peripheral marker for childhood-onset obsessive-compulsive disorder and Tourette's syndrome. Am J Psychiatry 1997;154:402–407.

Németh AH, Mills KR, Elston JS, et al: Do the same genes predispose to Gilles de la Tourette syndrome and dystonia? Report of a new family and review of the literature. Mov Disord 1999;14:826–831.

Nestadt G, Bienvenu OJ, Cai G, et al: Incidence of obsessive-compulsive disorder in adults. J Nerv Ment Dis 1998;186:401–406.

Nuttin P, Cosyns P, Demeulemeester H, et al: Electrical stimulation in anterior limbs of internal capsules in patients with obsessive-compulsive disorder. Lancet 1999;354:1526.

Nuttin BJ, Gabriels L, van Kuyck K, Cosyns P: Electrical stimulation of the anterior limbs of the internal capsules in patients with severe obsessive-compulsive disorder: Anecdotal reports. Neurosurg Clin N Am 2003;14:267–274.

Obeso JA, Rothwell JC, Marsden CD: The neurophysiology of Tourette syndrome. Adv Neurol 1982;35:105–114.

Ogdie MN, Macphie IL, Minassian SL, et al: A genome wide scan for attention-deficit/hyperactivity disorder in an extended sample: Suggestive linkage on 17p11. Am J Hum Genet 2003;72:1268–1279.

Orth M, Amann B, Robertson MM, Rothwell JC: Excitability of motor cortex inhibitory circuits in Tourette syndrome before and after single dose nicotine. Brain 2005;128:1292–1300.

Pakstis AJ, Heutink P, Pauls DL, et al: Progress in the search for genetic linkage with Tourette syndrome: An exclusion map covering more than 50% of the autosomal genome. Am J Hum Genet 1991;48:281–294.

Palumbo D, Maughan A, Kurlan R: Hypothesis III: Tourette syndrome is only one of several causes of a developmental basal ganglia syndrome. Arch Neurol 1997;54:475–483.

Pantoni L, Poggesi L, Repice A, Inzitari D: Disappearance of motor tics after Wernicke's encephalopathy in a patient with Tourette's syndrome. Neurology 1997;48:381–383.

Papa SM, Artieda J, Obeso JA: Cortical activity preceding self-initiated and externally triggered voluntary movement. Mov Disord 1991;6:217–224.

Pappert EJ, Goetz CG, Louis ED, et al: Objective assessments of longitudinal outcome in Gilles de la Tourette's syndrome. Neurology 2003;61:936–940.

Paschou P, Feng Y, Pakstis AJ, et al: Indications of linkage and association of Gilles de la Tourette syndrome in two independent family samples: 17q25 is a putative susceptibility region. Am J Hum Genet 2004;75:545.

Patel PI: Quest for the elusive genetic basis of Tourette syndrome. Am J Hum Genet 1996;59:980–982.

Pauls DL, Cohen DJ, Kidd KK, Leckman JF: Tourette syndrome and neuropsychiatric disorders: Is there a genetic relationship? Am J Hum Genet 1988;43:206–209.

Pauls DL, Raymond CL, Stevenson JM, Leckman JF: A family study of Gilles de la Tourette syndrome. Am J Hum Genet 1991;48:154–163.

Pediatric OCD Treatment Study (POTS) Team: Cognitive-behavior therapy, sertraline, and their combination for children and adolescents with obsessive-compulsive disorder: The Pediatric OCD Treatment Study (POTS) randomized controlled trial. JAMA 2004;292:1969–1976.

Pellecchia MT, Valente EM, Cif L, et al: The diverse phenotype and genotype of pantothenate kinase-associated neurodegeneration. Neurology 2005;64:1810–1812.

Perlmutter SJ, Leitman SF, Garvey MA, et al: Therapeutic plasma exchange and intravenous immunoglobulin for obsessive-compulsive disorder and tic disorders in childhood. Lancet 1999;354:1153–1158.

Peterson B: Neuroimaging studies of Tourette syndrome: A decade of progress. In Cohen DJ, Jankovic J, Goetz CG (eds): Tourette Syndrome. Advances in Neurology, vol 85. Philadelphia, Lippincott Williams & Wilkins, 2001, pp 179–196.

Peterson B, Cohen DJ: The treatment of Tourette's syndrome: Multimodal, developmental intervention. J Clin Psychiatry 1998;59(suppl):62–72.

Peterson B, Leckman JF: The temporal dynamics of tics in Gilles de la Tourette syndrome. Biol Psychiatry 1998;44:1337–1348.

Peterson B, Leckman JF, Tucker D, et al: Preliminary findings of antistreptococcal antibody titers and basal ganglia volumes in tic, obsessive-compulsive, and attention deficit/hyperactivity disorders. Arch Gen Psychiatry 2000;57:364–372.

Peterson B, Riddle MA, Cohen DJ, et al: Reduced basal ganglia volumes in Tourette's syndrome using three-dimensional reconstruction techniques from magnetic resonance images. Neurology 1993;43:941–949.

Peterson B, Skudlarski P, Anderson AW, et al: A functional magnetic resonance imaging study of tic suppression in Tourette syndrome. Arch Gen Psychiatry 1998a;54:326–333.

Peterson B, Zhang H, Anderson GM, Leckman JF: A double-blind, placebo-controlled, crossover trial of an antiandrogen in the treatment of Tourette's syndrome. J Clin Psychopharmacol 1998b;18:324–331.

Piacentini J, Chang S: Behavioral treatment for Tourette syndrome and tic disorders. In Cohen DJ, Jankovic J, Goetz CG (eds): Tourette Syndrome. Advances in Neurology, vol 85. Philadelphia, Lippincott Williams & Wilkins, 2001, pp 319–332.

Picchietti DL, Underwood DJ, Farris WA, et al: Further studies on periodic limb movement disorder and restless legs syndrome in children with attention-deficit hyperactivity disorder. Mov Disord 1999;14:1000–1007.

Pidoplichko VI, DeBiasi M, Williams JT, Dani JA: Nicotine activates and desensitizes midbrain dopamine neurons. Nature 1997;390:401–404.

Pliszka SR: Non-stimulant treatment of attention-deficit/hyperactivity disorder. CNS Spectr 2003;8:253–258.

Pliszka SR, Browne RG, Olvera RL, Wynne SK: A double-blind, placebo-controlled study of Adderall and methylphenidate in the treatment of attention-deficit/hyperactivity disorder. J Am Acad Child Adolesc 2000;39:619–626.

Price RA, Leckman JF, Pauls DL, et al: Gilles de la Tourette syndrome. Tics and central nervous system stimulants in twins and non-twins. Neurology 1986;36:232–237.

Rapoport JL: The neurobiology of obsessive-compulsive disorder. JAMA 1988;260:2888–2890.

Rappley MD: Clinical practice. Attention deficit-hyperactivity disorder. N Engl J Med 2005;352:165–173.

Rauch SL, Savage CR, Alpert NM, et al: Probing striatal function in obsessive-compulsive disorder: A PET study of implicit sequence learning. J Neuropsychiatry Clin Neurosci 1997;9:568–573.

Research Unit on Pediatric Psychopharmacology Anxiety Study Group: Fluvoxamine for the treatment of anxiety disorders in children and adolescents. N Engl J Med 2001;344:1279–1285.

Research Units on Pediatric Psychopharmacology Autism Network: Risperidone in children with autism and serious behavioral problems. N Engl J Med 2002;347:314–321.

Richard MM, Finkel MF, Cohen MD: Preparing reports documenting attention deficit/hyperactivity disorder for students in postsecondary education: What neurologists need to know. Neurologist 1998;4:277–283.

Rickards H, Robertson MM: Vomiting and retching in Gilles de la Tourette syndrome: A report of ten cases and a review of the literature. Mov Disord 1997;12:531–535.

Riddle MA, Carlson J: Clinical psychopharmacology for Tourette syndrome and associated disorders. In Cohen DJ, Jankovic J, Goetz CG (eds): Tourette Syndrome. Advances in Neurology, vol 85. Philadelphia, Lippincott Williams & Wilkins, 2001, pp 343–354.

Ringman JM, Jankovic J: The occurrence of tics in Asperger syndrome and autistic disorder. J Child Neurol 2000;15:394–400.

Robertson M: The Gilles de la Tourette syndrome: The current status. Br J Psychiatry 1989;154:147–169.

Robertson M: Tourette syndrome, associated conditions and the complexities of treatment. Brain 2000;123:425–462.

Robertson M, Banerjee S, Fox Hiley PJ, Tannock C: Personality disorder and psychopathology in Tourette's syndrome: A controlled study. Br J Psychiatry 1997;171:283–286.

Robertson M, Banerjee S, Kurlan R, et al: The Tourette Syndrome Diagnostic Confidence Index: Development and clinical associations. Neurology 1999;53:2108–2112.

Robertson M, Doran M, Trimble M, Lees AJ: The treatment of Gilles de la Tourette syndrome by limbic leucotomy. J Neurol Neurosurg Psychiatry 1990;53:691–694.

Robertson M, Eapen V: Pharmacologic controversy of CNS stimulants in Gilles de la Tourette's syndrome. Clin Neuropharmacol 1992;15:408–425.

Robertson M, Scull DA, Eapen V, Trimble MR: Risperidone in the treatment of Tourette syndrome: A retrospective case note study. J Psychopharmacol 1996;10:317–320.

Romstad A, Dupont E, Krag-Olsen B, et al: Dopa-responsive dystonia and Tourette syndrome in a large Danish family. Arch Neurol 2003;60:618–622.

Rosa AL, Jankovic J, Ashizawa T: Screening for mutations in the MECP2 (Rett Syndrome) gene in Gilles de la Tourette syndrome. Arch Neurol 2003;60:502–503.

Rothenberger A, Kostanecka T, Kinkelbur J, et al: Sleep and Tourette syndrome. In Cohen D, Jankovic J, Goetz C (eds): Tourette Syndrome. Advances in Neurology, vol 85. Philadelphia, Lippincott Williams & Wilkins, 2001, pp 245–260.

Sadovnick D, Kurlan R: The increasingly complex genetics of Tourette's syndrome. Neurology 1997;48:801–802.

Saiki S, Hirose G, Sakai K, et al: Chorea-acanthocytosis associated with Tourettism. Mov Disord 2004;19:833–836.

Saint-Hilaire MH, Saint-Hilaire JM, Granger L: Jumping Frenchmen of Maine. Neurology 1986;36:1269–1271.

Sallee FR, Kurlan R, Goetz CG, et al: Ziprasidone treatment of children and adolescents with Tourette's syndrome: A pilot study. J Am Acad Child Adolesc Psychiatry 2000;39:292–299.

Sallee FR, Nesbit L, Jackson C, et al: Relative efficacy of haloperidol and pimozide in children and adolesents. Am J Psychiatry 1997;154:1057–1062.

Sanberg PR, Emerich DF, el-Etri MM, et al: Nicotine potentiation of haloperidol-induced catalepsy: Stritatal mechanisms. Pharmacol Biochem Behav 1993;46:303–307.

Sanberg PR, Shytle RD, Silver AA: Treatment of Tourette's syndrome with mecamylamine. Lancet 1998;352:705–706.

Sasson Y, Zohar J, Chopra M, et al: Epidemiology of obsessive-compulsive disorder: A world view. J Clin Psychiatry 1997;58(suppl 12):7–10.

Scahill L, Erenberg G, Berlin CM Jr, et al: Contemporary assessment and pharmacotherapy of Tourette syndrome. NeuroRx 2006; 3:192–206.

Scahill L, Leckman JF, Schultz RT, et al: A placebo-controlled trial of risperidone in Tourette syndrome. Neurology 2003;60:1130–1135.

Scahill L, Riddle MA, McSwiggin-Hardin M, et al: Children's Yale-Brown obsessive compulsive scale: Reliability and validity. J Am Acad Child Adolesc Psychiatry 1997;36:844–852.

Scahill L, Tanner C, Dure L: The epidemiology of tics and Tourette syndrome in children and adolescents. In Cohen DJ, Jankovic J, Goetz CG (eds): Tourette Syndrome. Advances in Neurology, vol 85. Philadelphia, Lippincott Williams & Wilkins, 2001, pp 261–272.

Schwabe MJ, Konkol RJ: Menstrual cycle-related fluctuations of tics in Tourette syndrome. Pediatr Neurol 1992;8:43–46.

Scott BL, Jankovic J, Donovan DT: Botulinum toxin into vocal cord in the treatment of malignant coprolalia associated with Tourette's syndrome. Mov Disord 1996;11:431–433.

Sedel F, Friderici K, Nummy K, et al: Atypical Gilles de la Tourette syndrome with ß-mannosidase deficiency. Arch Neurol 2006;63:129–131.

Serrien DJ, Nirkko AC, Loher TJ, et al: Movement control of manipulative taks in patients with Gilles de la Tourette syndrome. Brain 2002;125:290–300.

Shahed J, Poysky J, Kenney C, et al: GPi deep brain stimulation for Tourette syndrome improves tics and psychiatric comorbidities. Neurology 2007;68(2):159–160.

Shapiro A, Shapiro E: Treatment of Gilles de la Tourette's syndrome with haloperidol. Br J Psychiatry 1968;114:345–350.

Shapiro AK, Shapiro E: Evaluation of the reported association of obsessive-compulsive symptoms or disease with Tourette's disorder. Compr Psychiatry 1992;33:152–165.

Shapiro AK, Shapiro ES, Young JG, Feinberg TE: Gilles de la Tourette's Syndrome, 2nd ed. New York, Raven Press, 1988.

Silay Y, Jankovic J: Emerging drugs in Tourette syndrome. Expert Opin Emerg Drugs 2005;10:365–380.

Silva RR, Magee HJ, Friedhoff AJ: Persistent tardive dyskinesia and other neuroleptic-related dyskinesias in Tourette's disorder. J Child Adolesc Psychopharmacol 1993;3:137–144.

Silver AA, Shytle RD, Philipp MK, Sanberg PR: Case study: Long-term potentiation of neuroleptics with transdermal nicotine in Tourette's syndrome. J Am Acad Child Adolesc Psychiatry 1996;35:1631–1636.

Silver AA, Shytle RD, Sheehan D, et al: A multi-center, double blind placebo controlled safety and efficacy study of mecamylamine (Inversine®) monotherapy for Tourette syndrome. J Am Acad Child Adolesc Psychiatry 2001;40:1103–1110.

Silvestri R, DeDomenico P, DiRosa AE, et al: The effects of nocturnal physiologic sleep on various movement disorders. Mov Disord 1990;5:8–14.

Simkin B: Mozart's scatological disorder. BMJ 1992;305:1563–1567.

Simonic I, Nyholt DR, Gericke GS, et al: Further evidence for linkage of Gilles de la Tourette syndrome (GTS) susceptibility loci on chromosomes 2p11, 8q22 and 11q23-24 in South African Afrikaners. Am J Med Genet 2001;105:163–167.

Singer HS: Current issues in Tourette syndrome. Mov Disord 2000;15:1051–1063.

Singer HS: Tourette's syndrome: From behaviour to biology. Lancet Neurol 2005;4:149–159.

Singer HS, Brown J, Quaskey S, et al: The treatment of attention-deficit hyperactivity disorder in Tourette's syndrome: A double-blind placebo-controlled study with clonidine and desipramine. Pediatrics 1995;95:74–81.

Singer HS, Dela Cruz PS, Abrams AT, et al: A tourette-like syndrome following cardiopulmonary bypass and hypothermia: MRI volumetric measurements. Mov Disord 1997;12:588–592.

Singer HS, Giuliano JD, Hansen BH, et al: Antibodies against human putamen in children with Tourette syndrome. Neurology 1998; 50:1618–1624.

Singer HS, Hahn IH, Moran TH: Abnormal dopamine uptake sites in postmortem striatum from patients with Tourette's syndrome. Ann Neurol 1991;30:558–562.

Singer HS, Loiselle CR, Lee O, et al: Anti-basal ganglia antibodies in PANDAS. Mov Disord 2004;19:406–415.

Singer HS, Reiss AL, Brown JE, et al: Volumetric MRI changes in basal ganglia of children with Tourette's syndrome. Neurology 1993; 43:950–956.

Singer HS, Schuerholz LJ, Denckla MB: Learning difficulties in children with Tourette's syndrome. J Child Neurol 1995;10:558–561.

Singer HS, Szymanski S, Giuliano J, et al: Elevated intrasynaptic dopamine release in Tourette's syndrome measured by PET. Am J Psychiatry 2002;159:1329–1336.

Singer HS, Wendlandt J, Krieger M, Giuliano J: Baclofen treatment in Tourette syndrome: A double-blind, placebo-controlled, crossover trial. Neurology 2001;56:599–604.

Singh S, Jankovic J: Tardive dystonia in patients with Tourette's syndrome. Mov Disord 1988;3:274–280.

Siponmaa L, Kristiansson M, Jonson C, et al: Juvenile and young adult mentally disordered offenders: The role of child neuropsychiatric disorders. J Am Acad Psychiatry Law 2001;29:420–426.

Smalley SL, Fisher SE, Francks C, et al: Genome-wide scan in attention deficit hyperactivity disorders (ADHD) [abstract]. Am J Hum Genet 2001;69:535.

Smith SJ, Lees AJ: Abnormalities of the blink reflex in Gilles de la Tourette syndrome. J Neurol Neurosurg Psychiatry 1989;52: 895–898.

Snider LA, Seligman LD, Ketchen BR, et al: Tics and problem behaviors in school children: Prevalence, characterization, and associations. Pediatrics 2002;110:331–336.

Snider LA, Swedo SE: Pediatric obsessive-compulsive disorder. JAMA 2000;284:3104–3106.

Snider LA, Swedo SE: Post-streptococcal autoimmune disorders of the central nervous system. Curr Opin Neurol 2003;16:359–365.

Sowell ER, Thompson PM, Welcome SE, et al: Cortical abnormalities in children and adolescents with attention-deficit hyperactivity disorder. Lancet 2003;362:1699–1707.

Spencer T, Biederman J, Steingard R, Wilens T: Bupropion exacerbates tics in children with attention-deficit hyperactivity disorder and Tourette's syndrome. J Am Acad Child Adolesc Psychiatry 1993;32:211–214.

Spitz MC, Jankovic J, Killian JM: Familial tic disorder, parkinsonism, motor neuron disease, and acanthocytosis: A new syndrome. Neurology 1985;35:366–377.

Stahl SM: Using secondary binding properties to select or not so selective reuptake inhibitor. J Clin Psychiatry 1998;59:642–643.

Stahl SM, Shayegan DK: The psychopharmacology of ziprasidone: Receptor-binding properties and real-world psychiatric practice. J Clin Psychiatry 2003;64(suppl 19):6–12.

Stein DJ: Obsessive-compulsive disorder. Lancet 2002;360:397–405.

Stell R, Thickbroom GW, Mastaglia FL: The audiogenic startle response in Tourette's syndrome. Mov Disord 1995;10:723–730.

Stern E, Silbersweig DA, Chee K-Y, et al: A functional neuroanatomy of tics in Tourette syndrome. Arch Gen Psychiatry 2000;57:741–748.

Stone L, Jankovic J: The coexistence of tics and dystonia. Arch Neurol 1991;48:862–865.

Swanson JM, Sergeant JA, Taylor E, et al: Attention-deficit hyperactivity disorder and hyperactivity disorder. Lancet 1998;351:429–433.

Swedo S, Leonard H, Mittelman B, et al: Children with PANDAS (pediatric autoimmune neuropsychiatric disorders associated with strep infections) are identified by a marker associated with rheumatic fever. Am J Psychiatry 1997;154:110–112.

Swerdlow NR, Magulae M, Filion D, Zinner S: Visuospatial priming and latent inhibition in children and adults with Tourette's syndrome. Neuropsychology 1996;10:485–494.

Swoboda KJ, Jenike MA: Frontal abnormalities in a patient with obsessive-compulsive disorder: The role of structural lesions in obsessive-compulsive behavior. Neurology 1995;45:2130–2134.

Tannock R: Attention deficit hyperactivity disorder: Advances in cognitive, neurobiological, and genetic research. J Child Psychol Psychiatry 1998;39:65–99.

Taylor JR, Morshed SA, Parveen S, et al: An animal model of Tourette's syndrome. Am J Psychiatry 2002;159:657–660.

Taylor LD, Krizman DB, Jankovic J, et al: 9p monosomy in a patient with Gilles de la Tourette's syndrome. Neurology 1991;41:1513–1515.

Teitelbaum P, Teitelbaum O, Nye J, et al: Movement analysis in infancy may be useful for early diagnosis of autism. Proc Natl Acad Sci U S A 1998;95:13982–13987.

Temel Y, Visser-Vandewalle V: Surgery in Tourette syndrome. Mov Disord 2004;19:3–14.

Thase ME, Entsua AR, Rudolph RL: Remission rates during treatment with venlafaxine or selective serotonin reuptake inhibitors. Br J Psychiatry 2001;178:234–241.

Tijssen MAJ, Brown P, Morris HR, Lees A: Late onset startle induced tics. J Neurol Neurosurg Psychiatry 1999;67:782–784.

Tolosa E, Jankovic J: Tics and Tourette's syndrome. In Jankovic J, Tolosa E (eds): Parkinson's Disease and Movement Disorders, 3rd ed. Baltimore, Williams & Wilkins, 1998, pp 491–512.

Toren P, Laor N, Cohen DJ, et al: Ondansetron treatment in patients with Tourette's syndrome. Int Clin Psychopharmacol 1999;14:373–376.

Tourette Syndrome Association International Consortium on Genetics: A complete genome screen in sib-pairs affected by Gilles de la Tourette syndrome. Am J Hum Genet 1999;65:1428–1436.

Tourette Syndrome Classification Study Group: Definitions and classification of tic disorders. Arch Neurol 1993;50:1013–1016.

Tourette Syndrome Study Group: Treatment of ADHD in children with tics: A randomized controlled trial. Neurology 2002;58:527–536.

Toth E, Sershen H, Hashim A, et al: Effect of nicotine on extracellular levels of neurotransmitters assessed by microdialysis in various brain regions: Role of glutamic acid. Neurochem Res 1992;17:265–271.

Towbin KE: Obsessive-compulsive symptoms in Tourette's syndrome. In Cohen DJ, Bruun RD, Leckman JF (eds): Tourette's Syndrome and Tic Disorders. New York, John Wiley & Sons, 1988, pp 138–149.

Trifiletti RR, Packard AM: Immune mechanisms in pediatric neuropsychiatric disorders: Tourette's syndrome, OCD, and PANDAS. Child Adolesc Psychiatr Clin N Am 1999;8:767–775.

Tulen JHM, Azzolini M, De Vries JA, et al: Quantitative study of spontaneous eye blinks and eye tics in Gilles de la Tourette's syndrome. J Neurol Neurosurg Psychiatry 1999;67:800–802.

Turjanski N, Sawle GV, Playford ED, et al: PET studies of the presynaptic and postsynaptic dopaminergic system in Tourette's syndrome. J Neurol Neurosurg Psychiatry 1994;57:688–692.

Vaidya C, Austin G, Kirkorian G, et al: Selective effects of methylphenidate in attention deficit hyperactivity disorder: A functional magnetic resonance study. Proc Natl Acad Sci U S A 1998;95:14494–14499.

Vandewalle V, Van Der Linden C, Groenewegen HJ, Caemaert J: Stereotactic treatment of Gilles de la Tourette syndrome by high frequency stimulation of thalamus. Lancet 1999;353:724.

Vincent A: Encephalitis lethargica: Part of a spectrum of post-streptococcal autoimmune diseases? Brain 2004;127:2–3.

Voderholzer U, Müller N, Haag C, et al: Periodic limb movements during sleep are a frequent finding in patients with Gilles de la Tourette's syndrome. J Neurol 1997;244:521–520.

Volkmar FR, Pauls D: Autism. Lancet 2003;362:1133–1141.

Voon V: Repetition, repetition, and repetition: Compulsive and punding behaviors in Parkinson's disease. Mov Disord 2004;19:367–370.

Walkup JT, LaBuda MC, Singer HS, et al: Family study and segregation analysis of Tourette syndrome: Evidence for a mixed model of inheritance. Am J Hum Genet 1996;59:684–693.

Walters AS, McHale D, Sage JI, et al: A blinded study of the suppressibility of involuntary movements in Huntington's chorea, tardive dyskinesia, and L-Dopa-induced chorea. Clin Neuropharmacol 1990;13:236–240.

Whittington CJ, Kendall T, Fonagy P, et al: Selective serotonin reuptake inhibitors in childhood depression: Systematic review of published versus unpublished data. Lancet 2004;363:1341–1345.

Wilens TE, Biederman J, Spencer TJ, Prince J: Pharmacotherapy of adult attention deficit/hyperactivity disorder: A review. J Clin Psychopharmacol 1995;15:270–279.

Wilens TE, Faraone SV, Biederman J: Attention-deficit/hyperactivity disorder in adults. JAMA 2004;292:619–623.

Wilhelm S, Deckersbach T, Coffey BJ, et al: Habit reversal versus supportive psychotherapy for Tourette's disorder: A randomized controlled trial. Am J Psychiatry 2003;160:1175–1177.

Witelson SF: Clinical neurology as data for basic neuroscience: Tourette's syndrome and human motor system. Neurology 1993;43:859–861.

Wolf S, Jones DW, Knable MB, et al: Tourette syndrome: Prediction of phenotypic variation in monozygotic twins by caudate nucleus D2 receptor binding. Science 1996;273:1225–1227.

Woods DW, Twohig MP, Flessner CA, Roloff TJ: Treatment of vocal tics in children with Tourette syndrome: Investigating the efficacy of habit reversal. J Appl Behav Anal 2003;36:109–112.

Yeargin-Allsopp M, Rice C, Karapurkar T, et al: Prevalence of autism in a US metropolitan area. JAMA 2003;289:49–55.

Zametkin AJ, Ernst M: Problems in the management of attention-deficit-hyperactivity disorder. N Engl J Med 1999;340:40–46.

Ziemann U, Paulus W, Rothenberger A: Decreased motor inhibition in Tourette's disorder: Evidence from transcranial magnetic stimulation. Am J Psychiatry 1997;154:1277–1284.

Zuchner S, Cuccaro ML, Tran-Viet KN, et al: SLITRK1 mutations in trichotillomania. Mol Psychiatry 2006;11:888–889.

# APPENDIX 17-1

## Patient Organizations

### Tourette Syndrome Association (TSA)
42-40 Bell Boulevard
Bayside, NY 11361
Telephone: 718-224-2999
Website: http://neuro-www2.mgh.harvard.edu/tsa/tsamain.nclk

*Other Relevant Websites*
http://www.tsa.org.uk
http://www.ed.gov
http://www.nih.gov

http://www.wemove.org
http://www.cw.bc.ca/childrens/mhrev05/cats/catsdrug.html
http://www.medscape.com/LCM/InfMind/2001/02.01/infinitemind.html

*Obsessive Compulsive Foundation*
http://www.ocfoundation.org/

*Children and Adults with Attention-Deficit Disorder*
http://www.chadd.org/
http://www.ets.org/disability/adhdplcy.html

# Chapter 18

# Stereotypies

Stereotypies may be defined as involuntary or unvoluntary (in response to or induced by inner sensory stimulus or unwanted feeling), coordinated, patterned, repetitive, rhythmic, seemingly purposeless movements or utterances (Jankovic, 1994, Jankovic, 2005). Typical motor stereotypies include body rocking, head nodding, head banging, hand waving, repetitive and sequential finger movements, lip smacking, and chewing movements; phonic stereotypies include grunting, moaning, and humming. Stereotypies are usually either continuous, such as those seen in patients with tardive dyskinesia, mental retardation, or autism, or intermittent, such as the stereotypic tics seen in patients with Tourette syndrome (TS). They can be either continual or intermittent in patients with mental retardation or autism. Mannerisms, which are gestures that are peculiar or unique to the individual, may at times seem stereotypic (patterned), but they are usually not continual. There is often an overlap between stereotypies and self-injurious behavior, such as biting, scratching, and hitting (Jankovic et al., 1998; Schroeder et al., 2001; Lutz et al., 2003).

In addition to motor and phonic types, stereotypies can be classified as either simple (e.g., foot tapping, body rocking) or complex (e.g., complicated rituals, sitting down in and rising from a chair). Stereotypies can also be described according to the distribution of the predominant site of involvement (orolingual, hand, leg, truncal). The term *stereotypy* should be used to describe a phenomenologic, not an etiologic, category of hyperkinetic movement disorders. However, recognition of stereotypy as a distinct movement disorder can logically lead from a phenomenologic to an etiologic diagnosis (Box 18-1). It is well known that stereotypies often accompany a variety of behavioral disorders, such as anxiety, obsessive-compulsive disorders (OCD), TS, schizophrenia, autism, mental retardation, akathisia, restless legs syndrome, and a variety of neurodegenerative disorders, including frontotemporal dementia (Nyatsanza et al., 2003), and postinfectious disorders such as subacute sclerosing panecephalitis (SSPE) (Jankovic et al., 1998) (Video 18-1). Thus, stereotypy is a motor-behavioral disorder that is found most frequently in patients who are in the borderland between neurology and psychiatry.

## PATHOPHYSIOLOGY OF STEREOTYPIES

There is no clear anatomic-clinical correlation for stereotypies, although it is believed that both cortical and subcortical structures are involved. While dysfunction in the basal ganglia has been implicated in the pathogenesis of certain stereotypies, some studies have also provided evidence for the role of the mesolimbic system, particularly the nucleus accumbens–amygdala pathway, in the pathogenesis of stereotypic movements. Stereotypies with or without associated obsessive-compulsive behavior have been observed in patients with

structural lesions in different anatomic areas, including bilateral lesions of the medial frontoparietal cortices (Sato et al., 2001; Kwak and Jankovic, 2002) and cerebellum (Hottinger-Blanc et al., 2002).

Stereotypic behavior is common in animals in lower species up to and including the primates and is particularly common in farm and zoo animals that are housed in restraining environments with low stimulation (Garner et al., 2003; Lutz et al., 2003) (Video 18-2). Self-injurious behavior, observed in 14% of housed monkeys, may be viewed as a form of stereotypy (Novak, 2003). Therefore, stereotypy has been viewed as either a self-generating sensory stimulus or a motor expression of underlying tension and anxiety. The repetitive and ritualistic behavior that some animals display has been used as an experimental model of OCD. Indeed, studies of animal and human stereotypies have provided important insights into relationships between motor function and behavior. Some veterinarian scientists have even suggested changing the nomenclature of stereotypies to *obsessive-compulsive behaviors*; however, there is little evidence to indicate that the stereotypic behavior that is observed in animals is driven by underlying obsessions and represents compulsive behavior (Garner et al., 2003; Low, 2003).

Most studies of stereotypic behavior in experimental animals have focused on the role of dopaminergic systems in the basal ganglia and limbic structures. Intrastriatal injection of dopamine and systemic administration of both presynaptically active dopaminergic drugs, such as amphetamine, and postsynaptically active dopamine agonists, such as apomorphine, in rats produce dose-related repetitive sniffing, gnawing, licking, biting, rearing, head bobbing, grooming, and other stereotypic learned activities.

The observation that self-biting behavior induced by dopaminergic drugs in 6-hydroxydopamine rats and monkeys with a unilateral lesion in the ventral medial tegmentum can be blocked by a selective $D_1$ antagonist SCH 23390 suggests that self-injurious behavior is mediated primarily by the $D_1$ receptors (Schroeder et al., 2001). Selective dopamine receptor agonists and antagonists have been used in experimental models to study different effects of $D_1$ and $D_2$ receptors on stereotypic behavior. SKF 38393, a $D_1$ agonist, produced no stereotypic behavior in normal rats, but it did enhance stereotypy induced by apomorphine, a mixed $D_1$ and $D_2$ agonist (Koller and Herbster, 1988). This suggests that the $D_2$ dopamine receptors mediate stereotypic behavior and that activation of the $D_1$ receptors potentiates these $D_2$-mediated effects. Additional evidence for the role of $D_2$ dopamine receptors in the pathogenesis of stereotypies is the observation that upregulation of $D_2$ receptors (e.g., with haloperidol, a selective $D_2$ antagonist) but not of $D_1$ receptors (e.g., with SCH 23390, a selective $D_1$ antagonist), enhanced apomorphine-induced stereotypies (Chipkin et al., 1987). Drug-induced models of

Box 18-1 Etiologic classification of stereotypies

**Physiologic**
Normal child development
Stress-related
Sensory deprivation, including restraining, blindness, deafness

**Pathologic**
Mental retardation
Autism (including Kanner syndrome, infantile autism, Asperger syndrome)
Rett syndrome
Neuroacanthocytosis
Schizophrenia
Catatonia
Obsessive-compulsive disorder (OCD)
Tourette syndrome (TS)
Tardive and other dyskinesias
Akathisia
Restless legs syndrome
Frontotemporal dementia
Epileptic automatism
Psychogenic

stereotypy, however, might not accurately reflect spontaneous or disease-related repetitive behaviors. Using several selective dopaminergic agonists (apomorphine, SKF81297, and quinpirole) as well as intrastriatal administration of the D2 receptor antagonist raclopride to study stereotypic behaviors in the deer mouse model of spontaneous and persistent stereotypy showed that spontaneously emitted and drug-induced stereotypies may have different mechanisms (Presti et al., 2004). Nevertheless, these studies suggest that the striatal dopaminergic system is significantly involved in stereotypic behaviors. Oral and forelimb stereotypies can be induced in the rat with injections of amphetamine into the ventrolateral striatum (Canales et al., 2000)), and certain genes can be activated in the striasomes with these drugs when they are administered orally (Canales and Graybiel, 2000). These studies provide further support for a basal ganglia involvement in stereotypies. Although there is experimental evidence from rodent and primate studies to support the notion that differential activation of striosomes in the basal ganglia plays an important role in pathophysiology of stereotypies (Saka and Graybiel, 2003), some recent studies found that motor stereotypies do not require enhanced activation of striosomes (Glickstein and Schmauss, 2004). In addition to the basal ganglia, the pontine tegmentum has been implicated in certain stereotypies, particularly repetitive involuntary leg movements that are somewhat similar to the leg movement in patients with restless legs syndrome (Lee et al., 2005).

Besides the classic neurotransmitters, evidence is accumulating in support of involvement of neuropeptides as modulators of stereotypic behavior. For example, microinjection of cholecystokinin and neurotensin into the medial nucleus accumbens markedly potentiated apomorphine-induced stereotypy (Blumstein et al., 1987). Since injection of these peptides into the striatum had no effect on the apomorphine-induced stereotypy, these studies provide additional evidence for the involvement of the limbic system in the pathogenesis

of this movement disorder. Improvement in self-injurious behavior observed in autistic children after administration of the opiate blockers naloxone and naltrexone has been interpreted as evidence for the role of endogenous opiates (e.g., β-endorphins) in this abnormal behavior (Sandman, 1988). Additional support for the role of endorphins in self-injurious and stereotypic behavior is the finding of elevated plasma and cerebrospinal fluid levels of β-endorphins in autistic patients with these behavioral abnormalities (Sandman, 1988). More recently, the emphasis has shifted to the serotonin system, supported by the observation that certain animal behaviors improve with serotonin uptake inhibitors (Hugo et al., 2003).

## PHYSIOLOGIC STEREOTYPIES

Certain stereotypies, such as tapping of the feet, adduction-abduction, and crossing-uncrossing and other repetitive movements of the legs, may be part of a repertoire of movements seen in otherwise normal individuals. In infants and children, there seems to be a progression of normal stereotypies (Castellanos et al., 1996). For example, thumb sucking and hand sucking in infancy are later replaced by body rocking, head rolling, and head banging. Some infants demonstrate head stereotypies that resemble bobble-head doll syndrome, sometimes associated with ataxia but without any other neurologic deficit and normal subsequent development (Hottinger-Blanc et al., 2002). A review of 40 "normal" children, aged 9 months to 17 years, with complex hand and arm stereotypies, such as flapping, shaking, clenching, posturing, and other "ritual" movements, showed that the movements can be temporarily suppressed in nearly all when cued (Mahone et al., 2004). Although the children were classified as "normal," 25% had comorbid attention deficit-hyperactivity disorder, and 20% had learning disability, probably due to referral bias, since this group is also known for their work in TS. This was supported by a relatively high family history of sterereotypies (25%) and tics (33%). A variety of stereotypies can be observed in children (Castellanos et al., 1996; Tan et al., 1997) and young adults (Niehaus et al., 2000) without any other neurologic deficits. Otherwise normal children have been observed with persistent head stereotypies similar to the bobble-head syndrome but without abnormal neuroimaging studies. Stereotypies may also occur during development of otherwise normal children who are congenitally blind (Troster et al., 1991) or deaf (Bachara and Phelan, 1980). Patients with Williams syndrome, a hypersociable behavior associated with hemizygous deletion in chromosome band 7q11.23, including the gene for elastin, also can present with slow, complex, persistent head stereotypies (Doyle et al., 2004; Meyer-Lindenberg et al., 2006) (Video 18-3). Head banging is seen in up to 15% of normal children (Sallustro and Atwell, 1978). Some girls exhibit stereotypic crossing and extending of legs, which actually represents a self-gratifying or masturbatory behavior (Mink and Neil, 1995) (Video 18-4). Otherwise normal children can also develop bruxism, nail biting, trichotillomania, and other stereotypic behaviors. These behaviors have been often attributed to underlying generalized anxiety disorder or OCD. However, when stereotypy is accompanied by other behavioral and neurologic findings, it usually indicates the presence of a serious underlying neurologic and/or psychiatric disorder (see Box 18-1).

## MENTAL RETARDATION

It is beyond the scope of this chapter to review the current notions about the clinical features and pathogenesis of mental retardation, but the reader is referred to a review of this topic (Nokelainen and Flint, 2002). In one study of 102 institutionalized mentally retarded people, with a mean age of 35 years (range: 21 to 68 years), 34% exhibited at least one type of stereotypy (rhythmic movement, 26%; bizarre posturing, 13%; object manipulation, 7%; and others) (Dura et al., 1987). In another study, 100 individuals with severe or profound intellectual disability were randomly selected and followed for 26 years (Thompson and Reid, 2002). Their behavior was recorded through career and psychiatrist ratings using the Modified Manifest Abnormality Scale of the Clinical Interview Schedule. The follow-up evaluations found that stereotypies, emotional abnormalities, eye avoidance, and other behavioral symptoms persist. Although there seems to be an inverse correlation between stereotypies and IQ, stereotypic behavior may be seen even in the mildly retarded. In some mental retardation disorders, typically Lesch-Nyhan syndrome, stereotypies are associated with self-injurious behavior (Videos 18-5 and 18-6). Supersensitivity of $D_1$ receptors, possibly in response to abnormal arborization of dopamine neurons in the striatum, has been postulated as a possible mechanism of self-injurious behavior in Lesch-Nyhan syndrome (Jankovic et al., 1988).

## AUTISM

Autism is a type of pervasive developmental disorder (PDD), sometimes referred to as autistic spectrum disorders, with onset during infancy or childhood, characterized by impairment in reciprocal social and interpersonal interactions, impairment in verbal and nonverbal communication, markedly restricted repertoire of activities and interests, and stereotyped movements (Bodfish et al., 2001; Gritti et al., 2003). Earlier studies have suggested that about 0.1% of all children are autistic (Sugiyama and Abe, 1989); however, more recent epidemiologic studies have estimated the prevalence of autistic disorders and related pervasive developmental disorders to range between 0.3% (Yeargin-Allsopp et al., 2003) and 0.6% (Chakrabarti and Fombonne, 2001). In children and adults with autism of any cause, stereotypies and other self-stimulatory activities constitute the most recognizable symptoms. Typical stereotypies that are seen in autistic individuals include facial grimacing, staring at flickering light, waving objects in front of the eyes, producing repetitive sounds, arm flapping, rhythmic body rocking, repetitive touching, feeling and smelling objects, jumping, walking on toes, and unusual hand and body postures. The motor manifestations are often associated with insensitivity or excessive sensitivity to sensory stimuli including pain and extremes of temperature, preoccupations with perceptual sensations such as lights or odors, insistence on preservation of sameness, and absence of fear or other emotional reactions. Self-stimulatory and self-injurious behaviors, such as self-biting and head banging, are also common. In addition to these and other behavioral and developmental abnormalities, some autistic individuals have isolated areas of remarkable and sometimes spectacular mental skills, the so-called savant syndrome (Miller, 1999; Treffert, 1999).

There are many causes of autism, including fragile X syndrome and a variety of eponymically classified types such as Kanner, Heller, Asperger, Down, and Rett syndromes (Ringman and Jankovic, 2000). Asperger syndrome is one of the most common forms of autism, found in 1 to 3 children in 1000 (Gillberg, 1989). Characterized by social isolation in combination with odd and eccentric behavior, Asperger syndrome shares many features with infantile autism. Several studies have indeed noted an overlap in various clinical and demographic characteristics between Asperger syndrome and infantile autism (Szatmari et al., 1989). In one study of 23 patients, the children with Asperger syndrome seemed to have relatively poor motor skills and had a stiff and awkward gait (without armswing), and their speech development was delayed, although they acquired better expressive speech than did the children with infantile autism. In contrast to infantile autism, Asperger syndrome usually does not become fully manifest until 30 to 36 months of age, but some children may have their first symptoms in infancy. A study of seven patients with the combination of Asperger syndrome and TS showed magnetic resonance imagine (MRI) evidence of cortical and subcortical abnormalities in five of these patients (Berther et al., 1993). Because children with Asperger syndrome are generally brighter than those with TS, it has been suggested that Asperger syndrome merely represents a mild variant of autism. Ringman and Jankovic (2000) studied eight patients with Asperger syndrome and an additional four with other forms of pervasive developmental disorder who were referred to their movement disorders clinic for evaluation of tics. All patients exhibited stereotypic movements; in addition, seven had tics, and six of these met inclusion diagnostic criteria for TS. Of the six patients with clinical features of both Asperger syndrome and TS, three had severe congenital sensory deficits, suggesting that sensory deprivation contributes to the development of adventitious movements in this population. Other autistic children also show features of TS (Rapin, 2001)

In patients with mental retardation and autism, irrespective of etiology, stereotypies are often associated with self-injurious behavior. This is particularly true for patients with body-rocking movements, a stereotypy that is most often associated with self-hitting (Rojahn, 1986). While head banging and other self-injurious behavior may occur in normal children, this type of behavior is usually abnormal and is particularly common in patients who also exhibit stereotypic behavior.

Some studies in autistic children reported that stereotypy interfered with learning, suggesting that treatment of stereotypies in patients with autism facilitates learning (Koegel and Covert, 1972) and implied that controlling stereotypic behavior was a necessary precondition for learning. Drugs that block postsynaptic dopamine and serotonin receptors, such as risperidone, have been found to be effective in the treatment of tantrums, aggression, and self-injurious behaviors in patients with autistic disorders (Research Units on Pediatric Psychopharmacology Autism Network, 2002; Gagliano et al., 2004). These benefits, however, must be weighed against potential side effects, such as sedation, weight gain, and parkinsonism. Other agents that are used in the treatment of autistic disorders include central nervous system stimulants, anticonvulsants, naltrexone, lithium, anxiolytics, and other treatments, but well-controlled, double-blind studies are lacking (Owley, 2002). The pathogenesis of autism is still unknown; one hypothesis suggests that in autistic children, the normal high brain serotonin synthesis capacity is somehow disrupted during early development (Chugani and Chugani, 2000), which might explain the beneficial effects of selective serotonin uptake inhibitors in some patients with autism (DeLong, 1999).

## NEUROIMAGING AND NEUROPATHOLOGIC STUDIES IN AUTISM

Dysfunction of the frontal-parietal cortex, neostriatum, thalamus, and cerebellum in autistic patients has been suggested by various cerebral metabolic and imaging studies. MRI studies have found left frontal and brainstem atrophy in some autistic patients (Hashimoto et al., 1989), but other studies have failed to find any characteristic abnormalities on MRI scans of autistic children (Kleiman et al., 1992). More recent MRI studies have found white matter enlargement in patients with autism (Herbert et al., 2004). Other imaging studies have shown that autistic children have a reversal of asymmetry in frontal language-related cortex (De Fosse et al., 2004). Neuropathologic studies have not found consistent abnormalities, but most have found increased cell density and smaller neuronal size in the limbic system, decreased number of Purkinje cells in the cerebellum, and cerebellar cortical dysgenesis, but additional studies utilizing new techniques are needed before a consistent picture will emerge (Palmen et al., 2004).

## Rett Syndrome

Although the genes for most autistic disorders have yet to be identified, many researchers investigating the cause of autism believe that most of the "idiopathic" forms of autism are genetic in origin (Muhle et al., 2004). Rett syndrome is an autistic disorder that occurs almost exclusively in girls and is manifested clinically by stereotypic movements and other movement disorders (Fitzgerald et al., 1990a; Percy, 2002) (Videos 18-7 and 18-8).  The prevalence has been reported to range between 1 in 10,000 and 1 in 28,000 (Kozinetz et al., 1993). In contrast to infantile autism and mental retardation, patients with Rett syndrome tend to have normal development until 6 to 18 months of age; this is then followed by gradual regression of both motor and language skills. Usually between the ages of 9 months and 3 years, there is a gradual social withdrawal and psychomotor regression with loss of acquired communication skills. Acquired finger and hand skills are gradually replaced by stereotypic hand movements, including hand clapping, wringing, clenching, washing, patting, rubbing, picking, and mouthing (Fig. 18-1).

Additionally, girls with Rett syndrome often exhibit body-rocking movements and shifting of weight from one leg to the other. Although most girls with Rett syndrome are able to walk, they tend to walk on their toes; their gait is usually broad-based and apraxic and associated with retropulsion and loss of balance. Other motor disturbances include respiratory dysregulation with episodic hyperventilation and breath holding, bruxism, ocular deviations, dystonia, myoclonus, athetosis, tremor, jerky truncal and gait ataxia, and parkinsonian findings. A study of 32 patients with Rett syndrome, ages 30 months to 28 years, suggested that the occurrence of the different motor disorders seemed to be age-related (Fitzgerald et al., 1990b). The hyperkinetic disorders were more common in younger girls, while bradykinetic disorders seemed more prominent in the older patients.

The pathophysiologic basis of the motor disturbances in Rett syndrome has not been fully elucidated (Akbarian 2003).

**Figure 18-1** A collage of hand and mouthing stereotypies exhibited by girls with Rett syndrome. (See Color Plate 14.)

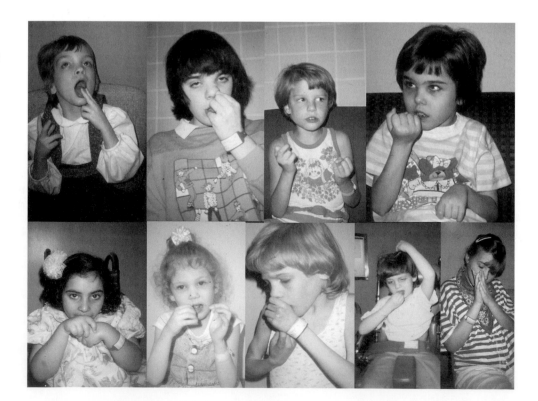

MRI studies have shown generalized brain and bilateral caudate atrophy (Reiss et al., 1993). Electroencephalographic recordings show age-related progressive deterioration characterized by slowing, loss of normal sleep characteristics, and the appearance of epileptiform activity. In a few postmortem examinations of brains of people with Rett syndrome, besides marked reduction in both gray and white matter volume, particularly involving the caudate nucleus (Subramaniam et al., 1997), some studies also found spongy degeneration of cerebral and cerebellar white matter, deposition of lipofuscin, and depigmentation of the substantia nigra and locus coeruleus (Hagberg, 1989). The various neuropathologic findings have been interpreted as a failure in the proper development or maintenance of synaptic connections. Since there is no evidence of a neurodegenerative process, there is a possibility of a therapeutic intervention that might not only alter the symptoms but also favorably modify the natural course of the disease.

The major advance in understanding the biology of Rett syndrome has come with the discovery of a gene that is responsible for most, but not all, cases of Rett phenotype. Since the initial discovery of the gene in 1999 (Amir et al., 1999), loss-of-function mutations of the X-linked gene encoding methyl-CpG binding protein 2 (MECP2) have been found to be responsible for more than 80% of Rett cases (Akbarian, 2003). The phenotypic spectrum of *MECP2* mutations is broadening, and it includes not only the classic Rett syndrome but also Rett variants, mentally retarded males, and autistic children (Neul and Zoghbi, 2004). The function of the MECP2 protein is still unknown, but it is expressed ubiquitously in neurons and binds primarily, but not exclusively, to methylated DNA; it is thought to regulate gene expression, chromatin composition, and chromosomal architecture and might be important for maintenance of neuronal chromatin during late development and in adulthood. The MECP2 protein is expressed exclusively in neurons at the time when they are starting to form synapses. In the cerebellum, the Purkinje cells, which are born early, strongly express MECP2 soon after birth, but granule cells, which mature later, do not express the protein until several weeks after birth (Fig. 18-2). Thus, the protein is not turned on until it is needed for the formation of synapses. Furthermore, selective knockout of the gene in mice results in a Rett-like phenotype, including a reduction in brain atrophy and neuronal dystrophy. Rett syndrome appears to be a disorder of synapse formation and proliferation.

A broad range of mutations associated with MECP2 have been described involving not only girls and women but also males; they include a variety of autistic spectrum disorders, such as Angelman syndrome, learning disability, mental retardation, and fatal encephalopathy (Percy, 2002). Although stereotypies are sometimes present in patients with TS, Rosa and colleagues (2003) excluded mutations in the *MECP2* gene in their population of patients with TS. There is no known treatment for Rett syndrome, but tamoxifen appeared to reverse or prevent these symptoms in a transgenic mouse model (Guy et al., 2007).

## Schizophrenia and Catatonia

Various stereotypies were described in schizophrenic patients long before neuroleptics were first introduced for the treatment of psychotic disorders. Since stereotypies in untreated childhood schizophrenia have not been well studied, the discussion of this topic is beyond the scope of this review (Ihara et al., 2002).

## Obsessive-Compulsive Disorder and Tic Disorders

Stereotypies can be encountered in various tic disorders, including TS and neuroacanthocytosis, both of which can also be associated with OCD. TS is discussed elsewhere in this volume (see Chapter 17); therefore, only a brief discussion of other tic disorders and OCD follows. Also, the reader is referred to recent reviews on this topic (Jankovic, 2001a, 2001b; Jenike, 2004).

Progression from a hyperkinetic to a bradykinetic movement disorder, as seen in Rett syndrome, may also be encountered in neuroacanthocytosis, another disorder that is manifested by stereotypic and self-injurious (e.g., lip and tongue biting) behavior. Symptoms usually first begin in the third and fourth decades but may start during childhood, with lip and tongue biting followed by orolingual ("eating")

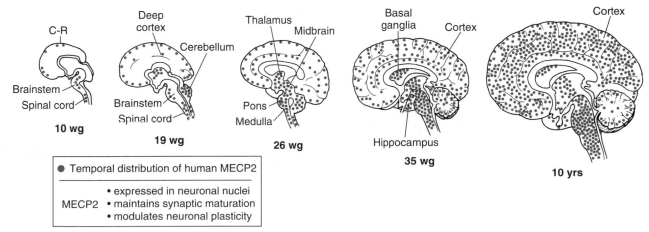

C-R = Cajal-Retzius cortical neurons

**Figure 18-2** During human development, MECP2 is initially expressed in the spinal cord, followed by the midbrain, thalamus, cerebellum, deep cortical neurons, basal ganglia, hypothalamus, hippocampus, and superficial cortical layers. (Reprinted with permission from Zoghbi HY: Postnatal neurodevelopmental disorders: Meeting at the synapse? Science 2003;302:826–830.)

dystonia, motor and phonic tics, generalized chorea, distal and body stereotypies, parkinsonism, vertical ophthalmoparesis, and seizures. Other features include cognitive and personality changes, dysphagia, dysarthria, amyotrophy, areflexia, evidence of axonal neuropathy, and elevated serum creatine kinase without evidence of myopathy. Besides movement disorders, other associated features included dysarthria; absent or reduced reflexes; dementia; psychiatric problems, such as depression, anxiety, and OCD; dysphagia; seizures; muscle weakness and wasting; and elevated creatine phosphokinase. Magnetic resonance volumetry and fluorodeoxyglucose PET show striatal atrophy in patients with neuroacanthocytosis (Jung et al., 2001).

Although autosomal-dominant, X-linked-recessive, and sporadic forms of neuroacanthocytosis have been reported, the majority of the reported families indicate autosomal-recessive inheritance. Genomewide scan for linkage in 11 families with autosomal-recessive inheritance showed a linkage to a marker on chromosome 9q21, indicating a single locus for the disease. Sequencing has identified a polyadenylation site with a protein with 3096 amino acid residues, which has been named Chorein, and subsequent studies have identified multiple mutations in the *CHAC* gene (Rampoldi et al., 2001).

Another psychiatric disorder that is frequently accompanied be stereotypic movements is OCD (Jenike, 2004). Foot tapping, crossing and uncrossing the legs, tapping fingers on a chair arm, and similar stereotypic behaviors may be associated with obsessive-compulsive symptoms (Niehaus et al., 2000). OCD was once considered a rare psychiatric disorder, but recent epidemiologic studies indicate that the lifetime prevalence of OCD is approximately 2.5% (Snider and Swedo, 2000). Compulsions might be difficult to differentiate from stereotypies. In contrast to stereotypies, compulsions are usually preceded by or associated with feelings of inner tension or anxiety and a need to perform the same act repeatedly in the same manner. Examples of compulsions are ritualistic hand washing; repetitively touching the same place; evening up; and arranging and checking doors, locks, and appliances. Reports of focal striatal lesions giving rise to severe OCD and the frequent association of OCD with basal ganglia disorders such as TS, Parkinson disease, and Sydenham disease (Church et al., 2002; Kwak and Jankovic, 2002) provide additional support for the link between abnormal behavior, such as OCD, and extrapyramidal dysfunction (Cummings, 1993; Rosario-Campos et al., 2001).

## Tardive Dyskinesia

Repetitive and patterned movements, phenomenologically identical to stereotypy, are characteristically seen in patients with tardive dyskinesia (Jankovic, 1995). All types of movement disorders, including parkinsonism, tremor, chorea, dystonia, tics, myoclonus, and stereotypy, can result from the use of dopamine receptor–blocking drugs (neuroleptics) both acutely and chronically (tardive). See Chapter 20 in this volume for a detailed review. The most typical form of tardive dyskinesia, the orofacial-lingual-masticatory movement, is one of the best examples of a stereotypic movement disorder (Miller and Jankovic, 1990). Tardive dystonia tends to occur more frequently in younger patients, although it is quite rare in children. Tardive stereotypy is more typically observed in

middle-aged or elderly patients, particularly women, and this is a very rare complication in children. However, there is a report of a 1-year-old girl who developed orofacial-lingual stereotypy at age 2 months after a 17-day treatment with metoclopramide for gastroesophageal reflux (Mejia and Jankovic, 2005). The stereotypy, documented by sequential videos, persisted for at least 9 months after the drug was discontinued. This patient, perhaps the first documented case of tardive dyskinesia in an infant, draws attention to the possibility that this disorder is frequently unrecognized in young children.

Akathisia—a combination of complex stereotypies, such as hair and face rubbing, picking at clothes, crossing and uncrossing legs, adduction-abduction and up-and-down leg pumping, sitting down and standing up, marching in place, pacing and shifting weight, and feelings of restlessness—is typically a manifestation of tardive dyskinesia but may also be seen in patients with Parkinson disease, in patients with various forms of mental retardation and autism (Bodfish et al., 1997), and as part of tardive dyskinesia (Video 18-9). In some  individuals, particularly those who abuse amphetamines or cocaine and patients with Parkinson disease taking levodopa, certain stereotypic behaviors, called punding are seen (Fernandez and Friedman, 1999; Evans et al., 2004; Voon, 2004). These include compulsive sorting of objects, nail polishing, shoe shining, hair dressing, and intense fascination with repetitive handling and examining of mechanical objects, such as picking at oneself or taking apart watches and radios, or sorting and arranging of common objects, such as lining up pebbles, rocks, or other small objects. This stereotypic behavior has not been previously described in children, even in those taking central nervous system stimulants for attention deficit-hyperactivity disorder, although no studies specifically designed to study punding in children have been reported.

With the advent of atypical neuroleptics, the incidence of tardive dyskinesia may be decreasing, but its frequency in children has not been well studied. Campbell and colleagues (1997), in their 15-year-long prospective double blind, placebo-controlled study of autistic children exposed to haloperidol reported that tardive dyskinesia developed in 9 of 118 children (7.6%). An analysis of five studies of tardive dyskinesia involving 392 children, ages 2.3 to 18 years, with multiple psychiatric diagnoses, autism, and mental retardation was carried out (Mejia and Jankovic, 2007). Tardive dyskinesia developed in 50 of the 392 (12.7%) patients, but these were not designed as epidemiologic studies; therefore, the true incidence and prevalence of tardive dyskinesia is unknown.

The most important step in the management of tardive dyskinesia is prevention; dopamine receptor–blocking drugs, particularly the typical neuroleptics, should be used only if other drugs do not adequately control the behavior or neurologic disorder, such as TS. Atypical antipsychotics might be better alternative medications with less risk of causing tardive dyskinesia and should be considered whenever possible. Drugs that have been found to be useful in the treatment of tardive dyskinesia include clonazepam and other benzodiazepines and dopamine depletors such as tetrabenazine (Jankovic and Beach, 1997; Vuong et al., 2004; Kenney and Jankovic, 2006). Beta-blockers and opioids have also been found effective in some patients with akathisia.

# References

Akbarian S: The neurobiology of Rett syndrome. Neuroscientist 2003;9:57–63.

Amir RE, Van den Veyver IB, Wan M, et al: Rett syndrome is caused by mutations in X-linked MECP2, encoding methyl-CpG-binding protein 2. Nat Genet 1999;23:185–188.

Bachara GH, Phelan WJ: Rhythmic movement in deaf children. Percept Mot Skills 1980;50(3, pt 1):933–934.

Berther ML, Bayes A, Tolosa ES: Magnetic resonance imaging in patients with concurrent Tourette's disorder and Asperger's syndrome. J Am Acad Child Adolesc Psychiatry 1993;32:633–639.

Blumstein LK, Crawley JN, Davis LG, Baldino F: Neuropeptide modulation of apomorphine-induced stereotyped behavior. Brain Res 1987;404:293–300.

Bodfish JW, Newell KM, Sprague RL, et al: Akathisia in adults with mental retardation: Development of the Akathisia Ratings of Movement Scale (ARMS). Am J Ment Retard 1997;101:413–423.

Bodfish JW, Parker DE, Lewis MH, et al: Stereotypy and motor control: Differences in the postural stability dynamics of persons with stereotyped and dyskinetic movement disorders. Am J Ment Retard 2001;106:123–134.

Campbell M, Armenteros JL, Malone RP, et al: Neuroleptic-related dyskinesias in autistic children: A prospective, longitudinal study. J Am Acad Child Adolesc Psychiatry 1997;36:835–843.

Canales JJ, Gilmour G, Iversen SD: The role of nigral and thalamic output pathways in the expression of oral stereotypies induced by amphetamine injections into the striatum. Brain Res 2000;856:176–183.

Canales JJ, Graybiel AM: A measure of striatal function predicts motor stereotypy. Nat Neurosci 2000;3:377–383.

Castellanos FX, Ritchie GF, Marsh WL, Rapoport JL: DSM-IV stereotypic movement disorder: Persistence of stereotypies of infancy in intellectually normal adolescents and adults. J Clin Psychiatry 1996;57:116–122.

Chakrabarti S, Fombonne E: Pervasive developmental disorders in preschool children. JAMA 2001;285:3093–3099.

Chipkin RE, McQuade RD, Iorio LC: D1 and D2 dopamine binding site up-regulation and apomorphine-induced stereotypy. Pharmacol Biochem Behav 1987;28:477–482.

Chugani DC, Chugani HT: PET: Mapping of serotonin synthesis. Adv Neurol 2000;83:165–171.

Church AJ, Cardoso F, Dale RC, et al: Anti-basal ganglia antibodies in acute and persistent Sydenham's chorea. Neurology 2002;59:227–231.

Cummings JL: Frontal sub-cortical circuits and human behaviour. Arch Neurol 1993;50:873–880.

De Fosse L, Hodge SM, Makris N, et al: Language-association cortex asymmetry in autism and specific language impairment. Ann Neurol 2004;56:757–766.

DeLong RG: Autism: New data suggest a new hypothesis. Neurology 1999;52:911–916.

Doyle TF, Bellugi U, Korenberg JR, Graham J: "Everybody in the world is my friend": Hypersociability in young children with Williams syndrome. Am J Med Genet 2004;124A:263–273.

Dura JR, Mulick JA, Rasnake LK: Prevalence of stereotypy among institutionalized nonambulatory profoundly mentally retarded people. Am J Ment Defic 1987;91:548–549.

Evans AH, Katzenschlager R, Paviour D, et al: Punding in Parkinson's disease: Its relation to the dopamine dysregulation syndrome. Mov Disord 2004;19:397–405.

Fernandez HH, Friedman JH: Punding on l-dopa. Mov Disord 1999;14:836–838.

Fitzgerald PM, Jankovic J, Glaze DG, et al: Extrapyramidal involvement in Rett's syndrome. Neurology 1990a;40:293–295.

Fitzgerald PM, Jankovic J, Percy AK: Rett syndrome and associated movement disorders. Mov Disord 1990b;5:195–203.

Gagliano A, Germano E, Pustorino G, et al: Risperidone treatment of children with autistic disorder: Effectiveness, tolerability, and pharmacokinetic implications. J Child Adolesc Psychopharmacol 2004;14:39–47.

Garner JP, Meehan CL, Mench JA: Stereotypies in caged parrots, schizophrenia and autism: Evidence for a common mechanism. Behav Brain Res 2003;145:125–134.

Gillberg C: The borderland of autism and Rett syndrome: Five case histories to highlight diagnostic difficulties. J Autism Dev Disord 1989;19:545–559.

Glickstein SB, Schmauss C: Focused motor stereotypies do not require enhanced activation of neurons in striosomes. J Comp Neurol 2004;469:227–238.

Gritti A, Bove D, Di Sarno AM, et al: Stereotyped movements in a group of autistic children. Funct Neurol 2003;18:89–94.

Guy J, Gian J, Selfridge J, Bird A: Reversal of neurological defects in a mouse model of Rett syndrome. Science 2007 (in press).

Hagberg BA: Rett syndrome: Clinical peculiarities, diagnostic approach, and possible cause. Pediatr Neurol 1989;5:75–83.

Hashimoto T, Tayama M, Mori F, et al: Magnetic resonance imaging in autism: Preliminary report. Neuropediatrics 1989;20:142–146.

Herbert MR, Ziegler DA, Makris N, et al: Localization of white matter volume increase in autism and developmental language disorder. Ann Neurol 2004;55:530–540.

Hottinger-Blanc PM, Ziegler AL, Deonna T: A special type of head stereotypies in children with developmental (?cerebellar) disorder: Description of 8 cases and literature review. Eur J Paediatr Neurol 2002;6:143–152.

Hugo C, Seier J, Mdhluli C, et al: Fluoxetine decreases stereotypic behavior in primates. Prog Neuropsychopharmacol Biol Psychiatry 2003;27:639–643.

Ihara M, Kohara N, Urano F, et al: Neuroleptic malignant syndrome with prolonged catatonia in a dopa-responsive dystonia patient. Neurology 2002;59:1102–1104.

Jankovic J, Armstrong D, Low NL, Goetz CG: What is it? Case 2: Congenital mental retardation and juvenile parkinsonism. Mov Disord 1988;3:352–335.

Jankovic J: Stereotypies. In Marsden CD, Fahn S (eds): Movement Disorders, 3rd ed. London, Butterworth Heinemann, 1994, pp 503–517.

Jankovic J: Tardive syndromes and other drug-induced movement disorders. Clin Neuropharmacol 1995;18:197–214.

Jankovic J: Differential diagnosis and etiology of tics. In Cohen DJ, Jankovic J, Goetz CG (eds): Tourette Syndrome. Advances in Neurology, vol 85. Philadelphia, Lippincott Williams & Wilkins, 2001a, pp 15–29.

Jankovic J: Tourette's syndrome. N Engl J Med 2001b;345:1184–1192.

Jankovic J: Tics and stereotypies. In Freund HJ, Jeannerod M, Hallett M, Leiguarda R (eds): Higher-Order Motor Disorders. Oxford, England, Oxford University Press, 2005, pp 383–396.

Jankovic J, Beach J: Long-term effects of tetrabenazine in hyperkinetic movement disorders. Neurology 1997;48:358–362.

Jankovic J, Caskey TC, Stout JT, Butler I: Lesch-Nyhan syndrome: A study of motor behavior and CSF monoamine turnover. Ann Neurol 1988;23:466–469.

Jankovic J, Sekula SL, Milas D: Dermatological manifestations of Tourette's syndrome and obsessive-compulsive disorder. Arch Dermatol 1998;134:113–114.

Jenike MA: Obsessive-compulsive disorder. N Engl J Med 2004;350:259–265.

Jung HH, Hergerberg M, Kneifel S, et al: McLeod syndrome: A novel mutation, predominant psychiatric manifestations, and distinct striatal imaging findings. Ann Neurol 2001;49:384–392.

Kenney C, Jankovic J: Tetrabenazine in the treatment of hyperkinetic movement disorders. Expert Rev Neurotherapeutics 2006;6:7–17.

Kleiman MD, Neff S, Rosman NP: The brain in infantile autism: Are posterior fossa structures abnormal? Neurology 1992;42:753–760.

Koegel RL, Covert A: The relationship of self-stimulation to learning in autistic children. J Appl Behav Anal 1972:5:381–387.

Koller WC, Herbster G: D1 and D2 dopamine receptor mechanisms in dopaminergic behaviors. Clin Neuropharmacol 1988;11:221–231.

Kozinetz CA, Skender ML, MacNaughton N, et al: Epidemiology of Rett syndrome: A population-based registry. Pediatrics 1993; 91:445–450.

Kwak C, Jankovic J: Tourettism and dystonia after subcortical stroke. Mov Disord 2002;17:821–825.

Lee PH, Lee JS, Yong SW, Huh K: Repetitive involuntary leg movements in patients with brainstem lesions involving the pontine tegmentum: Evidence for a pontine inhibitory region in humans. Parkinsonism Relat Disord 2005;11:105–110.

Low M: Stereotypies and behavioural medicine: Confusions in current thinking. Aust Vet J 2003;81:192–198.

Lutz C, Well A, Novak M: Stereotypic and self-injurious behavior in rhesus macaques: A survey and retrospective analysis of environment and early experience. Am J Primatol 2003;60:1–15.

Mahone EM, Bridges D, Prahme C, Singer HS: Repetitive arm and hand movements (complex motor stereotypies) in children. J Pediatr 2004;145:391–395.

Mejia N, Jankovic J: Metoclopramide-induced tardive dyskinesia in an infant. Mov Disord 2005;20:86–89.

Mejia N, Jankovic J: Tardive dyskinesia and withdrawal emergent in children. Arch Dis Child 2007 (in press).

Meyer-Lindenberg A, Mervis CB, Berman KF: Neural mechanisms in Williams syndrome: A unique window to genetic influences on cognition and behaviour. Nat Neurosci 2006;7:380–391.

Miller LG, Jankovic J: Neurological approach to drug-induced movement disorders: A study of 125 patients. South Med J 1990;83:525–535.

Miller LK: The savant syndrome: Intellectual impairment and exceptional skill. Psychol Bull 1999;125:31–46.

Mink JW, Neil JJ: Masturbation mimicking paroxysmal dystonia or dyskinesia in a young girl. Mov Disord 1995;10:518–520.

Muhle R, Trentacoste SV, Rapin I: The genetics of autism. Pediatrics 2004;113:472–486.

Neul JL, Zoghbi HY: Rett syndrome: A prototypical neurodevelopmental disorder. Neuroscientist 2004;10:118–128.

Niehaus DJ, Emsley RA, Brink P, Stein DJ: Stereotypies: Prevalence and association with compulsive and impulsive symptoms in college students. Psychopathology 2000;33:31–35.

Nokelainen P, Flint J: Genetic effects on human cognition: Lessons from the study of mental retardation syndrome. J Neurol Neurosurg Psychiatry 2002;72:287–296.

Novak MA: Self-injurious behavior in rhesus monkeys: New insights into its etiology, physiology, and treatment. Am J Primatol 2003; 59:3–19.

Nyatsanza S, Shetty T, Gregory C, et al: A study of stereotypic behaviours in Alzheimer's disease and frontal and temporal variant frontotemporal dementia. J Neurol Neurosurg Psychiatry 2003;74:1398–1402.

Owley T: The pharmacological treatment of autistic spectrum disorders. CNS Spectr 2002;7:663–669.

Palmen SJ, van Engeland H, Hof PR, Schmitz C: Neuropathological findings in autism. Brain 2004;127(pt 12):2572–2583.

Percy AK: Rett syndrome: Current status and new vistas. Neurol Clin N Am 2002;20:1125–1141.

Presti MF, Gibney BC, Lewis MH: Effects of intrastriatal administration of selective dopaminergic ligands on spontaneous stereotypy in mice. Physiol Behav 2004;80:433–439.

Rampoldi L, Dobson-Stone C, Rubio JP, et al: A conserved sorting-associated protein is mutant in chorea-acanthocytosis. Nat Genet 2001;28:119–120.

Rapin I: Autism spectrum disorders: Relevance to Tourette syndrome. Adv Neurol 2001;85:89–101.

Reiss AL, Faruque F, Naidu S, et al: Neuroanatomy of Rett syndrome: A volumetric imaging study. Ann Neurol 1993;34:227–237.

Research Units on Pediatric Psychopharmacology Autism Network: Risperidone in children with autism and serious behavioral problems. N Engl J Med 2002;347:314–321.

Ringman JM, Jankovic J: Occurrence of tics in Asperger's syndrome and autistic disorder. J Child Neurol 2000;15:394–400.

Rojahn J: Self-injurious and stereotypic behavior of noninstitutionalized mentally retarded people: Prevalence and classification. Am J Ment Defic 1986;91:268–276.

Rosa AL, Jankovic J, Ashizawa T: Screening for mutations in the MECP2 (Rett syndrome) gene in Gilles de la Tourette syndrome. Arch Neurol 2003;60:502–503.

Rosario-Campos MC, Leckman JF, Mercadante MT, et al: Adults with early-onset obsessive-compulsive disorder. Am J Psychiatry 2001;158:1899–1903.

Saka E, Graybiel AM: Pathophysiology of Tourette's syndrome: Striatal pathways revisited. Brain Dev 2003;25(suppl 1):S15–S19.

Sallustro A, Atwell CW: Body rocking, head banging, and head rolling in normal children. J Pediatr 1978;93:704–708.

Sandman CA: β-Endorphin disregulation in autistic and self-injurious behavior: A neurodevelopmental hypothesis. Synapse 1988; 2:193–199.

Sato S, Hashimoto T, Nakamura A, Ikeda S: Stereotyped stepping associated with lesions in the bilateral medial frontoparietal cortices. Neurology 2001;51:711–713.

Schroeder SR, Oster-Granite ML, Berkson G, et al: Self-injurious behavior: Gene-brain-behavior relationships. Ment Retard Dev Disabil Res Rev 2001;7:3–12.

Snider LA, Swedo SE: Pediatric obsessive-compulsive disorder. JAMA 2000;284:3104–3106.

Subramaniam B, Naidu S, Reiss AL: Neuroanatomy in Rett syndrome: Cerebral cortex and posterior fossa. Neurology 1997;2:399–407.

Sugiyama T, Abe T: The prevalence of autism in Nagoya, Japan: A total population study. J Autism Dev Dis 1989;19:87–96.

Szatmari P, Bremner R, Nagy J: Asperger syndrome: A review of clinical features. Can J Psychiatry 1989;34:554–560.

Tan A, Salgado M, Fahn S: The characterization and outcome of stereotypical movements in nonautistic children. Mov Disord 1997;12:47–52.

Thompson CL, Reid A: Behavioural symptoms among people with severe and profound intellectual disabilities: A 26-year follow-up study. Br J Psychiatry 2002;181:67–71.

Treffert DA: The Savant syndrome and autistic disorder. CNS Spectr 1999;4:57–60.

Troster H, Brambring M, Beelmann A: Prevalence and situational causes of stereotyped behaviors in blind infants and preschoolers. J Abnorm Child Psychol 1991;19:569–590.

Voon V: Repetition, repetition, and repetition: Compulsive and punding behaviors in Parkinson's disease. Mov Disord 2004; 19:367–370.

Vuong K, Hunter C, Mejia N, Jankovic J: Safety and efficacy of tetrabenazine in childhood hyperkinetic movement disorders. Mov Disord 2004;19(suppl 9):S422.

Yeargin-Allsopp M, Rice C, Karapurkar T, et al: Prevalence of autism in a US metropolitan area. JAMA 2003;289:49–55.

# Chapter 19

# Tremors
## Diagnosis and Treatment

## CLASSIFICATION

Tremor is a rhythmic, oscillatory movement produced by alternating or synchronous contractions of antagonist muscles. It is the most common form of involuntary movement, but only a small fraction of those who shake seek medical attention. Indeed, in one epidemiologic study of normal controls, 96% were found to have clinically detectable postural tremor, and 28% had a postural tremor of "moderate amplitude" (Louis, Ottman, et al., 1998).

Tremors can be classified according to their phenomenology, distribution, frequency, or etiology (Hallett, 1991; Lou and Jankovic, 1991b; Bain, 1993; Findley, 1993; Deuschl, Bain, et al., 1998; Jankovic, 2000; Deuschl et al., 2001). Phenomenologically, tremors are divided into two major categories: rest tremors and action tremors. Rest tremor is present when the affected body part is fully supported against gravity and not actively contracting; rest tremor is diminished or absent during voluntary muscle contraction and during movement. Action tremors occur with voluntary contraction of muscles, and they can be subdivided into postural, kinetic, task-specific or position-specific, and isometric tremors. Postural tremor is evident during maintenance of an antigravity posture, such as holding the arms in an outstretched horizontal position in front of the body. Some parkinsonian patients exhibit postural tremor that emerges after a latency of a few seconds. This tremor, referred to here as reemergent tremor, probably represents a rest tremor that has been "reset" during posture holding (Jankovic et al., 1999). The relationship of this reemergent tremor to the typical rest tremor is supported by the observation that this reemergent repose tremor shares many characteristics with the typical rest tremor; it has the same 3- to 6-Hz frequency, and it also responds to dopaminergic therapy (Video 19-1). Kinetic tremor can be seen when the voluntary movement starts (initial tremor), during the course of the movement (dynamic tremor), and as the affected body part approaches the target, such as while performing the finger-to-nose or the toe-to-finger maneuver (terminal tremor, also called intention tremor). Task-specific tremors occur only during, or are markedly exacerbated by, a certain task, such as while writing (primary handwriting tremor) (Video 19-2) or while speaking or singing (voice tremor) (Rosenbaum and Jankovic, 1988; Soland et al., 1996b). Besides being sometimes triggered during writing, task-specific tremors may be triggered during other activities, such as while playing golf, particularly when putting (Video 19-3). Position-specific tremors occur while holding a certain posture (e.g., the "wing-beating" position or holding a spoon or a cup close to the mouth). One example of a task- or position-specific tremor is the tremor that occurs in performing the dot test, during which the subject, seated at the desk with elbow elevated to a 90-degree shoulder abduction, is asked to hold the tip of the pen as close to a dot on a horizontal paper as possible without touching the dot. Patients with essential tremor (ET) or other action tremor usually exhibit exacerbation of the tremor during this specific task. A variant of this tremor occurs in performing the modified finger-nose-finger test, during which the subject stands in front of a paper mounted on a wall and is asked to mark the center of the drawn target and to make a mark with a felt-tipped pen five times (Louis, Applegate, et al., 2005). Isometric tremor occurs during a voluntary contraction of muscles that is not accompanied by a change in position of the body part, such as maintaining a tightly squeezed fist or while standing (e.g., orthostatic tremor; see later).

Tremors can also be classified according to their anatomic distribution —for example, head, tongue, voice, and trunk. Because of the complexity of limb tremors, it is best to describe them according to the joint about which the oscillation is most evident—for example, metacarpal-phalangeal joints, wrist, elbow, and ankle tremor. In most tremors, the frequency ranges between 4 and 10 Hz, but the cerebellar tremors may be slower, with a frequency of 2 to 3 Hz. The "slow" tremors (frequency: 1 to 3 Hz) are sometimes referred to as myorhythmia and are usually associated with brainstem pathology (Masucci et al., 1984; Cardoso and Jankovic, 1996). The "fast" tremors (frequency: 11 to 20 Hz) may be distinct tremor disorders, such as orthostatic tremor, or may represent harmonics of other tremors. The clinical characteristics of tremors provide the most important clues to their etiology (Box 19-1).

## ASSESSMENT OF TREMORS

There have been many attempts to quantitate tremor, but it is not apparent whether electromyographic (EMG), accelerometric, or other methods of measuring tremor correlate with clinical rating scales. Indeed, one study suggested that assessments of spirography and handwriting correlate better with overall functional tremor-related disability than do the electrophysiologic methods (Bain et al., 1993). However, because the physiologic measurements and the clinical ratings were not performed simultaneously and because of other technical problems, interpretation of the study is difficult. Elble and colleagues (1996) described the use of a digitizing tablet in quantification of tremor during writing and drawing. Although relatively good intertrial correlations were obtained with this method, the tablet does not capture the speed of writing or the amount of effort exerted by the patient in an attempt to control the tremor while writing. One study found high interobserver reliability using a diagnostic protocol for ET (Louis, Ford, Bismuth, 1998). The investigators also found

Box 19-1 Classification and differential diagnosis of tremors

**A. Rest tremors**
1. Parkinson disease (PD)
2. Other parkinsonian syndromes
   a. Multiple-system atrophies (SND, SDS, OPCA)
   b. Progressive supranuclear palsy
   c. Cortical-basal-ganglionic degeneration
   d. Parkinsonism-dementia-ALS of Guam
   e. Diffuse Lewy body disease
   f. Progressive pallidal atrophy
3. Heredodegenerative disorders
   a. Huntington disease
   b. Wilson disease
   c. Neuroacanthocytosis
   d. Hallervorden-Spatz disease
   e. Gerstmann-Strausler-Scheinker disease
   f. Ceroid lipofuscinosis
4. Secondary parkinsonism
   a. Toxic: MPTP, CO, Mn, methanol, cyanide, $CS_2$
   b. Drug-induced: dopamine receptor blocking drugs, neuroleptics ("rabbit syndrome"), dopamine-depleting drugs (reserpine, tetrabenazine), lithium, flunarizine, cinnarizine
   c. Vascular: multi-infarct, Binswanger, "lower body parkinsonism"
   d. Trauma: pugilistic encephalopathy, midbrain injury
   e. Tumor and paraneoplastic
   f. Infectious: postencephalitic, fungal, AIDS, SSPE, Creutzfeldt-Jakob disease
   g. Metabolic: hypoparathyroidism, chronic hepatic degeneration, mitochondrial cytopathies
   h. Normal pressure hydrocephalus
5. Severe essential tremor (ET)
6. Midbrain (rubral) tremor
7. Tardive tremor
8. Myorhythmia
9. Spasmus nutans

**B. Action tremors**
1. Postural tremors
   a. Physiologic tremor
   b. Enhanced physiologic tremor:
      1) Stress-induced: emotion, exercise, fatigue, anxiety, fever
      2) Endocrine: hypoglycemia, thyrotoxicosis, pheochromocytoma, adrenocorticosteroids
      3) Drugs: b-agonists (e.g., theophylline, terbutaline, epinephrine), dopaminergic drugs (levodopa, dopamine agonists), stimulants (amphetamines), psychiatric drugs (lithium, neuroleptics, tricyclics), methylxanthines (coffee, tea), valproic acid, cyclosporine, interferon
      4) Toxins: Hg, Pb, As, Bi, Br, alcohol withdrawal
   c. ET
      1) Autosomal-dominant
      2) Sporadic
      3) Myoclonus
   d. Postural tremor associated with
      1) Dystonia
      2) Parkinsonism
      3) Myoclonus
      4) Hereditary motor-sensory neuropathy (Roussy-Levy)
      5) Kennedy syndrome (X-linked spinobulbar atrophy)
   e. PD and other parkinsonian syndromes
   f. Tardive tremor
   g. Midbrain (rubral) tremor
   h. Cerebellar hypotonic tremor (titubation)
   i. Neuropathic tremor: motor neuron disease, peripheral neuropathy, peripheral nerve injury, reflex sympathetic dystrophy
2. Kinetic (intention, dynamic, termination) tremors
   a. Cerebellar disorders (cerebellar outflow): multiple sclerosis, trauma, stroke, Wilson disease, drugs and toxins
   b. Midbrain lesions
3. Task- or position-specific tremors
   a. Handwriting
   b. Orthostatic
   c. Other (e.g., occupational) task-specific tremors
4. Isometric
   a. Muscular contraction during sustained exertion
   b. Miscellaneous tremors and other rhythmic movements
      1) Myoclonus: rhythmic segmental myoclonus (e.g., palatal), oscillatory myoclonus, asterixis, mini-polymyoclonus
      2) Dystonic tremors
      3) Cortical tremors
      4) Epilepsia partialis continua
      5) Nystagmus
      6) Clonus
      7) Fasciculation
      8) Shivering
      9) Shuddering attacks
      10) Head bobbing (third ventricular cysts)
      11) Aortic insufficiency with head titubation

high specificity and sensitivity of a screening questionnaire when compared to the physician's examination in patients with definite and probable ET, but actual examination of the subjects is necessary to detect mild ET (Louis, Ford, Lee, and Andrews, 1998). In another study, the authors concluded that when a limited number of tests is available in large epidemiologic surveys, a test such as the finger-nose maneuver may be used to screen populations for ET, whereas to exclude normal subjects, the spiral drawing test, water pouring test, or arm extension test may be utilized (Louis et al., 1999a). A performance-based test for ET has been validated and compared to other measures of tremor (Louis et al., 1999b). Although this performance-based test was thought to objectively assess functional capacity in patients with ET, the test seems somewhat cumbersome to perform because it requires a variety of props, such as a milk carton, a glass, a soup spoon, a bowl, a saucer, a wallet, coins, an electrical socket, a thread and needle, a strip of buttons, and a telephone. Using another instrument, the modified Klove-Matthews Motor Steadiness Battery and the Nine-Hole Steadiness Tester, Louis, Yousefzadeh, and colleagues (2000) showed that these portable instruments provide a reliable and valid means of collecting objective quantitative data on tremor severity. A Tremor Disability Questionnaire has been developed and found to reliably correlate with multiple measures of tremor severity (Louis, Barnes, et al., 2000). A simple, user-friendly clinical tool is needed to assess tremors in the clinic and in the field. A teaching videotape for assessment of ET was developed to improve the uniform application of the Washington Heights–Inwood Genetic Study of Essential Tremor (Louis, Barnes, et al., 2001). Using a clinical evaluation (interview and videotaped examination) and an electrophysiologic evaluation (quantitative computerized tremor analysis using accelerometry and EMG), Louis and Pullman (2001) found a very high concordance rate between the two methods in 51 of 54 (94%) subjects, suggesting that using either technique would arrive at a similar diagnosis. Although not yet validated, the Unified Tremor Rating Assessment developed by the Tremor Research Group has been used in a number of clinical, therapeutic trials (Bain, 1993; Jankovic et al., 1996). The other scale, also not yet validated, that has been used in several tremor studies is the Tremor Rating Scale (Fahn et al., 1993).

## PATHOPHYSIOLOGIC MECHANISMS OF TREMORS

Current understanding of mechanisms that are involved in generation of tremors has been facilitated by the development of neurophysiologic and other quantitative techniques such as EMG recordings and uniaxial and triaxial accelerometers and by the application of computer technology to analyze the frequency spectra and other tremor-related physiologic variables (Elble and Koller, 1990; Gresty and Buckwell, 1990; Elble et al., 1994; Pullman, 1998; Louis, Dure, et al., 2001). A frequency of 6 Hz is usually the maximum rate of oscillation produced by a voluntary effort. During a voluntary contraction, motor units usually start firing at 8 Hz, and tetanic fusion frequency is reached at 15 to 20 Hz. Different parts of the human limb have mechanical characteristics (inertia and stiffness) that determine its natural resonant frequency. Such frequency is inversely related to the mass of the body part: finger, 25 Hz; wrist, 9 Hz; and elbow, 2 Hz.

A growing body of evidence supports the notion that central oscillators are important in the generation of physiologic and pathologic tremors (Pare et al., 1990; Plenz and Kitai, 1999; McAuley and Marsden, 2000; Brown, 2003). Using microelectrode recordings in awake or decerebrate monkeys who have been curarized and whose limbs were deafferented by sectioning C2 to T4 dorsal roots, Lamarre (1984) demonstrated spontaneous 3- to 6-Hz rhythmic discharges in the ventral thalamus and 7- to 12-Hz activity in the olivocerebellar system. Deafferenting the thalamus by a lesion in the ventromedial tegmentum of the midbrain

facilitates synchronization of thalamic neurons, which is ultimately expressed as a spontaneous, 3- to 6-Hz, parkinsonian rest tremor. The amplitude of these discharges and associated tremors is markedly enhanced by the tremorgenic drug harmaline, a potent reversible monoamine oxidase inhibitor. There are two types of harmaline-induced tremors, both of which appear to originate in the inferior olivary nucleus: an 8- to 12-Hz tremor in normal animals (analogous to physiologic tremor) and a 6- to 8-Hz tremor in monkeys with lesions in the dentate nucleus. Single-unit recordings from patients with parkinsonian tremors showed that neurons in the thalamic ventral nuclear group show rhythmic activity that correlated with EMG activity. Some, but not all, of these cells responded to somatosensory activity, indicating the importance of peripheral modulation (Lenz et al., 1994). In addition to the thalamus, there are other subcortical nuclei—particularly the subthalamic nucleus (STN) and globus pallidus externus (GPe)—that contain neuronal populations that produce synchronized oscillating bursts at 0.4, 0.8, and 1.8 Hz in a cell-culture environment (Plenz and Kitai, 1999). In addition to the low-frequency (<10 Hz) oscillations, there are 11- to 30-Hz and >60-Hz oscillatory activities within the subthalamopallidal-thalamocortical circuit (Brown, 2003). Furthermore, there is evidence that as a result of dopaminergic deficiency, the normal independent firing of pallidal neurons changes to both low-frequency (4 to 7 Hz) and high-frequency (10 to 16 Hz) oscillatory activity, which can also be recorded from the STN, and these oscillations often correlate with arm tremor (Bergman et al., 1998). This pacemaker could be responsible for the generation of tremor under pathologic conditions such as dopaminergic deficiency in Parkinson disease (PD). Therefore, surgical treatments of PD, such as lesion or stimulation of the globus pallidus internus (GPi) or STN, might act by desynchronizing the oscillatory basal ganglia–thalamocortical network activity. Such microelectrode-guided stereotactic operations in PD allow for single-cell recordings in the globus pallidus, thalamic nuclei, and other subcortical structures, leading to hypotheses about the normal and abnormal function of the basal ganglia. One such study, for example, found tremor locked cells in the center median-parafascicular complex of the thalamus with low-threshold calcium spike type bursts in central lateral nucleus and the paralamellar division of mediodorsal nucleus of the thalamus (Magnin et al., 2000).

Intracellular recordings from brainstem sections have demonstrated that neurons in the inferior olive have spontaneous oscillatory activity (Llinas, 1988; Kepler et al., 1990; Bevan et al., 2002). The autorhythmic properties of these neurons make this brainstem nucleus a prime candidate as a neuronal generator for tremor. In the olivary neurons, low-threshold $Ca^{2+}$ conductance at the somatic membrane enables these neurons to generate action potentials (low-threshold spike) even at subthreshold depolarization. A fast-action potential, generated by $Na^+$ current into the cell body, is followed by a slow, high-threshold $Ca^{2+}$ spike that activates prolonged (80 to 100 msec), $K^+$-mediated hyperpolarization. This is followed by an abrupt rebound response, generated by low-threshold $Ca^{2+}$ conductance, often large enough to generate a second, $Na^+$-dependent, action potential, and the cycle repeats itself. In addition to the olivary nucleus, there are other areas of the brain, particularly the STN and globus pallidus, that display spontaneous rhythmic activities. In the STN neurons, voltage-gated Na⁺ channels inactivate slowly during the depolarizing phase of the oscillation. In addition, Ca²⁺-dependent K⁺ current is activated by Ca²⁺ entry through high-voltage Ca²⁺ channels that open briefly during each Na⁺ action potential (Bevan et al., 2002). Harmaline enhances normal hyperpolarization, which is terminated by Ca²⁺ influx and rebound excitation, leading to rhythmic activation of the neurons. Besides harmaline, many toxins can produce tremors in animals and provide useful models for the study of tremors (Wilms et al., 1999). Microelectrode-guided single-cell recordings in patients with PD showed that the average firing rate in the GPi was 91 ± 52 Hz, and that in the globus pallidus externus was 60 ± 21 Hz (Magnin et al., 2000). In addition, rhythmic, low-threshold calcium spike bursts are often recorded in the pallidum and medial thalamus; some, but not all, are synchronous (in phase) with the typical rest tremor. It has been postulated that the low-threshold calcium spike bursts contribute to rigidity and dystonia by activating the supplementary motor area.

Physiologic tremor is present in all humans. It is an asymptomatic oscillation of a body part, resulting from a complex interaction between local mechanical-reflex mechanisms and central oscillators (McAuley and Marsden, 2000) (Fig. 19-1). The mechanical-reflex component is determined partly by the ballistocardiogram, mechanical properties of the muscle, motor neuron firing characteristics, stretch reflex and muscle spindle feedback, supraspinal influences, and state of activation of the muscle beta receptors (Marsden, 1984). The frequency of this component is inversely proportional to the mass and stiffness of the limb; thus, increasing the external mass load decreases the tremor frequency (Elble and Koller,

1990). Besides this variable frequency component, which is determined largely by the mechanical properties of the oscillating body part, spectral analyses of normal physiologic tremor show another, generally smaller, component with a relatively consistent frequency peak at about 10 (8 to 12) Hz. This 10-Hz frequency component is independent of peripheral influence, and it persists even after deafferentation, suggesting that this component of physiologic tremor is centrally generated. Supraspinal influence on physiologic tremor is supported by the observation that the loss of visual input when eyes are closed reduces or abolishes this tremor. The amplitude of physiologic tremor is determined largely by the degree of synchronization of motor unit discharges, modulated by muscle spindle Ia afferents. This process is exaggerated during anxiety, exercise, fatigue, and other conditions that are known to enhance peripheral β-adrenergic activity, and it may result in a visible tremor called enhanced physiologic tremor (see Box 19-1).

In most pathologic tremors, such as the rest or reemergent tremor of PD (Jankovic et al., 1999), the central oscillators are thought to drive the tremor, and the peripheral mechanisms are thought to merely modify or modulate its amplitude (Marsden, 1984; Britton et al., 1992a, 1992b). Magnetic brain stimulation can also modify certain pathologic tremors, providing further evidence that these tremors are centrally generated (Britton et al., 1993). The motor pathways that are involved in transmission of signals from these central generators are not well understood. Inhibition of tremor by lesions in the basal ganglia outflow nuclei and in the thalamus suggests that these subcortical nuclei are involved in the pathophysiology of tremors. In parkinsonian states, as a result of nigrostriatal dopamine depletion, excessive γ-aminobutyric acid (GABA)–mediated inhibition of the globus pallidus externus within the indirect striatopallidal pathway leads to a disinhibition of the STN and enhanced glutamate-mediated excitatory drive to the basal ganglia output nucleus (GPi) (DeLong, 1990). This increased drive from the output nuclei is reinforced by reduced inhibitory input to the GPi through the direct pathway. The typical 3- to 6-Hz rest tremor of PD possibly results from increased inhibition of the thalamic neurons that normally suppress the oscillators or from hyperpolarization of the oscillator neurons. In PD, the increased inhibitory output from the GPi leads to deafferentiation of the thalamus, particularly the reticular nucleus, and synchronization of local neuronal networks with intrinsic properties to spontaneously discharge (Lamarre, 1984; Huntsman et al., 1999). This spontaneous bursting is transmitted via the thalamocortical-spinal circuitry to the motor neurons in the spinal cord, causing synchronization of motor unit discharges, ultimately expressed as an oscillatory movement. In support of the role of the thalamus in the generation of parkinsonian rest tremor is the observation that the ventral thalamus of patients with PD contains a population of neurons that fire spontaneously and rhythmically and that their firing frequency correlates relatively well with the frequency of tremor, recorded by EMG in the contralateral limb (Lenz et al., 1988). Furthermore, a lesion in the nucleus ventralis intermedius (Vim) or electrical stimulation of the nucleus, so-called deep brain stimulation (DBS), abolishes contralateral rest tremor (Kelly et al., 1987; Benabid et al., 1991, 1996; Hubble et al., 1997; Koller et al., 1997; Ondo et al., 1998; Limousin et al., 1999). That parkinsonian tremor

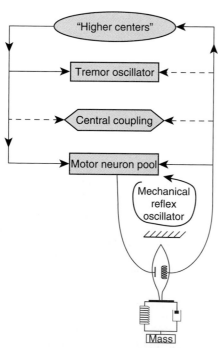

**Figure 19-1** Tremor results from a complex interaction of central oscillators, normally inhibited by "higher centers." When coupled and synchronized with the motor neuron pool, modified by peripheral mechanical reflex oscillator, the rhythmic discharges result in tremor.

is centrally driven is supported by the observation that complete paralysis of extensor forearm muscles as a result of radial nerve palsy actually increased the amplitude of the tremor without changing its frequency (Pullman et al., 1994). Volkmann and colleagues (1996) used magnetoencephalography to study parkinsonian resting tremor, and on the basis of these studies, they concluded that the typical 3- to 6-Hz parkinsonian tremor is generated by the same central mechanisms that are involved in voluntary rapid alternating movements. They proposed the following sequence of events for typical parkinsonian rest tremor: increased inhibitory output from GPi → hyperpolarization and activation of low-threshold calcium conductance in anterior ventrolateral nucleus (VLa) → 5 to 10 msec → activation of lateral premotor and motor cortex → 25 to 30 msec → EMG activity → 100 msec → activation of the central sulcus (reafferent input from muscle spindle to area 3a) → second activation of the somatosensory cortex by the antagonist contraction. The study of pacemaker neuronal networks as well as fast and slow oscillations within the basal ganglia circuitry will undoubtedly provide important insights into the pathophysiology of rhythmic involuntary movements such as tremors (Plenz and Kitai, 1999; Ruskin et al., 1999).

It has been suggested that the postural tremor of ET arises from spontaneous firing of the inferior olivary nucleus, which drives the cerebellum and its outflow pathways via the thalamus to the cerebral cortex and then to the spinal cord (Deuschl and Elble, 2000). In contrast to physiologic tremor, the frequency of ET does not decrease with mass loading, indicating a primary role of central mechanisms in ET (Elble and Koller, 1990). On the other hand, local cooling may significantly reduce the amplitude of ET, without changing its frequency (Lakie et al., 1994). Abnormal triphasic pattern with a delayed second agonist burst and other kinematic problems in response to a ballistic movement further support impaired cerebellar function in patients with ET (Koster et al., 2002). The involvement of the olivocerebellar-thalamocortical circuitry in ET is supported by changes in the cerebellar blood flow as measured by positron emission tomography (PET) during inhalation of $C^{15}$-labeled $O_2$ (Jenkins et al., 1993). Using this technique, the authors compared the cerebellar and cerebral blood flow in patients with ET and normal controls. They found that when the control subjects were holding one arm outstretched (in the absence of tremor), there was increased blood flow in the contralateral sensorimotor cortex and the supplementary motor area. In contrast, unilateral postural arm tremor in patients with ET was associated with markedly increased blood flow to *both cerebellar hemispheres*; in both premotor cortices; and to the contralateral striatal, thalamic, and sensorimotor cortex (but not the supplementary motor area). Passive and voluntary flexion-extension movements of the wrist significantly increased the blood flow only in the ipsilateral cerebellum. The investigators suggested that the increased flow in the cerebellum reflected increased activity of neurons involved in generation of tremor and that ET was due to oscillation within the olivocerebellar pathways, relayed by way of the thalamus and motor cortex to the spinal cord. Using a higher-resolution camera, the investigators were additionally able to demonstrate bilateral midbrain activation in the region of the red nuclei during tremor, but there was no change in the activity of the inferior olive either at rest or during postural tremor (Wills et al., 1994). Additional evidence of

increased activation of the cerebellum and red nucleus in ET has been provided by functional magnetic resonance imaging (MRI) studies (Bucher et al., 1997). The preponderance of evidence, based on PET and functional magnetic resonance imaging studies, indicates that the inferior olive probably does not play an important role in the generation of ET. This is in contrast to one previous study that indicated the involvement of the inferior olive in ET, suggested by the finding of glucose hypermetabolism during activation (finger-to-nose) of tremor in patients with ET (Dubinsky and Hallett, 1987). The absence of activity in the inferior olive and the bilateral overactivity of cerebellar-rubral-thalamic connections suggest that the tremor generator for ET is located in the cerebellum rather than the inferior olive. This conclusion is further supported by the finding of abnormal bilateral overactivity of cerebellar connections, as measured by rCBF determined by PET with $^{15}O$-labeled water, in patients with primary writing tremor and primary orthostatic tremor (Wills et al., 1995, 1996). Furthermore, alcohol has been found to suppress cerebellar synaptic overactivity in patients with ET, which in turn increases afferent input to the inferior olive (Boecker et al., 1996). In one study, 25% of ET patients were found to have moderate or severe kinetic tremor and other elements of cerebellar dysfunction (Deuschl et al., 2000). The demonstration by magnetic resonance spectroscopy of reduced N-acetyl-L-aspartate/creatine and N-acetyl-L-aspartate/choline ratios in the cerebellum of patients with ET compared to controls provides additional evidence for cerebellar dysfunction in ET (Pagan et al., 2003). Cerebellar pathology has also been described in some brains of patients with ET (Louis et al., 2006). Other abnormalities that are found in patients with ET include high blood levels of β-carboline alkaloids. Interestingly, these endogenous compounds, also found in plant-derived foods, increase the synchrony of neuronal firing in the inferior olive and cause tremor in experimental animals and humans. Some investigators have suggested that a loss of $GABA_A$ receptors may impair signaling by cerebellar Purkinje cells and cause tremor, as has been demonstrated in mice in which the gene coding for the $GABA_A$ receptor α1 subunit has been knocked out (Jankovic and Noebels, 2005; Kralic et al., 2005). Mutations in the coding region of the *GABRA1* gene, however, do not seem to be a major genetic cause of ET (Deng et al., 2006, 2007).

In addition to cerebellar involvement in ET, there is some evidence that cerebral cortex plays a role in the generation of ET (McAuley, 2001). Using simultaneous electroencephalogram (EEG)–EMG recordings, Hellwig and colleagues (2001) showed significant corticomuscular coherences in five of nine patients with ET. This is in contrast to a previous study that used magnetoencephalography (Halliday et al., 2000). That study found that in contrast to PD rest tremor, which is associated with marked disruption to the organization of the descending motor signals, there was no coherence between the magnetoencephalogram and EMG in patients with ET. However, the interpretation of the study that primary motor cortex does not contribute to the generation or maintenance of ET has been challenged because of possible insensitivity of the method (Elble, 2000c). The limitations of the various methods that were used in these studies have been pointed out by McAuley (2001), who also noted that electroencephalogram (EEG)–EMG coherence does not necessarily establish cortical origin of the tremor. Some patients with ET have abnormal vibration-induced illusion of movement, suggesting abnormal sensorimotor processing (Frima and Grunewald, 2005).

Cerebellar dysfunction in ET is also suggested by abnormalities in tandem gait, noted in 50% of ET patients (Singer et al., 1994; Stolze et al., 2001), and by mild postural instability (Henderson et al., 1996; Overby et al., 1996). This gait ataxia improves with alcohol at a blood level of 0.45% (Klebe et al., 2005). Posturographic analysis in patients with ET showed that balance control is only minimally impaired in ET, but patients with head tremor and longer disease duration may have slightly reduced postural stability (Bove et al., 2006). ET patients also show eye movement abnormalities indicative of cerebellar dysfunction, such as impaired smooth pursuit initiation and pathologic suppression of the vestibular-ocular reflex time constant by head tilts (otolith dumping) (Helmchen et al., 2003). Further evidence of cerebellar involvement in ET is suggested by a delay in second agonist EMG burst during rapid wrist movements (Britton et al., 1994). That the cerebellum might be involved in ET is also supported by the report of a 71-year-old man with ET in whom postural tremor disappeared on the right side after an ipsilateral cerebellar infarct (Dupuis et al., 1989). Since the amplitude of ET can be substantially reduced by thalamic lesions or thalamic stimulation (Benabid et al., 1991) and close correlation has been demonstrated between thalamic neuronal activity and forearm EMG in patients with ET (Hua et al., 1998), it is likely that the thalamus also plays an important role in the generation or transmission of ET. The possibility of additional cochlear involvement in ET is supported by the observation of high occurrence of partial or complete deafness in patients with ET (Ondo et al., 2003). Among 250 patients with ET, 42 (16.8%) wore hearing aids, compared to only 2 of 127 (1.6%) PD patients and 1 of 127 (0.8%) controls ($P < .0001$). Pure tone audiometry demonstrated age-dependent higher-frequency loss among patients with ET as compared to the general population. Although mental functioning is usually intact in patients with ET, detailed testing of cognitive performance has found some subtle abnormalities on tests of verbal fluency, naming, mental set-shifting, verbal working memory, and other tests of cognitive function (Benito-Leon et al., 2006b), and elderly patients with ET may possibly have an increased risk of dementia compared to those without ET (Benito-Leon et al., 2006a). Furthermore, higher levels of depression have been suggested to occur in patients with ET (this is similar to the control group with PD) (Lombardi et al., 2001). These deficits have been interpreted as suggesting involvement of frontocerebellar circuits. In a cross-sectional study of personality, patients with ET were found to have a tendency to have increased levels of pessimism, fearfulness, shyness, anxiety, and easy fatigability, but none of these traits correlated with the severity of the tremor (Chatterjee et al., 2004).

Rarely, postural tremor that occurs during sustained isometric muscle contraction can be a manifestation of cortical reflex myoclonus (Toro et al., 1993). This "cortical tremor," with or without seizures, usually starts between 19 and 30 years of age as tremulous finger movements, with a benign course and marked response to anticonvulsants, possibly cognitive decline, and a family history suggestive of ET (Okuma et al., 1998; van Rootselaar et al., 2005). It is characterized physiologically by an 8- to 15-Hz, synchronous, agonist-antagonist, EMG burst lasting less than 50 msec (10 to 50 msec). The condition shares neurophysiologic features with myoclonus, including giant somatosensory evoked responses and C-reflexes, and it responds well to anticonvulsants such as clonazepam, primidone, and valproate but not to beta blockers (Okuma et al., 1998). Since the EMG pattern can be influenced by transcranial magnetic and electrical stimulation but not by peripheral nerve stimulation, the rhythmic movement is thought to arise from central, possibly cortical, generators. Jerk-locked back-averaging revealed a positive electroencephalogram wave 15 msec preceding the EMG burst of the wrist extensor muscle (Okuma et al., 1998). In contrast to ET, strong corticomuscular and intermuscular coherence in the 8- to 30-Hz range was demonstrated in patients with familial cortical myoclonic tremor with epilepsy (van Rootselaar et al., 2006). The syndrome of autosomal-dominant cortical tremor, myoclonus, and epilepsy has been linked to genetic markers on 8q24 and 2p11.1–q12.2 (Striano et al., 2005). The term *familial cortical myoclonic tremor* with epilepsy has been suggested for this disorder, which has been reported in over 50 Japanese and European families (van Rootselaar et al., 2005).

Clinical-anatomic correlations indicate that kinetic tremor is usually associated with lesions in the cerebellar outflow pathways (Lou and Jankovic, 1993). Lesions of the dentate nucleus or the superior cerebellar peduncle proximal to the decussation correlate with kinetic tremor ipsilateral to the side of the lesion, whereas lesions that are distal to the decussation result in kinetic tremor contralateral to the side of the lesion (Carrea and Mettler, 1955). Lesions in the cerebellar hemisphere tend to produce kinetic tremors with a variable frequency ranging from 5 to 11 Hz; high brainstem lesions are usually associated with tremor frequency in the range of 5 to 7 Hz; and lower brainstem lesions produce faster tremors, ranging from 8 to 11 Hz (Cole et al., 1988). In contrast, the frequency of classic midbrain (red nucleus) tremor is relatively slow, at 2 to 3 Hz. In one study of patients with multiple sclerosis, two types of action tremors were identified. One group of patients had pure kinetic tremor with a frequency of 5 to 8 Hz and an EMG burst duration of 75 to 100 msec; the other group had coexisting kinetic and postural tremor. In contrast to kinetic tremor, postural tremor had a slower (2.5- to 4-Hz) frequency and a higher amplitude with a longer burst duration (125 to 200 msec) (Sabra and Hallett, 1984). The postural tremor was thought to result from a lesion in the cerebellar outflow pathway. Cerebellar kinetic tremor is associated with errors in timing and amplitude of the EMG activities of agonists and antagonists (Flament and Hore, 1986; Hore and Flament, 1986). The important role of peripheral reflex mechanisms in the pathogenesis of cerebellar kinetic tremor is supported by the observation that the character of the tremor can be altered by mechanical loading to the tremulous limb (Sanes et al., 1988) and by improvement in writing after 3 to 5 min of compressive ischemia of the affected arm (Dash, 1995). Lakie and colleagues (2004) showed that reduction of tremor by ischemia may be due to an accumulation of interstitial potassium in the muscle. The frequency of the tremor can be increased by increasing the spring stiffness and by decreasing the mass.

# REST TREMORS

## Diagnosis

Rest tremor is most typically present in patients with PD. In one study, all 34 patients with pathologically proven cases of idiopathic (Lewy body) parkinsonism demonstrated typical rest tremor sometime during the course of their illness (Rajput et al., 1991). Although this study suggests that parkinsonian patients who do not exhibit rest tremor probably do not have idiopathic parkinsonism, another study, involving 100 pathologically proven cases of PD, found that 32% of all patients apparently never manifested tremor during the course of their disease (Hughes et al., 1993).

Several studies have suggested that the natural course of PD is in part related to the presence or absence of tremor (Hughes et al., 1993). The tremor-dominant PD may be associated with earlier age at onset, less cognitive decline, and slower progression than the type of PD that is dominated by postural instability and gait difficulty (PIGD) (Jankovic et al., 1990). Clinical-pathologic correlations are needed to answer the question as to whether the tremor-dominant form and the PIGD-dominant form represent different diseases or merely variants of one disease, namely, PD. In support of the former is the finding that only 27% of patients with the PIGD form of idiopathic parkinsonism had Lewy bodies at autopsy (Rajput et al., 1993). In another clinical-pathologic study, Hirsch and colleagues (1992) demonstrated that patients with PD and prominent tremor have degeneration of a subgroup of midbrain (A8) neurons, whereas this area is spared in PD patients without tremor. This observation supports the hypothesis that differential damage of subpopulations of neuronal systems is responsible for the diversity of phenotypes seen in PD and other parkinsonian disorders. It is unclear whether the occasional patients with long-standing unilateral tremor and minimal or no other parkinsonian findings have a benign form of PD, as is suggested by PET scans showing low fluorodopa uptake in the contralateral putamen (Brooks et al., 1992), or whether this condition represents a separate disease entity. In contrast to patients with the PIGD form of PD, patients with tremor-dominant PD have increased metabolic activity in the pons, thalamus, and motor association cortices (Antonini et al., 1998). When rest tremors involve the fingers, hands, lips, jaw, and tongue in the same individual, they share a common frequency, suggesting that they are of central origin (Hunker and Abbs, 1990). This pattern, however, changes during sleep in that non–rapid eye movement (REM) sleep transforms the alternating tremor that is typically seen in the awake patient into subclinical repetitive muscle contractions of variable frequency and duration during sleep stages I to IV, and the tremor disappears during rapid eye movement sleep (Askenasy and Yahr, 1990).

Rest tremor has other causes besides PD and related parkinsonian disorders (see Box 19-1). Patients with severe ET may have tremor at rest and prominent kinetic tremor. It is not known whether the ET patients with rest tremor have associated PD, whether they later develop other features of PD, or whether the rest tremor is a feature of ET (Jankovic, 1989). Some patients with lesions in the cerebellar outflow pathways, particularly in the superior cerebellar peduncle near the red nucleus (cerebellar outflow, midbrain or "rubral" tremor),

also have tremor at rest, probably due to an interruption of the nigrostriatal pathway (Remy et al., 1995). The affected arm or leg may also be ataxic and may be associated with third nerve palsy (Benedikt syndrome) (Video 19-4). The cerebellar outflow tremor is most often caused by trauma, stroke, multiple sclerosis, and Wilson disease (Lou and Jankovic, 1993; Krauss et al., 1995; Miwa et al., 1996; Alarcon et al., 2004). Strokes involving the posterior circulation may involve the thalamus, producing slow (1- to 3-Hz) rest and postural tremors, sometimes referred to as myorhythmia (Masucci et al., 1984; Cardoso and Jankovic, 1996; Miwa et al., 1996).

Myorhythmia is a slow (1- to 3-Hz) frequency, continuous or intermittent, relatively rhythmic movement that is present at rest but may persist during activity (Masucci et al., 1984; Cardoso and Jankovic, 1996). It may be associated with palatal myoclonus, and it disappears with sleep. Except for the slower frequency, the presence of flexion-extension rather than the typical supination-pronation pattern, and the absence of associated parkinsonian findings, myorhythmia resembles a parkinsonian tremor. In the cases that were examined at autopsy, the sites of maximum pathology involved chiefly the brainstem (particularly the substantia nigra and the inferior olive) and the cerebellum. The etiology for myorhythmia includes brainstem stroke, cerebellar degeneration, Wilson disease, and Whipple disease (Masucci et al., 1984; Tison et al., 1992; Cardoso and Jankovic, 1996).

Palatal myoclonus, sometimes referred to as palatal tremor, has some features of tremor, but in contrast to tremor that is produced by alternating or synchronous contractions of antagonist muscles, the palatal movement is produced by rhythmic contractions of agonist muscles; thus, the term *myoclonus* is preferred, despite the arguments raised against this nosology (Zadikoff et al., 2006). Palatal myoclonus, a form of segmental myoclonus, is manifested by rhythmic contractions of the soft palate, resulting from acute or chronic lesions involving the Guillain-Mollaret triangle linking the dentate nucleus with the red nucleus via the central tegmental tract to the inferior olivary nucleus. Symptomatic palatal myoclonus usually persists during sleep, whereas essential palatal myoclonus, frequently associated with an ear-clicking sound, disappears with sleep. In essential palatal myoclonus, the muscle agonist is the tensor veli palatini, which opens the Eustachian tube and is innervated by the trigeminal nerve. In symptomatic palatal myoclonus, the palatal movement is due to contractions of the levator veli palatine, innervated by the facial nucleus and nucleus ambiguous. When the tensor muscle contracts, as in essential palatal myoclonus, the entire soft palate moves, whereas only the edges of the soft palate move when the levator muscle contracts in symptomatic palatal myoclonus. Symptomatic, but not essential, palatal myoclonus is often associated with hypertrophy of the inferior olive (Goyal et al., 2000).

Treatment with neuroleptics can also cause persistent tremor, referred to as tardive tremor (Stacy and Jankovic, 1992). This rest, postural, and kinetic tremor, with a frequency of 3 to 5 Hz, is aggravated by, and persists after, neuroleptic withdrawal and improves after treatment with the dopamine-depleting drug tetrabenazine. The tremor may be accompanied by other tardive movement disorders, including akathisia, chorea, dystonia, myoclonus, and stereotypy. There is usually no family history or other explanation for the tremor.

Spasmus nutans is characterized by the triad of nystagmus; abnormal head position; and irregular, multidirectional head nodding that disappears during sleep. This self-limited and often familial condition is first noted between the ages of 4 and 12 months, and it usually disappears within a year or two.

## Treatment

The treatment of rest tremors is similar to that of parkinsonism (Jankovic and Marsden, 1998; also see Chapter 6). Secondary and potentially curable causes should be excluded, particularly when there are associated features to suggest disorders other than PD (see Box 19-1). Anticholinergic and dopaminergic drugs provide the most effective relief of rest tremors. Clozapine, an atypical neuroleptic that does not significantly exacerbate parkinsonism but can cause potentially serious side effects such as agranulocytosis, has been shown to be effective in the treatment of parkinsonian tremor (and ET) (Bonuccelli et al., 1997; Friedman et al., 1997; Ceravolo et al., 1999). Ethosuximide, an anticonvulsant that blocks low-threshold $Ca^{2+}$ conductance in the thalamus, has been shown to reduce tremor in MPTP monkeys and to potentiate the effects of a D2 agonist (Gomez-Mancilla et al., 1992). However, ethosuximide was found ineffective in a pilot study of six PD patients with drug-resistant tremor (Pourcher et al., 1992). Mirtazapine (Remeron), a novel antidepressant that enhances noradrenergic and serotonergic transmission and acts as a presynaptic alpha-2, $5-HT_2$, and $5-HT_3$ receptor antagonist, has been reported to improve rest tremor (Pact and Giduz, 1999). High-amplitude parkinsonian tremors and rest tremors caused by disorders other than PD usually do not improve with pharmacologic therapy. In some cases, botulinum toxin (BTX) injections in the involved muscles produce a satisfactory reduction in the tremor amplitude (Jankovic and Schwartz, 1991; Jankovic et al., 1996; Hou and Jankovic, 2002). A multicenter, randomized, double-blind, controlled trial confirmed the results of an earlier study (Jankovic et al., 1996) that BTX injections produces significant reduction in the postural hand tremor of ET and modest functional improvement (Brin et al., 2001).

Ventral lateral thalamotomy, particularly involving the Vim, was considered the neurosurgical treatment of choice for disabling, drug-resistant tremors until the later 1980s when the ablative procedure was replaced by high-frequency deep brain (thalamic) stimulation (DBS) (Benabid et al., 1991; Fox et al., 1991; Jankovic et al., 1995b; Zirh et al., 1999). Although effective in a majority of cases, the tremor recurs in about 20% of patients, and there is a considerable risk of contralateral hemiparesis, hemianesthesia, ataxia, speech disturbance, and other potential complications. These are compounded when the procedure is performed bilaterally. Thalamic DBS is now the surgical treatment of choice for patients with disabling tremors (Deiber et al., 1993; Benabid et al., 1996; Ondo, Almaguer, et al., 2001; Ondo, Vuong, et al., 2001; Pahwa and Koller, 2001; Pahwa et al., 2006) (see Chapter 7). This technique has been proposed for chronic treatment of parkinsonian, essential, and other tremors. Using high-frequency (100-Hz) stimulation, with the tip of a monopolar electrode implanted stereotactically in the Vim contralateral to the disabling tremor, Benabid and colleagues (1991) noted "complete relief" of contralateral tremor in 27 of 43 (63%) thalami that were stimulated and "major

improvement" in 11 (23%). The series included 26 patients with PD and 6 with ET, 7 of whom had previously been treated with thalamotomy. The benefit of thalamic stimulation was maintained for up to 29 months (mean follow-up: 13 months). The results were similar in their subsequent report of long-term effects of chronic Vim stimulation in 117 patients, 74 of whom had bilateral implantation (Benabid et al., 1996). The most robust tremor suppression was noted in patients with PD ($n = 80$), but patients with ET ($n = 20$) also benefited, although 18.5% deteriorated with time. Dysarthria and ataxia still occurred, but the patients were able to adjust the intensity of stimulation to ameliorate these side effects, though at the expense of increased tremor. Nevertheless, the investigators felt that the reversible nature of the side effects was the chief advantage of DBS over the permanent lesion produced by thalamotomy. To compare thalamic DBS with thalamotomy, Schuurman and colleagues (2000) conducted a prospective, randomized study of 68 patients with PD, 13 with ET, and 10 with multiple sclerosis. They found that the functional status improved more in the DBS group than in the thalamotomy group, and tremor was suppressed completely or almost completely in 30 of 33 (90.9%) patients in the DBS group and in 27 of 34 (79.4%) patients in the thalamotomy group. Although one patient in the DBS group died after an intracerebral hemorrhage, DBS was associated with significantly fewer complications than was thalamotomy. This procedure may also be advantageous in elderly patients and when bilateral effects are desirable (Blond et al., 1992). Bilateral thalamic DBS has been found to be more effective than unilateral DBS in controlling bilateral appendicular and midline tremors of ET and PD, and thalamic DBS does not seem to improve meaningfully any parkinsonian symptoms other than tremor (Ondo, Almaguer, et al., 2001). Moreover, Vim DBS produces modest improvement, rather than tremor augmentation as previously suggested, in ipsilateral tremor in patients with ET (Ondo, Vuong, et al., 2001) (Fig. 19-2). A review of long-term efficacy of Vim DBS in 39 patients (20 with PD and 19 with ET) showed that the benefits may be maintained for at least 6 months (Rehncrona et al., 2003).

In addition to improving distal tremor associated with PD and ET, Vim DBS can effectively control ET head tremor, which usually does not respond to conventional therapy (Koller et al., 1999). Other midline tremors, such as voice, tongue, and face tremor, also may improve with unilateral Vim DBS, although additional benefit can be achieved with contralateral surgery (Obwegeser et al., 2000). Chronic stimulation of the thalamus appears to be well tolerated, and the risk of local gliosis is minimal (Caparros-Lefebvre et al., 1994). Unfortunately, thalamic stimulation does not appear to be as effective in patients with predominantly kinetic and axial tremors, and it does not improve other parkinsonian features such as bradykinesia, rigidity, and levodopa-related motor complications. Therefore, DBS targeting either the STN or the GPi is the preferred surgical treatment of tremor in patients with PD (Limousin et al., 1998; Benabid et al., 2000) The mechanism of action of DBS is unknown, but "jamming" of low-frequency oscillatory inputs has been suggested as a possible mechanism for the antitremor effects of DBS. Regional cerebral blood flow, measured by PET scan, demonstrated that tremor suppression was associated with decreased cerebellar blood flow and, presumably, decreased synaptic activity in the cerebellum (Deiber et al., 1993).

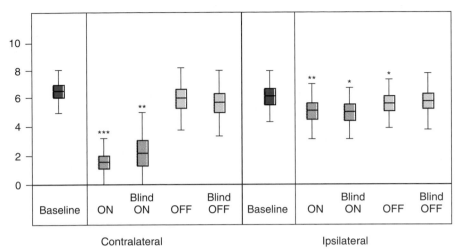

ARM TREMOR AND THALAMIC DBS IN ET
AT 3-MONTH FOLLOW-UP (n = 73)

**Figure 19-2** Thalamic DBS produces robust reduction in contralateral tremor and mild improvement in ipsilateral tremor. (Reprinted with permission from Ondo W, Almaguer M, Jankovic J, Simpson RK: Thalamic deep brain stimulation: Comparison between unilateral and bilateral placement. Arch Neurol 2001;58:218–222.)

**\*\*P < .005, \*\*\*P < .0001 ratings (mean, 95% mean CI, SD) include combined scores for rest, postural and action tremor on modified Tremor Rating Scale.**

In 1992, Laitinen of Stockholm, Sweden, reported the results of 90 pallidotomies in 86 patients with severe PD (Laitinen et al., 1992). The external, posteroventral portion of the medial GPi was the intended target for the stereotactically placed lesion. Nearly all patients had "marked improvement in tremor and akinesia." In addition, some patients apparently also noted improvement in their gait, speech, and pain. Only two patients suffered permanent visual field defect, and one had "minor stroke with hemiparesis." Several pallidotomy series have since confirmed the beneficial effects of pallidotomy on various parkinsonian symptoms, including tremor (Jankovic and Marsden, 1998). These results provide support for the notion that the GPi is "hyperactive" in PD and that surgical or chemical lesions of these structures may have a therapeutic value not only in controlling tremor but also in improving bradykinesia (Bergman et al., 1990; Aziz et al., 1991). Although some investigators (Subramanian et al., 1995) have suggested that posteroventral pallidotomy is as effective as thalamotomy in controlling parkinsonian tremor, others (Dogali et al., 1995) feel that pallidotomy provides only partial relief of tremor (see Chapter 7).

## POSTURAL TREMORS

### Diagnosis

Normal and enhanced physiologic tremors are the most common forms of postural tremor, but they rarely require medical attention. Postural tremors are clinically similar despite different etiologies. In contrast to ET, the frequency of physiologic tremor can be slowed by mass loading (Elble and Koller, 1990). Indeed, there appear to be two components to physiologic tremor: variable frequency (peak: 8 Hz), which is dependent on loading, and consistent frequency (peak: 10 Hz), which is independent of peripheral influence. Another feature that is helpful in differentiating ET from other postural tremors is that the amplitude of ET is less dependent on

the position of the tested limb than is the amplitude of the other postural tremors (Sanes and Hallett, 1990). While the amplitude of ET tends to increase with age, the tremor frequency decreases with age (Elble et al., 1994; Elble, 2000b).

Despite the frequently used modifier "benign," ET can produce physical and psychosocial disability (Busenbark et al., 1991; Jankovic, 2000; Sullivan et al., 2004; Louis, 2005) (see Appendix 19-1). Community-based epidemiologic studies have found the prevalence of ET to range between 0.4% and 4% (Haerer et al., 1982; Louis et al., 1995; Louis, Ford, Pullman, et al., 1998; Dogu et al., 2003), but it may be as high as 5.5% in people over the age of 40 years (Rautakorpi et al., 1982) and 14% in people 65 years old or older (Moghal et al., 1994). In one epidemiologic study, 108 of 1056 (10%) nondemented individuals in upper Manhattan, age 65 years or older, reported "shaking" (Louis et al., 1996). Neurologic examination confirmed rest tremor in 8.3% and action tremor in 17.6%, and the prevalence of PD and ET was estimated to be 3.2% and 10.2%, respectively. In a door-to-door survey of people age 40 years or older in Mersin Province, Turkey, the prevalence of ET was found to be 4% (Dogu et al., 2003). In another population-based survey, involving 5278 subjects age 65 years or older in central Spain who were followed for a median of 3.3 years, the adjusted annual incidence was determined to be 616 per 100,000 person-years; 64 of the 83 (77.1%) incident cases had not been previously diagnosed, and only 4 (4.8%) were taking antitremor medications (Benito-Leon et al., 2005). These epidemiologic studies provide strong evidence that the prevalence and incidence of ET are higher than was previously recognized.

Although ET was described as early as the 19th century (Dana, 1887; Louis, 2000), there is still considerable controversy about the diagnostic criteria for ET (Chouinard et al., 1997; Louis, Ford, Lee, et al., 1998; Jankovic, 2000). This is partly due to a lack of a disease-specific marker for ET. No specific pathologic changes indicative of PD were noted in 20 brains of ET patients that were examined at autopsy (Rajput et al., 2004). However, this study is fundamentally flawed, since all patients who were selected for the study had a diagnosis of ET at the time of death and patients who started with ET and later developed PD would have been excluded (Jankovic, 2004). It is of interest that in one patient with severe ET that began at age 45 and no parkinsonian features at the time of her death at age 91 years had Lewy bodies localized to the locus coeruleus, providing further evidence of a connection between ET and Lewy body disease (Louis, Honig, et al., 2005). The controversy about the possible association of ET and PD should be clarified once the genetic basis and pathophysiology of ET are understood. Until then, the operational diagnostic criteria must rely on the presence of typical clinical characteristics. The presence or absence of certain clinical characteristics may be used to categorize ET into "definite," "probable," and "possible" (Box 19-2). The diagnostic criteria may be used or modified according to specific needs. For example, for genetic linkage studies, only "definite" ET may be acceptable, whereas in studies that are designed to explore the clinical spectrum of ET, including associated features, the "possible" ET category might be more appropriate (Box 19-3). Family history, alcohol sensitivity, and propranolol responsiveness, while characteristic of ET, should not be considered necessary for the diagnosis. More recently, core and secondary criteria were proposed to facilitate a practical approach to the diagnosis of ET (Elble, 2000a). Core criteria include bilateral action tremor of the hands and forearms (but not rest tremor), absence of other neurologic signs (except for the Froment sign), and isolated head tremor without signs of dystonia. Secondary criteria include long duration (>3 years), a positive family history, and a beneficial response to alcohol. There are diagnostic red flags that indicate a diagnosis other than ET, such as unilateral tremor, leg tremor, rigidity, bradykinesia, rest tremor, gait disturbance, focal tremor, isolated head tremor with abnormal posture (head tilt or turning), sudden or rapid onset, and drug treatment that may cause or exacerbate tremor.

A review of the clinical features in 350 consecutive patients who were referred to the Movement Disorders Clinic at Baylor College of Medicine and diagnosed with ET has shown that although tremor is clearly the most troublesome symptom, it is not necessarily the only symptom in patients with ET (Lou and Jankovic, 1991a) (Tables 19-1 and 19-2). This is supported by the reports of well-studied families in which some members have typical ET, while others have dystonia, parkinsonism, or a combination of all three disorders (Jankovic et al., 1997; Farrer et al., 1999; Bertoli-Avella, 2003; Yahr et al., 2003). One multigenerational family, 36 members in five generations, had an admixture of ET, PD, and dystonia (Yahr et al., 2003). Two brothers, twins, with ET and PD had the classic pathologic features of PD at autopsy. The authors concluded, "This unusual set of clinical and pathologic circumstances can hardly be attributed to chance occurrence and raise the question of a specific genetic mutation and/or clustering, which may link ET with PD." In another large family, originally from Cuba, manifested by parkinsonism and ET, the parkinsonism was linked to a marker on chromosome 19p13.3–q12, but it did not cosegregate with ET (Bertoli-Avella, 2003). Some studies have suggested that there is an association between ET and dystonia and between ET and parkinsonism (Jankovic, 1994; Jankovic et al., 1997; Yahr et al., 2003; Shahed and Jankovic, 2007). In addition to dystonic tremor, patients with dystonia frequently have postural ET-like tremor present in body parts distal to the dystonia, and they have a higher-than-expected family history of postural

**Box 19-2** Proposed classification of essential tremor

**A. Definite ET**
1. Inclusions
   a. Bilateral postural tremor with or without kinetic tremor involving hands or forearms, which is visible and persistent and is long-standing in duration (>5 years).
   b. Tremor involving body parts other than the upper limbs may be present, the tremor may be asymmetric, amplitude may fluctuate, and the tremor might or might not produce disability.

2. Exclusions
   a. Neurologic signs, except for Froment sign (a "cogwheel" phenomenon on passive movement of the affected limb with voluntary movement of the contralateral limb)
   b. Causes of enhanced physiologic tremor
   c. Concurrent or recent exposure to tremorgenic drugs
   d. Direct or indirect trauma to the central and peripheral nervous system
   e. Historical or clinical evidence of psychogenic origins of tremor
   f. Convincing evidence of sudden onset or evidence of stepwise deterioration

**B. Probable ET**
1. Inclusions: The same as for definite ET, but the tremor may be confined to body parts other than hands and the duration is greater than 3 years.

2. Exclusions
   a. Primary orthostatic tremor, which is an isolated, high-frequency (14- to 18-Hz), bilaterally synchronous leg tremor on standing or voluntary contraction of leg muscles
   b. Isolated voice, tongue, or chin tremors
   c. Position- and task-specific tremors

**C. Possible ET**
1. Inclusions
   a. Type 1. Satisfy criteria for definite or probable ET but exhibit other recognizable neurologic disorders:
      1) Parkinsonism, dystonia, myoclonus, peripheral neuropathy, or restless legs syndrome
      2) Other neurologic signs of uncertain significance not sufficient to make a diagnosis of a recognizable neurologic disorder, such as mild extrapyramidal signs (hypomimia, decreased armswing, and mild bradykinesia).
   b. Type 2. Monosymptomatic and isolated tremors of uncertain relationship to ET. This includes position- and task-specific tremors, such as occupational tremors (primary writing tremors); primary orthostatic tremor; isolated voice, chin, tongue, and leg tremor; and unilateral postural hand tremor.
2. Exclusions: Same as *a* to *f* for definite ET

Tremor Research and Investigation Group: M. Brin, C. Contant, R. Elble, L. Findley, J. Jankovic, W. Koller, P. LeWitt, A. Rajput.

From Findley LJ, Koller WC: Definitions and behavioral classifications. In Findley LJ, Koller WC (eds): Handbook of Tremor Disorders. New York, Marcel Dekker, 1995 pp 1-5.

**Box 19-3** NIH Essential Tremor Consortium diagnostic criteria for essential tremor

**Definite**
1. Bilateral arm tremor with 2+ amplitude rating in at least one arm and 1+ in the other arm.
or
2. Predominant cranial-cervical tremor with 2+ amplitude rating and 1+ rating in at least one arm. The head tremor is rhythmic, without directional preponderance, and without asymmetry of cervical muscles.
3. Exclude obvious secondary causes of tremor: for example, physiologic, drug-induced, CMT, PD. (Coexistent dystonia is allowed, but coexistent PD is not.)

**Probable**
1. 1+ arm tremor bilaterally
or
2. Isolated cranial-cervical tremor with 2+ amplitude rating
or
3. Convincing history of ET
4. Exclude obvious secondary causes of tremor: for example, physiologic, drug-induced, CMT. (Coexistent dystonia is allowed; coexistent PD is allowed if there is a convincing history of pre-existing ET.)

**Possible**
1. Isolated 1+ cranial-cervical tremor
2. Task/position specific hand/arm tremor
3. Unilateral arm tremor
4. Orthostatic tremor

Tremor rating: 0, none perceived; 1, slight (barely noticeable); 2, moderate, noticeable, probably not disabling (<2-cm excursions); 3, marked, probably partially disabling (2- to 4-cm excursions); 4, severe, coarse, disabling (>4-cm excursions).Participants in the July 1996 NIH meeting: J. Beach, S. B. Bressman, M.F. Brin, L., D. De Leon, Goldfarb, M. Hallett, J. Jankovic, W. Koller, D. Mirel, K. Wilhemsen.

From Brin MF, Koller W: Epidemiology and genetics of essential tremor. Mov Disord 1998;13(suppl 3):55–63.

**Table 19-1** Essential tremor

| Variable | n | % |
|---|---|---|
| Gender | 179 males/ 171 females | 350 |
| Age at evaluation (years) | 58.4 16.4 | 350 |
| Duration of symptom (years) | 18.7 17.5 | 326 |
| Family history | | 350 |
| First-degree relative(s) | 219 | (62.5%) |
| Other relatives | 25 | (7.1%) |
| Associated disorders | | 350 |
| Dystonia | 165 | (47.1%) |
| Cervical dystonia | 94 | (26.8%) |
| Writer's cramp | 48 | (13.7%) |
| Blepharospasm | 26 | (7.4%) |
| Laryngeal dystonia | 14 | (4.0%) |
| Others | 21 | (6.0%) |
| Parkinsonism | 72 | (20.2%) |
| Myoclonus | 8 | (2.2%) |
| Improvement with drugs | | |
| Alcohol | 96/144 | (66.7%) |
| Propranolol (n = 147)* | 22/32 | (68.0%) |
| | 13/18 | (72.1%) |

From Lou JS, Jankovic J: Essential tremor: Clinical correlates in 350 patients. Neurol 1991;41:234–238.

likely to develop head tremor than were men (Hardesty et al., 2004).

The ongoing debate as to whether ET is a monosymptomatic or heterogeneous disorder or a phenotypic manifestations of multiple entities will probably not be resolved until disease-specific physiologic, genetic, or other biologic markers are identified (Schrag et al., 2000; Elble, 2002; Jankovic, 2002). Postural tremor, similar to ET, has been reported to occur in as many as 93% of patients with PD and correlate with the ipsilateral rest tremor but not with age at onset or disease duration

tremor (Chan et al., 1991; Jankovic et al., 1991; Deuschl et al., 1997). Whether the hand tremor that is seen in 10% to 85% of patients with cervical dystonia represents an enhanced physiologic tremor, ET, dystonic tremor, or some other form of postural tremor is unknown (Jankovic et al., 1991; Deuschl et al., 1997).

The clinical heterogeneity of ET suggests that there may be different subtypes. Indeed, Louis, Ford, and colleagues (2000) found that patients with older onset (>60 years) and those without head tremor progressed more rapidly than did patients with young-onset tremor and those with head tremor. They also later found that head tremor was present four times more frequently in women than in men (Louis et al., 2003; Hardesty et al., 2004). Using the medical records linkage system of the Rochester Epidemiology Project, the authors identified ET patients who also had an autopsy report and found that women with ET were six times more

**Table 19-2** Anatomic distribution of tremor

| Baby Part | Isolated | Plus Other Body Parts | Total | |
|---|---|---|---|---|
| Hands | 145 | 169 | 314 | (89.7%) |
| Head | 24 | 119 | 143 | (40.8%) |
| Voice | 1 | 61 | 62 | (17.4%) |
| Leg | 1 | 47 | 48 | (13.7%) |
| Jaw | 1 | 24 | 25 | (7.1%) |
| Face | 0 | 8 | 8 | (2.9%) |
| Trunk | 1 | 5 | 6 | (1.7%) |
| Tongue | 0 | 5 | 5 | (1.4%) |
| Orthostatic | 0 | 2 | 2 | (0.6%) |

From Lou JS, Jankovic J: Essential tremor: Clinical correlates in 350 patients. Neurol 1991;41:234–238.

(Louis, Levy, et al., 2001). Phenomenologically similar to ET, the postural tremor of PD has been linked by some investigators to coexistent ET (Geraghty et al., 1985; Jankovic, 1989; Jankovic et al., 1997; Jankovic 2000). Others, however, believe that the coexistence of the two disorders simply "represents a chance occurrence of two common diseases" (Pahwa and Koller, 1993). On the basis of an analysis of 678 patients diagnosed as having ET, some by movement disorder specialists and others by private practice neurologists, 6.1% were found to have concomitant PD, and 6.9% had coexisting dystonia (Koller et al., 1994). The authors concluded that "the frequency of PD in ET is more than would be reported in the general population." The coexistence of ET and PD may be difficult to recognize because once a patient develops PD, the postural tremor is usually attributed to the disease, and it is therefore difficult to diagnose ET in a patient who already has symptoms of PD. The "postural tremor" that is seen in many patients with PD may represent an enhanced physiologic tremor (Forssberg et al., 2000), coexistent ET (Geraghty et al., 1985; Jankovic, 1995), or a reemergent classic rest tremor (Jankovic et al., 1999) with the same frequency and clinical characteristics as the typical rest tremor. This reemergent tremor is also often exacerbated during walking. In contrast to ET, which is seen immediately when patients outstretch their arms, the reemergent tremor of PD usually appears after a latency of several seconds (Jankovic et al., 1999). Furthermore, this PD-related tremor often responds to levodopa, whereas the postural tremor of ET does not (Kulisevsky et al., 1995). It is actually this action tremor that seems to correlate with motor disability rather than the typical rest tremor, which correlates chiefly with social handicap (Zimmermann et al., 1994). The clinical characteristics, however, may not always reliably differentiate between the two types of postural tremor (Henderson et al., 1995). There is a higher frequency of the 263bp allele of the NACP-Rep1 polymorphism not only in patients with PD (odds ratio: 3.86) but also in patients with ET (odds ratio: 6.42) but not in patients with Huntington disease, supporting a genetic link between PD and ET (Tan et al., 2000). Further evidence that ET and PD may be related is the observation that patients with ET have an olfactory deficit that is similar, although milder, than that noted in patients with PD (Louis et al., 2002; Louis and Jurewicz, 2003). Gimenez-Roldan and Mateo (1991) have noted that patients with ET seem to have a higher propensity toward neuroleptic-induced parkinsonism than do patients without ET, although a formal epidemiologic study is needed to confirm this clinical observation. To examine an ET-PD relationship, 22 patients with childhood-onset ET who later developed PD were evaluated (Jankovic et al., 2004; Shahed and Jankovic, 2007). Of 11 patients reporting asymmetric ET, PD symptoms began on the same side as the more severe ET tremor in 10 (90.9%, $\chi^2 = 0.66$, $P = .024$), with 68.2% reporting change in tremor as their first PD manifestation. These findings suggest that in some patients, childhood ET evolves into adult tremor-dominant PD, explaining the coexistence of ET and PD within the same patient and family. One can postulate that ET-related gene mutations may predispose some patients to subsequent development of PD. In a similar study involving 13 patients who presented originally with asymmetric postural tremor and no rest tremor for at least 10 years (mean: 19.2 years) and were initially diagnosed with ET, all patients subsequently developed evidence of PD (Ray Chaudhuri et al., 2005). The onset of levodopa-responsive PD

was manifested by rest tremor for a mean of 2.5 years before final presentation in the clinic. Furthermore, five patients who had β-CIT single photon emission computed tomography all showed reduced uptake in the contralateral striatum. It is not clear whether these patients with a long-standing history of asymmetric postural tremor have PD at onset, whether patients with unilateral postural tremor (isolated tremor) or asymmetric postural tremor (atypical ET) who later develop PD represent an overlap between ET and PD, or whether this type of postural tremor is an early marker for PD (Grosset and Lees, 2005).

ET appears to be a heterogeneous disorder, as is suggested by multiple gene loci that have so far been identified and by the frequent association with other disorders, such as parkinsonism, dystonia, and myoclonus (Jankovic et al., 1997; Jankovic, 2002; Yahr et al., 2003). Postmortem studies of patients with ET have not provided evidence for nigrostriatal pathology in ET, but patients who had a diagnosis of PD at time of death (even though ET might have preceded the onset of PD) would have been excluded from these clinical-pathologic studies (Jankovic, 2004; Rajput et al., 2004). Furthermore, there is indirect evidence suggesting nigrostriatal impairment in some patients with ET. Relatives of patients with PD have at least a 2.5 times higher (those with the combination of ET-PD: 10 times higher) frequency of tremor than did normal controls, providing additional support for the association of ET and PD (Jankovic et al., 1995a). Furthermore, about 20% of patients with ET have a rest tremor that has the clinical and physiologic characteristics of PD tremor (Cohen et al., 2003). Similarly, a fourfold increase in prevalence of isolated tremor among relatives of patients with PD as compared to controls was found by Payami and colleagues (1994). A 10% to 13% reduction in $^{18}$F-dopa uptake in the striatum of patients with ET as compared to controls (Brooks et al., 1992) suggests a physiologically important compromise of the dopaminergic system in patients with ET (Jankovic et al., 1993). Furthermore, $^{18}$F-dopa uptake constants ($K_i$) in 5 of 32 asymptomatic relatives of patients with PD who had isolated postural tremor were reduced on average by 23% ($P < .001$) (Piccini et al., 1997). The mean $K_i$ for the other 27 asymptomatic relatives was decreased by 17% ($P < .001$). Using $^{123}$I-IPT single photon emission computed tomography to image the striatal dopamine transporter, Lee and colleagues (1999) found the mean bilateral uptake in nine patients with isolated postural tremor (ET) to be slightly lower than that in normal control subjects (3.60 versus 3.80), but this did not reach statistical significance. Six other patients in whom rest tremor developed 4 to 18 years (mean: $11.5 \pm 6.7$) after the onset of postural tremor without other parkinsonian features, however, had a significant reduction in the dopamine transporter compared to normal controls (2.61 versus 3.83, $P < .05$) but lower than PD patients (1.97 contralateral and 2.35 ipsilateral). They concluded that some patients with postural tremor may acquire rest tremor in association with mild substantia nigra neuronal loss. These findings provide further support for the notion that some ET patients later develop parkinsonian signs. Interestingly, among 196 twins with postural or kinetic tremors, Tanner and colleagues (2001) found that 137 had PD or had a twin with PD.

Although the relatively frequent coexistence of ET and dystonia supports the notions that there is a pathogenetic link between the two disorders, linkage analysis has excluded the dystonia (*DYT1*) gene on chromosome 9 in hereditary ET (Conway et al., 1993; Dürr et al., 1993). This suggests that the genes for these two disorders are on separate loci or that the relationship between the two disorders is physiologic rather than genetic. Münchau and colleagues (2001) studied 11 patients with classic ET and compared them to 19 patients with cervical dystonia and arm tremor. They found that the latency of second agonist burst during ballistic wrist flexion movements was later in ET patients than in those with arm tremor associated with cervical dystonia. Furthermore, the latter group had a greater variability in reciprocal inhibition than did the ET group. Patients with normal presynaptic inhibition had onset of their arm tremor simultaneously with onset of their cervical dystonia (mean age: 40 years), whereas patients with reduced or absent presynaptic inhibition had an earlier age at onset (mean 14 years), and the interval between the onset of the tremor and the onset of cervical dystonia was longer (mean: 21 years). This suggests that the mechanisms of arm tremor in patients with ET and cervical dystonia are different. The association between ET, dystonia, and PD is suggested by reports of families with manifestations of these three disorders in different or same members of the families (Jankovic et al., 1997; Yahr et al., 2003).

ET-like tremor has been described in patients with hereditary myoclonus and with hereditary motor-sensory neuropathy (sometimes referred to as Roussy-Levy syndrome) (Cardoso and Jankovic, 1993). ET-like tremor occurs in other genetic diseases, the study of which may provide important insights into possible genetic heterogeneity in families with clinically similar tremor. For example, postural tremor similar to that seen in ET has been reported in patients with Kennedy disease, also called X-linked recessive spinal and bulbar muscular atrophy, which is caused by a mutation characterized by expansion of CAG repeats in the gene on the X chromosome (Sperfeld et al., 2002). ET may also be associated (with higher-than-expected frequency) with restless legs syndrome (Ondo and Lai, 2006). The validity and meaning of such associations, however, are disputed, and the controversies are not likely to be resolved until a disease-specific marker (e.g., an ET-linked genetic locus) is identified. A diagnostic marker for ET would also help to resolve the question as to whether site-, position-, and task-specific tremors, such as primary handwriting tremor and orthostatic tremor, are distinct entities or whether these tremors represent clinical variants of ET (Table 19-3; see

**Table 19-3** Treatment of tremor variants

| Variant | Treatment |
| --- | --- |
| Postural hand/arm tremor | P, PRI, A, B, TH, DBS |
| Kinetic hand/arm tremor | C, P, PRI, B, BU, TH, DBS |
| Rest tremor | T, L, B, TH, DBS |
| Task-specific tremor | T, P, PRI, B |
| Head tremor | C, PRI, P, B |
| Voice tremor | P, B |
| Facial/tongue tremor | P, PRI, L, B |
| Orthostatic tremor | G, C, PRI, PH, L |

A, Alprazolam; B, Botulinum toxin; BU, Buspirone; C, Clonazepam; DBS, Deep brain stimulation; G, Gabapentin; L, Levodopa; P, Propranolol; PH, Phenobarbital; PRI, Primidone; T, Trihexyphenidyl; TH, thalamus.

also Table 19-2) (Rosenbaum and Jankovic, 1988; FitzGerald and Jankovic, 1991; Britton et al., 1993; Danek, 1993; Soland et al., 1996b; Sander et al., 1998).

Orthostatic tremor, first described by Heilman in 1984 (Heilman, 1984), is a fast (14- to 16-Hz) tremor, involving mainly the legs and trunk, but cranial muscles may also be involved (Koster et al., 1999) (Video 19-5). The latter study suggests that supraspinal mechanisms are involved. This is further supported by the finding of high intermuscular coherence between both sides, providing evidence that the tremor originates from a common site (Lauk et al., 1999). The observation of a 16-Hz tremor in a man with complete paraplegia suggests that the spinal cord is the generator of the tremor (Norton et al., 2004). Some authors have suggested that orthostatic tremor merely unmasks 16-Hz central oscillators involved in postural tremor (McAuley et al., 2000). Present chiefly on standing, orthostatic tremor may be precipitated also by isometric contraction of the upper limbs as well as facial and jaw muscles (Boroojerdi et al., 1999; Koster et al., 1999). This suggests that the generation of orthostatic tremor is more likely related to isometric force control rather than to regulation of stance. Orthostatic tremor is often associated with a feeling of unsteadiness and calf cramps and is relieved by sitting, by lying down, or by initiating walking. Fung and colleagues (2001) postulated that "the sensation of unsteadiness arises from a tremulous disruption of proprioceptive afferent activity from the legs." The leg cramps are presumably due to a high-frequency (titanic) contraction of the calf muscles. The muscle contraction can be "heard" by auscultating over the thigh or calf and listening for the characteristic thumping sound (Brown, 1995). In support of the association between ET and orthostatic tremor is the relatively high occurrence of familial, postural, tremor in patients with orthostatic tremor (FitzGerald and Jankovic, 1991) and similar PET findings indicative of bilateral cerebellar (and contralateral lentiform and thalamic) dysfunction (Wills et al., 1996). Some studies have also suggested that there is a dopaminergic deficit in orthostatic tremor. Leg tremor, phenomenologically similar to orthostatic tremor, may be the initial manifestation of PD (Kim and Lee, 1993). Some patients with orthostatic tremor respond to levodopa (Wills et al., 1999) and dopamine agonists (Finkel, 2000). Furthermore, [$^{123}$I]-FP-CIT single photon emission computed tomography showed evidence of marked reduction of dopamine transporter in patients with orthostatic tremor (Katzenschlager et al., 2003).

The involvement of the cranial muscles and a high degree of EMG coherence between right and left muscle groups suggest that supraspinal mechanisms are involved in the generation of orthostatic tremor (Koster et al., 1999). This is in contrast to ET or PD tremors, in which there is no such left/right coherence, and these tremors are probably generated by more than one oscillator (Raethjen et al., 2000). Furthermore, in contrast to ET, orthostatic tremor responds well to clonazepam and gabapentin. In one study, five of nine patients with orthostatic tremor benefited from levodopa (Wills et al., 1999). Whether dopamine agonists and other antiparkinsonian treatments, including thalamotomy and Vim or STN/GPi DBS, will provide benefit to patients with orthostatic tremor remains to be determined. Tremor that is present predominantly or only on standing, but usually of much lower frequency than the classic orthostatic tremor, can also be seen in other conditions, including parkinsonism, head trauma, pontine lesions, and other disorders (Gabellini et al., 1990; Benito-Leon et al., 1997). In a review of 41 patients with orthostatic tremor, Gerschlager and colleagues (2004) found that 24 (58%) patients had associated postural arm tremor, and 10 (25%) had "orthostatic tremor plus"; 6 (15%) patients had parkinsonism. The response to medications was generally poor, but some, particularly those with associated parkinsonism, responded to dopaminergic therapy. A recent study has suggested that coherent high-frequency tremor in the legs may be a normal response to perceived unsteadiness when standing still and that orthostatic tremor may be an exaggeration of this response (Sharott et al., 2003).

The age at onset for ET showed a bimodal distribution with peaks in the second and sixth decades (Lou and Jankovic, 1991a). This was evident in both genders and in patients with and without dystonia and parkinsonism. Patients with early onset (<30 years) ET had significantly more hand involvement, were more likely to have associated dystonia, and were more likely to improve with alcohol than were those with later onset (>40 years) ET ($P < .05$). There were no significant differences in any clinical variables between patients with and those without a family history of tremor. The relative lack of important differences between subgroups (early versus late onset, familial versus sporadic, mild versus severe, low versus high frequency) suggests that ET represents a single disease entity with a variable clinical expression. This conclusion is supported by a recent study by Koller and colleagues (1992). In their clinical and physiologic study of 61 patients, they found a frequency below 7 Hz in 79% of the patients, a positive family history in 72%, an amelioration with alcohol in 75%, an amelioration with primidone in 71%, and an amelioration with propranolol in 46%. Since no significant correlations could be found to suggest any particular grouping, they concluded that "essential tremor cannot be classified into subtypes." In a series of 19 patients with childhood ET, Louis, Dure, and colleagues (2001) found male preponderance and paucity of head tremor, but otherwise, there were no major differences between childhood and adult tremor. Of 39 patients with childhood-onset ET with a mean age at onset of $8.8 \pm 5.0$ years and a mean age at evaluation of $20.3 \pm 14.4$ years, some had their initial symptoms as early as infancy. A family history of tremor was noted for 79.5% of the patients. Eighteen (46.2%) patients had some neurologic comorbidity, such as dystonia, which was noted in 11 (28.2%) patients. Only 24 (61.5%) patients were treated with a specific antitremor medication; 5 of the 12 patients who were treated with propranolol experienced improvement. Some investigators have suggested that "shuddering attacks" of infancy might be the initial manifestation of ET (Vanasse et al., 1976; Kanazawa, 2000).

Some isolated site-specific tremors, such as those involving the head and trunk (Rivest and Marsden, 1990) and some task- or position-specific tremors, might actually represent forms of dystonic tremor (Elble et al., 1990; Jedynak et al., 1991; Bain et al., 1995). Dystonic tremor is typically irregular and position sensitive, and when the patient is allowed to move the affected body into the position of the maximal "pull," the so-called null point, the tremor often ceases  (Videos 19-6 and 19-7). Although there is some overlap between primary writing tremor and dystonic writer's cramp, the former is not usually associated with an excessive overflow of EMG activity into the proximal musculature, and the

reciprocal inhibition of the median nerve H-reflex on radial nerve stimulation is normal (Bain et al., 1995; Modugno et al., 2002). The latter two features are typical of dystonia, and their presence in patients with task-specific tremors suggests that despite the absence of overt dystonia, these tremors represent forms of focal dystonia (Rosenbaum and Jankovic, 1988; Soland et al., 1996b). The overlap with primary handwriting tremor is supported by the observed activation of brain areas on functional magnetic resonance imaging that are commonly activated in ET and dystonic writer's cramp. Other causes of postural tremor include midbrain (rubral) lesions. In six patients with midbrain tremors, PET studies indicated dopaminergic striatal denervation, supported by markedly decreased fluorodopa uptake in the ipsilateral striatum (Remy et al., 1995). This nigrostriatal denervation, however, was not accompanied by striatal dopamine receptor supersensitivity, and the density of striatal D2 receptors did not change. Furthermore, the density of dopamine transporter is the same as that in normal controls (Antonini et al., 2001). Another form of postural tremor with bilateral high-frequency (14-Hz) synchronous discharges was reported in a patient with sporadic olivopontocerebellar atrophy (Manto et al., 2003).

## Genetics of Essential Tremor

A family history of tremor has been reported in 17% to 100% of patients with ET (Busenbark et al., 1996; Louis and Ottman, 1996; Deng et al., 2007). The reason for such a large discrepancy is that unless all the symptomatic and asymptomatic members of the family are examined, the number of affected relatives will be underascertained (Jankovic et al., 1997; Louis et al., 1999b). Tremor in relatives is often wrongly attributed to aging, stress, nervousness, PD, alcoholism, or an associated illness or medications. In a study of 169 relatives of 46 ET patients, 12 (7.5%) were diagnosed as having probable or definite ET, but only 2 were reported by probands to have tremor (sensitivity: 16.7%); only 1 of 136 normal relatives were reported to have tremor (specificity: 99.3%) (Louis et al., 1999b). In other studies, the investigators found that 23% of elderly individuals had ET, and relatives of ET patients were five times more likely to develop the disease than was a control population (Louis, Ford, Frucht, et al., 2001), and first-degree relatives were more likely to have tremor compared to relatives of controls than were second-degree relatives (Louis, Ford, Frucht, and Ottman, 2001). Factors that were associated with more accurate reporting were female informant, increased tremor severity, sibling relationship, and higher level of education. In a comprehensive study of 20 index patients with hereditary ET and their 93 first-degree relatives and 38 more distant relatives, Bain and colleagues (1994) examined 53 definite and 18 possible cases. Similar to the findings of Lou and Jankovic (1991b), the investigators found a bimodal distribution and autosomal-dominant inheritance with nearly complete penetrance by the age of 65 years. In contrast to some previous studies, they found no cases of dystonia, PD, task-specific tremors, or primary orthostatic tremors, but migraine headaches occurred with a higher-than-expected frequency of 26%. About 50% were alcohol-responsive, but there was marked heterogeneity of responsiveness between and within families. In contrast, in a study of 252 members in four large kindreds with ET, three of the kindreds had a total of 41 members with the combination of ET and dystonia, and two had associated parkinsonism (Jankovic et al., 1997). Besides the one kindred with "pure" ET without any associated disorders (Jankovic et al., 1997), another large kindred of 216 individuals with "pure" ET was subsequently studied. The observation of earlier age at onset in successive generations suggests the phenomenon of anticipation, although the relatively small number of subjects and the possibility of ascertainment bias preclude any definite conclusions. A genome scan of 16 ET Icelandic families containing 75 affected relatives with "definite" ET identified a marker for the familial ET gene, FET1 or ETM1, on chromosome 3q13 (Gulcher et al., 1997). An analysis of a large Czech-American family established linkage to a locus ETM2 on chromosome 2p22–p25 (Higgins et al., 1997). Two other families with "pure" ET and one with ET-parkinsonism-dystonia also mapped to the same locus (Higgins et al., 1998). On the basis of studies of genetically diverse populations of ET, the locus has been narrowed to 2p24.1 with a candidate interval to a 192-kilobase interval between the loci etm1231 and APOB (Higgins et al., 2004). More recently, a missense mutation (828C→G) in the *HS1-BP3* gene was identified in two American families with ET and was absent in 150 control samples (300 chromosomes) (Higgins et al., 2005, 2006). The 828C→G mutation causes a substitution of a glycine for an alanine residue in the *HS1-BP3* protein (A265G), which is normally highly expressed in motor neurons and Purkinje cells and regulates the $Ca^{2+}$/calmodulin-dependent protein kinase activation of tyrosine and tryptophan hydroxylase. Studies by Deng and colleagues (2005) of patients with ET and suitable controls, however, have led to the conclusion that the variant might not be pathogenic for ET and might simply represent a polymorphism in the *HS1-BP3* gene. A linkage to 6p23 with an LOD score ranging from 1.265 to 2.983 was identified in two ET families, but further studies are needed to determine whether this represents merely a susceptibility locus or whether this gene region contains a causative gene (Shatunov et al., 2006). Recently, variants in the coding region of the D3 receptor gene (DRD3), localized on 3q13.3, have been found to be associated with ET in some families and in a case-control study (Lucotte et al., 2006).

Another marker for ET has been mapped to chromosome 4p14–16.3 (MIM 168601) in a family with autosomal-dominant PD (Farrer et al., 1999, 2004). This family, however, was later found to have α-synuclein gene (SNCA) triplication, and this SNCA triplication segregated with parkinsonism but not the postural tremor (Singleton et al., 2003). This suggests that the postural tremor is a coincidental finding. Since not all families map to the three known loci (ETM1, ETM2, or the 4p locus) (Kovach et al., 2001), it is likely that familial tremor has not only marked phenotypic but also genetic heterogeneity and that additional gene loci will be identified in the near future (Deng et al., 2007).

In 1935, Minor (1935), a Russian neurologist, not only stated that "the older one is, the more likely one displays tremor (ET)," but also suggested "that a factor for longevity was also contained in the tremor gamete." In support of the latter hypothesis, he offered the description of 51 cases of "hereditary tremor" associated with longevity. The longevity was based on patients' parents and grandparents usually being older than 70 years. His "control group" consisted of 11 cases of parkinsonism in which "no example of longevity was found out." However, the author did not state who in the ET families had tremor, and he did not provide any details on his parkinsonian patients (clinical features, ages of the subjects and relatives), and normal controls were not examined. Supporting the clinical observation that patients with ET live longer than a controlled population, Jankovic and colleagues (1995a) found that parents of patients with ET who had tremor (presumably ET) lived on the average 9.2 years longer than did parents without tremor. The association of familial tremor with significantly increased longevity suggests that familial tremor confers some antiaging influence. Alternatively, patients with ET might have an underlying personality trait that encourages dietary, occupational, and physical habits that promote longevity. Furthermore, the small amounts of alcohol to calm the tremor might prolong life; and finally, the tremor itself might be viewed as a form of exercise that would have long-standing beneficial effects on general health. Despite the overwhelming evidence that ET is of genetic origin, some researchers have suggested that environmental factors might also play a role, particularly since concordance among monozygotic twins is only 60% (Louis, 2001; Tanner et al., 2001). However, in another study involving 92 twins with ET from the Danish twin registry, the concordance rate was 93% among monozygotic twins and 29% among dizygotic twins when the Tremor Research and Investigation Group consensus criteria were used (Lorenz et al., 2004).

## Treatment

In designing protocols to study the effects of a therapeutic intervention on tremor-related functional impairment and on the mean amplitude (and frequency) of tremor, it is important to take into account the marked intraindividual and interindividual and diurnal variations in physiologic and pathologic tremors (van Hilten et al., 1991). Factors such as anxiety, caffeine or alcohol intake, drugs, and even temperature (Lakie et al., 1994) can affect hour-to-hour variations in the amplitude of tremor. Even without tremor, the ET amplitude may vary by 30% to 50% from hour to hour (Koller and Royse, 1986). The antitremor drugs exert their ameliorating effects by reducing tremor amplitude without any effect on tremor frequency. Reduction of tremor amplitude, however, does not always translate into improvement in function. There are currently no uniformly accepted ET rating scales, but the Unified Tremor Rating Assessment developed by the Tremor Research and Investigation Group (Jankovic et al., 1996; Ondo et al., 2000) and the Tremor Rating Scale developed by the Tremor Research Group (Tintner and Tremor Research Group, 2004) have been used in several studies.

The treatment of postural tremor depends largely on its severity; many patients require nothing more than simple reassurance. Most patients who are referred to a neurologist, however, have troublesome tremors that require pharmacologic or surgical treatments (Ondo and Jankovic, 1996; Bain, 1997; Lyons et al., 2003). The large-amplitude and slow-frequency postural tremors usually do not respond to any pharmacologic therapy. Since alcohol reduces the amplitude of ET in about two thirds of patients, some use it regularly for its calming effect, and some use it prophylactically—for example, before an important engagement at which the presence of tremor could be a source of embarrassment. Although evidence concerning the risk of alcoholism among ET patients is contradictory, regular use of alcohol to treat ET is inadvisable. The mechanism by which alcohol reduces tremor (effective blood level is only <30 mg %) is unknown, but it is thought to act centrally, since infusion of alcohol into the brachial artery of a tremulous arm is ineffective (Growdon et al., 1975). Furthermore, the amplitude of the central but not peripheral components of ET is decreased after alcohol consumption (Zeuner et al., 2003a). Alcohol is known to affect multiple neurotransmitters, and it might stabilize neuronal membranes by potentiating GABA receptor–mediated chloride influx. A pilot trial ($n = 12$) of 1-octanol, a food additive approved by the FDA that was previously demonstrated to suppress harmaline tremor, found that it significantly decreased amplitude of ET for about 90 minutes after oral dose of 1 mg/kg (Bushara et al., 2004). The benefits and tolerance (except for unusual taste) of this drug were demonstrated in an open-label trial at doses up to 64 mg/kg (Shill et al., 2004).

Propranolol, a β-adrenergic blocker, remains the most effective drug for the treatment of ET and enhanced physiologic tremors, but other beta blockers may also ameliorate postural tremor (Caccia et al., 1989; Calzetti et al., 1990; Koller et al., 2000) (Table 19-4). Propranolol is less effective in head tremor than hand tremor (Calzetti et al., 1992). Although a central mechanism of action has been suggested for this group of drugs, some beta blockers exert potent antitremor activity even though they are not lipid soluble and hence do not cross the blood-brain barrier. This suggests that the therapeutic effect of beta blockers may be mediated, at least in part, by the peripheral β-adrenergic receptors (Guan and Peroutka, 1990). The major side effects of propranolol and, to a lesser degree, other beta blockers include fatigability, sedation, depression, and sexual impotence. A critical review of 42 articles, based on controlled trials, concluded that despite the conventional wisdom, "there is no significant increased risk of depressive symptoms and only small increased risk of fatigue and sexual dysfunction" associated with beta blocker therapy (Ko et al., 2002). These drugs are contraindicated in the presence of asthma, second-degree atrioventricular block, and insulin-dependent diabetes. Contrary to traditional recommendations, they may be used safely in patients with stable congestive heart failure due to left ventricular systolic dysfunction (Packer et al., 1999). The efficacy of sotalol, a nonselective β-antagonist, in reducing ET is comparable to that of propranolol and atenolol, even though both atenolol and sotalol have very low lipid solubility and therefore act mainly through peripheral mechanisms (Leigh et al., 1983). Arotinolol, an alpha and beta blocker that is used as an antiobesity drug, was found to be as effective as propranolol in a randomized crossover study (Lee et al., 2003).

Table 19-4 Beta blockers in essential tremor

| Generic Name | Maintenance Dose | Lipid Solubility | Efficacy |
|---|---|---|---|
| Propranolol | 80–240 BID | +++ | +++ |
| Sotalol | 80–160 BID | + | +++ |
| Metoprolol | 100–200 BID | ++ | ++ |
| Timolol | 10–20 BID | ++ | + |
| Nadolol | 80–240 QD | 0 | ++ |
| Atenolol | 50–100 QD | 0 | ++ |
| Pindolol | 10–30 BID | ++ | 0 |

The antitremor effect of primidone has been confirmed by several open trials and placebo-controlled studies (Koller and Royse, 1986). By starting primidone at a very low dose (25 mg at bedtime), the occasional idiosyncratic acute, toxic side effects (nausea, vomiting, sedation, confusion, and ataxia) can be prevented. Since there is little or no correlation between blood levels and tremolytic effects, the daily dosage should be gradually increased over a period of several weeks until the optimal therapeutic response is achieved. Dosages above 250 mg per day are only rarely necessary. The antitremor effect of primidone is largely attributed to the parent compound rather than to its metabolites, phenylethylmalonamide (PEMA) or phenobarbital (Sasso et al., 1991). In one study (Koller and Royse, 1986), primidone alone was found to decrease tremor more than did propranolol alone, but a combination of the two drugs might be more efficacious than either drug alone. In a double-blind, placebo-controlled, crossover study, Gorman and colleagues (1986) found that both propranolol and primidone significantly reduced tremor compared to placebo. There is no evidence that either one of these primary anti-ET drugs is more efficacious than the other, but acute adverse effects with primidone and chronic side effects of propranolol limit therapy. The combination of the two drugs might be more efficacious than monotherapy (Koller and Royse, 1986). Although the benefits are usually maintained, the dosages might have to be increased after the first year to sustain the antitremor effectiveness. A double-blind study of 87 patients with ET, however, showed that low doses of primidone (250 mg per day) were as effective as, or more effective than, high doses (750 mg per day) (Serrano-Duenas, 2003).

In addition to beta blockers and primidone, the benzodiazepine drugs, such as diazepam, lorazepam, clonazepam, and alprazolam (Gunal et al., 2000), as well as barbiturates, also may have some ameliorating effects on ET or its variants (Ondo and Jankovic, 1996). In a double-blind, crossover, placebo-controlled study, 22 patients with ET received in random order alprazolam, acetazolamide, primidone, and placebo for 4 weeks, each separated by a 2-week washout period. The study demonstrated that alprazolam was superior to placebo and equipotent to primidone, whereas there was no statistically significant difference between acetazolamide and placebo (Gunal et al., 2000). The mean effective daily dose of alprazolam was 0.75 mg, and no troublesome side effects were reported by the patients who took alprazolam. Clonazepam was shown to be ineffective in controlling ET in one double-blind study, but at a mean dose of 2.2 mg per day, it improved kinetic tremor (Biary and Koller, 1987). Methazolamide (Neptazane), a sulfonamide that is used in the treatment of glaucoma, was reported to be effective in the treatment of ET (Muenter et al., 1991). Ten of 28 patients apparently achieved moderate to complete relief of their tremor. The average maintenance dose was 129 mg per day, and reported side effects included sedation, nausea, epigastric discomfort, and parasthesias. Aplastic anemia, the most feared complication, did not occur during the 6-month (10 weeks to 29 months) follow-up. The beneficial effects of methazolamide suggested by this open trial, however, could not be confirmed by a double-blind controlled study (Busenbark et al., 1993). Although our personal experience with this drug has been disappointing, Jankovic (personal observations) found that up to 10% to 20% of patients who were previously unresponsive to other antitremor treatments noted a marked improvement in their tremor with methazolamide. Flunarizine, a calcium channel blocker, was reported to improve ET in 13 of 15 patients (Biary and Deeb, 1991). This drug, however, is not available for use in the United States, and it can produce parkinsonism and tardive dyskinesia. Another calcium channel blocker, nimodipine at 120 mg per day, was found to improve ET in 8 of 15 patients who completed a double-blind, placebo-controlled trial (Biary et al., 1995).

Despite some encouraging results with gabapentin based on pilot studies, subsequent double-blind controlled studies showed mixed results (Louis, 1999), ranging from no benefit (Pahwa et al., 1998) to modest improvement (Ondo et al., 2000) to a marked benefit comparable to that obtained with propranolol (Gironell et al., 1999). Topiramate, a broad-spectrum anticonvulsant, has also been reported to reduce ET in a double-blind, placebo-controlled trial at 400 mg per day dose (Connor, 2002). Although well tolerated, topiramate may cause parasthesias and weight loss and may adversely affect cognition (Thompson et al., 2000). Some patients who are unresponsive to conventional treatments do improve even with low-dose (50 mg per day) topiramate (Gatto et al., 2003). In a multicenter, double-blind, placebo-controlled trial involving 208 patients (topiramate, 108; placebo, 100) the final visit score (last observation carried forward) was lower in the topiramate group than in the placebo group ($P < .001$) (Ondo et al., 2006). The mean percentage improvement in overall Tremor Rating Scale scores was 29% with topiramate at a mean final dose of 292 mg per day and 16% with placebo ($P < .001$), and topiramate was associated with greater improvement in function and disability ($P = .001$). The most common adverse effects were parasthesias (28%), weight loss (22%), and taste perversion (19%), but only the following adverse effects resulted in discontinuation of the drug: paresthesia (5%), nausea (3%), concentration/attention difficulty (3%), and somnolence (3%). Overall, adverse events were treatment-limiting in 31.9% of topiramate patients and 9.5% of placebo patients. Thus, this multicenter study showed that topiramate was effective in the treatment of ET with an acceptable tolerability profile. In a pilot, open-label, crossover trial designed to compare zonisamide and arotinolol in 14 patients with ET using the Fahn-Tolosa-Marin clinical rating scale at baseline and 2 weeks after administration of each drug, both drugs were found to have significant and equal antitremor effect, but zonisamide was more effective for voice, face, tongue, and head tremors (Morita et al., 2005). Levetiracetam, another antiepileptic, was shown to have a significant antitremor effect in one double-blind, placebo-controlled trial at 1000 mg as a single dose (Bushara et al., 2005) but not in other studies (Handforth and Martin, 2004; Ondo et al., 2004).

Mirtazapine has been reported to improve rest tremor (Pact and Giduz, 1999), but in a double-blind, placebo-controlled trial, the drug was not found to exert a significant benefit in ET (Pahwa and Lyons, 2003). Finally, clozapine has been found to be effective in selected drug-resistant patients with ET (Ceravolo et al., 1999). Gabapentin (Onofrj et al., 1998); levodopa (Wills et al., 1999), primidone, clonazepam, and phenobarbital seem to be particularly useful in patients with orthostatic tremor (Cabrera-Valdivia et al., 1991; FitzGerald and Jankovic, 1991). Despite earlier reports, amantadine has not been found effective in patients with ET

in a randomized, placebo-controlled trial, and in some patients, it actually exacerbated the postural tremor (Gironell et al., 2006).

Other treatment modalities for postural tremors include injections of BTX into muscles that are involved in the production of the oscillatory movement and various surgical approaches. In one open trial of BTX treatment, 67% of 51 patients with various disabling tremors noted at least some improvement (Jankovic and Schwartz, 1991). The average duration of improvement was 10.5 weeks, and side effects were chiefly related to local muscle weakness; 40% of 42 patients who were injected in the neck muscles to control head tremor and 60% of 10 patients who were injected in the forearm muscles to control hand tremor improved. Other studies have demonstrated the usefulness of BTX in the treatment of hand tremor (Trosch and Pullman, 1994). A double-blind, placebo-controlled trial has demonstrated a mild to moderate efficacy of BTX injections in patients with severe hand ET (Jankovic et al., 1996) and in patients with ET involving the head (Pahwa et al., 1995; Wissel et al., 1997). Although in one study, only 20% to 30% of patients with voice tremor were found to benefit from vocal cord injections of BTX, a majority of patients benefited from a subjective reduction in vocal effort that might have been attributable to reduced laryngeal airway resistance (Warrick et al., 2000). BTX may also be effective in primary writing tremor, although a specially designed writing device might be a simpler and at least as effective treatment (Espay et al., 2005).

Peripheral deafferentiation with anesthetic is currently being re-explored as a potential treatment of focal dystonia and tremor (Rondot et al., 1968; Pozos and Iaizzo, 1992; Kaji et al., 1995). An injection of 5 to 10 mL of 0.5% lidocaine into the target muscle not only improved focal dystonia, but also reduced the amplitude of the postural tremor. This short effect (<24 hours) can be extended for up to several weeks if ethanol is injected simultaneously (Kaji, personal communication). In a study of 10 patients with ET, Gironell and colleagues (2002) reported a transient (<1 hour) improvement in tremor after transient magnetic stimulation of the cerebellum.

The neurosurgical treatments, including DBS, that were discussed in the section on rest tremors may also be efficacious in patients with action hand tremors (Benabid et al., 1991; Blond et al., 1992; Deiber et al., 1993; Jankovic et al., 1995b; Koller et al., 1997), head tremors (Koller et al., 1999), and even task-specific tremors (Racette et al., 2001). It is of interest that cerebellar lesions can abolish ET, but it is unlikely that this observation will lead to surgically induced cerebellar lesions as a therapeutic modality in patients with ET (Dupuis et al., 1989). On the other hand, chronic cortical stimulation has been reported to improve contralateral action tremor (Nguyen et al., 1998). The observation that muscimol injection into the Vim thalamus in patients with ET suggests that GABA agonists might be useful in the treatment of ET (Pahapill et al., 1999). On the basis of the observation that vagus nerve stimulation has a nonspecific calming effect in treated epileptics and that it suppresses harmaline-induced tremor in rats (Handforth and Krahl, 2001), a multicenter trial was conducted to study the effects of vagus nerve stimulation in patients with essential and parkinsonian tremor, but no meaningful benefit was demonstrated (Handforth et al., 2003).

# KINETIC TREMORS

## Diagnosis

Kinetic tremor is typically associated with lesions or diseases that involve the cerebellum or its outflow pathways. The term *kinetic tremor* more accurately describes the oscillation occurring with limb movement than does the classic term *intention tremor*, which is ambiguous because it implies tremors that are present when "contemplating, initiating, performing, or completing a movement" (Lou and Jankovic, 1993). It is important to recognize that kinetic tremor is not simply a consequence of cerebellar ataxia (Diener and Dichgans, 1992), hypotonia, dysmetria, or dysdiadochokinesia but that the different motor disorders may coexist, often causing severe functional disability (Sabra and Hallett, 1984). Although kinetic tremor was traditionally considered a predominantly proximal tremor, using wrist (distal) or whole-arm (proximal) visually guided tracking in patients with multiple sclerosis showed a major frequency component at 4 to 5 Hz, most of the action tremor being distal rather than proximal (Liu et al., 1999).

In addition to this action, kinetic tremor patients with cerebellar lesions often exhibit postural tremors and titubation. The term *titubation* simply refers to a rhythmic oscillation of the head or trunk, presumably caused by hypotonia of the axial muscles. Kinetic cerebellar outflow tremor might be a component of the thalamic ataxia syndrome characterized in addition to the tremor by contralateral ataxia, hemisensory loss, and transient hemiparesis caused by a lesion in the mid to posterior thalamus involving the dentatorubrothalamic and ascending sensory pathways (Solomon et al., 1994). Kinetic terminal and postural tremors have been reported to result from repetitive transcranial magnetic stimulation, possibly by interfering with cerebellar inflow to the motor cortex (Topka et al., 1999). Although kinetic tremors are more difficult to assess than are ET or PD tremors, by using handwriting, spirals, and other tests, objective assessments of kinetic tremors, such as those seen in multiple sclerosis, can be reliably obtained (Alusi et al., 2000). In a study of 100 patients with definite multiple sclerosis, Alusi, Worthington, and colleagues (2001) found 58 with tremor, but it was symptomatic in only 38 and incapacitating in 10. The authors concluded that multiple sclerosis tremors are usually related to involvement of the cerebellum.

## Treatment

Some causes of tremor, such as alcohol, phenytoin, and valproate toxicity (Nouzeilles et al., 1999) and cerebellar tumors and abscesses are specifically treatable. Tremor and ataxia in such cases can resolve after the underlying cause is removed. Some kinetic tremors can be reduced by attaching weights to the wrist, but this method provides only limited improvement in function (Aisen et al., 1993).

No drugs have been shown to reduce cerebellar tremor satisfactorily and reproducibly. Isoniazid was initially thought to improve cerebellar, postural tremor more than kinetic tremor (Sabra and Hallett, 1984), but the results of a double-blind trial were disappointing (Hallett et al., 1991). Sechi and colleagues (1989) reported that carbamazepine was effective in the treatment of cerebellar tremor, possibly by reducing hyperactivity in thalamic neurons. Ten patients, seven with multiple sclerosis and three with cerebrovascular disease, were followed for 2 to 24 months. All patients improved on a clinical rating scale and by accelerometric recording when given carbamazepine, 400 to 600 mg daily. There was no improvement with placebo. Trelles and colleagues (1984) reported that cerebellar kinetic tremor secondary to multiple sclerosis and to olivopontocerebellar degeneration responded to clonazepam treatment at a daily dose of 8 to 15 mg. Glutethimide, a piperidinedione derivative with sedative and anticholinergic effects, has recently been reported to be effective at doses of 750 to 1250 mg per day in action tremors, including ET, cerebellar tremors, and midbrain tremors (Aisen et al., 1991). The encouraging results from this open trial await confirmation by properly designed controlled studies. Even if it is found to be effective, however, the potential side effects of glutethimide, including respiratory depression, aplastic anemia, and physical and psychological dependence, will limit its usefulness. Buspirone, a serotonin (5-hydroxytryptamine$_{1A}$) agonist was reported to be useful in some patients with mild cerebellar ataxia, but placebo-controlled study is needed before it can be concluded that this drug is effective in cerebellar ataxia or tremor (Lou et al., 1995). Baker and colleagues (2000) found that cannabinoids control tremor in a mouse model of multiple sclerosis; however, the effects of tetrahydrocannabinol in patients with cerebellar outflow tremor are unknown.

Other causes of kinetic tremor, phenomenologically similar to ET, include premutation in the fragile X gene (FMR1) (Hagerman et al., 2001; Berry-Kravis et al., 2003; Jacquemont et al., 2003, 2004; Leehey et al., 2003; Hagerman and Hagerman, 2004; Jacquemont et al., 2007). While normal individuals have about 30 CGG repeats in the FMR1 gene, the carriers of this permutation syndrome have 55 to 200 repeats. In addition to the ET-like tremor and ataxia, this fragile X–associated tremor/ataxia syndrome (FXTAS) is also associated with mild cognitive impairment with frontal executive deficit, parkinsonism, dysautonomia, erectile dysfunction, peripheral neuropathy, and generalized brain atrophy, regardless of family history. Unusual bilateral T2 middle cerebellar hyperintensities have been identified on magnetic resonance imaging in some cases (Leehey et al., 2003). Although some features overlap with those of multiple-system atrophy, FXTAS is a rare cause of multiple-system atrophy (Biancalana et al., 2005). Patients with FXTAS and parkinsonism have been found to have normal dopamine transporter as determined by CIT–single photon emission computed tomography, indicating a post-synaptic dopaminergic deficit (Ceravolo et al., 2005). Postmortem studies on brains of four elderly permutation carriers showed eosinophilic intranuclear inclusions in both neuronal and astrocytic nuclei throughout the brain, particularly involving the hippocampus (Greco et al., 2002). Subsequent neuropathologic studies of patients with FXTAS showed: (1) cerebral and cerebellar white matter disease with spongiosis in the middle cerebellar peduncles, (2) astrocytic pathology with enlarged inclusion-bearing astrocytes, and (3) intranuclear inclusions in the brain and spinal cord, including the cranial nerve nucleus XII (Greco et al., 2006). The number of inclusions seems to correlate with the number of CGG repeats. The inclusions contain a variety of proteins, such as RNA binding proteins, but ubiquinated

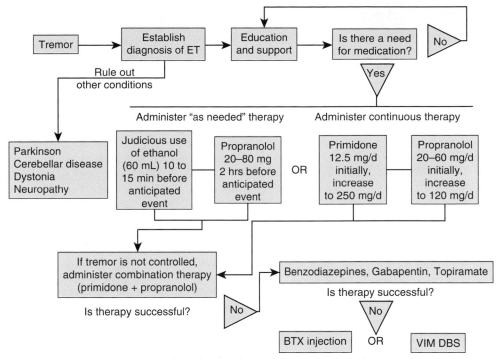

**Figure 19-3** Algorithm for the treatment of essential tremor.

proteins represent only a small portion of all the proteins, suggesting that breakdown of proteosomal degradation is not the main mechanism of the inclusions (Iwahashi et al., 2006). It has been postulated that premutation RNA is responsible for the observed neurodegeneration (Orr, 2004). Marked loss of Purkinje cells in the cerebellum, Purkinje axonal torpedoes, and Bergmann gliosis were also found. SCA12, a rare autosomal-dominant ataxia, may also present with ET-like tremor before other signs of ataxia become evident. This form of ataxia has been associated with CAG repeat expansion in the *PPP2R2B* gene (5q31–33) coding for protein phosphatase PP2A (Fujigasaki et al., 2001). The frequency of fragile X permutation, even in patients with tremor, parkinsonism, and ataxia, is so low that it is not cost-effective to routinely test for it even in an enriched movement disorders population (Arocena et al., 2004; Deng et al., 2004; Tan et al., 2004) Interestingly, the location of the CAG repeat expansion in the 5' region is similar to that of the CGG repeat in FMR1, in which an expansion results in CpG hypermethylation and disruption of transcription, resulting in the fragile X phenotype.

Stereotaxic thalamotomy has been reported to successfully relieve kinetic tremor in patients with multiple sclerosis and other etiologies (Andrew, 1984). Radiofrequency lesions in the Vim seem to provide the best control of tremor with the lowest risk of neurologic deficit (Speelman and Manen, 1984; Nagaseki et al., 1986; Alusi, Aziz et al., 2001), although thalamic DBS has also been reported to be useful in selected patients with cerebellar-outflow tremor due to multiple sclerosis or other causes (Whittle et al., 1998; Montgomery et al., 1999). A recent report of the Quality Standards Subcommittee of the American Academy of Neurology, based on a review of evidence-based publications, published the following practice parameters related to therapies for ET.

Propranolol and primidone reduce limb tremor (Level A); alprazolam, atenolol, gabapentin (monotherapy), sotalol, and topiramate are probably effective in reducing limb tremor (Level B); propranolol reduces head tremor (Level B); clonazepam, clozapine, nadolol, and nimodipine possibly reduce limb tremor (Level C); BTX type A may reduce limb, head, and voice tremor, but this treatment is limited by potential adverse effects (Level C); chronic DBS and thalamotomy are highly efficacious but potentially risky procedures (Level C); and there is insufficient evidence regarding surgical treatment of head and voice tremor and the use of gamma knife thalamotomy (Level U) (Zesiewicz et al., 2005) (Fig. 19-3).

## OTHER TREMORS

### Neuropathic Tremors

Tremor has been described in patients with various types of peripheral neuropathy (Said et al., 1982; Shahani, 1984). Distal postural tremor was noted in patients with chronic relapsing and dysgammaglobulinemic polyneuropathies (Bain et al., 1996). The amplitude was not related to the severity of weakness or proprioceptive sensory loss, and propranolol improved the tremor in some patients. Hereditary motor and sensory neuropathy is associated with tremor, clinically similar to ET, in nearly half of cases (Cardoso and Jankovic, 1993). The frequent association between tremor caused by peripheral nerve injury and reflex sympathetic dystrophy suggests that the sympathetic nervous system contributes to the pathogenesis of peripherally induced tremor (Jankovic and Van der Linden, 1988; Deuschl et al., 1991; Cardoso and Jankovic, 1995; Jankovic, 1994).

## Tremors Caused by Trauma or Stroke

Tremor can also occur after severe or even minimal head trauma (Biary et al., 1989; Goetz and Pappert, 1992; Jankovic, 1994; Krauss et al., 1995). Biary and colleagues (1989) described seven patients who developed postural and kinetic tremors involving various body parts up to several weeks after mild head injury without loss of consciousness. Ipsilateral predecussational dentatothalamic lesion was involved in the majority (56%) of 25 instances of severe posttraumatic tremor in 19 patients, followed by involvement of the contralateral predecussational dentatothalamic pathway (28%), dentate nucleus (4%), and thalamus (4%); no lesion was identified by neuroimaging in 2 (8%) patients (Krauss et al., 1995). Clonazepam was effective in reducing tremor in 3 patients, and propranolol was effective in 1. Posttraumatic midbrain tremor may improve with anticholinergic and dopaminergic drugs (Samie et al., 1990), but in general, this tremor only rarely responds satisfactorily to drug therapy. Many patients with posttraumatic tremors have benefited from Vim thalamotomy; additional patients may benefit from thalamic stimulation (Broggi et al., 1993). In addition to trauma, a variety of tremors can occur following ischemic or hemorrhagic strokes (Ferbert and Gerwig, 1993; Miwa et al., 1996).

Trauma can also cause injury to the peripheral nerves, producing a form of neuropathic tremor, which was discussed earlier. Traumatic neck injury may cause cervical radiculopathy, which may be associated with a postural tremor in the ipsilateral arm (Hashimoto et al., 2002). Loading and ischemic nerve block reduced the frequency of the tremor, suggesting a role of the mechanical reflex mechanism and stretch reflex loop in this peripherally induced tremor.

## Psychogenic Tremor

One of the most challenging tasks in the diagnosis of tremors is differentiating between psychogenic and neurogenic tremors. Koller and colleagues (1989) provided the following diagnostic criteria useful in the diagnosis of psychogenic tremors: (1) abrupt onset, (2) static course, (3) spontaneous remission, (4) difficulty in classifying (various combinations of rest, postural, and kinetic tremors), (5) selective disability, (6) changing amplitude and frequency, (7) unresponsiveness to antitremor drugs, (8) increasing of tremor with attention, (9) lessening of tremor with distractibility, (10) responsiveness to placebo, (11) absence of other neurologic signs, and  (12) remission with psychotherapy (Video 19-8). Deuschl, Koster, and colleagues (1998) found the following features particularly characteristic of psychogenic tremor: sudden onset and variable (rarely remitting) course, coactivation sign (fluctuations in muscle tone and in tremor during passive movements), and absent finger tremor. Although overt signs of hysteria were often lacking, evidence of depression and psychosomatic conditions were common. In another study of 70 patients with psychogenic tremor, 73% had an abrupt onset, and 46% had their maximal disability at onset (Kim et al., 1999). Additional features that were found helpful in confirming the diagnosis of psychogenic tremor included spread from a focal onset to generalized tremor, variability, and entrainment. Electrophysiologic studies are rarely helpful in differentiating organic tremor from psychogenic tremor

(McAuley et al., 1998). Using accelerometry, Zeuner and colleagues (2003b) demonstrated that in contrast to essential and parkinsonian tremor, patients with PT showed larger tremor frequency changes and higher individual variability while tapping. Longitudinal studies are needed to determine the natural history of psychogenic tremors. In one study, a 6-year follow-up of 64 patients with unexplained motor disorders, only 3 were later found to have an organic diagnosis (Crimlisk et al., 1998). In the Parkinson's Disease Center and Movement Disorders Clinic at the Baylor College of Medicine, psychogenic tremor is the most common of all psychogenic movement disorders, accounting for 4.1% of all patients (Jankovic and Thomas, 2006). Clinical information was obtained on 228 of 517 (44.1%) patients, who were followed for a mean of 3.4 ± 2.8 years. Among the 127 patients who were diagnosed with psychogenic tremor, 92 (72.4%) were female, the mean age at initial evaluation was 43.7 ± 14.1 years, and the mean duration of symptoms was 4.6 ± 7.6 years. The following clinical features were considered to be characteristic of psychogenic tremor: abrupt onset (78.7%), distractibility (72.4%), variable amplitude and frequency (62.2%), intermittent occurrence (35.4%), inconsistent movement (29.9%), and variable direction (17.3%). In the majority of patients, some precipitating event could be identified prior to the onset of tremor, including personal life stress (33.9%), physical trauma (23.6%), major illness (13.4%), surgery (9.4%), or reaction to a medical treatment or procedure (8.7%). Coexistent organic neurologic disorder was present in 37% of patients with psychogenic tremor; psychiatric comorbidities included depression in 50.7% and anxiety in 30.7%. Evidence of secondary gain was present in 32.3%, including maintenance of a disability status in 21.3%, pending compensation in 10.2%, and litigation in 9.4%. Improvement in tremor, reported on a global rating scale at last follow-up by 55.1%, was attributed chiefly to "effective treatment by physician" and "elimination of stressors." On the basis of the analysis of data in this largest longitudinal study of patients with psychogenic tremor, an accurate diagnosis should be based not only on exclusion of other causes but also be dependent on positive clinical criteria, the presence of which should avoid unnecessary investigation.

## Other Tremors

There are many other causes of tremors. The bobble-head doll syndrome is a form of slow (2- to 30Hz) oscillatory movement that is usually associated with cystic enlargement of the third ventricle, suprasellar arachnoid cysts, aqueductal stenosis, and other lesions involving the third ventricle (Goikhman, 1998; Bhattacharyya et al., 2003). Hereditary chin tremor, or hereditary geniospasm, is an autosomal-dominant disorder characterized by recurrent episodes of chin tremor (Soland et al.,  1996a) (Video 19-9). Usually a benign condition with a peak in mid-twenties (although it may be persistent in men), this condition has been mapped to a marker on chromosome 9q13–q21 (Jarman et al., 1997).

## References

Aisen ML, Arnold L, Baiges T, et al: The effect of mechanical damping loads on disabling action tremor. Neurology 1993;43:1346–1350.

Aisen ML, Holzer M, Rosen M, et al: Glutethimide treatment of disabling action tremor in patients with multiple sclerosis and traumatic brain injury. Arch Neurol 1991;48:513–515.

Alarcon F, Zijlmans JC, Duenas G, Cevallos N: Post-stroke movement disorders: Report of 56 patients. J Neurol Neurosurg Psychiatry 2004;75:1568–1574.

Alusi SH, Aziz TZ, Glickman S, et al: Stereotactic lesional surgery for the treatment of tremor in multiple sclerosis: A prospective case-controlled study. Brain 2001;124:1576–1589.

Alusi SH, Worthington J, Glickman S, et al: Evaluation of three different ways of assessing tremor in multiple sclerosis. J Neurol Neurosurg Psychiatry 2000;68:756–760.

Alusi SH, Worthington J, Glickman S, Bain PG: A study of tremor in mutiple sclerosis. Brain 2001;124:720–730.

Andrew J: Surgical treatment of tremor. In Findley LJ, Capildeo R (eds): Movement disorders: Tremor. New York, Oxford University Press, 1984, pp 339–351.

Antonini A, Moeller JR, Nakamura T, et al: The metabolic anatomy of tremor in Parkinson's disease. Neurology 1998;51:803–810.

Antonini A, Moresco RM, Gobbo C, et al: The status of dopamine nerve terminals in Parkinson's disease and essential tremor: A PET study with the tracer [11-C]FE-CIT. Neurol Sci 2001;22:47–48.

Arocena DG, Louis ED, Tassone F, et al: Screen for expanded FMR1 alleles in patients with essential tremor. Mov Disord 2004;19:930–933.

Askenasy JJM, Yahr MD: Parkinsonian tremor loses its alternating aspect during non-REM sleep and is inhibited by REM sleep. J Neurol Neurosurg Psychiatry 1990;53:749–753.

Aziz TZ, Peggs D, Sambrook MA, Crossman AR: Lesion of the subthalamic nucleus for the alleviation of 1-methyl-4-phenyl-1,2,3,6-tetrahydropyridine (MPTP)-induced parkinsonism in the primate. Mov Disord 1991;6:288–292.

Bain P: A combined clinical and neurophysiologic approach to the study of patients with tremor. J Neurol Neurosurg Psychiatry 1993;69:839–844.

Bain PG: The effectiveness of treatments for essential tremor. Neurologist 1997;3:305–321.

Bain PG, Britton TC, Jenkins IH, et al: Tremor associated with benign IgM paraproteinaemic neuropathy. Brain 1996;119:789–799.

Bain PG, Findley LJ, Atchison P, et al: Assessing tremor severity. J Neurol Neurosurg Psychiatry 1993;56:868–873.

Bain PG, Findley LJ, Britton TC, et al: Primary writing tremor. Brain 1995;118:1461–1472.

Bain PG, Findley LJ, Thompson PD, et al: A study of hereditary essential tremor. Brain 1994;117:805–824.

Baker D, Pryce G, Croxford JL, et al: Cannabinoids control spasticity and tremor in a multiple sclerosis model. Nature 2000;404:84–87.

Benabid AL, Koudsie A, Pollak P, et al: Future prospects of brain stimulation. Neurol Res 2000;22:237–246.

Benabid AL, Pollack P, Gao D, et al: Chronic electrical stimulation of the ventralis intermedius nucleus of the thalamus as a treatment of movement disorders. J Neurosurg 1996;84:203–214.

Benabid AL, Pollak P, Gervason C, et al: Long-term suppression of tremor by chronic stimulation of the ventral intermediate thalamic nucleus. Lancet 1991;1:403–406.

Benito-Leon J, Bermejo-Pareja F, Louis ED, Neurological Disorders in Central Spain (NEDICES) Study Group: Incidence of essential tremor in three elderly populations of central Spain. Neurology 2005;64:1721–1725.

Benito-Leon J, Rodriguez J, Orti-Pareja M, et al: Symptomatic orthostatic tremor in pontine lesions. Neurology 1997;49:1439–1441.

Benito-Leon J, Louis ED, Bermejo-Pareja F, Neurological Disorders in Central Spain Study Group: Elderly-onset essential tremor is associated with dementia. Neurology 2006a;66:1500–1505b.

Benito-Leon J, Louis ED, Bermejo-Pareja F, Neurological Disorders in Central Spain (NEDICES) Study Group: Population-based case-control study of cognitive function in essential tremor. Neurology 2006b;66:69–74a.

Bergman H, Feingold A, Nini A, et al: Physiological aspects of information processing in the basal ganglia of normal and parkinsonian primates. Trends Neurosci 1998;21:32–38.

Bergman H, Wichmann T, DeLong MR: Reversal of experimental parkinsonism by lesions of the subthalamic nucleus. Science 1990;249:1436–1438.

Berry-Kravis E, Lewin F, Wuu J, et al: Tremor and ataxia in fragile X premutation carriers: Blinded videotape study. Ann Neurol 2003;53:616–623.

Bertoli-Avella AM, Giroud-Benitez JL, Bonifati V, et al: Suggestive linkage to chromosome 19 in a large Cuban family with late-onset Parkinson's disease. Mov Disord 2003;18:1240–1249.

Bevan MD, Magill PJ, Terman D, et al: Move to the rhythm: Oscillations in the subthalamic nucleus-external globus pallidus network. Trends Neurosci 2002;25:525–531.

Bhattacharyya KB, Senapati A, Basu S, et al: Bobble-head doll syndrome: Some atypical features with a new lesion and review of the literature. Acta Neurol Scand 2003;108:216–220.

Biancalana V, Toft M, Le Ber I, et al: FMR1 premutations associated with fragile X-associated tremor/ataxia syndrome in multiple system atrophy. Arch Neurol 2005;62:962–966.

Biary N, Bahou Y, Sufi MA, et al: The effect of nimodipine on essential tremor. Neurology 1995;45:1523–1525.

Biary N, Cleeves L, Findley L, Koller W: Post-traumatic tremor. Neurology 1989;39:103–106.

Biary N, Deeb ASA: The effect of flunarizine on essential tremor. Neurology 1991;41:311–312.

Biary N, Koller W: Kinetic predominant essential tremor: Successful treatment with clonazepam. Neurology 1987;37:471–474.

Blond S, Caparros-Lefebvre D, Parker F, et al: Control of tremor and involuntary movement disorders by chronic stereotactic stimulation of the ventral intermediate thalamic nucleus. J Neurosurg 1992;77:62–68.

Boecker H, Wills AJ, Ceballos-Baumann A, et al: The effect of ethanol on alcohol-responsive essential tremor: A positron emission tomography study. Ann Neurol 1996;39:650–658.

Bonuccelli U, Ceravolo R, Salvetti S, et al: Clozapine in Parkinson's disease tremor: Effects of acute and chronic administration. Neurology 1997;49:1587–1590.

Boroojerdi B, Ferbert A, Foltys H, et al: Evidence for a non-orthostatic origin of orthostatic tremor. J Neurol Neurosurg Psychiatry 1999;66:284–288.

Bove M, Marinelli L, Avanzino L, et al: Posturographic analysis of balance control in patients with essential tremor. Mov Disord 2006;21:192–198.

Brin MF, Koller W: Epidemiology and genetics of essential tremor. Mov Disord 1998;13(suppl 3):55–63.

Brin MF, Lyons KE, Doucette J, et al: A randomized, double masked, controlled trial of botulinum toxin type A in essential hand tremor. Neurology 2001;56:1523–1528.

Britton TC, Thompson PD, Day BL, et al: Modulation of postural wrist tremors by magnetic stimulation of the motor cortex in patients with Parkinson's disease or essential tremor and in normal subjects mimicking tremor. Ann Neurol 1993;33:473–479.

Britton TC, Thompson PD, Day BL, et al: Rapid wrist movement in patients with essential tremor. The critical role of second agonist burst. Brain 1994;117:39–47.

Britton TC, Thompson PD, Rothwell JC, et al: "Resetting" of postural tremors at the wrist with mechanical stretches in Parkinson's disease, essential tremor, and normal subjects mimicking tremor. Ann Neurol 1992a;31:507–514.

Britton TC, Thompson PD, Van der Kamp W, et al: Primary orthostatic tremor: Current observations in six cases. J Neurol 1992b;239:209–217.

Broggi G, Brock S, Franzini A, Germiniani G: A case of posttraumatic tremor treated by chronic stimulation of the thalamus. Mov Disord 1993;8:206–208.

Brooks D, Playford ED, Ibanez V, et al: Isolated tremor and disruption of the nigrostriatal dopaminergic system: An 18F-dopa PET study. Neurology 1992;42:1554–1560.

Brown P: New clinical sign for orthostatic tremor. Lancet 1995; 346:306–307.

Brown P: Oscillatory nature of human basal ganglia activity: Relationship to the pathophysiology of Parkinson's disease. Mov Disord 2003;18:357–363.

Bucher SF, Seelos KC, Dodel RC, et al: Activation mapping in essential tremor with functional magnetic resonance imaging. Ann Neurol 1997;41:32–40.

Busenbark K, Barnes P, Lyons K, et al: Accuracy of reported family histories of essential tremor. Neurology 1996;47:264–265.

Busenbark K, Pahwa R, Hubble J, et al: Double-blind controlled study of methazolamide in the treatment of essential tremor. Neurology 1993;43:1045–1047.

Busenbark KL, Nash J, Nash S, et al: Is essential tremor benign? Neurology 1991;41:1982–1983.

Bushara KO, Goldstein SR, Grimes GJ Jr, et al: Pilot trial of 1-octanol in essential tremor. Neurology 2004;62:122–124.

Bushara KO, Malik T, Exconde RE: The effect of levetiracetam on essential tremor. Neurology 2005;64:1078–1080.

Cabrera-Valdivia F, Jimenez-Jimenez FJ, Albea EG, et al: Orthostatic tremor: Successful treatment with phenobarbital. Clin Neuropharmacol 1991;14:438–441.

Caccia MR, Osio M, Galimberti V, et al: Propranolol, clonidine, urapidil and trazodone infusion in essential tremor: A double-blind crossover trial. Acta Neurol Scand 1989;79:379–383.

Calzetti S, Sasso E, Baratti M, Fava R: Clinical and computer-based assessment of long-term efficacy of propranolol in essential tremor. Acta Neurol Scand 1990;81:392–396.

Calzetti S, Sasso E, Negrotti A, et al: Effect of propranolol in head tremor: quantitative study following single-dose and sustained drug administration. Clin Neuropharmacol 1992;15:470–476.

Caparros-Lefebvre D, Ruchoux MM, Blond S, et al: Long-term thalamic stimulation in Parkinson's disease: Postmortem anatomoclinical study. Neurology 1994;44:1856–1860.

Cardoso F, Jankovic J: Myorhythmia: A form of segmental myoclonus. Neurology 1996;46:A261.

Cardoso FC, Jankovic J: Hereditary motor-sensory neuropathy and movement disorders. Muscle Nerve 1993;16:904–910.

Cardoso FC, Jankovic J: Post-traumatic peripherally-induced tremor and parkinsonism. Arch Neurol 1995;52:263–270.

Carrea RME, Mettler FA: Function of the primate brachium conjunctivum and related structures. J Comp Neurol 1955;102: 151–322.

Ceravolo R, Antonini A, Volterrani D, et al: Dopamine transporter imaging study in parkinsonism occurring in fragile X premutation carriers. Neurology 2005;65:1971–1973.

Ceravolo R, Salvetti S, Piccini P, et al: Acute and chronic effects of clozapine in essential tremor. Mov Disord 1999;14:468–472.

Chan J, Brin MF, Fahn S: Idiopathic cervical dystonia: Clinical characteristics. Mov Disord 1991; 6:119–126.

Chatterjee A, Jurewicz EC, Applegate LM, Louis ED: Personality in essential tremor: Further evidence of non-motor manifestations of the disease. J Neurol Neurosurg Psychiatry 2004;75:958–961.

Chouinard S, Louis ED, Fahn S: Agreement among movement disorder specialists on the clinical diagnosis of essential tremor. Mov Disord 1997;12:973–976.

Cohen O, Pullman S, Jurewicz E, et al: Rest tremor in patients with essential tremor: Prevalence, clinical correlates, and electrophysiologic characteristics. Arch Neurol 2003;60:405–410.

Cole JD, Philip HI, Sedgwick EM: Stability and tremor in the fingers associated with cerebellar hemisphere and cerebellar tract lesions in man. J Neurol Neurosurg Psychiatry 1988;51:1558–1568.

Connor GS: A double-blind placebo-controlled trial of topiramate treatment for essential tremor. Neurology 2002;59:132–134.

Conway D, Bain PG, Warner TT, et al: Linkage analysis with chromosome 9 marker in herediatry essential tremor. Mov Disord 1993; 8:374–376.

Crimlisk HL, Bhatia K, Cope H, et al: Slater revisited: 6-year follow-up study of patients with medically unexplained motor symptoms. Br Med J 1998;31:582–586.

Dana CL: Hereditary tremor, a hitherto undescribed form of motor neurosis. Am J Med Sci 1887;94:386–393.

Danek A: Geniospasm: Hereditary chin trembling. Mov Disord 1993;8:335–338.

Dash MS: Role of peripheral inputs in cerebellar tremor. Mov Disord 1995;10:622–629.

Deiber M-P, Pollack P, Passingham R, et al: Thalamic stimulation and suppression of parkinsonian tremor: Evidence of cerebellar deactivation using positron emission tomography. Brain 1993;116: 267–279.

DeLong MR: Primate models of movement disorders of basal ganglia origin. Trends Neurosci 1990;13:281–285.

Deng H, Le W, Jankovic J: Premutation alleles associated with Parkinson disease and essential tremor. JAMA 2004;292:1685–1686.

Deng H, Le W, Jankovic J: Genetics of essential tremor. Brain 2007 (in press).

Deng H, Le WD, Guo Y, et al: Extended study of A265G variant of HS1BP3 in essential tremor and Parkinson's disease. Neurology 2005;65:651–652.

Deng H, Xie WJ, Le WD. et al: Genetic analysis of the GABRAI gene in patients with essential tremor. Neurosci Lett 2006;401:16–19.

Deuschl G, Bain P, Brin M, Ad Hoc Scientific Committee: Consensus statement of the Movement Disorder Society on Tremor. Mov Disord 1998;13(suppl 3):2–23.

Deuschl G, Blumberg H, Lücking CH: Tremor in reflex sympathetic dystrophy. Arch Neurol 1991;48:1247–1252.

Deuschl G, Elble RJ: The pathophysiology of essential tremor. Neurology 2000(suppl 4):S14–S20.

Deuschl G, Heinen F, Guschlbauer B, et al: Hand tremor in patients with spasmodic torticollis. Mov Disord 1997;12:547–552.

Deuschl G, Koster B, Lücking CH, Scheidt C: Diagnostic and pathophysiologic aspects of psychogenic tremors. Mov Disord 1998;13:294–302.

Deuschl G, Raethjen J, Lindemann M, Krack P: The pathophysiology of tremor. Muscle Nerve 2001;24:716–735.

Deuschl G, Wenzelburger R, Lögler K, et al: Essential tremor and cerebellar dysfunction: Clinical and kinematic analysis of intention tremor. Brain 2000;123:1568–1580.

Diener HC, Dichgans J: Pathophysiology of cerebellar ataxia. Mov Disord 1992;7:95–109.

Dogali M, Fazzini E, Kolodny E, et al: Stereotactic ventral pallidotomy for Parkinson's disease. Neurology 1995;45:753–761.

Dogu O, Sevim S, Camdeviren H, et al: Prevalence of essential tremor: Door-to-door neurologic exams in Mersin Province, Turkey. Neurology 2003;61:1804–1806.

Dubinsky R, Hallett M: Glucose hypermetabolism of the inferior olive in patients with essential tremor [abstract]. Ann Neurol 1987;22:118.

Dupuis MJM, Delwaide PJ, Boucquey D, Gonsette RE: Homolateral disappearance of essential tremor after cerebellar stroke. Mov Disord 1989;4:183–187.

Dürr A, Stevanin G, Jedynak CP, et al: Familial essential tremor and idiopathic torsion dystonia are different genetic entities. Neurology 1993;43;2212–2214.

Elble RJ: Diagnostic criteria for essential tremor and differential diagnosis. Neurology 2000a;54(suppl 4):S2–S6.

Elble RJ: Essential tremor frequency decreases with time. Neurology 2000b;55:1547–1551.

Elble RJ: Origins of tremor. Lancet 2000c;355:1113–1114.

Elble RJ: Essential tremor is a monosymptomatic disorder. Mov Disord 2002;17:633–637.

Elble RJ, Brilliant M, Leffler K, Higgins C: Quantification of essential tremor in writing and drawing. Mov Disord 1996;11:70–78.

Elble RJ, Higgins C, Leffler K, Hughes L: Factors influencing the amplitude and frequency of essential tremor. Mov Disord 1994; 9:589–596.

Elble RJ, Koller WC: The measurement and quantification of tremor. In Elble RJ, Koller WC (eds): Tremor. Baltimore, Johns Hopkins University Press, 1990, pp 10–36, 54–89.

Elble RJ, Moody C, Higgins C: Primary writing tremor: A form of focal dystonia? Mov Disord 1990;5:118–126.

Espay AJ, Hung SW, Sanger TD, et al: A writing device improves writing in primary writing tremor. Neurology 2005;64:1648–1650.

Fahn S, Tolosa E, Marin C: Clinical rating scale for tremor. In Jankovic J, Tolosa E (eds): Parkinson's Disease and Movement Disorders, 2nd ed. Baltimore, Williams & Wilkins, 1993, pp 271–280.

Farrer M, Gwinn-Hardy K, Muenter M, et al: A chromosome 4p haplotype segregating with Parkinson's disease and postural tremor. Hum Mol Genet 1999;8:81–85.

Farrer M, Kachergus J, Forno L, et al: Comparison of kindreds with parkinsonism and alpha-synuclein genomic multiplications. Ann Neurol 2004;55:174–179.

Ferbert A, Gerwig M: Tremor due to stroke. Mov Disord 1993;8:179–182.

Findley LJ: Tremors: Differential diagnosis and pharmacology. In Jankovic J, Tolosa E (eds): Parkinson's Disease and Movement Disorders, 2nd ed. Baltimore, Williams & Wilkins, 1993, pp 293–314.

Findley LJ, Koller WC: Definitions and behavioral classifications. In Findley LJ, Koller W (eds): Handbook of Tremor Disorders. New York, Marcel Dekker, 1995, pp 1–5.

Finkel MF: Pramipexole is a possible effective treatment for primary orthostatic tremor (shaky leg syndrome). Arch Neurol 2000;57:1519–1520.

FitzGerald PM, Jankovic J: Orthostatic tremor: An association with essential tremor. Mov Disord 1991;6:60–64.

Flament D, Hore J: Movement and electromyographic disorders associated with cerebellar dysmetria. J Neurophysiol 1986;55:1221–1233.

Forssberg H, Ingvarsson PE, Iwasaki N, et al: Action tremor during object manipulation in Parkinson's disease. Mov Disord 2000;15:244–254.

Fox MW, Ahlskog JE, Kelly PJ: Stereotactic ventrolateralis thalamotomy for medically refractory tremor in post-levodopa era Parkinson's disease patients. J Neurosurg 1991;75:723–730.

Friedman JH, Koller WC, Lannon MC, et al: Benztropine versus clozapine for the treatment of tremor in Parkinson's disease. Neurology 1997;48:1077–1081.

Frima N, Grunewald RA: Abnormal vibration induced illusion of movement in essential tremor: Evidence for abnormal muscle spindle afferent function. J Neurol Neurosurg Psychiatry 2005;76:55–57.

Fujigasaki H, Verma IC, Camuzat A, et al: SCA12 is a rare locus for autosomal dominant cerebellar ataxia: A study of an Indian family. Ann Neurol 2001;49:117–121.

Fung VSC, Sauner D, Day BL: A dissociation between subjective and objective unsteadiness in primary orthostatic tremor. Brain 2001;124:322–330.

Gabellini AS, Martinelli P, Gulli MR, et al: Orthostatic tremor: Essential and symptomatic cases. Acta Neurol Scand 1990;81:113–117.

Gatto EM, Roca MC, Raina G, Micheli F: Low doses of topiramate are effective in essential tremor: A report of three cases. Clin Neuropharmacol 2003;26:294–296.

Geraghty JJ, Jankovic J, Zetusky WJ: Association between essential tremor and Parkinson's disease. Ann Neurol 1985;17:329–333.

Gerschlager W, Munchau A, Katzenschlager R, et al: Natural history and syndromic associations of orthostatic tremor: A review of 41 patients. Mov Disord 2004;19:788–795.

Gimenez-Roldan S, Mateo D: Cinnarizine-induced parkinsonism: Susceptibility related to aging and essential tremor. Clin Neuropharmacol 1991;14:156–164.

Gironell A, Kulisevsky J, Barbanoj M, et al: A randomized placebo-controlled comparative trial of gabapentin and propranolol in essential tremor. Arch Neurol 1999;56:475–480.

Gironell A, Kulisevsky J, Lorenzo J, et al: Transcranial magnetic stimulation of the cerebellum in essential tremor: A controlled study. Arch Neurol 2002;59:413–417.

Gironell A, Kulisevsky J, Pascual-Sedano B, Flamarich D: Effect of amantadine in essential tremor: A randomized, placebo-controlled trial. Mov Disord 2006;21:441–445.

Goetz CG, Pappert EJ: Trauma and movement disorders. Neurol Clin 1992;10:907–919.

Goikhman I, Zelnik N, Peled N, Michowitz S: Bobble-head doll syndrome: A surgically treatable condition manifested as a rare movement disorder. Mov Disord 1998;13:192–194.

Gomez-Mancilla B, Latulippe J-F, Boucher R, Bedard PJ: Effect of ethosuximide on rest tremor in the MPTP monkey model. Mov Disord 1992;7:137–141.

Gorman WP, Cooper R, Pocock P, Campbell MJ: A comparison of primidone, propranolol, and placebo in essential tremor, using quantitative analysis. J Neurol Neurosurg Psychiatry 1986;49:64–68.

Goyal M, Versnick E, Tuite P, et al: Hypertrophic olivary degeneration: Metaanalysis of the temporal evolution of MR findings. Am J Neuroradiol 2000;21:1073–1077.

Greco CM, Berman RF, Martin RM, et al: Neuropathology of fragile X-associated tremor/ataxia syndrome (FXTAS). Brain 2006;129:243–255.

Greco CM, Hagerman RJ, Tassone F, et al: Neuronal intranuclear inclusions in a new cerebellar tremor/ataxia syndrome among fragile X carriers. Brain 2002;125:1760–1771.

Gresty M, Buckwell D: Spectral analysis of tremor: Understanding the results. J Neurol Neurosurg Psychiatry 1990;53:976–981.

Grosset DG, Lees AJ: Long duration asymmetric postural tremor in the development of Parkinson's disease. J Neurol Neurosurg Psychiatry 2005;76:9.

Growdon JH, Shahani BT, Young RR: The effect of alcohol on essential tremor. Neurology 1975;25:259–262.

Guan X-M, Peroutka SJ: Basic mechanisms of action of drugs used in the treatment of essential tremor. Clin Neuropharmacol 1990;13:210–223.

Gulcher JR, Jónsson P, Kong A, et al: Mapping of a familial essential tremor gene, FET1, to chromosome 3q13. Nat Genet 1997;17:84–87.

Gunal DI, Afsar N, Bekiroglu N, Aktan S: New alternative agents in essential tremor; double-blind placebo-controlled study of alprazolam and acetazolamide Neurol Sci 2000;21:315–317.

Haerer AF, Anderson DW, Schoenberg BS: Prevalence of essential tremor: Results from the Copiah County study. Arch Neurol 1982;39:750–751.

Hagerman PJ, Hagerman RJ: The fragile-X premutation: A maturing perspective. Am J Hum Genet 2004;74:805–816.

Hagerman RJ, Leehey M, Heinrichs W, et al: Intention tremor, parkinsonism, and generalized brain atrophy in male carriers of fragile X. Neurology 2001;57:127–130.

Hallett M: Classification and treatment of tremor. JAMA 1991;266:115–117.

Hallett M, Ravits J, Dubinsky RM, et al: A double-blind trial of isoniazid for essential tremor and other action tremors. Mov Disord 1991;6:253–256.

Halliday DM, Conway BA, Farmer SF, et al: Coherence between low-frequency activation of the motor cortex and tremor in patients with essential tremor. Lancet 2000;355:1149–1153.

Handforth A, Krahl SE: Suppression of harmaline-induced tremor in rats by vagus nerve stimulation. Mov Disord 2001;16:84–88.

Handforth A, Martin FC: Pilot efficacy and tolerability: A randomized, placebo-controlled trial of levetiracetam for essential tremor. Mov Disord 2004;19:1215–1221.

Handforth A, Ondo WG, Tatter S, et al: Vagus nerve stimulation for essential tremor: A pilot efficacy and safety trial. Neurology 2003;61:1401–1405.

Hardesty DE, Maraganore DM, Matsumoto JY, Louis ED: Increased risk of head tremor in women with essential tremor: Longitudinal data from the Rochester Epidemiology Project. Mov Disord 2004;19:529–533.

Hashimoto T, Sato H, Shindo M, et al: Peripheral mechanisms in tremor after traumatic neck injury. J Neurol Neurosurg Psychiatry 2002;73(5):585–587.

Heilman KM: Orthostatic tremor. Arch Neurol 1984;412:880–881.

Hellwig B, Häubler S, Schelter B, et al: Tremor-dominant cortical activity in essential tremor. Lancet 2001;357:519–523.

Helmchen C, Hagenow A, Miesner J, et al: Eye movement abnormalities in essential tremor may indicate cerebellar dysfunction. Brain 2003;126:1319–1332.

Henderson E, Overby A, Jankovic J: Postural control in essential tremor. Neurology 1996;46:A273.

Henderson JM, Einstein R, Jackson DM, et al: "Atypical" tremor. Eur Neurol 1995;35:321–326.

Higgins JJ, Lombardi RQ, Pucilowska J, et al: A variant in the *HS1-BP3* gene is associated with familial essential tremor. Neurology 2005;64:417–421.

Higgins JJ, Lombardi RQ, Pucilowska J, et al: *HS1-BP3* gene variant is common in familial essential tremor. Mov Disord 2006;21:306–309.

Higgins JJ, Lombardi RQ, Tan EK, et al: Haplotype analysis at the ETM2 locus in American and Singaporean populations with familial essential tremor. Clin Genet 2004;66:353–357.

Higgins JJ, Loveless JM, Jankovic J, Patel P: Evidence that a gene for essential tremor maps to chromosome 2p in four families. Mov Disord 1998;13:972–977.

Higgins JJ, Pho LT, Nee LE: A gene (ETM) for essential tremor maps to chromosome 2p22-p25. Mov Disord 1997;12:859–864.

Hirsch EC, Mouatt A, Faucheux B, et al: Dopamine, tremor, and Parkinson's disease [letter]. Lancet 1992;340:125–126.

Hore J, Flament D: Evidence that a disordered servo-like mechanism contributes to tremor in movements during cerebellar dysfunction. J Neurophysiol 1986;56:123–136.

Hou JG, Jankovic J: Botulinum toxin in the treatment of tremors. In Brin MF, Hallett M, Jankovic J (eds): Scientific and Therapeutic Aspects of Botulinum Toxin. Philadelphia, Lippincott Williams & Wilkins, 2002, pp 323–336.

Hua SE, Lenz FA, Zirh TA, et al: Thalamic neuronal activity correlated with essential tremor. J Neurol Neurosurg Psychiatry 1998;64:273–276.

Hubble JP, Busenbark KL, Wilkinson S, et al: Effects of thalamic deep brain stimulation based on tremor type and diagnosis. Mov Disord 1997;12:337–341.

Hughes AJ, Daniel SE, Blankson S, Lees AJ: A clinicopathologic study of 100 cases of Parkinson's disease. Arch Neurol 1993;50:140–148.

Hunker CJ, Abbs JH: Uniform frequency of parkinsonian resting tremor in the lips, jaw, tongue, and index finger. Mov Disord 1990;5:71–77.

Huntsman MM, Porcello DM, Homanics GE, et al: Reciprocal inhibitory connections and network synchrony in the mammalian thalamus. Science 1999;283:541–543.

Iwahashi CK, Yasui DH, An HJ, et al: Protein composition of the intranuclear inclusions of FXTAS. Brain 2006;129:256–271.

Jacquemont S, Hagerman RJ, Hagerman PJ, Leehey MA: Fragile-X syndrome and fragile X-associated tremor/ataxia syndrome: Two faces of FMR1. Lancet Neurol 2007;6:45–55.

Jacquemont S, Hagerman RJ, Leehey M, et al: Fragile X premutation tremor/ataxia syndrome: Molecular, clinical, and neuroimaging correlates. Am J Hum Genet 2003;72:869–878.

Jacquemont S, Hagerman RJ, Leehey MA, et al: Penetrance of the fragile X-associated tremor/ataxia syndrome in a permutation carrier population. JAMA 2004;291:460–469.

Jankovic J: Essential tremor and Parkinson's disease. Ann Neurol 1989;25:211.

Jankovic J: Posttraumatic movement disorders: Peripheral and central mechanisms. Neurology 1994;44:2008–2014.

Jankovic J: Essential tremor and other movement disorders. In Findley LJ, Koller W (eds): Handbook of Tremor Disorders. New York, Marcel Dekker, 1995, pp 245–262.

Jankovic J: Essential tremor: Clinical characteristics. Neurology 2000;54(suppl 4):S22–S26.

Jankovic J: Essential tremor: A heterogeneous disorder. Mov Disord 2002;17:638–644.

Jankovic J: Essential tremor course and disability: A clinicopathologic study of 20 cases. Neurology 2004;63:1541–1542.

Jankovic J, Beach J, Pandolfo M, Patel P: Familial essential tremor in four kindreds: Prospects for genetic mapping. Arch Neurol 1997;54:289–294.

Jankovic J, Beach J, Schwartz K, Contant C: Tremor and longevity in relatives of patients with Parkinson's disease, essential tremor and control subjects. Neurology 1995a;45:645–648.

Jankovic J, Cardoso F, Grossman RG, Hamilton WJ: Outcome after stereotactic thalamotomy for parkinsonian, essential and other types of tremor. Neurosurgery 1995b;45:1743–1746.

Jankovic J, Contant C, Perlmutter J: Essential tremor and Parkinson's disease. Neurology 1993;43:1447–1448.

Jankovic J, Leder S, Warner D, Schwartz K: Cervical dystonia: Clinical findings and associated movement disorders. Neurology 1991;41:1088–1091.

Jankovic J, Madisetty J, Vuong KD: Essential tremor among children. Pediatrics 2004;114:1203–1205.

Jankovic J, Marsden CD: Therapeutic strategies in Parkinson's disease. In Jankovic J, Tolosa E (eds): Parkinson's Disease and Movement Disorders, 3rd ed. Baltimore, Williams & Wilkins, 1998, pp 191–220.

Jankovic J, McDermott M, Carter J, et al: Variable expression of Parkinson's disease: A base-line analysis of the DATATOP cohort. Neurology 1990;40:1529–1534.

Jankovic J, Noebels JL: Genetic mouse models of essential tremor: Are they essential? J Clin Invest 2005;115:584–586.

Jankovic J, Schwartz K: Botulinum toxin treatment of tremors. Neurology 1991;41:1185–1188.

Jankovic J, Schwartz K, Clemence W, et al: A randomized, double-blind, placebo-controlled study to evaluate botulinum toxin type A in essential hand tremor. Mov Disord 1996;11:250–256.

Jankovic J, Schwartz, KS, Ondo W: Re-emergent tremor of Parkinson's disease. J Neurol Neurosurg Psychiatry 1999;67: 646–650.

Jankovic J, Thomas M: Psychogenic tremor and shaking. In Hallett M, Fahn S, Jankovic J, et al (eds): Psychogenic Movement Disorders: Neurology and Neuropsychiatry. Philadelphia, AAN Enterprises and Lippincott Williams & Wilkins, 2006, pp 42–47.

Jankovic J, Van der Linden C: Dystonia and tremor induced by peripheral trauma: Predisposing factors. J Neurol Neurosurg Psychiatry 1988;51:1512–1519.

Jarman PR, Wood NW, Davis MT, et al: Hereditary geniospasm: Linkage to chromosome 9q13-q21 and evidence for genetic heterogeneity. Am J Hum Genet 1997;61:928–933.

Jedynak CP, Bonnet AM, Agid Y: Tremor and idiopathic dystonia. Mov Disord 1991;6:230–236.

Jenkins IH, Bain PG, Colebatch JG, et al: A positron emission tomography study of essential tremor: Evidence for overactivity of cerebellar connections. Ann Neurol 1993;34:82–90.

Kaji R, Kohara N, Katayama M, et al: Muscle afferent block by intramuscular injection of lidocaine for the treatment of writer's cramp. Muscle Nerve 1995;18:234–235.

Kanazawa O: Shuddering attacks-report of four children. Pediatr Neurol 2000;23:421–424.

Katzenschlager R, Costa D, Gerschlager W, et al: [123I]-FP-CIT-SPECT demonstrates dopaminergic deficit in orthostatic tremor. Ann Neurol 2003;53:489–496.

Kelly PJ, Ahlskog JE, Daube JR, et al: Computer-assisted stereotactic ventralis lateralis thalamotomy with microelectrode recording control in patients with Parkinson's disease. Mayo Clin Proc 1987;62:655–664.

Kepler TB, Marder E, Abbott LF: The effect of electrical coupling on the frequency of model neuronal oscillators. Science 1990;240:83–85.

Kim JS, Lee MC: Leg tremor mimicking orthostatic tremor as an initial manifestation of Parkinson's disease. Mov Disord 1993;8:397–398.

Kim YJ, Pakiam ASI, Lang AE: Historical and clinical features of psychogenic tremor: A review of 70 cases. Can J Neurol Sci 1999;26:190–195.

Klebe S, Stolze H, Grensing K, et al: Influence of alcohol on gait in patients with essential tremor. Neurology 2005;65:96–101.

Ko DT, Hebert PR, Coffey CS, et al: Beta-blocker therapy and symptoms of depression, fatigue, and sexual dysfunction. JAMA 2002;288:351–357.

Koller EC, Hristova A, Brin M: Pharmacologic treatment of essential tremor. Neurology 2000;54(suppl 4):S30–S38.

Koller W, Lang A, Vetere-Overfield B, et al: Psychogenic tremors. Neurology 1989;39:1094–1099.

Koller W, Pahwa R, Busenbark K, et al: High-frequency unilateral thalamic stimulation in the treatment of essential and parkinsonian tremor. Ann Neurol 1997;42:292–299.

Koller WC, Busenbark K, Gray C, et al: Classification of essential tremor. Clin Neuropharmacol 1992;15:81–87.

Koller WC, Busenbark K, Miner K et al: The relationship of essential tremor to other movement disorders: Report on 678 patients. Ann Neurol 1994;35:717–723.

Koller WC, Lyons KE, Wilkins SB, Pahwa R: Efficacy of unilateral deep brain stimulation of the VIM nucleus of the thalamus for essential head tremor. Mov Disord 1999;14:847–850.

Koller WC, Royse VL: Efficacy of primidone in essential tremor. Neurology 1986;36:121–124.

Koster B, Deuschl G, Lauk M, et al: Essential tremor and cerebellar dysfunction: Abnormal ballistic movements. J Neurol Neurosurg Psychiatry 2002;73:400–405.

Koster B, Lauk M, Timmer J, et al: Involvement of cranial muscles and high intermuscular coherence in orthostatic tremor. Ann Neurol 1999;45:384–388.

Kovach MJ, Ruiz J, Kimonis K, et al: Genetic heterogeneity in autosomal dominant essential tremor. Genet Med 2001;3:197–199.

Kralic JE, Criswell HE, Osterman JL, et al: Genetic essential tremor in gamma-aminobutyric acid A receptor alpha1 subunit knockout mice. J Clin Invest 2005;115:774–779.

Krauss JK, Wakhloo AK, Nobbe F, et al: Lesion of dentatothalamic pathways in severe post-traumatic tremor. Neurol Res 1995;17: 409–416.

Kulisevsky J, Avila A, Barbanoj M, et al: Levodopa does not aggravate postural tremor in Parkinson's disease. Clin Neuropharmacol 1995;18:435–442.

Laitinen LV, Bergenheim AT, Hariz MI: Leksell's posteroventral pallidotomy in the treatment of Parkinson's disease. J Neurosurg 1992;76:53–61.

Lakie M, Walsh EG, Arblaster LA, et al: Limb temperature and human tremors. J Neurol Neurosurg Psychiatry 1994;57:35–42.

Lakie MD, Hayes NR, Combes N, Langford N: Is postural tremor size controlled by interstitial potassium concentration in muscle? J Neurol Neurosurg Psychiatry 2004;75:1013–1018.

Lamarre Y: Animal models of physiological, essential and parkinsonian-like tremors. In Findley LJ, Capildeo R (eds): Movement Disorders: Tremor. New York, Oxford University Press, 1984, pp 183–194.

Lauk M, Koster B, Timmer J, et al: Side-to-side correlation of muscle activity in physiological and pathological human tremors. Clin Neurophysiol 1999;110:1774–1783.

Lee KS, Kim JS, Kim JW, et al: A multicenter randomized crossover multiple-dose comparison study of arotinolol and propranolol in essential tremor. Parkinsonism Relat Disord 2003;9: 341–347.

Lee MS, Kim YD, Im JH, et al: $^{125}$I-IPT brain SPECT study in essential tremor and Parkinson's disease. Neurology 1999;52: 1422–1426.

Leehey MA, Munhoz RP, Lang AE, et al: The fragile X permutation presenting as essential tremor. Arch Neurol 2003;60:117–121.

Leigh PN, Jefferson D, Twomey A, Marsden CD: Beta-adrenoreceptor mechanisms in essential tremor; a double-blind placebo controlled trial of metoprolol, sotalol and atenolol. J Neurol Neurosurg Psychiatry 1983;46:710–715.

Lenz FA, Kwan HC, Martin RL, et al: Single unit analysis of the human ventral thalamic nuclear group. Tremor-related activity in functionally identified cells. Brain 1994;117:531–543.

Lenz FA, Tasker RR, Kwan HC, et al: Single unit analysis of the human ventral thalamic nuclear group: Correlation of thalamic "tremor cells" with the 3-6 Hz component of parkinsonian tremor. J Neurol Sci 1988;8:754–764.

Limousin P, Krack P, Pollak P, et al: Electrical stimulation of the subthalamic nucleus in advanced Parkinson's disease. N Engl J Med 1998;339:1105–1111.

Limousin P, Speelman JD, Gielen F, et al: Multicenter European study of thalamic stimulation in parkinsonian and essential tremor. J Neurol Neurosurg Psychiatry 1999;66:289–296.

Liu X, Miall RC, Aziz T, et al: Distal versus proximal arm tremor in multiple sclerosis assessed by visually guided tracking tasks. J Neurol Neurosurg Psychiatry 1999;66:43–47.

Llinas RR: The intrinsic electrophysiological properties of mammalian neurons: Insights into central nervous system function. Science 1988;242:1654–1664.

Lombardi WJ, Woolston DJ, Roberts JW, Cross RE: Cognitive deficits in patients with essential tremor. Neurology 2001;57:785–790.

Lorenz D, Frederiksen H, Moises H, et al: High concordance for essential tremor in monozygotic twins of old age. Neurology 2004;62:208–211.

Lou JS, Goldfarb L, McShane L, et al: Use of buspirone for treatment of cerebellar ataxia. An open-label study. Arch Neurol 1995;52:982–988.

Lou JS, Jankovic J: Essential tremor: Clinical correlates in 350 patients. Neurology 1991a;41:234–238.

Lou JS, Jankovic J: Tremors. In Appel SH (ed): Current Neurology, vol 11. Chicago, Mosby Year Book, 1991b, pp 199–232.

Lou JS, Jankovic J: Origin and treatment of tremor in cerebellar disease. In Lechtenberg R (ed): The Handbook of Cerebellar Disease, New York, Marcel Dekker, 1993, 45–63.

Louis ED: A new twist for stopping the shakes?: Revisiting GABAergic therapy for essential tremor. Arch Neurol 1999;56:807–808.

Louis ED: Essential tremor. Arch Neurol 2000;57:1522–1524.

Louis ED: Etiology of essential tremor: Should we be searching for environmental causes? Mov Disord 2001;16:822–829.

Louis ED: Essential tremor. Lancet Neurol 2005;4:100–110.

Louis ED, Applegate LM, Borden S, et al: Feasibility and validity of a modified finger-nose-finger test. Mov Disord 2005;20:636–639.

Louis ED, Barnes LF, Wendt K, et al: Validity and test-retest reliability of a disability questionnaire for essential tremor. Mov Disord 2000;15:516–523.

Louis ED, Barnes L, Wendt KJ, et al: A teaching videotape for the assessment of essential tremor. Mov Disord 2001;16:89–93.

Louis ED, Bromley SM, Jurewicz EC, Watner D: Olfactory dysfunction in essential tremor: A deficit unrelated to disease duration or severity. Neurology 2002;59:1631–1633.

Louis ED, Dure LS, Pullman S: Essential tremor in childhood: A series of nineteen cases. Mov Disord 2001;16:921–923.

Louis ED, Ford B, Barnes LF: Clinical subtypes of essential tremor. Arch Neurol 2000;57:1194–1198.

Louis ED, Ford B, Bismuth B: Reliability between two observers using a protocol for diagnosing essential tremor. Mov Disord 1998;13:287–293.

Louis ED, Ford B, Frucht S: Factors associated with increased risk of head tremor in essential tremor: A community-based study in northern Manhattan. Mov Disord 2003;18:432–436.

Louis ED, Ford B, Frucht S, et al: Risk of tremor and impairment from tremor in relatives of patients with essential tremor: A community-based family study. Ann Neurol 2001;49:761–769.

Louis ED, Ford B, Frucht S, Ottman R: Mild essential tremor in relatives of patients with essential tremor. What does this tell us about the penetrance of the disease? Arch Neurol 2001;58:1584–1589.

Louis ED, Ford B, Lee H, Andrews H: Does a screening questionnaire for essential tremor agree with the physician's examination? Neurology 1998;50:1351–1357.

Louis ED, Ford B, Lee H, et al: Diagnostic criteria for essential tremor. A population perspective. Arch Neurol 1998;55:823–828.

Louis ED, Ford B, Pullman S, Baron K: How normal is "normal"? Mild tremor in a multiethnic cohort of normal subjects. Arch Neurol 1998;55:222–227.

Louis ED, Ford B, Wendt KJ, et al: A comparison of different bedside tests for essential tremor. Mov Disord 1999a;14:462–467.

Louis ED, Ford B, Wendt KJ, Ottman R: Validity of family history data on essential tremor. Mov Disord 1999b;14:456–461.

Louis ED, Honig LS, Vonsattel JP, et al: Essential tremor associated with focal nonnigral Lewy bodies: A clinicopathologic study. Arch Neurol 2005;62:1004–1007.

Louis ED, Jurewicz EC: Olfaction in essential tremor patients with and without isolated rest tremor. Mov Disord 2003;18:1387–1389.

Louis ED, Levy G, Cote LJ, et al: Clinical correlates of action tremor in Parkinson disease. Arch Neurol 2001;58:1630–1634.

Louis ED, Marder K, Cote L, et al: Differences in the prevalence of essential tremor among elderly African-Americans, Caucasians, and Hispanics in Northern Manhattan. Arch Neurol 1995;52:1201–1205.

Louis ED, Marder K, Cote L, et al: Prevalence of a history of shaking in persons 65 years of age and older: Diagnostic and functional correlates. Mov Disord 1996;11:63–69.

Louis ED, Ottman R: How familial is familial tremor?: The genetic epidemiology of essential tremor. Neurology 1996;46:1200–1205.

Louis ED, Ottman R, Hauser WA: How common is the most common adult movement disorder?: Estimates of the prevalence of essential tremor throughout the world. Mov Disord 1998;13:5–10.

Louis ED, Pullman SL: Comparison of clinical vs electrophysiological methods of diagnosing of essential tremor. Mov Disord 2001;16:668–673.

Louis ED, Vonsattel JP, Honig LS, et al: Essential tremor associated with pathologic changes in the cerebellum. Arch Neurol 2006;63:1189–1193.

Louis ED, Yousefzadeh E, Barnes LF, et al: Validation of a portable instrument for assessing tremor severity in epidemiologic field studies. Mov Disord 2000;15:95–102.

Lucotte G, Lagarde JP, Funalot B, Sokoloff P: Linkage with the Ser9Gly DRD3 polymorphism in essential tremor families. Clin Genet 2006;69:437–440.

Lyons K, Pahwa R, Comella C, et al: Benefits and risks of pharmacological treatments for essential tremor. Drug Saf 2003;26:461–481.

Magnin M, Morel A, Jeanmonod D: Single-unit analysis of the pallidum, thalamus and subthalamic nucleus in parkinsonian patients. Neuroscience 2000;96:549–564.

Manto MU, Pandolfo M, Moore J: Bilateral high-frequency synchronous discharges: A new form of tremor in humans. Arch Neurol 2003;60:416–422.

Marsden CD: Origins of normal and pathological tremor. In Findley LJ, Capildeo R (eds): Movement Disorders: Tremor. New York, Oxford University Press, 1984, pp 37–84.

Masucci EF, Kurtzke JF, Saini N: Myorhythmia: A widespread movement disorder. Clinical-pathological correlations. Brain 1984;107:53–79.

McAuley JH: Does essential tremor originate in the cerebral cortex? Lancet 2001;357:492–494.

McAuley JH, Britton TC, Rothwell JC, et al: The timing of primary orthostatic tremor bursts has a task-specific plasticity. Brain 2000;123:254–266.

McAuley JH, Marsden CD: Physiologic and pathological tremors and rhythmic central motor control. Brain 2000;123:1545–1567.

McAuley JH, Rothwell JC, Marsden CD, et al: Electrophysiological aids in distinguishing organic from psychogenic tremor. Neurology 1998;50:1882–1884.

Minor VL: Heredo-familiare Nervenkrankheiten ohne anatomischen Befund. Das erbliche Zittern. In Bumke O (ed): Handbuch der Neurologie, vol 17. Berlin, J Springer, 1935, pp 976–1005.

Miwa H, Hatori K, Kondo T, et al: Thalamic tremor: Case reports and implications of the tremor-generating mechanism. Neurology 1996;46:75–79.

Modugno N, Nakamura Y, Bestmann S, et al: Neurophysiological investigations in patients with primary writing tremor. Mov Disord 2002;17:1336–1340.

Moghal S, Rajput AH, D'Arcy C, Rajput R: Prevalence of movement disorders in elderly community residents. Neuroepidemiology 1994;13:175–178.

Montgomery EB, Baker KB, Kinkel RP, Barnett G: Chronic thalamic stimulation for the tremor of multiple sclerosis. Neurology 1999;53:625–628.

Morita S, Miwa H, Kondo T: Effect of zonisamide on essential tremor: A pilot crossover study in comparison with arotinolol. Parkinsonism Relat Disord 2005;11:101–103.

Muenter MD, Daube JR, Caviness JN, Miller PM: Treatment of essential tremor with methazolamide. Mayo Clin Proc 1991;66:991–997.

Münchau A, Schrag A, Chuang C, et al: Arm tremor in cervical dystonia differs from essential tremor and can be classified by onset age and spread of symptoms. Brain 2001;124:1765–1776.

Nagaseki Y, Shibazaki T, Hirai T, et al: Long term follow-up results of selective VIM-thalamotomy. J Neurosurg 1986;65:296–302.

Nguyen J-P, Pollin B, Feve A, et al: Improvement of action tremor by chronic cortical stimulation. Mov Disord 1998;13:84–88.

Norton JA, Wood DE, Day BL: Is the spinal cord the generator of 16-Hz orthostatic tremor? Neurology 2004;62:632–634.

Nouzeilles M, Garcia M, Rabinowicz A, Merello M: Prospective evaluation of parkinsonism and tremor in patients treated with valproate. Parkinsonism Relat Disord 1999;5:67–68.

Obwegeser AA, Uiti RJ, Turk MF, et al: Thalamic stimulation for the treatment of midline tremors in essential tremor patients. Neurology 2000;54:2342–2344.

Okuma Y, Shimo Y, Shimura H, et al: Familial cortical tremor with epilepsy: An under-recognized familial tremor. Clin Neurol Neurosurg 1998;100:75–78.

Ondo W, Almaguer M, Jankovic J, Simpson RK: Thalamic deep brain stimulation: Comparison between unilateral and bilateral placement. Arch Neurol 2001;58:218–222.

Ondo W, Jankovic J: Essential tremor: Treatment options. CNS Drugs 1996;6:178–191.

Ondo W, Jankovic J, Schwartz K, et al: Unilateral thalamic deep brain stimulation for refractory essential tremor and Parkinson's disease tremor. Neurology 1998;51:1063–1069.

Ondo W, Vuong K, Almaguer M, et al: Thalamic deep brain stimulation: Effects on the nontarget limbs and rebound phenomenon. Mov Disord 2001;16:1137–1142.

Ondo WG, Hunter C, Schwartz K, Jankovic J: Gabapentin for essential tremor: Double-blind, placebo controlled trial. Mov Disord 2000;15:678–682.

Ondo WG, Jankovic J, Connor GS, et al: Topiramate in essential tremor: A double-blind, placebo-controlled trial. Neurology 2006;66:672–677.

Ondo WG, Jimenez JE, Vuong KD, Jankovic J: An open-label pilot study of levetiracetam for essential tremor. Clin Neuropharmacol 2004;27:274–277.

Ondo WG, Lai D: Association between restless legs syndrome and essential tremor. Mov Disord 2006;21:515–518.

Ondo WG, Sutton L, Dat Vuong K, et al: Hearing impairment in essential tremor. Neurology 2003;61:1093–1097.

Onofrj M, Thomas A, Paci C, D'Andreamatteo G: Gabapenting in orthostatic tremor: Results of a double-blind crossover with placebo in four patients. Neurology 1998;51:880–882.

Orr HT: RNA gains a new function: A mediator of neurodegeneration. Trends Neurosci 2004;27:233–234.

Overby A, Henderson N, Jankovic J: Lower extremity posture-evoked responses in persons with essential tremor. Neurology 1996;46:A142.

Packer M, Cohn JN, Abraham WT, et al: Consensus recommendations for the management of chronic heart failure. Am J Cardiol 1999;83:1A–38A.

Pact V, Giduz T: Mirtazapine treats resting tremor, essential tremor, and levodopa-induced dyskinesias. Neurology 1999;53:1154.

Pagan FL, Butman JA, Dambrosia JM, Hallett M: Evaluation of essential tremor with multi-voxel magnetic resonance spectroscopy. Neurology 2003;60:1344–1347.

Pahapill PA, Levy R, Dostrovsky J, et al: Tremor arrest with thalamic microinjections of muscimol in patients with essential tremor. Ann Neurol 1999;46:249–252.

Pahwa R, Busenbark K, Swanson-Hyland EF, et al: Botulinum toxin treatment of essential head tremor. Neurology 1995;45:822–824.

Pahwa R, Koller WC: Is there a relationship between Parkinson's disease and essential tremor? Clin Neuropharmacol 1993; 16:30–35.

Pahwa R, Koller WC: Thalamic stimulation for treatment of essential tremor. In Krauss JK, Jankovic J, Grossman RG (eds): Surgery for Parkinson's Disease and Movement Disorders. Philadelphia, Lippincott Williams & Wilkins, 2001, pp 278–281.

Pahwa R, Lyons KE: Mirtazapine in essential tremor: A double-blind, placebo-controlled pilot study. Mov Disord 2003;18:584–587.

Pahwa R, Lyons K, Hubble JP, et al: Double-blind controlled trial of gabapentin in essential tremor. Mov Disord 1998;13:465–467.

Pahwa R, Lyons KE, Wilkinson SB, et al: Long-term evaluation of deep brain stimulation of the thalamus. J Neurosurg 2006;104:506–512.

Pare D, Curro-Dossi R, Steriade M: Neuronal basis of the parkinsonian resting tremor: A hypothesis and its implications for treatment. Neuroscience 1990;35:217–226.

Payami H, Larsen K, Bernard S, Nutt J: Increased risk of Parkinson's disease in parents and siblings of patients. Ann Neurol 1994; 36:659–661.

Piccini P, Morrish PK, Tujanski N, et al: Dopaminergic function in familial Parkinson's disease: A clinical and $^{18}$F-dopa positron emission tomography study. Ann Neurol 1997;41:222–229.

Plenz D, Kitai S: A basal ganglia pacemaker formed by the subthalamic nucleus and external globus pallidus. Nature 1999;400: 677–681.

Pourcher E, Gomez-Mancilla B, Bedard PJ: Ethosuximide and tremor in Parkinson's disease: A pilot study. Mov Disord 1992;7:132–136.

Pozos RS, Iaizzo PA: Effects of topical anesthesia on essential tremor. Electromyogr Clin Neurophysiol 1992;32:369–372.

Pullman SL: Spiral analysis: A new technique for measuring tremor with a digitizing tablet. Mov Disord 1998;13(suppl 3):85–89.

Pullman SL, Elibol B, Fahn S: Modulation of parkinsonian tremor by radial nerve palsy. Neurology 1994;44:1861–1864.

Racette BA, Dowling J, Randle J, Mink JW: Thalamic stimulation for primary writing tremor. J Neurol 2001;248:380–382.

Raethjen J, Linde A, Schmaljohann H, et al: Multiple oscillators are causing parkinsonian and essential tremor. Mov Disord 2000;15: 84–94.

Rajput A, Robinson CA, Rajput AH: Essential tremor course and disability: A clinicopathologic study of 20 cases. Neurology 2004; 62:932–936.

Rajput AH, Pahwa R, Pahwa P: Prognostic significance of the onset mode in parkinsonism. Neurology 1993;43:829–830.

Rajput AH, Rozdilsky B, Ang L: Occurrence of resting tremor in Parkinson's disease. Neurology 1991;41:1298–1299.

Rautakorpi I, Takala J, Martilla RJ, et al: Essential tremor in a Finnish population. Acta Neurol Scand 1982;66:58–67.

Ray Chaudhuri KR, Buxton-Thomas M, Dhawan V, et al: Long duration asymmetrical postural tremor is likely to predict development of Parkinson's disease and not essential tremor: Clinical follow up study of 13 cases. J Neurol Neurosurg Psychiatry 2005;76:115–117.

Rehncrona S, Johnels B, Widner H, et al: Long-term efficacy of thalamic deep brain stimulation for tremor: Double-blind assessments. Mov Disord 2003;18:163–170.

Remy P, de Recondo A, Defer G, et al: Peduncular "rubral" tremor and dopaminergic denervation: A PET study. Neurology 1995;45: 472–477.

Rivest J, Marsden CD: Trunk and head tremor as isolated manifestations of dystonia. Mov Disord 1990;5:60–65.

Rondot P, Korn H, Scherrer J: Suppression of an entire limb tremor by anesthetizing a selective muscular group. Arch Neurol 1968;19:421–429.

Rosenbaum F, Jankovic J: Task-specific focal dystonia and tremor: Categorization of occupational movement disorders. Neurology 1988;38:522–527.

Ruskin DN, Bergstrom DA, Kaneoke Y, et al: Multisecond oscillations in firing rate in the basal ganglia: Robust modulation by dopamine receptor activation and anesthesia. J Neurophysiol 1999;81:2046–2055.

Sabra AF, Hallett M: Action tremor with alternating activity in antagonist muscles. Neurology 1984;34:151–156.

Said G, Bathien N, Cesaro P: Peripheral neuropathies and tremor. Neurology 1982;32:480–485.

Samie MR, Selhorst JB, Koller W: Post-traumatic midbrain tremors. Neurology 1990;40:62–66.

Sander HW, Masdeu J, Tavoulareas G, et al: Orthostatic tremor: An electrophysiological analysis. Mov Disord 1998;13:735–748.

Sanes JN, Hallett M: Limb positioning and magnitude of essential tremor and other pathological tremors. Mov Disord 1990;5: 304–309.

Sanes JN, LeWitt PA, Mauritz K-H: Visual and mechanical control of postural and kinetic tremor in cerebellar system disorders. J Neurol Neurosurg Psychiatry 1988;51:934–943.

Sasso E, Perucca E, Fava R, Calzetti S: Quantitative comparison of barbiturates in essential hand and head tremor. Mov Disord 1991;6:65–68.

Schrag A, Munchau A, Bhatia KP, et al: Essential tremor: An over-diagnosed condition? J Neurol 2000;247:955–959.

Schuurman PR, Bosch A, Bossuyt PMM, et al: A comparison of continuous thalamic stimulation and thalamotomy for suppression of severe tremor. N Engl J Med 2000;342:461–468.

Sechi GP, Zuddas M, Piredda M, et al: Treatment of cerebellar tremors with carbamazepine: A controlled trial with long term follow-up. Neurology 1989;39:1113–1115.

Serrano-Duenas M: Use of primidone in low doses (250 mg/day) versus high doses (750 mg/day) in the management of essential tremor: Double-blind comparative study with one-year follow-up. Parkinsonism Relat Disord 2003;10:29–33.

Shahani BT: Tremor associated with peripheral neuropathy. In Findley LJ, Capildeo R (eds): Movement Disorders: Tremor. New York, Oxford University Press, 1984, pp 389–398.

Shahed J, Jankovic J: Exploring the relationship between essential tremor and Parkinson's disease. Parkinsonism Relat Disord 2007;13(2):67–76.

Sharott A, Marsden J, Brown P: Primary orthostatic tremor is an exaggeration of a physiological response to instability. Mov Disord 2003;18:195–199.

Shatunov A, Sambuughin N, Jankovic J, et al: Genomewide scans in North American families reveal genetic linkage of essential tremor to a region on chromosome 6p23. Brain 2006;129(pt 9)2318–2331.

Shill HA, Bushara KO, Mari Z, et al: Open-label dose-escalation study of oral 1-octanol in patients with essential tremor. Neurology 2004;62:2320–2322.

Singer C, Sanchez-Ramos J, Weiner WJ: Gait abnormality in essential tremor. Mov Disord 1994;9:193–196.

Singleton AB, Farrer M, Johnson J, et al: alpha-Synuclein locus triplication causes Parkinson's disease. Science 2003;302:841.

Soland VL, Bhatia KP, Sheean GL, et al: Hereditary geniospasm: Two new families. Mov Disord 1996a;11:744–761.

Soland VL, Bhatia KP, Volonte MA, Marsden CD: Focal task-specific tremors. Mov Disord 1996b;11:665–670.

Solomon DH, Barohn RJ, Bazan C, Grissom J: The thalamic ataxia syndrome. Neurology 1994;44:810–814.

Speelman JD, Manen JV: Stereotactic thalamotomy for the relief of intention tremor of multiple sclerosis. J Neurol Neurosurg Psychiatry 1984;47:596–599.

Sperfeld AD, Karitzky J, Brummer D, et al: X-linked bulbospinal neuronopathy: Kennedy Disease. Arch Neurol 2002; 59: 1921–1926.

Stacy M, Jankovic J: Tardive tremor. Mov Disord 1992;7:53–57.

Stolze H, Petersen G, Raethjen J, et al: The gait disorder of advanced essential tremor. Brain 2001;124:2278–2286.

Striano P, Zara F, Striano S: Autosomal dominant cortical tremor, myoclonus and epilepsy: Many syndromes, one phenotype. Acta Neurol Scand 2005;111:211–217.

Subramanian T, Vitek J, Watts RL, et al: Microelectrode-guided stereotactic selective thalamotomy improves tremor but not bradykinesia in a young Parkinson's disease (PD) patient. Neurology 1995;45(suppl 4):A376.

Sullivan KL, Hauser RA, Zesiewicz TA: Essential tremor. Epidemiology, diagnosis, and treatment. Neurologist 2004;10:250–258.

Tan EK, Matsuura T, Nagamitsu S, et al: Polymorphism of NACP-Rep 1 in Parkinson's disease: An etiologic link with essential tremor? Neurology 2000;54:1195–1198.

Tan EK, Zhao Y, Puong KY, et al: Fragile X premutation alleles in SCA, ET, and parkinsonism in an Asian cohort. Neurology 2004;63: 362–363.

Tanner CM, Goldman SM, Lyons KE, et al: Essential tremor in twins. An assessment of genetic vs environmental determinants of etiology. Neurology 2001;57:1389–1391.

Thompson PJ, Baxendale SA, Duncan JS, Sander JWAS. Effects of topiramate on cognitive function. J Neurol Neurosurg Psychiatry 2000;69:636–641.

Tintner R, Tremor Research Group: The Tremor Rating Scale. Mov Disord 2004;19:1131.

Tison F, Louvet-Giendaj L, Henry P, et al: Permanent bruxism as a manifestation of the oculo-facial syndrome related to systemic Whipple's disease. Mov Disord 1992;7:82–85.

Topka H, Mescheriakov S, Boose A, et al: Cerebellar-like terminal and postural tremor induced in normal man by transcranial magnetic stimulation. Brain 1999;122:1551–1562.

Toro C, Pascual-Leone A, Deuschl G, et al: Cortical tremor: A common manifestation of cortical myoclonus. Neurology 1993;43: 2346–2353.

Trelles L, Trelles JO, Castro C: Successful treatment of two cases of intention tremor with clonazepam. Ann Neurol 1984;16:621.

Trosch RM, Pullman SL: Botulinum toxin A injections for the treatment of hand tremors. Mov Disord 1994;9:601–609.

Van Hilten JJ, van Dijk JG, Dunnewold RJW, et al: Diurnal variation of essential and physiological tremor. J Neurol Neurosurg Psychiatry 1991;54:516–519.

Van Rootselaar AF, Maurits NM, Koelman JH, et al: Coherence analysis differentiates between cortical myoclonic tremor and essential tremor. Mov Disord 2006;21:215–222.

Van Rootselaar AF, van Schaik IN, van den Maagdenberg AM, et al: Familial cortical myoclonic tremor with epilepsy: A single syndromic classification for a group of pedigrees bearing common features. Mov Disord 2005;20:665–673.

Vanasse M, Bedard P, Andermann F: Shuddering attacks in children: An early clinical manifestation of essential tremor. Neurology 1976;26:1027–1030.

Volkmann J, Joliot M, Mogilner A, et al: Central motor loop oscillations in parkinsonian resting tremor revealed by magnetoencephalography. Neurology 1996;46:1359–1370.

Warrick P, Dromey C, Irish JC, et al: Botulinum toxin for essential tremor of the voice with multiple anatomical sites of tremor: A crossover design study of unilateral versus bilateral injection. Laryngoscope 2000;110:1366–1374.

Whittle IR, Hooper J, Pentland B: Thalamic deep-brain stimulation for movement disorders due to mulptiple sclerosis. Lancet 1998;351:109–110.

Wills AJ, Brusa L, Wang HC, et al: Levodopa may improve orthostatic tremor: Case report and trial of treatment. J Neurol Neurosurg Psychiatry 1999;66:681–684.

Wills AJ, Jenkins IH, Thompson PD, et al: Red nuclear and cerebellar but no olivary activation associated with essential tremor: A positron emission tomographic study. Ann Neurol 1994;36: 636–642.

Wills AJ, Jenkins IH, Thompson PD, et al: A positron emission tomography study of cerebellar activation associated with essential and writing tremor. Arch Neurol 1995;52:299–305.

Wills AJ, Thompson PD, Findley LJ, Brooks DJ: A positron emission tomography study of primary orthostatic tremor. Neurology 1996;46:747–752.

Wilms H, Sievers J, Deuschl G: Animal models of tremor. Mov Disord 1999;14:557–571.

Wissel J, Masuhr F, Schelosky L, et al: Quantitative assessment of botulinum toxin treatment in 42 patients with head tremor. Mov Disord 1997;12:722–726.

Yahr MD, Orosz D, Purohit DP: Co-occurrence of essential tremor and Parkinson's disease: Clinical study of a large kindred with autopsy findings. Parkinsonism Relat Disord 2003,9:225–231.

Zadikoff C, Lang AE, Klein C: The "essentials" of essential palatal tremor: A reappraisal of the nosology. Brain 2006;129:832–840.

Zesiewicz TA, Elble R, Louis EE, et al: Practice parameter: Therapies for essential tremor. Report of the Quality Standards Subcommittee of the American Academy of Neurology. Neurology 2005;64:2008–2020.

Zeuner KE, Molloy FM, Shoge RO, et al: Effect of ethanol on the central oscillator in essential tremor. Mov Disord 2003a;18: 1280–1285.

Zeuner KE, Shoge RO, Goldstein SR, et al: Accelerometry to distinguish psychogenic from essential or parkinsonian tremor. Neurology 2003b;61:548–550.

Zimmermann R, Deutschl G, Horning A, et al: Tremors in Parkinson's disease: Symptom analysis and rating. Clin Neuropharmacol 1994;17:303–314.

Zirh A, Reich SG, Dougherty PM, Lenz FA: Stereotactic thalamotomy in the treatment of essential tremor of the upper extremity: Reassessment including a blinded measure of outcome. J Neurol Neurosurg Psychiatry 1999;66:772–775.

## APPENDIX 19-1

**International Essential Tremor Foundation (IETF)**
7046 W. 105th Street
Overland Park, KS 66212-1803
Telephone: 913-341-3880
Fax: 913-341-1296
E-mail: IntTremorFnd@worldnet.att.net
Website: www.essentialtremor.org

## Chapter 20

# The Tardive Syndromes
## Phenomenology, Concepts on Pathophysiology and Treatment, and Other Neuroleptic-Induced Syndromes

## OVERVIEW

The topic of tardive dyskinesia syndromes is very broad, covering different phenomenologies. This is also the appropriate chapter in which to cover nontardive neuroleptic-induced movement disorders, further extending the scope of material to review. Because of the volume of material to cover, the essential features of the tardive dyskinesia syndromes are highlighted in this summary section to allow the reader to understand the most pertinent material in a simple fashion.

1. The term *neuroleptic* was coined when reserpine (a dopamine-depleting drug) and then the antipsychotic drugs that block dopamine receptors were found to induce parkinsonism. Drug-induced parkinsonism correlates with the dosage of the neuroleptic and disappears when the drug is withdrawn.

2. The tardive dyskinesia syndromes are the result of treatment with dopamine receptor–blocking agents (DRBAs). These disorders tend to appear late in the course of treatment, hence the term *tardive*. Syndromes with similar clinical phenomenology in the absence of a reliable history of having received such medications exclude this diagnosis. Tardive syndromes have not been caused by dopamine depletors and only rarely by the atypical neuroleptics, such as clozapine. Some DRBAs are marketed for gastrointestinal problems (e.g., metoclopramide [Reglan]), for depression (e.g., amoxapine [Asendin]; perphenazine/amitriptyline [Triavil]), and for cough (e.g., promethazine [Phenergan]).

3. The tardive dyskinesia syndromes tend to persist and can remain permanently. It is generally believed that the sooner the offending drugs are withdrawn, the more likely it is that the syndrome will fade away with time. But evidence is lacking that prolonging the use of the drugs will increase the severity of the dyskinesia.

4. The tardive dyskinesia syndromes can occur when the patient is taking these drugs or within a period of time after stopping the drugs. The criteria should be set for the longest acceptable time after stopping the drugs that the disorder can still be considered to be due to the drugs.

5. Withdrawing the offending drugs often exacerbates the severity of the movements because of removal of dopamine receptor blockade. Increasing the dosage of these drugs often ameliorates the movements because of increasing the blockade.

6. The tardive dyskinesia syndromes present in a variety of phenomenologies. The most common is the pattern of repetitive, almost rhythmic, movements that can be labeled as stereotypic. This pattern often occurs in the oral-buccal-lingual (O-B-L) region, usually presenting as complex chewing movements with occasional popping out of the tongue and with writhing movements of the tongue when it should be at rest in the mouth. Other parts of the body may also express rhythmic movements, such as the hands, feet, and trunk. Respiration may also be affected, with an altered rhythmic pattern. This pattern of dyskinesia goes by the name *classic tardive dyskinesia* or *tardive dyskinesia* (TD). Because the individual movements may have the speed and brevity of choreoathetosis, the name *chorea* has been attached by some clinicians, but this only serves to confuse because the movements of classic chorea and athetosis are random or flowing and not rhythmic. Other names that have been used are *tardive stereotypy* and *rhythmic chorea*. In this chapter, the strikingly characteristic movement pattern is simply called classic tardive dyskinesia, or TD. It is exceedingly rare for such a pattern to be caused by any condition besides DRBA; it can sometimes be seen with levodopa, with brainstem strokes, and as an idiopathic disorder. There are other patterns of oral dyskinesias; they should not be confused with the pattern that is seen in TD. The most common idiopathic and spontaneous oral dyskinesia is oromandibular dystonia.

7. TD is often accompanied by a feeling of inner restlessness (akathisia), which can be whole-body restlessness or uncomfortable sensations in a specific part of the body. Such focal akathisia is extremely uncomfortable and is often expressed by the patient as a burning sensation; the mouth and vaginal regions are the most common sites of such focal akathisias. Generalized akathisia is often accompanied by a pattern of movement that appears to be executed in an attempt to relieve the abnormal uncomfortable sensations. These movements are often rhythmic, repetitive, and stereotypic, such as body rocking, crossing and uncrossing of the legs, and caressing of the scalp. Sometimes, these characteristic movement patterns are present without the patient's being able to express the presence of a feeling of restlessness. The discomfort of generalized akathisia can lead to constant moaning by the patient.

8. Akathisia can also occur in the early phase of treatment with DRBAs; this is called acute akathisia in contrast to the *tardive akathisia* described earlier. Acute akathisia is not persistent and will disappear on discontinuing the DRBA.

9. The third most common phenomenology in the tardive dyskinesia syndromes is dystonia, which can mimic idiopathic torsion dystonia, usually focal or segmental. Some differences include an increased tendency for tardive dystonia to cause retrocollis and opisthotonic posturing, accompanied by internal rotation of the shoulders, extension of the elbows, and flexion of the wrists. Focal dystonias are usually cranial in location, particularly affecting the jaw, tongue, and facial muscles. Tardive dystonia may also be

accompanied by tardive akathisia and by classic TD. The presence of classic TD or akathisia in a patient with dystonia who has had exposure to DRBA makes the diagnosis of tardive dystonia extremely likely. Tardive dystonia can occur at all ages, whereas classic TD is more common in the elderly.

10. In addition to tardive dystonia, which is usually persistent, children tend to get classic chorea, called withdrawal emergent syndrome, which is self-limiting, eventually disappearing over several weeks if the offending drugs are withdrawn.

11. Other clinical phenomenology has been described in the spectrum of the tardive dyskinesia syndromes. These include myoclonus, tremor, oculogyric crisis, and tics. Some cases that have been reported as tardive tics might have actually been the movements of tardive akathisia that were mistaken for tic-like movements.

12. The atypical antipsychotic agents, ranked in order of clozapine, quetiapine, and olanzapine, are less tightly bound to the D2 receptor than are the typical antipsychotic agents. This pharmacologic characteristic probably accounts for these atypical agents being much less likely to induce drug-induced parkinsonism, acute dystonic reactions, acute akathisia, neuroleptic malignant syndrome (NMS), or the tardive syndromes, but there are some case reports of these complications from these drugs.

13. At the present time, clozapine is the gold standard for the atypical antipsychotics, quetiapine being a close second. The third-ranking drug is olanzapine. Newer so-called atypical antipsychotics need to be in use clinically before their full side-effect profile can be known. Although risperidone has been labeled an atypical antipsychotic, it readily induces and worsens parkinsonism and can induce TD; it should be removed from this classification. Clozapine and quetiapine have been reported to be successful in some patients to reduce the severity of TD and tardive dystonia, but there remains uncertainty whether symptoms are reduced (1) because of D2 blocking activity with high doses, (2) because there is no such activity and tincture of time has resolved the tardive symptoms, or (3) because these drugs have some other action that can reduce TD. By and large, these two drugs are ineffective in reducing tardive symptoms. Drugs that deplete dopamine or block D2 receptors have been the most effective medications in reducing tardive disorders.

## FUNDAMENTALS AND DEFINITIONS

A variety of neurologic adverse effects are seen with drugs that block dopamine D2 receptors. Because these complications are mainly movement disorders and likely relate to the D2 receptors in the striatum and limbic system, they are usually called extrapyramidal reactions. These are listed in Box 20-1 and are covered in the clinical sections that follow.

The term *tardive syndromes* refers to a group of disorders that fit all of the following essential criteria: (1) Phenomenologically, the clinical features are that of a movement disorder—that is, abnormal involuntary movements or a sensation of restlessness that often causes "unvoluntary" movements; (2) the disorder is caused by the patient's having been exposed to at least one DRBA within 6 months of the onset of symptoms (in exceptional cases, exposure could be up to 12 months); and (3) the

**Box 20-1** Neurologic adverse effects of dopamine receptor antagonists

1. Acute reactions
   a. Acute dystonia
   b. Acute (subacute) akathisia
2. Toxicity state (overdosage)
   a. Drug-induced parkinsonism
3. Neuroleptic malignant syndrome (NMS)
4. Tardive syndromes
   a. Withdrawal emergent syndrome
   b. Classic tardive dyskinesia
   c. Tardive dystonia
   d. Tardive akathisia
   e. Tardive myoclonus
   f. Tardive tremor
   g. Tardive tics
   h. Tardive chorea
   i. (?) Tardive parkinsonism

Adapted from Fahn S: The tardive dyskinesias. In Matthews WB, Glaser GH (eds): Recent Advances in Clinical Neurology, vol 4, Edinburgh, Churchill Livingstone, 1984, pp 229–260.

disorder persists for at least 1 month after stopping the offending drug (Fahn, 1984a; Stacy and Jankovic, 1991). The question arises as to what to call persistent dyskinesias that are induced by drugs other than DRBAs. For example, Miller and Jankovic (1992) described such a patient who had been exposed to flecainide, a drug not known to be a DRBA. Another drug, buspirone, an azospirone compound, is an anxiolytic that is not known to have any dopamine receptor–blocking activity. Yet there is now a report of two patients who had persistent movement disorders after prolonged treatment with this drug (LeWitt et al., 1993). One patient had cervical-cranial dystonia, and the other had an exacerbation of pre-existing spasmodic torticollis and TD. It is possible, however, that future laboratory investigation will reveal flecainide and buspirone or one of their metabolites actually to be a DRBA.

Although there are several phenomenologically distinct types of tardive disorders, the collective group is referred to as tardive dyskinesia for historical reasons. Unfortunately, the term *tardive dyskinesia* is often used also to refer to a phenomenologically specific type of tardive syndrome, so the literature is often confusing; this note of caution is particularly important in trying to understand whether the author of a paper is referring to the tardive syndromes collectively or to a specific tardive syndrome. Since there could be different pathophysiologic mechanisms and treatments for the different forms of tardive syndromes, it is best that they be divided phenomenologically (Table 20-1). In this review, the tardive syndromes as a whole are referred to as tardive dyskinesia, and the specific type that was historically and initially labeled tardive dyskinesia is referred to as classic TD. Other names have been used for classic TD (see Table 20-1). The phenomenologically essential component of classic TD is the presence of repetitive, almost rhythmic movements. These are almost always present in the mouth region and therefore are also called O-B-L dyskinesias.

Thus, tardive dyskinesia is an iatrogenic syndrome of persistent abnormal involuntary movements that occur as a

Table 20-1 Terminology of the tardive syndromes

| Descriptions | Equivalent Common Names |
|---|---|
| Tardive syndromes as a group | Tardive syndrome<br>Tardive dyskinesia |
| Repetitive, rhythmic movements, usually in the oral-buccal-lingual region | Classic tardive dyskinesia (TD)<br>Oral-buccal-lingual (O-B-L) dyskinesias<br>Tardive stereotypy<br>Rhythmic chorea |
| Dystonic movements and postures | Tardive dystonia |
| Restlessness and the movements that occur as a result | Tardive akathisia |
| Myoclonus | Tardive myoclonus |
| Tremor | Tardive tremor |
| Tics | Tardive tics<br>Tardive tourettism |
| Chorea | Withdrawal emergent syndrome<br>Tardive chorea |
| Oculogyria | Tardive oculogyric crisis |
| Parkinsonism | Tardive parkinsonism (if it exists) |

complication of drugs that competitively block dopamine receptors, particularly the D2 receptor but possibly also the D3 receptor, which is in the D2 family of receptors.

TD was first described in patients who were treated for schizophrenic psychosis with antipsychotics (Schonecker, 1957; Sigwald et al., 1959). These disorders tend to appear late in the course of treatment, in contrast to acute dystonic reactions and drug-induced parkinsonism, which had previously been recognized as complications from antipsychotics—hence the term *tardive*. The offending antipsychotics are now known to block the D2 dopamine receptor; that is, these drugs are DRBAs. Since the first descriptions, TD has also been noted in patients without psychiatric disorders who had other indications for using dopamine receptor antagonists, such as those with gastrointestinal complaints (Casey, 1983), with Tourette syndrome (Riddle et al., 1987), or with dystonia (Greene and Fahn, 1988).

Dopamine receptor antagonists produce many undesirable side effects, most of which occur relatively early in the course of treatment and are reversible on discontinuation of the medication. However, disfiguring and disabling abnormal involuntary movements were also noted to often occur late in the course of treatment, and these were often noted to persist even after discontinuation of the medication. Hence, the term *tardive* was coined, referring to the late and insidious onset (Faurbye et al., 1964). Initially, the term *tardive dyskinesia* was equated with stereotypic repetitive movements of oral, buccal, and lingual distribution (Schonecker, 1957), but subsequently, other types of movements have been recognized (Burke et al., 1982; Fahn, 1984a). As such, the concept of tardive dyskinesia has evolved and has been modified considerably since the initial recognition of the syndrome.

The prevalences of drug-induced parkinsonism and the various tardive syndromes have been compared by van Harten and colleagues (1996b) on the island of Curaçao, which has only one psychiatric facility. In 194 in-patients, the prevalence for classic TD was 39.7%, that for parkinsonism was 36.1%,

that for tardive dystonia was 13.4%, and that for akathisia was 9.3%. Combinations of two or more of these phenomenologies occurred in 30% of patients (van Harten et al., 1997). The use of antipsychotic medications is a strong predictor of developing subsequent PD, and in one study patients taking neuroleptics have been found to be 5.4 times more likely to begin antiparkinsonian medications than nonusers (Noyes et al., 2006).

## DOPAMINE RECEPTORS AND THEIR ANTAGONISTS

Since TD is an iatrogenic disorder and the most constant feature of the syndrome is the pharmacologic class of the responsible etiologic agent, it is important to understand the nature of the drugs that produce TD (Table 20-2). Although models of abnormal basal ganglia circuitry have been proposed to explain the mechanism of TD (Marchand and Dilda, 2006), the pathophysiology is still poorly understood. Dopamine receptors are classified into five subtypes, based on the genetics of the receptors; they are labeled D1, D2, D3, D4, and D5 (Kebabian and Calne, 1979; Sokoloff et al., 1990). Table 20-3 characterizes the five dopamine receptors. It is the dopamine D2 receptor–blocking action of drugs that has been linked to the tardive syndromes and other neuroleptic drug-induced movement disorders (described later and listed in Table 20-4).

Recently introduced drugs in Table 20-2 (e.g., iloperidone [Jain, 2000], ziprasidone [Hirsch et al., 2002] and amisulpride [Curran and Perry, 2002]) need to be in clinical use for several years before their full potential in causing tardive dyskinesia syndromes can be known. In Table 20-2, the calcium channel blockers deserve comment. Cinnarizine [1-diphenylmethyl-4-(3-phenyl-2-propenyl) piperazine] and its difluorinated derivative flunarizine inhibit the MgATP-dependent generation of a transmembrane proton electrochemical gradient and dopamine vesicular uptake (Terland and Flatmark, 1999). Whether either of these mechanisms, rather than a proposed DRBA action, is responsible for its neuroleptic activity is uncertain. In regard to melatonin, there is a case report of withdrawal-emergent O-B-L dyskinesias associated with akathisia that occurred with sudden discontinuation of chronic melatonin use (Giladi and Shabtai, 1999). Such withdrawal syndromes are typical of drugs that block dopamine receptors. On resumption of melatonin, the patient's O-B-L dyskinesia and akathisia cleared. Sudden cessation of the drug again brought on the symptoms; slow taper over 2 months was effective without incident. This case suggests that either the melatonin product the patient was taking was impure and was contaminated with a DRBA or melatonin itself has dopamine receptor antagonist properties. In support of the latter is the result of a blinded crossover study showing some suppression of the tardive dyskinesia with melatonin (Shamir et al., 2001).

Some drugs that block dopamine D2 receptors are promoted for medical problems other than psychosis, but these drugs can cause drug-induced parkinsonism, acute dystonic reactions, tardive syndromes, and NMS, just like the drugs that are promoted for the treatment of psychosis. Metoclopramide (Ganzini et al., 1993) and clebopride (Sempere et al., 1994) are used mainly for dyspepsia and as antiemetic agents. Amoxapine has a tricyclic structure and is marketed as an antidepressant drug, but a metabolite has dopamine receptor–blocking activity and has

**Table 20-2** Drugs that can produce tardive syndromes

| Class of Drug | Examples of Drugs in Each Class |
| --- | --- |
| Phenothiazines | |
|   Aliphatic | Chlorpromazine (Thorazine), triflupromazine (Vesprin) |
|   Piperidine | Thioridazine (Mellaril), mesoridazine (Serentil) |
|   Piperazine | Trifluoperazine (Stelazine), prochlorperazine (Compazine), perphenazine (Trilafon), fluphenazine (Prolixin), perazine |
| Thioxanthenes | |
|   Aliphatic | Chlorprothixene (Tarctan) |
|   Piperazine | Thiothixene (Navane) |
| Butyrophenones | Haloperidol (Haldol), droperidol (Inapsine) |
| Diphenylbutylpiperidine | Pimozide (Orap) |
| Dibenzazepine | Loxapine (Loxitane) |
| Dibenzodiazepines | Clozapine (Clozaril), quetiapine (Seroquel) |
| Thienobenzodiazepine | Olanzapine (Zyprexa) |
| Pyrimidinone | Risperidone (Risperidal) |
| Benzisothiazole | Ziprasidone (Geodon) |
| Benzisoxazole | Iloperidone (Zomaril) |
| Substituted benzamides | Metoclopramide (Reglan), tiapride, sulpiride, clebopride, remoxipride, veralipride, amisulpride |
| Indolones | Molindone (Moban) |
| Quinolinone | Aripiprazole (Abilify) |
| Tricyclic | Amoxapine (Asendin) |
| Calcium channel blockers | Flunarizine (Sibelium), cinnarizine (Stugeron) |
| N-acetyl-4-methoxytryptamine | Melatonin |

been implicated in producing TD (Kang et al., 1986; Sa et al., 2001). Veralipride is a substituted benzamide that is used for the treatment of menopausal hot flushes (Masmoudi et al., 1995). Pimozide is marketed for the treatment of Tourette syndrome. Some commercial preparations contain dopamine receptor antagonists in combination with other drugs, and this can lead to inadvertent use of these drugs. A popular combination is that of perphenazine and amitriptyline, marketed as Triavil and Etrafon. Risperidone is commercially promoted with the suggestion that it might have less risk of drug-induced complications, but this appears not to be the case. Parkinsonism and TD have been noted in association with the calcium channel antagonists flunarizine and cinnarizine (Micheli et al., 1987). Both of these medications have mild dopamine receptor antagonist activity, which is thought be the mechanism for their complications (Micheli et al., 1989). Recognition of these drugs is essential not only in making the diagnosis of TD but also in preventing the occurrence of TD by being able to avoid using them.

Clozapine is a special drug that is discussed more thoroughly later in the chapter; it has greater affinity for blocking the D4 receptor than the D2 receptor and deserves the classification as an atypical antipsychotic because it rarely causes parkinsonism

or worsens Parkinson disease (PD). The newer antipsychotic quetiapine also qualifies as an atypical antipsychotic with just slightly more propensity to induce parkinsonism than does clozapine. Olanzapine has more propensity to induce parkinsonism and worsen PD. Many agents that are promoted as atypical antipsychotics should not be classified as such.

The D1 and D5 receptors were both previously known as D1 receptors; both are distinct in activating adenyl cyclase. The D2, D3, and D4 receptors were all previously lumped together as the D2 receptor and are still considered in the D2 family of receptors.

The D1 and D2 receptors are found mainly in the striatum and nucleus accumbens as well as in the substantia nigra, amygdala, cingulate cortex, and entorhinal area. The anterior lobe of the pituitary gland has only D2 receptors, and the thalamus and cerebral cortex outside of the cingulate and entorhinal area contain D1 receptors only (De Keyser et al., 1988). D2 receptor affinities of dopamine receptor antagonists correlate closely with antipsychotic and antiemetic properties of the drugs (Creese et al., 1976). Dopamine receptor antagonists are often referred to as neuroleptics or antipsychotics; the former term indicates the effect of drugs in producing par-

**Table 20-3** Characteristics of dopamine receptors

| Feature | D1 | D2 | D3 | D4 | D5 |
| --- | --- | --- | --- | --- | --- |
| Chromosome | 5q31–34 | 11q22–23 | 3q13.3 | 11p | 4p16.3 |
| Region | Striatum | Striatum | Accumbens | Frontal cortex | Hippocampus |
| DA affinity | μmolar | μmolar | nmolar | Subμmolar | Subμmolar |
| Agonist | SKF-82526 | Bromocriptine | 7-OH-DPAT | ? | SKF-82526 |
| Antagonist | SCH-23390 | Haloperidol | UH 232 | Clozapine | SCH-23390 |
| Adenyl cyclase | Stimulates | Inhibits | ? | Inhibits | Stimulates |

**Table 20-4** A brief listing of receptor binding profiles of "atypical" antipsychotic agents

| Drug | D1 | D2 | 5-HT$_{2A}$ | M2 | α1 | H1 |
|------|-----|-----|------|--------|----|-----|
| Clozapine | 85 | 125 | 2 | 1.9 | 7 | 6 |
| Quetiapine | 455 | 160 | 220 | 120 | 7 | 11 |
| Olanzapine | 31 | 11 | 4 | 1.9 | 19 | 7 |
| Risperidone | 75 | 3 | 0.6 | >10,000 | 2 | 155 |

Data are Ki (nM). The lower the number, the greater is the affinity of the drug for the receptor.
D1, dopamine D1; D2, dopamine D2; 5-HT$_{2A}$, serotonin 2A; H1, histamine type 1 receptors; M2, muscarinic type 2, α1, alpha NE type 1.

Data from Worrel JA, Marken PA, Beckman SE, Ruehter VL: Atypical antipsychotic agents: A critical review. Am J Health Syst Pharm 2000;57:238–255; Schmidt AW, Lebel LA, Howard HR Jr, Zorn SH: Ziprasidone: A novel antipsychotic agent with a unique human receptor binding profile. Eur J Pharmacol 2001;425:197–201.

kinsonism, and the latter indicates the effect of controlling psychosis.

The D3 receptor, another target of neuroleptics, is found chiefly in the mesolimbic areas. Because it is involved in emotional behaviors, it may be involved in tardive akathisia. Clozapine, an atypical neuroleptic, which has a low potential to induce parkinsonism or tardive syndromes, is primarily a D4 receptor antagonist. However, it has some D2-blocking action, which increases with higher doses.

## "ATYPICAL" ANTIPSYCHOTICS

The label *atypical* refers to a lower propensity of the antipsychotic agent to induce parkinsonism or a variety of other movement disorders described later (and listed in Table 20-4); that is, these agents have a lower propensity to be neuroleptics. A number of epidemiologic studies have found that the atypicals are less likely to induce tardive dyskinesia and other movement disorder problems (Tarsy and Baldessarini, 2006). Dolder and Jeste (2003) found that the atypicals reduced the incidence of tardive dyskinesia by half.

### Dopamine and Serotonin (5-HT) Receptor Antagonism

Although drugs that are labeled as atypical antipsychotic agents block dopamine D2 receptors, they also block serotonin 5-HT$_{2A}$ receptors, and some investigators attribute their antipsychotic effect to this mechanism and recommend research and drug development on newer agents that block other 5-HT receptors (Meltzer, 1999).

How tightly drugs bind to the D2 receptor (their occupancy rate) is currently considered to be important in a drug having neuroleptic potential in direct proportion. Seeman and Tallerico (1998) found that the atypical antipsychotic drugs bind more loosely than classic antipsychotic drugs (neuroleptics) to the D2 receptors. Kapur and colleagues (1999) measured D2 and 5-HT$_2$ receptor occupancies by positron emission tomography

(PET) scan for patients receiving clozapine, risperidone, or olanzapine. Clozapine showed a much lower D2 occupancy (16% to 68%) than did risperidone (63% to 89%) and olanzapine (43% to 89%); all three showed greater 5-HT$_2$ occupancy than D2 occupancy at all doses, although the difference was greatest for clozapine. In their PET study, Moresco and colleagues (2004) found that striatal D2 receptor occupancy was significantly higher with olanzapine than with clozapine. All these studies support the relationship between receptor occupancy and the clinical observations that clozapine and quetiapine are the most atypical, with the least propensity to cause parkinsonism, tardive syndromes, or other neuroleptic drug reactions.

A comparison of the receptor-binding profile of quetiapine, clozapine, olanzapine, and risperidone is presented in Table 20-4. Both quetiapine and clozapine have poor affinity for the dopamine D2 receptor, which probably accounts for the low incidence of inducing parkinsonism and tardive syndromes. Risperidone has the highest affinity for the D2 receptor resembling haloperidol (Table 20-5) and is therefore more of a typical than an atypical antipsychotic.

In one PET study, striatal D1 and D2 receptor occupancies were evaluated (Tauscher et al., 2004). D1 occupancy ranged from 55% with clozapine to 12% with quetiapine (rank order: clozapine > olanzapine > risperidone > quetiapine). The striatal D2 occupancy ranged from 81% with risperidone to 30% with quetiapine (rank order: risperidone > olanzapine > clozapine > quetiapine). The ratio of striatal D1/D2 occupancy was significantly higher for clozapine (0.88) relative to olanzapine (0.54), quetiapine (0.41), or risperidone (0.31).

## Clozapine

Clozapine was the first agent to be labeled as an atypical antipsychotic and deservedly so, although rare case reports do exist of drug-induced parkinsonism (Kurz et al., 1995), but it has been reported not to induce rigidity, and it rarely induces parkinsonian tremor (Gerlach and Peacock, 1994). It has also caused rare cases of acute akathisia (Friedman, 1993; Safferman et al., 1993), acute dystonic reaction (Kastrup et al., 1994; Thomas et al., 1994), tardive syndromes (Dave, 1994), tardive dystonia (Bruneau and Stip, 1998; Molho and Factor, 1999a), tardive akathisia (Kyriakos et al., 2005), and NMS (Sachdev et al., 1995; Benazzi, 1999; Lara et al., 1999; Gambassi et al., 2006). There are also parkinsonian features that are seen with clozapine. In a prospective study, seven out of 25 patients on clozapine developed TD (Bunker et al., 1996). In a retrospective study, comparison of clozapine and typical antipsychotics showed no lower prevalence of tardive dyskinesia in the clozapine group (Modestin, 2000). But it is not clear that the patients in the clozapine group had not been previously exposed to typical antipsychotics and had not developed TD while receiving them. What is clear from this study is that the conversion to using clozapine has not markedly reduced the prevalence of extrapyramidal syndromes; this finding supports the realization that clozapine does not effectively treat TD once it has developed. How effective its use would be in preventing TD in the first place still needs to be verified. For patients with PD, the low propensity to augment existing parkinsonism makes clozapine very useful in treating patients who have dopaminergic drug-induced psychosis (Factor and Friedman, 1997; Friedman et al., 1999).

Table 20-5 A more complete listing of antipsychotic affinities for human receptors and rat transporters

| Receptor | Haloperidol | Clozapine | Quetiapine | Olanzapine | Risperidone | Ziprasidone |
|---|---|---|---|---|---|---|
| Dopamine D1 | 15 | 53 | 390 | 10 | 21 | 9.5 |
| Dopamine D2 | 0.82 | 36 | 39 | 2.1 | 0.44 | 2.8 |
| Dopamine D3 | 2.5 | 22 | >500 | 17 | 13 | 28 |
| 5-HT$_{1A}$ | 2600 | 710 | >830 | 7100 | 21 | 37 |
| 5-HT$_{2A}$ | 28 | 4.0 | 82 | 1.9 | 0.39 | 0.25 |
| 5-HT$_{2C}$ | 1500 | 5.0 | 1500 | 2.8 | 6.4 | 0.55 |
| 5-HT$_6$ | 6600 | 9.5 | 33 | 10 | 2400 | not tested |
| 5-HT$_7$ | 80 | 21 | 290 | 120 | 1.6 | 4.9 |
| α1-adrenoceptor | 7.3 | 3.7 | 4.5 | 7.3 | 0.69 | 1.9 |
| α2-adrenoceptor | 1600 | 51 | 1100 | 140 | 1.8 | 390 |
| Histamine H1 | >730 | 17 | 21 | 5.6 | 88 | 510 |
| Muscarinic M1 | 570 | 0.98 | 56 | 2.1 | >5000 | >10,000 |

Receptor bindings are presented as Ki values (nmol/L).

Data are from Horacek J: Novel antipsychotics and extrapyramidal side effects: Theory and reality. Pharmacopsychiatry 2000;33:34–42; Schmidt AW, Lebel LA, Howard HR Jr, Zorn SH: Ziprasidone: A novel antipsychotic agent with a unique human receptor binding profile. Eur J Pharmacol 2001;425:197–201.

A single photon emission computed tomography (SPECT) study measuring dopamine D2 receptor binding reveals lower binding with clozapine than with typical neuroleptics (Broich et al., 1998). In animal studies, rats that have been pretreated with haloperidol for 4 weeks develop vacuous chewing movements (VCMs) after treatment with a dopaminergic, whereas rats that have been pretreated with clozapine do not (Ikeda et al., 1999).

The problem with clozapine is that weekly blood counts are required because there is a 1% to 2% incidence of leukopenia, which is reversible if the drug is withdrawn within 1 to 2 weeks. Granulocyte colony–stimulating factor can be an effective means to treat the agranulocytosis (Sperner-Unterweger et al., 1998). Other common adverse effects are drowsiness, drooling, weight gain, and seizures. An unusual adverse affect with clozapine was a case of myokymia (David and Sharif, 1998).

## Quetiapine

After clozapine, quetiapine is the most favorable in being least likely to induce parkinsonism, NMS (Stanley and Hunter, 2000), or tardive syndromes. D2 receptor antagonism is relatively selective for limbic than striatal receptors for clozapine and sertindole, followed by quetiapine, ziprasidone, olanzapine, and remoxipride, whereas risperidone in many respects has a profile that resembles that of haloperidol (Arnt and Skarsfeldt, 1998). Like clozapine, quetiapine easily induces drowsiness, so when it is used to treat dopa-induced psychosis, it should be taken at bedtime. The major advantage over clozapine is that it does not require blood tests because it does not induce agranulocytosis, however. There is a possibility that quetiapine has a risk of causing agranulocytosis (Ruhe et al., 2001). Since its introduction, there have been reports of acute dystonic reactions (Jonnalagada and Norton, 2000; Desarker and Sinha, 2006), acute akathisia (Prueter et al., 2003), and TD (Ghaemi and Ko, 2001). It is important to wait and see what other movement disorders develop with more widespread use.

In a SPECT study using the D2/D3 ligand [123I]-epidepride, the percent occupancy of receptors in the limbic system (temporal lobe) and striatal receptors while patients were receiving quetiapine was 60% and 32%, respectively, which is similar to results for clozapine (Stephenson et al., 2000). In another SPECT study, quetiapine was shown to occupy 5-HT$_{2A}$ receptors in the frontal and temporal cortex (Jones et al., 2001).

## Olanzapine

In contrast to clozapine and quetiapine, olanzapine more readily increases parkinsonian symptoms in patients with PD (Jimenez-Jimenez et al., 1998; Granger and Hanger, 1999; Molho and Factor, 1999b) but does so less readily than risperidone and conventional antipsychotics. Drug-induced parkinsonism, including rabbit syndrome, is seen with olanzapine (Durst et al., 2000). It can induce acute akathisia (Kurzthaler et al., 1997; Jauss et al., 1998) and TD but less so than does haloperidol (Tollefson et al., 1997; Wood, 1998). It can also induce NMS (Filice et al., 1998; Moltz and Coeytaux, 1998; Burkhard et al., 1999; Levenson, 1999; Margolese and Chouinard, 1999; Sierra-Biddle et al., 2000; Abu-Kishk et al., 2004; Zaragoza Fernandez and Torres Garcia, 2006), tardive dyskinesia (Herran and Vazquez-Barquero, 1999), and tardive dystonia (Dunayevich and Strakowski, 1999). Acute dystonic reactions also occur (Beasley et al., 1997; Landry and Cournoyer, 1998; Vena et al., 2006).

A direct comparison with chlorpromazine showed similar parkinsonism and acute akathisia for the two drugs (Conley et al., 1998). A double-blind comparison with haloperidol by Beasley and colleagues (1999) showed a much lower risk of developing tardive dyskinesia with olanzapine. After 1 year of exposure, 0.52% of patients developed TD with olanzapine and 7.45% developed TD with haloperidol. An open-label comparison with conventional antipsychotics after a 9-month follow-up after discharge from the hospital favored olanzapine, with TD being present in 2.3% for olanzapine

(2/87) and 16.7% (12/72) for the conventional treatment (Mari et al., 2004). There are case reports of agranulocytosis induced by olanzapine (Meissner et al., 1999; Naumann et al., 1999; Tolosa-Vilella et al., 2002), including a patient who previously had had agranulocytosis with clozapine (Benedetti et al., 1999). This has been attributed to some similar structural and pharmacologic properties of clozapine. A case of restless legs syndrome with periodic movements in sleep has been attributed to olanzapine (Kraus et al., 1999).

Olanzapine has relative regional mesolimbic dopaminergic selectivity and a broad-based binding affinity for serotonin (all 5-HT$_2$ receptor subtypes and the 5-HT$_6$ receptor), dopamine (D2, D3, and D4 receptors), muscarinic, and $\alpha_1$-adrenergic receptors (Bymaster et al., 1999). A PET study in schizophrenic patients being treated with olanzapine revealed that this drug is a potent 5-HT$_2$ blocker but also a blocker of D2 dopamine receptors similar to risperidone and less so than clozapine (Kapur et al., 1998). Patients on olanzapine were also studied with IBZM SPECT; the D2 receptor was occupied 60% and 83% of the time at doses of 5 mg per day and 10 mg per day, respectively (Raedler et al., 1999). Such high rates of occupancy probably account for olanzapine's tendency to worsen parkinsonism and induce DRBA-complications, because, as was noted earlier, D2 receptor occupancy rates are directly related to neuroleptic potential.

## Risperidone

With the success of clozapine, there is a commercial advantage for pharmaceutical companies to tout other antipsychotics as atypical. Such has been claimed for risperidone, but this drug can readily induce parkinsonism, including rabbit syndrome (Levin and Heresco-Levy, 1999), tardive syndromes (Haberfellner, 1997; Silberbauer, 1998; Hong et al., 1999; Ananth et al., 2000) and NMS (Newman et al., 1997). The prevalence of parkinsonism from risperidone is usually considered to be less than that with conventional neuroleptics, but it was observed in 42% compared to 29% in those on haloperidol (Knable et al., 1997). Tardive dyskinesia and tardive dystonia occurred in a patient who was exposed only to risperidone (Bassitt and Garcia, 2000). The annual incidence of TD in patients taking risperidone has been estimated to be 0.3%, compared to an annual incidence in patients taking conventional neuroleptics of 5% to 10% (Gutierrez-Esteinou and Grebb, 1997). However, in an open-label prospective study of 255 institutionalized patients with dementia who were treated with risperidone, the 1-year cumulative incidence of TD was 2.6% (Jeste et al., 2000).

Like conventional neuroleptics, risperidone induces acute dystonic reactions in marmosets, in contrast to clozapine, which does not (Fukuoka et al., 1997). In a recent report of an open-label comparison with haloperidol, Rosebush and Mazurek (1999) found the two drugs to have a similar side effect profile. In a prospective follow-up of first-episode schizophrenics treated with risperidone, movement disorders developed in more than one third of these patients, who had previously never been exposed to antipsychotic drugs (Lang et al., 2001). When risperidone was compared with low-potency antipsychotics, such as thioridazine, no difference was discerned in the rates of developing movement disorders (Schillevoort et al., 2001).

In a SPECT study, dopamine receptor binding with IBZM showed risperidone to have effects between those of haloperidol and clozapine, with a dose-response curve for risperidone showing greater similarity to that of haloperidol (Dresel et al., 1998). Clearly, risperidone is not an atypical antipsychotic agent. Risperidone's occupancy of the 5-HT$_2$ receptors is about 90%, and its occupancy of the D2 receptors is between 50% and 80%, but the latter correlates with the extrapyramidal side effects (Yamada et al., 2002).

## Ziprasidone

This benzisothiazole was approved by the FDA in 2001, and there are already case reports of acute dystonic reactions (Weinstein et al., 2006; Yumru et al., 2006), NMS, and rhabdomyolysis and pancreatitis (Murty et al., 2002; Yang and McNeely, 2002; Gray, 2004). It has been reported to cause tardive dyskinesia (Mendhekar, 2005) and tardive dystonia (Papapetropoulos et al., 2005). Although it is a potent 5-HT$_{2A}$ antagonist (like risperidone, olanzapine, and clozapine), it is also a D2 antagonist in humans as detected by PET scan (Bench et al., 1993, 1996). But in vitro studies reveal much lower affinity for the D2 receptor than for the 5-HT$_{2A}$ receptor (Seeger et al., 1995), and ziprasidone also binds less tightly to the D2 receptor than does dopamine (Seeman, 2002). Ziprasidone has two other unique features compared to other antipsychotic agents: (1) It is a potent 5-HT$_{1A}$ agonist and thus inhibits dorsal raphe serotonergic cell firing (Sprouse et al., 1999) and increases cortical dopamine release (Rollema et al., 2000), and (2) it inhibits neuronal uptake of 5-HT and norepinephrine in a manner comparable to the antidepressant imipramine (Schmidt et al., 2001). What these unique actions might contribute to antipsychotic activity or to propensity for or against extrapyramidal reactions is unclear.

## Aripiprazole

This quinolinone derivative has a novel mechanism of action. Like a number of other atypical antipsychotics, it is an antagonist at the 5-HT$_{2A}$ receptors. What is novel is that it is a partial agonist at the dopamine D2 receptor. It has a higher affinity for the presynaptic autoreceptor than for the postsynaptic receptor. Hence, it reduces dopamine synthesis and release through an agonist action at the dopamine autoreceptor (Tamminga and Carlsson, 2002). It is also a 5-HT$_{1A}$ partial agonist (Jordan et al., 2002). Because of its novel action as a partial D2 agonist, it is anticipated that it might cause fewer extrapyramidal adverse effects, and clinical trials reported favorable results (Kane et al., 2002). But until it faces much wider use, it is too early to be certain of its safety profile. But there have already been reports of NMS (Chakraborty and Johnston, 2004; Hammerman et al., 2006) and acute dystonic reactions (Desarkar et al., 2006; Fountoulakis et al., 2006).

## Amisulpride

Amisulpride, a substituted benzamide, is a highly selective antagonist for dopamine D2 and D3 receptors in the limbic region, which would predict potent antipsychotic activity with a low potential to cause extrapyramidal symptoms (Lecrubier, 2000). It binds less tightly to the D2 receptor than do the

**Table 20-6** Adverse effect profile of "atypical" neuroleptics

| Adverse Effect | Haloperidol | Clozapine | Quetiapine | Olanzapine | Risperidone |
|---|---|---|---|---|---|
| Sedation | + | +++ | ++ | + | + |
| Seizures | + | +++ | + | + | + |
| Hypotension | + | +++ | ++ | ++ | ++ |
| Increased prolactin | +++ | 0 | 0 | ++ | + |
| Weight gain | + | +++ | ++ | +++ | ++ |

0, none; +, mild; ++, moderate; +++, severe.

Data from Worrel JA, Marken PA, Beckman SE, Ruehter VL: Atypical antipsychotic agents: A critical review. Am J Health Syst Pharm 2000;57:238–255.

## Adverse Effects from Atypical Antipsychotics

Aside from the D2-blocking effects described previously, the four drugs in Table 20-4 have a number of other adverse effects. Sedation is a particular problem that is seen with each of them but particularly clozapine and quetiapine. Table 20-6 lists the common adverse effects of these drugs, along with haloperidol, for comparison.

It is not likely that drug-induced tardive syndromes will disappear, because use of both typical and atypical agents continues. In a survey in Lombardy (Italy), 35,363 individuals over age 65 were prescribed an antipsychotic prescription (2.18 subjects per 100 inhabitants, with two thirds receiving first-generation agents (Percudani et al., 2004). Although there may be a lower risk of developing these disorders with atypicals, these drugs can induce them (Table 20-7). It is even possible that if physicians consider atypicals safe to use, their use will increase even in situations in which the risk from typicals might have precluded their use. In the United States, the prevalence of atypical antipsychotic use was found to be 267.1 per 100,000 subjects aged 19 years and younger and was more than twice as high for male patients as for female patients (Curtis et al., 2005).

## NEUROLOGIC SIDE EFFECTS OF DOPAMINE D2 RECEPTOR ANTAGONISTS

To better understand the tardive syndromes, it is important to recognize the variety of other movement disorders that are induced by the dopamine receptor antagonists at different points in the course of treatment. These movement disorders are often lumped together as extrapyramidal syndromes, but the lumping often hinders the effort to sort out the clinical characteristics and pathophysiology of separate syndromes. It is better to subdivide them into their phenomenologic types (see Box 20-1). Movements that may be seen include acute dystonia, acute akathisia, parkinsonism, tardive syndromes, and NMS. Both dystonia and akathisia also occur as subtypes of tardive syndromes and are discussed in more detail in the section on tardive syndromes.

## Acute Dystonia

The earliest abnormal involuntary movement to appear after initiation of dopamine receptor antagonist therapy is an acute dystonic reaction. In about half of the cases, this reaction occurs within 48 hours, and in 90% of cases, it occurs by 5 days after starting the therapy (Ayd, 1961; Garver et al., 1976). The reaction may occur after the first dose (Marsden et al., 1975).

Dystonic movements are sustained muscle contractions, frequently causing twisting and repetitive movements or abnormal postures (Fahn, 1988). In a series of 3775 patients, Ayd (1961) found that acute dystonia is the least frequent side effect, affecting about 2% to 3% of patients, with males and younger patients being more susceptible. The incidence rate increases to beyond 50% with highly potent dopamine receptor blockers such as haloperidol (Boyer et al., 1987). In one prospective study, Aguilar and colleagues (1994) reported that 23 of 62 patients developed acute dystonia after haloperidol was introduced, that anticholinergic pretreatment significantly prevents this, and that younger age and severity of psychosis were risk factors. In the prospective study by Kondo and colleagues (1999), 20 (51.3%) of 39 patients placed on nemonapride had dystonic reactions, onset occurring within 3 days after the initiation of treatment in 90%. As in other series, the incidence of acute dystonia was significantly higher

**Table 20-7** Extrapyramidal adverse effects reported with "atypical" neuroleptics

| Adverse Effect | Haloperidol | Clozapine | Quetiapine | Olanzapine | Risperidone |
|---|---|---|---|---|---|
| Parkinsonism | Yes | Yes | Not yet | Yes | Yes |
| Acute akathisia | Yes | Yes | Yes | Yes | Yes |
| Acute dystonia | Yes | Yes | Yes | Yes | Yes |
| Neuroleptic malignant syndrome | Yes | Yes | Not yet | Yes | Yes |
| Tardive syndrome | Yes | Yes | Yes | Yes | Yes |

in males than in females (77.8% versus 28.6%, $P < .05$), and younger males ($\leq$30 years) had an extremely high incidence (91.7%). The incidence is much lower with the so-called atypical antipsychotics; Raja and Azzoni (2001) observed only 41 cases out of 1337 newly admitted patients treated with antipsychotics, which included 8 treated with risperidone, 1 with olanzapine, and 1 with quetiapine.

All agents that block D2 receptors can induce acute dystonic reactions, including risperidone (Brody, 1996; Simpson and Lindenmayer, 1997) and clozapine (Kastrup et al., 1994). One child developed an acute dystonic reaction after ingestion of a dextromethorphan-containing cough syrup (Graudins and Fern, 1996). Dextromethorphan has several different known pharmacologic actions, but D2 receptor blockade is not one of them. Serotonergic agents have also been reported to induce acute dystonic reactions (Lopez-Alemany et al., 1997; Madhusoodanan and Brenner, 1997; Olivera, 1997). The mechanism could relate to inadequate release of dopamine from the nerve terminals in the striatum owing to the inhibitory effect of serotonin on dopamine neurons in the substantia nigra pars compacta. The opioid $\sigma_1$ and $\sigma_2$ receptors have also been implicated (Matsumoto and Pouw, 2000).

Acute dystonic reactions most often affect the ocular muscles (oculogyric crisis), face, jaw, tongue, neck, and trunk and less often the limbs. Oculogyric crisis has previously been noted to occur as a common feature of postencephalitic parkinsonism (Duvoisin and Yahr, 1965). A typical acute dystonic reaction may consist of head tilt backward or sideways with tongue protrusion and forced opening of the mouth, often with arching of the trunk and ocular deviation upward or laterally (Rupniak et al., 1986). The forcefulness of the muscle contractions can be extremely severe and led to autoamputation of the tongue in one patient (Pantanowitz and Berk, 1999).

Mazurek and Rosebush (1996) studied the timing in the development of an acute dystonic reaction in 200 patients who were taking a neuroleptic medication for the first time. The neuroleptic was given twice daily, and over 80% of the episodes of acute dystonia occurred between 12:00 noon and 11:00 P.M.

Reserpine and $\alpha$-methyl-para-tyrosine, which deplete presynaptic monoamines, have not been associated with acute dystonic reactions (Duvoisin, 1972; Marsden et al., 1975; Walinder, 1976). However, another dopamine depletor, tetrabenazine (TBZ), has been reported to induce acute dystonic reactions (Burke et al., 1985). One possible explanation for this difference is that in addition to depleting dopamine, TBZ blocks dopamine receptors (Reches et al., 1983).

It is important to mention the case described by Wolf (1973) of a patient who developed an oral dyskinesia while taking reserpine. Figure 1 in his paper clearly shows a dystonic phenomenon and not the complex, rapid, stereotypic movements of classic TD. This development appeared too late after initiation of reserpine to be considered an acute dystonic reaction, however. Whether this could be an example of tardive dystonia is not clear, since the phenomenology of tardive dystonia is identical to that of naturally occurring primary dystonia; therefore, the patient could have had a coincidental case of spontaneous, idiopathic oromandibular dystonia (Fahn, 1984b). Thus, there is no absolute evidence that reserpine induces acute dystonic reactions, classic TD, or tardive dystonia. In fact, symptoms of these three tardive syndromes can be suppressed by reserpine, and eventually, reserpine can be withdrawn successfully in many patients without exacerbation of the symptoms

(Fahn, 1983). Furthermore, the long time that reserpine has been available without a clear-cut case of tardive syndromes can be compared to the much shorter duration of use of metoclopramide, in which there are already cases of acute dystonic reactions, classic TD, and tardive dystonia as a consequence of its use (Casteels-Van Daele et al., 1970; Gatrad, 1976; Pinder et al., 1976; Reasbeck and Hossenbocus, 1979; Miller and Jankovic, 1989; Lang, 1990).

Of 452 patients who were given high-dose oral metoclopramide to control emesis, Kris and colleagues (1983) observed 14 who developed acute dystonic reactions. However, there was a distinct preponderance of the reactions occurring in children (6 of 22) compared to adults (8 of 430). Intravenous metoclopramide is more likely to induce it than is oral administration (Pinder et al., 1976). In a study at a Veterans Administration hospital comparing patients treated with metoclopramide and controls, the relative risk for TD was 1.67, and the relative risk for drug-induced parkinsonism was 4.0 (Ganzini et al., 1993).

The available biochemical explanations for the acute dystonic reaction are unsatisfactory, but several observations contribute to the understanding of the phenomena, relating it to dopamine, muscarinic, and sigma receptors. Acute neuroleptic administration produces sudden increase of dopamine release and increased turnover lasting for 24 to 48 hours after a single dose (O'Keefe et al., 1970; Marsden and Jenner, 1980). This effect is blocked by anticholinergics consistent with their efficacy in treatment of acute dystonic reactions (O'Keefe et al., 1970). Moreover, in baboons that were pretreated with reserpine and $\alpha$-methyl-para-tyrosine, which markedly reduces presynaptic dopamine concentration, haloperidol-induced acute dystonic reaction is abolished or greatly reduced (Meldrum et al., 1977). On the other hand, blockade of the postsynaptic receptor fades in about 12 hours after a single dose of antipsychotics, and supersensitivity of receptors begins to develop. Therefore, presynaptic dopaminergic excess in combination with the emerging supersensitive postsynaptic dopamine receptors could result in markedly increased striatal dopaminergic activity at about 20 to 40 hours after a neuroleptic dose. This period corresponds to the critical time for acute dystonic reactions in human subjects who were given a single dose of butaperazine (Garver et al., 1976). However, extrapolating the data from experimental animals to the clinical situation has its limitations, including the fact that rats do not develop acute dystonic reactions. Further data on human cerebrospinal fluid (CSF) dopamine metabolites as an indicator of presynaptic function might prove to be of value in pursuing the hypothesis. Jeanjean and colleagues (1997) suggested that the $\sigma_2$ receptors could be involved in the acute dystonic reaction. They found a correlation between the clinical incidence of neuroleptic-induced acute dystonia and binding affinity of drugs for the sigma receptor.

Another animal model of acute dystonia is the common marmoset that is treated with haloperidol (Fukuoka et al., 1997). But it takes at least 6 weeks of such treatment to develop this reaction. The dystonia subsides, only to reappear when haloperidol treatment is restarted; other neuroleptics, including risperidone, can also make the dystonia reappear, but clozapine was without such an effect. In this animal model, the anticholinergic agent trihexyphenidyl inhibited the induction of acute dystonia.

In patients with acute dystonic reactions, symptoms can be relieved within minutes after parenteral anticholinergics or antihistaminics (Paulson, 1960; Waugh and Metts, 1960; Smith and Miller, 1961). Diphenhydramine 50 mg and benztropine mesylate or biperiden 1 to 2 mg is given intravenously and can be repeated if the effect is not seen in 30 minutes. Intravenous diazepam has also been shown to be effective and can be used as an alternative therapy (Korczyn and Goldberg, 1972; Gagrat et al., 1978; Rainer-Pope, 1979). If untreated, the majority of cases still resolve spontaneously in 12 to 48 hours after the last dose of the dopamine receptor antagonists. Dopamine receptor antagonists with high anticholinergic activities have low incidence rates of acute dystonic reactions (Swett, 1975). Therefore, prophylactic use of anticholinergics (Arana et al., 1988) and benztropine (Goff et al., 1991) have been studied and reported to be helpful in reducing the risk of acute dystonic reactions, especially in young patients on high-potency drugs. The response of acute dystonic reactions to anticholinergics is so characteristic that it is difficult to explain the report of a few cases that are apparently due to amitriptyline, which has considerable anticholinergic activity and no known DRBA activity (Ornadel et al., 1992).

A case of an acute dystonic reaction occurring in an elderly person with bipolar disorder taking the serotonin uptake inhibitor paroxetine has been reported (Arnone et al., 2002). Speculation about the risk due to previous exposure to neuroleptics was raised. This class of drug can reduce the firing rate of nigral dopaminergic neurons owing to their inhibition by serotonin.

## Acute Akathisia

The term *akathisia*, from the Greek, meaning "unable to sit down," was coined by Haskovec in 1903 (cited by Shen, 1981), long before antipsychotic drugs were introduced. Akathisia was seen in some patients with advanced parkinsonism, and in others, it was frequently thought to be functional. Akathisia refers to an abnormal state of excessive restlessness, a feeling of the need to move about, with relief of this symptom on actually moving. Today, it is most frequently encountered as a side effect of neuroleptic drugs.

Two major issues of akathisia remain in confusion. First, there is no consensus about diagnostic criteria. Some authors consider akathisia to be an abnormal subjective state and regard the movements as an expression of the subjective state but not a necessary feature for the diagnosis (Van Putten, 1975). Others recognize the characteristic patterns of restless movements and consider the presence of movements to be sufficient for the diagnosis (Munetz and Cornes, 1982; Barnes et al., 1983; Gibb and Lees, 1986). A second point of confusion is that akathisia occurs not only in an early-onset, self-limited form (acute akathisia) but also in a late-onset, persistent form (tardive akathisia). Much of the literature on akathisia does not distinguish between acute and tardive akathisia, which makes interpretation of the literature difficult. The recognition of tardive akathisia as a distinct subsyndrome of tardive syndromes has been more recent (Fahn, 1978, 1983; Braude and Barnes, 1983; Weiner and Luby, 1983). For the discussion of the clinical features of akathisia, acute and tardive akathisia are lumped together, since they are similar, but their treatments and most likely their pathophysiologies are distinct.

The subjective aspect of akathisia is characterized by inner tension and aversion to remaining still. Patients complain of vague inner tension, emotional unease, or anxiety with vivid phrases such as "jumping out of my skin" or "about to explode." Subjective descriptions, however, can be nonspecific. Inner restlessness and inability to remain still can be present in a significant number of psychiatric patients without akathisia and in control subjects without psychiatric problems (Braude et al., 1983). In an attempt to clarify the issue, Braude and colleagues (1983) systematically surveyed the frequency of various complaints and found that inability to keep the legs still was the most characteristic complaint and was present in over 90% of patients with akathisia in contrast to about 20% of those with other psychiatric disturbances. Others noted more conservative estimation of the frequency of complaints related to the legs from 27% (Gibb and Lees, 1986) to 57% (Burke et al., 1989). Various authors also described atypical features such as "acting out," suicidal ideation, disruptive behaviors, homicidal violence, sexual torment, terror, and exacerbation of psychosis as akathitic phenomena (Van Putten and Marder, 1987). Evaluation of the subjective aspect also depends on patients' ability to describe their feelings. Those with psychosis, dementia, or mental retardation are often unable to provide useful descriptions for diagnosis. Although akathisia may manifest itself as subjective feeling alone, lack of specific subjective feeling and variable expression by patients pose a diagnostic dilemma. Therefore, the presence of the motor phenomenon is very helpful for the diagnosis.

Akathisia can present as focal pain or burning, usually in the oral or genital region (Ford et al., 1994). The symptom of moaning may be a verbal expression of the subjective feeling of akathisia. Some patients may moan as part of a generalized akathitic state and have other motor evidence of akathisia, such as marching in place, inability to sit still accompanied by walking about, inability to lie quietly associated with writhing and rolling movements, and making stereotypic caressing or rocking movements. The differential diagnosis of moaning includes parkinsonism, akathisia, levodopa usage (Fahn et al., 1996), dementia, pain, and other syndromes of phonation, such as tics, oromandibular dystonia, and Huntington disease, as discussed by Fahn (1991).

The motor aspect of akathisia (akathitic movements) is generally described as excessive movements that are complex, semipurposeful, stereotypic, and repetitive. Braude and colleagues (1983) found that rocking from foot to foot, walking on the spot, and coarse tremor and myoclonic jerks of the feet were characteristic of akathitic movements. Others agree that various leg and feet movements are more common in patients with akathisia than in those with TD (Gibb and Lees, 1986; Burke et al., 1989). However, they also noted that these did not distinguish akathisia from the group that did not meet criteria for akathisia (Gibb and Lees, 1986), and movements involving other parts of the body, such as trunk rocking, respiratory grunting, face rubbing, and shifting weight while sitting, were also frequent (Burke et al., 1989). Although there are not enough data and consensus on the diagnostic movements of akathisia, these movements seem to be characteristic enough to be recognized by different authors who have independently documented similar phenomena.

Akathisia is seen in patients with PD (Lang and Johnson, 1987), in patients abusing cocaine (Daras et al., 1994), and as an adverse effect of selective serotonin reuptake inhibitors (Poyurovsky et al., 1995). Acute akathisia occurs not only as an adverse effect of DRBAs but also fairly commonly as an acute adverse effect of the dopamine depletors reserpine, TBZ, and α-methyl-tyrosine (Marsden and Jenner, 1980).

In Ayd's review (1961), half of the cases of acute akathisia occurred within 25 days of drug treatment, and 90% occurred within 73 days. Acute akathisia was the most common side effect of DRBAs, occurring in 21.2% of patients in that study (Ayd, 1961). In a more recent study by Sachdev and Kruk (1994) of 100 consecutive patients placed on neuroleptics, mild akathisia developed in 41%, and moderate-to-severe akathisia developed in 21%. In a literature review, Sachdev (1995b) reported that incidence rates for acute akathisia with conventional neuroleptics vary from 8% to 76%, 20% to 30% being a conservative estimate. Sachdev stated that preliminary evidence suggests that the newer atypical antipsychotic drugs are less likely to produce acute akathisia. Using the criterion that both subjective and objective phenomena are required for the diagnosis of acute akathisia, Miller and colleagues (1997) found an incidence rate of 22.4%, 75% of which occurred within the first 3 days of exposure to a neuroleptic. Muscettola and colleagues (1999) found a prevalence rate of 9.4%.

The potency of neuroleptics has been associated with incidence of akathisia, ranging from 0.5% for reserpine (Marsden and Jenner, 1980) to 75% for haloperidol (Van Putten et al., 1984). Other risk factors are neuroleptic dose, the rate of dosage increase, and the development of drug-induced parkinsonism (Sachdev and Kruk, 1994).

As with acute dystonic reactions, akathisia has also been induced by serotonergic agents (Chong, 1996; Lopez-Alemany et al., 1997). The mechanism was discussed in the section on acute dystonia.

As was noted previously, akathisia needs to be distinguished from other conditions, such as agitated depression; restless legs syndrome, in which similar subjective sensations may be described by patients but are mainly localized to legs and are present particularly at night (Blom and Ekbom, 1961); or complex motor tics with preceding aura, which show more variety of abnormal movements and complex vocal tics (Jankovic and Fahn, 1986). Akathisia can also be obscured by other psychiatric disorders, or it could be mistaken for a psychiatric disease. For example, when patients with psychosis develop akathisia after withdrawal from antipsychotic drugs, it may be mistaken for recurrence of psychosis. Paradoxical dystonia (see Chapter 13) in which dystonic movements are relieved by movement can be mistaken for akathisia.

The pathophysiology of acute akathisia remains poorly understood. On the basis of the observation in rats that show increased locomotor activity after blockade of the mesocortical dopamine system (Carter and Pycock, 1978), reduction of this dopaminergic projection was suggested to be responsible for akathisia (Marsden and Jenner, 1980). However, tardive akathisia cannot be explained by this hypothesis because dopamine depletors can ameliorate those symptoms. The observation that acute akathisia can occur with a serotonin uptake inhibitor (Altshuler et al., 1994) indicates that inhibiting dopamine neurons in the substantia nigra by such drugs could link the dopamine system with akathisia. These types of drugs have been reported to increase parkinsonism in patients with PD (Meco et al., 1994). One attractive possibility is that akathisia might reflect an alteration of the dopaminergic mesolimbic system.

Because propranolol has been reported to be beneficial in treating acute akathisia, another suggestion is that acute akathisia results from alterations in the cingulate cortex, the piriform cortex, or area 1 of the parietal cortex based on effects of propranolol in these regions in haloperidol-treated rats (Ohashi et al., 1998).

Ayd (1961) noted that acute akathisia is self-limited, disappearing on discontinuation of neuroleptics, and is well controlled by anticholinergics despite continuation of neuroleptics. Others have noted that only patients with concomitant parkinsonism improve significantly with anticholinergics (Kruse, 1960; Braude et al., 1983). Amantadine may also help, but patients can develop a tolerance (Zubenko et al., 1984a). Beta blockers at relatively low doses, below 80 mg per day of propranolol, have been noted to be effective in many studies including one with a double-blind design (Lipinski et al., 1984; Zubenko et al., 1984b; Adler et al., 1986; Dupuis et al., 1987). Nonlipophilic beta blockers that have poor penetration to the central nervous system are not as effective (Lipinski et al., 1984; Dupuis et al., 1987). Selective beta blockers might not be as effective as nonselective ones (Zubenko et al., 1984b); however, when two equally lipophilic beta blockers, propranolol and betaxolol, were compared, they were equally effective in treating acute akathisia (Dumon et al., 1992) although the former is a beta-2 blocker and the latter is a beta-1 blocker. In a rat model of acute akathisia (neuroleptic-induced defecation), a lipophilic beta-1 blocker was found to be effective in reducing the phenomenon (Sachdev and Saharov, 1997)

Clonidine also reduces central noradrenergic activity by stimulating central alpha-2 receptors and has been noted to be effective in a small number of studies. The sedating effect is pronounced, however (Adler et al., 1987). Nicotine patches have been reported to reduce akathisia (Anfang and Pope, 1997). Weiss and colleagues (1995) reported cyproheptadine, an antiserotonergic agent, to be effective in ameliorating akathisia. In a small placebo-controlled trial, mianserin, a $5-HT_2$ antagonist, was found to reduce the severity of acute akathisia (Poyurovsky et al., 1999). Trazadone has also been reported to be beneficial (Stryjer et al., 2003). Poyurovsky and Weizman (2001) discuss the potential of serotonin agents in akathisia.

## Parkinsonism

Neuroleptic-induced parkinsonism (usually referred to as extrapyramidal syndrome by psychiatrists and as drug-induced parkinsonism by neurologists) is a dose-related side effect and is indistinguishable phenomenologically from idiopathic PD, including high frequency of tremor and asymmetric signs (Hardie and Lees, 1988). SPECT imaging of the dopamine transporter, however, may be helpful in determining whether the neuroleptic-induced parkinsonism is entirely drug-induced or an exacerbation of subclinical PD (Lorberboym et al., 2006). It develops with use of both DRBAs and dopamine-depleting drugs such as reserpine and TBZ. Some authors have noted perioral tremor and termed this rabbit syndrome, which is a localized form of parkinsonian tremor (Decina et al., 1990). The incidence of parkinsonism varies. Korczyn and Goldberg (1976) found it to be 61%, while Muscettola and colleagues (1999) found it to be 19.4%. Women are affected almost twice as frequently as are men, which is the reverse of the ratio in idiopathic PD. Neuroleptic-induced parkinsonism also occurs increasingly with advanced age (Ayd, 1961; Hardie and Lees, 1988) in parallel with the incidence of idiopathic PD.

Blockade of dopamine receptors by antagonists or depletion of presynaptic monoamines by drugs such as reserpine mimics the deficient dopamine state in PD. All DRBAs can induce parkinsonism except clozapine (Factor and Friedman, 1997) (there are actually only rare reports with clozapine). Risperidone can do so (Gwinn and Caviness, 1997; Simpson and Lindenmayer, 1997), as well as olanzapine and, only rarely, quetiapine. Parkinsonism from neuroleptics is typically reversible when the medication is reduced or discontinued. Sometimes, the reversal can take many months; an interval of up to 18 months has been noted in the literature (Fleming et al., 1970).

Some patients show persisting parkinsonism despite prolonged discontinuation of neuroleptics (Stephen and Williamson, 1984; Hardie and Lees, 1988), giving rise to consideration of a proposed condition of tardive parkinsonism. A study of 8-week exposure of rats to haloperidol found a highly significant 32% to 46% loss of tyrosine hydroxylase (TH) immunoreactive neurons in the substantia nigra, and 20% contraction of the TH-stained dendritic arbor (Mazurek et al., 1998). Perhaps such pathologic changes account for some cases of prolonged drug-induced parkinsonism in humans. Several cases in the literature had initial resolution of parkinsonism and later reappearance of the symptoms without re-exposure to neuroleptics (Hardie and Lees, 1988). Two cases that had complete resolution of drug-induced parkinsonism after withdrawal of neuroleptics showed evidence of mild PD at autopsy (Rajput et al., 1982). Although one assumes that these patients had subclinical PD, the effect of neuroleptics on the disease progression is unknown. The use of the term *tardive parkinsonism* to refer to cases of persistent parkinsonism remains an enigma. Some are due to concurrent development of progressive PD, and there have been no autopsied proven examples of non-PD. Therefore, this suggests that there is as yet no evidence of tardive parkinsonism.

With the introduction of selective serotonin reuptake inhibitors to treat depression, it has been noticed that these drugs can sometimes worsen parkinsonism in patients with PD (Meco et al., 1994) and occasionally can induce parkinsonism in patients who never had symptoms of PD (Coulter and Pillans, 1995; DiRocco et al., 1998). In an intensive monitoring program in New Zealand of the selective serotonin reuptake inhibitor fluoxetine over a 4-year period, there were 15 reports of parkinsonism in 5555 patients who were exposed to the drug (Coulter and Pillans, 1995). Of these 15, four patients were also on a neuroleptic, and one was on metoclopramide. The explanation for inducing or enhancing parkinsonism is that increased serotonergic activity in the substantia nigra will inhibit dopamine-containing neurons, thus causing functional dopamine deficiency in the nigrostriatal pathway (Baldessarini and Marsh, 1992).

The possibility of the existence of tardive parkinsonism comes up from time to time because some patients have continued parkinsonism despite long-term discontinuation of the DRBA (Melamed et al., 1991). However, there is always the possibility that the patient had preclinical PD prior to developing drug-induced parkinsonism. Then, when the DRBA is withdrawn, the parkinsonism persists because of progressively worsening PD. One would need to show that there are no Lewy bodies or that the PET scan shows no loss of fluorodopa uptake in patients believed to have tardive parkinsonism.

Anticholinergics can be effective in reducing the severity of the parkinsonism induced by DRBAs, whereas dopaminergic drugs (that activate the dopamine receptors) are ineffective, probably because they are not able to displace the DRBA from its binding to the receptor. L-dopa up to 1000 mg in combination with a peripheral dopa decarboxylase inhibitor had no significant effect (Hardie and Lees, 1988), nor did apomorphine, a dopamine receptor agonist (Merello, 1996). On the other hand, levodopa can effectively reverse parkinsonism induced by dopamine depletors, such as reserpine. In fact, the discovery of the dopamine hypothesis for parkinsonism was based on this observation (Carlsson et al., 1957; Carlsson, 1959). Treatment is usually initiated with anticholinergics or amantadine (Mindham et al., 1972; Johnson, 1978; Konig et al., 1996).

## Neuroleptic Malignant Syndrome

NMS is an idiosyncratic reaction that can sometimes be life-threatening. The clinical triad consists of (1) hyperthermia, usually with other autonomic dysfunctions such as tachycardia, diaphoresis, and labile blood pressure; (2) extrapyramidal signs, usually increased muscle tone of rigidity or dystonia, often with accompanying elevation of muscle enzymes; and (3) alteration of mental status, such as agitation, inattention, and confusion. Fever is not an essential symptom (Peiris et al., 2000). The syndrome begins abruptly while the patient is on therapeutic, not toxic, dosages of medication. In a review of 340 clinical reports of NMS in the literature (Velamoor et al., 1994), changes in either mental status or rigidity were the initial manifestations of NMS in 82.3% of cases with a single presenting sign. All the symptoms are fully manifest within 24 hours and reach a maximum within 72 hours. There does not seem to be any relationship with the duration of therapy. NMS can develop soon after the first dose or at any time after prolonged treatment. Recovery usually occurs within 1 to several weeks but can be fatal in 20% to 30% of cases (Henderson and Wooten, 1981; Gute and Baxter, 1985). Even with awareness of the potential of fatality in modern medicine, death still occurs (van Maidegem et al., 2002). Muscle biopsies have shown swelling and edema, with 10% to 50% of fibers involved with vacuoles but scanty mononuclear infiltration (Behan et al., 2000).

All agents that block D2 receptors can induce NMS, including risperidone (Raitasuo et al., 1994; Webster and Wijeratne, 1994; Dave, 1995; Singer et al., 1995; Levin et al., 1996), clozapine (Miller et al., 1991; Amore et al., 1997; Dalkilic and Grosch, 1997), amisulpride (Bottlender et al., 2002), olanzapine (Kontaxakis et al., 2002; Kogoj and Velikonja, 2003), and phenothiazines with antihistaminic activity, such as alimemazine (van Maidegem et al., 2002). TBZ has been reported to cause NMS; this seems likely to be due to its D2-blocking activity (Reches et al., 1983) rather than to its dopamine-depleting action (by blocking the vesicular dopamine transporter). Reserpine has no known dopamine receptor antagonism, only dopamine-depleting activity (also by blocking the vesicular dopamine transporter), and has not been reported to cause NMS.

In a Japanese study, 10 of 564 (1.8%) patients who received antipsychotics developed NMS (Naganuma and Fujii, 1994), many more than the 12 of 9792 patients (0.1%) reported previously (Deng et al., 1990). Risk factors that were found were psychomotor excitement, refusal of food, weight loss, and oral administration of haloperidol at 15 mg per day or above (Naganuma and Fujii, 1994). Young males appear to be more predisposed to NMS (Gratz and Simpson, 1994), but the reason for this is uncertain. In a case-control study searching for risk factors, Sachdev and colleagues (1997) found that patients with NMS were more likely to be agitated or dehydrated, often needed restraint or seclusion, had received larger doses of neuroleptics, and more often had previous treatment with electroshock therapy before the development of the syndrome.

The pathophysiologic mechanism of NMS is not well understood. Autopsies failed to show any consistent findings (Itoh et al., 1977). A similar syndrome has been reported following abrupt withdrawal of levodopa (Friedman et al., 1985; Hirschorn and Greenberg, 1988; Keyser and Rodnitzky, 1991), suggesting a common mechanism of acute dopamine deficiency (Henderson and Wooten, 1981). There is also a report of a patient who developed the NMS syndrome following abrupt withdrawal of the combination of a long-acting neuroleptic and an anticholinergic agent (Spivak et al., 1996). Because it responded to procyclidine administration, it implicates a muscarinic overactivity. There are also reports of NMS-like syndromes following the sudden withdrawal of amantadine (has dopaminergic and antimuscarinic activity) (Ito et al., 2001) and following withdrawal of baclofen, in which case the patient recovered with reintroduction of baclofen (Turner and Gainsborough, 2001).

The idiosyncratic nature and rarity of the syndrome remain unexplained. Ram and colleagues (1995) evaluated the structure of the D2 receptor gene in 12 patients who had a history of NMS. One patient was found to have a nucleotide substitution of an exon of the D2 gene. The A1 allele of the *TaqIA* polymorphism of the dopamine D2 receptor gene appears to occur more commonly in patients who developed NMS (Suzuki et al., 2001). IBZM SPECT in one patient showed the dopamine receptor to be blocked in the acute phase of NMS, but the patient had been receiving a D2 blocker, which would be expected to result in this finding (Jauss et al., 1996).

Treatment of NMS consists of discontinuing the antipsychotic drugs and providing supportive measures. Rapid relief of symptoms has been reported with the use of dantrolene, bromocriptine, or L-dopa (Granato et al., 1982; Gute and Baxter, 1985). Nisijima and colleagues (1997) found L-dopa to be more effective than dantrolene, but Tsujimoto and colleagues (1998) found intravenous dantrolene plus hemodialysis to be effective. Subcutaneous apomorphine has been found to be effective as a solo treatment (Wang and Hsieh, 2001). Gratz and Simpson (1994) recommended using anticholinergics in an attempt to reverse rigidity prior to utilizing bromocriptine. Carbamazepine was dramatically effective in two patients (with recurrence on withdrawal of the drug) (Thomas et al., 1998). Steroids added to standard therapy have been reported to speed recovery time (Sato et al., 2003). Re-exposure to dopamine receptor antagonists does not necessarily lead to recurrence of NMS (Singh and Albaranzanchi, 1995; Singh and Hambidge, 1998). Residual catatonia that can last weeks to months has been reported, with some cases responding to electroshock therapy (Caroff et al., 2000).

## TARDIVE SYNDROMES

The first use of dopamine receptor antagonists for psychiatric disorders was in the early 1950s, and credit for the first report of TD is given to Schonecker (1957), who reported four patients with TD induced by chlorpromazine. Sigwald and colleagues (1959) provided the first detailed descriptions of the syndrome and divided it into acute, subacute, and chronic subtypes. Uhrbrand and Faurbye (1960) published the first systematic review of the complication among 500 psychiatric patients and noted 29 patients with the disorder. Faurbye and colleagues (1964) later coined the term *tardive dyskinesia* and emphasized the increased incidence of the syndrome with chronic exposure. Despite numerous reports of the classic O-B-L repetitive stereotypic movements, establishment of this disorder as a distinct clinical entity took decades of epidemiologic studies (American Psychiatric Association, 1980; Jeste and Wyatt, 1982b; Kane and Smith, 1982). Confusion arose in part from the difficulty of characterizing and communicating the exact type of movements these patients develop and distinguishing these from the ones that occur spontaneously. It should be noted that these drug-induced movements can be variable in duration; they may be short lasting and fade slowly after discontinuation of the medication, suppressed by the medication itself, or may be persistent.

Rigorous epidemiologic data are available only for classic TD (Jeste and Wyatt, 1982b; Kane and Smith, 1982), but tardive dystonia and tardive akathisia warrant separate recognition beyond their differences in clinical phenomenology because prognosis, at-risk population, and treatment are different. Some authors have noted chronic vocal and motor tics resembling Tourette syndrome (Klawans et al., 1978; Bharucha and Sethi, 1995), and others noted myoclonic movements (Little and Jankovic, 1987; Tominaga et al., 1987) as a chronic persistent problem of neuroleptic therapy, but further studies are necessary to establish them as distinct entities. More recently, a combination of resting, postural, and action tremor has been reported in five patients that persisted despite withdrawal of the offending DRBAs and that improved with treatment with the antidopaminergic TBZ (Stacy and Jankovic, 1992). The tremor was accompanied by other tardive phenomenology, and the authors suggested that this is another tardive syndrome, calling it tardive tremor. Tardive tremor has been reported with metoclopramide (Tarsy and Indorf, 2002).

## Withdrawal Emergent Syndrome

Withdrawal emergent syndrome was first described in children who had been on antipsychotic drugs for a long period of time and then were withdrawn abruptly from their medication (Polizos et al., 1973). The movements are choreic and resemble those of Sydenham disease (Videos 20-1 and 20-2). The abnormal movements are brief and flow from one muscle to another in a seemingly random way. They differ from the movements of classic TD, which are brief but stereotypic and repetitive.  The movements in withdrawal emergent syndrome involve mainly the limbs, trunk, and neck and rarely the oral region, which is the most prevalent site in classic TD. The dyskinetic movements disappear spontaneously within several weeks after withdrawal of the DRBA. For immediate suppression of movements, dopamine receptor antagonists can be reinstituted and withdrawn gradually without recurrence of the withdrawal emergent syndrome (Fahn, 1984a). A withdrawal reaction from melatonin with O-B-L dyskinesia and akathisia was reported by Giladi and Shabtai (1999) and was described earlier in the chapter.

Withdrawal emergent syndrome is analogous to the classic TD that is seen in adults except that the course is more benign and movements are more generalized, resembling the choreic movements of Sydenham disease. In fact, most cases of tardive dyskinesia that have been reported in children have a benign course, and the phenomenology has been reported to be more generalized choreic movements rather than stereotypic repetitive movements of oral, buccal, and lingual distribution. Acute withdrawal of chronic antipsychotic drugs in adults can also lead to transient tardive dyskinesia, which disappears within 3 months. This type of movement has been labeled withdrawal dyskinesia (Gardos et al., 1978; Schooler and Kane, 1982).

On the other hand, acute withdrawal of DRBA can precipitate a persistent akathisia (Poyurovsky et al., 1996; Rosebush et al., 1997) or dyskinesia (i.e., tardive akathisia and other tardive syndromes). Acute withdrawal should be avoided because of the propensity to induce TD, and a slow taper and withdrawal should be substituted. Abrupt withdrawal of risperidone therapy in one elderly person resulted in a near-fatal development of respiratory dyskinesia (Komatsu et al., 2005).

## Classic Tardive Dyskinesia

*Dyskinesia* is a general term referring to abnormal involuntary movements. The term *tardive dyskinesia* has been used to refer to abnormal movements that are seen as a complication of long-term dopamine receptor antagonist therapy, mainly the type that presents with rapid, repetitive, stereotypic movements involving the oral, buccal, and lingual areas. However, over the years, other types of movements have been noted as complications of dopamine receptor antagonist therapy. These movements have more specific terminologies, such as *dystonia* and *akathisia*. Therefore, some authors refer to the type of movements that were originally described as classic TD for lack of a more specific and distinct name for the movements (Fahn, 1989). Some have called them tardive stereotypy (Stacy and Jankovic, 1991; Jankovic, 1994) because of their repetitive, rather than random, nature. However, the stereotypic movements in classic TD are so characteristic and resemble those seen in almost all patients with this disorder, in contrast to other types of stereotypies that are seen in patients with mental retardation, autism, and psychosis, that the term *tardive stereotypy* does not convey this uniqueness and therefore seems unsatisfactory. Stereotyped hand clasping appears to be a rare form for the presentation of classic TD (Kaneko et al., 1993).

On the other hand, some have used the term *tardive dyskinesia* as equivalent to any oral dyskinesia. It therefore needs to be emphasized that the term *tardive* has become synonymous with chronic neuroleptic complications and should be reserved for these disorders. Sustained dystonic movements of the lower face must be distinguished from classic TD. Frequently, patients on anticholinergics or other medications develop oral dyskinesia with dryness of mouth. Other movements such as myokymia, myoclonus, and tics must be distinguished. The differential diagnosis of oral dyskinesia is summarized in Box 20-2, whereas Table 20-8 compares clinical features of tardive dyskinesia, Huntington disease, and oromandibular dystonia, the three most common forms of oral dyskinesias.

---

### Box 20-2 Differential diagnosis of oral dyskinesias

1. Chorea, rhythmic, stereotypic (see also Kurlan and Shoulson, 1988)
   a. Encephalitis lethargica: postencephalitic
   b. Drug-induced
      1) Dopamine receptor antagonists (classic TD)
      2) Levodopa
      3) Anticholinergic drugs
      4) Phenytoin intoxication
      5) Antihistamines
      6) Tricyclic antidepressants
      7) Lithium
   c. Huntington disease
   d. Hepatocerebral degeneration
   e. Cerebellar infarction
   f. Edentulous malocclusion
   g. Brainstem infarcts
   h. Idiopathic
2. Dystonia
   a. Idiopathic cranial dystonia (Meige syndrome)
   b. Symptomatic dystonias
      1) Dopamine receptor antagonists (acute dystonia, tardive dystonia)
      2) other secondary dystonias (see Calne and Lang, 1988)
3. Tics
4. Tremor
   a. Parkinsonian tremor of jaw, tongue, and lips
   b. Essential tremor of neck and jaw
   c. Cerebellar tremor of neck and jaw
   d. Idiopathic tremor of neck, jaw, tongue, or lips
5. Myoclonus
   a. Facial myoclonus of central origin
6. Others
   a. Hemifacial spasm
   b. Myokymia
   c. Facial nerve synkinesis
   d. Bruxism
   e. Epilepsia partialis continua

Adapted from Fahn S: The tardive dyskinesias. In Matthews WB, Glaser GH (eds): Recent Advances in Clinical Neurology, vol 4, Edinburgh, Churchill Livingstone, 1984, pp 229–260.

---

### CLINICAL FEATURES OF CLASSIC TARDIVE DYSKINESIA

The clinical features of classic TD are quite distinct from the features of other movement disorders (Fahn, 1984a). The principal site is the face, particularly around the mouth, typically called O-B-L dyskinesias. The limbs and trunk are affected less often than the mouth. Even when they are involved, it is usually in addition to involvement of the mouth. The forehead and eyebrows are seldom involved unless tardive dystonia is also present; this is in contrast to Huntington disease, in which chorea of the forehead and eyebrows is more common than choreic movements of the oral musculature. In TD, the mouth tends to show a pattern of repetitive, complex chewing motions (Video 20-3; see also Video 1-73), occasion-

Table 20-8 Clinical features of classic tardive dyskinesia, oromandibular dystonia, and Huntington disease

| Clinical Signs | Tardive Dyskinesia | Oromandibular Dystonia | Huntington Disease |
|---|---|---|---|
| Type of involuntary movements | Stereotypic | Dystonic | Choreic |
| Flowing movements | 0 | 0 | +++ |
| Repetitive movements | +++ | + | ∀ |
| Sustained contractions | + | +++ | ∀ |
| Movements of mouth | +++ | +++ | + |
| Blepharospasm | + | +++ | ∀ |
| Forehead chorea | ∀ | ∀ | ++ |
| Platysma | ∀ | +++ | ∀ |
| Masticatory muscles | +++ | +++ | ∀ |
| Nuchal muscles | + | ++ | ∀ |
| Trunk, legs | ++ | 0 | +++ |
| Akathisia | ++ | 0 | 0 |
| Marching in place | ++ | 0 | 0 |
| Truncal rocking | ++ | 0 | + |
| Motor impersistence (tongue, grip) | 0 | 0 | +++ |
| Stuttering-ataxic gait | ∀ | 0 | +++ |
| Postural instability | 0 | 0 | +++ |
| Effect of: | | | |
| Antidopaminergics | Decrease | Decrease | Decrease |
| Anticholinergics | Increase | Decrease | ∀ |
| Effect on: | | | |
| Talking, chewing | ∀ | +++ | + |
| Swallowing | 0 | ++ | +++ |

0, not seen; ∀ may be seen; +, occasionally seen; ++, usually seen; +++, almost always seen.

Data from Fahn S, Burke RE: Tardive dyskinesia and other neuroleptic-induced syndromes. In Rowland LP (ed): Merritt's Textbook of Neurology, 11th ed. Philadelphia, Lippincott Williams & Wilkins, 2005.

ally with smacking and opening of the mouth, tongue protrusion (flycatcher tongue) (Video 20-4), lip pursing, sucking movements, and fish-like lip puckering movements. The rhythmicity and coordinated pattern of movement are striking. This stereotypic pattern is in contrast to the dyskinesias that are seen in Huntington disease, in which the movements are without a predictable pattern. Usually, the limb involvement is limited to the distal part. Like the mouth region, the movements of the distal limbs show a repetitive pattern, earning the label of piano-playing fingers and toes. When the patient is sitting, the legs often move repeatedly, with flexion and extension movements of the toes and foot tapping. When the patient is lying down, flexion and extension of thighs may be seen. Rhythmic truncal rocking can be seen when the patient is lying, sitting, or standing (Video 20-5). The respiratory pattern can be involved with dyskinesia, causing hyperventilation at times and hypoventilation at other times (Yassa and Lai, 1986). In a study of the breathing pattern in patients with TD, patients had an irregular tidal breathing pattern, with a greater variability in both tidal volume and time of the total respiratory cycle (Wilcox et al., 1994). The presence of respiratory dyskinesia never causes a medical problem, although it might look alarming. Esophageal (associated with lingual) dyskinesias have also been reported, resulting in increased intraesophageal pressure and death due to asphyxiation in one patient (Horiguchi et al., 1999).

The involuntary movements of the mouth in classic TD are readily suppressed by patients when they are asked to do so. Furthermore, the movements cease as the patient is putting food in the mouth, when talking, or when a finger is placed on the lips. Since the movements do not interfere with basic functions, patients are often unaware of their movements. When the patient is asked to keep the tongue at rest inside the mouth, the tongue tends to assume a continual writhing motion of athetoid side-to-side and coiling movements. The constant lingual movements might lead to tongue hypertrophy, and macroglossia is a common clinical sign. On command, however, most patients with TD can keep the tongue protruded out, without its darting back into the mouth, for more than half a minute; patients with the chorea of Huntington disease typically cannot maintain a protruded tongue. This inability to sustain a voluntary contraction is called motor impersistence, which is not seen in TD.

## ABNORMAL MOVEMENTS IN SCHIZOPHRENIA IN THE ABSENCE OF EXPOSURE TO DOPAMINE RECEPTOR–BLOCKING AGENTS

Tardive dyskinesia as an entity induced by dopamine receptor blockers has been challenged by reports claiming that spontaneous movements are sometimes encountered in patients with schizophrenia who have never been exposed to neuroleptic agents (see the review by Boeti et al., 2003). McCreadie and colleagues (2002) evaluated 37 schizophrenic patients never treated with antipsychotics and followed for 18 months. Nine (24%) had dyskinesia on both occasions, 12

(33%) on one occasion, and 16 (43%) on neither occasion. Twenty-one (57%) had dyskinesia on at least one occasion. Thirteen patients (35%) had parkinsonism on at least one occasion. It is critical that the quality of the dyskinesia be reported, because the classic O-B-L dyskinesias are very distinct and almost specific for tardive dyskinesia, whereas many other types of movements could represent a different disorder. The presence of parkinsonism, though, suggests that the patients had been exposed to neuroleptics but that the investigators were clueless as to the exposure.

Many authors noted the existence of spontaneous oral dyskinesia occurring in untreated populations and in untreated schizophrenics. McCreadie and colleagues (1996) examined 308 elderly individuals in Madras, India, looking for abnormal movements and found them in 15%. The prevalence of spontaneous dyskinesia has been reported to be as high as 20% in psychiatric or nursing home patients (Brandon et al., 1971), but the average rate is about 5% (Jeste and Wyatt, 1982a; Kane and Smith, 1982). Others noted increasing prevalence of spontaneous dyskinesia with age (Klawans and Barr, 1982). Some studies looking at healthy elderly populations estimate the prevalence rate to be about 1% (Lieberman et al., 1984; D'Alessandro et al., 1986). Blanchet and colleagues (2004) evaluated 1018 (69.3% women) noninstitutionalized, frail elderly subjects attending day care centers to document the prevalence and phenomenology of spontaneous oral dyskinesia (SOD). The prevalence rate for spontaneous oral dyskinesia was 3.7% (4.1% for women and 2.9% for men). They reported more frequent ill-fitting dental devices, oral pain, and a lower rate of perception of good oral health compared to nondyskinetics.

The true prevalence rate of spontaneous oral dyskinesia that can mimic TD may be even lower, considering the fact that many other identifiable oral dyskinesias listed in Box 20-2 such as oromandibular dystonia can be difficult to distinguish from classic TD and may be counted as spontaneous dyskinesia in epidemiologic studies. On the other hand, spontaneous oral dyskinesia resembling the stereotypic O-B-L dyskinesia of classic TD has been reported in an aged cynomolgus monkey (Rupniak et al., 1990). Some patients with oral dyskinesias resembling those of TD and unexposed to DRBAs would seemingly be idiopathic in origin, but careful workup might reveal other etiologies (see Box 20-2), including treatment with lithium (Meyer-Lindenberg and Krausnick, 1997) and brainstem infarcts (Fahn et al., 1986).

Reports of oral dyskinesias occurring in schizophrenic patients who have never been exposed to neuroleptics raise the question as to how specifically the O-B-L movements should be attributed to DRBAs and whether or not they could be due to the schizophrenia. Fenn and colleagues (1996) examined 22 never-medicated schizophrenics in Casablanca, Morocco. Three had abnormal movements that are said to be characteristic of TD. Fenton and colleagues (1997) compared the prevalence of spontaneous oral dyskinesias among drug-naïve schizophrenics and patients with other psychiatric disorders. They found that dyskinetic movements were more common in the former group. Gervin and colleagues (1998) reported 6 (7.6%) out of 79 first-episode schizophrenics to have spontaneous dyskinesias. Until movement disorder experts can evaluate the movement phenomenology, it is possible that these individuals have some disorder other than TD.

Moreover, it is possible that the history of nondrug exposure is faulty. The overwhelming evidence is that the abnormal movements that are seen with DRBAs are due to these drugs.

As was mentioned earlier, a major concern in diagnosing spontaneous oral dyskinesias is the distinction between the stereotypic movements of TD and the movements of oromandibular dystonia. Authors should publish the videotape demonstrations of the abnormal movements so that the medical community can judge whether the movements do indeed fit the phenomenologic criteria of movements seen in TD.

## EPIDEMIOLOGY, RISK FACTORS, AND NATURAL HISTORY

Epidemiologic studies looking into the prevalence of TD have been confounded by the factors that affect the detection of the abnormal involuntary movements as well as the variables that affect the prognosis of the movements. Therefore, it is not surprising to find a wide range of prevalence estimations, from 0.5% to 65% in the literature (Jeste and Wyatt, 1982a; Kane and Smith, 1982). The prevalence of TD has been noted to have increased from 5% before 1965 to 25% in the late 1970s (Jeste and Wyatt, 1982a; Kane and Smith, 1982). Mean prevalence rates calculated by two different reviewers, however, agree well at around 20% (Jeste and Wyatt, 1982a; Kane and Smith, 1982).

The prevalence rates of spontaneous dyskinesias and dyskinesias in people who have been exposed to neuroleptics have been compared. In the study by Woerner and colleagues (1991), the overall prevalence of spontaneous dyskinesias was 1.3% in 400 healthy elderly people and 4.8% in elderly inpatients, with a range from 0 to 2% among psychiatric patients who had never been exposed to neuroleptics. These investigators reported a prevalence of TD of 13.3% and 36.1% in voluntary and state psychiatric hospitals, respectively. There was an interplay between age and gender. Among younger patients, men had higher rates; among subjects over age 40 years, rates were higher in women. Van Os and colleagues (1999) also found an increased risk for men in the younger population.

In one prospective study examining development of TD with low-dose haloperidol, the 12-month incidence of probable or persistent tardive dyskinesia was 12.3% (Oosthuizen et al., 2003). In a much larger study, the annual incidence rates ranged from 5% in a younger population (mean age 28) (Kane et al., 1986) to 12% in an older group (mean age 56) (Barnes et al., 1983). Kane and colleagues' data (1986) also show that the cumulative incidence of TD increases linearly with increasing duration of neuroleptic exposure at least for the first 4 to 5 years of such exposure. In a subsequent study by these authors, Chakos and colleagues (1996) studied prospectively 118 patients in their first episode of psychosis who were treatment-naïve and were then followed for up to 8.5 years while they were on neuroleptics. The cumulative incidence of presumptive TD was 6.3% after 1 year of follow-up, 11.5% after 2 years, 13.7% after 3 years, and 17.5% after 4 years. Persistent TD had a cumulative incidence of 4.8% after 1 year, 7.2% after 2 years, and 15.6% after 4 years. Thus, the earlier findings of Kane and colleagues (1986) of about 5% a year cumulative incidence seem to have been confirmed.

Jeste and colleagues (1999) looked at the cumulative incidence of tardive dyskinesia after exposure to neuroleptics in patients over the age of 45 years. The mean cumulative incidence was 3.4%, 5.9%, and 22.3% at 1, 3, and 12 months, respectively. Woerner and his colleagues (1998) studied patients over the age of 54 when first exposed to neuroleptics. The cumulative rates of tardive dyskinesia were 25%, 34%, and 53% after 1, 2, and 3 years of cumulative antipsychotic treatment. A greater risk of tardive dyskinesia was associated with a history of electroshock therapy treatment, higher mean daily and cumulative antipsychotic doses, and the presence of extrapyramidal signs early in treatment. Fron both these studies, the incidence rates for patients beginning treatment with conventional antipsychotics in their fifth decade or later arc three to five times what has been found for younger patients, despite treatment with lower doses.

Studies have been carried out in other countries. A prospective study of 11 psychiatric facilities in Japan found the prevalence of TD to be 7.6%, the annual incidence rate to be 3.7%, and an annual remission rate to be 28.7% (Inada et al., 1991). On the other hand, Hayashi and colleagues (1996) reported a prevalence of 22.1% in 258 patients receiving neuroleptics. A study in Austria reported the follow-up of the 270 patients still in a psychiatric hospital after 10 years out of an original population of 861 patients; the prevalence rate of TD was 3.7% in 1982 and 12.7% in 1992; the major risk factor for TD was advanced age (Miller et al., 1995). Jeste and colleagues (1995) followed 266 patients over the age of 45 years to determine incidence and prevalence rates of tardive dyskinesia following exposure to neuroleptics, using electromechanical sensors to detect the presence of movements. Cumulative incidence of TD was 26%, 52%, and 60% after 1, 2, and 3 years, respectively. These rates, which are higher than those found by Kane and his colleagues, might reflect the sensitive sensors used, and these could possibly give false-positive findings. The same group compared the development of abnormal movements in the orofacial and limb-truncal areas in these 266 middle-aged and elderly patients treated with neuroleptics and found that the cumulative incidence of orofacial TD was 38.5% and 65.7% after 1 and 2 years, respectively, whereas that of limb-truncal TD was 18.6% and 32.6% after 1 and 2 years, respectively (Paulsen et al., 1996).

Host and treatment factors affect the development, severity, and persistence of TD, thereby resulting in different prevalence rates. Age of the patient has been the most consistent factor that adversely affects the incidence, prognosis, and severity of tardive dyskinesia (Smith and Baldessarini, 1980; Jeste and Wyatt, 1982a; Kane and Smith, 1982; Kane et al., 1986). Possibly the youngest individual who developed O-B-L tardive dyskinesia was a 2-month old girl after a 17-day treatment with metoclopramide for gastroesophageal reflux (Mejia and Jankovic, 2005). The movements persisted for at least 9 months after the drug was discontinued. This patient is the first documented case of tardive dyskinesia in an infant.

Female sex has been associated with increased prevalence of TD, especially in the older population (Jeste and Wyatt, 1982a; Kane and Smith, 1982; Kane et al., 1988). Several authors noted increased incidence and prevalence among patients with affective disorders compared to schizophrenia or schizoaffective disorders (Gardos and Casey, 1983). Other host factors such as presence of previous brain damage as noted by increased ventricular size remain controversial (Jeste and Wyatt, 1982a; Kane and Smith, 1982). Some noted poor treatment response of schizophrenia to drug treatment as a risk factor for development of tardive dyskinesia (Chouinard et al., 1986). The parameters of drug exposures such as dose, duration, type of neuroleptics, and drug-free intervals have been very difficult to correlate with risk of TD partly because accurate history concerning the drug treatment is usually not available, and the drug itself can affect the detection of TD by masking or uncovering it.

Ethnicity has been found to be another important risk factor in both the development and prognosis of tardive dyskinesia, African-Americans being more susceptible than European-Americans (Wonodi et al., 2004b).

Prospective studies have noted that the total cumulative drug exposure correlates with incidence of withdrawal tardive dyskinesia (Kane et al., 1985) and development of TD five years later in patients who did not have TD initially (Chouinard et al., 1986). Continued use of DRBAs after the appearance of TD also adversely affects subsequent prognosis (Kane et al., 1986). Drug holidays were once advocated to decrease the risk of TD, but an increased number of drug-free intervals was found to worsen the prognosis after withdrawal (Jeste et al., 1979). The risk of developing TD is three times as great for patients with more than two neuroleptic interruptions as for patients with two or fewer interruptions (van Harten et al., 1998). Other than reduced risk with clozapine, olanzapine, and quetiapine, no other particular type of neuroleptic, including depot preparations, has been clearly identified as a risk factor (Yassa et al., 1988). The effect of other drugs, such as anticholinergics, on the incidence and prevalence of TD is controversial, although anticholinergics may increase its severity (Yassa, 1988). Lithium may decrease the chance of TD development (Kane et al., 1986). Development of parkinsonism tends to predispose patients to TD (Chouinard et al., 1986; Kane et al., 1986). Substance abuse has also been reported to be a risk factor (Bailey et al., 1997). Lacking the cytochrome P450 enzyme required for metabolism exogenous toxins because of nonfunctional alleles of the CYP2D6 gene appears to be a risk factor for developing both TD and drug-induced parkinsonism (Andreassen et al., 1997).

A review of the literature by Correll and colleagues (2004) found a lower incidence with the newer generation of antipsychotics (Table 20-9). A European consortium of investigators looking at 6-month results came to a similar conclusion

Table 20-9 Annual incidence of tardive dyskinesia comparing the second-generation antipsychotics with haloperidol

| Population | Second-Generation Antipsychotics | Haloperidol |
|---|---|---|
| Children | 0% | |
| Adults | 0.8% | 5.4% |
| Mixture of adults and elderly | 6.8% | |
| Older than 53 years | 5.3% | |

Data from Correll CU, Leucht S, Kane JM: Lower risk for tardive dyskinesia associated with second-generation antipsychotics: A systematic review of 1-year studies. Am J Psychiatry 2004;161 (3):414–425.

(Tenback et al., 2005). In their review of the literature, Tarsy and Baldessarini (2006) also suggest that there may be a declining incidence of TD as the second-generation antipsychotics are being more regularly used. On the other hand, in a survey on elderly demented patients treated with older or newer generation antipsychotics, no statistical difference was found in the development of nonparkinsonian movement disorders in relation to treatment class (Lee et al., 2005).

Although the majority of TD occurs while patients are on chronic treatment with DRBAs or shortly after discontinuing them, many cases have been reported in which the TD occurred after only a short interval of treatment and persisted. Some authors define TD arbitrarily as dyskinesias that occur after a minimum of 3 months of dopamine receptor antagonist therapy (Schooler and Kane, 1982), but it appears that there is no safe low-incidence period right after the initiation of treatment with DRBAs, nor is there any particularly high-risk period. The overall risk appears to accumulate as time goes on, although whether it continues to increase linearly even after the first several years of exposure is not clear from available data. Kang and colleagues' (1986) retrospective data also show that the cumulative number of patients who developed tardive dystonia increased almost linearly from the first few months.

Probably, most patients with TD have mild cases that could improve and disappear over time if the offending DRBAs were withdrawn. In an attempt to look at risk factors for the severe forms of TD, Caligiuri and colleagues (1997) conducted a longitudinal prospective study to determine the incidence of severe TD in middle-aged and elderly psychiatric patients. The cumulative incidence of severe TD was 2.5% after 1 year, 12.1% after 2 years, and 22.9% after 3 years. Risk factors for severe TD were higher daily doses of neuroleptics at study entry, greater cumulative amounts of prescribed neuroleptic, and greater severity of worsening negative psychiatric symptoms.

Once established, TD does not frequently become more severe even though the DRBA is continued (Labbate et al., 1997). Fernandez and colleagues (2001) evaluated the dyskinesia of TD and the clinical features of parkinsonism in 53 patients residing in a state psychiatric hospital over a 14-year period. TD improved and parkinsonism worsened in patients who continued to receive neuroleptic drugs. But the natural history of TD is not easy to determine because the DRBAs that cause the movement disorders also tend to suppress the movements, while they can cause drug-induced parkinsonism.

Movements that disappear with increasing dose or resumption of DRBAs have been called masked TD (Schooler and Kane, 1982). Conversely, movements of TD typically increase after discontinuation of the DRBAs. Transient dyskinesias that appear after withdrawal of DRBAs have been called withdrawal dyskinesias (Gardos et al., 1978). The term *covert dyskinesia* has also been used for dyskinesia that is not detectable during drug administration and is first noted during drug reduction or withdrawal and becomes permanent (Gardos et al., 1978). Therefore, the difference between withdrawal and covert dyskinesia is in duration. In fact, the spectrum of TD ranges from mild transient withdrawal dyskinesia to severe irreversible TD, which can occur during or after discontinuation of the antipsychotic drugs. These examples illustrate the complexity in the detection of TD in the presence of DRBAs. In an attempt to estimate the false-negative rate of detection for TD in patients taking DRBAs, Kane and colleagues (1988) withdrew the drug from patients who showed no evidence of TD while taking DRBAs. Withdrawal TD was seen in 34% of 70 subjects, with persistence beyond 3 months in 7 of them.

## PATHOPHYSIOLOGY

Although tardive dyskinesia is an iatrogenic condition with an established etiologic connection to dopamine receptor antagonism, the pathophysiology is not well understood. Any proposed mechanism for tardive dyskinesia will have to explain (1) the cumulative increase of risk with increasing duration of treatment, (2) frequent persistence of the condition despite discontinuation of the treatment, (3) increasing risk with age and other individual dispositions that leave only a portion of the population affected, (4) increased risk with intermittent exposure to DRBAs, and (5) clinical pharmacology of tardive dyskinesia (i.e., improvement of the condition by drugs that depress dopaminergic activity and worsening by increasing dopaminergic activity with L-dopa or amphetamine).

### Anatomic Pathology: Human and Animal Models

Postmortem pathologic studies are few and show nonspecific findings in the striatonigral system, which might be due to aging or other uncontrolled factors (Christensen et al., 1970). Jellinger (1977) found swollen large (i.e., cholinergic) neurons in the rostral caudate nucleus in 46% of neuroleptic-treated patients. In a review of the literature, Harrison (1999) notes other studies in which cholinergic neurons are affected by these drugs. In a magnetic resonance imaging (MRI) study, 2-year exposure to neuroleptics in schizophrenic patients resulted in an increase in caudate and lenticular nucleus volume, while in those who were similarly exposed to atypical antipsychotics, there was a decrease in volume (Corson et al., 1999).

Since TD is etiologically related to DRBAs and since the clinical pharmacology is most consistent with dopaminergic hyperactivity, many studies have been directed to the dopamine system (Klawans, 1973). Chronic dopamine receptor antagonist treatment in rats shows evidence of cell loss in the ventrolateral striatum (Nielson and Lyon, 1978), changes in synaptic patterns in the striatum at the electron microscopic level (Benes et al., 1985), and increases in glutamatergic synapses in the striatum (Meshul et al., 1994). In the accumbens in rats who developed VCMs, the dendritic surface area is reduced, and dynorphin-positive terminals contact more spines and form more asymmetric specializations than do those in animals without the syndrome (Meredith et al., 2000). Andreassen and colleagues (2001) found electron microscopic changes in rats who developed haloperidol-induced VCMs. The nerve terminal area in the striatum was increased but with a lower density of glutamate immunoreactivity. These results suggest that striatal glutamatergic transmission is affected in association with haloperidol-induced VCMs.

### Anatomic Pathology: In Vitro Models

Galili-Mosberg and colleagues (2000) exposed neuronal and PC-12 cultures to haloperidol and its three metabolites. These induced cell death by apoptosis, which was protected by the antioxidants vitamin E and N-acetylcysteine. Marchese and colleagues (2002) found a shrinkage of TH-immunostaining (TH-IM) cell bodies in the substantia nigra pars compacta and reticulata and a reduction of TH-immunostaining in the striatum of haloperidol-treated rats with the arising of VCMs. No differences were observed in TH-IM neurons of the ventral tegmental area and nucleus accumbens versus control rats.

## Rodent Models: Dopamine and Other Neurotransmitter Biochemistry

In experimental animals, a short-term treatment of dopamine receptor antagonist can increase striatal dopamine synthesis and turnover that revert to normal level within a few days despite continuing treatment (Asper et al., 1973). Receptor binding increases in 2 days and persists for up to a week (Asper et al., 1973; Klawans, 1973; Muller and Seeman, 1977). The change in receptor state correlates well with stereotypic gnawing movements by rats that are induced by dopamine agonists such as apomorphine (Clow et al., 1980). Chronic treatment for a year in rats produces an increase in receptor-binding sites between 1 and 6 months of treatment and overcomes the effects of the continued presence of a dopamine receptor antagonist drug. The increase of receptor binding and functional hypersensitivity takes about 6 months to return to baseline after withdrawal of drug treatment. Increased response of striatal adenylate cyclase to dopamine still persists at 6 months (Clow et al., 1980). The significance of this finding is not clear. Extrapolating from this rodent model of dopaminergic supersensitivity to patients with TD has limitations. Rats do not usually develop spontaneous movements such as TD, but they do demonstrate increased sensitivity to exogenously administered dopamine agonists and can develop VCMs.

The receptor supersensitivity in rodents develops in all the animals that are treated relatively early in the course of dopamine antagonist treatment and is completely reversible in 100% of animals shortly after withdrawal. This is clearly at odds with human TD, in which large individual variations and susceptibility factors are important and the disorder often starts late in the course of treatment and becomes persistent. Nonetheless, this model has been most useful for quick screening of potential neuroleptics that are likely to cause TD from those that are not. Calabresi and colleagues (1992) suggested that hypersensitivity of the D2 presynaptic receptors located on terminals of glutamatergic corticostriatal fibers in animals with chronic treatment with haloperidol would inhibit glutamate release in the striatum, thereby reducing the gamma-aminobutyric acid (GABA) output from postsynaptic striatal neurons. Dopamine D2 receptor occupancy appears to be a contributing factor in the development of the rodent model (Turrone et al., 2002). Andreassen and Jorgensen (2000) review the possible role of increased striatal glutamatergic activity in the rat model as an etiologic factor and suggest that excitoxicity is a possible cause of TD. Anatomic changes found by these authors were presented in the previous section.

## Rodent Models: Behavioral Changes

A common rodent model is that based on the increased rate of VCMs in rats, which develops after several months of dopamine receptor antagonist treatment (Gunne et al., 1982). The movement persists for several months after neuroleptic withdrawal. The behavioral syndrome is spontaneous, in contrast to the stereotypic gnawing movement that requires apomorphine to induce. The pharmacologic response is similar to that seen with TD in that acute haloperidol alleviates the behavioral syndrome. In these aspects, this model is closer to the characteristics of human TD than are models that are based on dopamine receptor supersensitivity.

The VCMs that persist after withdrawal of dopamine receptor antagonist do so at the time when the receptor-binding studies show no supersensitivity (Waddington et al., 1983). Blocking N-methyl-D-aspartate (NMDA) receptors with memantine while the rats are receiving treatment with haloperidol allowed these rats to lose the VCMs sooner than did those animals who did not receive memantine (Andreassen et al., 1996). This result supports the concept that excessive NMDA receptor stimulation might be a mechanism underlying the development of persistent dyskinesias in humans. Opioid receptor antagonists were also shown to block VCMs in rats, suggesting that increases in dynorphin in the direct striatonigral pathway and enkephalin in the indirect striatopallidal pathway following chronic neuroleptic administration are both likely to contribute to tardive dyskinesia (McCormick and Stoessl, 2002).

In one study of chronic haloperidol treatment in the rat, the animals that developed VCMs were compared with those that did not develop the movements (Shirakawa and Tamminga, 1994). Whereas all animals showed an increase in the dopamine D2 family receptor binding in the striatum and in the nucleus accumbens and an increase in GABA-A receptors in the substantia nigra pars reticulata (SNr), only those with VCMs had a significant decrease in dopamine D1 receptor density in the substantia nigra pars reticulata. One explanation is that increased dopamine release from dendrites in the substantia nigra pars reticulata downregulates the D1 receptor. But how this would produce dyskinesias is not clear. In dorsal striatal neurons, however, there was no change in D1 receptor mRNA, nor was there a change in cell counts in rats with neuroleptic-induced VCMs (Petersen et al., 2000).

Stereotyped behavior was evaluated in rats that were treated chronically with haloperidol, followed by D1 and D2 agonists. Somatostatin levels were then measured. The results suggested that somatostatin—but not enkephalin-containing striatal neurons—contribute to the expression of haloperidol-induced stereotypies (Marin et al., 1996).

Other neurotransmitters in the striatum may also be involved. Chronic haloperidol treatment in rats increases preproenkephalin messenger RNA in striatal neurons but fails to do so in rats that develop VCMs (Andreassen, Finsen, et al., 1999). Some authors noted that decreases of glutamic acid decarboxylase (GAD) and GABA in the substantia nigra correlate with increased VCM rates (Gunne and Haggstrom, 1983). Others noted no consistent change in GAD and choline acetyltransferase levels (Mithani et al., 1987). However, Delfs and colleagues (1995) reported that rats that were treated with haloperidol for up to 12 months showed a decrease of GAD mRNA in the external globus pallidus. This result suggests that there is reduced GABAergic transmission in the projection neurons of the external pallidum. Blocking NMDA receptors with memantine while the rats are receiving treatment with haloperidol allowed these rats to lose the VCMs sooner than did animals that did not receive memantine (Andreassen et al., 1996). This result supports the concept that excessive NMDA receptor stimulation could be a mechanism underlying the development of persistent dyskinesias in humans. Lesioning the subthalamic nuclei (and thus its glutamatergic efferents) eliminates VCMs after 1 to 3 weeks (Stoessl and Rajakumar, 1996). The 5-HT$_3$ receptor antagonist ondansetron reverses haloperidol-induced VCMs in rats (Naidu and Kulkarni, 2001).

As a test for the oxidative stress hypothesis in causing TD, rats were cotreated with coenzyme Q10 (CoQ10) along with haloperidol. Cotreatment with CoQ10 did not attenuate the development of the VCMs (Andreassen, Weber, et al., 1999). CoQ10 was absorbed, as detected in the serum, but there was no increase of CoQ10 in the brain.

### Primate Models with Behavioral Changes

The model that best resembles human tardive dyskinesia is that induced in nonhuman primates by DRBAs (Klintenberg et al., 2002). Primates show delayed onset of dyskinesia during the course of treatment, and only a fraction of the population that is treated is affected by dyskinesia. The behavioral effect is spontaneous and bears resemblance to human TD. The dyskinesia also persists after withdrawal of the DRBAs. Unfortunately, neuropathologic and biochemical data from this model are limited. One group suggested that the best neurochemical correlate of dyskinesia induced by DRBAs has been a decrease in GABA and GAD activity in the substantia nigra, subthalamic nucleus, and medial globus pallidus compared to control animals without drug treatment or animals with drug treatment but without dyskinesia (Gunne et al., 1984). This finding correlates with postmortem biochemical studies on humans with TD (see the next section) and with a recent 2-deoxyglucose study in primates with TD. In the latter study, Mitchell and colleagues (1992) reported that primates with TD had a reduced glucose metabolism in the medial globus pallidus and in the VA and VL nuclei of the thalamus. These findings correlate with other, similar studies of chorea and ballism and suggest a reduced subthalamopallidal output, so that the medial pallidum is not activated. Such a finding would be seen in the hemiballistic animal.

In a 5-year study of fluphenazine treatment of *Cebus apella* monkeys, re-exposure following 91 weeks of withdrawal increased dyskinesias and dystonias by 300% (Linn et al., 2001). This observation correlates with earlier clinical studies that found that intermittent treatment with neuroleptics can dramatically increase the incidence of dystonias and dyskinesias.

In a study looking for a proposed mitochondrial dysfunction in TD, baboons were treated for 41 weeks with haloperidol, producing TD; the animals were followed for another 17 weeks following withdrawal of haloperidol, during which the TD persisted (Eyles et al., 2000). Striatal mitochondria were examined by electron microscopy and showed no difference in either size or number between treated and control animals.

### Human Biochemistry

#### POSTMORTEM ANALYSIS

In a study that was well controlled for the premortem state of patients, a significant decrease in GAD activity was found in the subthalamic nucleus of five tardive dyskinesia patients compared to age-matched controls (Andersson et al., 1989). Dopamine receptor binding is not increased in postmortem brains of tardive dyskinesia patients (Crow et al., 1982; Cross et al., 1985; Kornhuber et al., 1989). One study noted increased homovanillic acid levels in the putamen and nucleus accumbens of the postmortem brain (Cross et al., 1985).

#### CEREBROSPINAL FLUID

CSF GABA concentration was found to be significantly lower in five patients with chronic schizophrenia and TD than in five patients with chronic schizophrenia without TD who were matched for age, duration of schizophrenia, and duration of neuroleptic therapy (Thaker et al., 1987). CSF cyclic-AMP is thought to reflect the dopamine receptor function and is not significantly elevated in patients with TD. CSF dopamine metabolite studies do not show significant elevation of homovanillic acid (Bowers et al., 1979; Nagao et al., 1979). CSF studies also showed a higher concentration of excitatory amino acid neurotransmitters and markers of oxidative stress in patients with TD, supporting the hypothesis of oxidative stress due to enhanced striatal glutamatergic neurotransmission by blocking presynaptic dopamine receptors (Tsai et al., 1998).

#### PET AND SPECT

PET data on the postsynaptic receptor status have failed to show an elevation of striatal receptor density compared to normal controls, but there was a positive correlation with severity of TD (Blin et al., 1989). No increase in dopamine transporter binding in striatum was found in a SPECT study, indicating no loss on dopaminergic nerve terminals (Lavalaye et al., 2001). A prospective study was carried out by using FDG PET in patients receiving antipsychotic drugs. Those who later developed TD had a relative hypermetabolism in temporolimbic, brainstem, and cerebellar regions and hypometabolism in parietal and cingulate gyrus (Szymanski et al., 1996).

Dopamine release studies using amphetamine following raclopride binding of the D2 receptor showed no differences between subjects with and without TD, indicating that dopamine release does not seem to be a factor (Adler et al., 2002).

#### GENETICS

Steen and colleagues (1997) reported that a specific allelic variation of the dopamine D3 receptor gene is found at a higher frequency (22% to 24%) of homozygosity among patients with TD compared with the relative underrepresentation (4% to 6%) of this genotype in patients with no TD. Subsequent studies (Segman et al., 1999; Liao et al., 2001) supported and extended an association between D3 receptor gene and TD in schizophrenia patients. A serine to glycine polymorphism in the first exon of the DRD3 gene appears to be a risk factor for developing TD (Liao et al., 2001; Ozdemir et al., 2001). Lerer and colleagues (2002) also found that the presence of the glycine allele carries a higher risk for developing TD. On the other hand, Chong and colleagues (2003) found the serine allele to have a higher risk. A meta-analysis of genetic studies supports the view that a serine to glycine polymorphism in the D3 receptor gene has a higher risk (odds ratio = 1.17) for developing TD (Bakker et al., 2006). Kishida and colleagues (2004) found that patients with NMS had a higher association with a polymorphism in the D2 receptor gene.

Polymorphisms of the CYP2D6 gene, which encodes the cytochrome P450 enzyme debrisoquine/spartein hydroxylase, has been reported to possibly be associated with an increased susceptibility to developing TD (Kapitany et al., 1998; Ohmori et al., 1998; Vandel et al., 1999).

Searches for polymorphisms in the $HTR_{2A}$ receptor gene did not find any significant differences among patients with or without TD (Basile et al., 2001; Segman et al., 2001), but this has been inconsistent (Tan et al., 2001).

#### NEUROENDOCRINE

Assessment of tuberoinfundibular dopaminergic sensitivity as a general indicator of dopamine supersensitivity shows lack of hyperresponsiveness of growth hormone and prolactin to dopamine agonist (Tamminga et al., 1977). Although these data on human TD are preliminary and indirect, the evidence for dopaminergic hypersensitivity has not been confirmed in human studies (Jeste and Wyatt, 1981; Fibiger and Lloyd, 1984).

### PHENYLALANINE LOADING

In a double-blind study, 100 mg/kg of phenylalanine or placebo was given orally to 10 patients with TD (Mosnik et al., 1997); the dyskinesia was exacerbated after ingestion of phenylalanine, confirming earlier reports. Impaired phenylalanine metabolism was found in men but not in women (Richardson et al., 1999)

## Human Imaging

Results of imaging studies are inconsistent. In one magnetic resonance imaging study, Buchanan and colleagues (1994) found no difference between schizophrenic patients who had tardive dyskinesia and those who did not when measuring volumes of the caudate, putamen, and pallidum. In contrast, Brown and colleagues (1996) reported larger caudate nuclei, particularly the right, in schizophrenic patients with TD compared to those without TD. To confuse this subject more, a computed tomography study using special statistical methods found that the left caudate nucleus was smaller and the temporal sulci were enlarged (Dalgalarrondo and Gattaz, 1994). Brain iron levels were found to be normal in the basal ganglia in a magnetic resonance imaging study (Elkashef et al., 1994).

Hoffman and Casey (1991) reviewed the literature on reports on computed tomographic evaluation of patients with tardive dyskinesia. They found that there is a trend toward larger cerebral ventricles in TD patients but that the overall difference from controls is small. Mion and colleagues (1991) compared magnetic resonance imaging scans in young TD patients versus controls and found that the volumes of the caudate nuclei were significantly smaller in the TD patients than in normal controls and in patients on neuroleptics without TD. But covariate analysis failed to show a significant difference.

## Oxidative Stress and Excitotoxicity

Maurer and Moller (1997) studied the effect on mitochondria of neuroleptics added to normal human brain cortex in vitro. Complex I activity was inhibited by all neuroleptics in the following order: haloperidol > chlorpromazine > risperidone >> clozapine. Haloperidol increases reactive oxygen species (generated from mitochondria) in rat cortical cell lines (Sagara, 1998). Erythrocyte Cu,Zn-superoxide dismutase activity was found to be reduced in patients on neuroleptics with TD compared to those without TD (Yamada et al., 1997). There were no differences in plasma vitamin E levels between TD and non-TD schizophrenic patients who were treated with neuroleptics (Brown et al., 1998). The CSF results mentioned earlier support the notion that by blocking presynaptic dopamine receptors, antipsychotics increase striatal glutamatergic transmission and subsequently excitotoxic stress (Tsai et al., 1998). Finding striatal changes in glutamate terminals in a rodent model lends support to the concept of excitotoxicity as a possible mechanism for developing TD (Andreassen et al., 2001) (see the section entitled "Anatomic Pathology: Human and Animal Models").

## Developing Tardive Dyskinesia in the Presence of Dopamine Deficiency States

If dopamine receptor supersensitivity plus active dopamine release from nerve terminals with activation of these supersensitive receptors plays any role in the pathogenesis of TD, then one might anticipate that a state of deficiency of dopamine storage would be incompatible with the development of TD. There appears to be some merit to this concept. Fahn and Mayeux (1980) presented the first report of a patient with PD who developed TD. Their patient had unilateral PD, was treated with a dopamine receptor blocker, and subsequently developed classic TD on the contralateral side of the body. There was no TD on the side with the parkinsonism. In essence, this case supports the notion that a marked deficiency of dopamine release renders the development of TD unlikely, as is seen in the parkinsonian half of the body. The other side probably had partial reduction of dopamine stores and reduced release of dopamine, but it was still capable of developing TD. So perhaps this suggests a quantitative requirement (i.e., a threshold of dopamine availability before an individual could develop TD). This concept is compatible with observations that patients with TD who are treated with dopamine-depleting agents, such as reserpine, can substitute the excessive movements with a parkinsonian state.

The second case was a patient with dopa-responsive dystonia who developed TD on long-term haloperidol therapy (de la Fuente-Fernandez, 1998). In dopa-responsive dystonia, there is a reduction of dopamine stores, but not a complete depletion. So again, if the quantity of dopamine available is the critical factor, a state of dopa-responsive dystonia seems to be quantitatively sufficient with dopamine.

## Pathophysiology: Summary

The biochemical basis of TD is still unclear, and the explanation involving dopamine receptor supersensitivity alone does not seem to be sufficient. There is little dispute that the primary and early effect of dopamine receptor antagonist is on the dopaminergic system with presynaptic and postsynaptic hypersensitivity. However, the changes do not seem to distinguish patients who develop TD from those who do not. Gerlach (1991) suggested that TD might be due to an increased ratio of D1/D2 receptor activity. The typical neuroleptics block presynaptic and postsynaptic D2 receptors, leaving D1 receptors spared. Thus, it is proposed that an increased D1 receptor activation would lead to the dyskinesias.

The effect of DRBAs is not restricted to the dopaminergic system, and the influence on other interconnected systems such as cholinergic, GABAergic, and peptidergic system needs to be studied. Clinical response to antidopaminergic drugs does not necessarily indicate a central pathophysiologic process in that system either. A good example is treatment of PD with anticholinergics, which does not directly reflect the dopaminergic deficiency of the disease. Moreover, changes may occur at the ultrastructural level, such as altered synaptic patterns between subsets of dopaminergic neurons and other interconnected neurons. Findings similar in humans and primate models of TD of decreased GABA activity in the subthalamic nucleus lend support to involvement of this nucleus in TD.

Oxyradicals have been implicated in the pathogenetic mechanism for the tardive syndromes (Lohr, 1991). This is based on the concept that DRBAs cause an increase in dopamine turnover, resulting in an increased synthesis of hydrogen peroxide, a metabolite of oxidative deamination of dopamine. Hydrogen peroxide, if not rapidly metabolized, will form oxyradicals, which can damage cell membranes and other cellular components. This hypothesis has received support from a study in which simultaneous administration of tocopherol to chronic haloperidol treatment in rats prevented the development of behavioral supersensitivity to apomorphine (Gattaz et al., 1993).

Additional studies and new approaches are needed to understand the pathophysiology of classic TD.

## Tardive Dystonia

Dystonia is most often an idiopathic disorder and can occur at all ages. Persistent dystonic movement as a complication of DRBA therapy has long been noted (Druckman et al., 1962). However, it has not been studied systematically to show that this represents a distinct syndrome until reported by Burke and colleagues (1982). Tardive dystonia has a different epidemiology and pharmacologic response from those of classic TD. Although secondary dystonia can be caused by many neurologic disorders (Calne and Lang, 1988), tardive dystonia is one of the most common causes (Kang et al., 1986). A rigorous epidemiologic study is not available for tardive dystonia, but the prevalence of tardive dystonia in chronic psychiatric inpatients has been estimated to be 1.5% to 2% (Friedman et al., 1986; Yassa et al., 1986). When mild forms of dystonia were evaluated, 27 of 125 patients on chronic antipsychotic medications had some form of dystonia (Sethi et al., 1990), indicating that the prevalence could be higher than was initially realized. Idiopathic torsion dystonia is a much less common condition with one of the most generous estimations of prevalence at around 1 per 3000 population (Nutt et al., 1988). Therefore, dystonic movements seem to be much more frequent in patients who have been exposed to DRBAs.

In primary dystonia, patients at a younger age of onset tend to develop generalized dystonia, and those with onset in adulthood are more likely to have craniocervical focal or segmental dystonia. Kang and colleagues (1986) and Kiriakakis and colleagues (1998) have reviewed large series of cases of tardive dystonia and found a similar correlation between distribution of dystonia and age at onset. They found a correlation between the site and age of onset; the site of onset ascended from the lower limbs to the face as the mean age of onset increased. But tardive dystonia rarely affects legs alone even in youngsters (Kang et al., 1986). Regardless of age at onset, tardive dystonia usually progresses over months or years from a focal onset to become more widespread; only 17% remain focal at the time of maximum severity (Kiriakakis et al., 1998). As in primary dystonia, tardive dystonia in adults tends to remain focal or segmental and tends to involve the craniocervical region.

The onset of tardive dystonia can be from days to years after exposure to a DRBA (Kang et al., 1986). Kiriakakis and colleagues (1998) found the range to extend from 4 days to 23 years of exposure (median: 5, mean: $6.2 \pm 5.1$ years) in their series of 107 patients, with a mean (standard deviation) age at onset of 38.3 (13.7) years (range: 13 to 68 years). There is no period that is safe from development of tardive dystonia; one patient in the series by Burke and colleagues (1982) developed it after a one-day exposure. Men are significantly younger than women at onset of dystonia, and it develops after shorter exposure in men (Kiriakakis et al., 1998). Yassa and colleagues (1989) found that severe tardive dystonia was more common in young men, while severe classic TD was more common in older women.

The phenomenology of tardive dystonia can be indistinguishable from that of idiopathic dystonia, including the improvement with sensory tricks (*geste antagoniste*), which can be used to advantage in creating mechanical devices to reduce the severity of the dystonia (Krack et al., 1998). Focal dystonias, such as tardive cervical dystonia (Molho et al., 1998) and tardive blepharospasm (Sachdev, 1998), can resemble primary focal dystonias. A comparison of tardive and primary oromandibular dystonia showed similar demographics, both occurring predominantly in women, with jaw-closing dystonia being the most common form (Tan and Jankovic, 2000). Primary oromandibular dystonia patients were more likely to have coexistent cervical dystonia, and the two types of dystonia responded equally well to botulinum toxin injections. Limb stereotypies, akathisia, and respiratory dyskinesia were seen only in the tardive oromandibular dystonia. Virtually any type of dystonia can occur in tardive dystonia, including focal, segmental (Video 20-6), and generalized, although the last is very uncommon and is seen only in children with tardive dystonia.

There are some dystonias that are more characteristic of tardive dystonia than of primary dystonia. For example, when the neck is involved, it is common for cervical dystonia to present as retrocollis in tardive dystonia (Video 20-7), whereas retrocollis is an infrequent manifestation of primary cervical dystonia, in which turning and tilting of the head are more common. One clinical presentation of tardive dystonia that is particularly more characteristic of tardive dystonia is the combination of retrocollis, trunk arching backward (opisthotonus), internal rotation of the arms, extension of the elbows, and flexion of the wrists (Video 20-8) (Kang et al., 1986), whereas patients with idiopathic dystonia more often have lateral torticollis and twisting of the trunk laterally. The presence of lightning-like (myoclonic) movements in association with dystonia may be more common in tardive dystonia than in primary dystonia (Video 20-9). Reduction of dystonic movements with voluntary action such as walking is often seen in tardive dystonia. This is distinctly unusual in idiopathic dystonia, in which the dystonic movements are usually exacerbated by voluntary action. It can be severe enough to jeopardize patients by causing life-threatening dysphagia (Samie et al., 1987; Hayashi et al., 1997)

Tardive dystonia tends to occur in all ages without predilection for any particular age range. The mean age of onset in the literature is about 40 years. This is in contrast to idiopathic dystonia, which shows a bimodal distribution with one early peak in childhood and another later peak in adulthood (Fahn, 1988). Tardive dystonia affects both sexes equally, and men have a younger age of onset than do women. Duration of exposure to dopamine receptor antagonist at the onset of tardive dystonia can range from as short as 3 weeks to close to 40 years. The mean duration is 7 years, and as many as 20% of cases develop within a year of the therapy. If the cumulative percentage of patients is plotted against the duration of exposure, the data show a linear line extrapolated to the origin of the graph at zero. This suggests that the risk of developing tardive dystonia starts at the initiation of therapy without any safe minimum period of exposure (Kang et al., 1986).

Wojcik and colleagues (1991) reviewed 32 patients with tardive dystonia and found that most were men but that women had a shorter exposure time to DRBAs. None of their patients had a complete remission, and the condition causes notable disability.

Many patients with tardive dystonia also have classic TD at some point in their course (Kang et al., 1986; van Harten et al.,

1997). It is not clear why some develop dystonia whereas others develop classic TD or why some develop both. When patients have both types, dystonic symptoms are usually much more pronounced and disabling (Kang et al., 1986; Gardos et al., 1987).

The dystonia can be so severe that complications can occur. One patient with powerful retrocollis fractured the odontoid process (Konrad et al., 2004).

## Tardive Akathisia

Originally, akathisia was mainly thought of as an acute to subacute side effect of dopamine receptor antagonists. Various authors, however, noted different variants of akathisia that occurred late in the course of the neuroleptic therapy and/or persisted despite discontinuation of neuroleptic therapy (Braude and Barnes, 1983; Fahn, 1983; Weiner and Luby, 1983). Concomitant or subsequent development of TD was also noted (Munetz and Cornes, 1982; Burke et al., 1989). Barnes and Braude (1985) made a systematic attempt to classify the complex variety of akathisia syndromes. They defined the disorder by the presence of both the subjective and objective features and confirmed that there are acute and chronic variants of akathisia (see Video 1-35). They also distinguished two types of chronic akathisia: one that occurred early in the course at the time of increasing neuroleptic dose and persisted (acute persistent akathisia) and one that occurred during long-term therapy, sometimes during reduction of the neuroleptic dose (tardive akathisia). Burke and colleagues (1989) reviewed experience with 30 patients with persistent akathisia who met both subjective and objective criteria. They found it difficult to distinguish between acute persistent and tardive akathisia in many cases owing to imprecise information about the onset of the disorder relative to initiation of therapy. It is not clear whether these are distinct syndromes or simply two ends of a continuum. Therefore, some researchers prefer to lump them together as tardive akathisia in line with other persistent movement disorders from dopamine receptor antagonists (Burke et al., 1989). Some attempts to classify akathisia syndromes are complex (Lang, 1994; Sachdev, 1995a); a simple method is to consider persistent neuroleptic-induced akathisia to be the tardive akathisia and withdrawal, transient akathisia to be acute akathisia, as is done here.

The clinical phenomenology of tardive akathisia is thought to be same as that of acute akathisia. Moaning (Video 20-10; see also Video 1-36) and focal pain are more common in tardive akathisia than in acute akathisia. In Burke and colleagues' study (1989), the mean age at onset of tardive akathisia was 58 years with a range from 21 to 82 years, similar to the age range of classic TD. The mean duration of dopamine receptor antagonist exposure before the onset was 4.5 years, with a range from 2 weeks to 22 years. Over half of the patients had onset within 2 years. Again the risk of developing tardive akathisia seems to start at the initiation of the drug therapy, as in other tardive syndromes. In tardive akathisia, there is a strong likelihood that there will be accompanying tardive dyskinesia (Video 20-11) or tardive dystonia (Video 20-12) movements. All of the patients with tardive akathisia in the study by Burke and colleagues (1989) also had either tardive dyskinesia (93%) or tardive dystonia (33%) or both (27%) at the same time. But isolated tardive akathisia

can exist as well. The pathophysiology of akathisia is not understood.

## TREATMENT OF TARDIVE SYNDROMES

The most important point to remember in the management of tardive syndromes is that they are iatrogenic disorders. One should avoid using a DRBA if possible. Patients should be forewarned of the risk of a tardive dyskinesia syndrome before being placed on the drug. In a survey of 520 psychiatrists, only 54% of them disclose this risk (Kennedy and Sanborn, 1992). A study of the impact of informed consent based on questionnaires showed that patients did retain the information both at 4 weeks and at 2 years (Kleinman et al., 1996). Another study comparing patients' knowledge of TD by a questionnaire revealed that those who were educated about the disorder had more knowledge about it 6 months later (Chaplin and Kent, 1998).

Once a tardive syndrome has been encountered, removal of the etiologic agent must be seriously considered as the first consideration. If it is to be discontinued, a slow taper appears to be safer than sudden withdrawal; the latter might exacerbate the severity of the syndrome. In classic TD, prospective data show 33% remission in 2 years following elimination of the DRBA (Kane et al., 1986). In retrospective studies, the remission rates were 12% for tardive dystonia and 8% for tardive akathisia (Kang et al., 1986; Burke et al., 1989). Some of these patients remitted only after at least 5 years of abstinence from DRBAs (Klawans and Tanner, 1983; Kang et al., 1986). Younger age is associated with a better chance of remission (Smith and Baldessarini, 1980), and earlier detection and discontinuation of dopamine receptor antagonists were more favorable for remission (Quitkin et al., 1977). In a study involving chronic schizophrenics, only 1 of 49 patients who discontinued the antipsychotic drugs had a lasting recovery, but 10 others had some improvement 1 year later (Glazer et al., 1990).

There are necessary indications for long-term use of DRBAs, such as chronic psychotic disorders (American Psychiatric Association, 1980). When patients are not able to discontinue antipsychotic medications, the concern is whether their TD will inexorably get worse, requiring higher and higher doses of antipsychotics to suppress the symptoms, but there are no data to indicate a worsening in most patients (Labbate et al., 1997), and the majority of patients show improvement over time (Gardos et al., 1988). Casey and colleagues (1986) noted that those with decreased neuroleptic doses showed no change in their dyskinesia score, and those with stable doses and increased doses showed a mean decrease in their dyskinesia scores at 3- to 11-year follow-up. Although these data do not answer whether the symptoms were simply masked or whether the disease itself has improved in its natural course, at least it appears that continuing antipsychotics does not necessarily aggravate the symptoms.

Therefore, a prudent approach is to keep the patients at the minimum dose of the drug necessary for their control of psychosis and add other forms of therapy for tardive dyskinesia. Many patients who are withdrawn from DRBAs still require symptomatic suppression of their movements when remission is not achieved or while waiting for remission. Since the clinical pharmacology is different in each subsyndrome, they are discussed separately.

## Treatment of Classic Tardive Dyskinesia

### DOPAMINE DEPLETORS

The concept of employing dopamine-depleting drugs, such as reserpine and TBZ (a synthetic benzoquinolizine), is that these agents effectively reduce dopaminergic synaptic activity, thereby reducing the TD symptoms without exposing the brain to an offending DRBA. This allows the possibility that over time, the brain will heal itself and completely eliminate the TD. In contrast, DRBAs can effectively decrease TD symptoms, but the brain continues to be exposed to the same pathogenetic mechanism that caused the TD in the first place, so the brain cannot recover. Both reserpine and TBZ inhibit the vesicular monoamine transporter. By preventing monoamines to be sequestered in the nerve terminal's vesicles, they allow the monoamines to be exposed to monoamine oxidase and catabolized, thus being markedly depleted in the nerve terminals.

Dopamine-depleting drugs have rarely, if ever, been noted to produce TD. In fact, among 17 patients with TD who were treated with reserpine by Fahn (1985), 4 remitted eventually while taking reserpine and were able to come off all treatment. Reserpine depletes catecholamine stores in sympathetic nerve terminals as well as in the central nervous system. Side effects include parkinsonism, apathy, depression, lethargy, and orthostatic hypotension. Some patients might require fairly high doses; significant improvement was reported with up to 5 to 8 mg per day (Sato et al., 1971; Fahn, 1985), whereas others who used lower doses reported less dramatic responses. Reserpine has a slow onset and a prolonged duration of action, and this must be taken into consideration when doses are changed. Once control of dyskinesia has been obtained, the dosage might need readjustment because of delayed onset of the catecholamine-depleting effect of reserpine with the induction of drug-induced parkinsonism. It is usually a question of balancing benefit and this adverse effect. Sixty-four percent of 96 patients in the literature had at least 50% improvement (Jeste and Wyatt, 1982b). One of the most notable results was that of a double-blind placebo-controlled study by Huang and colleagues (1980) that showed 50% improvement on reserpine 0.75 to 1.5 mg per day. Fahn's long-term study (1985) showed that 13 of 17 patients had moderate to marked benefit on higher doses up to 8 mg per day. Nine of the patients who improved also took α-methyl-para-tyrosine. Alpha-methyl-para-tyrosine is a competitive inhibitor of TH, the rate-limiting step in catecholamine synthesis. It is not very effective when used alone but can be a very powerful antidopaminergic drug when used with other presynaptically acting drugs.

TBZ has a quicker onset and shorter duration of action and has fewer peripheral catecholamine-depleting effects than reserpine. Like reserpine, TBZ has not been implicated in causing TD. However, in contrast to reserpine, TBZ does have some dopamine receptor–blocking activity (Reches et al., 1983), which probably accounts for the few reported cases of acute dystonic reaction that have been encountered clinically (Burke et al., 1985). In contrast to reserpine, remission of TD has not been reported during the treatment of TD with TBZ, although it has been seen in one of our patients (Fahn, personal observation). It would seem, therefore, that reserpine has the theoretical advantage of being more likely to allow for a remission of the TD, compared to TBZ. TBZ's major advantage is the quicker onset and fewer side effects compared to reserpine. TBZ is rapidly absorbed after oral administration and extensively metabolized during the first pass through the liver and/or the gut. One of the major metabolites, dihydrotetrabenazine, has pharmacologic actions similar to those of TBZ, although its ability to pass through the blood-brain barrier is unclear. Large individual variations are noted, and patients with hepatic dysfunction might expect alteration of pharmacokinetics (Mehvar et al., 1987). The dose has to be clinically titrated for each patient.

TBZ, clinically available in many countries, is now considered the treatment of choice for TD (Kenney and Jankovic, 2006). Improvement with TBZ was noted in 68% of 38 patients in the literature at a mean daily dose of 138 mg (Jeste and Wyatt, 1982a). Fahn (1985) reported improvement in five of six patients at doses of 75 to 300 mg per day in a long-term study. Kazamatsuri and colleagues (1972) noted that 54% of patients improved by at least 50% in a 6-week trial of TBZ compared to placebo treatment. Jankovic and Beach (1997) reported that 90% of patients had a marked improvement. Ondo and colleagues (1999) blindly rated videotapes taken of patients before and after TBZ treatment (mean duration: 20 weeks) and showed improvement in their dyskinesias. A major problem with TBZ therapy is with long-duration exposure. Most patients initially improve dramatically; then while maintained on the original dose, some begin to develop features of parkinsonism. Lowering the dose reduces this unwanted effect, but the TD then is less well controlled. Both reserpine and TBZ can induce acute akathisia and depression, so one needs to monitor for these adverse effects and treat them if they should occur. In some cases, however, depression actually improves after the introduction of TBZ, possibly as a result of abolishment of the involuntary movements (Kenney et al, 2006). Antidepressants, including monoamine oxidase inhibitors, can be used effectively to treat the depression. The selective norepinephrine reuptake inhibitor reboxetine has been found to rapidly reverse TBZ-induced depression (Schreiber et al., 1999).

### ATYPICAL ANTIPSYCHOTICS

By definition, the atypical antipsychotics have a reduced propensity to induce extrapyramidal adverse effects, tardive dyskinesia included. However, a range of the degree of adverse effects is encountered in use of the variety of drugs that have at one time or another been labeled as atypical neuroleptics. Today, the dibenzodiazepines clozapine and quetiapine are strong candidates for this labeling, and the thienobenzodiazepine olanzapine is less so. But originally, the *atypical* label was applied to the benzamine derivatives, such as sulpiride, metoclopramide, and tiapride. However, all three compounds have been reported to induce tardive dyskinesia or NMS (Casey, 1983; Achiron et al., 1990; Miller and Jankovic, 1990; Duarte et al., 1996). Similarly, risperidone has been touted as atypical, but it more resembles a typical antipsychotic, causing parkinsonism and inducing tardive dyskinesia (Buzan, 1996). The typical antipsychotics, including sulpiride, tiapride, and risperidone, by blocking and occupying dopamine D2 receptors, are effective in reducing the severity of tardive dyskinesia (Chouinard, 1995). But so do even stronger DRBAs, such as phenothiazines and haloperidol. The problem with using typical antipsychotics to treat TD is that they are in the class of the offending drugs and hence will prolong the exposure of the patient to the drugs that cause TD.

The question is whether the true atypical antipsychotics, such as clozapine and quetiapine, can reduce the symptoms of TD and still allow the healing process in the brain to proceed to eventually eliminate the pathophysiologic causation of the symptoms. There are reports of clozapine successfully reducing the abnormal movements of tardive dyskinesia and tardive akathisia (Huang et al., 1980; Wirshing et al., 1990; Bassitt and Neto, 1998) and in some patients with tardive dystonia (Lieberman et al., 1989, 1991; Van Putten et al., 1990; Friedman, 1994; Trugman et al., 1994; Wolf and Mosnain, 1994; Raja et al., 1996; van Harten et al., 1996a; Bassitt and Neto, 1998). But the response rate is lower than that with typical antipsychotics, such as haloperidol. Clozapine permitted the dyskinesia to disappear in about half the cases in one report (Gerlach and Peacock, 1994). In another, 8 of the 20 patients with TD improved after an average time of $261 \pm 188$ days of treatment (Bunker et al., 1996). With an average dose of approximately 400 mg per day, Bassitt and Neto (1998) obtained a 50% lessening of dyskinesia. It is still not clear whether the reduction of dyskinesia is due to the small amount of D2 blocking effect or whether actual healing of the TD can take place in the presence of clozapine. The proof of the latter and preferred category would be the lack of reappearance when clozapine is withdrawn. There has not yet been a report of such a case. Without that evidence, it is likely that the reductions of tardive dyskinesia and tardive dystonia are due to the small amount of D2 blocking activity by clozapine.

There is a case report of TD improving on quetiapine 600 mg per day (Vesely et al., 2000). The patient was not withdrawn from the drug. A large randomized study on high-dose quetiapine also found quetiapine to be effective (Emsley et al., 2004), but high doses of the atypical antipsychotics become typical by blocking D2 receptors, so the reduction of TD can be due solely to further D2 receptor blockade.

The questions that were raised from clozapine apply here as well: Is the reduction of dyskinesias due to its D2 blocking effect that would occur at high doses? If so, then withdrawal of the drug would be associated with a return of the dyskinesias. Is the reduction of dyskinesias due to a natural healing process, as has been demonstrated mainly with reserpine and somewhat with TBZ? If so, then withdrawal of the drug would not be associated with a return of the dyskinesias. The advantage of dopamine depletors, such as reserpine and TBZ, is that they allow symptomatic benefit and still allow the brain to heal spontaneously, so withdrawal of medication might be possible some day.

However, clozapine and quetiapine could substitute for a typical antipsychotic in a patient with a tardive syndrome who also has psychosis, thereby controlling the psychosis and possibly still allowing a chance for a complete remission to occur. Such a remission would not take place in the presence of the typical antipsychotic. Like clozapine, quetiapine needs to be tested. Olanzapine has successfully reduced the symptoms of TD (Littrell et al., 1998). But olanzapine is not a true atypical antipsychotic, and the reduction of the symptoms and signs is probably obtained by blockading D2 receptors. This would convey no advantage over using the more classic and conventional typical antipsychotics.

## DOPAMINE AGONISTS

Some investigators have tried to activate the presynaptic dopamine receptors by using low doses of a dopamine agonist, which in turn would reduce the biosynthesis and release of dopamine. Another approach by Alpert and Friedhoff (1980) was the use of levodopa in an attempt to desensitize the postsynaptic dopamine receptors. This can cause initial worsening of symptoms before eventual improvement is expected after discontinuation of levodopa. Unfortunately, dopaminergic drugs can also lead to overt recurrence of underlying psychosis (Fahn, 1983). This approach has theoretical merit but is very difficult to carry out in many patients and has not been widely used since the initial reports.

Amantadine has been reported to have some benefit (Angus et al., 1997), but it may be due to its glutamate receptor blocking effect rather than its dopaminergic effect.

## NONDOPAMINERGIC MEDICATIONS

Although neuroleptics are most effective in controlling the abnormal movements, some patients do not respond to the treatment. Numerous investigators (Jeste and Wyatt, 1982a; Jeste et al., 1988) have attempted nondopaminergic treatments. Agents that enhance GABA transmission have been tried because of GABA's inhibitory effect on the dopaminergic system and experimental data indicating changes in the GABA system in patients and animals that have been treated with chronic neuroleptics. Use of benzodiazepines, baclofen, valproate, and γ-vinyl GABA have met with limited success, partly owing to tolerance and side effects, such as worsening of psychosis. Some improvement was found with clonazepam (Thaker et al., 1990). Propranolol, fusaric acid, and clonidine decrease the noradrenergic activity and have been reported to be useful but require further study to clarify their role in treating tardive dyskinesia. Use of cholinergic drugs was based on the reciprocal dopamine-acetylcholine balance in the basal ganglia. Despite a flurry of reports in the 1970s, this modality has been quite limited and should be reconsidered now that some adequate cholinergic drugs are available. Anticholinergics, lithium, pyridoxine, tryptophan, cyproheptadine, vasopressin, naloxone, morphine, and estrogen were reported to be of no benefit. But in a controlled clinical trial involving 15 patients, pyridoxine was found to reduce the severity of TD (Lerner et al., 2001). Buspirone has been reported to be beneficial (Moss et al., 1993), but it is not clear that this drug does not have dopamine receptor-blocking activity. Calcium channel blockers have been reported to reduce the severity of TD (Kushnir and Ratner, 1989; Duncan et al., 1990; Suddath et al., 1991) but not in all studies (Loonen et al., 1992). A combination of acetazolamide and thiamine was found to reduce both TD and drug-induced parkinsonism (Cowen et al., 1997).

A review of randomized clinical trials was presented by Soares and McGrath (1999) with a meta-analysis when more than one randomized clinical trial had been carried out. Meta-analysis showed that baclofen, deanol, and diazepam were no more effective than was a placebo. Single randomized clinical trials demonstrated a lack of evidence of any effect for bromocriptine, ceruletide, clonidine, estrogen, gamma-linolenic acid, hydergine, lecithin, lithium, progabide, selegiline, and tetrahydroisoxazolopyridinol. Meta-analysis found that five interventions were effective: levodopa, oxypertine, sodium valproate, tiapride, and vitamin E; neuroleptic reduction was marginally significant. Vitamin E is more thoroughly discussed in the next paragraph. Data from single randomized clinical trials revealed that insulin, α-methyldopa and reserpine were more effective than a placebo. Meta-analysis found that 37.3% of placebo-treated subjects improved.

A role for antioxidants has been raised (Cadet and Lohr, 1989; Behl et al., 1995). Treatment with vitamin E has been found to reduce the severity of tardive dyskinesia (Elkashef et al., 1990; Dabiri et al., 1994; Adler et al., 1998; Sajjad, 1998) or have no effect (Lam et al., 1994). The meta-analysis mentioned earlier showed effectiveness. A small clinical trial of 41 subjects comparing 1200 IU per day of vitamin E and placebo found the former to better reduce severity of abnormal involuntary movements (45.9% versus 4.3%) (Zhang et al., 2004). However, the largest double-blind study, carried out by the Veterans Administration multicenter, placebo-controlled clinical trial (Adler et al., 1999), found vitamin E not to be effective. As a potential prophylactic agent, vitamin E (3200 IU per day) was found not to protect against development of drug-induced parkinsonism (Eranti et al., 1998). Nor was vitamin E treatment able to prevent neuroleptic-induced VCMs in rats (Sachdev et al., 1999). In a small open-label trial combining vitamins E and C, improvement in TD was seen (Michael et al., 2003).

There continue to be reports of TD responding to open-label trials. Gabapentin (Hardoy et al., 1999, 2003), pyridoxine (Lerner et al., 1999), and branched-chain amino acids (Richardson et al., 2003) are such compounds. Levetiracetam was helpful in a small trial (Konitsiotis et al., 2006).

Injections of botulinum toxin into the muscles causing oral dyskinesia have been reported to be effective in reducing the movements (Rapaport et al., 2000).

Sporadic reports noted efficacy of electroconvulsive therapy in refractory cases of TD (Price and Levin, 1978), but Yassa and colleagues (1990) reported success in only one of nine patients.

### CONCLUSIONS ON CLASSIC TARDIVE DYSKINESIA

By blocking D2 receptors or depleting dopamine from synaptic terminals, neuroleptics are effective in reducing the abnormal involuntary movements of TD. Depletors do not cause TD and are therefore preferred; their use, while controlling symptoms, allows the brain to heal spontaneously. Avoiding side effects, particularly drug-induced parkinsonism, is a major limiting factor. DRBAs, while controlling symptoms, are the culprits causing TD; the brain does not heal, and one cannot be certain that TD continues to worsen in the presence of these agents. If one needs to utilize an antipsychotic, it seems safer to use one that is suspected of having less ability to induce tardive dyskinesia, such as clozapine and quetiapine. Olanzapine comes closer to being a typical, rather than an atypical, antipsychotic. When clozapine and quetiapine occasionally reduce dyskinesias, the doses that are used suggest the response is from their D2-blocking activity.

Figures 20-1 and 20-2 are flowcharts that provide a useful algorithm for treating TD.

## Tardive Dystonia

As with classic TD, the most effective medications for tardive dystonia are also antidopaminergic drugs (Kang et al., 1986), but the percentage of patients who improve is smaller. Reserpine and TBZ each produce improvement in about 50% of patients. Some patients who do not respond or have intoler-

able side effects to one might respond to the other. DRBAs are more effective in suppressing the movements (77%). Symptomatically, those who remained on DRBAs after the onset of tardive dystonia and those who were withdrawn from them do not have a significant difference in their improvement rate. This again is in agreement with the data on classic TD, in which continued use of DRBAs does not necessarily lead to aggravation of the movements (Casey et al., 1986; Gardos et al., 1988). The atypical antipsychotic clozapine has been helpful in some patients with tardive dystonia (Lieberman et al., 1989, 1991; Van Putten et al., 1990; Friedman, 1994; Trugman et al., 1994; Wolf and Mosnaim, 1994; Raja et al., 1996; van Harten et al., 1996a). There are reports of quetiapine's effectiveness as well (Gourzis et al., 2005). It is likely that its treatment of tardive dystonia in some situations is due to its D2 receptor–blocking activity resulting in a masking of the symptoms, because withdrawal would exacerbate the dystonia (Krack et al., 1994). The combination of clozapine and clonazepam has been effective in some patients when either drug alone was much less satisfactory (Shapleske et al., 1996).

In tardive dystonia, antimuscarinics are almost as effective as antidopaminergic drugs. This is different from classic TD, which may get worse with antimuscarinics (Yassa, 1988). Kang and colleagues (1986) reported a 46% improvement rate on antimuscarinics such as trihexyphenidyl and ethopropazine. Central nervous system side effects of the antimuscarinics include forgetfulness, lethargy, psychosis, dysphoria, and personality changes; elderly patients are more susceptible to these. Peripheral side effects include blurred vision, dry mouth, constipation, urinary retention, and orthostatic dizziness. Those who develop side effects to one anticholinergic drug may tolerate another anticholinergic better. Although there is no evidence that one anticholinergic is more efficacious than the others, ethopropazine may produce fewer central nervous system side effects in elderly patients. Although peripheral pharmacokinetics show relatively short half-lives, their central effects have a very slow onset of action, and several weeks are often required before benefit is noticed. Therefore, the medications are started at a low dose, 2.5 mg of trihexyphenidyl or 25 mg of ethopropazine, and increased slowly by 2.5 mg of trihexyphenidyl or 25 mg of ethopropazine weekly until sufficient control of dystonia or intolerable side effects are achieved. As in idiopathic dystonia, many patients respond only to a high dose of anticholinergics. Therefore, every attempt must be made to control side effects so that high-dose anticholinergics may be tried. Kang and colleagues (1986) reported use of a maximum of 450 mg ethopropazine or 32 mg of trihexyphenidyl, and higher doses may be tolerated in young patients if judiciously used. Peripheral side effects are often controlled by peripheral cholinergic drugs, such as oral pyridostigmine and pilocarpine eye drops.

The clinical pharmacology of tardive dystonia indicates two subtypes: one group that responds to antidopaminergic drugs like the other tardive syndromes and one that responds to anticholinergics like idiopathic dystonia. Analysis of clinical characteristics of patients who respond to antidopaminergic drugs and those who respond to anticholinergic drugs has not shown any significant difference (Kang et al., 1986). However, the data from Kang and colleagues (1986) are retrospective, and the treatment choice between the two classes of drugs was rather arbitrary, partly based on anticipated side effects. For example, patients who were elderly or who had dementia were treated with dopamine-depleting drugs first, because these

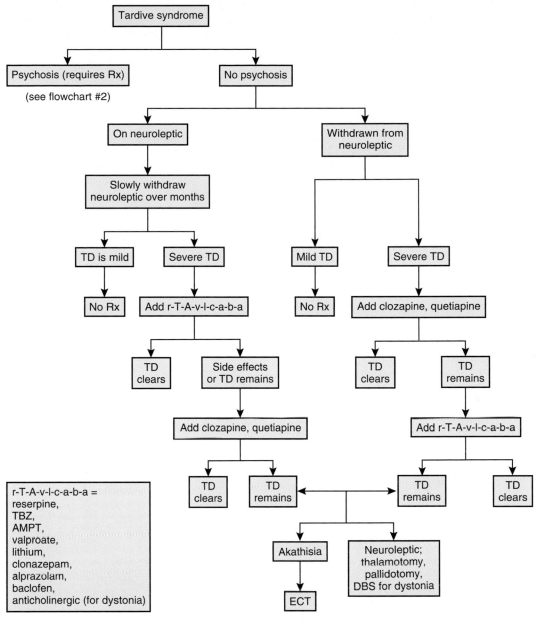

**Figure 20-1** Flowchart for treating tardive dyskinesia in the absence of psychosis. AMPT, α-methyl-para-tyrosine; DBS, deep brain stimulation; ECT, electroconvulsive therapy; TBZ, tetrabenazine.

patients have greater risk for anticholinergic side effects such as memory loss and confusion. Patients with depression might have relapse of their symptoms on dopamine-depleting drugs and were treated preferentially with anticholinergics. This is a reasonable clinical approach, but characterization of subtypes will require a controlled study with random assignment of the treatment. If either a dopamine depletor or antimuscarinic is ineffective by itself, the combination should be tried.

Benzodiazepines are mainly helpful as adjunctive therapy with dopamine-depleting or anticholinergic drugs. Minimal success with propranolol, levodopa, carbamazepine, and baclofen has been noted. Bromocriptine, deanol, clonidine, lisuride, amantadine, and valproate were reported with mixed results. The calcium channel blocker verapamil was reported to be effective in one patient (Abad and Ovsiew, 1993). Opioids do not have lasting value in suppressing tardive dys-

tonia (Berg et al., 2001). But one study found the combination of naltrexone and clonazepam to offer some benefit (Wonodi et al., 2004a).

If any residual dystonia remains that is localized to one or a few parts of the body, then injections of botulinum toxin into the affected parts, such as the orbicularis oculi, masseters, or cervical muscles, might be useful (Chatterjee et al., 1997; Tarsy et al., 1997; Kanovsky et al., 1999).

Electroconvulsive therapy might be effective in intractable cases (Yoshida et al., 1996), as would deep brain stimulation (Franzini et al., 2005) and intrathecal baclofen (Dressler et al., 1997). Surgery is not always effective, and it does pose risks of complications (Trottenberg et al., 2001).

A centrally acting muscle relaxant, eperisone, was successful in treating one patient with tardive dystonia (Nisijima et al., 1998). Eperisone is a beta-aminopropiophenone derivative.

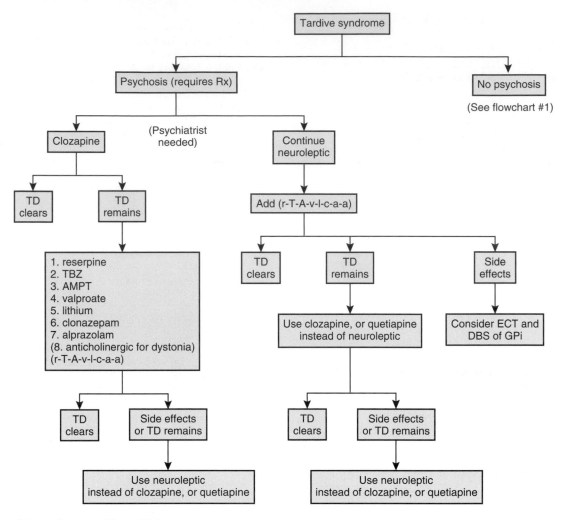

Abbreviations, see Figure 20-1

**Figure 20-2** Flowchart for treating tardive syndromes in the presence of psychosis.

Figures 20-1 and 20-2 depict flowcharts for therapy that can be applied to tardive dystonia as well as to classic TD.

## Tardive Akathisia

As was noted earlier, variants of akathisia have been the source of confusion in the literature. Most of the papers do not distinguish between acute and tardive akathisia or usually refer to acute akathisia and not tardive akathisia. Very few studies have been focused on the treatment of tardive akathisia.

Tardive akathisia is difficult to treat and does not respond to anticholinergics, which have been reported to help acute akathisia. It and tardive dystonia are the most distressing and disabling features of the tardive symptoms, and their treatment is important. In the study of tardive akathisia by Burke (1989), all of the patients noted that the subjective sensations were distressing. The same study reported that 87% of patients improved on reserpine up to 5 mg per day and 58% on TBZ up to 175 mg per day. In one third of these patients, the movements were completely suppressed. In this respect the clinical pharmacology is more like that of classic TD than that of acute akathisia. Opioids were reported to be beneficial

(Walters et al., 1986), but the effect has not been persistent (Burke et al., 1989). Electroconvulsive treatment can be effective in those patients whose akathisia has proved to be intractable (Hermesh et al., 1992).

Figures 20-1 and 20-2 depict flowcharts on therapy that can also be applied to tardive akathisia.

## TREATMENT SUMMARY

Box 20-3 summarizes a useful approach to treat tardive syndromes in general. The approach to treatment should be earmarked according to whether the patient is psychotic and requires antipsychotic medication, or is not psychotic. For detailed, step-by-step decisions in the treatment of the tardive syndromes, the flowcharts of Figures 20-1 and 20-2 should be helpful.

In summary, since the initial description of tardive dyskinesia as an iatrogenic complication of dopamine receptor antagonist, considerable progress has been made in understanding the risks, epidemiology, and clinical subtypes of the condition. However, pathogenesis and characteristics of distinct subtypes

Box 20-3 Treatment for tardive dyskinesia syndromes

1. Taper and slowly eliminate causative agents if clinically possible. Avoid sudden cessation of these drugs, which could exacerbate the tardive syndrome.
2. Avoid drugs, if possible (i.e., wait for spontaneous recovery). This is possible only if the dyskinesia is not severe or there is no accompanying tardive akathisia or tardive dystonia. Akathisia and dystonia are more distressing and disabling than is classic TD.
3. If necessary to treat the symptoms, first use dopamine–depleting drugs: reserpine, tetrabenazine (TBZ), α-methyl-para-tyrosine. Attempt to overcome the adverse effects of depression and parkinsonism with antidepressants and antiparkinsonism drugs, respectively.
4. Consider melatonin on the basis of one report (Shamir et al., 2001).
5. Next, consider the true atypical antipsychotic agents clozapine and quetiapine.
6. If these fail, consider tiny doses of a dopamine receptor agonist to activate only the presynaptic dopamine receptor and reduce the biosynthesis of dopamine.
7. For tardive dystonia, consider antimuscarinics.
8. For intractable tardive akathisia, consider electroconvulsive therapy.
9. Typical antipsychotic agents can be used to control the dyskinesias when all the previously mentioned approaches fail. Combining this with a dopamine depletor may increase the potency of the antidyskinetic effect and may theoretically protect against a worsening of the underlying tardive pathology.
10. Thalamotomy, pallidotomy, and deep brain stimulation of the thalamus and pallidum have been performed for tardive dystonia with success. Deep brain stimulation of the pallidum appears to be the preferred surgical procedure if the symptoms remain severe and all medication trials fail.

are still poorly understood. Management of tardive syndromes must be based on proper understanding of these aspects of the disorder. The only effective and safe antipsychotic agents that do not produce, or rarely produce, tardive dyskinesia appear to be clozapine and quetiapine. Meanwhile, prevention is possible by avoiding indiscriminate use of DRBAs and limiting their use to disorders for which no other type of medication is available or effective. When prevention and withdrawal of the offending drugs for eventual remission fail, symptomatic suppression can be achieved in many patients with pharmacologic treatments. New approaches are needed, and prospective controlled clinical trials with particular attention to clinical subtypes are necessary for better management of these conditions.

# References

Abad V, Ovsiew F: Treatment of persistent myoclonic tardive dystonia with verapamil. Br J Psychiatry 1993;162:554–556.

Abu-Kishk I, Toledano M, Reis A, et al: Neuroleptic malignant syndrome in a child treated with an atypical antipsychotic. J Toxicol Clin Toxicol 2004;42(6):921–925.

Achiron A, Zoldan Y, Melamed E: Tardive dyskinesia induced by sulpiride. Clin Neuropharmacol 1990;13:248–252.

Adler CM, Malhotra AK, Elman I, et al: Amphetamine-induced dopamine release and post-synaptic specific binding in patients with mild tardive dyskinesia. Neuropsychopharmacology 2002;26 (3):295–300.

Adler L, Angrist B, Peselow E, et al: A controlled assessment of propranolol in the treatment of neuroleptic-induced akathisia. Br J Psychiatry 1986;149:42–45.

Adler L, Angrist B, Peselow E, et al: Clonidine in neuroleptic-induced akathisia. Am J Psychiatry 1987;144:235–236.

Adler LA, Edson R, Lavori P, et al: Long-term treatment effects of vitamin E for tardive dyskinesia. Biol Psychiatry 1998;43:868–872.

Adler LA, Rotrosen J, Edson R, et al: Vitamin E treatment for tardive dyskinesia. Arch Gen Psychiatry 1999;56:836–841.

Aguilar EJ, Keshavan MS, Martinez-Quiles MD, et al: Predictors of acute dystonia in first-episode psychotic patients. Am J Psychiatry 1994;151:1819–1821.

Alpert M, Friedhoff A: Clinical application of receptor modification treatment. In Fann WE, Smith RC, Davis JM, Domino EF (eds): Tardive dyskinesia: Research and treatment. New York, SP Medical and Scientific Books, 1980, pp 471–474.

Altshuler LL, Pierre JM, Wirshing WC, Ames D: Sertraline and akathisia. J Clin Psychopharmacol 1994;14:278–279.

American Psychiatric Association: Task force on late neurological effects of antipsychotics. Tardive dyskinesia. Washington, DC, American Psychiatric Association, 1980.

Amore M, Zazzeri N, Berardi D: Atypical neuroleptic malignant syndrome associated with clozapine treatment. Neuropsychobiology 1997;35:197–199.

Ananth JJ, Burgoyne K, Aquino S: Meige's syndrome associated with risperidone therapy. Am J Psychiatry 2000;157:149.

Andersson U, Haggstrom J-E, Levin ED, et al: Reduced glutamate decarboxylase activity in the subthalamic nucleus in patients with tardive dyskinesia. Mov Disord 1989;4:37–46.

Andreassen OA, Aamo TO, Jorgensen HA: Inhibition by memantine of the development of persistent oral dyskinesias induced by long-term haloperidol treatment of rats. Br J Pharmacol 1996;119:751–757.

Andreassen OA, Finsen B, Ostergaard K, et al: The relationship between oral dyskinesias produced by long-term haloperidol treatment, the density of striatal preproenkephalin messenger RNA and enkephalin peptide, and the number of striatal neurons expressing preproenkephalin messenger RNA in rats. Neuroscience 1999;88:27–35.

Andreassen OA, Jorgensen HA: Neurotoxicity associated with neuroleptic-induced oral dyskinesias in rats: Implications for tardive dyskinesia? Prog Neurobiol 2000;61:525–541.

Andreassen OA, MacEwan T, Gulbrandsen AK, et al: Nonfunctional CYP2D6 alleles and risk for neuroleptic-induced movement disorders in schizophrenic patients. Psychopharmacology 1997;131: 174–179.

Andreassen OA, Meshul CK, Moore C, Jorgensen HA: Oral dyskinesias and morphological changes in rat striatum during long-term haloperidol administration. Psychopharmacology 2001;157:11–19.

Andreassen OA, Weber C, Jorgensen HA: Coenzyme Q10 does not prevent oral dyskinesias induced by long-term haloperidol treatment of rats. Pharmacol Biochem Behav 1999;64:637–642.

Anfang MK, Pope HG: Treatment of neuroleptic-induced akathisia with nicotine patches. Psychopharmacology 1997;134:153–156.

Angus S, Sugars J, Boltezar R, et al: A controlled trial of amantadine hydrochloride and neuroleptics in the treatment of tardive dyskinesia. J Clin Psychopharmacol 1997;17:88–91.

Arana GW, Goff DC, Baldessarini RJ, Keepers GA: Efficacy of anticholinergic prophylaxis for neuroleptic-induced acute dystonia. Am J Psychiatry 1988;145:993–996.

Arnone D, Hansen L, Kerr JS: Acute dystonic reaction in an elderly patient with mood disorder after titration of paroxetine: Possible mechanisms and implications for clinical care. J Psychopharmacol 2002;16(4):395–397.

Arnt J, Skarsfeldt T: Do novel antipsychotics have similar pharmacological characteristics? A review of the evidence. Neuropsychopharmacology 1998;18:63–101.

Asper H, Baggiolini M, Burke HR, et al: Tolerance phenomena with neuroleptics: Catalepsy, apomorphine stereotypies and striatal dopamine metabolism in the rat after single and repeated administration of loxapine and haloperidol. Eur J Pharmacol 1973;22:287–294.

Ayd FJ: A survey of drug-induced extrapyramidal reactions. JAMA 1961;175:1054–1060.

Bailey L, Maxwell S, Brandabur MM: Substance abuse as a risk factor for tardive dyskinesia: A retrospective analysis of 1,027 patients. Psychopharmacol Bull 1997;33:177–181.

Bakker PR, van Harten PN, van Os J: Antipsychotic-induced tardive dyskinesia and the Ser9Gly polymorphism in the DRD3 gene: A meta analysis. Schizophr Res 2006;83(2–3):185–192.

Baldessarini RJ, Marsh E: Fluoxetine and side effects. Arch Gen Psychiatry 1992;47:191–192.

Barnes TRE, Braude WM: Akathisia variants and tardive dyskinesia. Arch Gen Psychiatry 1985;42:874–878.

Barnes TRE, Kidger T, Gore SM: Tardive dyskinesia: A 3-year follow-up study. Psychol Med 1983;13:71–81.

Basile VS, Ozdemir V, Masellis M, et al: Lack of association between serotonin-2A receptor gene (HTR2A) polymorphisms and tardive dyskinesia in schizophrenia. Mol Psychiatry 2001;6:230–234.

Bassitt DP, Garcia LDL: Risperidone-induced tardive dyskinesia. Pharmacopsychiatry 2000;33:155–156.

Bassitt DP, Neto MRL: Clozapine efficacy in tardive dyskinesia in schizophrenic patients. Eur Arch Psychiatry Clin Neurosci 1998;248:209–211.

Beasley CM, Dellva MA, Tamura RN, et al: Randomised double-blind comparison of the incidence of tardive dyskinesia in patients with schizophrenia during long-term treatment with olanzapine or haloperidol. Br J Psychiatry 1999;174:23–30.

Beasley CM Jr, Tollefson GD, Tran PV: Safety of olanzapine. J Clin Psychiatry 1997;58(suppl 10):13–17.

Behan WMH, Madigan M, Clark BJ, et al: Muscle changes in the neuroleptic malignant syndrome. J Clin Pathol 2000;53:223–227.

Behl C, Rupprecht R, Skutella T, Holsboer F: Haloperidol-induced cell death—mechanism and protection with vitamin E in vitro. Neuroreport 1995;7:360–364.

Benazzi F: Clozapine-induced neuroleptic malignant syndrome not recurring with olanzapine, a structurally and pharmacologically similar antipsychotic. Hum Psychopharmacol Clin Exp 1999;14:511–512.

Bench CJ, Lammertsma AA, Dolan RJ, et al: Dose dependent occupancy of central dopamine D2 receptors by the novel neuroleptic CP-88,059-01: A study using positron emission tomography and 11C-raclopride. Psychopharmacology (Berl) 1993;112:308–314.

Bench CJ, Lammertsma AA, Grasby PM, et al: The time course of binding to striatal dopamine D2 receptors by the neuroleptic ziprasidone (CP-88,059-01) determined by positron emission tomography. Psychopharmacology (Berl) 1996;124:141–147.

Benedetti F, Cavallaro R, Smeraldi E: Olanzapine-induced neutropenia after clozapine-induced neutropenia. Lancet 1999;354:567.

Benes FM, Paskevich PA, Davidson J, Domesick VB: The effects of haloperidol on synaptic patterns in the rat striatum. Brain Res 1985;329:265–274.

Berg D, Becker G, Naumann M, Reiners K: Morphine in tardive and idiopathic dystonia. J Neural Transm 2001;108:1035–1041.

Bharucha KJ, Sethi KD: Tardive tourettism after exposure to neuroleptic therapy. Mov Disord 1995;10:791–793.

Blanchet PJ, Abdillahi O, Beauvais C, et al: Prevalence of spontaneous oral dyskinesia in the elderly: A reappraisal. Mov Disord 2004;19(8):892–896.

Blin J, Baron JC, Cambon H, et al: Striatal dopamine D2 receptors in tardive dyskinesia: PET study. J Neurol Neurosurg Psychiatry 1989;52:1248–1252.

Blom S, Ekbom KA: Comparison between akathisia developing on treatment with phenothiazine derivatives and the restless leg syndrome. Acta Med Scand 1961;170:689–694.

Boeti C, Black DN, Waddington JL: Dyskinesia in patients with schizophrenia never treated with antipsychotics. In Bedard M-A, Agid Y, Chouinard S, et al (eds): Mental and Behavioral Dysfunction in Movement Disorders. Totowa, NJ, Humana Press, 2003, pp 489–498.

Bottlender R, Jager M, Hofschuster E, et al: Neuroleptic malignant syndrome due to atypical neuroleptics: Three episodes in one patient. Pharmacopsychiatry 2002;35(3):119–121.

Bowers MB, Moore D, Tarsy D: Tardive dyskinesia: A clinical test of the supersensitivity hypothesis. Psychopharmacology 1979;61:137–141.

Boyer WF, Bakalar NH, Lake CR: Anticholinergic prophylaxis of acute haloperidol-induced acute dystonic reactions. J Clin Psychopharmacol 1987;7:164–166.

Brandon S, McClelland HA, Protheroe C: A study of facial dyskinesia in a mental hospital population. Br J Psychiatry 1971;118:171–184.

Braude WM, Barnes TRE: Late-onset akathisia—an indicant of covert dyskinesia: Two case reports. Am J Psychiatry 1983;140:611–612.

Braude WM, Barnes TRE, Gore SN: Clinical characteristics of akathisia: A systematic investigation of acute psychiatric inpatient admissions. Br J Psychiatry 1983;143:139–150.

Brody AL: Acute dystonia induced by rapid increase in risperidone dosage. J Clin Psychopharmacol 1996;16:461–462.

Broich K, Grunwald F, Kasper S, et al: D-2-dopamine receptor occupancy measured by IBZM-SPECT in relation to extrapyramidal side effects. Pharmacopsychiatry 1998;31:159–162.

Brown K, Reid A, White T, et al: Vitamin E, lipids, and lipid peroxidation products in tardive dyskinesia. Biol Psychiatry 1998;43:863–867.

Brown KW, White T, Wardlaw JM, et al: Caudate nucleus morphology in tardive dyskinesia. Br J Psychiatry 1996;169:631–636.

Bruneau MA, Stip E: Metronome or alternating Pisa syndrome: A form of tardive dystonia under clozapine treatment. Int Clin Psychopharmacol 1998;13:229–232.

Buchanan RW, Gellad F, Munson RC, Breier A: Basal ganglia pathology in schizophrenia and tardive dyskinesia: An MRI quantitative study. Am J Psychiatry 1994;151:752–755.

Bunker MT, Sommi RW, Stoner SC, Switzer JL: Longitudinal analysis of abnormal involuntary movements in long-term clozapine-treated patients. Psychopharmacol Bull 1996;32:699–703.

Burke RE, Fahn S, Jankovic J, et al: Tardive dystonia: Late-onset and persistent dystonia caused by antipsychotic drugs. Neurology 1982;32:1335–1346

Burke RE, Kang UJ, Jankovic J, et al: Tardive akathisia: An analysis of clinical features and response to open therapeutic trials. Mov Disord 1989;4:157–175.

Burke RE, Reches A, Traub MM, et al: Tetrabenazine induces acute dystonic reactions. Ann Neurol 1985;17:200–202.

Burkhard PR, Vingerhoets FJG, Alberque C, et al: Olanzapine induced neuroleptic malignant syndrome. Arch Gen Psychiatry 1999;56:101–102.

Buzan RD: Risperidone-induced tardive dyskinesia. Am J Psychiatry 1996;153:734–735.

Bymaster F, Perry KW, Nelson DL, et al: Olanzapine: A basic science update. Br J Psychiatry 1999;174:36–40.

Cadet JL, Lohr BJ: Possible involvement of free radicals in neuroleptic-induced movement disorders: Evidence from treatment of tardive dyskinesia with vitamin E. Ann N Y Acad Sci 1989; 528:176–185.

Calabresi P, De Murtas M, Mercuri NB, Bernardi G: Chronic neuroleptic treatment: D2 dopamine receptor supersensitivity and striatal glutamatergic transmission. Ann Neurol 1992;31:366–373.

Caligiuri MP, Lacro JP, Rockwell E, et al: Incidence and risk factors for severe tardive dyskinesia in older patients. Br J Psychiatry 1997; 171:148–153.

Calne DB, Lang AE: Secondary dystonia. In Fahn S, Marsden CD, Calne DB (eds): Dystonia 2: Advances in Neurology, vol 50. New York, Raven Press, 1988, pp 9–34.

Carlsson A: The occurrence, distribution and physiological role of catecholamines in the nervous system. Pharmacol Rev 1959;11:490–493.

Carlsson A, Lindqvist M, Magnusson T: 3,4-Dihydroxyphenylalanine and 5-hydroxytryptophan as reserpine antagonists. Nature 1957; 180:1200.

Caroff SN, Mann SC, Keck PE, Francis A: Residual catatonic state following neuroleptic malignant syndrome. J Clin Psychopharmacol 2000;20:257–259.

Carter CJ, Pycock CJ: Studies on the role of catecholamines in the frontal cortex. Br J Pharmacol 1978;42:402.

Casey DE: Metoclopramide side effects. Ann Intern Med 1983;98: 673–674.

Casey DE, Povlsen UJ, Meidahl B, Gerlach J: Neuroleptic-induced tardive dyskinesia and parkinsonism: Changes during several years of continuing treatment. Psychopharmacol Bull 1986;22:250–253.

Casteels-Van Daele M, Jaeken J, Van Der Schueren P, et al: Dystonic reactions in children caused by metoclopramide. Arch Dis Child 1970;45:130–133.

Chakos MH, Alvir JMJ, Woerner MG, et al: Incidence and correlates of tardive dyskinesia in first episode of schizophrenia. Arch Gen Psychiatry 1996;53:313–319.

Chakraborty N, Johnston T: Aripiprazole and neuroleptic malignant syndrome. Int Clin Psychopharmacol 2004;19(6):351–353.

Chaplin R, Kent A: Informing patients about tardive dyskinesia: Controlled trial of patient education. Br J Psychiatry 1998;172: 78–81.

Chatterjee A, Gordon MF, Giladi N, Trosch R: Botulinum toxin in the treatment of tardive dystonia. J Clin Psychopharmacol 1997;17: 497–498.

Chong SA: Fluvoxamine and akathisia. J Clin Psychopharmacol 1996;16:334–335.

Chong SA, Tan EC, Tan CH, et al: Polymorphisms of dopamine receptors and tardive dyskinesia among Chinese patients with schizophrenia. Am J Med Genet 2003;116B(1):51–54.

Chouinard G: Effects of risperidone in tardive dyskinesia: An analysis of the Canadian multicenter risperidone study. J Clin Psychopharmacol 1995;15:S36–S44.

Chouinard G, Annable L, Mercier P, Ross-Couinard A: A five-year follow-up study of tardive dyskinesia. Psychopharmacol Bull 1986;22:259–263.

Christensen E, Moller JE, Faurbye A: Neuropathological investigation of 28 brains from patients with dyskinesia. Acta Psychiatr Scand 1970;46:14–23.

Clow A, Theodorou A, Jenner P, Marsden CD: Cerebral dopamine function in rats following withdrawal from one year of continuous neuroleptic administration. Eur J Pharmacol 1980;63: 145–157.

Conley RR, Tamminga CA, Bartko JJ, et al: Olanzapine compared with chlorpromazine in treatment-resistant schizophrenia. Am J Psychiatry 1998;155:914–920.

Correll CU, Leucht S, Kane JM: Lower risk for tardive dyskinesia associated with second-generation antipsychotics: A systematic review of 1-year studies. Am J Psychiatry. 2004;161(3):414–425.

Corson PW, Nopoulos P, Miller DD, et al: Change in basal ganglia volume over 2 years in patients with schizophrenia: Typical versus atypical neuroleptics. Am J Psychiatry 1999;156:1200–1204.

Coulter DM, Pillans PI: Fluoxetine and extrapyramidal side effects. Am J Psychiatry 1995;152:122–125.

Cowen MA, Green M, Bertollo DN, Abbott K: A treatment for tardive dyskinesia and some other extrapyramidal symptoms. J Clin Psychopharmacol 1997;17:190–193.

Creese I, Burt DR, Snyder SH: Dopamine receptor binding predicts clinical and pharmacological potencies of antischizophrenic drugs. Science 1976;192:481–483.

Cross AJ, Crow TJ, Ferrier IN, et al: Chemical and structural changes in the brain in patients with movement disorder. In Casey DE, Chase TN, Chritine AV, Gerlach J (eds): Dyskinesia: Research and treatment. New York, Springer-Verlag, 1985, pp 104–110.

Crow TJ, Cross AJ, Johnstone EC, et al: Abnormal involuntary movements in schizophrenia: Are they related to the disease process or its treatment? Are they associated with changes in dopamine receptors? J Clin Psychopharmacol 1982;2:336–340.

Curran MP, Perry CM: Spotlight on amisulpride in schizophrenia. CNS Drugs 2002;16:207–211.

Curtis LH, Masselink LE, Ostbye T, et al: Prevalence of atypical antipsychotic drug use among commercially insured youths in the United States. Arch Pediatr Adolesc Med 2005;159(4):362–366.

Dabiri LM, Pasta D, Darby JK, Mosbacher D: Effectiveness of vitamin E for treatment of long-term tardive dyskinesia. Am J Psychiatry 1994;151:925–926.

D'Alessandro R, Benassi G, Cristina E, et al: The prevalence of lingual-facial-buccal dyskinesia in the elderly. Neurology 1986;36: 1350–1351.

Dalgalarrondo P, Gattaz WF: Basal ganglia abnormalities in tardive dyskinesia: Possible relationship with duration of neuroleptic treatment. Eur Arch Psychiatry Clin Neurosci 1994;244:272–277.

Dalkilic A, Grosch WN: Neuroleptic malignant syndrome following initiation of clozapine therapy. Am J Psychiatry 1997;154:881–882.

Daras M, Koppel BS, Atosradzion E: Cocaine-induced choreoathetoid movements (crack dancing). Neurology 1994;44:751–752.

Dave M: Clozapine-related tardive dyskinesia. Biol Psychiatry 1994;35:886–887.

Dave M: Two cases of risperidone-induced neuroleptic malignant syndrome. Am J Psychiatry 1995;152:1233–1234.

David WS, Sharif AA: Clozapine-induced myokymia. Muscle Nerve 1998;21:827–831.

De Keyser J, Claeys A, De Backer J-P, et al: Autoradiographic localization of D1 and D2 dopamine receptors in the human brain. Neurosci Lett 1988;91:142–147.

de la Fuente-Fernandez R: Tardive dyskinesia in dopa-responsive dystonia: A reappraisal of the dopamine hypothesis of tardive dyskinesia. Neurology 1998;50:1134–1135.

Decina P, Caracci G, Scapicchio PL: The rabbit syndrome. Mov Disord 1990;5:263.

Delfs JM, Ellison GD, Mercugliano M, Chesselet MF: Expression of glutamic acid decarboxylase mRNA in striatum and pallidum in an animal model of tardive dyskinesia. Exp Neurol 1995;133:175–188.

Deng MZ, Chen GQ, Phillips MR: Neuroleptic malignant syndrome in 12 of 9,792 Chinese inpatients exposed to neuroleptics: A prospective study. Am J Psychiatry 1990;147:1149–1155.

Desarker P, Sinha VK: Quetiapine-induced acute dystonia and akathisia. Aust N Z J Psychiatry 2006;40(6):607–608.

Desarkar P, Thakur A, Sinha VK: Aripiprazole-induced acute dystonia. Am J Psychiatry 2006;163(6):1112–1113.

DiRocco A, Brannan T, Prikhojan A, Yahr MD: Sertraline induced parkinsonim: A case report and an in-vivo study of the effect of sertraline on dopamine metabolism. J Neural Transm 1998;105: 247–251.

Dolder CR, Jeste DV: Incidence of tardive dyskinesia with typical versus atypical antipsychotics in very high risk patients. Biol Psychiatry 2003;53(12):1142–1145.

Dresel S, Tatsch K, Dahne I, et al: Iodine-123-iodobenzamide SPECT assessment of dopamine D-2 receptor occupancy in risperidone-treated schizophrenic patients. J Nucl Med 1998;39:1138–1142.

Dressler D, Oeljeschlager RO, Ruther E: Severe tardive dystonia: Treatment with continuous intrathecal baclofen administration. Mov Disord 1997;12:585–587.

Druckman R, Seelinger D, Thulin B: Chronic involuntary movements induced by phenothiazines. J Nerv Ment Dis 1962;135:69–76.

Duarte J, Campos JM, Cabezas C, et al: Neuroleptic malignant syndrome while on tiapride treatment. Clin Neuropharmacol 1996; 19:539–540.

Dumon J-P, Catteau J, Lanvin F, Dupuis BA: Randomized, double-blind, crossover, placebo-controlled comparison of propranolol and betaxolol in the treatment of neuroleptic-induced akathisia. Am J Psychiatry 1992;149:647–650.

Dunayevich E, Strakowski SM: Olanzapine-induced tardive dystonia. Am J Psychiatry 1999;156:1662.

Duncan E, Adler L, Angrist B, Rotrosen J: Nifedipine in the treatment of tardive dyskinesia. J Clin Psychopharmacol 1990;10:414–416.

Dupuis B, Catteau J, Dumon J-P, et al: Comparison of propranolol, sotalol, and betaxolol in the treatment of neuroleptic-induced akathisia. Am J Psychiatry 1987;144:802–805.

Durst R, Katz G, Zislin J, et al: Rabbit syndrome treated with olanzapine. Br J Psychiatry 2000;176:193.

Duvoisin RC: Reserpine for tardive dyskinesia. N Engl J Med 1972; 286:611.

Duvoisin RC, Yahr MD: Encephalitis and parkinsonism. Arch Neurol 1965;12:227–239.

Elkashef AM, Egan MF, Frank JA, et al: Basal ganglia iron in tardive dyskinesia: An MRI study. Biol Psychiatry 1994;35:16–21.

Elkashef AM, Ruskin PE, Bacher N, Barrett D: Vitamin E in the treatment of tardive dyskinesia. Am J Psychiatry 1990;147:505–506.

Emsley R, Turner HJ, Schronen J, et al: A single-blind, randomized trial comparing quetiapine and haloperidol in the treatment of tardive dyskinesia. J Clin Psychiatry 2004;65(5):696–701.

Eranti VS, Gangadhar BN, Janakiramaiah N: Haloperidol induced extrapyramidal reaction: Lack of protective effect by vitamin E. Psychopharmacology 1998;140:418–420.

Eyles DW, Pond SM, Vander-Scyf CJ, Halliday GM: Mitochondrial ultrastructure and density in a primate model of persistent tardive dyskinesia. Life Sci 2000;66:1345–1350.

Factor SA, Friedman JH: The emerging role of clozapine in the treatment of movement disorders. Mov Disord 1997;12:483–496.

Fahn S: Tardive dyskinesia and akathisia. New Engl J Med 1978;299: 202–203.

Fahn S: Treatment of tardive dyskinesia: Use of dopamine-depleting agents. Clin Neuropharmacol 1983;6:151–158.

Fahn S: The tardive dyskinesias. In Matthews WB, Glaser GH (eds): Recent Advances in Clinical Neurology, vol 4. Edinburgh, Churchill Livingstone, 1984a, pp 229–260.

Fahn S: The varied clinical expressions of dystonia. Neurol Clin 1984b;2:541–554.

Fahn S: A therapeutic approach to tardive dyskinesia. J Clin Psychiatry 1985;46:19–24.

Fahn S: Concept and classification of dystonia. In Fahn S, Marsden CD, Calne DB (eds): Dystonia 2: Advances in Neurology, vol 50. New York, Raven Press, 1988, pp 1–8.

Fahn S: The medical treatment of movement disorders. In Crossman A, Sambrook MA (eds): Neural Mechanism in Disorders of Movement. London, John Libbey, 1989, pp 249–267.

Fahn S: Discussion of differential diagnosis in Micheli F, Fernandez Pardal M, Giannaula R, Fahn S: What Is It? Case 3, 1991: Moaning in a man with parkinsonian signs. Mov Disord 1991;6:376–378.

Fahn S, Brin MF, Dwork AJ, et al: Case 1, 1996: Rapidly progressive parkinsonism, incontinence, impotency, and levodopa-induced moaning in a patient with multiple myeloma. Mov Disord 1996; 11:298–310.

Fahn S, Burke RE: Tardive dyskinesia and other neuroleptic-induced syndromes. In Rowland LP (ed): Merritt's Textbook of Neurology, 10th ed. Philadelphia, Lippincott Williams & Wilkins, 2000, pp 696–699.

Fahn S, Jankovic J, Lang AE: What Is It? Case 5, 1986: A man with oral-buccal-lingual dyskinesia. Mov Disord 1986;1:309–318.

Fahn S, Mayeux R: Unilateral Parkinson's disease and contralateral tardive dyskinesia: A unique case with successful therapy that may explain the pathophysiology of these two disorders. J Neural Transm 1980;16(suppl):179–185.

Faurbye A, Rasch PJ, Peterson PB, et al: Neurological symptoms in pharmacotherapy of psychoses. Acta Psychiatrica Scand 1964;40:10–27.

Fenn DS, Moussaoui D, Hoffman WF, et al: Movements in never-medicated schizophrenics: A preliminary study. Psychopharmacology 1996;123:206–210.

Fenton WS, Blyler CR, Wyatt RJ, McGlashan TH: Prevalence of spontaneous dyskinesia in schizophrenic and non-schizophrenic psychiatric patients. Br J Psychiatry 1997;171:265–268.

Fernandez HH, Krupp B, Friedman JH: The course of tardive dyskinesia and parkinsonism in psychiatric inpatients: 14-year follow-up. Neurology 2001;56:805–807.

Fibiger HC, Lloyd KG: Neurobiological biological substrates of tardive dyskinesia: The GABA hypothesis. Trends Neurosci 1984;7: 462–464.

Filice GA, McDougall BC, Ercan Fang N, et al: Neuroleptic malignant syndrome associated with olanzapine. Ann Pharmacotherapy 1998; 32:1158–1159.

Fleming P, Makar H, Hunter FR: Levodopa in drug-induced extrapyramidal disorders. Lancet 1970;ii:1186.

Ford B, Greene P, Fahn S: Oral and genital tardive pain syndromes. Neurology 1994;44:2115–2119.

Fountoulakis KN, Siamouli M, Kantartzis S, et al: Acute dystonia with low-dosage aripiprazole in Tourette's disorder. Ann Pharmacother 2006;40(4):775–777.

Franzini A, Marras C, Ferroli P, et al: Long-term high-frequency bilateral pallidal stimulation for neuroleptic-induced tardive dystonia: Report of two cases. J Neurosurg 2005;102(4):721–725.

Friedman J, Lannon M, Comella C, et al: Low-dose clozapine for the treatment of drug-induced psychosis in Parkinson's disease. N Engl J Med 1999;340:757–763.

Friedman JH: Clozapine treatment of psychosis in patients with tardive dystonia: Report of three cases. Mov Disord 1994;9:321–324.

Friedman JH, Feinberg SS, Feldman RG: A neuroleptic malignant-like syndrome due to levodopa therapy withdrawal. JAMA 1985; 254:2792–2795.

Friedman JH, Kucharski LT, Wagner RL: Tardive dystonia in a psychiatric hospital. J Neurol Neurosurg Psychiatry 1986;50:801–803.

Fukuoka T, Nakano M, Kohda A, et al: The common marmoset (Callithrix jacchus) as a model for neuroleptic-induced acute dystonia. Pharmacol Biochem Behav 1997;58:947–953.

Gagrat D, Hamilton J, Belmaker RH: Intravenous diazepam in the treatment of neuroleptic-induced acute dystonia and akathisia. Am J Psychiatry 1978;135:1232–1233.

Galili-Mosberg R, Gil-Ad I, Weizman A, et al: Haloperidol-induced neurotoxicity: Possible implications for tardive dyskinesia. J Neural Transm 2000;107:479–490.

Gambassi G, Capurso S, Tarsitani P, et al: Fatal neuroleptic malignant syndrome in a previously long-term user of clozapine following its reintroduction in combination with paroxetine. Aging Clin Exp Res 2006;18(3):266–270.

Ganzini L, Casey DE, Hoffman WF, McCall AL: The prevalence of metoclopramide-induced tardive dyskinesia and acute extrapyramidal movement disorders. Arch Intern Med 1993;153: 1469–1475.

Gardos G, Casey D (eds): Tardive Dyskinesia and Affective Disorders. Washington, DC, American Psychiatric Press, 1983.

Gardos G, Cole JO, Haskell D, et al: The natural history of tardive dyskinesia. J Clin Psychopharmacol 1988;8:31S–37S.

Gardos G, Cole JO, Salomon M, Schniebolk S: Clinical forms of severe tardive dyskinesia. Am J Psychiatry 1987;144:895–902.

Gardos G, Cole JO, Tarsy D: Withdrawal syndromes associated with antipsychotic drugs. Am J Psychiatry 1978;135:1321–1324.

Garver DL, Davis JM, Dekermejian H, et al: Dystonic reactions following neuroleptics: Time course and proposed mechanism. Psychopharmacology 1976;47:199–201.

Gatrad AR: Dystonic reactions to metoclopramide. Dev Med Child Neurol 1976;18:767–769.

Gattaz WF, Emrich A, Behrens S: Vitamin E attenuates the development of haloperidol-induced dopaminergic hypersensitivity in rats: Possible implications for tardive dyskinesia. J Neural Transm Gen Sect 1993;92:197–201.

Gerlach J: Current views on tardive dyskinesia. Pharmacopsychiatry 1991;24:47–48.

Gerlach J, Peacock L: Motor and mental side effects of clozapine. J Clin Psychiatry 1994;55(suppl B):107–109.

Gervin M, Browne S, Lane A, et al: Spontaneous abnormal involuntary movements in first-episode schizophrenia and schizophreniform disorder: Baseline rate in a group of patients from an Irish catchment area. Am J Psychiatry 1998;155:1202–1206.

Ghaemi SN, Ko JY: Quetiapine-related tardive dyskinesia. Am J Psychiatry 2001;158:1737.

Gibb WRG, Lees AJ: The clinical phenomenon of akathisia. J Neurol Neurosurg Psychiatry 1986;49:861–866.

Giladi N, Shabtai H: Melatonin-induced withdrawal emergent dyskinesia and akathisia. Mov Disord 1999;14:381–382.

Glazer WM, Morgenstern H, Schooler N, et al: Predictors of improvement in tardive dyskinesia following discontinuation of neuroleptic medication. Br J Psychiatry 1990;157:585–592.

Goff DC, Arana GW, Greenblatt DJ, et al: The effect of benztropine on haloperidol-induced dystonia, clinical efficacy and pharmacokinetics: A prospective, double-blind trial. J Clin Psychopharmacol 1991;11:106–112.

Gourzis P, Polychronopoulos P, Papapetropoulos S, et al: Quetiapine in the treatment of focal tardive dystonia induced by other atypical antipsychotics: A report of 2 cases. Clin Neuropharmacol 2005; 28(4):195–196.

Granato JE, Stern BJ, Ringel A, et al: Neuroleptic malignant syndrome: Successful treatment with dantrolene and bromocriptine. Ann Neurol 1982;14:89–90.

Granger AS, Hanger HC: Olanzapine: Extrapyramidal side effects in the elderly. Aust N Z J Med 1999;29:371–372.

Gratz SS, Simpson GM: Neuroleptic malignant syndrome: Diagnosis, epidemiology and treatment. CNS Drugs 1994;2:429–439.

Graudins A, Fern RP: Acute dystonia in a child associated with therapeutic ingestion of a dextromethorphan containing cough and cold syrup. J Toxicol Clin Toxicol 1996;34:351–352.

Gray NS: Ziprasidone-related neuroleptic malignant syndrome in a patient with Parkinson's disease: A diagnostic challenge. Hum Psychopharmacol Clin Exp 2004;19(3):205–207.

Greene P, Fahn S: Tardive complications in patients with idiopathic dystonia treated with dopamine blocking agents. Neurology 1988;38(Suppl 1):131.

Gunne LM, Growdon J, Glaaeser B: Oral dyskinesia in rats following brain lesions and neuroleptic drug administration. Psychopharmacology 1982;77:134–139.

Gunne LM, Haggstrom JE: Reduction of nigral glutamic acid decarboxylase in rats with neuroleptic-induced oral dyskinesia. Psychopharmacology 1983;81:191–194.

Gunne LM, Haggstrom JE, Sjoquist B: Association with persistent neuroleptic-induced dyskinesia of regional changes in brain GABA synthesis. Nature 1984;309:347–349.

Gute BH, Baxter LR: Neuroleptic malignant syndrome. New Engl J Med 1985;313:163–166.

Gutierrez-Esteinou R, Grebb JA: Risperidone: An analysis of the first three years in general use. Int Clin Psychopharmacol 1997;12: S3–S10.

Gwinn KA, Caviness JN: Risperidone-induced tardive dyskinesia and parkinsonism. Mov Disord 1997;12:119–121.

Haberfellner EM: Tardive dyskinesia during treatment with risperidone. Pharmacopsychiatry 1997;30:271.

Hammerman S, Lam C, Caroff SN: Neuroleptic malignant syndrome and aripiprazole. J Am Acad Child Adolesc Psychiatry 2006; 45(6):639–641.

Hardie RJ, Lees AJ: Neuroleptic-induced Parkinson's syndrome: Clinical features and results of treatment with levodopa. J Neurol Neurosurg Psychiatry 1988;51:850–854.

Hardoy MC, Carta MG, Carpiniello B, et al: Gabapentin in antipsychotic-induced tardive dyskinesia: Results of 1-year follow-up. J Affect Disord 2003;75(2):125–130.

Hardoy MC, Hardoy MJ, Carta MG, Cabras PL: Gabapentin as a promising treatment for antipsychotic-induced movement disorders in schizoaffective and bipolar patients. J Affect Disord 1999; 54:315–317.

Harrison PJ: The neuropathological effects of antipsychotic drugs. Schizophr Res 1999;40:87–99.

Hayashi T, Nishikawa T, Koga I, et al: Prevalence of and risk factors for respiratory dyskinesia. Clin Neuropharmacol 1996;19:390–398.

Hayashi T, Nishikawa T, Koga I, et al: Life-threatening dysphagia following prolonged neuroleptic therapy. Clin Neuropharmacol 1997;20:77–81.

Henderson VW, Wooten GF: Neuroleptic malignant syndrome: A pathogenetic role for dopamine receptor blockade. Neurology 1981;31:132–137.

Hermesh H, Aizenberg D, Friedberg G, et al: Electroconvulsive therapy for persistant neuroleptic-induced akathisia and parkinsonism: A case report. Biol Psychiatry 1992;31:407–411.

Herran A, Vazquez-Barquero JL: Tardive dyskinesia associated with olanzapine. Ann Intern Med 1999;131:72.

Hirsch SR, Kissling W, Bauml J, et al: A 28-week comparison of ziprasidone and haloperidol in outpatients with stable schizophrenia. J Clin Psychiatry 2002;63:516–523.

Hirschorn KA, Greenberg HS: Successful treatment of levodopa-induced myoclonus and levodopa withdrawal-induced neuroleptic malignant syndrome: A case report. Clin Neuropharmacol 1988;2:278–281.

Hoffman WF, Casey DE: Computed tomographic evaluation of patients with tardive dyskinesia. Schizophr Res 1991;5:1–12.

Hong KS, Cheong SS, Woo JM, Kim E: Risperidone induced tardive dyskinesia. Am J Psychiatry 1999;156:1290.

Horiguchi J, Shingu T, Hayashi T, et al: Antipsychotic-induced life-threatening "esophageal dyskinesia." Int Clin Psychopharmacol 1999;14:123–127.

Huang CC, Wang RIH, Hasegawa A, Alverno L: Evaluation of reserpine and alpha-methyldopa in the treatment of tardive dyskinesia. Psychopharmacol Bull 1980;16:41–43.

Ikeda H, Adachi K, Hasegawa M, et al: Effects of chronic haloperidol and clozapine on vacuous chewing and dopamine-mediated jaw movements in rats: Evaluation of a revised animal model of tardive dyskinesia. J Neural Transm 1999;106:1205–1216.

Inada T, Ohnishi K, Kamisada M, et al: A prospective study of tardive dyskinesia in Japan. Eur Arch Psychiatry Clin Neurosci 1991; 240:250–254.

Ito T, Shibata K, Watanabe A, Akabane J: Neuroleptic malignant syndrome following withdrawal of amantadine in a patient with influenza A encephalopathy. Eur J Pediatr 2001;160:401.

Itoh M, Ohtsuka N, Ogita K, et al: Malignant neuroleptic syndrome: Its present status in Japan and clinical problems. Folia Psychiatr Neurol Jpn 1977;31:565–576.

Jain KK: An assessment of iloperidone for the treatment of schizophrenia. Expert Opin Investig Drugs 2000;9:2935–2943.

Jankovic J: Stereotypies. In Marsden CD, Fahn S (eds): Movement Disorders 3. Oxford, Butterworth-Heinemann, 1994, pp 503–517.

Jankovic J, Beach J: Long-term effects of tetrabenazine in hyperkinetic movement disorders. Neurology 1997;48:358–362.

Jankovic J, Fahn S: The phenomenology of tics. Mov Disord 1986;1: 17–26.

Jauss M, Krack P, Franz M, et al: Imaging of dopamine receptors with [I-123]iodobenzamide single-photon emission-computed tomography in neuroleptic malignant syndrome. Mov Disord 1996;11:726–728.

Jauss M, Schroder J, Pantel J, et al: Severe akathisia during olanzapine treatment of acute schizophrenia. Pharmacopsychiatry 1998;31:146–148.

Jeanjean AP, Laterre EC, Maloteaux JM: Neuroleptic binding to sigma receptors: Possible involvement in neuroleptic-induced acute dystonia. Biol Psychiatry 1997;41:1010–1019.

Jellinger K: Neuropathological findings after neuroleptic long-term therapy. In Roizin L, Shiraki H, Grcevic N (eds): Neurotoxicology. New York, Raven Press, 1977, pp 25–42.

Jeste DV, Caligiuri MP, Paulsen JS, et al: Risk of tardive dyskinesia in older patients: A prospective longitudinal study of 266 outpatients. Arch Gen Psychiatry 1995;52:756–765.

Jeste DV, Lacro JP, Palmer B, et al: Incidence of tardive dyskinesia in early stages of low-dose treatment with typical neuroleptics in older patients. Am J Psychiatry 1999;156:309–311.

Jeste DV, Lohr JB, Clark K, Wyatt RJ: Pharmacological treatment of tardive dyskinesia in the 1980s. J Clin Psychopharmacol 1988;8:38S–48S.

Jeste DV, Okamoto A, Napolitano J, et al: Low incidence of persistent tardive dyskinesia in elderly patients with dementia treated with risperidone. Am J Psychiatry 2000;157:1150–1155.

Jeste DV, Potkin SG, Sinha S, et al: Tardive dyskinesia: Reversible and persistent. Arch Gen Psychiatry 1979; 36(5):585–590.

Jeste DV, Wyatt RJ: Dogma disputed: Is tardive dyskinesia due to postsynaptic dopamine receptor supersensitivity? J Clin Psychiatry 1981;42:455–457.

Jeste DV, Wyatt RJ: Therapeutic strategies against tardive dyskinesia: Two decades of experience. Arch Gen Psychiatry 1982a;39:803–816.

Jeste DV, Wyatt RJ: Understanding and Treating Tardive Dyskinesia. New York, Guilford Press, 1982b.

Jimenez-Jimenez FJ, Tallon-Barranco A, Ortipareja M, et al: Olanzapine can worsen parkinsonism. Neurology 1998;50:1183–1184.

Johnson DAW: Prevalence and treatment of drug-induced extrapyramidal syndromes. Br J Psychiatry 1978;132:27–30.

Jones HM, Travis MJ, Mulligan R, et al: In vivo 5-HT2A receptor blockade by quetiapine: An R91150 single photon emission tomography study. Psychopharmacology 2001;157:60–66.

Jonnalagada JR, Norton JW: Acute dystonia with quetiapine. Clin Neuropharmacol 2000;23:229–230.

Jordan S, Koprivica V, Chen R, et al: The antipsychotic aripiprazole is a potent, partial agonist at the human 5-HT1A receptor. Eur J Pharmacol 2002;441(3):137–140.

Kane JM, Carson WH, Saha AR, et al: Efficacy and safety of aripiprazole and haloperidol versus placebo in patients with schizophrenia and schizoaffective disorder. J Clin Psychiatry 2002;63(9):763–771.

Kane JM, Smith JM: Tardive dyskinesia: Prevalence and risk factors. Arch Gen Psychiatry 1982;39:473–481.

Kane JM, Woerner M, Borenstein M, et al: Integrating incidence and prevalence of tardive dyskinesia. Psychopharmacol Bull 1986;22:254–258.

Kane JM, Woerner M, Lieberman J: Tardive dyskinesia: Prevalence, incidence, and risk factors. J Clin Psychopharmacol 1988;8:52S–56S.

Kane JM, Woerner MW, Lieberman JA, et al: The prevalence of tardive dyskinesia. Psychopharmacol Bull 1985;21:136–139.

Kaneko K, Yuasa T, Miyatake T, Tsuji S: Stereotyped hand clasping: An unusual tardive movement disorder. Mov Disord 1993;8:230–231.

Kang UJ, Burke RE, Fahn S: Natural history and treatment of tardive dystonia. Mov Disord 1986;1:193–208.

Kanovsky P, Streitova H, Bares M, Hortova H: Treatment of facial and orolinguomandibular tardive dystonia by botulinum toxin A: Evidence of a long-lasting effect. Mov Disord 1999;14:886–888.

Kapitany T, Meszaros K, Lenzinger E, et al: Genetic polymorphisms for drug metabolism (CYP2D6) and tardive dyskinesia in schizophrenia. Schizophr Res 1998;32:101–106.

Kapur S, Zipursky RB, Remington G: Clinical and theoretical implications of 5-HT2 and D-2 receptor occupancy of clozapine, risperidone, and olanzapine in schizophrenia. Am J Psychiatry 1999;156:286–293.

Kapur S, Zipursky RB, Remington G, et al: 5-HT2 and D-2 receptor occupancy of olanzapine in schizophrenia: A PET investigation. Am J Psychiatry 1998;155:921–928.

Kastrup O, Gastpar M, Schwarz M: Acute dystonia due to clozapine. J Neurol Neurosurg Psychiatry 1994;57:119.

Kazamatsuri H, Chien C, Cole JO: Treatment of tardive dyskinesia. Arch Gen Psychiatry 1972;27:95–99.

Kebabian JW, Calne DB: Multiple receptors for dopamine. Nature 1979;277:93–96.

Kennedy NJ, Sanborn JS: Disclosure of tardive dyskinesia: Effect of written policy on risk disclosure. Psychopharmacol Bull 1992;28:93–100.

Kenney C, Hunter C, Mejia N, Jankovic J: Tetrabenazine: Is history of depression a contraindication to treatment with tetrabenazine? Clin Neuropharmacol 2006;29(5):259–264.

Kenney C, Jankovic J: Tetrabenazine in the treatment of hyperkinetic movement disorders. Expert Rev Neurotherapeutics 2006;6:7–17.

Keyser DL, Rodnitzky RL: Neuroleptic malignant syndrome in Parkinson's disease after withdrawal or alteration of dopaminergic therapy. Arch Intern Med 1991;151:794–796.

Kiriakakis V, Bhatia KP, Quinn NP, Marsden CD: The natural history of tardive dystonia: A long-term follow-up study of 107 cases. Brain 1998;121:2053–2066.

Kishida I, Kawanishi C, Furuno T, et al: Association in Japanese patients between neuroleptic malignant syndrome and functional polymorphisms of the dopamine D-2 receptor gene. Mol Psychiatry 2004;9(3):293–298.

Klawans HL: The pharmacology of tardive dyskinesia. Am J Psychiatry 1973;130:82–86.

Klawans HL, Barr A: Prevalence of spontaneous lingual-facial-buccal dyskinesia in the elderly. Neurology 1982;39:473–481.

Klawans HL, Falk DK, Nausieda PA, Weiner WJ: Gilles de la Tourette syndrome after long-term chlorpromazine therapy. Neurology 1978;28:1064–1068.

Klawans HL, Tanner CM: The reversibility of "permanent" tardive dyskinesia. Neurology 1983;33(suppl 2):163.

Kleinman I, Schachter D, Jeffries J, Goldhamer P: Informed consent and tardive dyskinesia: Long-term follow-up. J Nerv Ment Dis 1996;184:517–522.

Klintenberg R, Gunne L, Andren PE: Tardive dyskinesia model in the common marmoset. Mov Disord 2002;17(2):360–365.

Knable MB, Heinz A, Raedler T, Weinberger DR: Extrapyramidal side effects with risperidone and haloperidol at comparable D2 receptor occupancy levels. Psychiat Res Neuroimag 1997;75:91–101.

Kogoj A, Velikonja I: Olanzapine induced neuroleptic malignant syndrome: A case review. Hum Psychopharmacol 2003;18(4):301–309.

Komatsu S, Kirino E, Inoue Y, Arai H: Risperidone withdrawal-related respiratory dyskinesia: A case diagnosed by spirography and fibroscopy. Clin Neuropharmacol 2005;28(2):90–93.

Kondo T, Otani K, Tokinaga N, et al: Characteristics and risk factors of acute dystonia in schizophrenic patients treated with nemonapride, a selective dopamine antagonist. J Clin Psychopharmacol 1999;19:45–50.

Konig P, Chwatal K, Havelec L, et al: Amantadine versus biperiden: A double-blind study of treatment efficacy in neuroleptic extrapyramidal movement disorders. Neuropsychobiology 1996;33:80–84.

Konitsiotis S, Pappa S, Mantas C, Mavreas V: Levetiracetam in tardive dyskinesia: An open label study. Mov Disord 2006;21(8):1219–1221.

Konrad C, Vollmer-Haase J, Gaubitz M, et al: Fracture of the odontoid process complicating tardive dystonia. Mov Disord 2004;19(8):983–985.

Kontaxakis VP, Havaki-Kontaxaki BJ, Christodoulou NG, Paplos KG: Olanzapine-associated neuroleptic malignant syndrome. Prog Neuropsychopharmacol Biol Psychiatry 2002;26(5):897–902.

Korczyn AD, Goldberg GJ: Intravenous diazepam in drug-induced dystonic reactions. Br J Psychiatry 1972;121:75–77.

Korczyn AD, Goldberg GJ: Extrapyramidal effects of neuroleptics. J Neurol Neurosurg Psychiatry 1976;39:866–869.

Kornhuber J, Riederer P, Reynolds GP, et al: 3H-Spiperone binding sites in post-mortem brains from schizophrenic patients: Relationship to neuroleptic drug treatment, abnormal movements, and positive symptoms. J Neural Transm 1989;75:1–10.

Krack P, Schneider S, Deuschl G: Geste device in tardive dystonia with retrocollis and opisthotonic posturing. Mov Disord 1998;13:155–157.

Krack P, Teschendorf W, Dorndorf W: Clozapine treatment of psychosis can worsen preexisting tardive dystonia. Mov Disord 1994;9(suppl 1):54.

Kraus T, Schuld A, Pollmacher T: Periodic leg movements in sleep and restless legs syndrome probably caused by olanzapine. J Clin Psychopharmacol 1999;19:478–479.

Kris MG, Tyson LB, Gralla RJ, et al: N Engl J Med 1983;309:433.

Kruse W: Treatment of drug-induced extrapyramidal symptoms. Dis Nerv Syst 1960;21:79–81.

Kurlan R, Shoulson I: Differential diagnosis of facial chorea. In Jankovic J, Tolosa E (eds): Facial dyskinesias. Advances in Neurology, vol 49. New York, Raven Press, 1988, pp 225–238.

Kurz M, Hummer M, Oberbauer H, Fleischhacker WW: Extrapyramidal side effects of clozapine and haloperidol. Psychopharmacology 1995;118:52–56.

Kurzthaler I, Hummer M, Kohl C, et al: Propranolol treatment of olanzapine-induced akathisia. Am J Psychiatry 1997;154:1316.

Kushnir SL, Ratner JT: Calcium channel blockers for tardive dyskinesia in geriatric psychiatric patients. Am J Psychiatry 1989;146:1218–1219.

Kyriakos D, Bozikas VP, Garyfallos G, et al: Tardive nocturnal akathisia due to clozapine treatment. Int J Psychiatry Med 2005;35(2):207–211.

Labbate LA, Lande RG, Jones F, Oleshansky MA: Tardive dyskinesia in older out-patients: A follow-up study. Acta Psychiatr Scand 1997;96:195–198.

Lam LCW, Chiu HFK, Hung SF: Vitamin E in the treatment of tardive dyskinesia: A replication study. J Nerv Ment Dis 1994;182:113–114.

Landry P, Cournoyer J: Acute dystonia with olanzapine. J Clin Psychiatry 1998;59:384.

Lang AE: Clinical differences between metoclopramide- and antipsychotic-induced tardive dyskinesias. Can J Neurol Sci 1990;17:137–139.

Lang AE: Withdrawal akathisia: Case reports and a proposed classification of chronic akathisia. Mov Disord 1994;9:188–192.

Lang AE, Johnson K: Akathisia in idiopathic Parkinson's disease. Neurology 1987;37:477–481.

Lang DJ, Kopala LC, Vandorpe RA, et al: An MRI study of basal ganglia volumes in first-episode schizophrenia patients treated with rispcridone. Am J Psychiatry 2001;158:625–631.

Lara DR, Wolf AL, Lobato MI, et al: Clozapine-induced neuroleptic malignant syndrome: An interaction between dopaminergic and purinergic systems? J Psychopharmacol 1999;13:318–319.

Lavalaye J, Sarlet A, Booij J, et al: Dopamine transporter density in patients with tardive dyskinesia: A single photon emission computed tomography study. Psychopharmacology 2001;155:107–109.

Lecrubier Y: Is amisulpride an "atypical" atypical antipsychotic agent? Int Clin Psychopharmacol 2000;15:S21–S26.

Lee PE, Sykora K, Gill SS, et al: Antipsychotic medications and drug-induced movement disorders other than parkinsonism: A population-based cohort study in older adults. J Am Geriatr Soc 2005;53(8):1374–1379.

Lerer B, Segman RH, Fangerau H, et al: Pharmacogenetics of tardive dyskinesia: Combined analysis of 780 patients supports association with dopamine D3 receptor gene Ser9Gly polymorphism. Neuropsychopharmacology 2002;27(1):105–119.

Lerner V, Kaptsan A, Miodownik C, Kotler M: Vitamin B6 in treatment of tardive dyskinesia: A preliminary case series study. Clin Neuropharmacol 1999;22:241–243.

Lerner V, Miodownik C, Kaptsan A, et al: Vitamin B-6 in the treatment of tardive dyskinesia: A double-blind, placebo-controlled, crossover study. Am J Psychiatry 2001;158:1511–1514.

Levenson JL: Neuroleptic malignant syndrome after the initiation of olanzapine. J Clin Psychopharmacol 1999;19:477–478.

Levin GM, Lazowick AL, Powell HS: Neuroleptic malignant syndrome with risperidone. J Clin Psychopharmacol 1996;16:192–193.

Levin T, Heresco-Levy U: Risperidone-induced rabbit syndrome: An unusual movement disorder caused by an atypical antipsychotic. Eur Neuropsychopharmacol 1999;9:137–139.

LeWitt PA, Walters A, Hening W, McHale D: Persistent movement disorders induced by buspirone. Mov Disord 1993;8:331–334.

Liao DL, Yeh YC, Chen HM, et al: Association between the Ser9Gly polymorphism of the dopamine D3 receptor gene and tardive dyskinesia in Chinese schizophrenic patients. Neuropsychobiology 2001;44:95–98.

Lieberman J, Johns C, Cooper T, et al: Clozapine pharmacology and tardive dyskinesia. Psychopharmacology (Berl) 1989;99(suppl):S54–S59.

Lieberman J, Kane JM, Woerner M: Prevalence of tardive dyskinesia in elderly samples. Psychopharmacol Bull 1984;20:22–26.

Lieberman JA, Saltz BL, Johns CA, et al: The effects of clozapine on tardive dyskinesia. Br J Psychiatry 1991;158:503–510.

Linn GS, Lifshitz K, O'Keeffe RT, et al: Increased incidence of dyskinesias and other behavioral effects of re-exposure to neuroleptic treatment in social colonies of Cebus apella monkeys. Psychopharmacology 2001;153:285–294.

Lipinski JF, Zubenko GS, Cohen BM, Barriera PJ: Propranolol in the treatment of neuroleptic-induced akathisia. Am J Psychiatry 1984;141:412–415.

Little JT, Jankovic J: Tardive myoclonus. Mov Disord 1987;2:307–311.

Littrell KH, Johnson CG, Littrell S, Peabody CD: Marked reduction of tardive dyskinesia with olanzapine. Arch Gen Psychiatry 1998;55:279–280.

Lohr JB: Oxygen radicals and neuropsychiatric illness: Some speculations. Arch Gen Psychiatry 1991;48:1097–1106.

Loonen AJM, Verwey HA, Roels PR, et al: Is diltiazem effective in treating the symptoms of (tardive) dyskinesia in chronic psychiatric inpatients? A negative, double-blind, placebo-controlled trial. J Clin Psychopharmacol 1992;12:39–42.

Lopez-Alemany M, Ferrer-Tuset C, Bernacer-Alpera B. Akathisia and acute dystonia induced by sumatriptan. J Neurol 1997;244:131–132.

Lorberboym M, Treves TA, Melamed E, et al: [123I]-FP/CIT SPECT imaging for distinguishing drug-induced parkinsonism from Parkinson's disease. Mov Disord 2006;21:510–514.

Madhusoodanan S, Brenner R: Reversible choreiform dyskinesia and extrapyramidal symptoms associated with sertraline therapy. J Clin Psychopharmacol 1997;17:138–139.

Marchand WR, Dilda V: New models of frontal-subcortical skeletomotor circuit pathology in tardive dyskinesia. Neuroscientist 2006;12(3):186–198.

Marchese G, Casu MA, Bartholini F, et al: Sub-chronic treatment with classical but not atypical antipsychotics produces morphological changes in rat nigro-striatal dopaminergic neurons directly related to "early onset" vacuous chewing. Eur J Neurosci 2002;15(7):1187–1196.

Margolese HC, Chouinard G: Olanzapine-induced neuroleptic malignant syndrome with mental retardation. Am J Psychiatry 1999;156:1115–1116.

Mari JDJ, Lima MS, Costa AN, et al: The prevalence of tardive dyskinesia after a nine month naturalistic randomized trial comparing olanzapine with conventional treatment for schizophrenia and related disorders. Eur Arch Psychiatry Clin Neurosci 2004;254 (6):356–361.

Marin C, Engber TM, Bonastre M, et al: Effect of long-term haloperidol treatment on striatal neuropeptides: Relation to stereotyped behavior. Brain Res 1996;731:57–62.

Marsden CD, Jenner P: The pathophysiology of extrapyramidal side-effects of neuroleptic drugs. Psychol Med 1980;10:55–72.

Marsden CD, Tarsy D, Baldessarini RJ: Spontaneous and drug induced movement disorders in psychotic patients. In Benson DF, Blumer D (eds): Psychiatric Aspects of Neurological Disease. New York, Grune & Stratton, 1975, pp 219–266.

Masmoudi K, Decocq G, Chetaille E, et al: Extrapyramidal side effects of veralipride: Five cases. Therapie 1995;50:451–454.

Matsumoto RR, Pouw B: Correlation between neuroleptic binding to sigma(1) and sigma(2) receptors and acute dystonic reactions. Eur J Pharmacol 2000;401:155–160.

Maurer I, Moller HJ: Inhibition of complex I by neuroleptics in normal human brain cortex parallels the extrapyramidal toxicity of neuroleptics. Mol Cell Biochem 1997;174:255–259.

Mazurek MF, Rosebush PI: Circadian pattern of acute, neuroleptic-induced dystonic reactions. Am J Psychiatry 1996;153:708–710.

Mazurek MF, Savedia SM, Bobba RS, et al: Persistent loss of tyrosine hydroxylase immunoreactivity in the substantia nigra after neuroleptic withdrawal. J Neurol Neurosurg Psychiatry 1998;64:799–801.

McCormick SE, Stoessl AJ: Blockade of nigral and pallidal opioid receptors suppresses vacuous chewing movements in a rodent model of tardive dyskinesia. Neuroscience 2002;112(4):851–859.

McCreadie RG, Padmavati R, Thara R, Srinivasan TN: Spontaneous dyskinesia and parkinsonism in never-medicated, chronically ill patients with schizophrenia: 18-month follow-up. Br J Psychiatry 2002;181:135–137.

McCreadie RG, Thara R, Kamath S, et al: Abnormal movements in never-medicated Indian patients with schizophrenia. Br J Psychiatry 1996;168:221–226.

Meco G, Bonifati V, Fabrizio E, Vanacore N: Worsening of parkinsonism with fluvoxamine: Two cases. Hum Psychopharmacol Clin Exp 1994;9:439–441.

Mehvar R, Jamali F, Watson MW, Skelton D: Pharmacokinetics of tetrabenazine and its major metabolite in man and rat: Bioavailability and dose dependency studies. Drug Metab Dispos 1987;15:250–255.

Meissner W, Schmidt T, Kupsch A, et al: Reversible leucopenia related to olanzapine. Mov Disord 1999;14:872–873.

Mejia NI, Jankovic J: Metoclopramide-induced tardive dyskinesia in an infant. Mov Disord 2005;20(1):86–89.

Melamed E, Achiron A, Shapira A, Davidovicz S: Persistent and progressive parkinsonism after discontinuation of chronic neuroleptic therapy: An additional tardive syndrome. Clin Neuropharmacol 1991;14:273–278.

Meldrum BS, Anlezark GM, Marsden CD: Acute dystonia as an idiosyncratic response to neuroleptic drugs in baboons. Brain 1977; 100:313–326.

Meltzer HY: The role of serotonin in antipsychotic drug action. Neuropsychopharmacology 1999;21:S106–S115.

Mendhekar DN: Ziprasidone-induced tardive dyskinesia. Can J Psychiatry 2005;50(9):567–568.

Meredith GE, DeSouza IEJ, Hyde TM, et al: Persistent alterations in dendrites, spines, and dynorphinergic synapses in the nucleus accumbens shell of rats with neuroleptic-induced dyskinesias. J Neurosci 2000;20:7798–7806.

Merello M, Starkstein S, Petracca G, et al: Drug-induced parkinsonism in schizophrenic patients: Motor response and psychiatric changes after acute challenge with L-dopa and apomorphine. Clin Neuropharmacol 1996;19:439–443.

Meshul CK, Stallbaumer RK, Taylor B, Janowsky A: Haloperidol-induced morphological changes in striatum are associated with glutamate synapses. Brain Res 1994;648:181–195.

Meyer-Lindenberg A, Krausnick B: Tardive dyskinesia in a neuroleptic-naive patient with bipolar-I disorder: Persistent exacerbation after lithium intoxication. Mov Disord 1997;12:1108–1109.

Michael N, Sourgens H, Arolt V, Erfurth A: Severe tardive dyskinesia in affective disorders: Treatment with vitamin E and C. Neuroradiology 2003;46:28–30.

Micheli F, Fernandez Pardal M, Gatto M, et al: Flunarizine- and cinnarizine-induced extrapyramidal reactions. Neurology 1987;37: 881–884.

Micheli FE, Fernandez Pardal MMF, Giannaula R, et al: Movement disorders and depression due to flunarizine and cinnarizine. Mov Disord 1989;4:139–146.

Miller CH, Hummer M, Oberbauer H, et al: Risk factors for the development of neuroleptic induced akathisia. Eur Neuropsychopharmacol 1997;7:51–55.

Miller CH, Simioni I, Oberbauer H, et al: Tardive dyskinesia prevalence rates during a ten-year follow-up. J Nerv Ment Dis 1995; 183:404–407.

Miller DD, Sharafuddin MJA, Kathol RG: A case of clozapine-induced neuroleptic malignant syndrome. J Clin Psychiatry 1991; 52:96–101.

Miller LG, Jankovic J: Metoclopramide-induced movement disorders: Clinical findings with a review of the literature. Arch Intern Med 1989;149:2486–2492.

Miller LG, Jankovic J: Sulpiride-induced tardive dystonia. Mov Disord 1990;5:83–84.

Miller LG, Jankovic J: Persistent dystonia possibly induced by flecainide. Mov Disord 1992;7:62–63.

Mindham RHS, Gaind R, Anstee BH, Rimmer L: Comparison of amantadine, orphenadrine, and placebo in the control of phenothiazine-induced parkinsonism. Psychol Med 1972;2:406–413.

Mion CC, Andreasen NC, Arndt S, et al: MRI abnormalities in tardive dyskinesia. Psychiat Res 1991;40:157–166.

Mitchell IJ, Crossman AR, Liminga U, et al: Regional changes in 2-deoxyglucose uptake associated with neuroleptic-induced tardive dyskinesia in the Cebus monkey. Mov Disord 1992;7:32–37.

Mithani S, Atmadja S, Baimbridge KG, Fibiger HC: Neuroleptic-induced oral dyskinesia: Effects of progabide and lack of correlation with regional changes in glutamic acid decarboxylase and choline acetyltransferase activities. Psychopharmacology 1987;93: 94–100.

Modestin J, Stephan PL, Erni T, Umari T: Prevalence of extrapyramidal syndromes in psychiatric inpatients and the relationship of clozapine treatment to tardive dyskinesia. Schizophr Res 2000; 42:223–230.

Molho ES, Factor SA: Possible tardive dystonia resulting from clozapine therapy. Mov Disord 1999a;14:873–874.

Molho ES, Factor SA: Worsening of motor features of parkinsonism with olanzapine. Mov Disord 1999b;14:1014–1016.

Molho ES, Feustel PJ, Factor SA: Clinical comparison of tardive and idiopathic cervical dystonia. Mov Disord 1998;13:486–489.

Moltz DA, Coeytaux RR: Case report: Possible neuroleptic malignant syndrome associated with olanzapine. J Clin Psychopharmacol 1998;18:485–486.

Moresco RM, Cavallaro R, Messa C, et al: Cerebral D-2 and 5-HT2 receptor occupancy in schizophrenic patients treated with olanzapine or clozapine. J Psychopharmacol 2004;18(3):355–365.

Mosnik DM, Spring B, Rogers K, Baruah S: Tardive dyskinesia exacerbated after ingestion of phenylalanine by schizophrenic patients. Neuropsychopharmacology 1997;16:136–146.

Moss LE, Neppe VM, Drevets WC: Buspirone in the treatment of tardive dyskinesia. J Clin Psychopharmacol 1993;13:204–209.

Muller P, Seeman P: Brain neurotransmitter receptors after long-term haloperidol. Life Sci 1977;21:1751–1758.

Munetz MR, Cornes CL: Akathisia, pseudoakathisia and tardive dyskinesia: Clinical examples. Compr Psychiatry 1982;23:345–352.

Murty RG, Mistry SG, Chacko RC: Neuroleptic malignant syndrome with ziprasidone. J Clin Psychopharmacol 2002;22(6):624–626.

Muscettola G, Barbato G, Pampallona S, et al: Extrapyramidal syndromes in neuroleptic-treated patients: Prevalence, risk factors, and association with tardive dyskinesia. J Clin Psychopharmacol 1999;19:203–208.

Naganuma H, Fujii I: Incidence and risk factors in neuroleptic malignant syndrome. Acta Psychiatr Scand 1994;90:424–426.

Nagao T, Ohshimo T, Mitsunobu K, et al: Cerebrospinal fluid monoamine metabolites and cyclic nucleotides in chronic schizophrenic patients with tardive dyskinesia or drug-induced tremor. Biol Psychiatry 1979;14:509–523.

Naidu PS, Kulkarni SK: Reversal of neuroleptic-induced orofacial dyskinesia by 5-HT3 receptor antagonists. Eur J Pharmacol 2001; 420:113–117.

Naumann R, Felber W, Heilemann H, Reuster T: Olanzapine-induced agranulocytosis. Lancet 1999;354:566–567.

Newman M, Anjee A, Jampala C: Atypical neuroleptic malignant syndrome associated with risperidone treatment. Am J Psychiatry 1997;154:1475.

Nielson EB, Lyon M: Evidence for cell loss in corpus striatum after long-term treatment with a neuroleptic drug (flupenthixol) in rats. Psychopharmacology 1978;59:85–89.

Nisijima K, Noguti M, Ishiguro T: Intravenous injection of levodopa is more effective than dantrolene as therapy for neuroleptic malignant syndrome. Biol Psychiatry 1997;41:913–914.

Nisijima K, Shimizu M, Ishiguro T: Treatment of tardive dystonia with an antispastic agent. Acta Psychiatr Scand 1998;98:341–343.

Noyes K, Liu H, Holloway RG: What is the risk of developing parkinsonism following neuroleptic use? Neurology 2006;66:941–943.

Nutt JG, Muenter MD, Aronson A, et al: Epidemiology of focal and generalized dystonia in Rochester, Minnesota. Mov Disord 1988;3:188–194.

Ohashi K, Hamamura T, Lee Y, et al: Propranolol attenuates haloperidol-induced Fos expression in discrete regions of rat brain: Possible brain regions responsible for akathisia. Brain Res 1998;802:134–140.

Ohmori O, Suzuki T, Kojima H, et al: Tardive dyskinesia and debrisoquine 4-hydroxylase (CYP2D6) genotype in Japanese schizophrenics. Schizophr Res 1998;32:107–113.

O'Keefe R, Sharman DF, Vogt M: Effect of drugs used in psychoses on cerebral dopamine metabolism. Br J Pharmacol 1970;38:287–304.

Olivera AA: Sertraline and akathisia: Spontaneous resolution. Biol Psychiatry 1997;41:241–242.

Ondo WG, Hanna PA, Jankovic J: Tetrabenazine treatment for tardive dyskinesia: Assessment by randomized videotape protocol. Am J Psychiatry 1999;156:1279–1281.

Oosthuizen PP, Emsley RA, Maritz JS, et al: Incidence of tardive dyskinesia in first-episode psychosis patients treated with low-dose haloperidol. J Clin Psychiatry 2003;64(9):1075–1080.

Ornadel D, Barnes EA, Dick DJ: Acute dystonia due to amitriptyline. J Neurol Neurosurg Psychiatry 1992;55:414.

Ozdemir V, Basile VS, Masellis M, Kennedy JL: Pharmacogenetic assessment of antipsychotic-induced movement disorders: Contribution of the dopamine D3 receptor and cytochrome P450 1A2 genes. J Biochem Biophys Methods 2001;47:151–157.

Pantanowitz L, Berk M: Auto-amputation of the tongue associated with flupenthixol induced extrapyramidal symptoms. Int Clin Psychopharmacol 1999;14:129–131.

Papapetropoulos S, Wheeler S, Singer C: Tardive dystonia associated with ziprasidone. Am J Psychiatry 2005;162(11):2191.

Paulsen JS, Caligiuri MP, Palmer B, et al: Risk factors for orofacial and limbtruncal tardive dyskinesia in older patients: A prospective longitudinal study. Psychopharmacology 1996;123:307–314.

Paulson G: Procyclidine for dystonia caused by phenothiazine derivatives. Dis Nerv Syst 1960;21:447–448.

Peiris DTS, Kuruppuarachchi KALA, Weerasena LP, et al: Neuroleptic malignant syndrome without fever: A report of three cases. J Neurol Neurosurg Psychiatry 2000;69:277–278.

Percudani M, Barbui C, Fortino I, Petrovich L: Antipsychotic drug prescribing in the elderly is cause for concern. Int Clin Psychopharmacol 2004;19(6):347–350.

Petersen R, Finsen B, Andreassen OA, et al: No changes in dopamine D-1 receptor mRNA expressing neurons in the dorsal striatum of rats with oral movements induced by long-term haloperidol administration. Brain Res 2000;859:394–397.

Pinder RM, Brogden RF, Sawyer PR, et al: Metoclopramide: A review of its pharmacological properties and clinical use. Drugs 1976;12:81–131.

Polizos P, Engelhardt DM, Hoffman SP, Waizer J: Neurological consequences of psychotropic drug withdrawal in schizophrenic children. J Autism Child Schizophr 1973;3:247–253.

Poyurovsky M, Hermesh H, Weizman A: Severe withdrawal akathisia following neuroleptic discontinuation successfully controlled by clozapine. Int Clin Psychopharmacol 1996;11:283–286.

Poyurovsky M, Meerovich I, Weizman A: Beneficial effect of low-dose mianserin on fluvoxamine-induced akathisia in an obsessive-compulsive patient. Int Clin Psychopharmacol 1995;10:111–114.

Poyurovsky M, Shardorodsky M, Fuchs C, et al: Treatment of neuroleptic-induced akathisia with the 5-HT2 antagonist mianserin: Double-blind, placebo-controlled study. Br J Psychiatry 1999;174:238–242.

Poyurovsky M, Weizman A: Serotonin-based pharmacotherapy for acute neuroleptic-induced akathisia: A new approach to an old problem. Br J Psychiatry 2001;179:4–8.

Price TRP, Levin R: The effects of electroconvulsive therapy on tardive dyskinesia. Am J Psychiatry 1978;112:983–987.

Prueter C, Habermeyer B, Norra C, Kosinski CM: Akathisia as a side effect of antipsychotic treatment with quetiapine in a patient with Parkinson's disease. Mov Disord 2003;18(6):712–713.

Quitkin F, Rifkin A, Gochfeld L, Klein DF: Tardive dyskinesia: Are first signs reversible? Am J Psychiatry 1977;134:84–87.

Raedler TJ, Knable MB, Lafargue T, et al: In vivo determination of striatal dopamine D-2 receptor occupancy in patients treated with olanzapine. Psychiat Res 1999;90:81–90.

Rainer-Pope CR: Treatment with diazepam of children with drug-induced extrapyramidal symptoms. S Afr Med J 1979;55:328.

Raitasuo V, Vataja R, Elomaa E: Risperidone-induced neuroleptic malignant syndrome in young patient. Lancet 1994;344:1705.

Raja M, Azzoni A: Novel antipsychotics and acute dystonic reactions. Int J Neuropsychopharmacol 2001;4(4):393–397.

Raja M, Maisto G, Altavista MC, Albanese A: Tardive lingual dystonia treated with clozapine. Mov Disord 1996;11:585–586.

Rajput AH, Rozdilsky B, Hornykiewicz O, et al: Reversible drug-induced parkinsonism: Clinical pathologic study of two cases. Arch Neurol 1982;39:644–646.

Ram A, Cao QH, Keck PE, et al: Structural change in dopamine D-2 receptor gene in a patient with neuroleptic malignant syndrome. Am J Med Genet 1995;60:228–230.

Rapaport A, Sadeh M, Stein D, et al: Botulinum toxin for the treatment of oro-facial-lingual-masticatory tardive dyskinesia. Mov Disord 2000;15(2):352–355.

Reasbeck PG, Hossenbocus A: Death following dystonic reaction to oral metoclopramide. Br J Clin Pract 1979;33:31–33.

Reches A, Burke RE, Kuhn CM, et al: Tetrabenazine, an amine-depleting drug, also blocks dopamine receptors in rat brain. J Pharmacol Exp Ther 1983;225:515–521.

Richardson MA, Bevans ML, Read LL, et al: Efficacy of the branched-chain amino acids in the treatment of tardive dyskinesia in men. Am J Psychiatry 2003;160(6):1117–1124.

Richardson MA, Reilly MA, Read LL, et al: Phenylalanine kinetics are associated with tardive dyskinesia in men but not in women. Psychopharmacology 1999;143:347–357.

Riddle MA, Hardie MT, Towbin KE, et al: Tardive dyskinesia following haloperidol treatment in Tourette's syndrome. Arch Gen Psychiatry 1987;44:98–99.

Rollema H, Lu Y, Schmidt AW, et al: 5-HT(1A) receptor activation contributes to ziprasidone-induced dopamine release in the rat prefrontal cortex. Biol Psychiatry 2000;48:229–237.

Rosebush PI, Kennedy K, Dalton B, Mazurek MF: Protracted akathisia after risperidone withdrawal. Am J Psychiatry 1997;154:437–438.

Rosebush PI, Mazurek MF: Neurologic side effects in neuroleptic-naive patients treated with haloperidol or risperidone. Neurology 1999;52:782–785.

Ruhe HG, Becker HE, Jessurun P, et al: Agranulocytosis and granulo-cytopenia associated with quetiapine. Acta Psychiatr Scand 2001;104:311–313.

Rupniak NMJ, Jenner P, Marsden CD: Acute dystonia induced by neuroleptic drugs. Psychopharmacology 1986;88:403–419.

Rupniak NMJ, Tye SJ, Steventon MJ, et al: Spontaneous orofacial dyskinesias in a captive cynomolgus monkey: Implications for tardive dyskinesia. Mov Disord 1990;5:314–318.

Sa DS, Kapur S, Lang AE: Amoxapine shows an antipsychotic effect but worsens motor function in patients with Parkinson's disease and psychosis. Clin Neuropharmacol 2001;24:242–244.

Sachdev P: The classification of akathisia. Mov Disord 1995a;10:235.

Sachdev P: The epidemiology of drug-induced akathisia. 1. Acute akathisia. Schizophr Bull 1995b;21:431–449.

Sachdev P: Tardive blepharospasm. Mov Disord 1998;13:947–951.

Sachdev P, Kruk J: Clinical characteristics and predisposing factors in acute drug-induced akathisia. Arch Gen Psychiatry 1994;51:963–974.

Sachdev P, Kruk J, Kneebone M, Kissane D: Clozapine-induced neuroleptic malignant syndrome: Review and report of new cases. J Clin Psychopharmacol 1995;15:365–371.

Sachdev P, Mason C, Hadzi-Pavlovic D: Case-control study of neuroleptic malignant syndrome. Am J Psychiatry 1997;154:1156–1158.

Sachdev P, Saharov T, Cathcart S: The preventative role of antioxidants (selegiline and vitamin E) in a rat model of tardive dyskinesia. Biol Psychiatry 1999;46:1672–1681.

Sachdev PS, Saharov T: The effects of beta-adrenoceptor antagonists on a rat model of neuroleptic-induced akathisia. Psychiatry Res 1997;72:133–140.

Safferman AZ, Lieberman JA, Pollack S, Kane JM: Akathisia and clozapine treatment. J Clin Psychopharmacol 1993;13:286–287.

Sagara Y: Induction of reactive oxygen species in neurons by haloperidol. J Neurochem 1998;71:1002–1012.

Sajjad SHA: Vitamin E in the treatment of tardive dyskinesia: A preliminary study over 7 months at different doses. Int Clin Psychopharmacol 1998;13:147–155.

Samie MR, Dannenhoffer MA, Rozek S: Life-threatening tardive dyskinesia caused by metoclopramide. Mov Disord 1987;2:125–129.

Sato S, Daly R, Peters H: Reserpine therapy of phenothiazine induced dyskinesia. Dis Nerv Syst 1971;32:680–685.

Sato Y, Asoh T, Metoki N, Satoh K: Efficacy of methylprednisolone pulse therapy on neuroleptic malignant syndrome in Parkinson's disease. J Neurol Neurosurg Psychiatry 2003;74(5):574–576.

Schillevoort I, deBoer A, Herings RMC, et al: Antipsychotic-induced extrapyramidal syndromes: Risperidone compared with low- and high-potency conventional antipsychotic drugs. Eur J Clin Pharmacol 2001;57:327–331.

Schmidt AW, Lebel LA, Howard HR Jr, Zorn SH: Ziprasidone: A novel antipsychotic agent with a unique human receptor binding profile. Eur J Pharmacol 2001;425:197–201.

Schonecker VM: Ein eigentumliches Syndrom im oralen Bereich bei Megaphenapplikation. Nervenarzt 1957;28:35–43.

Schooler NR, Kane JM: Research diagnoses for tardive dyskinesia. Arch Gen Psychiatry 1982;39:486–487.

Schreiber W, Krieg JC, Eichhorn T: Reversal of tetrabenazine induced depression by selective noradrenaline (norepinephrine) reuptake inhibition. J Neurol Neurosurg Psychiatry 1999;67:550.

Seeger TF, Seymour PA, Schmidt AW, et al: Ziprasidone (CP-88,059): A new antipsychotic with combined dopamine and serotonin receptor antagonist activity. J Pharmacol Exp Ther 1995;275:101–113.

Seeman P: Atypical antipsychotics: Mechanism of action. Can J Psychiatry 2002;47:27–38.

Seeman P, Tallerico T: Antipsychotic drugs which elicit little or no parkinsonism bind more loosely than dopamine to brain D2 receptors, yet occupy high levels of these receptors. Mol Psychiatry 1998;3:123–134.

Segman R, Neeman T, Heresco-Levy U, et al: Genotypic association between the dopamine D3 receptor and tardive dyskinesia in chronic schizophrenia. Mol Psychiatry 1999;4:247–253.

Segman RH, Heresco-Levy U, Finkel B, et al: Association between the serotonin 2A receptor gene and tardive dyskinesia in chronic schizophrenia. Mol Psychiatry 2001;6:225–229.

Sempere AP, Duarte J, Palomares JM, et al: Parkinsonism and tardive dyskinesia after chronic use of clebopride. Mov Disord 1994;9:114–115.

Sethi KD, Hess DC, Harp RJ: Prevalence of dystonia in veterans on chronic antipsychotic therapy. Mov Disord 1990;5:319–321.

Shamir E, Barak Y, Shalman I, et al: Melatonin treatment for tardive dyskinesia. A double-blind, placebo-controlled, crossover study. Arch Gen Psychiatry 2001;58:1049–1052.

Shapleske J, McKay AP, McKenna PJ: Successful treatment of tardive dystonia with clozapine and clonazepam. Br J Psychiatry 1996;168:516–518.

Shen WW: Akathisia: An overlooked, distressing, but treatable condition. J Nerv Ment Dis 1981;169:599–600.

Shirakawa O, Tamminga CA: Basal ganglia GABA(A) and dopamine D-1 binding site correlates of haloperidol-induced oral dyskinesias in rat. Exp Neurol 1994;127:62–69.

Sierra-Biddle D, Herran A, Diez-Aja S, et al: Neuroleptic malignant syndrome and olanzapine. J Clin Psychopharmacol 2000;20:704–705.

Sigwald J, Bouttier D, Raymondeaud C, Piot C: Quatre cas de dyskinesie facio-bucco-linguo-masticatrice a l'evolution prolongee secondaire a un traitement par les neuroleptiques. Rev Neurol (Paris) 1959;100:751–755.

Silberbauer C: Risperidone-induced tardive dyskinesia. Pharmacopsychiatry 1998;31:68–69.

Simpson GM, Lindenmayer JP: Extrapyramidal symptoms in patients treated with risperidone. J Clin Psychopharmacol 1997;17:194–201.

Singer S, Richards C, Boland RJ: Two cases of risperidone-induced neuroleptic malignant syndrome. Am J Psychiatry 1995;152:1234.

Singh AN, Albaranzanchi AJ: Neuroleptic rechallenge after neuroleptic malignant syndrome in a 73-year-old woman with schizophrenia: Four years' follow-up. J Drug Dev Clin Pract 1995;7:63–65.

Singh AN, Hambidge DM: Successful use of risperidone after neuroleptic malignant syndrome (NMS): A 1-year follow-up. Hum Psychopharmacol Clin Exp 1998;13:65–66.

Smith JM, Baldessarini RJ: Changes in prevalence, severity, and recovery in tardive dyskinesia with age. Arch Gen Psychiatry 1980;37:1368–1373.

Smith MJ, Miller MM: Severe extrapyramidal reaction to perphenazine treated with diphenhydramine. New Eng J Med 1961;264:396–397.

Soares KVS, McGrath JJ: The treatment of tardive dyskinesia: A systematic review and meta-analysis. Schizophr Res 1999;39:1–16.

Sokoloff P, Giros B, Martres M, et al: Molecular cloning of a novel dopamine receptor (D3) as a target for neuroleptics. Nature 1990;347:146–151.

Sperner-Unterweger B, Czeipek I, Gaggl S, et al: Treatment of severe clozapine-induced neutropenia with granulocyte colony-stimulating factor (G-CSF): Remission despite continuous treatment with clozapine. Br J Psychiatry 1998;172:82–84.

Spivak B, Gonen N, Mester R, et al: Neuroleptic malignant syndrome associated with abrupt withdrawal of anticholinergic agents. Int Clin Psychopharmacol 1996;11:207–209.

Sprouse JS, Reynolds LS, Braselton JP, et al: Comparison of the novel antipsychotic ziprasidone with clozapine and olanzapine: Inhibition of dorsal raphe cell firing and the role of 5-HT1A receptor activation. Neuropsychopharmacology 1999;21:622–631.

Stacy M, Jankovic J: Tardive dyskinesia. Curr Opin Neurol Neurosurg 1991;4:343–349.

Stacy M, Jankovic J: Tardive tremor. Mov Disord 1992;7:53–57.

Stanley AK, Hunter J: Possible neuroleptic malignant syndrome with quetiapine. Br J Psychiatry 2000;176:497.

Steen VM, Lovlie R, Macewan T, McCreadie RG: Dopamine D3-receptor gene variant and susceptibility to tardive dyskinesia in schizophrenic patients. Mol Psychiatry 1997;2:139–145.

Stephen PJ, Williamson J: Drug-induced parkinsonism in the elderly. Lancet 1984;2:1082–1083.

Stephenson CME, Bigliani V, Jones HM, et al: Striatal and extra-striatal D-2/D-3 dopamine receptor occupancy by quetiapine in vivo: [I-123]-epidepride single photon emission tomography (SPET) study. Br J Psychiatry 2000;177:408–415.

Stoessl AJ, Rajakumar N: Effects of subthalamic nucleus lesions in a putative model of tardive dyskinesia in the rat. Synapse 1996;24:256–261.

Stryjer R, Strous RD, Bar F, et al: Treatment of neuroleptic-induced akathisia with the 5-HT2A antagonist trazodone. Clin Neuropharmacol 2003;26(3):137–141.

Suddath RL, Straw GM, Freed WJ, et al: A clinical trial of nifedipine in schizophrenia and tardive dyskinesia. Pharmacol Biochem Behav 1991;39:743–745.

Suzuki A, Kondo T, Otani K, et al: Association of the TaqI A polymorphism of the dopamine D-2 receptor gene with predisposition to neuroleptic malignant syndrome. Am J Psychiatry 2001;158:1714–1716.

Swett C: Drug-induced dystonia. Am J Psychiatry 1975;132:532–534.

Szymanski S, Gur RC, Gallacher F, et al: Vulnerability to tardive dyskinesia development in schizophrenia: An FDG-PET study of cerebral metabolism. Neuropsychopharmacology 1996;15:567–575.

Tamminga CA, Carlsson A: Partial dopamine agonists and dopaminergic stabilizers, in the treatment of psychosis. Curr Drug Targets CNS Neurol Disord 2002;1(2):141–147.

Tamminga CA, Smith RC, Pandey G, et al: A neuroendocrine study of supersensitivity in tardive dyskinesia. Arch Gen Psychiatry 1977;34:1199–1203.

Tan EC, Chong SA, Mahendran R, et al: Susceptibility to neuroleptic-induced tardive dyskinesia and the T102C polymorphism in the serotonin type 2A receptor. Biol Psychiatry 2001;50:144–147.

Tan EK, Jankovic J: Tardive and idiopathic oromandibular dystonia: A clinical comparison. J Neurol Neurosurg Psychiatry 2000;68:186–190.

Tarsy D, Baldessarini RJ: Epidemiology of tardive dyskinesia: Is risk declining with modern antipsychotics? Mov Disord 2006;21(5):589–598.

Tarsy D, Indorf G: Tardive tremor due to metoclopramide. Mov Disord 2002;17(3):620–621.

Tarsy D, Kaufman D, Sethi KD, et al: An open-label study of botulinum toxin A for treatment of tardive dystonia. Clin Neuropharmacol 1997;20:90–93.

Tauscher J, Hussain T, Agid O, et al: Equivalent occupancy of dopamine D-1 and D-2 receptors with clozapine: Differentiation from other atypical antipsychotics. Am J Psychiatry 2004;161(9):1620–1625.

Tenback DE, van Harten PN, Slooff CJ, et al: Effects of antipsychotic treatment on tardive dyskinesia: A 6-month evaluation of patients from the European Schizophrenia Outpatient Health Outcomes (SOHO) Study. J Clin Psychiatry 2005;66(9):1130–1133.

Terland O, Flatmark T: Drug-induced parkinsonism: Cinnarizine and flunarizine are potent uncouplers of the vacuolar H+-ATPase in catecholamine storage vesicles. Neuropharmacology 1999;38:879–882.

Thaker GK, Nguyen JA, Strauss ME, et al: Clonazepam treatment of tardive dyskinesia: A practical GABA-mimetic strategy. Am J Psychiatry 1990;147:445–451.

Thaker GK, Tamminga CA, Alps LD, et al: Brain gamma-aminobutyric acid abnormality in tardive dyskinesia. Arch Gen Psychiatry 1987;44:522–529.

Thomas P, Lalaux N, Vaiva G, Goudemand M: Dose-dependent stuttering and dystonia in a patient taking clozapine. Am J Psychiatry 1994;151:1096.

Thomas P, Maron M, Rascle C, et al: Carbamazepine in the treatment of neuroleptic malignant syndrome. Biol Psychiatry 1998;43:303–305.

Tollefson GD, Beasley CM, Tamura RN, et al: Blind, controlled, long-term study of the comparative incidence of treatment-emergent tardive dyskinesia with olanzapine or haloperidol. Am J Psychiatry 1997;154:1248–1254.

Tolosa-Vilella C, Ruiz-Ripoll A, Mari-Alfonso B, Naval-Sendra E: Olanzapine-induced agranulocytosis—a case report and review of the literature. Prog Neuropsychopharmacol Biol Psychiatry 2002;26(2):411–414.

Tominaga H, Fukuzako H, Izumi K, et al: Tardive myoclonus. Lancet 1987:322.

Trottenberg T, Paul G, Meissner W, et al: Pallidal and thalamic neurostimulation in severe tardive dystonia. J Neurol Neurosurg Psychiatry 2001;70:557–559.

Trugman JM, Leadbetter R, Zalis ME, et al: Treatment of severe axial tardive dystonia with clozapine: Case report and hypothesis. Mov Disord 1994;9:441–446.

Tsai GC, Goff DC, Chang RW, et al: Markers of glutamatergic neurotransmission and oxidative stress associated with tardive dyskinesia. Am J Psychiatry 1998;155:1207–1213.

Tsujimoto S, Maeda K, Sugiyama T, et al: Efficacy of prolonged large-dose dantrolene for severe neuroleptic malignant syndrome. Anesth Analg 1998;86:1143–1144.

Turner MR, Gainsborough N: Neuroleptic malignant-like syndrome after abrupt withdrawal of baclofen. J Psychopharmacol 2001;15:61–63.

Turrone P, Remington G, Nobrega JN: The vacuous chewing movement (VCM) model of tardive dyskinesia revisited: Is there a relationship to dopamine D-2 receptor occupancy? Neurosci Biobehav Rev 2002;26(3):361–380.

Uhrbrand L, Faurbye A: Reversible and irreversible dyskinesia after treatment with perphenazine, chlorpromazine, reserpine, and electroconvulsive therapy. Psychopharmacologia 1960;1:408–418.

van Harten PN, Hoek HW, Matroos GE, et al: The inter-relationships of tardive dyskinesia, parkinsonism, akathisia and tardive dystonia: The Curacao Extrapyramidal Syndromes Study. 2. Schizophr Res 1997;26:235–242.

van Harten PN, Hoek HW, Matroos GE, et al: Intermittent neuroleptic treatment and risk for tardive dyskinesia: Curacao extrapyramidal syndromes study. III. Am J Psychiatry 1998;155:565–567.

van Harten PN, Kamphuis DJ, Matroos GE: Use of clozapine in tardive dystonia. Prog Neuropsychopharmacol Biol Psychiatry 1996a;20:263–274.

van Harten PN, Matroos GE, Hoek HW, Kahn RS: The prevalence of tardive dystonia, tardive dyskinesia, parkinsonism and akathisia: The Curacao Extrapyramidal Syndromes Study: 1. Schizophr Res 1996b;19:195–203.

van Maidegem BT, Smit LME, Touw DJ, Gemke RJBJ: Neuroleptic malignant syndrome in a 4-year-old girl associated with alimemazine. Eur J Pediatr 2002;161(5):259–261.

van Os J, Walsh E, van Horn E, et al: Tardive dyskinesia in psychosis: Are women really more at risk? Acta Psychiatr Scand 1999;99:288–293.

Van Putten T: The many faces of akathisia. Compr Psychiatry 1975;16:43–47.

Van Putten T, Marder SR: Behavioral toxicity of antipsychotic drugs. J Clin Psychiatry 1987;48(suppl);13–19.

Van Putten T, May PRA, Marder SR: Akathisia with haloperidol and thiothixene. Arch Gen Psychiatry 1984;41:1036–1039.

Van Putten T, Wirshing WC, Marder SR: Tardive Meige syndrome responsive to clozapine. J Clin Psychopharmacol 1990;10:381–382.

Vandel P, Haffen E, Vandel S, et al: Drug extrapyramidal side effects. CYP2D6 genotypes and phenotypes. Eur J Clin Pharmacol 1999; 55:659–665.

Velamoor VR, Norman RMG, Caroff SN, et al: Progression of symptoms in neuroleptic malignant syndrome. J Nerv Ment Dis 1994; 182:168–173.

Vena J, Dufel S, Paige T: Acute olanzapine-induced akathisia and dystonia in a patient discontinued from fluoxetine. J Emerg Med 2006;30(3):311–317.

Vernaleken I, Siessmeier T, Buchholz HG, et al: High striatal occupancy of D-2-like dopamine receptors by amisulpride in the brain of patients with schizophrenia. Int J Neuropsychopharmacol 2004;7(4):421–430.

Vesely C, Kufferle B, Brucke T, Kasper S: Remission of severe tardive dyskinesia in a schizophrenic patient treated with the atypical antipsychotic substance quetiapine. Int Clin Psychopharmacol 2000;15:57–60.

Waddington JL, Cross AJ, Gamble SJ, Bourne RC: Spontaneous orofacial dyskinesia and dopaminergic function in rats after 6 months of neuroleptic treatment. Science 1983;220:530–532.

Walinder J, Skott A, Carlsson A, Roos B-E: Potentiation by metyrosine of thioridazine effects in chronic schizopherenics. Arch Gen Psychiatry 1976;33:501–505.

Walters A, Hening W, Chokroverty S, Fahn S: Opioid responsiveness in patients with neuroleptic-induced akathisia. Mov Disord 1986;1:119–127.

Wang HC, Hsieh Y: Treatment of neuroleptic malignant syndrome with subcutaneous apomorphine monotherapy. Mov Disord 2001;16:765–767.

Waugh WH, Metts JC Jr: Severe extrapyramidal motor activity induced by prochlorperazine. New Eng J Med 1960;262:353–354.

Webster P, Wijeratne C: Risperidone-induced neuroleptic malignant syndrome. Lancet 1994;344:1228–1229.

Weiner WJ, Luby ED: Persistent akathisia following neuroleptic withdrawal. Ann Neurol 1983;13:466–467.

Weinstein SK, Adler CM, Strakowski SM: Ziprasidone-induced acute dystonic reactions in patients with bipolar disorder. J Clin Psychiatry 2006;67(2):327–328.

Weiss D, Aizenberg D, Hermesh H, et al: Cyproheptadine treatment in neuroleptic-induced akathisia. Br J Psychiatry 1995;167:483–486.

Wilcox PG, Bassett A, Jones B, Fleetham JA: Respiratory dysrhythmias in patients with tardive dyskinesia. Chest 1994;105:203–207.

Wirshing WC, Phelan CK, Van Putten T, et al: Effects of clozapine on treatment-resistant akathisia and concomitant tardive dyskinesia. J Clin Psychopharmacol 1990;10:371–373.

Woerner MG, Alvir JMJ, Saltz BL, et al: Prospective study of tardive dyskinesia in the elderly: Rates and risk factors. Am J Psychiatry 1998;155:1521–1528.

Woerner MG, Kane JM, Lieberman JA, et al: The prevalence of tardive dyskinesia. J Clin Psychopharmacol 1991;11:34–42.

Wojcik JD, Falk WE, Fink JS, et al: A review of 32 cases of tardive dystonia. Am J Psychiatry 1991;148:1055–1059.

Wolf ME, Mosnaim AD: Improvement of axial dystonia with the administration of clozapine. Int J Clin Pharmacol Ther 1994; 32:282–283.

Wolf SM: Reserpine: Cause and treatment of oral-facial dyskinesia. Bull Los Angeles Neurol Soc 1973;38:80–84.

Wonodi I, Adami H, Sherr J, et al: Naltrexone treatment of tardive dyskinesia in patients with schizophrenia. J Clin Psychopharmacol 2004a;24(4):441–445.

Wonodi I, Adami HM, Cassady SL, et al: Ethnicity and the course of tardive dyskinesia in outpatients presenting to the Motor Disorders Clinic at the Maryland Psychiatric Research Center. J Clin Psychopharmacol 2004b;24(6):592–598.

Wood A: Clinical experience with olanzapine, a new atypical antipsychotic. Int Clin Psychopharmacol 1998;13:S59–S62.

Yamada K, Kanba S, Anamizu S, et al: Low superoxide dismutase activity in schizophrenic patients with tardive dyskinesia. Psychol Med 1997;27:1223–1225.

Yamada Y, Ohno Y, Nakashima Y, et al: Prediction and assessment of extrapyramidal side effects induced by risperidone based on dopamine D-2 receptor occupancy. Synapse 2002;46(1):32–37.

Yang SH, McNeely MJ: Rhabdomyolysis, pancreatitis, and hyperglycemia with ziprasidone. Am J Psychiatry 2002;159(8):1435.

Yassa R: Tardive dyskinesia and anticholinergic drugs. L'Encephale 1988;14:233–239.

Yassa R, Hoffman H, Canakis M: The effect of electroconvulsive therapy on tardive dyskinesia: A prospective study. Convuls Ther 1990;6:194–198.

Yassa R, Iskandar H, Ally J: The prevalence of tardive dyskinesia in fluphenazine-treated patients. J Clin Psychopharmacol 1988;8: 17S–20S.

Yassa R, Lai S: Respiratory irregularity and tardive dyskinesia. Acta Psychiatr Scand 1986;73:506–510.

Yassa R, Nair V, Dimitry R: Prevalence of tardive dystonia. Acta Psychiatr Scand 1986;73:629–633.

Yassa R, Nair V, Iskandar H: A comparison of severe tardive dystonia and severe tardive dyskinesia. Acta Psychiatr Scand 1989;80: 155–159.

Yoshida K, Hasebe T, Higuchi H, et al: Marked improvement of tardive dystonia in a schizophrenic patient after electroconvulsive therapy. Hum Psychopharmacol Clin Exp 1996;11:421–423.

Yumru M, Savas HA, Selek S, Savas E: Acute dystonia after initial doses of ziprasidone: A case report. Prog Neuropsychopharmacol Biol Psychiatry 2006;30(4):745–747.

Zaragoza Fernandez M, Torres Garcia E: Olazapine induced neuroleptic malignant syndrome. Actas Esp Psiquiatr 2006;34(2):144–145.

Zhang XY, Zhou DF, Cao LY, et al: The effect of vitamin E treatment on tardive dyskinesia and blood superoxide dismutase: A double-blind placebo-controlled trial. J Clin Psychopharmacol 2004; 24(1):83–86.

Zubenko GS, Barreira P, Lipinski JF: Development of tolerance to the therapeutic effect of amantadine on akathisia. J Clin Psychopharmacol 1984a;4:218–219.

Zubenko GS, Lipinski JF, Cohen BM, Barriera PJ: Comparison of metoprolol and propranolol in the treatment of akathisia. Psychiatry Res 1984b;11:143–148.

# Chapter 21

# Myoclonus
## Phenomenology, Etiology, Physiology, and Treatment

Literally, *myoclonus* means "a quick movement of muscle." Sudden, brief jerks may be caused not only by active muscle contractions (positive myoclonus) but also by sudden, brief lapses of muscle contraction in active postural muscles (negative myoclonus or asterixis) (Shibasaki, 1995).

The history of myoclonus has been described by Marsden and colleagues (1982), Hallett (1986), and Fahn (2002). Friedreich first defined myoclonus as a discrete entity in a case report published in 1881 of a patient with essential myoclonus. He wanted to separate the involuntary movement that he saw from epileptic clonus, a single jerk in patients with epilepsy, and chorea, which was the only previously described type of involuntary movement. For the next 10 to 20 years, many other types of involuntary movements, such as tic and myokymia, were also called myoclonus, but in 1903, Lundborg proposed a classification of myoclonus that cleared up much of the confusion. Lundborg classified myoclonus into three groups: symptomatic myoclonus, essential myoclonus, and familial myoclonic epilepsy.

Myoclonus is distinguished from tics because the latter can be controlled by an effort of will, at least temporarily, whereas myoclonus cannot. In addition, many tics are complex movements that are accompanied by a conscious urge to move and by relief of tension after the tic has occurred. Many of the individual movements of chorea may be myoclonic jerks, but in chorea the movements continue in a constant flow, randomly distributed over the body and randomly distributed in time. Many patients with dystonia have brief muscle spasms, sometimes repetitively (myoclonic dystonia), but these drive the body part into distinctive dystonic postures. Sometimes myoclonic jerks may be rhythmic, giving a superficial impression of tremor.

Myoclonus is a common movement disorder. Caviness and colleagues (1999) reviewed the record linkage system for Olmstead County at the Mayo Clinic in Rochester, Minnesota, from 1976 to 1990 and found an average annual incidence of myoclonus of 1.3 cases per 100,000 and a prevalence in 1990 of 8.6 cases per 100,000.

## CLASSIFICATION OF MYOCLONUS

Myoclonus can be classified on the basis of its clinical characteristics, its pathophysiology, or its cause (Box 21-1) (Marsden et al., 1982; Hallett et al., 1987; Fahn, 2002).

### Clinical Features

The whole body, or most of it, may be affected in a single jerk (generalized myoclonus); many different parts of the body may be affected, not necessarily at the same time (multifocal myoclonus); or myoclonus may be confined to one particular region of the body (focal or segmental myoclonus) (Video 21-1). Myoclonic jerks may occur repetitively and rhythmically or irregularly. They may be evident at rest, on maintaining a posture, or on movement (action myoclonus). Jerks may be triggered by external stimuli (reflex myoclonus), which can be visual, auditory, or somesthetic (touch, pinprick, muscle stretch). Myoclonus can also be a paroxysmal lapse of tonic electromyographic (EMG) activity; this is called negative myoclonus or asterixis. While by definition it is always present during action, it may be triggered by sensory stimuli just like positive myoclonus (reflex negative myoclonus) (Video 21-2).

## Pathophysiology

The clinical features of myoclonus and the results of electrophysiologic investigation allow a relatively precise prediction as to its site of origin in the nervous system. On this basis, myoclonus may be shown to arise in the cerebral cortex (cortical myoclonus); in the brainstem (brainstem myoclonus); or in the spinal cord (spinal myoclonus). Rarely, lesions of spinal roots, nerve plexi, or peripheral nerves can cause myoclonus (peripheral myoclonus). Hemifacial spasm might be considered a form of peripheral myoclonus, due most often to neurovascular compression.

Cortical myoclonus, in which the abnormal activity originates in the sensorimotor cortex and is transmitted down the spinal cord in pyramidal pathways, may manifest as focal jerks, sometimes repetitive (epilepsia partialis continua), which can propagate into focal motor seizures, with or without secondary generalization (Hallett et al., 1979; Shibasaki, 2000; Ugawa et al., 2002).

Myoclonus arising in the brainstem can take different forms (Hallett, 2002). One employs the pathways that are responsible for the startle reflex, causing exaggerated startle syndromes and the hyperekplexias. Another is independent of startle mechanisms but causes generalized muscle jerks (brainstem reticular myoclonus). A third is the palatal myoclonus (tremor) syndrome.

In the spinal cord, two forms of myoclonus are now recognized: Spinal segmental myoclonus affects a restricted body part, involving a few spinal segments; propriospinal myoclonus produces generalized axial jerks, usually beginning in the abdominal muscles. Rarely, local lesions of peripheral nerves, the plexi, or nerve roots may produce segmental myoclonus.

Finally, one pathophysiologic type of essential myoclonus takes the form of spontaneous or action-induced ballistic EMG bursts in muscles, with inappropriate overflow into other muscles (ballistic movement overflow myoclonus) (Hallett et al., 1977b).

Box 21-1  Classification schemes for myoclonus

**Clinical**
Spontaneous
Action
Reflex
—
Focal
Axial
Multifocal
Generalized
—
Irregular
Repetitive
Rhythmic
—

**Pathophysiology**
Cortical
  Focal
  Multifocal
  Generalized
  EPC
—
Thalamic
—
Brainstem
  Reticular
  Startle
  Palatal
—
Spinal
  Segmental
  Propriospinal
—
Peripheral
—
Ballistic

**Etiology**
Physiologic
—
Essential
—
Epileptic
—
Symptomatic
  Storage diseases
  Cerebellar degenerations
  Basal ganglia degenerations
  Dementias
  Viral encephalopathies
  Metabolic encephalopathies
  Toxic encephalopathies
  Hypoxia
  Focal damage

## Cause

With regard to etiology, so many neurologic conditions may produce myoclonus that such a classification runs to a textbook of neurology (Box 21-2) (Marsden et al., 1982; Hallett et al., 1987; Fahn, 2002). It is, however, useful to consider several broad categories.

Physiologic myoclonus refers to muscle jerks that occur in certain circumstances in normal subjects. These include sleep jerks (hypnic jerks) and hiccup. Essential myoclonus consists of multifocal myoclonus in which there is no other neurologic deficit or abnormality on investigation. Epileptic myoclonus refers to conditions in which the major clinical problem is one of epilepsy, but one of the manifestations of the epileptic attacks is myoclonic jerks. Symptomatic generalized myoclonus refers to those many conditions in which generalized or multifocal muscle jerking is a manifestation of an underlying identifiable neurologic disease. Psychogenic myoclonus refers to myoclonus that is produced as a conversion symptom or as "voluntary" or "simulated" myoclonus (Thompson et al., 1992; Monday and Jankovic, 1993).

In the survey by Caviness and colleagues (1999), symptomatic myoclonus was most common, followed by epileptic myoclonus and essential myoclonus. Dementing illnesses were the most common cause of symptomatic myoclonus.

## NEUROPHYSIOLOGIC ASSESSMENT

Polymyography (recording the duration, distribution, and stimulus sensitivity of EMG activity in affected muscles) is the first step in assessing a patient with myoclonus (Shibasaki, 1988, 2000; Toro and Hallett, 1997; Hallett, 1999, 2000a; Shibasaki and Hallett, 2005). Most myoclonic jerks are due to brief EMG bursts of 10- to 50-msec duration. EMG bursts in the 100-msec range are seen in some situations such as essential myoclonus. Longer jerks of more than 100 ms are likely to be dystonic. Agonists and antagonists usually fire synchronously (Fig. 21-1).

The distribution of muscles involved may suggest that it arises as a result of a lesion of a peripheral nerve, part of a plexus, a spinal root, or a restricted number of segments of the spinal cord (*segmental myoclonus*). Myoclonic muscle jerks affecting axial muscles (neck, shoulders, trunk, and hips) may arise in the brainstem as an exaggerated startle response or brainstem reticular myoclonus or in the spinal cord as propriospinal myoclonus. In *brainstem myoclonus*, there is no preceding cortical discharge. Cranial nerve muscles are usually activated from the XI nucleus up the brainstem; limb and axial muscles are activated in descending order. In propriospinal myoclonus, the first muscles that are activated are usually in the thoracic cord, with slow upward and downward spread. *Cortical myoclonus* is indicated when somatosensory-evoked potentials (SEPs) produced by peripheral nerve stimulation are pathologically enlarged, and a cortical correlate can be back-averaged in the ongoing electroencephalogram (EEG) by triggering from the EMG of the muscle jerk (Hallett et al., 1979; Obeso et al., 1985; Shibasaki, 2000; Shibasaki and Hallett, 2005). Stimuli that generate giant SEPs often provoke a subsequent EMG burst of myoclonic activity (the C reflex) at a latency that is compatible with conduction through fast corticomotoneuron pathways from the motor cortex to muscle. The giant SEPs usually consist of an enlarged $P_{25}/N_{33}$ component; the first major cortical negative peak ($N_{20}$), reflecting arrival of the

**Box 21-2** Etiologic classification of myoclonus

---

I. **Physiologic Myoclonus (Normal Subjects)**
   A. Sleep jerks (hypnic jerks)
   B. Anxiety-induced
   C. Exercise-induced
   D. Hiccough (singultus)
   E. Benign infantile myoclonus with feeding

II. **Essential Myoclonus No Known Cause Other Than Genetic and No Other Gross Neurologic Deficit)**
   A. Hereditary (autosomal dominant)
   B. Sporadic

III. **Epileptic Myoclonus (Seizures Dominate and No Encephalopathy, at Least Initially)**
   A. Fragments of epilepsy
      Isolated epileptic myoclonic jerks
      Photosensitive myoclonus
      Myoclonic absences in petit mal
      Epilepsia partialis continua
   B. Childhood myoclonic epilepsies
      Infantile spasms
      Myoclonic astatic epilepsy (Lennox-Gastaut)
      Cryptogenic myoclonus epilepsy (Aicardi)
      Juvenile myoclonus epilepsy (JME) of Janz
   C. Benign familial myoclonic epilepsy (Rabot)
   D. Progressive myoclonus epilepsy (Unverricht-Lundborg)

IV. **Symptomatic Myoclonus (Progressive or Static Encephalopathy Dominates)**
   A. Storage disease
      Lafora body disease
      Lipidoses (e.g., GM1 and GM2 gangliosidosis, Krabbe)
      Ceroid-lipofuscinosis (Batten)
      Sialidosis ("cherry-red spot")
   B. Spinocerebellar degeneration
      Unverricht-Lundborg disease
      Ataxia telangiectasia
      Adult-onset cerebellar ataxias
      ADCA Type I
      Sporadic OPCA
      Celiac disease
   C. Basal ganglia degenerations
      Wilson disease
      Dystonia
      Hallervorden-Spatz disease

Progressive supranuclear palsy
Multiple-system atrophy
Huntington disease
Corticobasal ganglionic degeneration
Dentatorubro-pallidoluysian atrophy
Parkinson disease
   D. Dementias
      Creutzfeldt-Jakob disease
      Alzheimer disease
   E. Viral encephalopathies
      Subacute sclerosing panencephalitis (SSPE)
      Encephalitis lethargica
      Arbor virus encephalitis
      Herpes simplex encephalitis
      Postinfectious encephalitis
      Opsoclonus-myoclonus syndrome
      Whipple disease
      AIDS
   F. Metabolic
      Hepatic failure
      Renal failure
      Dialysis syndrome
      Hyponatremia
      Hypoglycemia
      Infantile myoclonic encephalopathy
      Nonketotic hyperglycaemia
      Mitochondrial encephalomyopathy
      Multiple carboxylase deficiency
      Biotin deficiency
   G. Toxic encephalopathies
      Bismuth
      Heavy-metal poisons
      Methyl bromide, DDT
      Drugs, including levodopa
      Serotonin syndrome (e.g., SSRIs)
   H. Physical encephalopathies
      Posthypoxic (Lance-Adams)
      Posttraumatic
      Heat stroke
      Electric shock
      Decompression injury
   I. Focal CNS damage
      Poststroke
      Postthalamotomy
      Tumor
      Trauma
      Dentato-olivary lesions (palatal myoclonus/tremor)

---

sensory volley in the cortex, usually is of normal size. The motor volleys in cortical myoclonus activate the cranial and limb musculature in descending order via fast conducting corticospinal pathways. Abnormal corticomuscular and intermuscular coupling can also be a sensitive physiologic feature in cortical myoclonus (Grosse et al., 2003). Cortical reflex myoclonus usually consists of positive EMG discharges, but negative cortical reflex myoclonus also occurs (Shibasaki, 1995; Tassinari et al., 1998), in which a giant somatosensory cortical

potential is time-locked to EMG silence. Subcortical myoclonus is suggested when reflex myoclonus triggered by peripheral stimuli occurs after a latency that is too short to involve cortical pathways (Thompson et al., 1994; Cantello et al., 1997).

Psychogenic myoclonus is suggested if stimulus-evoked jerks are of very variable latency and longer than a voluntary reaction time (Thompson et al., 1992) and when the Bereitschaftspotential is evident prior to EMG bursts on jerk-locked back-averaging of the EEG, as in voluntary movement

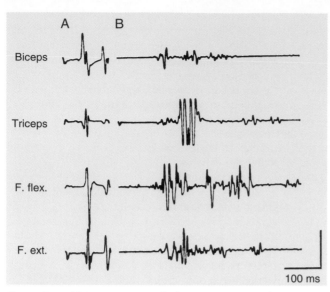

**Figure 21-1** EMG patterns underlying two types of myoclonus. **A** represents a patient with posthypoxic myoclonus; **B** represents a patient with a type of essential myoclonus (ballistic movement overflow myoclonus). The time scale is the same for both; vertical calibration is 1 mV for **A** and 0.5 mV for **B**. In **A,** the EMG burst is very short and synchronous in antagonist muscles, whereas in **B,** the EMG bursts are longer and asynchronous. (Reprinted with permission from Chadwick D, Hallett M, Harris R, et al: Clinical, biochemical, and physiologic features distinguishing myoclonus responsive to 5-hydroxytryptophan, tryptophan with a monoamine oxidase inhibitor, and clonazepam. Brain 1977;100:455–487.)

(Terada et al., 1995). Monday and Jankovic (1993) reported the clinical features of 18 such patients (13 women and 5 men with an age range of 22 to 75 years). The myoclonus was present for 1 to 110 months; and it was segmental in 10 patients, generalized in 7 patients, and focal in 1 patient. Stress precipitated or exacerbated the myoclonic movements in 15 patients; 14 patients had a definite increase in myoclonic activity during periods of anxiety. The following findings helped to establish the psychogenic nature of the myoclonus: clinical features incongruous with "organic" myoclonus, evidence of underlying psychopathology, an improvement with distraction or placebo, and the presence of incongruous sensory loss or false weakness. Over half of all patients with adequate follow-up improved after gaining insight into the psychogenic mechanisms of their movement disorder.

## MAKING THE DIAGNOSIS

It is convenient to consider myoclonus according to its clinical distribution, for this is how neurologists first assess the patient. Therefore, described here first is focal myoclonus that is restricted to one body part (e.g., a limb or brainstem-innervated muscles). Then axial (neck, trunk, and proximal limb muscles) myoclonus is described, followed by generalized multifocal myoclonus.

## FOCAL MYOCLONUS

Jerking of one body part may arise anywhere from the peripheral nerve to the motor cortex (Table 21-1). Spontaneous rhythmic

**Table 21-1** Causes of focal myoclonus

| Category | Source | Etiology |
| --- | --- | --- |
| Peripheral lesions | Peripheral nerve plexus | Trauma |
| | | Tumor |
| | Nerve roots | Electrical injury |
| | | Surgery |
| e.g., hemifacial spasm | Seventh nerve | Vascular compression or tumor |
| Spinal lesions | a) Spinal segmental myoclonus | Trauma |
| | | Inflammation |
| | | Infection |
| | | Demyelination |
| | | Tumor |
| | | A-V malformation |
| | | Ischemic myelopathy |
| | | Spondylitic myelopathy |
| | | Spinal anesthesia |
| | | Idiopathic |
| | b) Propriospinal myoclonus | Trauma |
| | | Tumor |
| | | Idiopathic |
| Brainstem lesions | Palatal myoclonus | See Table 21-2 |
| Cortical lesions | Sensorimotor cortex | See Table 21-3 |
| Idiopathic | | |

focal myoclonus is likely to be epilepsia partialis continua, or spinal segmental myoclonus. Stimulus-sensitive myoclonus, particularly affecting the distal limbs, is most likely to arise in the cerebral cortex. Polymyography, SEPs, and back-averaging from spontaneous jerks will usually suffice to define the site of origin.

A variety of lesions of the peripheral nerve and spinal cord have been described as causing focal myoclonus (Frenken et al., 1976; Jankovic and Pardo, 1986). These include peripheral nerve tumors, trauma or radiation, spinal cord trauma, tumor, vascular lesions, multiple sclerosis, and other inflammatory myelitis. Such spinal segmental myoclonus characteristically is rhythmic (0.5 to 3 Hz), is confined to muscles innervated by a few spinal segments, and persists during sleep (Fig. 21-2 and Video 21-3). Spinal segmental myoclonus appears to be due to loss of inhibitory interneurons in the posterior horns, which may be demonstrated physiologically (Di Lazzaro et al., 1996). As a result, there is spontaneous bursting of groups of anterior horn cells. Usually, it is not stimulus-sensitive, but it can be (Davis et al., 1981). Clonazepam is most likely to help. One case was responsive to topiramate (Siniscalchi et al., 2004).

Palatal myoclonus (alternately referred to as palatal tremor) describes the syndrome of rhythmic palatal movements at about 1.5 to 3 Hz, sometimes synchronously affecting the eyes, face, tongue, and larynx and even the head, trunk, intercostal muscles, and diaphragm (Deuschl et al., 1990, 1994a, 1994b). The movements usually are bilateral and symmetric, occurring between 100 and 150 times per minute, and persist during sleep in some circumstances. There are two forms: essential palatal myoclonus and symptomatic palatal myoclonus (Box 21-3; Video 21-4). The main troublesome symptom that these movements cause, seen only in the essential form, is clicking in the ear (see Video 1-63) due to rhythmic contractions of tensor veli palatini, which opens the Eustachian tube. The tensor veli palatini is innervated by the trigeminal nerve.

In many cases, a focal brainstem lesion can be identified (symptomatic palatal myoclonus/tremor), usually a stroke, encephalitis, multiple sclerosis, tumor, trauma, or degenerative disease (Table 21-2). Often the palatal myoclonus appears some months after the acute lesion. Such patients will have symptoms appropriate to the brainstem damage and to the underlying cause, in addition to the palatal myoclonus. They also may have pendular vertical nystagmus (ocular myoclonus) (see Video 1-64), as well as facial, intercostal, and diaphragmatic jerks in synchrony with the palatal myoclonus. The pathology in symptomatic palatal myoclonus damages the dentato-olivary pathway, often in the brainstem central tegmental tract (Fig. 21-3); the resulting denervation of the inferior olive leads to hypertrophy (Fig. 21-4), which can be seen on brain magnetic resonance imaging (Deuschl et al., 1994b). In this situation, the palatal movement is due to contractions of the levator veli palatini (innervated by the nucleus ambiguous). Only rarely can the ear clicking be caused by spontaneous contractions of the levator veli palatini (Jamieson et al., 1996).

In other cases, no cause is evident (essential palatal myoclonus/tremor). The complaint of these patients is of the ear clicking; the eye and other structures are not involved; and there are no other symptoms or signs. These patients tend to be younger and do not appear to go on to develop other diseases. Clonazepam, anticholinergics, or carbamazepine may help some patients with palatal myoclonus (Sakai and Murakami, 1981; Jabbari et al., 1987). Sumatriptan can be effective (Scott et al., 1996) but not in patients with symptomatic palatal myoclonus. Ear clicking can be relieved by injection of botulinum toxin into the appropriate muscles (Deuschl et al., 1991; Jamieson et al., 1996). Ear clicking occasionally may be due to simple partial seizures (Ebner and Noachtar, 1995).

Cortical myoclonus produces spontaneous muscle jerks (spontaneous cortical myoclonus), jerks triggered by external stimuli (cortical reflex myoclonus), or jerks on movement (cortical action myoclonus) (Hallett et al., 1979; Obeso et al., 1985). Such patients have neurophysiologic evidence of an abnormal discharge in the sensory motor cortex generating the myoclonic jerks via fast conducting corticomotoneuron pathways (Figs. 21-5 and 21-6). Myoclonus arising in the cerebral cortex can be focal affecting one body part, such as a hand or foot, but multiple cortical discharges can cause multifocal

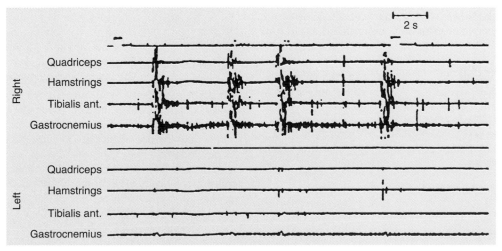

**Figure 21-2** Spinal segmental myoclonus. Myoclonic jerking of the right leg: surface recording of EMG activity in both legs. This 75-year-old man developed involuntary jerking of the right leg 8 days prior to investigation. He had an abdominal aortic aneurysm and died 3 months later. Autopsy showed ischemic loss of interneurons in the thoracolumbar cord. (Reprinted with permission from Davis SM, Murray NM, Diengdoh JV, et al: Stimulus-sensitive spinal myoclonus. J Neurol Neurosurg Psychiatry 1981;44:884–888.)

Box 21-3 Differences between essential and symptomatic palatal myoclonus

> **Essential Palatal Myoclonus**
> Ear click may be present
> Tensor veli palatini muscle (CN5): Elevates the roof of the soft palate and opens the Eustachian tube
> Stops during sleep
> Hypertrophy of the inferior olive is NOT found
>
> **Symptomatic Palatal Myoclonus**
> Levator veli palatini muscle (CN7 or CN9): Lifts and pulls back the soft palate
> May be accompanied by synchronous activity of adjacent muscles
> Continues during sleep
> Exerts remote effect on limb muscles
> Associated with ipsilateral cerebellar dysfunction
> Contralateral hypertrophy of inferior olive

jerks, each jerk being due to a discrete discharge in one part of the motor cortex. In addition, cortical discharges can cause generalized muscle jerks, either by intracortical and transcallosal spread to activate both motor cortices (Brown, Day, et al., 1991; Brown and Marsden, 1996; Brown et al., 1996) or by corticoreticular pathways activating brainstem myoclonic generators. Such multifocal and generalized cortical myoclonus is discussed later. Patients with focal cortical myoclonus also exhibit epilepsia partialis continua (Juul-Jensen and Denny-Brown, 1966), partial motor seizures, and secondary generalization with tonic-clonic grand mal seizures (Cowan et al., 1986) (Fig. 21-7). Focal slow-frequency repetitive transcranial magnetic stimulation has suppressed focal cortical myoclonus in a patient with cortical dysplasia (Rossi et al., 2004).

Epilepsia partialis continua is defined clinically as a syndrome of continuous focal jerking of a body part, usually localized to a distal limb, occurring over hours, days, or even years, due to a cerebral cortical abnormality (Cockerell et al., 1996) (Fig. 21-8). The most common etiologies now are Rasmussen encephalitis and cerebrovascular disease. Most, but not all, patients are found to have epileptic or other EEG abnormalities, and over

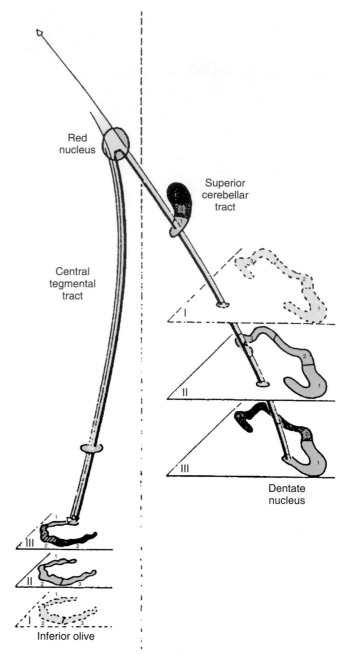

Figure 21-3 Palatal myoclonus. Dentato-olivary somatotopic relationships in humans are crossed in both horizontal and vertical planes; somatotopic relationships between the dentate nucleus and homolateral superior cerebellar peduncle are direct. The dentato-olivary pathway (*continuous dark line*) passes from the dentate nucleus through the superior cerebellar peduncle and joins the contralateral central tegmental tract on its way to the inferior olive; in the red nucleus region, this pathway passes by the internal and dorsal surfaces of this structure. (Modified with permission from Lapresle J: Palatal myoclonus. Adv Neurol 1986; 43:265–273.)

Table 21-2 Causes of palatal myoclonus in 287 patients

| Condition | Number |
|---|---|
| A) Primary (essential) palatal myoclonus | 77 |
| B) Secondary (symptomatic) palatal myoclonus | 210 |
| 1. Vascular disease | 115 |
| 2. Trauma | 23 |
| 3. Tumor (brainstem) | 19 |
| 4. Multiple sclerosis | 9 |
| 5. Degenerations | 7 |
| 6. Encephalitis | 5 |
| 7. Other (e.g., arteriovenous malformation, herpes zoster) | 32 |

Data from Deuschl G, Mischke G, Schenck E, et al: Symptomatic and essential rhythmic palatal myoclonus. Brain 1990;113:1645–1672.)

half have identifiable cortical lesions on brain magnetic resonance imaging. A similar clinical picture can occur with subcortical lesions, in which case it is suggested that the term *myoclonia continua* be employed (Cockerell et al., 1996). Cortical myoclonus sometimes is so rhythmic as to produce a

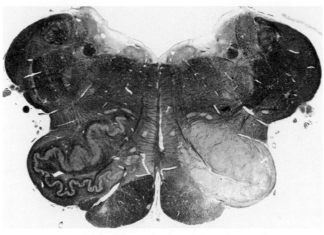

**Figure 21-4** Unilateral hypertrophy of the inferior olive in a patient with unilateral symptomatic palatal myoclonus. (Reprinted with permission from Deuschl G, Toro C, Valls-Solé J, et al: Symptomatic and essential palatal tremor: 1. Clinical, physiological, and MRI analysis. Brain 1994;117:775–788.)

tremor (Ikeda et al., 1990; Toro et al., 1993) (Video 21-5). A focal cortical lesion produces focal myoclonus in the opposite appropriate body part. Such lesions include those due to vascular disease, tumor, granulomas, and focal encephalitis (Table 21-3) (Thomas et al., 1977; Cockerell et al., 1996). Chronic, prolonged focal myoclonic jerking in children suggests the possibility of Rasmussen encephalitis.

Rasmussen encephalitis is a disorder of childhood and adolescence in which a unilateral focal seizure disorder is accompanied by a progressive hemiplegia due to focal cortical inflammation and destruction (Antel and Rasmussen, 1996). The seizures are severe, often with epilepsia partialis continua, partial motor seizures, and secondary generalization. The EEG may show focal epileptiform activity, periodic lateralized discharges, or both. In addition to the progressive hemiplegia, there often is cognitive decline. The cause is uncertain, but viral invasion (cytomegalovirus and herpes simplex type 1) has been claimed by using polymerase chain reaction techniques in brain biopsy specimens (Jay et al., 1995). An alternative hypothesis is that the chronic encephalitis is due to an autoimmune process, specifically to the glutamate receptor (GluR) 3 subunit, with such antibodies acting as a glutamate receptor agonist to cause an excitotoxic cascade (Rogers et al., 1994; Twyman et al., 1995; Gahring et al., 2001). Immunotherapy (steroids, plasmaphoresis, or human IVIG) might help some, but hemispherectomy might be necessary.

## AXIAL MYOCLONUS

Typically, axial myoclonus consists of neck and trunk flexion with abduction of the arms and flexion of the hips.

Axial myoclonic jerks may arise in the spinal cord or brainstem. Propriospinal myoclonus involves long propriospinal fibers in the spinal cord distributed to axial muscles (Brown, Thompson, and Rothwell, 1991b) (Fig. 21-9). The most prominent movement of propriospinal myoclonus is truncal flexion, and it can be either spontaneous or stimulus induced (Video 21-6). The etiology of many of these cases is not clear, although

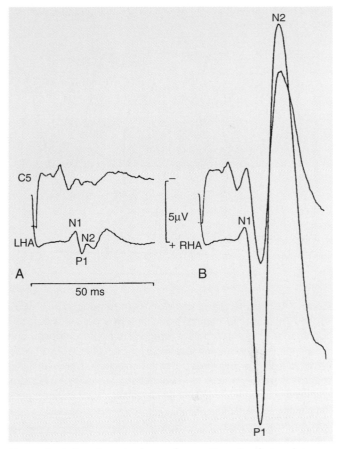

**Figure 21-5** Focal cortical myoclonus. Details of short-latency components of SEPs in cervical (*C5* [*top traces*]) and cortical hand area of the left and right hands. (*LHA, RHA* [*bottom traces*]) following electrical stimulation of the index finger of the left hand (**A**) and right hand (**B**). The patient, J.B., a 34-year-old woman, had an undiagnosed left hemisphere lesion. For some 6 years, she had experienced rare grand mal seizures but continuous flexor jerking of the right hand and forearm while awake. These jerks occurred spontaneously, on action, or in response to touch with the fingers or a tap with a tendon hammer. On examination, apart from the focal myoclonus of the right hand, there were no other neurologic signs. Brain imaging was normal, as was a carotid arteriogram and CSF examination. Routine EEG showed a focal abnormality over the region of the left sensorimotor area, with spike-sharp-wave discharges. The early cervical potentials, with a peak latency of 13 ms, and the first major cortical response (*N1*), with a latency of 20 ms, are the same size on both sides. The later components are much enlarged after right hand stimulation (**B**). Traces are the average of 999 sweeps, with the stimulation given at the beginning of the sweep. Electrodes referred to a reference at Fz. The apparent large late responses recorded at the cervical electrode in **B** are due to activity at the Fz reference. (Reprinted with permission from Rothwell JC, Obeso JA, Marsden CD: Electrophysiology of somatosensory reflex myoclonus. Adv Neurol 1986;43:385–398.)

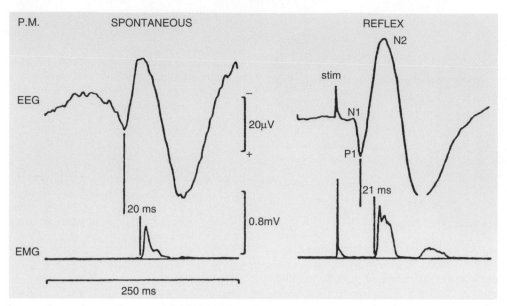

**Figure 21-6** Focal cortical myoclonus. Average (of 128) EMG and EEG events associated with spontaneous (*left traces*) and reflex-evoked (*right traces*) cortical myoclonus in a patient with focal dysplastic lesion of the right sensorimotor cortex. The EEG during spontaneous jerks was back-averaged from a trigger point on the rectified EMG record. Reflex jerks were elicited by giving electrical stimuli (*stim*) to the left forefinger, 50 ms after the start of the recording sweep. The time interval between the large P1 positive wave in the EEG and the start of the myoclonic EMG burst is indicated. EMG was taken from the left first dorsal interosseous; EEG records were taken from the contralateral sensorimotor hand area, referred to a linked mastoid reference. (Reprinted with permission from Rothwell JC, Obeso JA, Marsden CD: On the significance of giant SEPs in cortical myoclonus. J Neurol Neurosurg Psychiatry 1984;47:33–42.)

**Figure 21-7** Cortical myoclonus. The various manifestations of spike discharges in the motor cortex and their interrelationships are depicted. The physiologic correlate of the focal cortical myoclonic jerk is a cortical positive wave (an interictal spike), which represents a volley of pyramidal cell discharge in motor cortex. This can occur spontaneously, on voluntary movement, or in response to stimuli. Multiple spikes can cause multifocal myoclonus. The cortical discharge can also spread throughout the motor strip and, via the corpus callosum, to the opposite motor cortex to cause multifocal or generalized cortical myoclonus. If the spike discharge occurs repetitively, the result is epilepsia partialis continua. If it propagates locally, it may cause a simple Jacksonian motor seizure, or if it becomes secondarily generalized, a tonic-clonic grand mal seizure occurs.

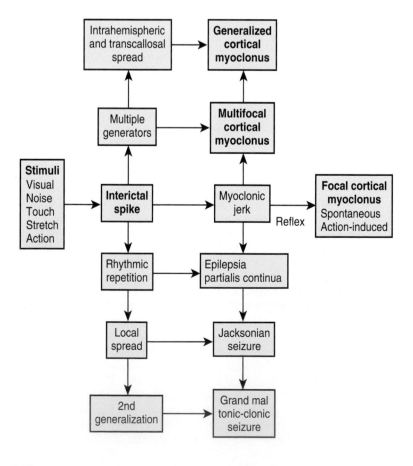

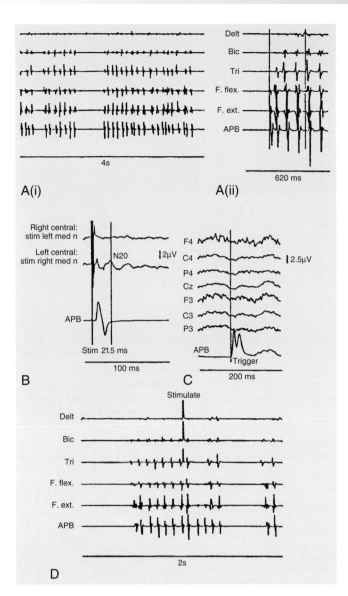

**Figure 21-8** Epilepsia partialis continua. **A (i),** Pattern of spontaneous jerking in the left arm of a case due to cerebral infarction. Hypersynchronous bursts of EMG activity occur at the same time in virtually all muscles of the arm. (APB, abductor pollicis brevis; Bic, biceps; Delt, deltoid; F. ext, extensor muscles in the forearm; F. flex, flexor muscles in the forearm; Tri, triceps.) The jerks occur in short runs with pauses of 0.5 s or so between each. **A (ii)** shows the start of a run of activity after one of these pauses. Note that the first jerk of the run occurs only in forearm and hand muscles; the second jerk involves most of the muscles of the left arm. **B,** Lack of enlarged SEP and reflex muscle jerk following stimulation of the left median nerve at the elbow. The top two traces are average (of 256 trials) EEG records from the right central (C4) and left central (C3) electrodes, referenced to linked earlobes. The bottom trace is the EMG from the abductor pollicis brevis (APB). The N20 component of the SEP is present and of normal size and latency. **C,** Lack of any back-averaged EEG correlate preceding spontaneous jerks of the left APB muscle (rectified EMG record in bottom trace); 350 trials were averaged. Linked earlobe reference. **D,** Effect of a submotor threshold magnetic stimulus over the right motor cortex on an ongoing run of spontaneous jerking. The stimulus occurs at the time of the stimulus artifact. No short-latency muscle response is evident (on this time scale, it would merge into the stimulus artifact). A spontaneous jerk of all arm muscles follows the stimulus, but then the upper arm muscles pause for the following two jerks. (Reprinted with permission from Cockerell OC, Rothwell J, Thompson PD, et al: Clinical and physiological features of epilepsia partialis continua: Cases ascertained in the UK. Brain 1996;119: 393–407.)

injury to the spinal cord from trauma, infection, tumor, and disc herniation has been described (Capelle et al., 2005). Note that the EMG pattern of propriospinal myoclonus can be mimicked voluntarily, indicating that psychogenic myoclonus should be in the differential diagnosis in these cases (Kang and Sohn, 2006).

Brainstem reticular myoclonus (Box 21-4 and Fig. 21-10) may follow cerebral anoxia and probably is responsible for the generalized muscle jerks that occur in a number of toxic myoclonic syndromes, as, for example, in uremia and other metabolic disturbances, as well as those precipitated by drugs. It is characterized by a generalized axial myoclonic jerk that starts in muscles innervated by the lower brainstem, then spreads up the brainstem and down the spinal cord (Hallett et al., 1977a). There is no time-locked cortical correlate, and sensory-evoked potentials are normal. Such brainstem reticular myoclonus may occur after cerebral anoxia and can be seen in some patients with stiff-person syndrome (Leigh et al., 1980). Brainstem lesions, such as occur in multiple sclerosis, also may be responsible (Smith and Scheinberg, 1990).

Exaggerated startle syndromes (hyperekplexia) consist of an excessive motor response, or jump, to unexpected auditory and, sometimes, somesthetic and visual stimuli (Box 21-5; see also Box 21-4) (Suhren et al., 1966; Andermann and Andermann, 1988; Brown, Rothwell, et al., 1991; Matsumoto et al., 1992; Matsumoto and Hallett, 1994; Bakker et al. 2006). The jump consists of a blink, contortion of the face, flexion of the neck and trunk, and abduction and flexion of the arm (Fig. 21-11). Such patients jump in response to sound and crash to the ground, injuring themselves. There is no loss of consciousness. An exaggerated startle syndrome may be due to local brainstem pathology (anoxia, inflammatory lesions including sarcoidosis and multiple sclerosis, and hemorrhage) and also occurs as an inherited condition (hereditary hyperekplexia), transmitted as an autosomal-dominant trait (Video-21-7). The first abnormal gene identified for this disorder is a point mutation in the alpha-1 subunit of the glycine-receptor (Shiang et al., 1993, 1995; Tijssen et al., 1995). This may lead to altered ligand binding or disturbance of the chloride ion channel part of the receptor. Subsequently other mutations were found in the glycine receptor and glycine receptor complex. Additionally, responsible mutations are also found presynaptically in the glycine transporter 2 (Rees et al., 2006). Glycine is an inhibitory neurotransmitter in several spinal interneurons, including Renshaw cells, Ia

Table 21-3 Causes of focal cortical myoclonus and epilepsia partialis continua

| | Number | |
| Etiology | Thomas et al.[*] | Cockerell et al.[†] |
|---|---|---|
| Infarct or cerebral hemorrhage | 8 | 9 |
| Tumor | 5 | 4 |
|   Astrocytoma | | |
|   Hemangioma | | |
|   Lymphoma | | |
|   Uncertain | | |
| Encephalitis (including Rasmussen's encephalitis) | 5 | 7 |
| Trauma | 2 | 1 |
| Hepatic encephalopathy | 2 | — |
| Subarachnoid hemorrhage | 1 | — |
| Unknown | 9 | 9 |
| **Total** | **32** | **30** |
| **Others** | | |
|   Subdural hematoma | | |
|   Absess | | |
|   Granuloma (T.B.) | | |
|   Multiple sclerosis | | |
|   Meningitis | | |
|   Nonketotic hyperglycemia | | |
|   Focal gliosis | | |
|   Spinocerebellar degeneration | | |
|   Mitochondrial disease | | |

*Thomas JE, Reagan TJ, Klass DW: Epilepsia partialis continua: A review of 32 cases. Arch Neurol 1977;34:266–275.
†Cockerell OC, Rothwell J, Thompson PD, et al: Clinical and physiological features of epilepsia partialis continua: Cases ascertained in the UK. Brain 1996;119:393–407.

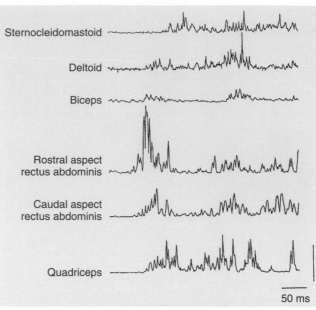

Figure 21-9 Propriospinal myoclonus. EMG record of a single spontaneous jerk in a patient with propriospinal myoclonus. Muscles are sternocleidomastoid, deltoid, biceps, rostral aspect of rectus abdominis, caudal aspect of rectus abdominis, and quadriceps. EMG activity occurred first in rectus abdominis. Contraction of the sternocleidomastoid, rectus abdominis, and quadriceps occurred in all jerks, but activity in the deltoid and biceps (evident here) was variable. Vertical calibration line = 200 μV and 100 μV for the bottom and top three channels, respectively. (Reprinted with permission from Brown P, Thompson PD, Rothwell JC, et al: Axial myoclonus of propriospinal origin. Brain 1991;114: 197–214.)

inhibitory interneurons, and some Ib inhibitory interneurons. Physiologic studies suggest normal recurrent inhibition, but abnormal Ia reciprocal inhibition in hyperekplexia (Floeter et al., 1996). Affected babies are hypertonic and stiff when handled and have difficulty subsequently with walking. They develop excessive startles, which take two forms. The minor form is a simple brief startle jerk; the major form is a more prolonged tonic startle spasm. In these situations, the normal startle reflex is exaggerated, both in amplitude and in its failure to rapidly habituate (Brown, Rothwell, et al., 1991; Matsumoto et al., 1992; Matsumoto and Hallett, 1994). The afferent and efferent systems of the startle reflex in hyperekplexia are identical to those of the normal startle response, involving a similar or the same generator in the lower brainstem, probably in the medial bulbopontine reticular formation. However, there might be differences between the minor form and the major form of hyperekplexia. First, only the major form appears to be linked to 5q33–q35 (Tijssen et al., 1995, 2002). Second, the physiologic abnormalities in the minor and major forms appear to differ (Tijssen et al., 1996, 1997). Treatment with clonazepam may be very effective in some patients (Matsumoto and Hallett, 1994). Others have responded to sodium valproate or piracetam.

An exaggerated startle response might be responsible for the initial motor manifestation of jumping Frenchmen and

other culturally determined startle syndromes (Andermann and Andermann, 1988; Brown, Rothwell, et al., 1991; Matsumoto and Hallett, 1994). In these syndromes the startle is followed by stereotyped behaviors such as a vocalization or striking out (Video 21-8). Hyperekplexia must be distinguished from startle-evoked epileptic seizures (Matsumoto and Hallett, 1994; Manford et al., 1996).

Box 21-4 Two types of brainstem reticular myoclonus

In both types, the myoclonus originates in the caudal brainstem, and muscles are activated up the brainstem and down the spinal cord. The myoclonus is generalized and mainly axial to cause neck flexion, shoulder elevation, and trunk and knee extension.

1. **Exaggerated Startle Response**
   Bulbospinal pathways are slow conducting
   Evoked by sudden noise or light or by sensory stimuli to the mantle area
   Spontaneous jerks not prominent

2. **Reticular Reflex Myoclonus**
   Bulbospinal pathways are fast conducting
   Stimulus sensitivity is greatest over the limbs
   Spontaneous jerks are common

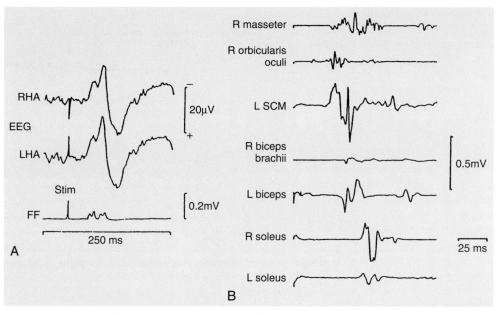

**Figure 21-10** Brainstem reticular myoclonus. **A,** Average of 128 EEG and EMG responses to electrical stimulation (stim) of the index finger of the right hand in a patient with reticular reflex myoclonus. The EEG was recorded monopolarly from over the sensorimotor hand area (LHA, left-hand area; RHA, right-hand area) referred to a linked mastoid reference. Rectified EMG from surface electrodes was placed over the flexor carpi radialis (FF). No enlargement of the EEG response is evident preceding the myoclonic muscle jerk. The bilateral late response is probably produced by movement artifact from the generalized muscle jerk. **B,** The order of muscle activation on a single generalized myoclonic jerk in the same patient, produced by a light tap with a tendon hammer to the forehead at the start of the sweep. The jerk begins in the sternocleidomastoid (SCM) and travels up the cranial nerves and down the spinal cord. This 41-year-old man developed increasing generalized muscle stiffness and jerks over a period of about 1 year. Eventually, he became bedridden with severe rigidity but remained alert and, according to his relatives, suitably responsive. On examination, although alert, he was severely dysarthric, and he could not move voluntarily. His limbs were held in flexion and exhibited extreme rigidity. Tendon reflexes were brisk, and the plantar responses were flexor. Any stimulus, including visual menace, load noise, light touch, or a tap with a tendon hammer, evoked massive generalized muscle jerking. All investigations failed to reveal a pathologic diagnosis, although clinically it was suspected that he had a diffuse encephalomyelitis. (Reprinted with permission from Rothwell JC, Obeso JA, Marsden CD: Electrophysiology of somatosensory reflex myoclonus. Adv Neurol 1986;43:385–398.)

## MULTIFOCAL AND GENERALIZED CORTICAL MYOCLONUS

Multifocal myoclonus of cortical origin typically affects many parts of the body bilaterally but not synchronously. Each myoclonic jerk involves only a few adjacent muscles. The movements of the fingers or toes may be small twitches (minipolymyoclonus) (Wilkins et al., 1985); those of more proximal and axial muscles cause bigger movements. Multifocal cortical myoclonus is due to a generalized excitability of the cerebral cortex, particularly of the sensorimotor cortex. The EEG may show multifocal spike discharges, and back-averaging reveals the typical cortical correlate to each focal myoclonic jerk. SEPs often are enlarged. The jerks are frequently stimulus sensitive.

Many patients with multifocal cortical myoclonus also exhibit generalized myoclonic jerks, synchronous in many muscles at the same time. Some of these originate in the brainstem (brainstem reticular myoclonus), perhaps driven by a cortical origin. However, discharge in the sensorimotor cortex may produce a generalized jerk as a result of transcallosal and intracortical spread (Brown, Day, et al., 1991).

Many conditions cause multifocal and generalized cortical myoclonus. These include epileptic myoclonus, in which epilepsy dominates and there is no progressive disease of the brain; progressive myoclonus epilepsy and progressive myoclonic ataxia; postanoxic myoclonus; viral encephalopathies; metabolic disease; and toxic encephalopathies (see Box 21-2).

Epileptic myoclonus refers to those epilepsies characterized exclusively or predominantly by brief myoclonic, atonic, or tonic seizures. Epileptic myoclonus can be positive (with active muscle contractions) or negative (lapses of postural tone) (Guerrini et al., 1993; Tassinari et al., 1995, 1998). Conditions that are subsumed under this category include infantile spasms, Lennox-Gastaut syndrome, cryptogenic myoclonic epilepsy, the myoclonus associated with petit mal, and juvenile myoclonic epilepsy (JME) of adolescence (Janz). The key features of these various conditions are summarized in Box 21-6 (Aicardi, 1986).

Of these conditions, JME is the most frequent epileptic syndrome presenting with myoclonus, usually in adolescence. The main symptom is myoclonic jerks, usually without loss of consciousness, predominantly in the morning after awakening from sleep. Generalized tonic clonic seizures also tend to occur in the morning. Linkage studies are identifying genetic loci for some patients with JME and other myoclonic epilepsies (Delgado-Escueta et al., 1999; Serratosa et al., 1999a).

**Box 21-5** Causes of the startle syndrome

**A. Pathologic Exaggeration of the Normal Startle Reflex**
1. Hereditary hyperekplexia
2. Idiopathic hyperekplexia
3. Symptomatic startle syndromes
   Static encephalopathies
   a. Static perinatal encephalopathy with tonic spasms
   b. Postanoxic encephalopathy
   c. Posttraumatic encephalopathy
   Brainstem encephalitis
   a. Sarcoidosis
   b. Viral encephalomyelitis
   c. Encephalomyelitis with rigidity
   d. Multiple sclerosis

   e. Paraneoplastic
   Structural
   a. Brainstem hemorrhage/infarct
   b. Cerebral abscess
**B. Brainstem Reticular Reflex Myoclonus**
   Postanoxic Encephalopathy
**C. Unknown Physiology**
1. Hexosaminidase A deficiency
2. Static perinatal encephalopathy with epileptic tonic spasms (startle epilepsy)
3. Gilles de la Tourette syndrome
4. Jumping, Latah, and Myriachit
5. Hysterical jumps

Data from Brown P, Rothwell JC, Thompson PD, et al: The hyperekplexias and their relationship to the normal startle reflex. Brain 1991;114:1903–1928.

In one family with JME, the abnormal gene has been identified in the alpha-1 subunit of the gamma-aminobutyric acid (GABA) receptor (Cossette et al., 2002).

Progressive myoclonus epilepsy refers to a combination of severe myoclonus (spontaneous, action, and stimulus-sensitive), severe generalized tonic-clonic and other seizures, and progressive neurologic decline, particularly dementia and ataxia (Marseille Consensus Group, 1990; Berkovic and Andermann, 1986; Berkovic et al., 1986). Progressive myoclonic ataxia (sometimes known as Ramsay-Hunt syndrome) (Marsden et al., 1990) is distinguished from progressive

myoclonus epilepsy by seizures being mild or absent and dementia being mild or nonexistent, but myoclonus and ataxia are the major problems (Fig. 21-12).

The differential diagnosis of progressive myoclonus epilepsy (Table 21-4) and progressive myoclonic ataxia (Box 21-7) is dominated by five main conditions.

Lafora body disease and neuronal ceroid lipofuscinosis generally produce severe neurologic decline with dementia or regression, along with myoclonus and fits (Rapin, 1986). Lafora body disease (EPM2), inherited as an autosomal-recessive trait, is characterized by polyglucosan acid–Schiff–positive

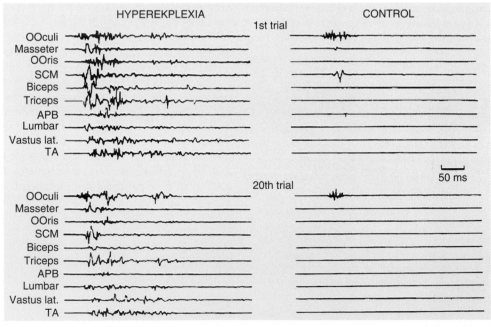

**Figure 21-11** EMG in hereditary hyperekplexia. Multichannel surface EMG recordings of startle responses in a 13-year-old girl with hereditary hyperekplexia compared with a normal subject. *Top left:* An initial 103-dB acoustic stimulus given at the onset of the trace is followed by a generalized EMG startle response. Note the early activation of the orbicularis oculi followed by the sterno-cleidomastoid (SCM). *Bottom left:* The 20th startle response after repetitive acoustic stimuli given at 1-minute intervals shows little habituation. The control subject's recordings on the right show a much more subdued response that reveals marked habituation at the 20th trial. (Reprinted with permission from Matsumoto J, Hallett M: Startle syndromes. In Marsden CD and Fahn S [eds]: Movement Disorders 3. Oxford, UK, Butterworth-Heinemann, 1994, pp 418–433.)

**Box 21-6** Characteristics of major primary epileptic myoclonus syndromes

**Cryptogenic Myoclonic Epilepsy**
1. Massive myoclonic jerks as the only or major seizure type
2. Bursts of bilateral irregular slow spike/wave at 2.5 Hz or more
3. Onset 6 months to 5 years
4. No signs of brain damage prior to seizures
5. Tonic-clonic seizures but no tonic seizures
6. Relatively good prognosis

**Juvenile Myoclonic Epilepsy (Janz)**
1. Myoclonus, mainly in the arms, especially in the morning
2. Spikes, polyspikes, and slow waves in EEG
3. Onset around puberty
4. No signs of brain damage
5. Tonic-clonic seizures, especially at night; absences in 10%
6. Very good response to sodium valproate

**Eyelid Myoclonus with Absences**
1. Photosensitive attacks
2. Marked eyelid jerking, with upward eye deviation, during absences

3. Irregular 3-Hz spike/wave in EEG

**Absences in Petit Mal**
1. Eyelid myoclonus and, more rarely, massive myoclonic jerks, with absences
2. 3-Hz spike/wave in EEG

**Infantile Spasms**
1. Flexor (extensor) spasms
2. Hypsarrhythmic EEG
3. Onset in first year of life
4. Many causes recognized
5. Mental retardation

**Lennox-Gastaut Syndrome**
1. Massive myoclonic jerks, tonic spasms, and atonic attacks
2. Atypical slow (less than 2.5 Hz) spike/wave in EEG
3. Onset after infantile spasms and other brain insults around 2 to 8 years of age
4. Tonic-clonic and other seizures
5. Poor prognosis

---

inclusions in cells of the brain, liver, muscle, and skin (eccrine sweat glands). Onset is usually in childhood, with behavioral and cognitive change, dementia, and seizures, as well as myoclonus; late-onset forms with a more benign onset also occur (Footitt et al., 1997). The gene that is responsible in about 75% of cases has been localized to chromosome 6q and

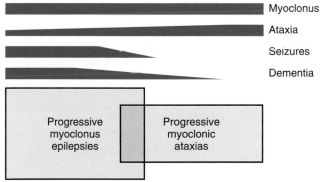

Figure 21-12 Schematic representation of the clinical features and relationship of the syndromes of progressive myoclonic epilepsy (PME) and of progressive myoclonic ataxia (PMA). The bars (*upper part*) give a general indication of the prominence of the key clinical signs in the PME and PMA syndromes. Initial recognition of either syndrome then demands an attempt to reach a specific diagnosis. A specific diagnosis can now usually be made in patients with PME, whereas a larger proportion of cases with PMA remain undiagnosed. Previous authors have used the term *Ramsay Hunt syndrome* to describe different groups of patients within this spectrum. (Reprinted with permission from Marsden CD, Harding AE, Obeso JA, Lu CS: Progressive myoclonic ataxia (the Ramsay Hunt syndrome). Arch Neurol 1990;47:1121–1125.)

has now been identified (Minassian et al., 1999) as encoding a protein tyrosine phosphatase (Minassian et al., 1998; Serratosa et al., 1999b). The protein, called laforin (or EPM2A), localizes at the plasma membrane and the endoplasmic reticulum (Minassian et al., 2001). Laforin presumably metabolizes polyglucosans, preventing their aggregation (Chan et al., 2004a). A second gene is associated with Lafora body disease, NHLRC1 (also called EPM2B), which encodes malin, a putative E3 ubiquitin ligase with a RING finger domain and six NHL motifs (Chan et al., 2003; Ganesh et al., 2006). Laforin is a substrate for malin (Gentry et al., 2005). Both laforin and malin colocalize to the ER, suggesting that they operate in a related pathway, protecting against polyglucosan accumulation. A third locus is predicted on a basis of a family without linkage to the two known sites (Chan et al., 2004b). There is a mouse model of the disorder (Ganesh et al., 2002). Zonisamide has been described as being very useful for the myoclonus and epilepsy in these patients (Yoshimura et al., 2001).

Neuronal ceroid lipfuscinosis (Batten disease), inherited as an autosomal-recessive condition, also presents with seizures and myoclonus with cognitive impairment and dementia, along with blindness in the late infantile and juvenile forms. The adult form is often dominated by psychiatric and cognitive impairment. Lipopigment accumulates in lysosomes in the brain, eccrine glands, skin, muscle, and gut with characteristic inclusions (curvilinear bodies and fingerprint profiles). Both Lafora body disease and neuronal ceroid lipofuscinosis usually can be diagnosed in axillary skin biopsies with electromicroscopy.

Unverricht-Lundborg disease (EPM1) is characterized by stimulus-sensitive myoclonus, tonic-clonic seizures, a characteristic EEG (paroxysmal generalized spike-wave activity, and photosensitivity), and a progressive course with ataxia but only mild intellectual decline (Eldridge et al., 1983;

Table 21-4 Major causes of progressive myoclonus epilepsy

| Condition | Age at Onset (years) | Diagnostic Features | | |
|-----------|---------------------|--------------------|--|--|
| | | Clinical | Laboratory | Diagnostic Test |
| Unverricht-Lundborg disease | 6–15 | Severe myoclonus Dementia absent or mild | EEG | Clinical |
| Lafora body disease | 11–18 | Occipital seizures | EEG | Lafora bodies (skin, liver, brain) |
| | | Dementia | | |
| Neuronal ceroid Lipofuscinosis (Batten) Late-infantile (Jansky-Bielschowsky) | 2.5–4 (dead by 6–10) | Severe seizures | EEG | EM of skin, muscle |
| | | Rapid regression Macular degeneration | ERG VER | Rectum or brain |
| Juvenile (Spielmeyer-Vogt) | 4–10 (dead by 15–25) | Visual failure Macular degeneration | Dolichols | |
| Adults (Kufs) | 12–50 (long course) | Behavioral change Dementia | | |
| Sialidosis Type I | 8–20 | Cherry-red spot | Storage in lymphocytes, etc. | alpha-N-acetyl- neuraminidase |
| Type II | 10–30 | Cherry-red spot | Urinary sialyl-oligo- saccharides | |
| | | Dysmorphic | | |
| Mitochondrial enceph- alomyopathy (MERRF) | 5–42 | Short stature | Blood and CSF Lactate | "Ragged-red" fibers on muscle biopsy |
| | | Deafness | | |
| | | | | DNA tests |

EEG, electroencephalogram; ERG, electroretinogram; MERRF, myoclonus epilepsy and ragged-red fibers; VEP, visual evoked responses.

Adapted from Berkovic SF, Andermann F: The progressive myoclonic epilepsies. In Pedley TA, Meldrum BS (eds): Recent Advances in Epilepsy 3. Edinburgh, Churchill Livingstone, 1986, pp 157–187.

Box 21-7 Causes of progressive myoclonic ataxia

**Major Causes**
Unverricht-Lundborg disease
Mitochondrial encephalomyopathy
Sialidosis
Lafora body disease*
Neuronal ceroid lipofuscinosis*
Spinocerebellar degenerations

**Rarer Causes**
Gaucher disease (noninfantile neuronopathic form)
GM$_2$ gangliosidosis*
Biotin-responsive encephalopathy
Neuroaxonal dystrophy (juvenile form)*
Hallervorden-Spatz disease*
Atypical inclusion-body disease
Action myoclonus-renal failure syndrome
Dentatorubro-pallidoluysian atrophy
PME and deafness (May-White syndrome)
PME and lipomas
Celiac disease
Whipple disease

*Dementia often prominent, so not typical of progressive myoclonic ataxia.

Koskiniemi, 1986; Lehesjoki and Koskiniemi, 1998, 1999). It is inherited as an autosomal-recessive trait, with onset around the age of 6 to 15 years and occurs worldwide. Autopsy shows widespread degeneration, with prominent loss of cerebellar Purkinje cells without storage material. The gene for Unverricht-Lundborg disease has now been linked to the long arm of chromosome 21q22.3 in a number of Finnish and Mediterranean families, and the gene involved codes for cystatin B, a small protein that is a member of a superfamily of cysteine protease inhibitors (Lehesjoki and Koskiniemi, 1998, 1999). The most common mutation is an unstable expansion of a dodecamer minisatellite repeat unit in the promoter region of the cystatin B gene. The exact role of cystatin B is not known, but it has been found primarily localized in the nucleus (Riccio et al., 2001). Cystatin B interacts with a variety of proteins, and these multiprotein complexes are found in the cerebellum (Di Giaimo et al., 2002). An animal model has been developed (Shannon et al., 2002). In an Arab family with similar clinical appearance, a cystatin B mutation was ruled out, linkage was identified on chromosome 12, and the disorder was named EPM1B (Berkovic et al., 2005).

It is of critical importance in these cases to recognize that phenytoin treatment may be associated with worsening of the condition (Eldridge et al., 1983). Patients can be treated successfully with other anticonvulsants as described later.

Mitochondrial encephalomyopathy presents in many guises. One phenotype is the myoclonus epilepsy and ragged-red fiber syndrome (MERRF) (Traff et al., 1995; Canafoglia et al., 2001). Symptoms typically commence in the second decade, but onset as late as the age of 40 has been described. Myoclonus and ataxia are typical features, while tonic-clonic seizures and dementia often also occur. Deafness and short stature may be a clue to the diagnosis. Muscle weakness is variable. A raised blood or cerebrospinal fluid (CSF) lactate concentration might suggest the diagnosis. Muscle biopsy reveals the characteristic "ragged-red" fibers. Maternal inheritance can sometimes be evident, and a number of mutations of mitochondrial genes have been identified.

Sialidosis (cherry-red spot myoclonus syndrome) also is inherited as an autosomal-recessive condition with onset in childhood or adolescence (Rapin, 1986). The sialidoses are lysosomal storage disorders associated with a deficiency of alpha-N-acetylneuraminidase and, in some, with additional deficiency of alpha-galactosidase.

In adults, another group of conditions, namely, spinocerebellar degenerations, might cause myoclonus. For example, one presentation of dentatorubro-pallidoluysian atrophy is with myoclonus and epilepsy (Becher et al., 1997). Some patients with the autosomal-dominant cerebellar ataxias, including Type 1, also may have prominent myoclonus. So may patients with multiple-system atrophy, in whom the myoclonus tends to affect the fingers and toes and is stimulus-sensitive (Rodriguez et al., 1994).

There is an interesting but unexplained association between progressive myoclonic ataxia and celiac disease (Lu et al., 1986; Bhatia et al., 1995). The onset of the neurologic syndrome may follow the gastrointestinal and other manifestations of celiac disease even while on a gluten-free diet, in the absence of overt features of malabsorption or nutritional deficiency. The neurologic syndrome was dominated by action and stimulus-sensitive myoclonus of cortical origin with mild ataxia and infrequent seizures. The condition may progress despite strict adherence to diet. No treatment is known.

Action myoclonus-renal failure syndrome is a distinctive form of progressive myoclonus epilepsy associated with renal dysfunction. Badhwar and colleagues (2004) have described 15 individuals who presented with either renal or neurologic features. Segregation analyses suggested autosomal-recessive inheritance. Tremor (onset age 17 to 26 years), action myoclonus (onset age 14 to 29 years), infrequent generalized seizures (onset age 20 to 28 years), and cerebellar features were characteristic. Brain autopsy in two patients revealed extraneuronal pigment accumulation. Proteinuria, detected between ages 9 and 30 years in all cases, progressed to renal failure in most patients within 8 years. Renal biopsies showed collapsing glomerulopathy, a severe variant of focal glomerulosclerosis. Dialysis and renal transplantation were effective for the renal features but not for the neurologic features, which continued to progress even when kidney function was improved.

Other causes of progressive myoclonus epilepsy and progressive myoclonic ataxia are much rarer (see Box 21-7). Investigation of patients with these clinical syndromes should include neurophysiology, white cell enzyme assays, and muscle and axillary skin biopsy.

Myoclonus after cerebral anoxia is usually the result of an anesthetic accident, cardiac arrest, or respiratory failure often due to asthma (Lance and Adams, 1963; Werhahn et al., 1997; Frucht, 2002) (Table 21-5). In acute posthypoxic myoclonus,

there is an initial period of coma, sometimes with myoclonic storms. The first 3 days are crucial to long-term prognosis; generalized myoclonic status epilepticus carries a very poor prognosis (Wijdicks et al., 1994). In those who survive, spontaneous, action-induced and stimulus-sensitive myoclonus may emerge on recovery (Video 21-9). Intellect may be normal, but there might be additional cerebellar ataxia as well as the disabling myoclonus. Seizures may persist. Postanoxic myoclonus may consist of multifocal jerks of cortical origin, generalized jerks due to intrahemispheric and transcallosal spread, brainstem reticular myoclonus, or a mixture of all these types (Werhahn et al., 1997; Hallett, 2000b). Many patients have prominent negative myoclonus particularly of the legs, causing a bouncy gait and sudden falls (Video 21-10). An animal model has been developed that should be useful in understanding the pathophysiology of this disorder (Kanthasamy et al., 2000; Nguyen et al., 2000; Truong et al., 2000).

The clinical syndrome as reported by Lance and Adams noted the precipitating feature of action and the association with cerebellar ataxia, postural lapses, gait disturbance, and grand mal seizures. Werhahn and colleagues (1997) reported the clinical and neurophysiologic features of 14 patients with chronic posthypoxic myoclonus. All patients had a cardiorespiratory arrest, most caused by an acute asthmatic attack. All patients had multifocal action myoclonus, and 11 had additional stimulus-sensitive myoclonus. There was late improvement in the myoclonic syndrome and the level of disability in all but one patient. Cognitive deficits were found in 7 patients and were usually mild. Electrophysiologic investigation confirmed cortical action myoclonus in every case, although this could be combined with cortical reflex myoclonus, an exaggerated startle response, or brainstem reticular reflex myoclonus. The site of the responsible lesion in the brain is not certain, but there does appear to be a disorder of serotonin metabolism supported not only by the therapeutic response to 5-hydroxytryptophan but also by the reduction in CSF levels of 5-HIAA, which improves with successful therapy. A study using glucose positron emission tomography (PET) showed a bilateral hypermetabolism in the ventrolateral thalamus and pontine tegmentum relative to controls, but the significance of this is not clear (Frucht et al., 2004).

Multifocal and generalized myoclonus also may occur in a variety of acute encephalitic illnesses or postinfectious disseminated encephalomyelitis (Bhatia et al., 1992). It is characteristic of some of the slow viral encephalopathies, such as subacute sclerosing panencephalitis (SSPE) and

Table 21-5 Causes of posthypoxic myoclonus

| Cause | Number of Patients |
|---|---|
| Associated with anaesthesia and surgery | 32 |
| Myocardial infarct | 12 |
| Obstructed airway | 11 |
| Drug intoxication | 9 |
| Miscellaneous | 21 |
| Not stated | 3 |
| **Total** | **88** |

Data from Fahn S: Posthypoxic action myoclonus: Literature review update. Adv Neurol 1986;43:157–169.

Creutzfeldt-Jakob disease (Shibasaki et al., 1981; Brown et al., 1986). In SSPE, the myoclonus is often periodic at long intervals (Video 21-11). Carbamazepine might be considered for the myoclonus of SSPE (Yigit and Sarikaya, 2006). In these latter conditions, the myoclonus often has a characteristic hung-up jerk, and periodic EEG discharges are evident in the majority of patients. Myoclonus also is seen in patients with the AIDS-dementia complex (Maher et al., 1997).

The myoclonic encephalopathy of infants (opsoclonus-myoclonus, or dancing eyes–dancing feet syndrome) appears between the ages of 6 months and 18 months and often responds dramatically to steroid or adrenocorticotropic hormone treatment (Pranzatelli, 1992, 1996; Tate et al., 2005) (Box 21-8). The chaotic, large-amplitude, conjugate eye movements are a striking feature. Plasmapheresis might also be effective (Yiu et al., 2001). About half of such cases have an underlying neuroblastoma. An autoimmune origin seems likely, since it is associated with a distinctive pattern of serum IgM and IgG binding to neural tissues and antigens (Connolly et al., 1997). Reduced levels of the metabolites of serotonin (5HIAA) and dopamine (homovanillic acid) have been found in the CSF (Pranzatelli et al., 1995), and some patients may benefit from treatment with the serotonin precursor 5-hydroxy-L-tryptophan. The incidence of subsequent developmental or neurologic disturbance is high (Rudnick et al., 2001). A similar syndrome of opsoclonus and myoclonus may

occur in adults, whether inflammatory or paraneoplastic (Bataller et al., 2001) (Box 21-9, Video 21-12). The idiopathic cases have a more benign course than do those with cancer. If the cancer is treated, the opsoclonus-myoclonus might resolve. One defined syndrome is breast cancer and anti-Ri antibody (Weizman and Leong, 2004). A patient with large-cell carcinoma of the lung and ANNA-2 antibodies responded well to treatment of the tumor, and antibody levels declined (Erlich et al., 2004). Whipple disease also can produce such a clinical picture (Schwartz et al., 1986). Symptomatic therapy that should be considered includes steroids or adrenocorticotropic hormone. Plasmapheresis may be effective (Yiu et al., 2001). Trazadone may also be helpful.

Myoclonus and dementia in adults occur not only in Creutzfeldt-Jakob disease but also in Alzheimer disease (Wilkins et al., 1984). Parkinson disease rarely manifests myoclonus. While the myoclonus appears to be cortical in origin, there is no reflex myoclonus or a giant SEP (Caviness

---

**Box 21-8** The opsoclonus-myoclonus syndrome (dancing eyes and dancing feet)

Opsoclonus: Continuous, arrhythmic, multidirectional, large saccades
Myoclonus: Trunk, limbs, diaphragm, larynx, pharynx, and palate
Causes: Viral infections, postinfectious encephalitis, trauma, tumor (metabolic)
50% of children have a neuroblastoma (chest or abdomen)
Only 2% of those with a neuroblastoma have opsoclonus-myoclonus syndrome
20% of adults have an underlying cancer

---

**Box 21-9** Brainstem encephalitis

Subacute onset of ataxia, dysarthria, diplopia and ophthalmoplegia, nystagmus, opsoclonus, vertigo, deafness, and myoclonus
Viral infection (e.g., herpes simplex) bacterial infection (e.g., listeria), postinfectious, demyelination, vascular disease, tumor, or paraneoplastic syndromes
Paraneoplastic cases have normal imaging but often have an active CSF with oligoclonal bands. Many have anti-Purkinje cell (e.g., anti-Yo) or anti-Ri antibodies. Common cancers are of the ovary and lung.

---

et al., 1998, 2002). Myoclonus is a well-described feature of dopa-dyskinesias (Luquin et al., 1992), and this would be its most frequent cause in patients with Parkinson disease. Myoclonus is more common in multiple-system atrophy. Myoclonus can be seen in patients with dystonia, the myoclonus in this situation being a short "burst" of dystonia (Video 21-13). It may also be a feature of Huntington disease, and in one case, it was shown to be cortical myoclonus (Caviness and Kurth, 1997). Myoclonus is a prominent, characteristic feature of corticobasal degeneration (Kompoliti et al., 1998). The myoclonus is stimulus-sensitive with a short latency that may be helpful in differential diagnosis. Its pathophysiology is still debated as to whether it is cortical or subcortical in origin (Carella et al., 1997; Strafella et al., 1997).

A wide variety of drugs (Klawans et al., 1986) and toxins (Obeso et al., 1986) may provoke multifocal and generalized myoclonus, as may renal failure (Chadwick and French, 1979). Among drugs, antidepressants (particularly the selective serotonin reuptake inhibitors), anesthetics, anticonvulsants (particularly at toxic levels), withdrawal of benzodiazepines and propranolol, lithium (Caviness and Evidente, 2003), monoamine oxidase inhibitors, and levodopa can all cause myoclonus. Among toxins, bismuth, heavy metals, glue and gasoline sniffing, and toxic cooking oil in Spain can cause prominent myoclonus. Myoclonus is prominent in the "serotonin syndrome," along with confusion, agitation, diarrhea, fever, and sweating. This syndrome has been reported after treatment with tryptophan, monoamine oxidase inhibitors, selective serotonin reuptake inhibitors, and tricyclic antidepressants, alone or in combination (Mason et al., 2000). Myoclonus is also associated with the use of gabapentin but is generally mild and might not cause any symptomatic problem (Asconape et al., 2000).

Essential myoclonus refers to a syndrome of nonprogressive multifocal myoclonus, without other cognitive or neurologic symptoms or signs or fits. It may be inherited as an autosomal-dominant trait (Daube and Peters, 1966; Mahloudji and Pikielny, 1967; Korten et al., 1974; Fahn and Sjaastad, 1991). Essential myoclonus usually presents in the first or second decade of life, and the course is benign. There are no seizures, dementia, or ataxia, and the EEG is normal. In some patients with essential myoclonus, the physiologic abnormality appears to be that of overflow of ballistic movement patterns (Hallett et al., 1977b).

Sporadic cases of essential myoclonus also occur (Bressman and Fahn, 1986). In some families with essential myoclonus, there also are manifestations of dystonia; some individuals have both, and others have myoclonus or dystonia. The myoclonus in such families may be very responsive to alcohol, hence the description as alcohol-sensitive myoclonus dystonia (Quinn, 1996). Most families with myoclonus dystonia have an abnormal gene for epsilon-sarcoglycan (Zimprich et al., 2001). The clinical presentation is relatively homogeneous with this gene defect, with myoclonus predominantly of neck and upper limbs and dystonia presenting as cervical dystonia and/or writer's cramp (Asmus et al., 2002). In one family, however, epilepsy was also seen in affected members, so the phenotype may be broad (Foncke et al., 2003). There is clearly genetic heterogeneity (Grimes et al., 2002). See also Chapter 13 for more details on myoclonus-dystonia.

Myoclonus is a frequent presentation of a psychogenic movement disorder, and it is important to keep this in mind in the differential diagnosis (Video 21-14). Psychogenic movement disorders are discussed in Chapter 26, but in the context of discussing myoclonus, it is noteworthy that the clinical neurophysiology is distinctive and can help to resolve the differential diagnosis (Brown, 2006).

## DRUG TREATMENT OF GENERALIZED OR MULTIFOCAL MYOCLONUS

Myoclonus, particularly action myoclonus, can be very disabling. It distorts speech, interferes with manual function, and prevents walking. The drugs that are used to treat myoclonus generally possess anticonvulsant properties (Table 21-6) (Obeso et al., 1989; Brown, 1995; Obeso, 1995; Pranzatelli and Nadi, 1995; Frucht, 2000), usually by enhancing gamma-aminobutyric acid inhibitory activity. In epilepsy, it is currently fashionable to try to manage patients using a single drug rather than polytherapy. However, there are good reasons for the opposite approach in the treatment of myoclonus. Electrophysiologic evidence suggests that antimyoclonic

**Table 21-6** Appropriate dosages of agents for the treatment of myoclonus

| Drug | Dosage |
|---|---|
| Baclofen | 15–100 mg/day |
| Benztropine | 4–9 mg/day |
| Carbamazepine | 800–1600 mg/day |
| Clonazepam | Up to 15 mg/day |
| Diazepam | 5–30 mg/day |
| 5-Hydroxytryptophan | Up to 1.5 g/day* |
| Levetiracetam | 1000–3000 mg/day* |
| Phenobarbitol (phenobarbitone) | 60–180 mg/day |
| Phenytoin | 100–300 mg/day |
| Piracetam | 2.4–16.8 g/day |
| Primidone | 500–750 mg/day |
| Tetrabenazine | 50–200 mg/day |
| Trihexyphenidyl (benzhexol) | Up to 35 mg/day |
| Valproic acid (sodium valproate) | 1000–1500 mg/day |

*In combination with a peripheral aromatic amino acid decarboxylase inhibitor (such as carbidopa 100 to 300 mg/day).

Data modified from Brown P: Myoclonus: A practical guide to drug therapy. CNS Drugs 1995;3:22–29.

**Table 21-7** Drug treatment for specific types of myoclonus

| Type of Myoclonus | Drug(s) of First Choice | Other Agents |
|---|---|---|
| Cortical myoclonus | Valproic acid (sodium valproate or clonazepam | Primidone, phenobarbital, levetiracetam, piracetam, 5-HTP* |
| Brainstem reticular myoclonus | Valproic acid or clonazepam† | 5-HTP* |
| Hyperekplexia | Clonazepam | Carbamazepine, phenytoin |
| Ballistic overflow myoclonus | Benztropine or trihexyphenidyl (benzhexol) | Alcohol (ethanol), clonazepam, 5-HTP* |
| Palatal myoclonus | Phenytoin, carbamazepine, clonazepam, diazepam, trihexyphenidyl or baclofen† | 5-HTP,* sumatriptan |
| Propriospinal myoclonus | Clonazepam | |
| Segmental spinal myoclonus | Clonazepam | Diazepam, carbamazepine, tetrabenazine |

*Combined with a peripheral aromatic amino acid decarboxylase inhibitor (such as carbidopa). Usefulness limited by poor tolerability.
†Treatment with any agent is often unsuccessful.
5-HTP, 5-hydroxytryptophan.

drugs might exert different actions on the sequence of events that are responsible for myoclonus, at least for those who are concerned with cortical myoclonus. Some drugs that decrease cortical myoclonus increase the size of the giant sensory-evoked potential, while others have the opposite effect. Myoclonus thus often responds best to a combination of drugs (Obeso et al., 1989).

Table 21-7 summarizes the drugs that are used to treat specific types of myoclonus arising in the different parts of the neuraxis.

Epileptic myoclonus and cortical myoclonus respond best to drugs such as sodium valproate and clonazepam, which are often used in combination in maximum tolerated anticonvulsant doses (Obeso et al., 1989). Sodium valproate is the drug of choice for the treatment of JME. An alternative is acetazolamide (Resor and Resor, 1990).

It is conventional to start with sodium valproate in patients with severe myoclonus and then add clonazepam. If the disability is not adequately improved, piracetam or levetiracetam can then be added. The mechanism of action of piracetam is uncertain, but it undoubtedly possesses antimyoclonic activity (Obeso et al., 1988; Brown et al., 1993; Ikeda et al., 1996; Koskiniemi et al., 1998; Genton et al., 1999; Fedi et al., 2001). Levetiracetam, a molecule related to piracetam that has been approved for the treatment of epilepsy also is very effective for myoclonus (Genton and Gelisse, 2000, 2001; Genton and Van Vleymen, 2000; Frucht et al., 2001; Krauss et al., 2001; Schauer et al., 2002; Magaudda et al., 2004). There is one report of tizanidine helping two of three patients (Mukand and Giunti, 2004).

Primidone also may be of value as an additional drug in severely affected patients, as may clobazam and acetazolamide (Vaamonde et al., 1992). The potential antimyoclonic activity of newer anticonvulsants, such as vigabatrin, gabapentin, and lamotrigine, remains to be established. However, both vigabatrin and gabapentin may, paradoxically, worsen some types of myoclonus (Asconape et al., 2000). Milacemide, a glycine precursor, has been shown to be ineffective (Brown, Thompson, and Rothwell, 1991a; Gordon et al., 1993). One patient with alcohol-responsive posthypoxic myoclonus responded well to gamma-hydroxybutyric acid (Frucht et al., 2005).

Unfortunately, while spontaneous, action, and reflex-positive myoclonus often is helped by drug therapy, negative myoclonus frequently is resistant. As a result, disabling postural lapses in antigravity leg muscles usually persist to cause the typical bouncy unsteady stance and gait, often with falls. One patient was described who had an excellent response to levetiracetam (Gelisse et al., 2003). In the setting of childhood partial epilepsy, negative myoclonus can be effectively treated with ethosuximide (Oguni et al., 1998; Capovilla et al., 1999). It is not clear whether this treatment would be useful in other circumstances.

It has been claimed that the antioxidant N-acetylcysteine has considerable beneficial effect on the myoclonus in Unverricht-Lundborg disease (Hurd et al., 1996; Ben-Menachem et al., 2000). Alcohol also has been found to be a potent antimyoclonic agent in posthypoxic myoclonus as well as Unverricht-Lundborg disease (Genton and Guerrini, 1992).

Those with brainstem myoclonus seem to respond best to clonazepam. 5-Hydroxytryptophan with a peripheral decarboxylase inhibitor also has been used with some success, although gastrointestinal side effects might be prominent (Chadwick et al., 1977).

Spinal and other segmental myoclonus also responds best to treatment with clonazepam (Obeso, 1995; Devetag Chalaupka and Bernardi, 1999), but tetrabenazine and baclofen occasionally may be helpful. Levetiracetam can be useful (Keswani et al., 2002). One case responded to valproate and serotonergic therapy (Jimenez-Jimenez et al., 1991). If all else fails, botulinum toxin can be used (Lagueny et al., 1999).

Essential myoclonus sometimes improves with alcohol, a beta-blocker such as propranolol, or an anticholinergic agent (Duvoisin, 1984; Chokroverty et al., 1987). In myoclonus-dystonia syndrome, alcohol can be of benefit to the myoclonus but not to the dystonia with which it may be associated (Quinn, 1996). One patient with myoclonus-dystonia improved with bilateral deep brain stimulation of the globus pallidus internus (Cif et al., 2004).

## Acknowledgments

This chapter is the work of the U.S. government and is not copyrighted. This chapter has been extensively modified and updated from an original by C. D. Marsden.

## References

Aicardi J: Myoclonic epilepsies of infancy and childhood. Adv Neurol 1986;43:11–31.

Andermann F, Andermann E: Startle disorders of man: Hyperekplexia, jumping and startle epilepsy. Brain Dev 1988;10:214–222.

Antel JP, Rasmussen T: Rasmussen's encephalitis and the new hat. Neurology 1996;46:9–11.

Asconape J, Diedrich A, DellaBadia J: Myoclonus associated with the use of gabapentin. Epilepsia 2000;41:479–481.

Asmus F, Zimprich A, Tezenas Du Montcel S, et al: Myoclonus-dystonia syndrome: Epsilon-sarcoglycan mutations and phenotype. Ann Neurol 2002;52:489–492.

Badhwar A, Berkovic SF, Dowling JP, et al: Action myoclonus-renal failure syndrome: Characterization of a unique cerebro-renal disorder. Brain 2004;127:2173–2182.

Bakker MJ, van Dijk JG, van den Maagdenburg AMJM, et al: Startle syndromes. Lancet Neurology 2006;5:513–524.

Bataller L, Graus F, Saiz A, Vilchez JJ: Clinical outcome in adult onset idiopathic or paraneoplastic opsoclonus-myoclonus. Brain 2001;124:437–443.

Becher MW, Rubinsztein DC, Leggo J, et al: Dentatorubral and pallidoluysian atrophy (DRPLA). Clinical and neuropathological findings in genetically confirmed North American and European pedigrees. Mov Disord 1997;12:519–530.

Ben-Menachem E, Kyllerman M, Marklund S: Superoxide dismutase and glutathione peroxidase function in progressive myoclonus epilepsies. Epilepsy Res 2000;40:33–39.

Berkovic SF, Andermann F: The progressive myoclonic epilepsies. In Pedley TA, Meldrum BS (eds): Recent Advances in Epilepsy 3. Edinburgh, Churchill Livingstone, 1986, pp 157–187.

Berkovic SF, Andermann F, Carpenter S, Wolfe LD: Progressive myoclonic epilepsies: Specific causes and diagnosis. New Engl J Med 1986;315:296–305.

Berkovic SF, Mazarib A, Walid S, et al: A new clinical and molecular form of Unverricht-Lundborg disease localized by homozygosity mapping. Brain 2005;128:652–658.

Bhatia K, Thompson PD, Marsden CD: "Isolated" postinfectious myoclonus. J Neurol Neurosurg Psychiatry 1992;55:1089–1091.

Bhatia KP, Brown P, Gregory R, et al: Progressive myoclonic ataxia associated with coeliac disease: The myoclonus is of cortical origin, but the pathology is in the cerebellum. Brain 1995;118:1087–1093.

Bressman S, Fahn S: Essential myoclonus. Adv Neurol 1986;43:287–294.

Brown P: Myoclonus: A practical guide to drug therapy. CNS Drugs 1995;3:22–29.

Brown P: Clinical neurophysiology of myoclonus. In Hallett M, Fahn S, Jankovic J, et al (eds): Psychogenic Movement Disorders: Neurology and Neuropsychiatry. Philadelphia, Lippincott Williams & Wilkins, 2006, pp 262–264.

Brown P, Cathala F, Castaigne P, Gajdusek DC: Creutzfeldt-Jakob disease: Clinical analysis of a consecutive series of 230 neuropathologically verified cases. Ann Neurol 1986; 20: 597–602.

Brown P, Day BL, Rothwell JC, et al: Intrahemispheric and interhemispheric spread of cerebral cortical myoclonic activity and its relevance to epilepsy. Brain 1991;114:2333–2251.

Brown P, Marsden CD: Rhythmic cortical and muscle discharge in cortical myoclonus. Brain 1996;119:1307–1316.

Brown P, Ridding MC, Werhahn KJ, et al: Abnormalities of the balance between inhibition and excitation in the motor cortex of patients with cortical myoclonus. Brain 1996;119:309–317.

Brown P, Rothwell JC, Thompson PD, et al: The hyperekplexias and their relationship to the normal startle reflex. Brain 1991;114:1903–1928.

Brown P, Steiger MJ, Thompson PD, et al: Effectiveness of piracetam in cortical myoclonus. Mov Disord 1993;8:63–68.

Brown P, Thompson PD, Rothwell JC, et al: A therapeutic trial of milacemide in myoclonus and the stiff-person syndrome. Mov Disord 1991a;6:73–75.

Brown P, Thompson PD, Rothwell JC, et al: Axial myoclonus of propriospinal origin. Brain 1991b;114:197–214.

Canafoglia L, Franceschetti S, Antozzi C, et al: Epileptic phenotypes associated with mitochondrial disorders. Neurology 2001;56:1340–1346.

Cantello R, Gianelli M, Civardi C, Mutani R: Focal subcortical reflex myoclonus. A clinical and neurophysiological study. Arch Neurol 1997;54:187–196.

Capelle HH, Wohrle JC, Weigel R, et al: Propriospinal myoclonus due to cervical disc herniation. Case report. J Neurosurg Spine 2005;2:608–611.

Capovilla G, Beccaria F, Veggiotti P, et al: Ethosuximide is effective in the treatment of epileptic negative myoclonus in childhood partial epilepsy. J Child Neurol 1999;14:395–400.

Carella F, Ciano C, Panzica F, Scaioli V: Myoclonus in corticobasal degeneration. Mov Disord 1997;12:598–603.

Caviness JN, Adler CH, Beach TG, et al: Small-amplitude cortical myoclonus in Parkinson's disease: Physiology and clinical observations. Mov Disord 2002;17:657–662.

Caviness JN, Adler CH, Newman S, et al: Cortical myoclonus in levodopa-responsive parkinsonism. Mov Disord 1998;13:540–544.

Caviness JN, Alving LI, Maranganore DM, et al: The incidence and prevalence of myoclonus in Olmsted County, Minnesota. Mayo Clin Proc 1999;74:565–569.

Caviness JN, Evidente VG: Cortical myoclonus during lithium exposure. Arch Neurol 2003;60:401–404.

Caviness JN, Kurth M: Cortical Myoclonus in Huntington's disease associated with an enlarged somatosensory evoked potential. Mov Disord 1997;12:1046–1051.

Chadwick D, French AT: Uraemic myoclonus: An example of reticular reflex myoclonus? J Neurol Neurosurg Psychiatry 1979;42:52–55.

Chadwick D, Hallett M, Harris R, et al: Clinical, biochemical, and physiological features distinguishing myoclonus responsive to 5 hydroxytryptophan, tryptophan with a monoamine oxidase inhibitor, and clonazepam. Brain 1977;100:455–487.

Chan EM, Ackerley CA, Lohi H, et al: Laforin preferentially binds the neurotoxic starch-like polyglucosans, which form in its absence in progressive myoclonus epilepsy. Hum Mol Genet 2004a;13:1117–1129.

Chan EM, Omer S, Ahmed M, et al: Progressive myoclonus epilepsy with polyglucosans (Lafora disease): Evidence for a third locus. Neurology 2004b;63:565–567.

Chan EM, Young EJ, Ianzano L, et al: Mutations in NHLRC1 cause progressive myoclonus epilepsy. Nat Genet 2003;35:125–127.

Chokroverty S, Manocha MK, Duvoisin RC: A physiologic and pharmacologic study in anticholinergic-responsive essential myoclonus. Neurology 1987;37:608–615.

Cif L, Valente EM, Hemm S, et al: Deep brain stimulation in myoclonus-dystonia syndrome. Mov Disord 2004;19:724–727.

Cockerell OC, Rothwell J, Thompson PD, et al: Clinical and physiological features of epilepsia partialis continua: Cases ascertained in the UK. Brain 1996;119:393–407.

Connolly AM, Pestronk A, Mehta S, et al: Serum autoantibodies in childhood opsoclonus-myoclonus syndrome: An analysis of antigenic targets in neural tissues. J Pediatr 1997;130:878–884.

Cossette P, Liu L, Brisebois K, et al: Mutation of GABRA1 in an autosomal dominant form of juvenile myoclonic epilepsy. Nat Genet 2002;31:184–189.

Cowan JM, Rothwell JC, Wise RJ, Marsden CD: Electrophysiological and positron emission studies in a patient with cortical myoclonus, epilepsia partialis continua and motor epilepsy. J Neurol Neurosurg Psychiatry 1986;49:796–807.

Daube JR, Peters HA: Hereditary essential myoclonus. Arch Neurol 1966;15:587–594.

Davis SM, Murray NM, Diengdoh JV, et al: Stimulus-sensitive spinal myoclonus. J Neurol Neurosurg Psychiatry 1981;44:884–888.

Delgado-Escueta AV, Medina MT, Serratosa JM, et al: Mapping and positional cloning of common idiopathic generalized epilepsies: Juvenile myoclonus epilepsy and childhood absence epilepsy. Adv Neurol 1999;79:351–374.

Deuschl G, Löhle E, Heinen F, Lücking C: Ear click in palatal tremor: Its origin and treatment with botulinum toxin. Neurology 1991;41:1677–1679.

Deuschl G, Mischke G, Schenck E, et al: Symptomatic and essential rhythmic palatal myoclonus. Brain 1990;113:1645–1672.

Deuschl G, Toro C, Hallett M: Symptomatic and essential palatal tremor: 2. Differences of palatal movements. Mov Disord 1994a;9:676–678.

Deuschl G, Toro C, Valls-Solé J, et al: Symptomatic and essential palatal tremor: 1. Clinical, physiological, and MRI analysis. Brain 1994b;117:775–788.

Devetag Chalaupka F, Bernardi M: A case of segmental myoclonus in amputation stump: Evidence for spinal generator and physiopathogenetic hypothesis. Ital J Neurol Sci 1999;20:327–331.

Di Giaimo R, Riccio M, Santi S, et al: New insights into the molecular basis of progressive myoclonus epilepsy: A multiprotein complex with cystatin B. Hum Mol Genet 2002;11:2941–2950.

Di Lazzaro V, Restuccia D, Nardone R, et al: Changes in spinal cord excitability in a patient with rhythmic segmental myoclonus. J Neurol Neurosurg Psychiatry 1996;61:641–644.

Duvoisin RC: Essential myoclonus: Response to anticholinergic therapy. Clin Neuropharmacol 1984;7:141–147.

Ebner A, Noachtar S: Ear clicking as the initial symptom of simple partial seizures. J Neurol 1995;242:180–181.

Eldridge R, Iivanainen M, Stern R, et al: Baltic myoclonus epilepsy: Hereditary disorder of childhood made worse by phenytoin. Lancet 1983;2:838–842.

Erlich R, Morrison C, Kim B, et al: ANNA-2: An antibody associated with paraneoplastic opsoclonus in a patient with large-cell carcinoma of the lung with neuroendocrine features: Correlation of clinical improvement with tumor response. Cancer Invest 2004;22:257–261.

Fahn S: Overview, history and classification of myoclonus. In Fahn S, Frucht SJ, Hallett M, Truong DD (eds): Myoclonus and Paroxysmal Dyskinesias. Advances in Neurology, vol 89. Philadelphia, Lippincott Williams & Wilkins, 2002, pp 13–17.

Fahn S, Sjaastad O: Hereditary essential myoclonus in a large Norwegian family. Mov Disord 1991;6:237–247.

Fedi M, Reutens D, Dubeau F, et al: Long-term efficacy and safety of piracetam in the treatment of progressive myoclonus epilepsy. Arch Neurol 2001;58:781–786.

Floeter MK, Andermann F, Andermann E, et al: Physiological studies of spinal inhibitory pathways in patients with hereditary hyperekplexia. Neurology 1996;46:766–772.

Foncke EM, Klein C, Koelman JH, et al: Hereditary myoclonus-dystonia associated with epilepsy. Neurology 2003;60:1988–1990.

Footitt DR, Quinn N, Kocen RS, et al: Familial Lafora body disease of late onset: Report of four cases in one family and a review of the literature. J Neurol 1997;244:40–44.

Frenken CW, Notermans SL, Korten JJ, Horstink MW: Myoclonic disorders of spinal origin. Clin Neurol Neurosurg 1976;79:107–118.

Frucht S: Myoclonus. Curr Treat Options Neurol 2000;2:231–242.

Frucht SJ: The clinical challenge of posthypoxic myoclonus. Adv Neurol 2002;89:85–88.

Frucht SJ, Bordelon Y, Houghton WH: Marked amelioration of alcohol-responsive posthypoxic myoclonus by gamma-hydroxybutyric acid (Xyrem). Mov Disord 2005;20:745–751.

Frucht SJ, Louis ED, Chuang C, Fahn S: A pilot tolerability and efficacy study of levetiracetam in patients with chronic myoclonus. Neurology 2001;57:1112–1114.

Frucht SJ, Trost M, Ma Y, Eidelberg D: The metabolic topography of posthypoxic myoclonus. Neurology 2004;62:1879–1881.

Gahring L, Carlson NG, Meyer EL, Rogers SW: Granzyme B proteolysis of a neuronal glutamate receptor generates an autoantigen and is modulated by glycosylation. J Immunol 2001;166: 1433–1438.

Ganesh S, Delgado-Escueta AV, Sakamoto T, et al: Targeted disruption of the Epm2a gene causes formation of Lafora inclusion bodies, neurodegeneration, ataxia, myoclonus epilepsy and impaired behavioral response in mice. Hum Mol Genet 2002;11:1251–1262.

Ganesh S, Puri R, Singh S, et al: Recent advances in the molecular basis of Lafora's progressive myoclonus epilepsy. J Hum Genet 2006;51:1–8.

Gelisse P, Crespel A, Genton P, Baldy-Moulinier M: Dramatic effect of levetiracetam on epileptic negative myoclonus. Acta Neurol Scand 2003;107:302–303.

Genton P, Gelisse P: Antimyoclonic effect of levetiracetam. Epileptic Disord 2000;2:209–212.

Genton P, Gelisse P: Suppression of post-hypoxic and post-encephalitic myoclonus with levetiracetam. Neurology 2001;57: 1144–1145.

Genton P, Guerrini R: Effect of alcohol on action myoclonus in Lance-Adams syndrome and progressive myoclonus epilepsy. Mov Disord 1992;7:92.

Genton P, Guerrini R, Remy C: Piracetam in the treatment of cortical myoclonus. Pharmacopsychiatry 1999;32(suppl 1):49–53.

Genton P, Van Vleymen B: Piracetam and levetiracetam: Close structural similarities but different pharmacological and clinical profiles. Epileptic Disord 2000;2:99–105.

Gentry MS, Worby CA, Dixon JE: Insights into Lafora disease: Malin is an E3 ubiquitin ligase that ubiquitinates and promotes the degradation of laforin. Proc Natl Acad Sci U S A 2005;102: 8501–8506.

Gordon MF, Diaz-Olivo R, Hunt AL, Fahn S: Therapeutic trial of milacemide in patients with myoclonus and other intractable movement disorders. Mov Disord 1993;8:484–488.

Grimes DA, Han F, Lang AE, et al: A novel locus for inherited myoclonus-dystonia on 18p11. Neurology 2002;59:1183–1186.

Grosse P, Guerrini R, Parmeggiani L, et al: Abnormal corticomuscular and intermuscular coupling in high-frequency rhythmic myoclonus. Brain 2003;126:326–342.

Guerrini R, Dravet C, Genton P, et al: Epileptic negative myoclonus. Neurology 1993;43:1078–1083.

Hallett M: Early history of myoclonus. In Fahn S, Marsden CD, Van Woert MH (eds): Myoclonus, vol 43. New York, Raven Press, 1986, pp 7–10.

Hallett M: Electrophysiologic evaluation of movement disorders. In Aminoff MJ (ed): Electrodiagnosis in Clinical Neurology. New York, Churchill Livingstone, 1999, pp 365–380.

Hallett M: Electrodiagnosis in movement disorders. In Levin KH, Lüders HO (eds): Comprehensive Clinical Neurophysiology. Philadelphia, WB Saunders, 2000a, pp 281–294.

Hallett M: Physiology of posthypoxic myoclonus. Mov Disord 2000b;15(suppl 1):8–13.

Hallett M: Neurophysiology of brainstem myoclonus. Adv Neurol 2002;89:99–102.

Hallett M, Chadwick D, Adam J, Marsden CD: Reticular reflex myoclonus: A physiological type of human post-hypoxic myoclonus. J Neurol Neurosurg Psychiatry 1977a;40:253–264.

Hallett M, Chadwick D, Marsden CD: Ballistic movement overflow myoclonus a form of essential myoclonus. Brain 1977b;100: 299–312.

Hallett M, Chadwick D, Marsden CD: Cortical reflex myoclonus. Neurology 1979;29:1107–1125.

Hallett M, Marsden CD, Fahn S: Myoclonus. In Vinken PJ, Bruyn GW, Klawans HL (eds): Handbook of Clinical Neurology, vol 5. Amsterdam, Elsevier, 1987, pp 609–625.

Hurd RW, Wilder BJ, Helveston WR, Uthman BM: Treatment of four siblings with progressive myoclonus epilepsy of the Unverricht-Lundborg type with N-acetylcysteine. Neurology 1996;47: 1264–1268.

Ikeda A, Kakigi R, Funai N, et al: Cortical tremor: A variant of cortical reflex myoclonus. Neurology 1990;40:1561–1565.

Ikeda A, Shibasaki H, Tashiro K, et al: Clinical trial of piracetam in patients with myoclonus: Nationwide multiinstitution study in Japan. The Myoclonus/Piracetam Study Group. Mov Disord 1996;11:691–700.

Jabbari B, Rosenberg M, Scherokman B, et al: Effectiveness of trihexyphenidyl against pendular nystagmus and palatal myoclonus: Evidence of cholinergic dysfunction. Mov Disord 1987;2:93–98.

Jamieson DR, Mann C, O'Reilly B, Thomas AM: Ear clicks in palatal tremor caused by activity of the levator veli palatini. Neurology 1996;46:1168–1169.

Jankovic J, Pardo R: Segmental myoclonus: Clinical and pharmacological study. Arch Neurol 1986;43:1025–1031.

Jay V, Becker LE, Otsubo H, Cortez M, et al: Chronic encephalitis and epilepsy (Rasmussen's encephalitis): Detection of cytomegalovirus and herpes simplex virus 1 by the polymerase chain reaction and in situ hybridization. Neurology 1995;45: 108–117.

Jimenez-Jimenez FJ, Roldan A, Zancada F, et al: Spinal myoclonus: Successful treatment with the combination of sodium valproate and L-5-hydroxytryptophan. Clin Neuropharmacol 1991;14: 186–190.

Juul-Jensen P, Denny-Brown D: Epilepsia partialis continua. Arch Neurol 1966;15:563–578.

Kang SY, Sohn YH: Electromyography patterns of propriospinal myoclonus can be mimicked voluntarily. Mov Disord 2006;21: 1241–1244.

Kanthasamy AG, Nguyen BQ, Truong DD: Animal model of posthypoxic myoclonus: II. Neurochemical, pathologic, and pharmacologic characterization. Mov Disord 2000;15:31–38.

Keswani SC, Kossoff EH, Krauss GL, Hagerty C: Amelioration of spinal myoclonus with levetiracetam. J Neurol Neurosurg Psychiatry 2002;73:457–458.

Klawans HL, Carvey PM, Tanner CM, Goetz CG: Drug-induced myoclonus. Adv Neurol 1986;43:251–264.

Kompoliti K, Goetz CG, Boeve BF, et al: Clinical presentation and pharmacological therapy in corticobasal degeneration. Arch Neurol 1998;55:957–961.

Korten JJ, Notermans SL, Frenken CW, et al: Familial essential myoclonus. Brain 1974;97:131–138.

Koskiniemi ML: Baltic myoclonus. Adv Neurol 1986;43:57–64.

Koskiniemi M, Van Vleymen B, Hakamies L, et al: Piracetam relieves symptoms in progressive myoclonus epilepsy: A multicentre, randomised, double blind, crossover study comparing the efficacy and safety of three dosages of oral piracetam with placebo. J Neurol Neurosurg Psychiatry 1998;64:344–348.

Krauss GL, Bergin A, Kramer RE, et al: Suppression of post-hypoxic and post-encephalitic myoclonus with levetiracetam. Neurology 2001;56:411–412.

Lagueny A, Tison F, Burbaud P, et al: Stimulus-sensitive spinal segmental myoclonus improved with injections of botulinum toxin type A. Mov Disord 1999;14:182–185.

Lance JW, Adams RD: The syndrome of intention or action myoclonus as a sequel to hypoxic encephalopathy. Brain 1963;86:111–136.

Lehesjoki AE, Koskiniemi M: Clinical features and genetics of progressive myoclonus epilepsy of the Univerricht-Lundborg type. Ann Med 1998;30:474–480.

Lehesjoki AE, Koskiniemi M: Progressive myoclonus epilepsy of Unverricht-Lundborg type. Epilepsia 1999;40:23–28.

Leigh PN, Rothwell JC, Traub M, Marsden CD: A patient with reflex myoclonus and muscle rigidity: "Jerking stiff-man syndrome." J Neurol Neurosurg Psychiatry 1980;43:1125–1131.

Lu CS, Thompson PD, Quinn NP, et al: Ramsay Hunt syndrome and coeliac disease: A new association? Mov Disord 1986;1: 209–219.

Luquin MR, Scipioni O, Vaamonde J, et al: Levodopa-induced dyskinesias in Parkinson's disease: Clinical and pharmacological classification. Mov Disord 1992;7:117–124.

Magaudda A, Gelisse P, Genton P: Antimyoclonic effect of levetiracetam in 13 patients with Unverricht-Lundborg disease: Clinical observations. Epilepsia 2004;45:678–681.

Maher J, Choudhri S, Halliday W, et al: AIDS dementia complex with generalized myoclonus. Mov Disord 1997;12:593–597.

Mahloudji M, Pikielny RT: Hereditary essential myoclonus. Brain 1967;90:669–674.

Manford MR, Fish DR, Shorvon SD: Startle provoked epileptic seizures: Features in 19 patients. J Neurol Neurosurg Psychiatry 1996;61:151–156.

Marsden CD, Hallett M, Fahn S: The nosology and pathophysiology of myoclonus. In Marsden CD, Fahn S (eds): Movement Disorders: Neurology 2. London, Butterworth Scientific, 1982, pp 196–248.

Marsden CD, Harding AE, Obeso JA, Lu CS: Progressive myoclonic ataxia (the Ramsay Hunt syndrome). Arch Neurol 1990;47:1121–1125.

Marseille Consensus Group: Classification of progressive myoclonus epilepsies and related disorders. Ann Neurol 1990;28:113–116.

Mason PJ, Morris VA, Balcezak TJ: Serotonin syndrome: Presentation of 2 cases and review of the literature. Medicine (Baltimore) 2000;79:201–209.

Matsumoto J, Fuhr P, Nigro M, Hallett M: Physiological abnormalities in hereditary hyperekplexia. Ann Neurol 1992;32:41–50.

Matsumoto J, Hallett M: Startle syndromes. In Marsden CD, Fahn S (eds): Movement Disorders 3. Oxford, Butterworth-Heinemann, 1994, pp 418–433.

Minassian BA, Andrade DM, Ianzano L, et al: Laforin is a cell membrane and endoplasmic reticulum-associated protein tyrosine phosphatase. Ann Neurol 2001;49:271–275.

Minassian BA, Lee JR, Herbrick JA, et al: Mutations in a gene encoding a novel protein tyrosine phosphatase cause progressive myoclonus epilepsy. Nat Genet 1998;20:171–174.

Minassian BA, Sainz J, Serratosa JM, et al: Genetic locus heterogeneity in Lafora's progressive myoclonus epilepsy. Ann Neurol 1999;45:262–265.

Monday K, Jankovic J: Psychogenic myoclonus. Neurology 1993;43:349–352.

Mukand JA, Giunti EJ: Tizanidine for the treatment of intention myoclonus: A case series. Arch Phys Med Rehabil 2004;85:1125–1127.

Nguyen BQ, Kanthasamy AG, Truong DD: Animal models of myoclonus: An overview. Mov Disord 2000;15:22–25.

Obeso JA: Therapy of myoclonus. Clin Neurosci 1995;3:253–257.

Obeso JA, Artieda J, Quinn N, et al: Piracetam in the treatment of different types of myoclonus. Clin Neuropharmacol 1988;11:529–536.

Obeso JA, Artieda J, Rothwell JC, et al: The treatment of severe action myoclonus. Brain 1989;112:765–777.

Obeso JA, Rothwell JC, Marsden CD: The spectrum of cortical myoclonus: From focal reflex jerks to spontaneous motor epilepsy. Brain 1985;108:193–224.

Obeso JA, Viteri C, Martinez Lage JM, Marsden CD: Toxic myoclonus. Adv Neurol 1986;43:225–230.

Oguni H, Uehara T, Tanaka T, et al: Dramatic effect of ethosuximide on epileptic negative myoclonus: Implications for the neurophysiological mechanism. Neuropediatrics 1998;29:29–34.

Pranzatelli MR: The neurobiology of the opsoclonus-myoclonus syndrome. Clin Neuropharmacol 1992;15:186–228.

Pranzatelli MR: The immunopharmacology of the opsoclonus-myoclonus syndrome. Clin Neuropharmacol 1996;19:1–47.

Pranzatelli MR, Huang Y, Tate E, et al: Cerebrospinal fluid 5-hydroxyindoleacetic acid and homovanillic acid in the pediatric opsoclonus-myoclonus syndrome. Ann Neurol 1995;37:189–197.

Pranzatelli MR, Nadi NS: Mechanism of action of antiepileptic and antimyoclonic drugs. Adv Neurol 1995;67:329–360.

Quinn NP: Essential myoclonus and myoclonic dystonia. Mov Disord 1996;11:119–124.

Rapin I: Myoclonus in neuronal storage and Lafora diseases. Adv Neurol 1986;43:65–85.

Rees, MI, Harvey K, Pearce BR, et al: Mutations in the gene encoding GlyT2 (SLC6A5) define a presynaptic component of human startle disease. Nature Genetics 2006:38:801–806.

Resor SR Jr, Resor LD: Chronic acetazolamide monotherapy in the treatment of juvenile myoclonic epilepsy. Neurology 1990;40:1677–1681.

Riccio M, Di Giaimo R, Pianetti S, et al: Nuclear localization of cystatin B, the cathepsin inhibitor implicated in myoclonus epilepsy (EPM1). Exp Cell Res 2001;262:84–94.

Rodriguez ME, Artieda J, Zubieta JL, Obeso JA: Reflex myoclonus in olivopontocerebellar atrophy. J Neurol Neurosurg Psychiatry 1994;57:316–319.

Rogers SW, Andrews PI, Gahring LC, et al: Autoantibodies to glutamate receptor GluR3 in Rasmussen's encephalitis. Science 1994;265:648–651.

Rossi S, Ulivelli M, Bartalini S, et al: Reduction of cortical myoclonus-related epileptic activity following slow-frequency rTMS. Neuroreport 2004;15:293–296.

Rudnick E, Khakoo Y, Antunes NL, et al: Opsoclonus-myoclonus-ataxia syndrome in neuroblastoma: Clinical outcome and anti-neuronal antibodies—A report from the Children's Cancer Group Study. Med Pediatr Oncol 2001;36:612–622.

Sakai T, Murakami S: Palatal myoclonus responding to carbamazepine. Ann Neurol 1981;9:199–200.

Schauer R, Singer M, Saltuari L, Kofler M: Suppression of cortical myoclonus by levetiracetam. Mov Disord 2002;17:411–415.

Schwartz MA, Selhorst JB, Ochs AL, et al: Oculomasticatory myorhythmia: A unique movement disorder occurring in Whipple's disease. Ann Neurol 1986;20:677–683.

Scott BL, Evans RW, Jankovic J: Treatment of palatal myoclonus with sumatriptan. Mov Disord 1996;11:748–751.

Serratosa JM, Gardiner RM, Lehesjoki AE, et al: The molecular genetic bases of the progressive myoclonus epilepsies. Adv Neurol 1999a;79:383–398.

Serratosa JM, Gomez-Garre P, Gallardo ME, et al: A novel protein tyrosine phosphatase gene is mutated in progressive myoclonus epilepsy of the Lafora type (EPM2). Hum Mol Genet 1999b;8:345–352.

Shannon P, Pennacchio LA, Houseweart MK, et al: Neuropathological changes in a mouse model of progressive myoclonus epilepsy: Cystatin B deficiency and Unverricht-Lundborg disease. J Neuropathol Exp Neurol 2002;61:1085–1091.

Shiang R, Ryan SG, Zhu YZ, et al: Mutations in the alpha 1 subunit of the inhibitory glycine receptor cause the dominant neurologic disorder, hyperekplexia. Nat Genet 1993;5:351–358.

Shiang R, Ryan SG, Zhu YZ, et al: Mutational analysis of familial and sporadic hyperekplexia. Ann Neurol 1995;38:85–91.

Shibasaki H: AAEE minimonograph #30: Electrophysiologic studies of myoclonus. Muscle Nerve 1988;11:899–907.

Shibasaki H: Pathophysiology of negative myoclonus and asterixis. In Fahn S, Hallett M, Lüders HO, Marsden CD (eds): Negative Motor Phenomena, vol 67. Philadelphia, Lippincott-Raven, 1995, pp 199–209.

Shibasaki H: Electrophysiological studies of myoclonus. Muscle Nerve 2000;23:321–335.

Shibasaki H, Hallett M: Electrophysiological studies of myoclonus. Muscle Nerve 2005;31:157–174.

Shibasaki H, Motomura S, Yamashita Y, et al: Periodic synchronous discharge and myoclonus in Creutzfeldt-Jakob disease: Diagnostic application of jerk-locked averaging method. Ann Neurol 1981;9:150–156.

Siniscalchi A, Mancuso F, Russo E, et al: Spinal myoclonus responsive to topiramate. Mov Disord 2004;19:1380–1381.

Smith CR, Scheinberg L: Coincidence of myoclonus and multiple sclerosis: Dramatic response to clonazepam. Neurology 1990;40:1633–1634.

Strafella A, Ashby P, Lang AE: Reflex myoclonus in cortical-basal ganglionic degeneration involves a transcortical pathway. Mov Disord 1997;12:360–369.

Suhren O, Bruyn GW, Tuynman JA: Hyperexplexia: A hereditary startle syndrome. J Neurol Sci 1966;3:577–605.

Tassinari CA, Rubboli G, Parmeggiani L, et al: Epileptic negative myoclonus. In Fahn S, Hallett M, Lüders HO, Marsden CD (eds): Negative Motor Phenomena, vol 67. Philadelphia, Lippincott-Raven, 1995, pp 181–197.

Tassinari CA, Rubboli G, Shibasaki H: Neurophysiology of positive and negative myoclonus. Electroencephalogr Clin Neurophysiol 1998;107:181–195.

Tate ED, Allison TJ, Pranzatelli MR, Verhulst SJ: Neuroepidemiologic trends in 105 US cases of pediatric opsoclonus-myoclonus syndrome. J Pediatr Oncol Nurs 2005;22:8–19.

Terada K, Ikeda A, Van Ness PC, et al: Presence of Bereitschaftspotential preceding psychogenic myoclonus: Clinical application of jerk-locked back averaging. J Neurol Neurosurg Psychiatry 1995;58:745–747.

Thomas JE, Reagan TJ, Klass DW: Epilepsia partialis continua: A review of 32 cases. Arch Neurol 1977;34:266–275.

Thompson PD, Colebatch JG, Brown P, et al: Voluntary stimulus-sensitive jerks and jumps mimicking myoclonus or pathological startle syndromes. Mov Disord 1992;7:257–262.

Thompson PD, Day BL, Rothwell JC, et al: The myoclonus in corticobasal degeneration. Evidence for two forms of cortical reflex myoclonus. Brain 1994;117:1197–1207.

Tijssen MA, Padberg GW, van Dijk JG: The startle pattern in the minor form of hyperekplexia. Arch Neurol 1996;53:608–613.

Tijssen MA, Shiang R, van Deutekom J, et al: Molecular genetic reevaluation of the Dutch hyperekplexia family. Arch Neurol 1995;52:578–582.

Tijssen MA, Vergouwe MN, van Dijk JG, et al: Major and minor form of hereditary hyperekplexia. Mov Disord 2002;17:826–830.

Tijssen MA, Voorkamp LM, Padberg GW, van Dijk JG: Startle responses in hereditary hyperekplexia. Arch Neurol 1997;54:388–393.

Toro C, Hallett M: Pathophysiology of myoclonic disorders. In Watts RL, Koller WC (eds): Movement Disorders: Neurologic Principles and Practice. New York, McGraw-Hill, 1997, pp 551–560.

Toro C, Pascual-Leone A, Deuschl G, et al: Cortical tremor: A common manifestation of cortical myoclonus. Neurology 1993;43:2346–2353.

Traff J, Holme E, Ekbom K, Nilsson BY: Ekbom's syndrome of photomyoclonus, cerebellar ataxia and cervical lipoma is associated with the tRNA(Lys) A8344G mutation in mitochondrial DNA. Acta Neurol Scand 1995;92:394–397.

Truong DD, Kanthasamy A, Nguyen B, et al: Animal models of posthypoxic myoclonus: I. Development and validation. Mov Disord 2000;15:26–30.

Twyman RE, Gahring LC, Spiess J, Rogers SW: Glutamate receptor antibodies activate a subset of receptors and reveal an agonist binding site. Neuron 1995;14:755–762.

Ugawa Y, Hanajima R, Okabe S, Yuasa K: Neurophysiology of cortical positive myoclonus. Adv Neurol 2002;89:89–97.

Vaamonde J, Legarda I, Jimenez-Jimenez J, Obeso JA: Acetazolamide improves action myoclonus in Ramsay Hunt syndrome. Clin Neuropharmacol 1992;15:392–396.

Weizman DA, Leong WL: Anti-Ri antibody opsoclonus-myoclonus syndrome and breast cancer: A case report and a review of the literature. J Surg Oncol 2004;87:143–145.

Werhahn KJ, Brown P, Thompson PD, Marsden CD: The clinical features and prognosis of chronic posthypoxic myoclonus. Mov Disord 1997;12:216–220.

Wijdicks EF, Parisi JE, Sharbrough FW: Prognostic value of myoclonus status in comatose survivors of cardiac arrest. Ann Neurol 1994;35:239–243.

Wilkins DE, Hallett M, Berardelli A, et al: Physiologic analysis of the myoclonus of Alzheimer's disease. Neurology 1984;34:898–903.

Wilkins DE, Hallett M, Erba G: Primary generalised epileptic myoclonus: A frequent manifestation of minipolymyoclonus of central origin. J Neurol Neurosurg Psychiatry 1985;48:506–516.

Yigit A, Sarikaya S: Myoclonus relieved by carbamazepine in subacute sclerosing panencephalitis. Epileptic Disord 2006;8:77–80.

Yiu VW, Kovithavongs T, McGonigle LF, Ferreira P: Plasmapheresis as an effective treatment for opsoclonus-myoclonus syndrome. Pediatr Neurol 2001;24:72–74.

Yoshimura I, Kaneko S, Yoshimura N, Murakami T: Long-term observations of two siblings with Lafora disease treated with zonisamide. Epilepsy Res 2001;46:283–287.

Zimprich A, Grabowski M, Asmus F, et al: Mutations in the gene encoding epsilon-sarcoglycan cause myoclonus-dystonia syndrome. Nat Genet 2001;29:66–69.

# Chapter 22

# Ataxia
## Pathophysiology and Clinical Syndromes

Ataxia is the type of clumsiness that is produced by dysfunction of the cerebellum or cerebellar pathways. The pathophysiology of the signs and symptoms is detailed in the earlier chapter on motor control (Chapter 2). The core symptoms are difficulty with balance and gait, clumsiness of the hands, and dysarthria. The differential diagnosis of the ataxias is very long and includes all types of neurologic pathologic processes. While most patients presenting with ataxia will have a sporadic disorder, there has been increasing attention recently on the genetic ataxias because of the rapid advances in molecular genetics.

## SPORADIC ATAXIA

Box 22-1 lists the principal categories. A series of 112 patients with sporadic ataxia with the following criteria were studied: (1) progressive ataxia, (2) onset after 20 years, (3) informative and negative family history (no similar disorders in first- and second-degree relatives, parents older than 50 years), and (4) no established symptomatic cause (Abele et al., 2002). Thirty-two patients (29%) met the clinical criteria of possible (7%) or probable (22%) multiple-system atrophy (MSA). With genetic testing, Friedreich ataxia (FA) was found in 5 patients (4%), the spinocerebellar ataxia (SCA) type 2 mutation in 1 patient (1%), the SCA3 mutation in 2 patients (2%), and the SCA6 mutation in 7 patients (6%). The disease remained unexplained in 65 patients (58%). Antigliadin antibodies were present in 14 patients, 10 patients with unexplained ataxia (15%) and 4 patients with an established diagnosis (9%); this interesting aspect is discussed further later in the chapter.

### Degenerative Ataxia

MSA is likely the most common disorder, certainly in adults (Wenning et al., 1997, 2000). In addition to ataxia, patients have parkinsonism and autonomic dysfunction (including impotence). The disorder can also be called olivopontocerebellar atrophy when the emphasis is on ataxia, striatonigral degeneration when the emphasis is on bradykinesia and rigidity, and Shy-Drager syndrome when the emphasis is on autonomic dysfunction. Early falls are a prominent feature. Variable clinical features include pyramidal signs, tremor, dysarthria, dystonia, and mild dementia. There is typically a poor response to levodopa, but clearly, at times, there is some response, and this can be confusing. Responses are never dramatic and are typically unsustained. The response of bradykinesia to levodopa depends on whether this parkinsonian sign is due to loss of dopamine receptors in the striatum or only to loss of nigral dopaminergic neurons. The more the striatal localized dopamine receptors are involved, the smaller is the response to levodopa. The pathologic hallmark of the

disorder, in addition to neuronal cell loss, is the glial cytoplasmic inclusion (Dickson et al., 1999).

Laboratory findings of value are particularly autonomic abnormalities. Studies include the skin sympathetic response, the Valsalva maneuver, and heart rate variation. Rectal sphincter electromyography shows denervation, but this test must be done with caution. Women who have been through childbirth may have denervation secondary to their delivery. The specificity of this finding has been called into question. Magnetic resonance imaging (MRI) can show cerebellar and pontine atrophy. The hot cross bun sign in the pons is due to degeneration of corticocerebellar fibers. Magnetic resonance spectroscopy (MRS) can show decreased N-acetyl aspartate signal in the cerebellum, and positron emission tomography (PET) can show decreased cerebellar metabolism.

Another degenerative cause is progressive myoclonic epilepsy, since ataxia is typically a part of this syndrome. Often, myoclonus and ataxia become difficult to separate. These syndromes are described in Chapter 21.

### Strokes

A variety of strokes produce ataxia. These can be due to lesions of the cerebellum or the cerebellar pathways.

Ataxic hemiparesis is characterized by both weakness and incoordination. Lesions can be in the thalamus and posterior limb of the internal capsule, upper basis pontis and cerebral peduncle, parietal lobe, and (debated) anterior internal capsule and frontal lobe.

Hemisensory loss and hemiataxia is typically due to a thalamic lesion.

Isolated gait ataxia can be seen with a lesion of the pontomedullary junction.

Ataxia (hemiataxia and/or gait ataxia) with variable cranial nerve involvement can be seen with involvement of several arteries. The superior cerebellar artery affects the upper pontine tegmentum; the anterior inferior cerebellar artery leads to damage of the lateral pontomedullary junction; and the posterior inferior cerebellar artery gives rise to the well-known lateral medullary syndrome.

### Tumors

The tumors that commonly affect the cerebellum are listed in Box 22-2.

### Toxic/Metabolic Causes

Toxic damage to the cerebellum can be caused by alcohol, both acute and chronic. The acute effects of alcohol appear to cause a true ataxia as measured by physiologic studies. In the chronic state, there can be irreversible cerebellar damage, particularly to the cerebellar vermis and anterior lobe of the cerebellum (Victor and Adams, 1953), leading to particular difficulties with stance and gait. There is also a characteristic prominent anterior-posterior sway when standing.

Hypoxia damages the cerebellum with a particular propensity for the Purkinje cells. Patients with hypoxia may also get myoclonus. Hyperthermia is another cause for Purkinje cell loss.

The childhood hyperammonemias can cause intermittent ataxia.

Celiac disease or sprue is an interesting cause of ataxia and possibly myoclonus (Hadjivassiliou et al., 1998). Celiac disease itself is a gluten-sensitive enteropathy with malabsorption. The gastrointestinal disorder can be reversed with a gluten-free diet, but the cerebellar degeneration does not necessarily get better. Curiously, it is now clear that up to 40% of patients with sporadic ataxia have antigliadin antibodies but no sign of celiac disease (Pellecchia et al., 1999; Burk et al., 2001; Bushara et al., 2001; Hadjivassiliou et al., 2003). This has been disputed, but the power of that study might have been too low (Abele et al., 2003). Antigliadin antibodies are also seen in a similar percentage of patients with genetic ataxias (Bushara et al., 2001). This has also been disputed (Hadjivassiliou et al., 2003), but the percent abnormal might depend on the numbers of the specific SCA types. It is not clear what this means. In some of these patients, there are abnormalities of the white matter and prominent headache; at least these patients have some symptomatic response to a gluten-free diet (Hadjivassiliou et al., 2001). Antibodies to gangliosides were found in 64% of patients with mixed ataxias, suggesting that the increase in antigliadin antibodies may not be specific (Shill et al., 2003). In gluten-associated ataxia, there can also be antibodies

directed to type 2 tissue transglutaminase, and in one patient's brain at autopsy, these antibodies targeted the tissue around the blood vessels (Hadjivassiliou et al., 2006).

Vitamin deficiencies can cause cerebellar dysfunction including thiamine (vitamin $B_1$), vitamin $B_{12}$, and vitamin E. Zinc deficiency might also be a culprit.

In the endocrine area, hypothyroidism, hypoparathyroidism, and hypoglycemia (insulinoma) have been associated with ataxia.

Toxic drugs include thallium, bismuth subsalicylate, methyl mercury, methyl bromide, and toluene. Drugs include phenytoin, carbamazepine, barbiturates, lithium, cyclosporine, methotrexate, and 5-FU. Ataxia can be a component of the serotonin syndrome, from selective serotonin reuptake inhibitors. Overdosage of benzodiazepines can cause ataxia that clears with a lowering of the dose.

## Paraneoplastic Causes

The paraneoplastic causes are very important to keep in mind (Anderson et al., 1988; Bolla and Palmer, 1997). The clinical syndrome is often a rapidly progressive one over a relatively short period of time and then a plateau without further change. What appears to be happening is a rapid destruction of Purkinje cells. Even if the cancer is found and successfully treated, the disorder might well not improve because the cells are irreversibly damaged. Nevertheless, the best treatment is certainly treatment of the cancer.

In many cases, there will be detectable antibodies in the serum. These antibodies are markers of the cancer and are not specific for cerebellar syndromes. Some cases of paraneoplastic ataxia have no defined associated antibody.

There are three types of anti-Purkinje cell antibodies. Anti-Yo (PCA-1) is seen with tumors of breast, ovary, and adnexa. Atypical anticytoplasmic antibody (anti-Tr or PCA-Tr) is seen with Hodgkin disease and tumors of the lung and colon. Recently, PCA-2 has been identified mostly with lung tumors; 3 of 10 patients had ataxia (Vernino and Lennon, 2000).

There are three antineuronal antibodies. Anti-Hu (ANNA-1) can be seen in possible conjunction with encephalomyelitis (Lucchinetti et al., 1998). It is associated with small-cell lung tumor and tumors of breast, prostate, and neuroblastoma. Anti-Ri (ANNA-2) is found with tumors of the breast and ovary. Atypical Anti-Hu is seen with tumors of the lung and colon, adenocarcinoma, and lymphoma.

Anti-CV2 (CRMP) antibody is associated with a syndrome of ataxia and optic neuritis (de la Sayette et al., 1998). It has been seen with small-cell lung carcinoma. The CV2 antigen is expressed by oligodendrocytes. Interestingly, this is one syndrome in which improvement has been seen with removal of the tumor.

Antibodies directed to a serum protein, Ma1, have been seen in patients with testicular and other tumors (Dalmau et al., 1999; Gultekin et al., 2000). The antibodies are anti-Ma and anti-Ta (Ta is Ma2). These patients may also have limbic encephalitis. Ma1 is a phosphoprotein that is highly limited to the brain and testes.

Antibodies directed to amphiphysin have rarely been associated with a cerebellar syndrome (Saiz et al., 1999). This is a marker for small-cell lung carcinoma.

Antibodies against a glutamate receptor can be seen with cancer, and this causes a pure cerebellar syndrome (Sillevis

Smitt et al., 2000). Patients with Hodgkin disease can develop paraneoplastic cerebellar ataxia because of the generation of autoantibodies against mGluR1, and this is mediated by both functional and degenerative effects (Coesmans et al., 2003).

Tests that are currently commercially available include Hu, Ma, Ta, Yo, Ri, and CV2.

In a series of 50 patients with paraneoplastic cerebellar degeneration out of 137 with any neurologic syndrome, 19 had anti-Yo, 16 had anti-Hu, 7 had anti-Tr, 6 had anti-Ri and 2 had anti-mGluR1 (Shams'ili et al., 2003). While 100% of patients with anti-Yo, anti-Tr, and anti-mGluR1 antibodies had ataxia, 86% of anti-Ri patients and only 18% of anti-Hu patients had paraneoplastic cerebellar degeneration. In 42 patients (84%), a tumor was detected; the most common were gynecologic and breast cancer (anti-Yo and anti-Ri), lung cancer (anti-Hu), and Hodgkin lymphoma (anti-Tr and anti-mGluR1). All patients received antitumor therapy, and seven had some neurologic improvement. The functional outcome was best in the anti-Ri patients, with three out of six patients improving neurologically, and five patients were able to walk at the time of last follow-up or death. Survival was worse with anti-Yo and anti-Hu than with anti-Tr and anti-Ri.

## Autoimmune Causes

Ataxia has been seen in association with anti–glutamic acid decarboxylase antibodies (Saiz et al., 1997; Abele et al., 1999; Honnorat et al., 2001). There can be a pure ataxia syndrome and one with an associated peripheral neuropathy. In one series of 14 patients, 13 patients were women and 11 patients had late onset diabetes (Honnorat et al., 2001). Anti–glutamic acid decarboxylase antibodies are better known for the association with stiff-person syndrome, but the relationship is not clear. In one case with antibodies in the cerebrospinal fluid, the antibody blocked GABAergic transmission in the rat cerebellum (Mitoma et al., 2000). As with stiff-person syndrome, patients can exhibit other forms of autoimmunity.

## Infectious/Postinfectious Causes

Infectious causes include rubella and *Haemophilus influenzae*. Acute postinfectious cerebellitis is generally a childhood condition, occurring most commonly after varicella. Creutzfeldt-Jakob disease may have an ataxic form.

## Demyelination

Ataxia is common in multiple sclerosis. A patient with leucoencephalopathy with neuroaxonal spheroids, a rare disease of cerebral and cerebellar white matter, had a 14-year course of progressive neurologic decline consistent with a clinical diagnosis of probable MSA, with prominent cerebellar dysfunction and dysautonomia (Moro-De-Casillas et al., 2004).

## Other Syndromes

Other syndromes include Chiari malformation, abscess, hydrocephalus, and superficial central nervous system hemosiderosis.

## Ataxia of Noncerebellar Origin

What looks like cerebellar ataxia can come from dysfunction outside the cerebellum. The most common causes include neuropathies such as the Miller Fisher form of Guillain-Barré syndrome (O'Leary and Willison, 1997) and spinocerebellar tract lesions.

# GENETIC ATAXIA

One of the most active areas in movement disorders and genetics is in determining the genes for numerous types of hereditary ataxias. Additionally, we are beginning to understand some of the mechanisms of neurodegeneration. On the other hand, specific therapies are still in the future. Many of the genes can be tested commercially. This is helpful, but it is important to remember that genetic testing can have significant consequences, both emotionally and socially, not only for the individual who is tested but also for the family. Hence, testing should be done with care and clear informed consent (Tan and Ashizawa, 2001).

Moseley and colleagues (1998) determined the incidence of SCA types 1, 2, 3, 6, and 7 and FA among a large panel of ataxia families. They collected DNA samples and clinical data from patients representing 361 families with adult-onset ataxia of unknown etiology. Patients with a clinical diagnosis of FA were specifically excluded. Among the 178 dominant kindreds, they found SCA1 expansion at a frequency of 5.6%, SCA2 expansion at a frequency of 15.2%, SCA3 expansion at a frequency of 20.8%, SCA6 expansion at a frequency of 15.2%, and SCA7 expansion at a frequency of 4.5%. Among patients with apparently recessive or negative family histories of ataxia, 6.8% and 4.4%, respectively, tested positive for a CAG expansion at one of the dominant loci, and 11.4% and 5.2% of patients with apparently recessive or sporadic forms of ataxia, respectively, had FA expansions. Among the FA patients, the repeat sizes for one or both FA alleles were relatively small, the sizes for the smaller allele ranging from 90 to 600 GAA repeats. The clinical presentation for these patients was atypical for FA, including adult onset of disease, retained tendon reflexes, normal plantar response, and intact or partially intact sensation. The incidence of the SCAs has also been explored in other countries, such as Australia (Storey et al., 2000) and Taiwan (Soong et al., 2001).

A detailed compendium of the genetic ataxic disorders can be found at http://www.neuro.wustl.edu/neuromuscular/ataxia/aindex.html.

Here the principal disorders are reviewed. There are several good reviews, including those of Di Donato (1998), Subramony and colleagues (1999), Evidente and colleagues (2000), Klockgether (2000), Stevanin and colleagues (2000), Di Donato and colleagues (2001), and Schols and colleagues (2004).

## Dominant Ataxia

The dominant ataxias were divided into three clinical syndromes by Anita Harding (1982): the autosomal-dominant cerebellar ataxias (ADCAs), ADCA I, II, and III. ADCA I is a cerebellar syndrome plus other neurologic degenerations such as pyramidal, extrapyramidal, ophthalmoplegia, and dementia. ADCA II is a cerebellar syndrome with a pigmentary maculopathy. ADCA III is largely a pure cerebellar syndrome, with possible mild pyramidal signs. Subsequently, the genes were identified for these disorders, and they have been called the spinocerebellar ataxias, or SCAs. This terminology is much more common now in clinical use. The identified SCAs are growing rapidly, and clearly there are more to be determined (Devos et al., 2001).

Table 22-1 gives the identified SCAs and their known genetic disorder. Many of them are due to expanded trinucleotide repeats. SCA3 is identical to Machado-Joseph disease (MJD) and is often referred to as SCA3/MJD. Dentatorubro-pallidoluysian atrophy (DRPLA) is often included in such lists. It shares the mutation disorder of CAG expansion and may have prominent ataxia as part of its manifestation. Some details about the proteins are known, and these are listed in Table 22-2.

Commercial tests are available for SCA1, SCA2, SCA3, SCA6, SCA7, SCA8, SCA10, SCA12, SCA17, and dentatorubro-pallidoluysian atrophy (and this list is likely to expand).

Generally, the cerebellar syndrome is similar in the different disorders. Patients experience the gradual onset of balance and gait difficulty, dysarthria, and clumsiness of the hands. There may be visual symptoms, such as blurry vision or diplopia. The age of onset is highly variable. SCA12 might be unique in that it might have a presentation with an action tremor that may look like essential tremor (O'Hearn et al.,

2001). Other manifestations might help in predicting the genotype, but virtually any constellation of signs and symptoms can occur with any phenotype. Some guidelines are noted here.

Lining up the ADCAs and the SCAs gives a start (Table 22-3). Subramony has suggested some phenotypic clues (Subramony et al., 1999), and these are updated in Table 22-4.

Dentatorubro-pallidoluysian atrophy is most common in the Japanese. It is also known as Haw River syndrome from an African-American family in North Carolina. In addition to ataxia, there may be myoclonus, epilepsy, chorea, athetosis, dystonia, dementia, psychiatric disorders, and parkinsonism.

The pathophysiology of the triplet repeat ataxias has been under extensive study (Koeppen, 2005). It does appear that the mutated protein is toxic to the cell. In a mouse model of SCA1, the gene was made conditional; when the gene was turned off, the animals improved (Zu et al., 2004). Similarly, treatment of a mouse model of SCA1 with RNA interference can improve the disorder. Recombinant adeno-associated virus vectors expressing short hairpin RNAs were injected into the cerebellum with marked benefit (Xia et al., 2004).

Then there are the autosomal-dominant episodic ataxias (Table 22-5) (Evidente et al., 2000; Kullmann et al., 2001), known as EA-1, EA-2, and EA-3.

EA-1 is associated with interictal myokymia. There are brief attacks of ataxia and dysarthria lasting seconds to minutes,

**Table 22-1  The SCAs**

| Name | Chromosome | Mutation | Normal Repeat Number | Range of Repeats in the Disorder |
|---|---|---|---|---|
| SCA 1 | 6p | CAG expansion | 6–44 | 40–83 |
| SCA 2 | 12q | CAG expansion | 14–31 | 34–59 |
| SCA 3 | 14q | CAG expansion | 12–38 | 56–86 |
| SCA 4 | 16q | | | |
| SCA 5 | 11c | Deletion or point mutation | | |
| SCA 6 | 19p | CAG expansion | 4–20 | 21–31 |
| SCA 7 | 3p | CAG expansion | 7–17 | 38–>200 |
| SCA 8 | 13q | CTG expansion | 15–91 | 100–155 |
| (SCA 9) | Not Assigned | | | |
| SCA 10 | 22q | ATTCT repeat | 10–22 | 800–3800 |
| SCA 11 | 15q | | | |
| SCA 12 | 5q | CAG expansion | <29 | 66–93 |
| SCA 13 | 19q | | | |
| SCA 14 | 19q | Point mutation | | |
| SCA 15 | 3p | | | |
| SCA 16 | 8q | | | |
| SCA 17 | 6q | CAG expansion | 25–42 | 45–63 |
| SCA 18 | 7q | | | |
| SCA 19 | 1p-q | | | |
| SCA 20 (tentative) | 11 | Point mutation | | |
| SCA 21 | 7p | | | |
| SCA 22 | 1p-q | | | |
| SCA 23 | 20p | | | |
| (SCA 24) | Reserved | | | |
| SCA 25 | 2p | | | |
| SCA 26 | 19p | | | |
| SCA 27 | 13q | Point mutation | | |
| SCA 28 | 18p | | | |
| DRPLA | 12p | CAG expansion | 3–36 | 49–88 |

**Table 22-2** The proteins that are affected in the SCAs

| Name | Protein |
|---|---|
| SCA 1 | Ataxin-1 |
| SCA 2 | Ataxin-2 |
| SCA 3 (MJD) | Ataxin-3 |
| SCA 4 | |
| SCA 5 (also called Lincoln ataxia) | Beta III Spectrin (SPTBN2) |
| SCA 6 | α1a component of the voltage dependent calcium channel: CACNL1A4 |
| SCA 7 | Ataxin-7 |
| SCA 8 | (mutation is in noncoding region) |
| (SCA 9) | |
| SCA 10 | Ataxin-10 |
| SCA 11 | |
| SCA 12 | Protein phosphatase 2A, regulatory subunit B (PPP2R2B) |
| SCA 13 | |
| SCA 14 | Protein kinase Cγ (PRKCG) |
| SCA 15 | |
| SCA 16 | |
| SCA 17 | TATA binding protein |
| SCA 18 | |
| SCA 19 | |
| SCA 20 | |
| SCA 21 | |
| SCA 22 | |
| SCA 23 | |
| SCA 24 | |
| SCA 25 | |
| SCA 26 | |
| SCA 27 | Fibroblast growth factor 14 |
| SCA 28 | |
| DRPLA | Atrophin-1 or DRPLA protein |

**Table 22-4** Clues to the SCAs

| Clinical Feature | Genetic Forms |
|---|---|
| Age at onset | Young adult: SCA1, 2, 3, 21 |
| | Older adult: SCA 6 |
| | Childhood onset: SCA 7, 13, DRPLA |
| Prominent anticipation | SCA 7, DRPLA |
| Upper motor neuron signs | SCA 1, 3, 7,12 |
| | Some in SCA 6, 8 |
| | Rare in SCA 2 |
| Slow saccades | Early, prominent: SCA 2, 7, 12 |
| | Late: SCA 1, 3 |
| | Rare: SCA 6 |
| Extrapyramidal signs | Early chorea: DRPLA |
| | Akinetic-rigid, Parkinson: SCA 2, 3, 21 |
| Generalized areflexia | SCA 2, 4, 19, 21 |
| | Late: SCA 3 |
| | Rare: SCA 1 |
| Visual loss | SCA 7 |
| Dementia | Prominent: SCA 17, DRPLA |
| | Early: SCA 2, 7 |
| | Otherwise: rare |
| Myoclonus | SCA 2, 14 |
| Tremor | SCA 12, 16, 19 |
| Seizures | SCA 10 |

can also be effective (Strupp et al., 2004). The gene for EA-2 is the same as the gene for SCA6, but the nature of the mutation differs. A different missense or truncation mutation in this gene causes familial hemiplegic migraine. There can be phenotypic overlaps among all three conditions. Two patients have been described that progressed to a late-life dystonia (Spacey et al., 2005). Such patients may also have weakness and a disorder at the neuromuscular junction has been demonstrated with single-fiber electromyography (Jen et al., 2001; Maselli et al., 2003).

precipitated by exercise or startle. Onset is in childhood or early adolescence. The myokymia is prominent around the eyes or lips or in the fingers. The myokymia may respond to phenytoin and the ataxia to acetazolamide.

EA-2 has intermittent attacks of ataxia, dysarthria, nausea, vertigo, diplopia, and oscillopsia lasting minutes to days. There may be interictal nystagmus or mild ataxia. Episodes are provoked by stress and exercise but not by startle. About half of the patients also have migraine. The attacks may respond to acetazolamide. The potassium channel blocker 4-aminopyridine

**Table 22-3** Relationship between ADCAs and SCAs

| ADCA type | SCA type |
|---|---|
| I | 1, 2, 3, 4, 12, 16, 17, DRPLA |
| II | 7 |
| III | 5, 6, 8, 11, 14, 15, 22 |
| Ataxia and epilepsy | 10 |
| Early onset with mental retardation | 13 |

**Table 22-5** The episodic ataxias

| Name | Chromosome | Mutation | Protein |
|---|---|---|---|
| EA type 1 | 12p | Missense | Potassium channel, KCNA1 |
| EA type 2 | 19p | Missense | α1a component of the voltage dependent calcium channel: CACNL1A4 |
| EA type 3 | | | |
| EA type 4 | | | |
| EA with paroxysmal choreoathetosis and spasticity | 1p | | |
| EA type 5 | 2q | | CACNB4β4 |

EA-3, called periodic vestibulocerebellar ataxia, is an autosomal-dominant disorder characterized by defective smooth pursuit, gaze-evoked nystagmus, ataxia, and vertigo (Damji et al., 1996).

EA-4 is characterized by vestibular ataxia, vertigo, tinnitus, and interictal myokymia; attacks are diminished by acetazolamide (Steckley et al., 2001).

Episodic ataxia with paroxysmal choreoathetosis and spasticity has an age of onset of 2 to 15 years (Auburger et al., 1996). There are attacks of ataxia, with involuntary movements and dystonia of extremities, paresthesias, and headache. Episodes last about 20 minutes and occur twice per day to twice per year. Precipitating factors include alcohol, fatigue, emotional stress, and physical exercise. In some, there is spastic paraplegia that may persist between attacks. Treatment is with acetazolamide.

EA-5 has been identified in one family and is due to a mutation in a calcium channel gene (Escayg et al., 2000). In other families with a mutation in this gene, there is epilepsy.

## Recessive Ataxia

### FRIEDREICH ATAXIA

The major autosomal-recessive ataxia to consider is Friedreich ataxia (FA), the most common cause of hereditary ataxia, with a prevalence of 1 in 50,000 persons (Bradley et al., 2000; Evidente et al., 2000). Age of onset is generally before 20 years. The clinical features, in addition to ataxia, are dysarthria, sensory loss, and corticospinal tract signs with absent reflexes. There is an axon-loss peripheral neuropathy. There may be skeletal abnormalities, such as kyphoscoliosis, cardiomyopathy, and diabetes. The cardiomyopathy is hypertrophic with possible associated muscular subaortic stenosis or hypokinetic-dilated left ventricle. Abnormal electrocardiograms are common.

The genetic abnormality is usually an expanded trinucleotide repeat of GAA in a gene on chromosome 9q coding for the protein called frataxin, and a commercial genetic test is available. The normal repeat length is 6 to 28; FA patients have 66 to 1700. Six percent of the time, there is a point mutation. Frataxin is a mitochondrial protein encoded by nuclear DNA. It is believed that frataxin is involved in iron transport, and in FA, there is excessive iron accumulation in mitochondria. By using functional MRI, increased iron has been detected in patients in the dentate nucleus (Waldvogel et al., 1999). The excess iron may lead to toxin-free radical damage. There is significant reduction in the activities of complex I, complex II/III, and aconitase in FA heart muscle (Bradley et al., 2000).

In some trials, the free-radical scavenger idebenone has had some success in reducing heart size without clear effect on the ataxia (Rustin et al., 1999, 2002; Hausse et al., 2002; Buyse et al., 2003; Mariotti et al., 2003). One patient had improvement of heart failure with idebenone (Lerman-Sagie et al., 2001). Note, however, that there is also a negative study on cardiac function (Schols et al., 2001). In an open-label trial of nine patients, with an age range of 11 to 19 years, who were treated with idebenone at 5 mg/kg per day, there was a significant reduction in ataxia scores after 3 months of treatment (Artuch et al., 2002). The authors concluded that idebenone treatment at early stages of the disease might reduce the progression of cerebellar manifestations.

There are also some attempts at treatment using coenzyme Q10. Cardiac muscle 31P magnetic resonance spectroscopy has been demonstrated to improve with combination therapy with CoQ10 and vitamin E (Lodi et al., 2001).

Now that the gene can be identified, the phenotype has been widened in recent years. (1) Late-onset FA with an age of onset of more than 25 years characterized by a more benign course, (2) FA with retained reflexes, and (3) the Acadian or Louisiana form with slower progression (Evidente et al., 2000). FA can even present with peripheral neuropathy alone, without ataxia (Panas et al., 2002).

A second gene has been identified whose mutation can lead to classic FA. This has been localized to chromosome 9p (Christodoulou et al., 2001).

### ATAXIA WITH ISOLATED VITAMIN E DEFICIENCY

This is a rare but important disorder that has a phenotype similar to that of FA. Additionally, there can be ophthalmoplegia and retinitis pigmentosa. This disorder is due to a defect in the TTP1 gene coding for $\alpha$-tocopherol transfer protein. This protein incorporates $\alpha$-tocopherol into lipoproteins secreted by the liver. As in the conditions when vitamin E is deficient because of malabsorption, this disorder can be treated with vitamin E (Gabsi et al., 2001). It should not be missed!

### ABETALIPOPROTEINEMIA

Abetalipoproteinemia is a rare autosomal-recessive deficiency of apoB-containing lipoproteins caused by a microsomal triglyceride transfer protein deficiency. With onset in the teenage years or early adulthood, the syndrome is due to vitamin E deficiency. The main characteristics are ataxia and polyneuropathy, as well as acanthocytosis, celiac syndrome, and retinal degeneration (Triantafillidis et al., 1998). It should be treated with high doses of vitamin E.

### ATAXIA TELANGIECTASIA

This disorder is due to a mutation in the *ATM* gene that codes for a protein kinase that plays an important role in cell cycle control, apoptosis, and DNA double-strand break repair. This abnormality leads to an increased incidence of malignancy as well as neurodegeneration. The mutations are scattered over the gene. The disorder begins early in childhood, often age 1 to 2 years (Woods and Taylor, 1992; Di Donato et al., 2001). There is ataxia, truncal more than appendicular, and dysarthria. Oculomotor apraxia, difficulty in initiating saccades, occurs early. Many other features are associated, such as dystonia, masked facies, choreoathetosis, myoclonus, tremor, long tract signs, and, eventually, peripheral neuropathy and cognitive decline. There are the well-known oculocutaneous telangiectasias as well as immunodeficiencies with reduced immunoglobulins and T-cell deficiencies, recurrent sinopulmonary infections, and malignancies, particularly leukemia or lymphoma. Alpha-fetoprotein levels are elevated, and chromosome breaks can be identified.

## EARLY-ONSET ATAXIA WITH OCULAR MOTOR APRAXIA AND HYPOALBUMINEMIA

Two disorders that are recognized in Japan, early-onset ataxia with hypoalbuminemia and ataxia with ocular motor apraxia, are now considered to be the same clinical entity because of the identification of a common mutation in the aprataxin gene (*APTX*). In six patients from four families, cerebellar ataxia and peripheral neuropathy were noted in all patients, ocular motor apraxia was observed in five patients, and choreic movements of the limbs and mental deterioration were observed in five patients (Shimazaki et al., 2002). All patients had hypoalbuminemia and hypercholesterolemia, and brain MRI or computed tomography showed marked cerebellar atrophy. Nerve biopsy revealed depletion of large myelinated fibers in three of the five patients who were examined. This disorder is also common in Portugal but rare in Germany (Habeck et al., 2004). Genetic testing is available. Ataxia with oculomotor apraxia type 2 has also been identified with a similar clinical picture but with mutations in the *SETX* gene (Criscuolo et al., 2006).

## AUTOSOMAL-RECESSIVE SPASTIC ATAXIA OF CHARLEVOIX-SAGUENAY

This disorder of ataxia and pyramidal signs with a high prevalence in northeastern Quebec is due to a mutation in the gene *SACS*, which codes for a protein sacsin (Engert et al., 2000). Even in Quebec, the clinical syndrome is genetically heterogeneous (Thiffault et al., 2006). Although this entity has been thought to be geographically distinct, a family in Tunisia was identified with the disorder (Mrissa et al., 2000). Commercial genetic testing is available for this disorder.

## CAYMAN ATAXIA

Cayman ataxia is a recessive congenital ataxia that is restricted to one area of Grand Cayman Island and appears to be due to one of two mutations (Bomar et al., 2003). The gene *ATCAY* or *Atcay* encodes a neuron-restricted protein called caytaxin. Caytaxin contains a CRAL-TRIO motif that is common to proteins that bind small lipophilic molecules. Mutations in caytaxin are also responsible for the jittery mouse. Mutations in another protein containing a CRAL-TRIO domain, $\alpha$-tocopherol transfer protein, cause the vitamin E–responsive ataxia noted previously.

# OTHER FAMILIAL ATAXIAS

## Familial Cerebellar Ataxia with Muscle Coenzyme Q10 Deficiency

Six patients with muscle CoQ10 deficiency (26% to 35% of normal) presented with cerebellar ataxia, pyramidal signs, and seizures (Musumeci et al., 2001). All six patients responded to CoQ10 supplementation; strength increased, ataxia improved, and seizures became less frequent. In a study of muscle biopsies in 135 patients with undefined cerebellar ataxia, 13 were found to have deficient CoQ10 (Lamperti et al., 2003). The mutation in one family was in the aprataxin gene (Quinzii et al., 2005). This diagnosis is a potentially important cause of familial ataxia because it is at least partially treatable (Artuch et al., 2006).

## Fragile X–Associated Tremor/ Ataxia Syndrome

Recently, attention has been drawn to the fact that the fragile X premutation has been associated with tremor, with appearance similar to essential tremor (Leehey et al., 2003). Ataxia and executive dysfunction are also prominent in this disorder (Hagerman and Hagerman, 2004). Women can be affected as well as men (Hagerman et al., 2004). Fragile X–associated tremor/ataxia syndrome (FXTAS) has a clinical appearance similar to that of MSA, but in a review of 77 patients with an MSA diagnosis, only one person was identified with fragile X–associated tremor/ataxia syndrome (Biancalana et al., 2005), and in another review of 426 patients, only 4 patients had the premutation (Kamm et al., 2005). The neuropathology of this syndrome is characterized by intranuclear inclusions (Greco et al., 2006). An increased signal in the middle cerebellar peduncle can sometimes be seen by MRI.

# DIAGNOSTIC PLAN

In the evaluation of a patient with ataxia, Box 22-3 outlines a reasonable approach. After a good history and physical examination, laboratory tests should be done to follow up clinical suspicions.

# RECOVERY FROM CEREBELLAR INJURY, THERAPY

Chronic signs and symptoms of cerebellar injury differ from those of the acute phase, and signs may disappear entirely, especially when cerebellar damage is sustained early in life or is limited in extent. In general, recovery from lesions limited to regions of the cerebellar cortex, especially of the lateral hemispheres, is potentially greater than recovery from lesions that affect the deep nuclei. This may be due to plasticity at other sites within and outside of the cerebellum, combined with the fact that cerebral repercussions of cerebellar injury might not be especially apparent on conventional testing.

Weakness, deconditioning, and spasticity are often seen in conjunction with ataxia and contribute substantially to its morbidity. All other factors being equal, stronger, more athletic individuals tend to tolerate moderate ataxia better. Specific physical treatments for ataxia with the application of weights might be helpful. The use of added mass to treat certain tremors has a

---

**Box 22-3** Evaluation of the ataxic patient

Good history and physical examination, including a careful family history
Standard laboratory, including lipids and thyroid
Magnetic resonance imaging (and positron emission tomography and/or magnetic resonance spectroscopy if available)
Autonomic testing, sphincter electromyography
Genetic testing
Toxic screen, vitamin levels (especially E)
Paraneoplastic antibodies, antigliadin antibodies

sound mechanical basis. Because the addition of mass lowers the resonant frequency of a limb, it reduces its response to high-frequency oscillating driving signals. Indeed, Hewer and colleagues (1972) found better results in patients who had a tremor frequency greater than 7 Hz. In general, the more severe the tremor in terms of amplitude, the more weight was needed to obtain improvement. In regard to ataxia, up to a point, additional mass also improved ataxia of arm movement and of gait. However, beyond this, increased weight was associated with poorer performance. The optimal weight value varied by individual and was not clearly related to the severity of ataxia. Within the limits of fatigue tolerance, which unfortunately may pose a significant restriction, weight therapy remains a reasonable treatment option for some patients. It is also possible to use devices with incorporated viscous damping (Aisen et al., 1993).

Several agents have been reported to show some ataxia-ameliorating effects. Botez and colleagues (1996) found low levels of the dopamine metabolite homovanillic acid in the cerebrospinal fluid of patients with FA and olivopontocerebellar atrophy, and in a double-blind trial, amantadine produced significant improvements in both movement time and reaction time in patients. Unfortunately, this was not associated with functional improvement. Research, conducted largely in Japan, has emphasized the potential utility of thyrotropin-releasing hormone and many analogues in cerebellar ataxia (Sobue et al., 1983), but these results are generally not dramatic and have not been widely reproduced.

The dense and widespread distribution of serotonergic terminals throughout the cerebellum and spinocerebellar tracts suggests that serotonin plays a major role in regulating cerebellar functions. While some studies have shown benefit in ataxic patients from oral administration of L-5-hydroxytryptophan (L-5-HTP) (Trouillas et al., 1995), there have also been a number of negative results (Wessel et al., 1995). Moreover, L-5-HTP has been associated with a somewhat high rate of unpleasant gastrointestinal side effects, chiefly nausea and diarrhea, even when administered with a peripheral decarboxylase blocker. In addition, L-5-HTP has been associated with a syndrome that resembles eosinophilia-myalgia, although the possible role of contaminants in the preparation has not been fully determined (Michelson et al., 1994). Some attention has shifted toward trials of alternative serotonin agonists. Buspirone is a selective serotonin 1A receptor agonist that has been found by Lou and colleagues (1995) in an open-label study and Trouillas and colleagues (1997) both in an open study and in a randomized double-blind study to produce some small benefit. There has been a double-blind study at NINDS with negative results (S. Massaquoi and M. Hallett, unpublished). Another serotonin 1A receptor agonist, tandospirone, may have some beneficial effects for patients with SCA 3 (Takei et al., 2005). Ondansetron, a 5-HT$_3$ antagonist, may help some patients (Mandelcorn et al., 2004).

There have been reports of a small but persistent improvement in ataxia and possibly arrest of symptom progression in patients treated with physostigmine, either orally or via a transdermal patch (Aschoff et al., 1996), but double-blind studies have failed to demonstrate significant benefit (Wessel et al., 1997). In anecdotal reports (Helveston et al., 1996a, 1996b; Hurd et al., 1996), the antioxidant N-acetylcysteine has been reported to improve ataxia along with a number of other problems in different ataxias, but controlled trials have not been done. A double-blind crossover trial of branched-chain amino acid therapy has suggested some improvement over a 4-week period (Mori et al., 2002). The proposed explanation of efficacy is that this therapy improved glutamatergic transmission in the cerebellum. A small trial of D-cycloserine was successful (Ogawa et al., 2003), and one patient improved significantly on piracetam (Vural et al., 2003). In an open trial, 10 patients improved with gabapentin (Gazulla et al., 2004). Pharmacologic therapy has been reviewed (Ogawa, 2004).

Surgical ablation or high-frequency electrical stimulation of the ventral intermediate nucleus of the thalamus can be effective in reducing cerebellar tremor (Narabayashi, 1992; Nguyen and Degos, 1993); however, these procedures do not significantly lessen ataxia.

## Acknowledgment

This chapter is the work of the U.S. government and is not copyrighted.

## References

Abele M, Burk K, Schols L, et al: The aetiology of sporadic adult-onset ataxia. Brain 2002;125:961–968.

Abele M, Schols L, Schwartz S, Klockgether T: Prevalence of antigliadin antibodies in ataxia patients. Neurology 2003;60: 1674–1675.

Abele M, Weller M, Mescheriakov S, et al: Cerebellar ataxia with glutamic acid decarboxylase autoantibodies. Neurology 1999;52: 857–859.

Aisen ML, Arnold A, Baiges I, et al: The effect of mechanical damping loads on disabling action tremor. Neurology 1993;43:1346–1350.

Anderson NE, Rosenblum MK, Posner JB: Paraneoplastic cerebellar degeneration: Clinical-immunological correlations. Ann Neurol 1988;24:559–567.

Artuch R, Aracil A, Mas A, et al: Friedreich's ataxia: Idebenone treatment in early stage patients. Neuropediatrics 2002;33:190–193.

Artuch R, Brea-Calvo G, Briones P, et al.: Cerebellar ataxia with coenzyme Q(10) deficiency: Diagnosis and follow-up after coenzyme Q(10) supplementation. J Neurol Sci 2006;246:153–158.

Aschoff JC, Kailer NA, Walter K: [Physostigmine in treatment of cerebellar ataxia]. Nervenarzt 1996;67:311–318.

Auburger G, Ratzlaff T, Lunkes A, et al: A gene for autosomal dominant paroxysmal choreoathetosis/spasticity (CSE) maps to the vicinity of a potassium channel gene cluster on chromosome 1p, probably within 2 cM between D1S443 and D1S197. Genomics 1996;31:90–94.

Biancalana V, Toft M, Le Ber I, et al: FMR1 premutations associated with fragile X-associated tremor/ataxia syndrome in multiple system atrophy. Arch Neurol 2005;62:962–966.

Bolla L, Palmer RM: Paraneoplastic cerebellar degeneration: Case report and literature review. Arch Intern Med 1997;157:1258–1262.

Bomar JM, Benke PJ, Slattery EL, et al: Mutations in a novel gene encoding a CRAL-TRIO domain cause human Cayman ataxia and ataxia/dystonia in the jittery mouse. Nat Genet 2003;35: 264–269.

Botez MI, Botez-Marquard T, Elie R, et al: Amantadine hydrochloride treatment in heredodegenerative ataxias: A double blind study. J Neurol Neurosurg Psychiatry 1996;61:259–264.

Bradley JL, Blake JC, Chamberlain S, et al: Clinical, biochemical and molecular genetic correlations in Friedreich's ataxia. Hum Mol Genet 2000;9:275–282.

Burk K, Bosch S, Muller CA, et al: Sporadic cerebellar ataxia associated with gluten sensitivity. Brain 2001;124:1013–1019.

Bushara KO, Goebel SU, Shill H, et al: Gluten sensitivity in sporadic and hereditary cerebellar ataxia. Ann Neurol 2001;49:540–543.

Buyse G, Mertens L, Di Salvo G, et al: Idebenone treatment in Friedreich's ataxia: Neurological, cardiac, and biochemical monitoring. Neurology 2003;60:1679–1681.

Christodoulou K, Deymeer F, Serdaroglu P, et al: Mapping of the second Friedreich's ataxia (FRDA2) locus to chromosome 9p23-p11: Evidence for further locus heterogeneity. Neurogenetics 2001;3:127–132.

Coesmans M, Smitt PA, Linden DJ, et al: Mechanisms underlying cerebellar motor deficits due to mGluR1-autoantibodies. Ann Neurol 2003;53:325–336.

Criscuolo C, Chessa L, Di Giandomenico S, et al: Ataxia with oculomotor apraxia type 2: A clinical, pathologic, and genetic study. Neurology 2006;66:1207–1210.

Dalmau J, Gultekin SH, Voltz R, et al: Ma1, a novel neuron- and testis-specific protein, is recognized by the serum of patients with paraneoplastic neurological disorders. Brain 1999;122:27–39.

Damji KF, Allingham RR, Pollock SC, et al: Periodic vestibulocerebellar ataxia, an autosomal dominant ataxia with defective smooth pursuit, is genetically distinct from other autosomal dominant ataxias. Arch Neurol 1996;53:338–344.

de la Sayette V, Bertran F, Honnorat J, et al: Paraneoplastic cerebellar syndrome and optic neuritis with anti-CV2 antibodies: Clinical response to excision of the primary tumor. Arch Neurol 1998;55: 405–408.

Devos D, Schraen-Maschke S, Vuillaume I, et al: Clinical features and genetic analysis of a new form of spinocerebellar ataxia. Neurology 2001;56:234–238.

Di Donato S: The complex clinical and genetic classification of inherited ataxias: I. Dominant ataxias. Ital J Neurol Sci 1998;19:335–343.

Di Donato S, Gellera C, Mariotti C: The complex clinical and genetic classification of inherited ataxias. II. Autosomal recessive ataxias. Neurol Sci 2001;22:219–228.

Dickson DW, Lin W, Liu WK, Yen SH: Multiple system atrophy: A sporadic synucleinopathy. Brain Pathol 1999;9:721–732.

Engert JC, Bernbe P, Mercier J, et al: ARSACS, a spastic ataxia common in northeastern Quebec, is caused by mutations in a new gene encoding an 11.5-kb ORF. Nat Genet 2000;24:120–125.

Escayg A, De Waard M, Lee DD, et al: Coding and noncoding variation of the human calcium-channel beta4-subunit gene CACNB4 in patients with idiopathic generalized epilepsy and episodic ataxia. Am J Hum Genet 2000;66:1531–1539.

Evidente VG, Gwinn-Hardy KA, Caviness JN, Gilman S: Hereditary ataxias. Mayo Clin Proc 2000;75:475–490.

Gabsi S, Gouider-Khouja N, Belal S, et al: Effect of vitamin E supplementation in patients with ataxia with vitamin E deficiency. Eur J Neurol 2001;8:477–481.

Gazulla J, Errea JM, Benavente I, Tordesillas CJ: Treatment of ataxia in cortical cerebellar atrophy with the GABAergic drug Gabapentin: A preliminary study. Eur Neurol 2004;52:7–11.

Greco CM, Berman RF, Martin RM, et al: Neuropathology of fragile X-associated tremor/ataxia syndrome (FXTAS). Brain 2006;129: 243–255.

Gultekin SH, Rosenfeld MR, Voltz R, et al: Paraneoplastic limbic encephalitis: Neurological symptoms, immunological findings and tumour association in 50 patients. Brain 2000;123:1481–1494.

Habeck M, Zuhlke C, Bentele KH, et al: Aprataxin mutations are a rare cause of early onset ataxia in Germany. J Neurol 2004;251:591–594.

Hadjivassiliou M, Grunewald R, Sharrack B, et al: Gluten ataxia in perspective: Epidemiology, genetic susceptibility and clinical characteristics. Brain 2003;126:685–691.

Hadjivassiliou M, Grunewald RA, Chattopadhyay AK, et al: Clinical, radiological, neurophysiological, and neuropathological characteristics of gluten ataxia. Lancet 1998;352:1582–1585.

Hadjivassiliou M, Grunewald RA, Lawden M, et al: Headache and CNS white matter abnormalities associated with gluten sensitivity. Neurology 2001;56:385–388.

Hadjivassiliou M, Maki M, Sanders DS, et al: Autoantibody targeting of brain and intestinal transglutaminase in gluten ataxia. Neurology 2006;66:373–377.

Hagerman PJ, Hagerman RJ: The fragile-X premutation: A maturing perspective. Am J Hum Genet 2004;74:805–816.

Hagerman RJ, Leavitt BR, Farzin F, et al: Fragile-X-associated tremor/ataxia syndrome (FXTAS) in females with the FMR1 premutation. Am J Hum Genet 2004;74:1051–1056.

Harding AE: The clinical features and classification of the late onset autosomal dominant cerebellar ataxias: A study of 11 families, including descendants of "the Drew family of Walworth." Brain 1982;105:1–28.

Hausse AO, Aggoun Y, Bonnet D, et al: Idebenone and reduced cardiac hypertrophy in Friedreich's ataxia. Heart 2002;87:346–349.

Helveston W, Cibula JE, Hurd R, et al: Abnormalities of antioxidant metabolism in a case of Friedreich's disease. Clin Neuropharmacol 1996a;19:271–275.

Helveston W, Hurd R, Uthman B, Wilder BJ: Abnormalities of glutathione peroxidase and glutathione reductase in four patients with Friedreich's disease [letter]. Mov Disord 1996b;11:106–107.

Hewer RL, Cooper R, Morgan MH: An investigation into the value of treating intention tremor by weighting the affected limb. Brain 1972;95:579–590.

Honnorat J, Saiz A, Giometto B, et al: Cerebellar ataxia with anti-glutamic acid decarboxylase antibodies: Study of 14 patients. Arch Neurol 2001;58:225–230.

Hurd RW, Wilder BJ, Helveston WR, Uthman BM: Treatment of four siblings with progressive myoclonus epilepsy of the Unverricht-Lundborg type with N-acetylcysteine. Neurology 1996;47:1264–1268.

Jen J, Wan J, Graves M, et al: Loss-of-function EA2 mutations are associated with impaired neuromuscular transmission. Neurology 2001;57:1843–1848.

Kamm C, Healy DG, Quinn NP, et al: The fragile X tremor ataxia syndrome in the differential diagnosis of multiple system atrophy: Data from the EMSA Study Group. Brain 2005;128:1855–1860.

Klockgether T: Recent advances in degenerative ataxias. Curr Opin Neurol 2000;13:451–455.

Koeppen AH: The pathogenesis of spinocerebellar ataxia. Cerebellum 2005;4:62–73.

Kullmann DM, Rea R, Spauschus A, Jouvenceau A: The inherited episodic ataxias: How well do we understand the disease mechanisms? Neuroscientist 2001;7:80–88.

Lamperti C, Naini A, Hirano M, et al: Cerebellar ataxia and coenzyme Q10 deficiency. Neurology 2003;60:1206–1208.

Leehey MA, Munhoz RP, Lang AE, et al: The fragile X premutation presenting as essential tremor. Arch Neurol 2003;60:117–121.

Lerman-Sagie T, Rustin P, Lev D, et al: Dramatic improvement in mitochondrial cardiomyopathy following treatment with idebenone. J Inherit Metab Dis 2001;24:28–34.

Lodi R, Hart PE, Rajagopalan B, et al: Antioxidant treatment improves in vivo cardiac and skeletal muscle bioenergetics in patients with Friedreich's ataxia. Ann Neurol 2001;49:590–596.

Lou J-S, Goldfarb L, McShane L, et al: Use of buspirone for treatment of cerebellar ataxia: An open-label study. Arch Neurol 1995;52: 982–988.

Lucchinetti CF, Kimmel DW, Lennon VA: Paraneoplastic and oncologic profiles of patients seropositive for type 1 antineuronal nuclear autoantibodies. Neurology 1998;50:652–657.

Mandelcorn J, Cullen NK, Bayley MT: A preliminary study of the efficacy of ondansetron in the treatment of ataxia, poor balance and incoordination from brain injury. Brain Inj 2004;18:1025–1039.

Mariotti C, Solari A, Torta D, et al: Idebenone treatment in Friedreich patients: One-year-long randomized placebo-controlled trial. Neurology 2003;60:1676–1679.

Maselli RA, Wan J, Dunne V, et al: Presynaptic failure of neuromuscular transmission and synaptic remodeling in EA2. Neurology 2003;61:1743–1748.

Michelson D, Page SW, Casey R, et al: An eosinophilia-myalgia syndrome related disorder associated with exposure to L-5-hydroxytryptophan. J Rheumatol 1994;21:2261–2265.

Mitoma H, Song S, Ishida K, et al: Presynaptic impairment of cerebellar inhibitory synapses by an autoantibody to glutamate decarboxylase. J Neurol Sci 2000;175:40–44.

Mori M, Adachi Y, Mori N, et al: Double-blind crossover study of branched-chain amino acid therapy in patients with spinocerebellar degeneration. J Neurol Sci 2002;195:149–152.

Moro-De-Casillas ML, Cohen ML, Riley DE: Leucoencephalopathy with neuroaxonal spheroids (LENAS) presenting as the cerebellar subtype of multiple system atrophy. J Neurol Neurosurg Psychiatry 2004;75:1070–1072.

Moseley ML, Benzow KA, Schut LJ, et al: Incidence of dominant spinocerebellar and Friedreich triplet repeats among 361 ataxia families. Neurology 1998;51:1666–1671.

Mrissa N, Belal S, Hamida CB, et al: Linkage to chromosome 13q11-12 of an autosomal recessive cerebellar ataxia in a Tunisian family. Neurology 2000;54:1408–1414.

Musumeci O, Naini A, Slonim AE, et al: Familial cerebellar ataxia with muscle coenzyme Q10 deficiency. Neurology 2001;56:849–855.

Narabayashi H: Analysis of intention tremor. Clin Neurol Neurosurg 1992;94:S130–S132.

Nguyen JP, Degos JD: Thalamic stimulation and proximal tremor: A specific target in the nucleus ventrointermedius thalami. Arch Neurol 1993;50:498–500.

Ogawa M: Pharmacological treatments of cerebellar ataxia. Cerebellum 2004;3:107–111.

Ogawa M, Shigeto H, Yamamoto T, et al: D-Cycloserine for the treatment of ataxia in spinocerebellar degeneration. J Neurol Sci 2003;210:53–56.

O'Hearn E, Holmes SE, Calvert PC, et al: SCA-12: Tremor with cerebellar and cortical atrophy is associated with a CAG repeat expansion. Neurology 2001;56:299–303.

O'Leary CP, Willison HJ: Autoimmune ataxic neuropathies (sensory ganglionopathies). Curr Opin Neurol 1997;10:366–370.

Panas M, Kalfakis N, Karadima G, et al: Friedreich's ataxia mimicking hereditary motor and sensory neuropathy. J Neurol 2002;249:1583–1586.

Pellecchia MT, Scala R, Filla A, et al: Idiopathic cerebellar ataxia associated with celiac disease: Lack of distinctive neurological features [see comments]. J Neurol Neurosurg Psychiatry 1999;66:32–35.

Quinzii CM, Kattah AG, Naini A, et al: Coenzyme Q deficiency and cerebellar ataxia associated with an aprataxin mutation. Neurology 2005;64:539–541.

Rustin P, Rotig A, Munnich A, Sidi D: Heart hypertrophy and function are improved by idebenone in Friedreich's ataxia. Free Radic Res 2002;36:467–469.

Rustin P, von Kleist-Retzow JC, Chantrel-Groussard K, et al: Effect of idebenone on cardiomyopathy in Friedreich's ataxia: A preliminary study. Lancet 1999;354:477–479.

Saiz A, Arpa J, Sagasta A, et al: Autoantibodies to glutamic acid decarboxylase in three patients with cerebellar ataxia, late-onset insulin-dependent diabetes mellitus, and polyendocrine autoimmunity. Neurology 1997;49:1026–1030.

Saiz A, Dalmau J, Butler MH, et al: Anti-amphiphysin I antibodies in patients with paraneoplastic neurological disorders associated with small cell lung carcinoma. J Neurol Neurosurg Psychiatry 1999;66:214–217.

Schols L, Bauer P, Schmidt T, et al: Autosomal dominant cerebellar ataxias: Clinical features, genetics, and pathogenesis. Lancet Neurol 2004;3:291–304.

Schols L, Vorgerd M, Schillings M, et al: Idebenone in patients with Friedreich ataxia. Neurosci Lett 2001;306:169–172.

Shams'ili S, Grefkens J, de Leeuw B, et al: Paraneoplastic cerebellar degeneration associated with antineuronal antibodies: Analysis of 50 patients. Brain 2003;126:1409–1418.

Shill HA, Alaedini A, Latov N, Hallett M: Anti-ganglioside antibodies in idiopathic and hereditary cerebellar degeneration. Neurology 2003;60:1672–1673.

Shimazaki H, Takiyama Y, Sakoe K, et al: Early-onset ataxia with ocular motor apraxia and hypoalbuminemia: The aprataxin gene mutations. Neurology 2002;59:590–595.

Sillevis Smitt P, Kinoshita A, De Leeuw B, et al: Paraneoplastic cerebellar ataxia due to autoantibodies against a glutamate receptor. N Engl J Med 2000;342:21–27.

Sobue I, Takayanagi T, Nakanishi T, et al: Controlled trial of thyrotropin releasing hormone tartrate in ataxia of spinocerebellar degenerations. J Neurol Sci 1983;61:235–248.

Soong BW, Lu YC, Choo KB, Lee HY: Frequency analysis of autosomal dominant cerebellar ataxias in Taiwanese patients and clinical and molecular characterization of spinocerebellar ataxia type 6. Arch Neurol 2001;58:1105–1109.

Spacey SD, Materek LA, Szczygielski BI, Bird TD: Two novel CACNA1A gene mutations associated with episodic ataxia type 2 and interictal dystonia. Arch Neurol 2005;62:314–316.

Steckley JL, Ebers GC, Cader MZ, McLachlan RS: An autosomal dominant disorder with episodic ataxia, vertigo, and tinnitus. Neurology 2001;57:1499–1502.

Stevanin G, Durr A, Brice A: Clinical and molecular advances in autosomal dominant cerebellar ataxias: From genotype to phenotype and physiopathology. Eur J Hum Genet 2000;8:4–18.

Storey E, du Sart D, Shaw JH, et al: Frequency of spinocerebellar ataxia types 1, 2, 3, 6, and 7 in Australian patients with spinocerebellar ataxia. Am J Med Genet 2000;95:351–357.

Strupp M, Kalla R, Dichgans M, et al: Treatment of episodic ataxia type 2 with the potassium channel blocker 4-aminopyridine. Neurology 2004;62:1623–1625.

Subramony SH, Vig PJ, McDaniel DO: Dominantly inherited ataxias. Semin Neurol 1999;19:419–425.

Takei A, Hamada T, Yabe I, et al: Treatment of cerebellar ataxia with 5-HT1A agonist. Cerebellum 2005;4:211–215.

Tan E, Ashizawa T: Genetic testing in spinocerebellar ataxias: Defining a clinical role. Arch Neurol 2001;58:191–195.

Thiffault I, Rioux MF, Tetreault M, et al: A new autosomal recessive spastic ataxia associated with frequent white matter changes maps to 2q33-34. Brain 2006;129:2332–2340.

Triantafillidis JK, Kottaras G, Sgourous S, et al: A-beta-lipoproteinemia: Clinical and laboratory features, therapeutic manipulations, and follow-up study of three members of a Greek family. J Clin Gastroenterol 1998;26:207–211.

Trouillas P, Serratrice G, Laplane D, et al: Levorotatory form of 5-hydroxytryptophan in Friedreich's ataxia: Results of a double-blind drug-placebo cooperative study. Arch Neurol 1995:456–460.

Trouillas P, Xie J, Adeleine P, et al: Buspirone, a 5-hydroxytryptamine1A agonist, is active in cerebellar ataxia: Results of a double-blind drug placebo study in patients with cerebellar cortical atrophy. Arch Neurol 1997;54:749–752.

Vernino S, Lennon VA: New Purkinje cell antibody (PCA-2): Marker of lung cancer-related neurological autoimmunity. Ann Neurol 2000;47:297–305.

Victor M, Adams RD: The effect of alcohol on the nervous system. Res Publ Assoc Res Nerv Ment Dis 1953;32:526–573.

Vural M, Ozekmekci S, Apaydin H, Altinel A: High-dose piracetam is effective on cerebellar ataxia in patient with cerebellar cortical atrophy. Mov Disord 2003;18:457–459.

Waldvogel D, van Gelderen P, Hallett M: Increased iron in the dentate nucleus of patients with Friedrich's ataxia. Ann Neurol 1999; 46:123–125.

Wenning GK, Ben-Shlomo Y, Hughes A, et al: What clinical features are most useful to distinguish definite multiple system atrophy from Parkinson's disease? J Neurol Neurosurg Psychiatry 2000;68:434–440.

Wenning GK, Tison F, Ben Shlomo Y, et al: Multiple system atrophy: A review of 203 pathologically proven cases. Mov Disord 1997;12:133–147.

Wessel K, Hermsdorfer J, Deger K, et al: Double-blind crossover study with levorotatory form of hydroxytryptophan in patients with degenerative cerebellar diseases. Arch Neurol 1995;52:451–455.

Wessel K, Langenberger K, Nitschke MF, Kompf D: Double-blind crossover study with physostigmine in patients with degenerative cerebellar diseases. Arch Neurol 1997;54:397–400.

Woods CG, Taylor AM: Ataxia telangiectasia in the British Isles: The clinical and laboratory features of 70 affected individuals. Q J Med 1992;82:169–179.

Xia H, Mao Q, Eliason SL, et al: RNAi suppresses polyglutamine-induced neurodegeneration in a model of spinocerebellar ataxia. Nat Med 2004;10:816–820.

Zu T, Duvick LA, Kaytor MD, et al: Recovery from polyglutamine-induced neurodegeneration in conditional SCA1 transgenic mice. J Neurosci 2004;24:8853–8861.

# Chapter 23

# The Paroxysmal Dyskinesias

The overwhelming majority of individuals with hyperkinetic movement disorders have symptoms that are continuous or continual (e.g., chorea, dystonia, tardive dyskinesia), except for relief with sleep, and with some variation in intensity during periods of stress and relaxation or other factors such as voluntary movements (e.g., action dystonia, intention myoclonus, intention tremor) or maintaining certain postures (e.g., essential tremor). The symptoms and signs of dopa-responsive dystonia sometimes have a diurnal pattern, being absent or slight in the morning hours and becoming more pronounced as the day proceeds (see Chapter 13). Some dyskinesias (Box 23-1) are characterized as occurring intermittently, such as myoclonus (Fahn et al., 1986; Hallett et al., 1987) and startle syndromes (hyperekplexia) (Andermann and Andermann, 1986) that can be triggered by a variety of stimuli. Restless legs syndrome is best described as a diurnal disorder, manifesting itself primarily in the evenings with abnormal crawling sensations that are relieved when the patient moves about and during the night with periodic movements in sleep (Hening et al., 1986; Walters et al., 1991). Sandifer syndrome is a tilting downward of the head after eating a meal, occurring in boys and associated with gastroesophageal reflux (Menkes and Ament, 1988). Movements that occur as a result of akathisia relieve the sensation of inner restlessness. These movements occur intermittently and are usually complex (see Chapter 20). Stereotypies are also complex movements that appear largely in individuals with mental retardation, autism, and schizophrenia (Fahn, 1993). They are not always present but occur frequently and almost continually, but in some patients, they appear as intermittent bursts (Tan et al., 1997). The explanation as to why these patients make these movements is not known, but suggestions such as "being in touch with the environment" have been proposed. Perhaps the commonest dyskinesias that occur intermittently are tics, which are suppressible to varying degrees (Koller and Biary, 1989). Although tics and myoclonic jerks, since they commonly occur out of a normal background, could possibly be considered paroxysmal, this term is usually reserved for an entirely different set of hyperkinetic movement disorders, which is the topic of this chapter. The term *paroxysmal dyskinesia* has been applied to these disorders.

The common neurologic paroxysmal disorders are epilepsy and migraine. Movement disorders that turn up out of the blue and are transient and recurring are uncommon and often appear to the clinician as confusing diagnostic problems. Not uncommonly, the history that is provided by the patient often does not convey the information that the episodes of abnormal movements occur at intermittent intervals, and the clinician might overlook the category of paroxysmal dyskinesias. Therefore, if the examination does not reveal the presence of a movement disorder, the clinician needs to consider the possibility that he or she is dealing with a paroxysmal dyskinesia and thereby ask the appropriate questions that can lead to the proper diagnosis. To compound the problem, nonfamilial paroxysmal movement disorders are often psychogenic in etiology (Bressman et al., 1988); therefore, the clinician has the problem of determining the etiologic distinction of psychogenic versus organic.

The pathophysiology of paroxysmal dyskinesias is not understood, and "epilepsy of the basal ganglia" has been a serious consideration but difficult to prove. Some paroxysmal dyskinesias are supplementary sensorimotor seizures, including many of the hypnogenic variety (Lüders, 1996). The classification of the paroxysmal dyskinesias is still incomplete and evolving (Demirkiran and Jankovic, 1995), and treatment for many of them is often unsuccessful, but treatment for some can be highly successful. A most welcome burst of research on the genetics of the paroxysmal dyskinesias is shedding new light in the classification of these disorders (Nutt and Gancher, 1997), their diagnoses, and their mechanism of action as channelopathies (Griggs and Nutt, 1995) now that the genes that have so far been discovered for these disorders are those that code for some of the ion channels.

## DEFINITIONS: TRANSIENT, PAROXYSMAL, EPISODIC, AND PERIODIC

Some pediatric neurologists have utilized the term *transient* for a number of movement disorders in children, but the concept of paroxysmal dyskinesias is becoming more widely recognized among pediatric neurologists (Lotze and Jankovic, 2003). Excluding tic disorders, Fernandez-Alvarez (1998) reviewed the 356 movement disorder cases under the age of 18 years that had been seen in his department's clinic and reported that 19% of them were classified as transient dyskinesias (Box 23-2). Sometimes, these transient movements can be mistaken for seizures (Donat and Wright, 1990). An accurate diagnosis can be reassuring to the family because these movements are not seizures and are almost always benign. The diagnosis depends on the clinical features; diagnostic tests are normal and unnecessary.

Kotagal and colleagues (2002) evaluated their cases of paroxysmal nonepileptic events. These are reviewed in Chapter 26. These were most common in adolescents and the school-age group. In the preschool group, the most common diagnoses were stereotypies, hypnic jerks, parasomnias, and Sandifer syndrome.

It is not clear how the label paroxysmal became the most common terminology applied to the group of dyskinesias of the choreoathetotic and dystonic type and the label episodic became commonly used for the ataxic variety. According to *Dorland's Medical Dictionary*, a *paroxysm* is defined as (1) a

**Box 23-1** Classic movement disorders that usually appear in bursts or with specific actions but are not considered paroxysmal dyskinesias

---

The movements usually occur so frequently that they are not distinguished with a *paroxysmal* label.
Action and intention tremors
Action dystonia
Action myoclonus
Akathitic movements
Arrhythmic myoclonus
Hyperekplexia
Periodic movements in sleep
Restless legs syndrome
Sandifer syndrome
Stereotypies
Tics

---

sudden recurrence or intensification of symptoms and (2) a spasm or seizure. *Webster's Third International Dictionary* gives a similar definition. *Episodic* is not listed in Dorland's; Webster's defines *episodic* as occurring, appearing, or changing at usually irregular intervals. This definition is not very different from the definition of *paroxysmal* except that the latter includes the word *sudden*. Both terms are reasonable and acceptable.

The term *periodic* is defined by both Dorland's and Webster's as recurring at regular intervals of time. Since the paroxysmal dyskinesias do not recur at regular intervals, the term *periodic* would not be appropriate. Despite this, in neurology, this term is used for the condition of familial periodic paralysis (Rowland and Gordon, 2005) and familial periodic ataxia (Vighetto et al., 1988), even though muscle weakness and ataxia, respectively, in these disorders do not occur at regular intervals. Some authors (Griggs et al., 1978) had used the term *paroxysmal ataxia* in preference to *periodic ataxia*, and others use the term *episodic ataxia* (Zasorin et al., 1983). But the literature today uses *episodic ataxia*.

According to the dictionary definitions, either *paroxysmal* or *episodic* would be an appropriate term for the dyskinesias that are under discussion in this chapter. By common usage and with few exceptions (Margolin and Marsden, 1982), *paroxysmal* has been chosen in preference to *episodic* for the choreoathetotic and dystonic types and is used in this chapter. The term *episodic* is also applied here to the ataxias in keeping with the current trend in the literature. The term *paroxysmal*

**Box 23-2** Transient movement disorders in children seen at the Fernandez-Alvarez (1998) clinic

---

Benign myoclonus of infancy
Benign myoclonus of the newborn
Benign paroxysmal tonic upgaze
Benign paroxysmal torticollis in infancy
Jitteriness
Palatal essential myoclonus
Shuddering
Spasmus nutans
Transient idiopathic dystonia of infancy
Transient tic

---

has been utilized to indicate that the symptoms occur suddenly out of a background of normal motor behavior. It does not define the frequency, severity, duration, aggravating factors, or type of dyskinesia of the attack. These features vary and are important in the current nosology and classification of the paroxysmal dyskinesias.

## HISTORICAL ASPECTS

This is a condensed review of historical highlights of the paroxysmal and episodic dyskinesias. For a more complete discussion, see the review by Fahn (1994). A review of paroxysmal dyskinesias in the Japanese literature is available in English by Hishikawa and colleagues (1973).

### Earliest Descriptions: Reported as Epilepsy

Although Gowers (1885) is often credited with the first report of movement-induced seizures, it is possible that his cases actually represented paroxysmal dyskinesia. One of his patients was a boy whose attack lasted 15 seconds, but the boy was said to be unconscious during his initial attack. Later, he remained awake during the attacks. Another patient was a girl whose attacks started at the age of 11 years and occurred when she arose suddenly after prolonged sitting. But at least one of her attacks was said to be associated with a terrified expression, flushed facies, and dilated pupils. Subsequent to Gowers, a number of reports of "movement-induced seizures" appeared in the literature. Many of these reports have been published under the designation of reflex epilepsy and tonic seizures induced by movement. But unlike most motor convulsions, there was no alteration in the state of consciousness. Moreover, some of these reports had more than tonic contraction; that is, they included sustained twisting, athetosis, and chorea. These characteristics are today referred to as paroxysmal dystonia and paroxysmal choreoathetosis rather than convulsive seizures. Even the presence of choreoathetosis did not lead the earliest interpreters of these brief attacks to conclude they were a movement disorder; instead, they were considered to be a form of epilepsy, the cerebral site of these "seizures" being in the basal ganglia or in the subcortical region.

After the report of Gowers, the next report of movement-induced paroxysmal movements appears to be that of Spiller in 1927. Spiller described two patients with brief tonic spasms that were brought on by voluntary movement of the involved limbs and, in one of them, also by passive manipulation. Spiller called this subcortical epilepsy. Wilson (1930) described a 5-year-old boy who had brief attacks of unilateral torsion and tonic spasm that lasted up to 3 minutes and were precipitated by fright or excitement. There was no loss of consciousness. The attacks could be preceded by pain. Wilson considered this to be reflex tonic epilepsy and thought it also to be subcortical in origin. In more recent times, the concept that these attacks of tonic, often twisting, contractions without loss of consciousness are uncommon seizure disorders has continued (Whitty et al., 1964; Burger et al., 1972). It would appear that today these movement-induced involuntary movements would be considered paroxysmal choreoathetosis/dystonia rather than convulsive movements of the reflex epilepsy type. Differentiation of the attacks between cortical seizures and paroxysmal dyskinesias is sometimes difficult. Clouding of consciousness, if it occurs, would point to a seizure disorder.

By 1966 and 1967, when papers using the term *paroxysmal choreoathetosis* began to appear regularly (Stevens, 1966; Kertesz, 1967; Mushet and Dreifuss, 1967), particularly those cases induced by movements, there were still occasional papers referring to the condition as a seizure disorder. As is discussed later in the chapter, in the section "Paroxysmal Hypnogenic Dyskinesia," nocturnal epilepsy is now considered to be the leading cause.

## Reported as a Paroxysmal Disorder of Involuntary Movements

In 1940, Mount and Reback (1940) introduced a new concept: that of labeling attacks of tonic spasms plus choreic and athetotic movements as a paroxysmal type of movement disorder. They described a 23-year-old man who had had both large and small "spells" since infancy. Both types were preceded by a sensory aura of tightness in parts of the body or by a feeling of tiredness. The movements involved the arms and legs and were usually a combination of sustained twisted posturing and chorea and athetosis. The small attacks lasted from 5 to 10 minutes. Longer attacks were considered large and also involved the neck (retrocollis), eyes (upward gaze), face (ipsilateral to the limbs if the limb involvement was unilateral), and speech. These large attacks lasted for as long as 2 hours, and the movements were considered to resemble those seen in Huntington disease. There was never a loss of consciousness or clonic convulsive movements, biting of the tongue, or loss of sphincter control. Drinking alcohol, coffee, tea, or cola would usually bring on an attack. Fatigue, smoking, and concentrating were other precipitating factors. The attacks would clear more rapidly if the patient lay down and would be aborted by asleep. The patient had an average of one large and two small attacks a day. Between attacks, the neurologic examination was normal. Phenytoin and phenobarbital had no effect, and scopolamine was the only drug that was found to reduce the frequency, severity, and duration of the attacks. The family history revealed 27 other members who had had similar attacks; the pedigree showed autosomal-dominant inheritance with what appears to be complete penetrance. Mount and Reback called this disorder familial paroxysmal choreoathetosis.

Mount and Reback's paper became the seminal paper in the field of paroxysmal dyskinesias. Following its publication, most of the reports in the literature referenced it over the next five decades. However, the next report of a large family with similar attacks of muscle spasms did not refer to it. In 1961, Forssman (1961) described a family with autosomal-dominant inheritance in which there were attacks lasting from 4 minutes to 3 hours.

The next large family was described in 1963 by Lance (1963). Like Forssman (1961), Lance did not relate this to nor refer to Mount and Reback's report, nor did he mention the report by Forssman. In fact, Lance considered his patients to have a form of epilepsy. Later, Lance (1977) was to write one of the definitive papers in this field, containing a useful classification scheme in which he related his family to those of Mount and Reback (1940), Forssman (1961), and Richards and Barnett (1968).

Although there were reports of patients whose paroxysmal dyskinesias were induced by sudden movement, they were not denoted by any special terminology until 1967, when Kertesz (1967) introduced the label *paroxysmal kinesigenic choreoathetosis*. This label has developed into a most useful and widely accepted designation, since the kinesigenic feature has proved to be so characteristic. Kinesigenicity has an important place in the classification of the paroxysmal dyskinesias, and Demirkiran and Jankovic (1995) recommended that the term *paroxysmal kinesigenic dyskinesia* (PKD) be used instead because the movements can be other than choreoathetotic. That suggestion is followed in this chapter. As is pointed out later, the PKD designation can be applied to some patients who do not have the dyskinesias triggered by sudden movement (or startle).

Kertesz reported 10 new cases of paroxysmal dyskinesia and reviewed the literature. Among the important features of his paper, Kertesz differentiated the kinesigenic variety (induced by sudden movement) from that described by Mount and Reback, by Forssman, and by Lance, which were aggravated not by movement but by alcohol, caffeine, and fatigue. (It should be noted that Kertesz differentiated the kinesigenic type from that reported by Mount and Reback [1940] and by Lance [1963], but he failed to mention the paper by Forssman [1961].)

Although phenytoin was recognized earlier as a very useful agent for PKD, carbamazepine was later found to be as useful and was introduced as a treatment by Kato and Araki (1969). This drug currently appears to be the one that is most commonly used for this disorder.

After the 1963 paper by Lance, Richards and Barnett (1968) reported the next big family with the same type of paroxysmal dyskinesia as in Mount and Reback's case and thought that Lance's family (1963) represented a variant, since there were only tonic spasms and no movements in that family. Richards and Barnett emphasized the nonkinesigenic nature of the attacks and felt that the terms *rigidity, tremor, dystonia, torsions spasm, athetosis, chorea,* and *hemiballism* could all be used for such movements, often blending into each other. To emphasize the postural and increased tone, they added *dystonic* to the label. They recommended avoiding the term *epilepsy* until the pathophysiology is better known. Richards and Barnett coined the term *paroxysmal dystonic choreoathetosis* (PDC), which was later adopted by Lance in 1977. The terms *paroxysmal nonkinesigenic choreoathetosis* and *paroxysmal dystonia* are sometimes used instead of *PDC* (Bressman et al., 1988). The term *paroxysmal nonkinesigenic dyskinesia* (PNKD) proposed by Demirkiran and Jankovic (1995) is used here.

The original cases that were reported as PNKD were idiopathic and usually familial. It was not long before symptomatic cases began to be reported in which the attacks of movements were described as a PNKD: perinatal encephalopathy (Rosen, 1964), encephalitis (Mushet and Dreifuss, 1967), and head injury (Whitty et al., 1964; Robin, 1977). However, earlier reports of symptomatic PNKD had been described as a manifestation of multiple sclerosis but considered as a form of epilepsy (Matthews, 1958; Joynt and Green, 1962; Verheul and Tyssen, 1990). Many other etiologies have been reported since the cases in the 1950s and 1960s.

One of the most enlightening papers (Lance, 1977) achieved the following:

1. It discovered Forssman's (1961) paper.
2. It placed together as one syndrome the families that Mount and Reback (1940), Forssman (1961), Lance

(1963), and Richards and Barnett (1968) had reported, bringing them all in under the term *familial paroxysmal dystonic choreoathetosis* (PDC), which has a duration of attacks from 5 minutes to 4 hours.

3. It expanded the description of Lance's own previously reported (1963) family, which he now classified as having this disorder instead of the seizure disorder that he had originally considered.

4. It added another family with paroxysmal dyskinesia that had attacks induced by continuous exercise rather than by sudden movement that affected the legs, with a duration between 5 and 30 minutes. (These were the first cases of what is now recognized as paroxysmal exertional dyskinesia.)

5. It classified the paroxysmal dyskinesias into three groups separated primarily by duration of action (prolonged, intermediate, and brief attacks) and secondarily by precipitating factors.

6. It reported the therapeutic response to clonazepam in some patients with the prolonged attacks.

7. It mentioned normal autopsy findings in two individuals with the prolonged attacks.

8. It summarized the literature to that date.

9. It pointed out that the Forssman and Lance families with the prolonged attacks had dystonic postures without choreoathetosis, whereas the Mount and Reback and the Richards and Barnett families had choreoathetosis.

10. It explained that over time, patients with sustained spasms can eventually develop writhing movements, thereby linking these phenotypes together.

11. It commented that in all types of paroxysmal dyskinesias, males are more affected than females.

Instead of Lance's proposed classification (item 5 in the preceding list) based on duration of the attacks, the classification scheme that is adopted here is the one based on precipitating factors suggested by Demirkiran and Jankovic (1995).

The next historical advances were the recognition that idiopathic PNKD can occur sporadically and not just in families (Bressman et al., 1988) and that sporadic PNKD is often psychogenic in origin (Bressman et al., 1988; Fahn and Williams, 1988).

## Paroxysmal Hypnogenic Dyskinesia

Horner and Jackson (1969) described two families in which several members of the family had attacks of involuntary movement that occurred during sleep. These appear to be the first cases of paroxysmal hypnogenic dyskinesia (PHD) to be reported. Family W is of particular interest because some affected members had classic PKD, some had hypnogenic dyskinesia, and others had a combination. Case 3 in this family began with the hypnogenic variety at age 8. By age 11, daytime attacks also occurred, sometimes triggered by sudden movement. Gradually, the hypnogenic episodes disappeared, leaving the patient with kinesigenic dyskinesia that responded to anticonvulsants. Lugaresi and his colleagues (Lugaresi and Cirignotta, 1981; Lugaresi et al., 1986) independently rediscovered and eventually popularized the syndrome of PHDs.

In addition to these short-duration attacks, Lugaresi and colleagues (1986) reported long-duration hypnogenic attacks.

Such long-duration attacks occur in a minority of individuals with PHD. These longer attacks last from 2 to 50 minutes and do not respond to medication, including anticonvulsants, tricyclics, benzodiazepines, and antipsychotics.

There has long been considerable speculation as to whether the short-duration hypnogenic attacks could be a manifestation of epilepsy, since they respond so well to anticonvulsants. The lack of abnormal electroencephalographic findings during the attack has been used to argue against this concept. However, there is accumulating evidence that many PHDs are indeed due to seizures. Tinuper and colleagues (1990) described three patients with this disorder who had electroencephalographic evidence for frontal lobe seizures as a cause of the attacks. Sellal and colleagues (1991) and Meierkord and colleagues (1992) studied a series of patients with hypnogenic dystonia and concluded that these represent seizure disorders, particularly of frontal lobe epilepsy, because repeated nocturnal electroencephalographic recordings often reveal epileptic patterns of abnormalities. Seizures arising near the mesial posterior frontal supplementary sensorimotor area may be a particular culprit in inducing PHDs in children (Bass et al., 1995). These types of seizures tend to be brief, frequent, and with bilateral tonic posturing, gross proximal limb movements, and preserved consciousness. Dystonic and other dyskinetic features may result from spread of epileptic activity from the mesial frontal region to the basal ganglia because there are close anatomic connections between them. It appears that the short-lasting attacks of PHDs are most likely due to seizures, but the question remains whether patients without abnormal electroencephalograms (EEGs) and more prolonged hypnogenic attacks could have something more akin to the paroxysmal dyskinesias. In a family with autosomal-dominant nocturnal frontal lobe epilepsy, interictal EEGs were normal, but ictal video-electroencephalographic studies showed that the attacks were partial seizures with frontal lobe origin (Scheffer et al., 1995). Fish and Marsden (1994) have reviewed epilepsy masquerading as a movement disorder, and they concluded that most cases of hypnogenic dyskinesias are due to epilepsy, as did Lüders (1996), with a cyclic alternating electroencephalographic pattern believed to be a provocative factor (Terzano et al., 1997).

The genetics of hypnogenic dyskinesias/seizures is being explored. A large autosomal-dominant Australian family (Oldani et al., 1998) and a Norwegian family (Nakken et al., 1999) have been described with mutations in the nicotinic acetylcholine receptor alpha 4 subunit (*CHRNA4*) gene, located on chromosome 20q13.2–q13.3. A second acetylcholine receptor subunit, *CHRNB2*, is also associated with autosomal-dominant nocturnal frontal lobe epilepsy (Phillips et al., 2001). Another family with autosomal-dominant hypnogenic frontal lobe epilepsy has been mapped to 15q24 (Phillips et al., 1998).

In addition to epilepsy mimicking hypnogenic paroxysmal dyskinesias, there is a syndrome of infantile convulsions and paroxysmal dyskinesias, referred to as the infantile convulsions with choreoathetosis (ICCA) syndrome (Lee et al., 1998). The gene for this disorder has been mapped to the pericentromeric region of chromosome 16 (see the discussion in the section on PKD and the discussion in the section titled "Molecular Genetics of Paroxysmal Dyskinesias"). Single photon emission computed tomography (SPECT) studies revealed alterations in local cerebral perfusion in the sensorimotor cortex, the supplementary motor areas, and the pallidum (Thiriaux et al., 2002).

## Transient Paroxysmal Dyskinesias in Infancy

Snyder (1969) introduced a new type of paroxysmal dyskinesia that he called paroxysmal torticollis in infancy. He described 12 cases of intermittent head tilting in young infants. The age at onset was between 2 and 8 months of age, except for three cases in which the first attacks occurred at 14, 17, and 30 months. The attacks would occur about two to three times a month and last from 10 minutes to 14 days, usually 2 to 3 days. The head would tilt to either side and often rotate slightly to the opposite side. There is no distress unless a parent attempts to straighten the head, upon which the baby cries. In some cases, the head tilting is associated with vomiting, pallor, and agitation for a short period. The infant is normal between attacks, which disappear after months or years, usually around age 2 or 3 years. Subsequently, a number of similar cases have been described (Gourley, 1971; Sanner and Bergstrom, 1979; Bratt and Menelaus, 1992), including familial cases (Lipson and Robertson, 1978). Sanner and Bergstrom (1979) reported a patient whose father had a similar condition in early infancy, suggesting that this disorder is hereditary.

 The clinical picture of paroxysmal torticollis in infancy (Video 23-1) that has evolved is that the trunk can also be involved, with lateral curvature concave to the same side as the head tilting, and the ipsilateral leg can be flexed. Onset can be as early as the first months of life, and the symptoms can recur every couple of weeks until they disappear before the age of 2 years. Each attack can last a couple of hours to a couple of weeks. In between attacks, the child is normal. The main differential diagnosis is a posterior fossa tumor and Sandifer syndrome (Menkes and Ament, 1988).

In 1988, the clinical spectrum expanded with the report by Angelini and colleagues (1988) under the name *transient paroxysmal dystonia in infancy*. They described nine patients who had onset of the paroxysmal dyskinesias between 3 and 5 months of age, except for one patient who had an onset at age 1 month. Three had a history of perinatal brain damage; six did not. The attacks consisted of opisthotonus, increased muscle tone with twisting of the limbs, and, in three, neck and trunk twisting, thereby linking this with "paroxysmal torticollis in infancy." The attacks last several minutes, with a maximum of 2 hours in one patient. They would occur from several times per day (Video 23-2) to once a month. Remission occurred between the ages of 8 and 22 months, with two patients not yet having reached a remission.

Dunn (1981) described an infant with head turning and posturing of the right arm lasting from 45 minutes to 18 hours. There were six attacks from age 26 months to age 40 months. The author did not mention the possible diagnosis of paroxysmal torticollis in infancy and made a diagnosis of paroxysmal dystonic choreoathetosis instead. One should consider the possibility that PNKD may occur in infancy and disappear over several months. If so, then the paroxysmal torticollis in infancy of Snyder and the paroxysmal dystonia in infancy of Angelini may represent the lowest age spectrum of PNKD and a benign form of the disorder.

Some patients with benign paroxysmal torticollis of infancy come from kindreds with familial hemiplegic migraine linked to *CACNA1A* mutation, and after recovering from these episodes as they reach childhood, they might have migraines (Giffin et al., 2002).

Intrauterine cocaine exposure can be associated with multiple transient dyskinesias. Beltran and Coker (1995) described four infants who tested positive for cocaine metabolite at birth with subsequent transient dystonic reactions, beginning at 3 hours to 3 months of age and persisting for several months.

The syndrome of transient paroxysmal dyskinesia of infancy should not be confused with the syndrome referred to as benign paroxysmal tonic upgaze of childhood (Ouvrier and Billson, 1988; Deonna et al., 1990; Echenne and Rivier, 1992; Campistol et al., 1993), which is a sustained tonic conjugate upward deviation of the eyes that begins in infancy and eventually disappears in childhood. This appears to be an autosomal-dominant disorder (Guerrini et al., 1998). An infant with tonic upgaze was found to have a partial tetrasomy of 15q (Joseph et al., 2005). Ataxia may be present, and there can be clumsiness and delayed walking. The ocular deviations lessen in the morning hours and disappear with sleep. Acetazolamide is not effective; however, Campistol and colleagues (1993) reported levodopa to be effective. Perhaps *tonic upgaze with diurnal fluctuations* would be a better term than *paroxysmal*. Not all cases of infantile transient tonic upgaze disturbance are benign, although the mean age of offset is 2.5 years (Hayman et al., 1998). Ouvrier and Billson (2005) published a recent review of this disorder.

Another paroxysmal ocular disorder, known as paroxysmal ocular downward deviation, has been described in normal and brain-damaged infants (Yokochi, 1991; Miller and Packard, 1998). The ocular displacement was accompanied by closure of the upper eyelids, and the episodes lasted seconds.

The syndrome of benign myoclonus of infancy can be mistaken for infantile spasms, but the benign EEG and clinical course allow for a clear distinction. The movements are sudden myoclonic and shuddering episodes of the head and shoulders (Lombroso and Fejerman, 1977; Fejerman, 1984). The jerks often repeat in a series; consciousness remains intact.

Another benign paroxysmal disorder in infants is spasmus nutans. It consists of a slow (2.4-Hz) tremor of the head, usually horizontal, and often an associated pendular nystagmus (Antony et al., 1980). It tends to disappear within 6 months and must be differentiated from congenital nystagmus (Fernandez-Alvarez, 1998).

## Episodic (Paroxysmal) Ataxias and Tremor

Intermittent ataxia can be due to metabolic defects such as Hartnup disease (Baron et al., 1956), pyruvate decarboxylase deficiency (Lonsdale et al., 1969; Blass et al., 1970, 1971), and maple syrup urine disease (Dancis et al., 1967). Fever often triggers the attacks of ataxia. In one case with pyruvate decarboxylase deficiency (Blass et al., 1971), choreoathetosis tended to accompany the chorea. Paroxysmal ataxia and dysarthria have also been reported to occur in multiple sclerosis (Andermann et al., 1959; Espir et al., 1966; DeCastro and Campbell, 1967; Miley and Forster, 1974; Gorard and Gibberd, 1989), which, as noted previously, is a disorder that also can cause paroxysmal choreoathetosis/dystonia. The attacks of paroxysmal ataxia due to multiple sclerosis, which last seconds, are much shorter than the attacks described later and can respond to carbamazepine. Paroxysmal ataxia has also been reported in Behçet disease (Akmandemir et al., 1995).

In 1946, Parker described six patients in four families with idiopathic familial paroxysmal ataxia, which he labeled periodic ataxia. The age at onset ranged from 21 to 32 years. The attacks affected gait and speech and lasted from 30 seconds to 30 minutes. There could be several attacks per day, or there could be interval-free periods of several weeks. Vestibular symptoms occurred in some of the patients. Progressive cerebellar ataxia developed in some members.

In 1963, Farmer and Mustian reported a family from rural North Carolina with idiopathic paroxysmal ataxia. The major clinical differences from Parker's cases were the high frequency of accompanying vestibular symptoms of vertigo, diplopia, and oscillopsia and the lack of speech involvement. Farmer and Mustian labeled their family's disorder as vestibulocerebellar ataxia. The age at onset ranged from 23 to 42 years. The attacks ranged from a few minutes to 2 months in duration. The brief episodes could occur daily, but free intervals could last a year or more. Some affected members also developed progressive ataxia.

A second family from the same region in North Carolina also had ocular motility problems. These were abnormal smooth pursuit with normal saccades, dampened optokinetic nystagmus, inability to suppress the vestibulo-ocular reflex, gaze-evoked nystagmus, and episodic attacks of horizontal diplopia, oscillopsia, ataxia, nausea, vertigo, and tinnitus (Damji et al., 1996). This family's disorder was considered part of the same neurologic disorder that is referred to as periodic vestibulocerebellar ataxia, like Farmer and Mustian's family. Of special clinical significance is the lack of dysarthria. Genetic studies showed that the ataxia of this family is distinct from the two types of episodic ataxias (EA-1 and EA-2) that were previously characterized genetically (see later).

Hill and Sherman (1968) described another family, in which onset was in childhood in many of the affected members and there was no development of progressive ataxia. White (1969) described another family that experienced childhood onset and a benign course. All the families showed autosomal-dominant inheritance.

An important advance was the discovery by Griggs and colleagues (1978) that acetazolamide can effectively prevent attacks. These authors showed this benefit in one kindred with familial paroxysmal ataxia. The following year, Donat and Auger (1979) had similar results in another kindred. Fahn (1983, 1984) reported a woman who had paroxysmal tremor, both intention and resting, associated with ataxia and postural instability during the attack; acetazolamide eliminated the attacks. Factor and colleagues (1991) reported an infant who had three attacks of coarse tremor and an orofacial dyskinesia that resembled that seen with tardive dyskinesia. Each attack lasted several hours before spontaneously clearing. Tetrahydrobiopterin, the cofactor for the enzymes tyrosine hydroxylase and phenylalanine hydroxylase, was reduced. The child responded to levodopa.

Mayeux and Fahn (1982) reported a patient with PNKD in a background of hereditary ataxia. Onset of PNKD was at age 10; onset of ataxia was at age 19. During an attack, which could last from 10 minutes to 4 hours, there was an accompanying increase of ataxia. Initially, there was an 8-month response to acetazolamide. After the drug was no longer effective, the patient's PNKD responded to clonazepam. This patient might be a link between familial PNKD and paroxysmal ataxia.

Several other reports of acetazolamide-responsive familial paroxysmal ataxia have been reported (Aimard et al., 1983; Zasorin et al., 1983; Koller and Bahamon-Dussan, 1987). Although computed tomography (CT) has been normal, magnetic resonance imaging studies have revealed selective atrophy in the anterior cerebellar vermis (Vighetto et al., 1988).

Families with a combination of periodic ataxia and persistent, continuous electrical activity in several muscles, reported either as myokymia (Van Dyke et al., 1975; Hanson et al., 1977; Gancher and Nutt, 1986; Brunt and Van Weerden, 1990) or as neuromyotonia (Vaamonde et al., 1991), have been described. Description of the attacks, which are brief and are sometimes preceded by sudden movement, include dyskinetic movements and sustained posturing as well as ataxia, dysarthria, and vertigo. This type of paroxysmal ataxia is now called episodic ataxia 1 (EA-1)

In 1986, Gancher and Nutt (1986) classified the hereditary episodic ataxias into three syndromes. In one group are those cases associated with persistent myokymia or neuromyotonia (now called EA-1). They described the attacks as being precipitated by fatigue, excitement, stress, and physical trauma, but the family reported by Vaamonde and colleagues (1991) had attacks triggered by sudden movement, and kinesigenicity is now recognized as a feature. There is no dizziness or vertigo. The attacks last 2 minutes or less. Acetazolamide and anticonvulsants are usually ineffective. The gene for this type of paroxysmal ataxia has been located at chromosome 12p13 (Litt et al., 1994).

The second group (now known as EA-2) is featured by attacks of ataxia (with or without interictal nystagmus and with or without persistent ataxia), responding to acetazolamide or amphetamines. The attacks are precipitated by exercise, fatigue, or stress and occasionally by carbohydrate or alcohol ingestion. In addition to ataxia, the attacks are accompanied by vertigo, headache, nausea, and malaise. The attacks last for several hours or until the patient falls asleep. In recent years, additional families have been reported with these features (Bain et al., 1991; Baloh and Winder, 1991; Hawkes, 1992). The siblings reported by Bain and colleagues (1991) had persistent diplopia due to superior oblique paresis as part of the syndrome. Using [31P] nuclear magnetic resonance spectroscopy, Bain and his colleagues (1992) found the pH levels in the cerebellum to be increased in untreated subjects with acetazolamide-responsive paroxysmal ataxia; the pH dropped to normal with treatment. The gene for this type of paroxysmal ataxia has been mapped to chromosome 19p13 (Vahedi et al., 1995; Von Brederlow et al., 1995).

Gancher and Nutt (1986) listed a third group, which is kinesigenic. Typical PKD can occur in some members of the family. The attacks of ataxia last minutes to hours, whereas the PKD lasts seconds. The disorder can resolve with time. Acetazolamide appears to be ineffective, but phenytoin is effective for both the kinesigenic ataxia and the PKD. In their review, Griggs and Nutt (1995) place this third type with associated PKD in the first group of paroxysmal ataxias. Genotyping has now definitively placed this as EA-1 (Nutt and Gancher, 1997).

A case was reported in which a young girl had attacks of ataxia associated with fevers and accompanied by vertical supranuclear ophthalmoplegia (Nightingale and Barton, 1991). The ataxia and eye findings can last days.

## Miscellaneous Paroxysmal Disorders

Keane (1984) reported two patients with posttraumatic periodic, rhythmic movements of the tongue. The attacks occurred about every 20 seconds, and each attack lasted 10 seconds. They consisted of three undulations per second. Eventually, the movements diminished. Other cases of episodic lingual dyskinesias were associated with epilepsy (Jabbari and Coker, 1981) and pontine ischemia (Postert et al., 1997).

A few paroxysmal dyskinesias are mentioned here but are not discussed further. These are Sandifer syndrome (prolonged head tilting in children following eating, due to gastroesophageal reflux) (see the review by Menkes and Ament [1988]), hyperekplexia (excessive startle syndrome with complex movements) (see the review by Andermann and Andermann [1986] and Chapter 21), stereotypy (Duchowny et al., 1988; Tan et al., 1997), and paroxysmal bursts of myoclonus and tics. Classically, stereotypy, myoclonus, and tics are each recognized as a specific class of movement disorders, and they characteristically present as paroxysmal bursts of their type of movement. As a result, their discussion should be separated from discussion of conditions labeled as paroxysmal. Shuddering attacks in children (Holmes and Russman, 1986) are brief bursts of rapid shivering-like movements of the head and arms, occurring up to 100 times per day; they can begin in infancy or in older children, and they resolve over time. The attacks last several seconds without impairment of consciousness. The frequency of shuddering movements as seen on electromyography or EEG was similar to that of essential tremor (Kanazawa, 2000).

## CLASSIFICATION OF THE PAROXYSMAL DYSKINESIAS

Because the various movement phenomena in any of the paroxysmal dyskinesias can vary from chorea/ballism to the sustained contractions of dystonia in any given patient, Demirkiran and Jankovic (1995) suggested that these disorders be labeled with the more generic names paroxysmal kinesigenic dyskinesia (PKD), paroxysmal nonkinesigenic dyskinesia (PNKD) (whether short-lasting or long-lasting), and paroxysmal exertion-induced dyskinesia (PED) regardless of the duration of the attack. This classification system is used here, but the paroxysmal dyskinesias that last seconds and might not be induced by sudden movement are also included in the PKD category because of their otherwise similar short duration of attacks and response to anticonvulsants. "Exertion-induced" is also simplified here to "exertional" in PED.

The highlights of various categories of paroxysmal dyskinesias are presented in outline format.

## Paroxysmal Kinesigenic Dyskinesia

Duration: seconds to 5 minutes
Precipitant: sudden movement, startle, or hyperventilation
Treatment: responds well to anticonvulsants

### ETIOLOGY

Primary: familial, sporadic
Secondary

### GENETICS

The syndrome of infantile convulsions and PKD has been mapped to chromosome 16p11.2–q12.1.
The syndrome of PKD without infantile convulsions has been mapped to chromosome 16q13–q22.1. There is no overlap.

*Note:* The effectiveness of anticonvulsants correlates with brief duration of the paroxysms rather than their being triggered by sudden movement. New diagnostic criteria for PKD have been proposed (Bruno et al., 2004a).

**Variant:** A family of paroxysmal kinesigenic atonia has been reported (Fukuda et al., 1999). There was no alteration of consciousness or electroencephalographic findings of epilepsy. Anticonvulsants were effective in reducing the attacks.

## Paroxysmal Nonkinesigenic Dyskinesia (Mount-Reback Type)

Duration: 2 minutes to 4 hours
Precipitant: none
Aggravating factors: alcohol, caffeine, and fatigue
Treatment: not sensitive to anticonvulsants

### ETIOLOGY

Primary: familial, sporadic
Secondary
Alternating hemiplegia of childhood
Psychogenic

### GENETICS OF THREE FAMILIAL TYPES

Familial paroxysmal dyskinesia type 1 on 2q34; myofibrillogenesis regulator 1 (MR-1) gene
Choreoathetosis/spasticity episodica on 1p
Familial infantile convulsions on chromosome 16, called infantile convulsions with choreoathctosis (ICCA) with the gene identified as the sodium/glucose cotransporter

## Paroxysmal Exertional Dyskinesia

Duration: 5 to 30 minutes
Precipitant: continued exertion

### ETIOLOGY

Idiopathic: familial, sporadic
Symptomatic
Psychogenic

### GENETICS

Paroxysmal exertional dyskinesia and autosomal-recessive rolandic epilepsy, chromosome 16p12–11.2

## Paroxysmal Hypnogenic Dyskinesia

1. Brief attacks (many are due to supplementary/frontal lobe seizures)
2. Prolonged attacks

### GENETICS

Chromosome 20q13.2
Chromosome 15q24
Chromosome 1

## Benign Dyskinesias in Infancy and Childhood

1. Paroxysmal dystonia/torticollis in infancy
2. Paroxysmal tonic upgaze or downgaze
3. Paroxysmal myoclonus of infancy
4. Shuddering attacks
5. Spasmus nutans
6. Sandifer syndrome
7. Sterotypies

## Paroxysmal Dyskinesias and Epilepsy

1. PHDs as frontal lobe epilepsy (see earlier)
2. Infantile convulsions and paroxysmal dyskinesias (ICCA) on chromosomes 16p12–q12 and 16q13–q22.1.

## Paroxysmal Ataxia and Tremor

1. EA-1: With myokymia/neuromyotonia
   Attacks: ataxia, dysarthria, or behavioral changes or feeling strange
   Duration: brief, less than 2 minutes
   Precipitant: sudden movement or startle
   Treatment: sometimes sensitive to acetazolamide and to anticonvulsants
   Interictal: persistent myokymia/neuromyotonia
   Other feature: may be accompanied by PKD
   Genetics: point mutations on chromosome 12p13, involving the ion gated potassium channel
2. EA-2: With nystagmus
   Attacks: ataxia and dysarthria
   Duration: hours
   Precipitant: exercise, fatigue, stress, alcohol
   Treatment: sensitive to acetazolamide
   Interictal: nystagmus
   Other features: headache, malaise, may develop persistent ataxia
   Genetics: mapped to chromosome 19p
3. EA-3 with tinnitus and headache
   Attacks: ataxia, tinnitus, falling, headache, blurred vision, vertigo, nausea
   Duration: 10 to 30 minutes
4. EA-4 with ocular motility dysfunction
   Attacks: ataxia, diplopia, oscillopsia, vertigo, nausea, tinnitus
   Duration: minutes to hours
   Precipitants: sudden change in head position, fatigue, and an environment where objects are moving past the patient
   Treatment: lying quietly with eyes closed for 15 to 30 minutes; no response to acetazolamide
   Other features: The episodes become more frequent and then become constant with progressive ataxia.
   Genetics: genetically distinct from other episodic ataxias

Precipitants: none
Treatment: acetazolamide
Other features: myokymia
Genetics: genetically distinct from other episodic ataxias

## PAROXYSMAL KINESIGENIC DYSKINESIA

### Clinical Features

The attacks of PKD consist of any combination of dystonic postures, chorea, athetosis, and ballism (see Video 1-71). They can be unilateral—always on one side or on either side—or bilateral. Unilateral episodes can be followed by a bilateral episode. The attacks are brief, usually lasting only seconds, but rarely can last up to 5 minutes. They are precipitated by a sudden movement or a startle, usually after the patient has been sitting quietly for some time (Video 23-3). The attacks can be severe enough to cause a patient to fall down. There can be as many as 100 attacks per day. After an attack, there is usually a short refractory period before another attack can take place. Speech can sometimes be affected, with inability to speak due to dystonia, but there is never any alteration of consciousness. The attacks can sometimes be aborted if the patient stops moving or warms up slowly. Very often, patients report variable sensations at the beginning of the paroxysms. These can consist of paresthesias, a feeling of stiffness, crawling sensations, or a tense feeling.

Equivalent to PKD are equally brief attacks that are not precipitated by sudden movement or startle. Because the duration and therapeutic response are the same as in PKD, they are listed here under the PKD rubric rather than in an entirely new category. Often, these attacks, lasting a few seconds, can be triggered by hyperventilation.

Kinast and colleagues (1980) reported as Case 4 a patient with typical brief dyskinesias occurring many times a day, preceded by paresthesias, and responding to anticonvulsants but not induced by sudden movement. Although this was technically not PKD, because sudden movements did not trigger any attacks, the clinical features otherwise resemble the attacks that are seen in PKD. As was mentioned previously, this type of paroxysmal dyskinesia is placed in this category of PKD. Since the attacks of PNKD are usually so prolonged and because they do not ordinarily respond to anticonvulsants, this case does not fit into the PNKD category. See the later discussion on this classification of these brief attacks as symptomatic PKD.

Plant (1983) emphasized the focal and unilateral nature of PKD in many patients. Of the 73 cases of PKD in the literature reviewed by him, he found the following types of laterality:

Unilateral, one side only: 25
Unilateral, either side: 12
Unilateral and bilateral: 11
Bilateral only 22
Not stated: 3

### Primary Paroxysmal Kinesigenic Dyskinesia

The etiology of most case reports of PKD has been idiopathic and predominantly hereditary, inheritance being autosomal-dominant. For some unexplained reason males are more often affected than females, with a ratio of 3.75:1 (75 males and 20 females reported in Fahn, 1994). A large series of 150 cases was reported from a questionnaire in Japan. This gender imbalance was supported by the additional 26 cases reported by Houser and colleagues (1999), consisting of 23 men and 3 women, and another 150 cases from Japan (Nagamitsu et al., 1999). Adding all these cases together brings the total to 218 men and 53 women, or a ratio of 4.1:1. Age at onset shows a wide range, usually starting in childhood between the ages of 6 and 16 years, but can range from 6 months to 40 years (Frucht and Fahn, 1999; Li et al., 2005). Excluding the cases by Nagamitsu and colleagues (1999), the mean age at onset is 12 years; the median age is 12 years. Familial cases might be more common among the Japanese (Kishimoto, 1957; Fukuyama and Okada, 1967; Kato and Araki, 1969) and Chinese (Jung et al., 1973). The survey reported by Nagamitsu and colleagues (1999) found 53 sporadic cases and 97 familial ones.

There is one report of the development of PKD in a patient who had essential tremor (Nair et al., 1991). EEGs are generally normal, and CT scans are also normal (Goodenough et al., 1978; Kinast et al., 1980; Suber and Riley, 1980; Bortolotti and Schoenhuber, 1983; Lou, 1989) with a few exceptions, such as the case reported by Watson and Scott (1979) with suggested brainstem atrophy and the one by Gilroy (1982) with an ill-defined unilateral hemispheric lesion. However, Hirata and colleagues (1991) demonstrated an abnormal EEG with rhythmic 5-Hz discharges over the entire scalp during episodes of PKD, raising the possibility that the PKD might have an epileptogenic basis. A patient was reported who developed PKD shortly after initiation of therapy with methylphenidate for attention deficit/hyperactivity disorder. Attacks persisted long after methylphenidate was discontinued and responded to treatment with carbamazepine (Gay and Ryan, 1994). The authors believe that the patient had a hereditary susceptibility for PKD that was triggered by the drug.

The attacks tend to diminish with age. Fortunately, PKD responds dramatically to anticonvulsants. The early literature indicates that phenytoin was the most popular, followed by phenobarbital and primidone. Carbamazepine appears to be the drug that is most commonly used. Valproate has also been effective (Suber and Riley, 1980), although Hwang and colleagues (1998) report that both carbamazepine and phenytoin were superior to valproate. Other anticonvulsants are effective also, including oxcarbazepine (Gokcay and Gokcay, 2000), lamotrigine (Pereira et al., 2000; Uberall and Wenzel, 2000), levetiracetam (Chatterjee et al., 2002), oxcarbazepine (Tsao, 2004), and topiramate (Huang et al., 2005b). There is one report of response to levodopa (Loong and Ong, 1973) but another report of lack of effect with this drug (Garello et al., 1983). Analogously, there is one report of three patients with PKD worsening with haloperidol (Przuntek and Monninger, 1983), but Garello and colleagues (1983) reported no effect from this drug (as well as levodopa) in two brothers. The calcium channel blocker flunarizine, which is also a neuroleptic, was effective in a 7-year-old girl, who did not respond to carbamazepine or methylphenidate (Lou, 1989).

Homan and colleagues (1980) reported that children with PKD need doses of phenytoin that are similar to those used to treat epilepsy, whereas adults can respond to lower doses. These authors also describe a patient who might have had interictal chorea (the patient was described as fidgety) and suggested that this might represent a possible link to benign hereditary chorea. However, the fidgetiness that was described might not have

been chorea. On the other hand, these authors supported their notion with the report by Bird and colleagues (1978), in which a woman had anxiety-induced dystonia/choreoathetosis and random, adventitious small jerky movements when she was not having an attack (first reported by Perez-Borja et al., 1967); her daughter had delayed milestones and persistent choreoathetosis. However, it seems likely that the daughter's choreoathetosis is not idiopathic but secondary, so it seems that paroxysmal dyskinesias and hereditary benign chorea should not be linked on the basis of a couple of these cases.

The pathophysiology of PKD is still unclear, and its relationship with epilepsy remains speculative. Because movement-induced seizures can occur (e.g., the case of Falconer et al., 1963) and because PKD responds dramatically to anticonvulsants, these are not sufficient reasons to consider PKD a form of epilepsy. The retention of consciousness and lack of postictal phenomena, as well as the presence of dystonia and choreoathetosis, should be sufficient to disqualify PKD from the epilepsies. However, Beaumanoir and colleagues (1996) described a boy with PKD and normal EEGs and consciousness who later had a longer attack with clouding of consciousness and recording of postictal abnormalities on the EEG to support the diagnosis of reflex epilepsy. There is emerging a syndrome of infantile epilepsy followed by childhood paroxysmal dyskinesias, referred to as the ICCA syndrome, as was mentioned earlier in the chapter (Lee et al., 1998; Thiriaux et al., 2002).

Franssen and colleagues (1983) investigated the contingent negative variation in one patient with PKD. Contingent negative variation is a slow cerebral potential that follows a warning stimulus, which prepares the subject to expect an imperative stimulus requiring a decision or motor response. The slow negative wave component of the contingent negative variation was more pronounced than that in control subjects. It returned to normal after phenytoin treatment. Mir and colleagues (2005) later demonstrated reduced intracortical inhibition, reduced early phase transcallosal inhibition, and reduced first phase of spinal reciprocal inhibition in PKD patients; treatment with carbamazepine normalized the abnormality of transcallosal inhibition.

The differential diagnosis of PKD is focal epilepsy, tetany, hyperekplexia, tics, stereotypies, and hysteria, as was noted in the misdiagnosis of the case reported by Waller (1977). The clinical features are so distinctive, particularly if triggered by sudden movement, that there is little likelihood of not diagnosing the condition correctly once one is aware of its existence. Similarly, the markedly effective response to anticonvulsants sets PKD apart from the other disorders. One case of primary PKD has been observed to be the result of a consistent ictal discharge arising focally form the supplementary sensorimotor cortex, with a concomitant discharge recorded from the ipsilateral caudate nucleus without spread to other neocortical areas (Lombroso, 1995), which suggests that some primary PKDs could be epileptic in origin. The nonkinesigenic, brief attacks of hemidystonia, often precipitated by hyperventilation and controlled with anticonvulsants, have been considered a sign of epilepsy (Kotagal et al., 1989; Newton et al., 1992). So each case of such suspected nonkinesigenic paroxysmal dyskinesia needs to be evaluated for a convulsive disorder.

In addition to the cases of PKD described in the historical highlights earlier in the chapter, a number of other reports should be cited to make the review complete (Zacchetti et al., 1983; Boel and Casaer, 1984; Lang, 1984). One case of paroxysmal torticollis induced by sudden movement or stimulus appeared 5 years after the onset of classic spasmodic torticollis that had begun at age 20 years (Lagueny et al., 1993). After failing to respond to alcohol, tiapride, haloperidol, carbamazepine, clobazam, and valproate, the patient was treated effectively with injections of botulinum toxin.

There have been reports of two autopsies in PKD. Case 4 of Kertesz (1967) died, apparently by suicide, and a postmortem examination revealed no clear-cut abnormality in the brain, just the presence of some melanin pigment in macrophages in the locus coeruleus. Stevens (1966) had earlier reported the postmortem findings of one of his patients, which were also essentially normal, showing only a slight asymmetry of the substantia nigra.

SPECT scans measuring cerebral blood flow were studied in two children with PKD, revealing increased perfusion in the contralateral basal ganglia at the onset of an attack in one (Ko et al., 2001) and in the contralateral thalamus in the other (Shirane et al., 2001).

Three independent laboratories have mapped autosomal-dominant PKD with infantile convulsions (ICCA syndrome) to chromosome 16p11.2–q12.1 (Tomita et al., 1999; Bennett et al., 2000; Swoboda et al., 2000). A second locus on this chromosome at 16q13–q22.1 has been found in other families, referred to as EKD2 (Valente et al., 2000). This locus does not overlap with those of the other families. This family is distinct from the others by not having infantile convulsions. Evidence for a third locus, called EKD3, has been suggested because three families did not map to the two known ones on chromosome 16 (Spacey et al., 2002).

A familial atonic form of PKD has been reported (Fukuda et al., 1999).

# Secondary Paroxysmal Kinesigenic Dyskinesia

The overwhelming majority of reported cases of PKD are idiopathic or familial. Although not reported as often, symptomatic PKD is probably more common. Box 23-3 lists the most common causes of symptomatic PKD, the most common being associated with multiple sclerosis and head injury. Pseudohypoparathyroidism has recently been added to this list (Huang et al., 2005a). In one family with X-linked mutations in the thyroid hormone transporter gene *MCT8*, paroxysmal dyskinesias accompanied global mental retardation (Brockmann et al., 2005).

In symptomatic PKD, like primary PKD, attacks that last seconds are sometimes induced not by sudden movement but by hyperventilation. These also usually respond to anticonvulsants, such as carbamazepine, and are also seen in multiple sclerosis (Verheul and Tyssen, 1990; Sethi et al., 1992). Fahn (unpublished data) has encountered a patient who had attacks lasting seconds, induced by hyperventilation and without being induced by sudden movement, following a mild cerebral ischemic episode, that also responded to carbamazepine. These pharmacologic responses suggest that the briefness of the attack is more important than is the sudden movement to distinguish the classification of the paroxysmal dyskinesias. Sethi and colleagues (1992) reported success in treating three patients with paroxysmal dystonia (not induced by movement but triggered by hyperventilation and lasting many seconds) with acetazolamide with or without the addition of carbamazepine.

## MULTIPLE SCLEROSIS

Although few of the paroxysmal dyskinesias that are associated with multiple sclerosis are triggered by sudden movement, an occasional patient with multiple sclerosis manifests typical PKD (Matthews, 1958). In fact, the presenting symptom of multiple sclerosis can be PKDs, as in the case reported by Roos and colleagues (1991); these attacks were associated with a lesion in the caudate nucleus and responded to phenytoin. In three of the eight patients reported by Berger and colleagues (1984) with paroxysmal dyskinesia associated with multiple sclerosis, the attacks were induced by sudden movement; they were relieved by anticonvulsants. The patient with PKD with multiple sclerosis reported by Burguera and colleagues (1991) had a lesion in the left thalamus demonstrated by magnetic resonance imaging. The PKD was the presenting symptom, as in other cases of demyelinating disease. Gatto and colleagues (1996) reported medullary lesions in multiple sclerosis and bilateral paroxysmal dystonia.

## HEAD TRAUMA

Case 3 of Whitty and colleagues (1964) was a 13-year-old boy with onset 9 months after mild head trauma. Robin (1977) reported a 33-year-old man with severe head injury who developed PKD 8 months later. In two of the three cases of posttraumatic paroxysmal dyskinesias reported by Drake and colleagues (1986), the movements were induced by sudden movement of the affected body part. Richardson and colleagues (1987) reported another posttraumatic case. These posttraumatic cases of PKD responded to anticonvulsants, similar to idiopathic PKD. Attacks of dystonia lasting several seconds and induced by tactile stimulation were reported secondary to a head injury; they disappeared within 2 months without treatment (George et al., 1990). Nijssen and Tijssen (1992) reported another case of tactile-induced dyskinesias as a result of a thalamic infarct.

**Box 23-3** Symptomatic paroxysmal kinesigenic dyskinesia

Multiple sclerosis
Head injury
Perinatal hypoxic encephalopathy
Idiopathic hypoparathyroidism
Pseudohypoparathyroidism
Basal ganglia calcifications
Hemiatrophy
Putaminal infarct
Thalamic infarct
Moyamoya disease
Medullary lesion (hemorrhage, subarachnoid cyst)
HIV infection
Hyperglycemia in the presence of a lenticular vascular malformation
Progressive supranuclear palsy
Spinal cord lesion
Huntington disease

### PERINATAL HYPOXIC ENCEPHALOPATHY

Rosen (1964) appears to have been the first to report a case of PKD associated with perinatal hypoxic encephalopathy, with the onset at age 12. This boy's attacks were usually triggered by a combination of startle and body contact. Mushet and Dreifuss (1967) described a 9-year-old boy who developed brief attacks of athetosis and dystonia. They usually occurred when he was startled but also could occur following sudden movement. At age 6 months, he had a febrile illness, which was retrospectively thought to be encephalitis. He had considerable motor regression and was not able to walk, nor did he gain syntactical speech. His dyskinetic attacks were not suppressed by anticonvulsants but did respond to anticholinergics.

### BASAL GANGLIA CALCIFICATIONS

PKD has been reported to occur with basal ganglia calcifications with or without hypoparathyroidism (Arden, 1953). Subsequent cases of hypoparathyroidism were reported (Tabaee-Zadeh et al., 1972; Barabas and Tucker, 1988). The clinical syndrome resembles that of primary infantile convulsions and childhood PKD (Hattori and Yorifuji, 2000). Calciferol was effective in controlling these attacks. The case reported by Soffer and colleagues (1977) was not noted to have the attacks induced by sudden movement, but the briefness of the attack resembles that of PKD.

### HEMIATROPHY

Case 2 of the five cases described by Kinast and colleagues (1980) had attacks of left hemidystonia lasting 1 minute and occurring up to 50 times a day. The major precipitating factor was not sudden movement but stress and the anticipation of movement (also reported in one patient by Franssen et al., 1983). Technically, like their Case 4 described earlier, this patient does not fulfill the criterion of attacks induced by sudden movement. This is another example, because of the brief duration, the frequency of the attacks, and their response to phenytoin, that otherwise resembles PKD and again points out why such nonkinesigenic cases are placed under the PKD rubric in the classification scheme used here. Examination of this revealed left-sided hemiatrophy and hyperreflexia with a normal CT scan. Because the hemiatrophy syndrome can be associated with a delayed-onset movement disorder (Buchman et al., 1988), it seems reasonable to consider it an etiologic factor in this particular case.

Gilroy (1982) reported a 32-year-old man with an abnormal right hemisphere on CT scan who had had multiple daily brief attacks of left hemidystonia since the age of 5 that were typical of PKD. The speculation is that the PKD was secondary to pathology in the involved hemisphere. An arteriogram and cortical biopsy did not shed further light on the pathology.

### CEREBRAL INFARCTS AND HEMORRHAGES

With the advent of magnetic resonance imaging, more cases of PKD have been reported as a result of cerebral infarcts, with  putaminal infarct (Merchut and Brumlik, 1986), thalamic infarct (Video 23-4) (Camac et al., 1990; Nijssen and Tijssen, 1992; Milandre et al., 1993), an infarct probably in the cortex (Fuh et al., 1991), and medullary hemorrhage (LeDoux,

1997). As was mentioned earlier, the case of Nijssen and Tijssen (1992) had attacks stimulated by touch of the affected limb. The attacks secondary to infarcts (Merchut and Brumlik, 1986; Fuh et al., 1991) or to multiple sclerosis (Sethi et al., 1992) can be painful tonic spasms. Riley (1996) reported a case of paroxysmal attacks of tightening of his throat muscles and elevation of his tongue to the roof of his mouth associated with a remote hemorrhage in the medulla. Moyamoya disease has been reported to cause PKD (and PNKD) (Gonzalez-Alegre et al., 2003).

### OTHER ETIOLOGIES

PKD has also been reported to occur in a patient with progressive supranuclear palsy (Adam and Orinda, 1986), in hyperglycemia in the presence of a lenticular vascular malformation (Vincent, 1986), in spinal cord lesion (Cosentino et al., 1996), and in subacute sclerosing panencephalitis (Ondo and Verma, 2002). A case of PKD was reported in which it was the first symptom in a patient who developed Huntington disease (Scheidtmann et al., 1997). HIV infection has been reported to be associated with PKD and PNKD (Mirsattari et al., 1999). A lesion in the medulla has been associated with PKD (Jabbari et al., 1999).

## PAROXYSMAL NONKINESIGENIC DYSKINESIA

### Clinical Features

As with PKD, the attacks of PNKD consist of any combination of dystonic postures, chorea, athetosis, and ballism. They can be unilateral—always on one side or on either side—or bilateral. Unilateral episodes can be followed by a bilateral one. They can affect a single region of the body or be generalized. Involvement of the neck can be a combination of torticollis and head tremor (Hughes et al., 1991). The major distinctions from PKD are the longer duration of each attack (see Video 1-32), the smaller frequency of the attacks, and a host of different aggravating factors for the attacks. The attacks last minutes to hours, sometimes longer than a day. Usually, they range from 5 minutes to 4 hours (Video 23-5). They are primed by consuming alcohol, coffee, or tea; by psychological stress or excitement; and by fatigue. There are usually no more than three attacks per day, and attacks may be months apart. The attacks can be severe enough to cause a patient to fall down. Speech is often affected, with inability to speak due to dystonia, but there is never any alteration of consciousness. The attacks can sometimes be aborted if the patient goes to sleep. As with PKD, patients very often report variable sensations at the beginning of the paroxysms. These can consist of paresthesias, a feeling of stiffness, crawling sensations, or a tense feeling.

A form of PNKD known as intermediate PDC, and more recently as paroxysmal exertional dyskinesia, is triggered only by prolonged exercise and not the other precipitants. This was first described by Lance (1977) and subsequently reported in another family by Plant and colleagues (1984) and in a sporadic case by Nardocci and colleagues (1989). In the classification scheme of Demirkiran and Jankovic (1995), this form, which is discussed separately, is called paroxysmal exertional dyskinesia (PED).

## Primary Paroxysmal Nonkinesigenic Dyskinesia (Mount-Reback Syndrome)

The initial reports of PNKD were familial (Mount and Reback, 1940; Forssman, 1961; Lance, 1963; Weber, 1967; Richards and Barnett, 1968; Horner and Jackson, 1969; Lance, 1977; Tibbles and Barnes, 1980; Walker, 1981; Mayeux and Fahn, 1982; Przuntek and Monninger, 1983; Jacome and Risko, 1984), hereditary transmission being autosomal-dominant. Kinast and colleagues in 1980 (Case 4) and Dunn in 1981 each described a child with PNKD without a positive family history. Bressman and colleagues (1988) later described seven sporadic cases of PNKD, and Nardocci and colleagues (1989) added another one. The familial cases of idiopathic PNKD still greatly outnumber sporadic cases, according to the reports in the literature. However, the sporadic cases are much more difficult to diagnose, and they have the difficulty of the need to be differentiated from a psychogenic etiology (Bressman et al., 1988; Fahn and Williams, 1988). On the basis of the experience of Bressman and her colleagues (1988), the sporadic form might actually be more common than the familial form but is rarely reported.

For some unexplained reason, males are slightly more often affected than females, with a ratio of 1.4:1 (32 males and 23 females reported in the reviewed English literature) (see Fahn, 1994). Age at onset shows a wide range, usually in childhood between the ages of 6 and 16 years, but can range from 2 months to 30 years. The mean age at onset is 12 years; the median is 12 years. CT scans are normal (Mayeux and Fahn, 1982; Jacome and Risko, 1984).

The EEGs are generally normal, but the case of Jacome and Risko (1984) may be of interest. The patient had unilateral PNKD and had normal interictal EEGs. Photic stimulation at low frequencies induced paroxysmal lateralized epileptiform discharges from the contralateral hemisphere. From this, the authors suggest that the disorder might have some epileptogenic basis.

Sleep aborted the episodes in one family that had myokymia in addition to the PNKD (Byrne et al., 1991). The presence of myokymia links this particular family to several with paroxysmal ataxia, in which myokymia is a feature (Van Dyke et al., 1975; Vaamonde et al., 1991).

A family reported by Kurlan and colleagues (1987) had some atypical features for classic PNKD. The long-duration attacks were painful dystonic spasms that were not precipitated by alcohol, caffeine, or excitement but could follow exposure to cold or heat or result from exertional cramping. Other members of the family had only exertional cramping without PNKD. The authors suggested that exertional cramping might be a forme fruste of PNKD. It is also possible that the PNKD in this family falls into the category of the intermediate form of paroxysmal dyskinesia that was reported by Lance (1977) and Plant and colleagues (1984). Also unusual was the presence of some fixed dystonia, which had not been reported previously. Bressman and colleagues (1988) also described some sporadic cases of PNKD in which the patients had some interictal dystonia.

Lance (1977) mentioned that autopsies performed on two patients with PNKD revealed no pathology. His Case II.4 had normal macroscopic findings. His Case IV.2 died of sudden infant death syndrome; macroscopic and microscopic findings were normal.

The attacks can diminish spontaneously with age (Lance, 1977; Kinast et al., 1980; Bressman et al., 1988). Unfortunately, most patients have persistence of their attacks, and they are difficult to treat. As a general rule, PNKD does not respond to the same type of anticonvulsants that so effectively treat PKD. An occasional patient will respond to such agents as carbamazepine, valproate, and gabapentin (Chudnow et al., 1997). Clonazepam, as introduced for PNKD by Lance (1977), appears to be the most successful agent for both primary PNKD and symptomatic PNKD. A number of other drugs have been tried, sometimes with success. These include antimuscarinics (Mount and Reback, 1940), chlordiazepoxide (Perez-Borja et al., 1967; Walker, 1981), acetazolamide (Mayeux and Fahn, 1982; Bressman et al., 1988), oxazepam and other benzodiazepines (Kurlan and Shoulson, 1983; Kurlan et al., 1987), sublingual lorazepam (Dooley and Brna, 2004), and L-tryptophan, (Kurlan et al., 1987).

Kurlan and Shoulson (1983) treated one patient with familial PNKD on alternate-day oxazepam. He had marked benefit from diazepam but only for 4 weeks. Clonazepam and oxazepam gave relief for 2 to 3 weeks each. Eventually, he was placed on a regimen of 40 mg oxazepam given on alternate days. The concept was that the benzodiazepine receptors became desensitized on daily doses. Alternate-day administration prevented this desensitization.

Przuntek and Monninger (1983) and Coulter and Donofrio (1980) carried out trials of the dopamine receptor antagonist haloperidol and reported benefit. In the obverse, Przuntek and Monninger (1983) found that levodopa worsened one patient.

Chronic stimulation of the ventral intermediate nucleus of the thalamus was effective in reducing the frequency, duration, and intensity of attacks in one patient with PNKD (Loher et al., 2001). At least one patient with PNKD has been treated successfully with deep brain stimulation of the globus pallidus interna (Yamada et al., 2006).

In contrast to idiopathic PKD, which is so distinctive, the major difficulty in the diagnosis of sporadic PNKD is to differentiate it from a psychogenic movement disorder. The problem is that the disappearance of the movements with placebo or psychotherapy could be coincidental, since the attacks disappear spontaneously. However, if the paroxysms are frequent and the attacks are prolonged, then repeated trials with placebo can be informative. If such trials consistently produce remissions, then one can be convinced that the diagnosis is a psychogenic disorder (see Chapter 26).

Three different genetic mappings have been made for PNKD. The first type, originally described by Mount and Reback (1940), is referred to genetically as familial paroxysmal dyskinesia type 1, which was mapped to 2q33–35 (Fink et al., 1996; Fouad et al., 1996; Hofele et al., 1997; Matsuo et al., 1999). One of these families (Pzuntek and Monninger, 1983; Hofele et al., 1997) shows a fair response to diazepam. The second type of PNKD has additional clinical features, including perioral paresthesias, double vision, and headache during attacks, and some also have a constant spastic paraparesis; this type was mapped to chromosome 1p (Auburger et al., 1996) and has been called choreoathetosis/spasticity episodica. The third type of PNKD has been seen in familial infantile convulsions, in which the gene has been mapped to the pericentromeric region of chromosome 16 (Szepetowski et al., 1997). This has been called infantile convulsions with paroxysmal choreoathetosis (ICCA). The gene has been identified as the sodium/glucose cotransporter (Roll et al., 2002).

## Secondary Paroxysmal Nonkinesigenic Dyskinesia

The overwhelming majority of reported cases of PNKD are idiopathic or familial in etiology, but a number of cases of symptomatic PNKD have been reported. Box 23-4 lists the most common causes of symptomatic PNKD.

The most common cause of symptomatic PNKD, just like PKD, is multiple sclerosis (Matthews, 1958; Joynt and Green, 1962; Lance, 1963; Berger et al., 1984; Verheul and Tyssen, 1990; Sethi et al., 1992). In multiple sclerosis, the paroxysmal movements may only be ocular, lasting several minutes (MacLean and Sassin, 1973). One patient with paroxysmal hemidystonia associated with multiple sclerosis later developed psychogenic PNKD (Morgan et al., 2005).

The next two most common causes are perinatal encephalopathy (Lance, 1963; Erickson and Chun, 1987; Bressman et al., 1988) and psychogenic (Video 23-6) (Bressman et al., 1988; Fahn and Williams, 1988; Lang, 1995). A longer discourse of psychogenic PNKD is presented in Chapter 26.

Other causes of PNKD are encephalitis (Video 23-7) (Mushet and Dreifuss, 1967; Bressman et al., 1988), cystinuria (Cavanagh et al., 1974), hypoparathyroidism (Soffer et al., 1977; Yamamoto and Kawazawa, 1987; Dragasevic et al., 1997), basal ganglia calcifications without altered serum calcium (Micheli et al., 1986), thyrotoxicosis (Fischbeck and Layzer, 1979), transient ischemic attacks (Margolin and Marsden, 1982; Bennett and Fox, 1989), infantile hemiplegia (Huffstutter and Myers, 1983), head trauma (Perlmutter and Raichle, 1984; Drake et al., 1986), hypoglycemia (Newman and Kinkel, 1984; Winer et al., 1990; Schmidt and Pillay, 1993), AIDS (Nath et al., 1987), diabetes (Haan et al., 1988), anoxia (Bressman et al., 1988), brain tumor (Bressman et al., 1988), hypoglycemia induced by an insulinoma (Shaw et al., 1996), and poststreptococcal autoimmune neuropsychiatric disease (Dale et al., 2002). The patient with AIDS (Nath et al., 1987) had two attacks of dystonia, but details are lacking in regard to the duration or characteristics of the attacks. Moyamoya disease has been reported to cause PNKD (and PKD) (Gonzalez-Alegre et al., 2003).

There is a case report of one person who developed paroxysmal hemidystonia after starting fluoxetine, which cleared on discontinuing the drug (Dominguez-Moran et al., 2001). Related to transient ischemic attacks mentioned earlier is the case of one patient who had paroxysmal hemidystonia precipitated by assuming an upright position after sitting or lying, associated with occlusion of the contralateral internal carotid artery and near-total occlusion of the ipsilateral internal carotid artery (Sethi et al., 2002). The authors called this *orthostatic paroxysmal dystonia*. A SPECT study demonstrated decreased perfusion in the contralateral frontoparietal cortex during the typical dystonic spell. PNKD has now been reported in the antiphospholipid syndrome (Engelen and Tijssen, 2005). A series of 17 cases of secondary paroxysmal dyskinesias was reported by Blakeley and Jankovic (2002), who found that 9 patients had PNKD, 2 patients had PKD, 5 patients had mixed PKD/PNKD, and 1 patient had PHD.

PNKD caused by endocrine disorders responds to appropriate treatment. But in general, treatment of symptomatic PNKD is not often effective.

Micheli and colleagues (1987) reported an interesting case of a mentally retarded youth who had received dopamine receptor–blocking drugs since the age of 3. At age 16, he developed paroxysmal dystonia. The attacks could be precipitated by stress but not by movement, caffeine, cold, fatigue, or hyperventilation. The episodes lasted from 30 minutes to 3 hours. They did not respond to anticonvulsants but were abolished with trihexyphenidyl 20 mg per day. It is possible that the PNKD in this youth represented a variant of tardive dystonia (Burke et al., 1982; Kang et al., 1986).

A PET study was performed on one patient with posttraumatic paroxysmal hemidystonia (Perlmutter and Raichle, 1984). Decreased oxygen metabolism, decreased oxygen extraction, increased blood volume, and increased blood flow in the contralateral basal ganglia were found.

The syndrome commonly known as alternating hemiplegia of childhood typically contains periods of prolonged dystonic attacks, along with other elements of the syndrome (Bourgeois et al., 1993). The syndrome begins before 18 months of age. In addition to prolonged periods of dystonia, there are attacks of nystagmus, dyspnea, and autonomic phenomena. Episodes of quadriplegia appear either when a hemiplegia shifts from one side to the other or as an isolated manifestation. The episodes were often followed by developmental deterioration. Eventually, there is cognitive impairment and a choreoathetotic movement disorder. Sleep relieves the weakness and other paroxysmal phenomena, but they can reappear after awakening. The attacks can last from a few minutes to several days. Flunarizine is partially effective. Some infants manifest paroxysmal dystonia before the classic features of alternating hemiplegia develop (Andermann et al., 1994). Magnetic resonance spectroscopy was normal in the case reported by Nezu and colleagues (1997).

**Box 23-4** Symptomatic paroxysmal nonkinesigenic dyskinesia

Multiple sclerosis
Perinatal hypoxic encephalopathy
Psychogenic
Encephalitis
Idiopathic hypoparathyroidism
Basal ganglia calcifications
Thyrotoxicosis
Transient ischemic attacks
Infantile hemiplegia
Cystinuria
Head injury
Hypoglycemia
AIDS
Diabetes
Anoxia
Brain tumor
Tardive syndrome(?)
Alternating hemiplegia of childhood
Antiphospholipid syndrome
Moyamoya disease

## PAROXYSMAL EXERTIONAL DYSKINESIA

Lance (1977) was the first to describe what he called an intermediate form of PDC (now called PNKD). Today, this family would appear to have PED. The family had attacks that were briefer than those in classic PNKD, lasting from 5 to 30 minutes, and in which the attacks were precipitated by prolonged exercise and not by cold, heat, stress, ethanol, excitement, or anxiety. The spasms affected mainly the legs. Plant and colleagues (1984) reported a second family. In both families, the inheritance pattern was that of autosomal-dominant transmission. In neither family did anyone derive any benefit from barbiturate, levodopa, or clonazepam. Sporadic cases are also seen (Video 23-8), such as the case reported by Nardocci and colleagues (1989) (Case 3). This patient also had interictal chorea without any family history of a similar condition. This patient was helped by clonazepam. Wali (1992) reported another sporadic case; this was an 18-year-old man in whom attacks of right hemidystonia lasting about 10 minutes were precipitated by prolonged running (about 10 minutes) or by cold. The EEG and the CT scan were normal; anticonvulsants were not helpful. Demirkiran and Jankovic (1995) mentioned seeing five patients, three being females. The largest series of sporadic cases is that by Bhatia and colleagues (1997). Familial cases appear to be autosomal-dominant (Kluge et al., 1998). A large family with PED with four affected members had onset at 9 to 15 years of age and a male:female ratio of 3:1 (Munchau et al., 2000).

The 26 reported cases consisted of 13 women and 13 men. The age at onset ranged from 2 to 30 years, all but six beginning in childhood.

Some patients labeled as PKD (e.g., Cases 1 and 3 of Jung and colleagues [1973]) and PNKD (e.g., the family of Kurlan and associates [1987]) have attacks that occur after prolonged exercise. It is possible that such patients have a variant of PNKD or a combination of PNKD and one of the other paroxysmal dyskinesias. However, if the attacks last only seconds and respond to anticonvulsants, they fit clinically with these features of PKD.

The family reported by Schloesser and colleagues (1996) supports the notion that PED is a variant of PNKD. The father of the proband was affected by exertional cramping, and two other men in the family had PED. Women in the family had more prolonged attacks, fitting those of PNKD.

Ictal and interictal cerebral perfusion SPECT studies have been conducted (Kluge et al., 1998). During the motor attacks, decreased perfusion of the frontal cortex and increased cerebellar perfusion were observed. The perfusion of the basal ganglia also decreased. No cortical hyperperfusion indicative of an epileptic nature was seen. The authors conclude that PED represents a paroxysmal movement disorder rather than epilepsy. Posteroventral pallidotomy has been reported to ameliorate attacks of PED (Bhatia et al., 1998).

In a patient with familial PED, different stimuli and maneuvers in triggering dystonic attacks in the arm were studied. Motor paroxysms could be provoked by muscle vibration, passive movements, transcranial magnetic stimulation, magnetic stimulation of the brachial plexus, and electrical nerve stimulation but not by sham stimulation (Meyer et al., 2001). The authors conclude that dystonic attacks are triggered by proprioceptive afferents.

Guerrini and colleagues (1999) described a family with PED and autosomal-recessive rolandic epilepsy, with the gene mapped to chromosome 16p12–11.2 (That family's dystonia resembles the ICCA syndrome, and the genetic mapping overlaps with that syndrome.) Perniola and colleagues (2001) described another family with autosomal-dominant PED and epilepsy; fasting and stress were also precipitating factors.

In a study in which cerebrospinal fluid monoamine metabolites were measured before and after the attack, a twofold increase in the concentration of homovanillic acid and 5-hydroxyindoleacetic acid was detected after the attack (Barnett et al., 2002).

A case of PED foot dystonia in an adult was found to be due to the earliest symptom of Parkinson disease, as established by dopamine transporter binding and SPECT and effectively treated with dopaminergic medication (Katzenschlager et al., 2002). Two other adults (second cousins) who presented with paroxysmal exercise-induced dystonia later developed clinical features of Parkinson disease (Bruno et al., 2004b).

Table 23-1 lists the major distinguishing features of nonepileptic PKD, PNKD, and PED.

## EPISODIC ATAXIAS

The paroxysmal ataxias, called episodic ataxias, have been distinguished by their clinical features and by their genotypes. These characteristics are presented and summarized in Table 23-2.

The genes for two of the hereditary episodic ataxias have been determined. In one of them, EA-1, the type associated with myokymia or neuromyotonia, has been found to be due to point mutations in the gene $Kv1.1$ for the voltage-gated potassium channel ($KCNA1$) (Browne et al., 1994; Comu et al., 1996). The gene is located on chromosome 12p13 (Litt et al., 1994). Different mutations have been found in different families (D'Adamo et al., 1998; Zerr et al., 1998; Eunson et al., 2000). The attacks are brief, lasting seconds to minutes; myokymia is present during and between attacks. The attacks can be triggered by sudden movement (Nutt and Gancher, 1997), and these can respond to anticonvulsants. Some families have episodes of myokymia without ataxia (Eunson et al., 2000). In one family, mutations in the KCNA1 gene can cause severe neuromyotonia resulting in marked skeletal deformities without episodic ataxia, and others in the family had the ataxia (Kinali et al., 2004).

Another episodic ataxia, EA-2, is the type that has a vestibular component and does not have myokymia as an associated feature. The attacks last between 15 minutes and a few days and respond to acetazolamide. The gene was mapped to chromosome 19p13 (Vahedi et al., 1995; Von Brederlow et al., 1995) and mutations in the gene were found for the calcium channel CACNA1A (Spacey et al., 2005). Spontaneous mutations (Yue et al., 1998) as well as familial cases have been described. There is clinical heterogeneity, with attacks varying from pure ataxia to combinations of symptoms that suggest involvement of the cerebellum, brainstem, and cortex. Oculographic findings were localizing to the vestibulocerebellum and posterior vermis. Some affected individuals exhibited a progressive ataxia syndrome that is phenotypically indistinguishable from the dominantly inherited SCA syndromes. SCA6 has been found to be due to an expanded CAG repeat on the same gene (Zhuchenko et al., 1997). Two patients with childhood onset EA-2 developed adult-onset dystonia (Spacey et al., 2005). About one half of the affected individuals have migraine headaches, and several have episodes that are typical of basilar migraine (Baloh et al., 1997). Both familial hemiplegic migraine and EA-2 are caused by mutations in the $Ca^{2+}$ channel gene CACNL1A4 and can be considered as allelic channelopathies (Ophoff et al., 1996). When progressive

**Table 23-1** Symptomatic paroxysmal nonkinesigenic dyskinesia

| Feature | PKD | PNKD | PED |
|---|---|---|---|
| Male:female | 4:1 | 1.4:1 | 13:13 (n = 26) |
| Inheritance | AD | AD | AD |
| Genetic mapping | 1. 16p11.2–q12.1 (also designated as DYT10) | 1. Mount-Reback syndrome 2q34 (FDP1) (also designated as DYT8) myofibrillogenesis regulator 1 (MR-1) gene | With autosomal-recessive rolandic epilepsy; 16p12–11.2 |
| | 2. 16q13–q22.1, possibly identical with ICCA and the sodium/glucose cotransporter gene (see #3 in PNKD) | 2. With diplopia and spasticity (CSE); chromosome 1p21 (also designated as DYT9) | |
| | | 3. With familial infantile convulsions; ICCA, chromosome 16, pericentric, sodium/glucose cotransporter | |
| Age at onset | | | |
| Range: | <1–40 | <1–30 | 2–30 |
| Median: | 12 | 12 | 11.5 |
| Mean: | 12 | 12 | 12 |
| Attacks | | | |
| Duration | <5 minutes | 2 minutes–4 hours | 5 minutes–2 hours |
| Frequency | 100/day–1/month | 3/day–2/year | 1/day–2/month |
| Trigger | Sudden movement, startle, hyperventilation | nil | Prolonged exercise; muscle vibration; nerve stimulation; TMS of motor Cx. |
| Precipitant | Stress | ETOH, stress, caffeine, fatigue | Stress |
| Movement pattern | Any combination of dystonic postures, chorea, athetosis, and ballism; unilateral or bilateral | Any combination of dystonic postures, chorea, athetosis, and ballism; unilateral or bilateral | Any combination of dystonic postures, chorea, athetosis, and ballism; unilateral or bilateral |
| Treatment | Anticonvulsants | Clonazepam, benzodiazepines, acetazolamide, antimuscarinics | Acetazolamide, antimuscarinics, benzodiazepines |

AD, autosomal dominant; CSE, choreoathetosis/spasticty episodic; ETOH, ethanol; ICCA, infantile convulsions with choreathetosis; PED, paroxysmal exertional dyskinesia; PKD, paroxysmal kinesigenic dyskinesia; PNKD, paroxysmal nonkinesigenic dyskinesia; TMS, transcranial magnetic stimulation.

ataxia is present, there is cerebellar atrophy on magnetic resonance imaging scans, and not all cases have a CAG expansion (Yue et al., 1997). On the other hand, cases with the CAG expansion and cerebellar atrophy can also have EA-2 (Jodice et al., 1997). A family with the phenotype of EA-2 was found not to have a mutation of the CACNL1A gene on chromosome 19p13, indicating genetic heterogeneity for this disorder (Hirose et al., 2003).

Not all families with migraine and episodic vertigo could be linked to the EA-2 markers on chromosome 19p, indicating genetic heterogeneity for this type of episodic ataxia (Baloh et al., 1996).

A third type has also been described (Steckley et al., 2001). This autosomal-dominant episodic ataxia is manifested by vestibular ataxia, vertigo, tinnitus, and interictal myokymia; attacks are diminished by acetazolamide. EA-1 and EA-2 genetics were excluded. The fourth type of paroxysmal ataxia with ocular motility problems can be precipitated by sudden head movement. The gene for this fourth type of EA has not yet been mapped but is genetically distinct from EA-1 and EA-2.

Sporadic cases of episodic ataxias occur. Four patients with autopsies had ataxia resembling EA-2 but did not respond to acetazolamide, nor did their molecular genetics workup fit EA-2 (Julien et al., 2001).

## MOLECULAR GENETICS OF PAROXYSMAL DYSKINESIAS

PKD with infantile convulsions has been mapped to 16p11.2–q12.1 (Tomita et al., 1999; Bennett et al., 2000; Swoboda et al., 2000). PKD without convulsions has been mapped to 16q13–q22.1 with the gene referred to as *EKD2* (Valente et al., 2000). The ICCA syndrome has also been reported without linkage to these two loci (Spacey et al., 2002).

A family with infantile convulsions has an associated PNKD, and the abnormal gene has been mapped to chromosome 16 (Szepetowski et al., 1997). The gene in this region that appears to be responsible for ICCA is the sodium/glucose cotransporter gene (*KST1*) (Roll et al., 2002). It also appears to be responsible for benign familial infantile convulsions. Perhaps this disorder with its genetic mapping has been referred to by others as PKD with infantile convulsions (see the first paragraph in this section). Guerrini (2001) proposes that disparate reports of families suggest that the same gene could be responsible for rolandic epilepsy, PED, writer's cramp, and PNKD, with specific mutations accounting for each of these Mendelian disorders. Evidence is for a major gene or a cluster of genes for epilepsy and paroxysmal

**Table 23-2** Clinical and genetic features of episodic ataxias

| Type | Age at Onset | Acetazolamide | | Precipitant | Frequency/Duration | Interictal | Gene |
| | | Clinical | Response | | | | |
| --- | --- | --- | --- | --- | --- | --- | --- |
| Myokymia, neuromyotonia (EA-1) | 2–15 | Aura of weightless or weak, then ataxia, dysarthria, tremor, **facial twitching** | In some kindreds; **anticonvulsants** may help | **Startle, movement,** exercise, excitement, fatigue | **Up to 15 per day;** usually one or fewer per day; seconds to **minutes,** usually 2–10 minutes | **Myokymia,** shortened Achilles tendon; **PKD** | **12p13, K⁺ channel,** different point mutations in KCNA1 |
| Vestibular (EA-2) | 0–40, usually 5–15 | Ataxia, vertigo, **nystagmus,** dysarthria, HA, ptosis, ocular palsy, vermis atrophy | Very effective | Stress, alcohol, fatigue, exercise, caffeine | Daily to q 2 months; usually **hours;** 5 minutes to weeks | **Nystagmus,** mild **ataxia,** less common: dysarthria and progressive cerebellar | **19p13, Ca⁺ channel** CACNL1A4 familial hemiplegic migraine |
| Tinnitus (EA-3) (Steckley et al., 2001) | 1–41 | Ataxia, tinnitus, falling, headache, blurred vision, vertigo, nausea | Effective | None | Daily; 10–30 minutes | Myokymia; some with ataxia | 1q42 |
| Ocular (EA-4) (Damji et al., 1996) | 20–50 | Ataxia, diplopia, vertigo, nausea | No response | Sudden change in head position | Daily to year; **minutes to hours** | Symptoms gradually become constant | Unknown |

PKD, paroxysmal kinesigenic dyskinesia.

dyskinesia to the pericentromeric region of chromosome 16. These families need to be tested for the KST1 gene.

Two papers independently reported the mapping of a gene for PNKD to chromosome 2q31–36 (Fink et al., 1996; Fouad et al., 1996), and the region has been narrowed to 2q33–q35 by Fink and colleagues (1997). Another family was mapped by Raskind and colleagues (1998), who narrowed the region to 2q34. Jarman and colleagues (1997) mapped the gene to a large British family. Although a cluster of sodium channel genes is near the PNKD locus, the mutated gene has now been found to be the myofibrillogenesis regulator 1 (MR-1) (Lee et al., 2004). The mutations in this gene were associated with PNKD in 50 individuals from eight families; they cause changes (Ala to Val) in the N-terminal region of two MR-1 isoforms. The MR-1L isoform is specifically expressed in the brain and is localized to the cell membrane, while the MR-1S isoform is ubiquitously expressed and shows diffuse cytoplasmic and nuclear localization. The MR-1 gene is homologous to the hydroxyacylglutathione hydrolase gene, which functions in a pathway to detoxify methylglyoxal, a compound that is present in coffee and alcoholic beverages and is produced as a by-product of oxidative stress. The finding of the MR-1 gene locus suggests a mechanism whereby alcohol, coffee, and stress may act as precipitants of attacks in PNKD. However, there is genetic heterogeneity in PNKD, because there is a Canadian family without this mutation, with links to a separate locus at 2q31 instead (Spacey et al., 2006).

Auburger and colleagues (1996) studied a family with PNKD with associated spasticity; their mutated gene was mapped to a potassium channel gene cluster on chromosome 1p. The attacks are said to consist of dystonia of limbs, imbalance, dysarthria, diplopia, and sometimes headache. The attacks last about 20 minutes and can be precipitated by exercise, stress, lack of sleep, and alcohol consumption. Some affected members had persistent spastic paraparesis, which would make this family different from those with classic Mount-Reback syndrome. This condition has been called choreoathetosis/spasticity episodica.

A large Australian family with autosomal-dominant hypnogenic frontal lobe seizures/dystonia has been found to have a missense mutation in the second transmembrane domain of the nicotinic acetylcholine receptor alpha 4 subunit (CHRNA4) gene, located on chromosome 20q13.2–13.3 (Oldani et al., 1998). A second locus has been found on chromosome 15q24 (Phillips et al., 1998, 2001), and a third locus has been found on chromosome 1 in a large Italian family (Gambardella et al., 2000).

## MISCELLANY

There are probably a number of other types of paroxysmal dyskinesias that do not fit well into the classification scheme listed previously (Pourfar et al., 2005). For example, a case of truncal flexion spasms that persist repeatedly in attacks lasting several hours has been described (Brown et al., 1991). These were considered to have a spinal origin, presumably involving the propriospinal pathways. Multiple brief dystonic spasms, lasting seconds, have been seen in a woman following cardiac arrhythmias. These attacks have all the clinical features of symptomatic PKD, except that they were not precipitated by sudden movement or startle. Like PKD, they responded dramatically to low dosages of carbamazepine. Perhaps the major delimiter in classifying the paroxysmal dyskinesias should be not whether they are kinesigenic but the duration of the attacks. Like tics, stereotypies can occur episosidically (Video 23-9).

A syndrome in infant girls is self-stimulatory (previously called masturbatory) behavior that occurs episodically (Fleisher and Morrison, 1990; Mink and Neil, 1995; Nechay et al., 2004; Yang et al., 2005). The episodes appear between 3 and 14 months of age and consist of the child's applying her suprapubic region to a firm edge of furniture, such as the arm of a sofa (Video 23-10). There is often stiffening of the lower extremities. The episodes last less than a minute to hours at a time. Most commonly, this behavior is misdiagnosed as epilepsy or paroxysmal dystonia.

## SUMMARY

The paroxysmal dyskinesias are usually divided into kinesigenic dyskinesias (which are induced by sudden movement and are brief in duration, lasting seconds to 5 minutes), the nonkinesigenic dyskinesias (which are not induced by sudden movement), and the exertional dyskinesias. The duration of PNKD is usually prolonged (2 minutes to 4 hours, up to 2 days), and PED is intermediate in duration (5 to 30 minutes). PNKD is often induced by alcohol, cold, heat, fatigue, caffeine, and stress and is caused by mutations in a gene (MR-1) that is involved in a stress-response pathway.

The kinesigenic dyskinesias ordinarily respond extremely well to a variety of anticonvulsants, whereas these drugs are usually not beneficial in the other two types. PNKD is sometimes sensitive to clonazepam, benzodiazepines, acetazolamide, anticholinergics, and neuroleptics.

PKD, PNKD, and PED have all been reported also to occur with benign infantile epilepsy (ICCA syndrome); the genes have been mapped to the 16p12 region, and it appears that the involved gene for this syndrome is the sodium/glucose cotransporter gene (KST1).

Variants of these disorders are the paroxysmal dyskinesias that occur during sleep (PHDs), for which there is mounting evidence that they are supplementary sensorimotor area seizures, and the transient paroxysmal dystonias (particularly torticollis) in infants.

When the genes have been identified, they involve ion channels. It is likely that all the paroxysmal dyskinesias will be channelopathies.

## References

Adam AM, Orinda D: Focal paroxysmal kinesigenic choreoathetosis preceding the development of Steele-Richardson-Olszewski syndrome [letter]. J Neurol Neurosurg Psychiatry 1986;49:957–968.

Aimard G, Vighetto A, Trillet M, et al: Ataxie paroxystique familiale sensible a l'acetazolamide. Rev Neurol (Paris) 1983;139:251–257.

Akmandemir FG, Eraksoy M, Gurvit IH, et al: Paroxysmal dysarthria and ataxia in a patient with Behçet's disease. J Neurol 1995;242:344–347.

Andermann F, Andermann E: Excessive startle syndromes: Startle disease, jumping, and startle epilepsy. Adv Neurol 1986;43:321–338.

Andermann F, Cosgrove JBR, Lloyd-Smith D, et al: Paroxysmal dysarthria and ataxia in multiple sclerosis. Neurology 1959;9:211–215.

Andermann F, Ohtahara S, Andermann E, et al: Infantile hypotonia and paroxysmal dystonia: A variant of alternating hemiplegia of childhood. Mov Disord 1994;9:227–229.

Angelini L, Rumi V, Lamperti E, Nardocci N: Transient paroxysmal dystonia in infancy. Neuropediatrics 1988;19:171–174.

Antony JH, Ouvrier RA, Wise G: Spasmus nutans, a mistaken identity. Arch Neurol 1980;37:373–375.

Arden F: Idiopathic hypoparathyroidism. Med J Aust 1953;2:217–219.

Auburger G, Ratzlaff T, Lunkes A, et al: A gene for autosomal dominant paroxysmal choreoathetosis spasticity (CSE) maps to the vicinity of a potassium channel gene cluster on chromosome 1p, probably within 2 cM between D1S443 and D1S197. Genomics 1996;31:90–94.

Bain PG, Larkin GBR, Calver DM, Obrien MD: Persistent superior oblique paresis as a manifestation of familial periodic cerebellar ataxia. Br J Ophthalmol 1991;75:619–621.

Bain PG, O'Brien MD, Keevil SF, Porter DA: Familial periodic cerebellar ataxia: A problem of cerebellar intracellular pH homeostasis. Ann Neurol 1992;31:147–154.

Baloh RW, Foster CA, Yue Q, Nelson SF: Familial migraine with vertigo and essential tremor. Neurology 1996;46:458–460.

Baloh RW, Winder A: Acetazolamide-responsive vestibulocerebellar syndrome: Clinical and oculographic features. Neurology 1991; 41:429–433.

Baloh RW, Yue Q, Furman JM, Nelson SF: Familial episodic ataxia: Clinical heterogeneity in four families linked to chromosome 19p. Ann Neurol 1997;41:8–16.

Barabas G, Tucker SM: Idiopathic hypoparathyroidism and paroxysmal dystonic choreoathetosis [letter]. Ann Neurol 1988;24:585.

Barnett MH, Jarman PR, Heales SJR, Bhatia KP: Further case of paroxysmal exercise-induced dystonia and some insights into pathogenesis. Mov Disord 2002;17(6):1386–1387.

Baron DN, Dent CE, Harris H, et al: Hereditary pellagra-like skin rash with temporary cerebellar ataxia, constant renal aminoaciduria and other bizarre biochemical features. Lancet 1956;2: 421–428.

Bass N, Wyllie E, Comair Y, et al: Supplementary sensorimotor area seizures in children and adolescents. J Pediatr 1995;126:537–544.

Beaumanoir A, Mira L, van Lierde A: Epilepsy or paroxysmal kinesigenic choreoathetosis? Brain Dev 1996;18:139–141.

Beltran RS, Coker SB: Transient dystonia of infancy, a result of intrauterine cocaine exposure? Pediatr Neurol 1995;12:354–356.

Bennett DA, Fox JH: Paroxysmal dyskinesias secondary to cerebral vascular disease: Reversal with aspirin. Clin Neuropharmacol 1989;12:215–216.

Bennett LB, Roach ES, Bowcock AM: A locus for paroxysmal kinesigenic dyskinesia maps to human chromosome 16. Neurology 2000;54:125–130.

Berger JR, Sheremata WA, Melamed E: Paroxysmal dystonia as the initial manifestation of multiple sclerosis. Arch Neurol 1984;41: 747–750.

Bhatia KP, Marsden CD, Thomas DGT: Posteroventral pallidotomy can ameliorate attacks of paroxysmal dystonia induced by exercise. J Neurol Neurosurg Psychiatry 1998;65:604–605.

Bhatia KP, Soland VL, Bhatt MH, et al: Paroxysmal exercise-induced dystonia: Eight new sporadic cases and a review of the literature. Mov Disord 1997;12:1007–1012.

Bird TD, Carlson CB, Horning M: Ten year follow-up of paroxysmal choreoathetosis: A sporadic case becomes familial. Epilepsia 1978;19:129–132.

Blakeley J, Jankovic J: Secondary paroxysmal dyskinesias. Mov Disord 2002;17(4):726–734.

Blass JP, Avigan J, Uhlendorf BW: A defect in pyruvate decarboxylase in a child with an intermittent movement disorder. J Clin Invest 1970;49:423–432.

Blass JP, Kark RAP, Engel WK: Clinical studies of a patient with pyruvate decarboxylase deficiency. Arch Neurol 1971;25:449–460.

Boel M, Casaer P: Paroxysmal kinesigenic choreoathetosis. Neuropediatrics 1984;15:215–217.

Bortolotti P, Schoenhuber R: Paroxysmal kinesigenic choreoathetosis [letter]. Arch Neurol 1983;40:529.

Bourgeois M, Aicardi J, Goutieres F: Alternating hemiplegia of childhood. J Pediatr 1993;122:673–679.

Bratt HD, Menelaus MB: Benign paroxysmal torticollis of infancy. J Bone Joint Surg [Br] 1992;74:449–451.

Bressman SB, Fahn S, Burke RE: Paroxysmal non-kinesigenic dystonia. Adv Neurol 1988;50:403–413.

Brockmann K, Dumitrescu AM, Best TT, et al: X-linked paroxysmal dyskinesia and severe global retardation caused by defective MCT8 gene. J Neurol 2005;252:663–666.

Brown P, Thompson PD, Rothwell JC, et al: Paroxysmal axial spasms of spinal origin. Mov Disord 1991;6:43–48.

Browne DL, Gancher ST, Nutt TG, et al: Episodic ataxia/myokymia syndrome is associated with point mutations in the human potassium channel gene, KCNA1. Nat Genet 1994;8:136–140.

Bruno MK, Hallett M, Gwinn-Hardy K, et al: Clinical evaluation of idiopathic paroxysmal kinesigenic dyskinesia: New diagnostic criteria. Neurology 2004a;63:2280–2287.

Bruno MK, Ravina B, Garraux G, et al: Exercise-induced dystonia as a preceding symptom of familial Parkinson's disease. Mov Disord 2004b;19(2):228–230.

Brunt ERP, Van Weerden TW: Familial paroxysmal kinesigenic ataxia and continuous myokymia. Brain 1990;113:1361–1382.

Buchman AS, Goetz CG, Klawans HL: Hemiparkinsonism with hemiatrophy. Neurology 1988;38:527–530.

Burger LJ, Lopez RI, Elliott FA: Tonic seizures induced by movement. Neurology 1972;22:656–659.

Burguera JA, Catala J, Casanova B: Thalamic demyelination and paroxysmal dystonia in multiple sclerosis. Mov Disord 1991;6: 379–381.

Burke RE, Fahn S, Jankovic J, et al: Tardive dystonia: Late-onset and persistent dystonia caused by antipsychotic drugs. Neurology 1982;32:1335–1346.

Byrne E, White O, Cook M: Familial dystonic choreoathetosis with myokymia: A sleep responsive disorder. J Neurol Neurosurg Psychiatry 1991;54:1090–1092.

Camac A, Greene P, Khandji A: Paroxysmal kinesigenic dystonic choreoathetosis associated with a thalamic infarct. Mov Disord 1990;5:235–238.

Campistol J, Prats JM, Garaizar C: Benign paroxysmal tonic upgaze of childhood with ataxia — A neuroophthalmological syndrome of familial origin. Dev Med Child Neurol 1993;35:436–439.

Cavanagh NP, Bicknell J, Howard F: Cystinuria with mental retardation and paroxysmal dyskinesia in 2 brothers. Arch Dis Child 1974;49:662–664.

Chatterjee A, Louis ED, Frucht S: Levetiracetam in the treatment of paroxysmal kinesiogenic choreoathetosis. Mov Disord 2002; 17(3):614–615.

Chudnow RS, Mimbela RA, Owen DB, Roach ES: Gabapentin for familial paroxysmal dystonic choreoathetosis. Neurology 1997; 49:1441–1442.

Comu S, Giuliani M, Narayanan V: Episodic ataxia and myokymia syndrome: A new mutation of potassium channel gene Kv1.1. Ann Neurol 1996;40:684–687.

Cosentino C, Torres L, Flores M, Cuba JM: Paroxysmal kinesigenic dystonia and spinal cord lesion. Mov Disord 1996;11:453–455.

Coulter DL, Donofrio P: Haloperidol for nonkinesiogenic paroxysmal dyskinesia [letter]. Arch Neurol 1980;37:325–326.

D'Adamo MC, Liu ZP, Adelman JP, et al: Episodic ataxia type-1 mutations in the hKv1.1 cytoplasmic pore region alter the gating properties of the channel. EMBO J 1998;17:1200–1207.

Dale RC, Church AJ, Surtees RAH, et al: Post-streptococcal autoimmune neuropsychiatric disease presenting as paroxysmal dystonic choreoathetosis. Mov Disord 2002;17(4):817–820.

Damji KF, Allingham RR, Pollock SC, et al: Periodic vestibulocerebellar ataxia, an autosomal dominant ataxia with defective smooth pursuit, is genetically distinct from other autosomal dominant ataxias. Arch Neurol 1996;53:338–344.

Dancis J, Hutzler J, Rokkones T: Intermittent branched-chain ketonuria: Variant of maple-syrup-urine disease. N Engl J Med 1967;276:84–89.

DeCastro W, Campbell J: Periodic ataxia. JAMA 1967;200:892–894.

Demirkiran M, Jankovic J: Paroxysmal dyskinesias: Clinical features and classification. Ann Neurol 1995;38:571–579.

Deonna T, Roulet E, Meyer HU: Benign paroxysmal tonic upgaze of childhood: A new syndrome. Neuropediatrics 1990;21:213–214.

Dominguez-Moran JA, Callejo JM, Fernandez-Ruiz LC, Martinez-Castrillo JC: Acute paroxysmal dystonia induced by fluoxetine. Mov Disord 2001;16:767–769.

Donat JF, Wright FS: Episodic symptoms mistaken for seizures in the neurologically impaired child. Neurology 1990;40:156–157.

Donat JR, Auger R: Familial periodic ataxia. Arch Neurol 1979;36:568–569.

Dooley JM, Brna PM: Sublingual lorazepam in the treatment of familial paroxysmal nonkinesigenic dyskinesia. Pediatr Neurol 2004;30(5):365–366.

Dragasevic N, Petkovic-Medved B, Svetel M, et al: Paroxysmal hemiballism and idiopathic hypoparathyroidism. J Neurol 1997;244:389–390.

Drake ME Jr, Jackson RD, Miller CA: Paroxysmal choreoathetosis after head injury [letter]. J Neurol Neurosurg Psychiatry 1986;49:837–843.

Duchowny MS, Resnick TJ, Deray MJ, Alvarez LA: Video EEG diagnosis of repetitive behavior in early childhood and its relationship to seizures. Pediatr Neurol 1988;4:162–164.

Dunn DW: Paroxysmal dystonia. Am J Dis Child 1981;135:381–382.

Echenne B, Rivier F: Benign paroxysmal tonic upward gaze. Pediatr Neurol 1992;8:154–155.

Engelen M, Tijssen MAJ: Paroxysmal non-kinesigenic dyskinesia in antiphospholipid syndrome. Mov Disord 2005;20(1):111–113.

Erickson GR, Chun RW: Acquired paroxysmal movement disorders. Pediatr Neurol 1987;3:226–229.

Espir MLE, Watkins SM, Smith HV: Paroxysmal dysarthria and other transient neurological disturbances in disseminated sclerosis. J Neurol Neurosurg Psychiatry 1966;29:323–330.

Eunson LH, Rea R, Zuberi SM, et al: Clinical, genetic, and expression studies of mutations in the potassium channel gene KCNA1 reveal new phenotypic variability. Ann Neurol 2000;48:647–656.

Factor SA, Coni RJ, Cowger M, Rosenblum EL: Paroxysmal tremor and orofacial dyskinesia secondary to a biopterin synthesis defect. Neurology 1991;41:930–932.

Fahn S: Paroxysmal tremor. Neurology 1983;33(suppl 2):131.

Fahn S: Atypical tremors, rare tremors, and unclassified tremors. In Findley LJ, Capildeo R (eds): Movement Disorders: Tremor. New York, Oxford University, 1984, pp 431–443.

Fahn S: Motor and vocal tics. In Kurlan R (ed): Handbook of Tourette's Syndrome and Related Tic and Behavioral Disorders. New York, Marcel Dekker, 1993, pp 3–16.

Fahn S: The paroxysmal dyskinesias. In Marsden CD, Fahn S (eds): Movement Disorders 3. Oxford, UK, Butterworth-Heinemann, 1994, pp 310–345.

Fahn S, Marsden CD, Van Woert MH: Definition and clinical classification of myoclonus. Adv Neurol 1986;43:1–5.

Fahn S, Williams DT: Psychogenic dystonia. Adv Neurol 1988;50:431–455.

Falconer M, Driver M, Serafetinides E: Seizures induced by movement: Report of a case relieved by operation. J Neurol Neurosurg Psychiatry 1963;26:300–307.

Farmer TW, Mustian VM: Vestibulocerebellar ataxia. Arch Neurol 1963;8:471–480.

Fejerman N: Mioclonias benignas de la infancia temprana. An Esp Pediatr 1984;21:725–731.

Fernandez-Alvarez E: Transient movement disorders in children. J Neurol 1998;245(1):1–5.

Fink JK, Hedera P, Mathay JG, Albin RL: Paroxysmal dystonic choreoathetosis linked to chromosome 2q: Clinical analysis and proposed pathophysiology. Neurology 1997;49:177–183.

Fink JK, Rainier S, Wilkowski J, et al: Paroxysmal dystonic choreoathetosis: Tight linkage to chromosome 2q. Am J Hum Genet 1996;59:140–145.

Fischbeck KH, Layzer RB: Paroxysmal choreoathetosis associated with thyrotoxicosis. Ann Neurol 1979;6:453–454.

Fish DR, Marsden CD: Epilepsy masquerading as a movement disorder. In Marsden CD, Fahn S (eds): Movement Disorders 3. Oxford, UK, Butterworth-Heinemann, 1994, pp 346–358.

Fleisher DR, Morrison A: Masturbation mimicking abdominal pain or seizures in young girls. J Pediatr 1990;116:810–814.

Forssman H: Hereditary disorder charactrized by attacks of muscular contractions, induced by alcohol amongst other factors. Acta Med Scand 1961;170:517–533.

Fouad GT, Servidei S, Durcan S, et al: A gene for familial paroxysmal dyskinesia (FPD1) maps to chromosome 2q. Am J Hum Genet 1996;59:135–139.

Franssen H, Fortgens C, Wattendorff AR, van Woerkom TCAM: Paroxysmal kinesigenic choreoathetosis and abnormal contingent negative variation: A case report. Arch Neurol 1983;40:381–385.

Frucht S, Fahn S: Paroxysmal kinesigenic dyskinesia in infancy. Mov Disord 1999;14:694–695.

Fuh JL, Chang DB, Wang SJ, et al: Painful tonic spasms: An interesting phenomenon in cerebral ischemia. Acta Neurol Scand 1991;84:534–536.

Fukuda M, Hashimoto O, Nagakubo S, Hata A: A family with an atonic variant of paroxysmal kinesigenic choreoathetosis and hypercalcitoninemia. Mov Disord 1999;14:342–344.

Fukuyama S, Okada R: Hereditary kinesthetic reflex epilepsy: Report of five families of peculiar seizures induced by sudden movements. Adv Neurol Sci (Tokyo) 1967;11:168–197.

Gambardella A, Annesi G, DeFusco M, et al: A new locus for autosomal dominant nocturnal frontal lobe epilepsy maps to chromosome 1. Neurology 2000;55:1467–1471.

Gancher ST, Nutt JG: Autosomal dominant episodic ataxia: A heterogeneous syndrome. Mov Disord 1986;1:239–253.

Garello L, Ottonello GA, Regesta G, Tanganelli P: Familial paroxysmal kinesigenic choreoathetosis: Report of a pharmacological trial in 2 cases. Eur Neurol 1983;22:217–221.

Gatto EM, Zurru MC, Rugilo C: Medullary lesions and unusual bilateral paroxysmal dystonia in multiple sclerosis. Neurology 1996;46:847–848.

Gay CT, Ryan SG: Paroxysmal kinesigenic dystonia after methylphenidate administration. J Child Neurol 1994;9:45–46.

George MS, Pickett JB, Kohli H, et al: Paroxysmal dystonic reflex choreoathetosis after minor closed head injury. Lancet 1990;336:1134–1135.

Giffin NJ, Benton S, Goadsby PJ: Benign paroxysmal torticollis of infancy: Four new cases and linkage to CACNA1A mutation. Dev Med Child Neurol 2002;44(7):490–493.

Gilroy J: Abnormal computed tomograms in paroxysmal kinesigenic choreoathetosis. Arch Neurol 1982;39:779–780.

Gokcay A, Gokcay F: Oxcarbazepine therapy in paroxysmal kinesigenic choreoathetosis. Acta Neurol Scand 2000;101:344–345.

Gonzalez-Alegre P, Ammache Z, Davis PH, Rodnitzky RL: Moyamoya-induced paroxysmal dyskinesia. Mov Disord 2003;18(9):1051–1056.

Goodenough DJ, Fariello RG, Annis BL, Chun RW: Familial and acquired paroxysmal dyskinesias: A proposed classification with delineation of clinical features. Arch Neurol 1978;35:827–831.

Gorard DA, Gibberd FB: Paroxysmal dysarthria and ataxia—associated MRI abnormality. J Neurol Neurosurg Psychiatry 1989;52:1444–1445.

Gourley IM: Paroxysmal torticollis in infancy. Can Med Assoc J 1971;105:504–505.

Gowers WR: Epilepsy and Other Chronic Convulsive Diseases. Their Causes, Symptoms and Treatment. New York: William Wood, 1885. Reprint, New York, Dover, 1964.

Griggs RC, Moxley RT III, Lafrance RA, McQuillen J: Hereditary paroxysmal ataxia: Response to acetazolamide. Neurology 1978; 28:1259–1264.

Griggs RC, Nutt JG: Episodic ataxias as channelopathies. Ann Neurol 1995;37:285–287.

Guerrini R: Idiopathic epilepsy and paroxysmal dyskinesia. Epilepsia 2001;42:36–41.

Guerrini R, Belmonte A, Carrozzo R: Paroxysmal tonic upgaze of childhood with ataxia: A benign transient dystonia with autosomal dominant inheritance. Brain Dev 1998;20:116–118.

Guerrini R, Bonanni P, Nardocci N, et al: Autosomal recessive rolandic epilepsy with paroxysmal exercise-induced dystonia and writer's cramp: Delineation of the syndrome and gene mapping to chromosome 16p12-11.2. Ann Neurol 1999;45:344–352.

Haan J, Kremer HPH, Padberg G: Paroxysmal chreoathetosis as presenting symptom of diabetes mellitus. J Neurol Neurosurg Psychiatry 1988;52:133.

Hallett M, Marsden CD, Fahn S: Myoclonus. Handbook of Clinical Neurology, vol 49, Extrapyramidal Disorders. Amsterdam, Elsevier, 1987, pp 609–625.

Hanson PA, Martinez LB, Cassidy R: Contractures, continuous muscle discharges, and titubation. Ann Neurol 1977;1:120–124.

Hattori H, Yorifuji T: Infantile convulsions and paroxysmal kinesigenic choreoathetosis in a patient with idiopathic hypoparathyroidism. Brain Dev 2000;22:449–450.

Hawkes CH: Familial paroxysmal ataxia: Report of a family. J Neurol Neurosurg Psychiatry 1992;55:212–213.

Hayman M, Harvey AS, Hopkins IJ, et al: Paroxysmal tonic upgaze: A reappraisal of outcome. Ann Neurol 1998;43:514–520.

Hening W, Walters A, Kavey N, et al: Dyskinesias while awake and periodic movements in sleep in restless legs syndrome: Treatment with opioids. Neurology 1986;36:1363–1366.

Hill W, Sherman H: Acute intermittent familial cerebellar ataxia. Arch Neurol 1968;18:350–357.

Hirata K, Katayama S, Saito T, et al: Paroxysmal kinesigenic choreoathetosis with abnormal electroencephalogram during attacks. Epilepsia 1991;32:492–494.

Hirose H, Arayama T, Takita J, et al: A family of episodic ataxia type 2: No evidence of genetic linkage to the CACNA1A gene. Int J Mol Med 2003;11(2):187–189.

Hishikawa Y, Furuya E, Yamamoto J, Nan'no H: Dystonic seizures induced by movement. Arch Psychiatr Nervenkr 1973;217:113–138.

Hofele K, Benecke R, Auburger G: Gene locus FPD1 of the dystonic Mount-Reback type of autosomal-dominant paroxysmal choreoathetosis. Neurology 1997;49:1252–1257.

Holmes GL, Russman BS: Shuddering attacks: Evaluation using electroencephalographic frequency modulation radiotelemetry and videotape monitoring. Am J Dis Child 1986;140:72–73.

Homan RW, Vasko MR, Blaw M: Phenytoin plasma concentrations in paroxysmal kinesigenic choreoathetosis. Neurology 1980;30:673–676.

Horner FH, Jackson LC: Familial paroxysmal choreoathetosis. In Barbeau A, Brunette J-R (eds): Progress in Neuro-Genetics. Amsterdam, Excerpta Medica Foundation, 1969, pp 745–751.

Houser MK, Soland VL, Bhatia KP, et al: Paroxysmal kinesigenic choreoathetosis: A report of 26 patients. J Neurol 1999;246:120–126.

Huang CW, Chen YC, Tsai JJ: Paroxysmal dyskinesia with secondary generalization of tonic-clonic seizures in pseudohypoparathyroidism. Epilepsia 2005a;46(1):164–165.

Huang YG, Chen YC, Du F, et al: Topiramate therapy for paroxysmal kinesigenic choreoathetosis. Mov Disord 2005b;20(1):75–77.

Huffstutter WM, Myers GJ: Paroxysmal motor dysfunction. Ala J Med Sci 1983;20:311–313.

Hughes AJ, Lees AJ, Marsden CD: Paroxysmal dystonic head tremor. Mov Disord 1991;6:85–86.

Hwang WJ, Lu CS, Tsai JJ: Clinical manifestations of 20 Taiwanese patients with paroxysmal kinesigenic dyskinesia. Acta Neurol Scand 1998;98:340–345.

Jabbari B, Coker SB: Paroxysmal rhythmic lingua movements and chronic epilepsy. Neurology 1981;31:1364–1367.

Jabbari B, Khajevi K, Rao K: Medullary dystonia. Mov Disord 1999; 14:698–700.

Jacome DE, Risko M: Photic induced-driven PLEDs in paroxysmal dystonic choreoathetosis. Clin Electroencephalogr 1984;15:151–154.

Jarman PR, Davis MB, Hodgson SV, et al: Paroxysmal dystonic choreoathetosis: Genetic linkage studies in a British family. Brain 1997;120:2125–2130.

Jodice C, Mantuano E, Veneziano L, et al: Episodic ataxia type 2 (EA2) and spinocerebellar ataxia type 6 (SCA6) due to CAG repeat expansion in the CACNA1A gene on chromosome 19p. Hum Mol Genet 1997;6:1973–1978.

Joseph K, Avallone J, Difazio M: Paroxysmal tonic upgaze and partial tetrasomy of chromosome 15: A novel genetic association. J Child Neurol 2005;20(2):165–168.

Joynt RJ, Green D: Tonic seizures as a manifestation of multiple sclerosis. Arch Neurol 1962;6:293–299.

Julien J, Denier C, Ferrer X, et al: Sporadic late onset paroxysmal cerebellar ataxia in four unrelated patients: A new disease? J Neurol 2001;248:209–214.

Jung S-S, Chen K-M, Brody JA: Paroxysmal choreoathetosis: Report of Chinese cases. Neurology 1973;23:749–755.

Kanazawa O: Shuddering attacks: Report of four children. Pediatr Neurol 2000;23:421–424.

Kang UJ, Burke RE, Fahn S: Natural history and treatment of tardive dystonia. Mov Disord 1986;1:193–208.

Kato M, Araki S: Paroxysmal kinesigenic choreoathetosis: Report of a case relieved by carbamazepine. Arch Neurol 1969;20:508–513.

Katzenschlager R, Costa D, Gacinovic S, Lees AJ: [I-123]-FP-CIT-SPECT in the early diagnosis of PD presenting as exercise-induced dystonia. Neurology 2002;59(12):1974–1976.

Keane JR: Galloping tongue: Post-traumatic, episodic, rhythmic movements. Neurology 1984;34:251–252.

Kertesz A: Paroxysmal kinesigenic choreoathetosis: An entity within the paroxysmal choreoathetosis syndrome: Description of 10 cases, including 1 autopsied. Neurology 1967;17:680–690.

Kinali M, Jungbluth H, Eunson LH, et al: Expanding the phenotype of potassium channelopathy: Severe neuromyotonia and skeletal deformities without prominent episodic ataxia. Neuromuscular Disord 2004;14(10):689–693.

Kinast M, Erenberg G, Rothner AD: Paroxysmal choreoathetosis: Report of five cases and review of the literature. Pediatrics 1980; 65:74–77.

Kishimoto K: A novel case of conditionally responsive extrapyramidal syndrome. Annu Rep Res Inst Environ Med Nagoya Univ 1957;6:91–101.

Kluge A, Kettner B, Zschenderlein R, et al: Changes in perfusion pattern using ECD-SPECT indicate frontal lobe and cerebellar involvement in exercise-induced paroxysmal dystonia. Mov Disord 1998;13:125–134.

Ko CH, Kong CK, Ngai WT, Ma KM: Ictal Tc-99m ECD SPECT in paroxysmal kinesigenic choreoathetosis. Pediatr Neurol 2001; 24:225–227.

Koller W, Bahamon-Dussan J: Hereditary paroxysmal cerebellopathy: Responsiveness to acetazolamide. Clin Neuropharmacol 1987; 10:65–68.

Koller WC, Biary NM: Volitional control of involuntary movements. Mov Disord 1989;4:153–156.

Kotagal P, Costa M, Wyllie E, Wolgamuth B: Paroxysmal nonepileptic events in children and adolescents. Pediatrics 2002;110(4):E46.

Kotagal P, Luders H, Morris HH, et al: Dystonic posturing in complex partial seizures of temporal lobe onset: A new lateralizing sign. Neurology 1989;39:196–201.

Kurlan R, Behr J, Medved L, Shoulson I: Familial paroxysmal dystonic choreoathetosis: A family study. Mov Disord 1987;2:187–192.

Kurlan R, Shoulson I: Familial paroxysmal dystonic choreoathetosis and response to alternate-day oxazepam therapy. Ann Neurol 1983;13:456–457.

Lagueny A, Ellie E, Burbaud P, et al: Paroxysmal stimulus-sensitive spasmodic torticollis. Mov Disord 1993;8:241–242.

Lance JW: Sporadic and familial varieties of tonic seizures. J Neurol Neurosurg Psychiatry 1963;26:51–59.

Lance JW: Familial paroxysmal dystonic choreoathetosis and its differentiation from related syndromes. Ann Neurol 1977;2:285–293.

Lang AE: Focal paroxysmal kinesigenic choreoathetosis [letter]. J Neurol Neurosurg Psychiatry 1984;47:1057–1060.

Lang AE: Psychogenic dystonia: A review of 18 cases. Can J Neurol Sci 1995;22:136–143.

LeDoux MS: Paroxysmal kinesigenic dystonia associated with a medullary hemorrhage. Mov Disord 1997;12:819.

Lee HY, Xu Y, Huang Y, et al: The gene for paroxysmal non-kinesigenic dyskinesia encodes an enzyme in a stress response pathway. Hum Mol Genet 2004;13(24):3161–3170.

Lee WL, Tay A, Ong HT, et al: Association of infantile convulsions with paroxysmal dyskinesias (ICCA syndrome): Confirmation of linkage to human chromosome 16p12-q12 in a Chinese family. Hum Genet 1998;103:608–612.

Li Z, Turner RP, Smith G: Childhood paroxysmal kinesigenic dyskinesia: Report of seven cases with onset at an early age. Epilepsy Behav 2005;6:435–439.

Lipson EH, Robertson WC Jr: Paroxysmal torticollis of infancy: Familial occurrence. Am J Dis Child 1978;132:422–423.

Litt M, Kramer P, Browne D, et al: A gene for episodic ataxia/myokymia maps to chromosome 12p13. Am J Hum Genet 1994;55:702–709.

Loher TJ, Krauss JK, Burgunder JM, et al: Chronic thalamic stimulation for treatment of dystonic paroxysmal nonkinesigenic dyskinesia. Neurology 2001;56:268–270.

Lombroso CT: Paroxysmal choreoathetosis: An epileptic or non-epileptic disorder. Ital J Neurol Sci 1995;16:271–277.

Lombroso CT, Fejerman N: Benign myoclonus of early infancy. Ann Neurol 1977;1:138–143.

Lonsdale D, Faulkner WR, Price JW, et al: Intermittent cerebellar ataxia associated with hyperpyruvic acidemia, hyperalaninemia, and hyperalaninuria. Pediatrics 1969;43:1025–1034.

Loong SC, Ong YY: Paroxysmal kinesigenic choreoathetosis: Report of a case relieved by L-dopa. J Neurol Neurosurg Psychiatry 1973;36:921–924.

Lotze T, Jankovic J: Paroxysmal kinesigenic dyskinesias. Seminars Ped Neurol 2003;10:68–79.

Lou HC: Flunarizine in paroxysmal choreoathetosis. Neuropediatrics 1989;20:112.

Lüders HO: Paroxysmal choreoathetosis. Eur Neurol 1996;36:20–23.

Lugaresi E, Cirignotta F: Hypnogenic paroxysmal dystonia: Epileptic seizure or a new syndrome? Sleep 1981;4:129–138.

Lugaresi E, Cirignotta F, Montagna P: Nocturnal paroxysmal dystonia. J Neurol Neurosurg Psychiatry 1986;49:375–380.

MacLean JB, Sassin JF: Paroxysmal vertical ocular dyskinesia. Arch Neurol 1973;29(2):117–119.

Margolin DL, Marsden CD: Episodic dyskinesias and transient cerebral ischemia. Neurology 1982;32:1379–1380.

Matsuo H, Kamakura K, Saito M, et al: Familial paroxysmal dystonic choreoathetosis: Clinical findings in a large Japanese family and genetic linkage to 2q. Arch Neurol 1999;56:721–726.

Matthews WB: Tonic seizures in disseminated sclerosis. Brain 1958;81:193–206.

Mayeux R, Fahn S: Paroxysmal dystonic choreoathetosis in a patient with familial ataxia. Neurology 1982;32:1184–1186.

Meierkord H, Fish DR, Smith SJM, et al: Is nocturnal paroxysmal dystonia a form of frontal lobe epilepsy? Mov Disord 1992;7:38–42.

Menkes JH, Ament ME: Neurologic disorders of gastroesophageal function. Adv Neurol 1988;49:409–416.

Merchut MP, Brumlik J: Painful tonic spasms caused by putaminal infarction. Stroke 1986;17:1319–1321.

Meyer BU, Irlbacher K, Meierkord H: Analysis of stimuli triggering attacks of paroxysmal dystonia induced by exertion. J Neurol Neurosurg Psychiatry 2001;70:247–251.

Micheli F, Fernandez Pardal M, de Arbelaiz R, et al: Paroxysmal dystonia responsive to anticholinergic drugs. Clin Neuropharmacol 1987;10:365–369.

Micheli F, Fernandez Pardal MM, Casas Parera I, Giannaula R: Sporadic paroxysmal dystonic choreoathetosis associated with basal ganglia calcifications [letter]. Ann Neurol 1986;20:750.

Milandre L, Brosset C, Gabriel B, Khalil R: Mouvements involontaires transitoires et infarctus thalamiques. [Transient dyskinesias associated with thalamic infarcts: Report of five cases.] Rev Neurol 1993;149:402–406.

Miley CE, Forster FM: Paroxysmal signs and symptoms in multiple sclerosis. Neurology 1974;24:458–461.

Miller VS, Packard AM: Paroxysmal downgaze in term newborn infants. J Child Neurol 1998;13:294–295.

Mink JW, Neil JJ: Masturbation mimicking paroxysmal dystonia or dyskinesia in a young girl. Mov Disord 1995;10:518–520.

Mir P, Huang YZ, Gilio F, et al: Abnormal cortical and spinal inhibition in paroxysmal kinesigenic dyskinesia. Brain 2005;128:291–299.

Mirsattari SM, Berry MER, Holden JK, et al: Paroxysmal dyskinesias in patients with HIV infection. Neurology 1999;52:109–114.

Morgan JC, Hughes M, Figueroa RE, Sethi KD: Psychogenic paroxysmal dyskinesia following paroxysmal hemidystonia in multiple sclerosis. Neurology. 2005;65(6):E12.

Mount LA, Reback S: Familial paroxysmal choreoathetosis. Arch Neurol Psychiat 1940;44:841–847.

Munchau A, Valente EM, Shahidi GA, et al: A new family with paroxysmal exercise induced dystonia and migraine: A clinical and genetic study. J Neurol Neurosurg Psychiatry 2000;68:609–614.

Mushet GR, Dreifuss FE: Paroxysmal dyskinesia: A case responsive to benztropine mesylate. Arch Dis Child 1967;42:654–656.

Nagamitsu S, Matsuishi T, Hashimoto K, et al: Multicenter study of paroxysmal dyskinesias in Japan: Clinical and pedigree analysis. Mov Disord 1999;14:658–663.

Nair KR, Bhaskaran R, Marsden CD: Essential tremor associated with paroxysmal kinesigenic dystonia. Mov Disord 1991;6:92–93.

Nakken KO, Magnusson A, Steinlein OK: Autosomal dominant nocturnal frontal lobe epilepsy: An electroclinical study of a Norwegian family with ten affected members. Epilepsia 1999;40:88–92.

Nardocci N, Lamperti E, Rumi V, Angelini L: Typical and atypical forms of paroxysmal choreoathetosis. Dev Med Child Neurol 1989;31:670–674.

Nath A, Jankovic J, Pettigrew LC: Movement disorders and AIDS. Neurology 1987;37:37–41.

Nechay A, Ross LM, Stephenson JBP, O'Regan M: Gratification disorder ("infantile masturbation"): A review. Arch Dis Child 2004;89:225–226.

Newman RP, Kinkel WR: Paroxysmal choreoathetosis due to hypoglycemia. Arch Neurol 1984;41:341–342.

Newton MR, Berkovic SF, Austin MC, et al: Dystonia, clinical lateralization, and regional blood flow changes in temporal lobe seizures. Neurology 1992;42:371–377.

Nezu A, Kimura S, Ohtsuki N, et al: Alternating hemiplegia of childhood: Report of a case having a long history. Brain Dev 1997;19:217–221.

Nightingale S, Barton ME: Intermittent vertical supranuclear ophthalmoplegia and ataxia. Mov Disord 1991;6:76–78.

Nijssen PCG, Tijssen CC: Stimulus-sensitive paroxysmal dyskinesias associated with a thalamic infarct. Mov Disord 1992;7:364–366.

Nutt JG, Gancher ST: A 10-year follow up: Genotypic analysis disproves phenotypic classification. Mov Disord 1997;12:472.

Oldani A, Zucconi M, Asselta R, et al: Autosomal dominant nocturnal frontal lobe epilepsy: A video-polysomnographic and genetic appraisal of 40 patients and delineation of the epileptic syndrome. Brain 1998;121:205–223.

Ondo WG, Verma A: Physiological assessment of paroxysmal dystonia secondary to subacute sclerosing panencephalitis. Mov Disord 2002;17(1):154–157.

Ophoff RA, Terwindt GM, Vergouwe MN, et al: Familial hemiplegic migraine and episodic ataxia type-2 are caused by mutations in the Ca$^{2+}$ channel gene CACNL1A4. Cell 1996;87:543–552.

Ouvrier R, Billson F: Paroxysmal tonic upgaze of childhood: A review. Brain Dev 2005;27(3):185–188.

Ouvrier RA, Billson MD: Benign paroxysmal tonic upgaze of childhood. J Child Neurol 1988;3:177–180.

Parker HL: Periodic ataxia. Mayo Clin Proc 1946;38:642–645.

Pereira AC, Loo WJ, Bamford M, Wroe SJ: Use of lamotrigine to treat paroxysmal kinesigenic choreoathetosis. J Neurol Neurosurg Psychiatry 2000;68:796–797.

Perez-Borja C, Tassinari AC, Swanson AG: Paroxysmal choreoathetosis and seizure induced by movement (reflex epispsy). Epilepsia 1967;8:260–270.

Perlmutter JS, Raichle ME: Pure hemidystonia with basal ganglion abnormalities on positron emission tomography. Ann Neurol 1984;15:228–233.

Perniola T, Margari L, de Iaco MG, et al: Familial paroxysmal exercise-induced dyskinesia, epilepsy, and mental retardation in a family with autosomal dominant inheritance. Mov Disord 2001; 16:724–730.

Phillips HA, Favre I, Kirkpatrick M, et al: CHRNB2 is the second acetylcholine receptor subunit associated with autosomal dominant nocturnal frontal lobe epilepsy. Am J Hum Genet 2001;8:225–231.

Phillips HA, Scheffer IE, Crossland KM, et al: Autosomal dominant nocturnal frontal-lobe epilepsy: Genetic heterogeneity and evidence for a second locus at 15q24. Am J Hum Genet 1998;63: 1108–1116.

Plant G: Focal paroxysmal kinesigenic choreoathetosis. J Neurol Neurosurg Psychiatry 1983;46:345–348.

Plant GT, Williams AC, Earl CJ, Marsden CD: Familial paroxysmal dystonia induced by exercise. J Neurol Neurosurg Psychiatry 1984; 47:275–279.

Postert T, Amoiridis G, Pohlau D, et al: Episodic undulating hyperkinesias of the tongue associated with brainstem ischemia. Mov Disord 1997;12:619–621.

Pourfar M, Guerrini R, Parain D, Frucht SJ: Classification conundrums in paroxysmal dyskinesias: A new subtype or variations on classic themes? Mov Disord 2005;20:1047–1051.

Przuntek H, Monninger P: Therapeutic aspects of kinesigenic paroxysmal choreoathetosis and familial paroxysmal choreoathetosis of the Mount and Reback type. J Neurol 1983;230:163–169.

Raskind WH, Bolin T, Wolff J, et al: Further localization of a gene for paroxysmal dystonic choreoathetosis to a 5-cM region on chromosome 2q34. Hum Genet 1998;102:93–97.

Richards RN, Barnett HJ: Paroxysmal dystonic choreoathetosis: A family study and review of the literature. Neurology 1968;18: 461–469.

Richardson JC, Howes JL, Celinski MJ, Allman RG: Kinesigenic choreoathetosis due to brain injury. Can J Neurol Sci 1987;14: 626–628.

Riley DE: Paroxysmal kinesigenic dystonia associated with a medullary lesion. Mov Disord 1996;11:738–740.

Robin JJ: Paroxysmal choreoathetosis following head injury. Ann Neurol 1977;2:447–448.

Roll P, Massacrier A, Pereira S, et al: New human sodium/glucose cotransporter gene (KST1): Identification, characterization, and mutation analysis in ICCA (infantile convulsions and choreo-

athetosis) and BFIC (benign familial infantile convulsions) families. Gene 2002;285(1–2):141–148.

Roos R, Wintzen AR, Vielvoye G, Polder TW: Paroxysmal kinesiogenic choreoathetosis as presenting symptom of multiple sclerosis. J Neurol Neurosurg Psychiatry 1991;54:657–658.

Rosen JA: Paroxysmal choreoathetosis: Associated with perinatal hypoxic encephalopathy. Arch Neurol 1964;11:385–387.

Rowland LP, Gordon PH: Familial periodic paralysis. In Rowland LP: Merritt's Neurology, 11th ed. Philadelphia: Lippincott Williams & Wilkins, 2005, pp 911–915.

Sanner G, Bergstrom B: Benign paroxysmal torticollis in infancy. Acta Paediatr Scand 1979;68:219–223.

Scheffer IE, Bhatia KP, Lopes-Cendes I, et al: Autosomal dominant nocturnal frontal lobe epilepsy: A distinctive clinical disorder. Brain 1995;118:61–73.

Scheidtmann K, Schwarz J, Holinski E, et al: Paroxysmal choreoathetosis—a disorder related to Huntington's disease? J Neurol 1997;244:395–398.

Schloesser DT, Ward TN, Williamson PD: Familial paroxysmal dystonic choreoathetosis revisited. Mov Disord 1996;11:317–320.

Schmidt BJ, Pillay N: Paroxysmal dyskinesia associated with hypoglycemia. Can J Neurol Sci 1993;20:151–153.

Sellal F, Hirsch E, Maquet P, et al: Postures et mouvements anormaux paroxystiques au cours du sommeil: Dystonie paroxystique hypnogenique ou epilepsie partielle? [Abnormal paroxysmal movements during sleep: Hypnogenic paroxysmal dystonia or focal epilepsy?] Rev Neurol 1991;147:121–128.

Sethi KD, Hess DC, Huffnagle VH, Adams RJ: Acetazolamide treatment of paroxysmal dystonia in central demyelinating disease. Neurology 1992;42:919–921.

Sethi KD, Lee KH, Deuskar V, Hess DC: Orthostatic paroxysmal dystonia. Mov Disord 2002;17(4):841–845.

Shaw C, Haas L, Miller D, Delahunt J: A case report of paroxysmal dystonic choreoathetosis due to hypoglycaemia induced by an insulinoma. J Neurol Neurosurg Psychiatry 1996;61:194–195.

Shirane S, Sasaki M, Kogure D, et al: Increased ictal perfusion of the thalamus in paroxysmal kinesigenic dyskinesia. J Neurol Neurosurg Psychiatry 2001;71:408–410.

Snyder CH: Paroxysmal torticollis in infancy. Am J Dis Child 1969;117:458–460.

Soffer D, Licht A, Yaar I, Abramsky O: Paroxysmal choreoathetosis as a presenting symptom in idiopathic hypoparathyroidism. J Neurol Neurosurg Psychiatry 1977;40:692–694.

Spacey SD, Adams PJ, Lam PC, et al: Genetic heterogeneity in paroxysmal nonkinesigenic dyskinesia. Neurology 2006;66(10): 1588–1590.

Spacey SD, Materek LA, Szczgielski BI, Bird TD: Two novel CACNA1A gene mutations associated with episodic ataxia type 2 and interictal dystonia. Arch Neurol 2005;62:314–316.

Spacey SD, Valente EM, Wali GM, et al: Genetic and clinical heterogeneity in paroxysmal kinesigenic dyskinesia: Evidence for a third EKD gene. Mov Disord 2002;17(4):717–725.

Spiller WG: Subcortical epilepsy. Brain 1927;50:171–187.

Steckley JL, Ebers GC, Cader MZ, McLachlan RS: An autosomal dominant disorder with episodic ataxia, vertigo, and tinnitus. Neurology 2001;57:1499–1502.

Stevens H: Paroxysmal choreo-athetosis. Arch Neurol 1966;14: 415–420.

Suber DA, Riley TL: Valproic acid and normal computerized tomographic scan in kinesigenic familial paroxysmal choreoathetosis [letter]. Arch Neurol 1980;37:327.

Swoboda KJ, Soong BW, McKenna C, et al: Paroxysmal kinesigenic dyskinesia and infantile convulsions: Clinical and linkage studies. Neurology 2000;55:224–230.

Szepetowski P, Rochette J, Berquin P, et al: Familial infantile convulsions and paroxysmal choreoathetosis: A new neurological syndrome linked to the pericentromeric region of human chromosome 16. Am J Hum Genet 1997;61:889–898.

Tabaee-Zadeh MJ, Frame B, Kapphahn K: Kinesiogenic choreoathetosis and idiopathic hypoparathyroidism. N Engl J Med 1972; 286:762–763.

Tan A, Salgado M, Fahn S: The characterization and outcome of stereotypic movements in nonautistic children. Mov Disord 1997; 12:47–52.

Terzano MG, Monge-Strauss MF, Mikol F, et al: Cyclic alternating pattern as a provocative factor in nocturnal paroxysmal dystonia. Epilepsia 1997;38:1015–1025.

Thiriaux A, de St Martin A, Vercueil L, et al: Co-occurrence of infantile epileptic seizures and childhood paroxysmal choreoathetosis in one family: Clinical, EEG, and SPECT characterization of episodic events. Mov Disord 2002;17(1):98–104.

Tibbles JA, Barnes SE: Paroxysmal dystonic choreoathetosis of Mount and Reback. Pediatrics 1980;65:149–151.

Tinuper P, Cerullo A, Cirignotta F, et al: Nocturnal paroxysmal dystonia with short-lasting attacks: Three cases with evidence for an epileptic frontal lobe origin of seizures. Epilepsia 1990;31:549–556.

Tomita H, Nagamitsu S, Wakui K, et al: Paroxysmal kinesigenic choreoathetosis locus maps to chromosome 16p11.2-q12.1. Am J Hum Genet 1999;65:1688–1697.

Tsao CY: Effective treatment with oxcarbazepine in paroxysmal kinesigenic choreoathetosis. J Child Neurol 2004;19:300–301.

Uberall MA, Wenzel D: Effectiveness of lamotrigine in children with paroxysmal kinesigenic choreoathetosis. Dev Med Child Neurol 2000;42:699–700.

Vaamonde J, Artieda J, Obeso JA: Hereditary paroxysmal ataxia with neuromyotonia. Mov Disord 1991;6:180–182.

Vahedi K, Joutel A, van Bogaert P, et al: A gene for hereditary paroxysmal cerebellar ataxia maps to chromosome 19p. Ann Neurol 1995;37:289–293.

Valente EM, Spacey SD, Wali GM, et al: A second paroxysmal kinesigenic choreoathetosis locus (EKD2) mapping on 16q13-q22.1 indicates a family of genes which give rise to paroxysmal disorders on human chromosome 16. Brain 2000;123:2040–2045.

Van Dyke DH, Griggs RC, Murphy MJ, Goldstein MN: Hereditary myokymia and periodic ataxia. J Neurol Sci 1975;25:109–118.

Verheul GAM, Tyssen CC: Multiple sclerosis occurring with paroxysmal unilateral dystonia. Mov Disord 1990;5:352–353.

Vighetto A, Froment JC, Trillet M, Aimard G: Magnetic resonance imaging in familial paroxysmal ataxia. Arch Neurol 1988;45:547–549.

Vincent FM: Hyperglycemia-induced hemichoreoathetosis: The presenting manifestation of a vascular malformation of the lenticular nucleus. Neurosurgery 1986;18:787–790.

von Brederlow B, Hahn A, Koopman WJ, et al: Mapping the gene for acetazolamide responsive hereditary paryoxysmal cerebellar ataxia to chromosome 19p. Hum Mol Genet 1995;4:279–284.

Wali GM: Paroxysmal hemidystonia induced by prolonged exercise and cold. J Neurol Neurosurg Psychiatry 1992;55:236–237.

Walker ES: Familial paroxysmal dystonic choreoathetosis: A neurologic disorder simulating psychiatric illness. Johns Hopkins Med J 1981;148:108–113.

Waller DA: Paroxysmal kinesigenic choreoathetosis or hysteria? Am J Psychiatry 1977;134:1439–1440.

Walters AS, Hening WA, Chokroverty S: Review and videotape recognition of idiopathic restless legs syndrome. Mov Disord 1991;6: 105–110.

Watson RT, Scott WR: Paroxysmal kinesigenic choreoathetosis and brain-stem atrophy [letter]. Arch Neurol 1979;36:522.

Weber MB: Familial paroxysmal dystonia. J Nerv Ment Dis 1967;145: 221–226.

White JC: Familial periodic nystagmus, vertigo, and ataxia. Arch Neurol 1969;20:276–280.

Whitty CWM, Lishman WA, FitzGibbon JP: Seizures induced by movement: A form of reflex epilepsy. Lancet 1964;1:1403–1406.

Wilson SAK: The Morrison Lectures on nervous semeiology, with special reference to epilepsy: Lecture III. Symptoms indicating increase of neural function. Br Med J 1930;2:90–94.

Winer JB, Fish DR, Sawyers D, Marsden CD: A movement disorder as a presenting feature of recurrent hypoglycaemia. Mov Disord 1990;5:176–177.

Yamada K, Goto S, Soyama N, et al. Complete suppression of paroxysmal nonkinesigenic dyskinesia by globus pallidus internus pallidal stimulation. Mov Disord 2006;21:576–580.

Yamamoto K, Kawazawa S: Basal ganglion calcification in paroxysmal dystonic choreoathetosis [letter]. Ann Neurol 1987;22:556.

Yang ML, Fullwood E, Goldstein J, Mink JM: Masturbation in infancy and early childhood presenting as a movement disorder: 12 cases and a review of the literature. Pediatrics 2005;116:1427–1432.

Yokochi K: Paroxysmal ocular downward deviation in neurologically impaired infants. Pediatr Neurol 1991;7:426–428.

Yue Q, Jen JC, Nelson SF, Baloh RW: Progressive ataxia due to a missense mutation in a calcium-channel gene. Am J Hum Genet 1997;61:1078–1087.

Yue Q, Jen JC, Thwe MM, et al: De novo mutation in CACNA1A caused acetazolamide-responsive episodic ataxia. Am J Med Genet 1998;77:298–301.

Zacchetti O, Sozzi G, Zampollo A: Paroxysmal kinesigenic choreoathetosis: Case report. Ital J Neurol Sci 1983;3:345–347.

Zasorin NL, Baloh RW, Myers LB: Acetazolamide-responsive episodic ataxia syndrome. Neurology 1983;33:1212–1214.

Zerr P, Adelman JP, Maylie J: Episodic ataxia mutations in Kv1.1 alter potassium channel function by dominant negative effects or haploinsufficiency. J Neurosci 1998;18:2842–2848.

Zhuchenko O, Bailey J, Bonnen P, et al: Autosomal dominant cerebellar ataxia (SCA6) associated with small polyglutamine expansions in the alpha 1A-voltage-dependent calcium channel. Nat Genet 1997;15:62–69.

# Chapter 24

# Restless Legs Syndrome and Peripheral Movement Disorders

## RESTLESS LEGS SYNDROME AND PERIODIC MOVEMENTS OF SLEEP

The term *restless legs* has been applied to a number of conditions. Ekbom (1960) originally applied this term to unpleasant crawling sensations in the legs, particularly in sitting and relaxing in the evening, that disappeared on walking. The syndrome was probably first described by Thomas Willis in 1685. Restlessness is also a characteristic feature of akathisia, but here the feeling is of inner restlessness not specifically referred to the legs, although this inner feeling can be dissipated by activity. Inner tension is also a feature of the urge to tic, relieved by the involuntary movement.

Restless legs syndrome (RLS) is characterized by a deep, ill-defined discomfort or dysesthesia in the legs that arises during prolonged rest or when the patient is drowsy and trying to fall asleep, especially at night (Walters, 1995; Walters et al., 1996; Wetter and Pollmacher, 1997; Winkelmann et al., 2000; Bassetti et al., 2001). The disorder is truly diurnal; the symptoms are worse during the night even when the person tries to stay awake for long periods of time (Hening, Walters, et al., 1999; Trenkwalder et al., 1999). The discomfort may be difficult to describe; terms such as crawling, creeping, pulling, itching, drawing, or stretching are used, and the feeling usually is felt in the muscles or bones. These intolerable sensations are relieved by movement of the legs or by walking. The feeling is usually bilateral, and the arms are only rarely involved. Standardized criteria have been put forward by the International Restless Legs Syndrome Study Group (Box 24-1) (Allen et al., 2003). Complaints of restless legs are common, with an estimated prevalence of 3% to 10% (Phillips et al., 2000; Rothdach et al., 2000; Hening et al., 2004; Bjorvatn et al., 2005). A large population study (over 16,000 adults) showed a prevalence of any restless symptoms to be 7.2% and moderately or severely distressing symptoms to be 2.7% (Allen et al., 2005). RLS is generally a condition of middle to old age, but at least one third of patients experience their first symptoms before the age of 20 years (Walters et al., 1996; Kotagal and Silber, 2004). Most patients have mild symptoms to begin with, but these get worse with time, so that the patients seek aid in middle life. Remission is uncommon, occurring in about 15% of patients (Walters et al., 1996).

The majority of people with RLS also exhibit periodic movements of sleep (Lugaresi et al., 1986; Pollmacher and Schulz, 1993; Walters, 1995; Trenkwalder et al., 1996) (Box 24-2). These consist of brief (1- to 2-second) jerks of one or both legs, consisting of, at their simplest, dorsiflexion of the big toe and foot. Initially, there is a jerk, but subsequently, there is sustained tonic spasm. Such events tend to occur in runs every 20 seconds or so for minutes or hours. Sometimes, the whole leg or both legs flex (Fig. 24-1). The movement resembles a flexion reflex (Bara-Jimenez et al., 2000). Such

periodic movements often wake the sleeping partner and may cause disturbance of sleep in the affected individual, in which case there may be excessive daytime drowsiness. Generally, the movements appear during periods of arousal during sleep in stage I and II and decrease during stages III and IV; they are unusual during REM sleep. Sometimes, the flexion movements of one or both legs can occur in the waking subject, particularly when drowsy (Hening et al., 1986) (Video 24-1).  Note should be made that some patients with RLS have propriospinal myoclonus just before falling asleep (Vetrugno et al., 2005).

While most people with restless legs have periodic movements of sleep (at least in the sleep laboratory), there are patients with periodic movements of sleep who do not complain of restless legs. The combined syndrome of restless legs and periodic movements of sleep is an age-related condition; its incidence increases in adulthood and late life. It usually presents after the age of 30 years, and it is said to affect 5% of those between the ages of 30 and 50 years and as many as 30% of those over the age of 50 years. However, in a large proportion of cases, the periodic movements of sleep do not cause complaint and are found incidentally during sleep studies. In many with RLS, the condition is not disabling.

There is evidence to suggest that the complaint in many if not most patients is transmitted as an autosomal-dominant trait (Walters et al., 1996; Winkelmann et al., 2000). Linkage on 12q seems the best defined and has been designated RLS1 (Desautels et al., 2005). Linkage has been found on 14q for a few families and has been designated RLS2 (Bonati et al., 2003; Levchenko et al., 2004). Linkage on 9p24-22 has been designated RLS3 (Liebetanz et al., 2006; Winkelmann and Ferini-Strambi, 2006).

Some cases have been associated with anemia, pregnancy, chronic myelopathies and peripheral neuropathies, gastric surgery, uremia, and chronic lung disease (Ekbom, 1960; Ondo and Jankovic, 1996; Winkelmann et al., 2000). It is not uncommon in Parkinson disease (Ondo et al., 2002), and one epidemiologic study did find an increased prevalence compared with the general population (Krishnan et al., 2003), whereas another did not (Tan et al., 2002). These symptomatic cases of restless legs should be distinguished from the primary familial form of the condition. Occasionally, drugs (neuroleptics and antidepressants, lithium, and anticonvulsants) may precipitate intense restlessness of the legs.

Interestingly, in the idiopathic form of the disorder, Earley and colleagues (2000b) found low cerebrospinal ferritin levels and high transferrin levels. Further investigations by this group have shown that the cerebrospinal ferritin level is low only in the early-onset RLS patients and that levels are lower at night than during the day (Earley et al., 2005). There was no difference, however, in serum ferritin and transferrin levels. The findings suggest that there might be low brain iron in

**Box 24-1** Essential diagnostic criteria for restless legs syndrome

1. An urge to move the legs, usually accompanied or caused by uncomfortable and unpleasant sensations in the legs (Sometimes the urge to move is present with the uncomfortable sensations and sometimes the arms or other body parts are involved in addition to the legs)
2. The urge to move or unpleasant sensations begin or worsen during periods of rest or inactivity such as lying or sitting
3. The urge to move or unpleasant sensations are partially or totally relieved by movement, such as walking or stretching, at least as long as the activity continues
4. The urge to move or unpleasant sensations are worse in the evening or night than during the day or only occur in the evening or night (When symptoms are very severe, the worsening at night may not be noticeable but must have been previously present)

**Supportive Clinical Features of Restless Legs Syndrome**
***Family History***
The prevalence of restless legs syndrome (RLS) among first-degree relatives of people with RLS is 3 to 5 times greater than in people without RLS.

***Response to Dopaminergic Therapy***
Nearly all people with RLS show at least an initial response to either L-dopa or a dopamine-receptor agonist at doses considered to be very low in relation to the traditional doses of these medications used for the treatment of Parkinson disease. This initial response is not, however, universally maintained.

***Periodic Limb Movements (during Wakefulness or Sleep)***
Periodic limb movements in sleep (PLMS) occur in at least 85% of people with RLS; however, PLMS also commonly occur in other disorders and in the elderly. In children, PLMS are much less common than in adults.

Reprinted with permission from Allen RP, Picchietti D, Hening WA, et al: Restless legs syndrome: Diagnostic criteria, special considerations, and epidemiology: A report from the restless legs syndrome diagnosis and epidemiology workshop at the National Institutes of Health. Sleep Med 2003;4:101–119.

these patients. Neuroimaging studies of iron have been controversial, and a neuropathologic evaluation of seven brains has demonstrated decreased H-ferritin, but not iron, in the substantia nigra (Connor et al., 2003).

Periodic movements of sleep should be distinguished from hypnic jerks or "sleep starts," which consist of whole-body sudden jerks on falling asleep, and from fragmentary sleep myoclonus. The latter consists of multifocal myoclonus, which can commonly be observed in the dog asleep on the mat. Restless legs must be distinguished from the syndrome of painful legs and moving toes and from painful night cramps.

The pathophysiology of primary restless legs and periodic movements of sleep is unknown (Hening, 2004; Trenkwalder and Paulus, 2004). That dopaminergic mechanisms are involved is strongly suggested by the amelioration of symp-

toms with dopaminergic therapy. A critical role for the basal ganglia is suggested by the observation that pallidotomy or deep brain stimulation of the pallidum for Parkinson disease ameliorated the sensory symptoms of restless legs (Rye and DeLong, 1999; Okun et al., 2005). (In relation to surgery for Parkinson disease, some patients with deep brain stimulation of the subthalamic nucleus will develop RLS [Kedia et al., 2004]. This might be due to the fact that dopaminergic drug therapy is reduced, and this might unmask the disorder.) There is some evidence that D2 receptor binding in the striatum is low, while presynaptic dopamine function appears to be normal as indicated by dopamine transporter measurement (Michaud et al., 2002). Not all studies find this D2 receptor abnormality (Eisensehr et al., 2001). Interestingly, there is a strong relationship between iron and dopamine, iron deficiency causing a dopamine deficiency (Allen, 2004).

Opioid receptor availability evaluated with PET and [$^{11}$C]diprenorphine, a nonselective opioid receptor radioligand, showed no difference between patients and controls (von Spiczak et al., 2005). However, patients' symptoms were inversely proportional to the binding in the brain medial pain system.

RLS is characterized by abnormal sensations, and sensory testing reveals abnormalities of temperature sensation. Studies suggest that in idiopathic RLS, the abnormality is in the central processing (Schattschneider et al., 2004).

If the syndrome is distressing, drug treatment might be justified. A nocturnal dose of a levodopa preparation has been found to be beneficial (Kaplan et al., 1993; Hening, Allen, et al., 1999; Tan and Ondo, 2000; Trenkwalder et al., 2003). Dopamine agonists such as bromocriptine are also effective (Walters et al., 1988; Earley et al., 1998; Pieta et al., 1998), and there have been studies demonstrating the value of pergolide (Wetter et al., 1999; Stiasny et al., 2001), pramipexole (Montplaisir et al., 1999), and ropinirole (Ondo, 1999; Adler et al., 2004; Bogan et al., 2006). The use of dopaminergic therapy has been reviewed (Comella, 2002). Dopaminergic therapy has efficacy even in patients with complete spinal cord lesions, suggesting some action at the level of the spinal cord (de Mello et al., 1999). Alternatively, a nocturnal dose of an opiate such as propoxyphene (Hening et al., 1986) or codeine phosphate (Becker et al., 1993; Walters et al., 1993; Prinz, 1995) or of a benzodiazepine such as clonazepam may be of help. Carbamazepine also may help (Telstad et al., 1984), as may baclofen (Guilleminault and Flagg, 1984), clonidine (Wagner et al., 1996), and gabapentin (Garcia-Borreguero et al., 2002; Albanese and Filippini, 2003).

**Box 24-2** Periodic movements of sleep

Runs (every 20 seconds or so) of brief (1- to 2-second) jerks in one or both legs
Initial jerk followed by a tonic spasm
Dorsiflexion of the big toe and foot (or flexion of the whole leg)
Occurs during arousal (stage I and II sleep)
May occur in an awake, drowsy individual
Asymptomatic, may wake sleeping partner or sometimes the patient
Prevalence increases with age: rare in those under 30 years of age, 5% in those 30 to 50 years of age; 29% in those over 50 years of age

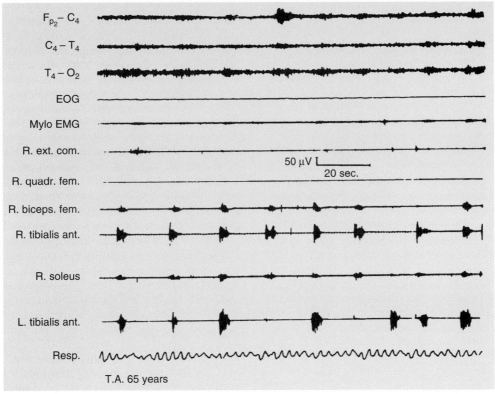

**Figure 24-1** Polysomnography recording from a patient with periodic limb movements in sleep (PLMS). Note the periodic electromyographic bursts in leg muscles coming about every 20 seconds. (Reprinted with permission from Lugaresi E, Cirignotta F, Coccagna G, Montagna P: Nocturnal myoclonus and restless legs syndrome. Adv Neurol 1986;43:295–307.)

Iron also has been recommended for therapy (Ekbom, 1960), and it has been suggested that it might act by virtue of its effect on dopamine and opiate receptors (Earley et al., 2000a), but one study has been negative (Davis et al., 2000). Another open-label study has evaluated the effects of a single 1000-mg intravenous infusion of iron dextran (Earley et al., 2004). Therapy significantly improved the mean global RLS symptom severity, total sleep time, hours with RLS symptoms, and PLMS, but on an individual basis, it failed to produce any response in 3 of the 10 subjects who were fully treated. Brain iron concentrations at 2 weeks postinfusion as determined by magnetic resonance imaging were increased in the substantia nigra and prefrontal cortex. In those who responded to the iron infusion, further iron infusions may maintain the effect, but this was not true for all patients (Earley et al., 2005). Iron is curative, of course, in cases associated with iron deficiency. It might be necessary to change from one drug to another if tolerance develops.

The literature on therapy for RLS has been reviewed and evaluated (Hening, Allen, et al., 1999), and guidelines have been proposed (Chesson et al., 1999). The American Academy of Sleep Medicine has published practice parameters (Littner et al., 2004). A useful algorithm has been developed (Silber et al., 2004).

## PERIPHERAL MOVEMENT DISORDERS

Abnormal involuntary movements (dyskinesias) usually are caused by brain damage or dysfunction. Occasionally, however, lesions of the spinal cord, spinal roots, cervical or lumbar plexus, or even peripheral nerves appear to cause a variety of dyskinesias (Box 24-3). Sometimes, the relationship between the trauma and the movement disorder is not definite, and there are no proven rules to relate them. Jankovic and colleagues have proposed some criteria that can be used as guidelines until more definitive rules are determined (Box 24-4) (Jankovic, 1994; Cardoso and Jankovic, 1995). An example of a definitive peripheral disorder is hemifacial spasm, in which compression of the facial nerve by a cerebellopontine angle mass lesion or by aberrant arteries in the posterior fossa produces repetitive clonic and tonic contractions of one side of the face. Local pathology in the spinal cord may lead to focal spinal segmental myoclonus. Similar focal myoclonus is sometimes

**Box 24-3** Peripheral movement disorders

Hemifacial spasm
Spinal segmental myoclonus
Root, plexus, nerve lesions
Reflex sympathetic dystrophy (RSD)
Causalgia-dystonia syndrome
Dystonia triggered by peripheral injury
Jumpy stumps
Belly dancer's dyskinesia
Painful legs and moving toes

**Box 24-4** Criteria for a movement disorder to be related to trauma

1. The injury must be severe enough to cause local symptoms that persist for at least 2 weeks or require medical evaluation within 2 weeks of the injury.
2. The onset of the movement disorder must have occurred within a few days or months (up to 1 year) after the injury.
3. The onset of the movement disorder must have been anatomically related to the site of the injury.

From Jankovic J: Post-traumatic movement disorders: Central and peripheral mechanisms. Neurology 1994;44:2006–2014; Cardoso F, Jankovic J: Peripherally induced tremor and parkinsonism. Arch Neurol 1995;52:263–270.

due to damage to spinal roots, the plexus, or peripheral nerves. Such lesions also rarely cause other dyskinesias, such as dystonia and other forms of muscle spasms, sometimes associated with causalgia and reflex sympathetic dystrophy (RSD). Finally, a peripheral injury may act as the trigger to the appearance of dyskinesias that are thought to arise in the brain, as is the case in a significant proportion of patients with primary dystonia. In some way, the peripheral injury alters central nervous system activity to generate involuntary movements.

## Hemifacial Spasm

Hemifacial spasm is characterized by synchronous spasms of one side of the face (Box 24-5). Most cases are primary, but some are secondary following recovery from facial nerve

**Box 24-5** Hemifacial spasm

Unilateral clonic jerks, with tonic spasm of all facial muscles
Starts around the eye, spreads to the mouth and platysma
Spasms lift the eyebrow
Irregular and unpredictable; triggered by facial movement; may occur in flurries
Mild facial weakness develops, with paradoxical synkinesis
Adults; females more than males (ratio: 3:2)
95% primary, due to vascular compression of the seventh nerve at the exit from the brainstem
5% secondary, due to postparalytic (Bell palsy) or cerebellopontine angle mass lesions (tumor or arteriovenous malformation) or, rarely, brainstem lesions (multiple sclerosis: tonic spasms or facial myokymia)
Remissions are rare.
Treatment:
Drugs usually do not help.
Botulinum toxin
Posterior fossa exploration and facial nerve protection

paresis (Colosimo et al., 2006). The spasms are usually very brief but can occur in runs and are occasionally tonic. The disorder typically begins around the eye, and this often is the most symptomatic aspect to the disorder (Fig. 24-2 and Video 24-2). The disorder can be bilateral, but then the two sides of the face do not spasm in synchrony. Cases do seem to be more common in people of Asian origin (Poungvarin et al., 1995). Twitching can be brought out by facial muscle contraction. The disorder clearly involves the facial nerve, and the etiology appears to be most frequently (94%) a compression of the nerve by a blood vessel just as the nerve leaves the brainstem (Tan and Chan, 2004). About 4% of cases are due to a tumor compressing the nerve. Biopsy of the compressed nerve shows demyelination. Definitive treatment can consist of surgery to decompress the nerve (Samii et al., 2002), although many patients prefer botulinum toxin treatment, which can be highly effective (Poungvarin et al., 1995; Jost and Kohl, 2001; Defazio et al., 2002) and can improve quality of life (Tan et al., 2004).

Although the etiology is relatively clear, the pathophysiology is still not certain. There are two main hypotheses, and there are good data to support each.

### NERVE ORIGIN HYPOTHESIS

The nerve origin hypothesis proposes that the abnormal discharges that produce the spasms come from the region of demyelinated nerve that is under compression (Nielsen,

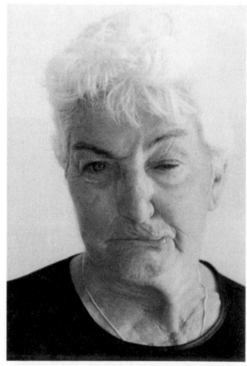

**Figure 24-2** Left-sided hemifacial spasm. Note the elevation of the left brow with the spasm due to contraction of the frontalis muscle. Elevation of the brow with closing of the eye is not easily possible voluntarily. The phenomenon was noted by Babinski and has been referred to as "the other Babinski's sign." (See Color Plate 15.) (Reprinted with permission from Devoize JL: "The other" Babinski's sign: Paradoxical raising of the eyebrow in hemifacial spasm. J Neurol Neurosurg Psychiatry 2001;70:516.)

1984a, 1984b; Nielsen and Jannetta, 1984). It is known that demyelinated nerve can produce spontaneous discharges, called ectopic discharges. In addition, there can be lateral transmission of activity between demyelinated nerve axons, called ephaptic transmission. Ephaptic transmission can be responsible for involvement of much of the face. It is also possible in activity in demyelinated axons with ephaptic transmission for trains of activity to be produced following a single action potential. These phenomena could well explain many of the clinical features.

Additionally, there are physiologic studies that are consistent. If a branch of the seventh nerve is stimulated, late responses will be seen in these patients in muscles that are innervated by other branches at latencies that are consistent with ephaptic transmission at the site of demyelination. This phenomenon is not influenced by botulinum toxin treatment (Geller et al., 1989). Studies of the variability of transmission of this effect, using the technique of jitter, are consistent with only the neuromuscular junction and no intervening synapses (Sanders, 1989).

The final argument in favor of the nerve origin hypothesis is the fact that the disorder very rapidly ameliorates following decompression.

### FACIAL NUCLEUS HYPOTHESIS

According to the facial nucleus hypothesis, the peripheral lesion leads to hyperexcitability of the facial nucleus and the discharges arise there. There is a rat model in which such a phenomenon has been demonstrated. Perhaps the most persuasive argument for this hypothesis is that there is hyperexcitability of the blink reflex in hemifacial spasm, and this must involve brainstem synaptic circuitry. By this theory, the late responses that are seen with stimulation of branches of the nerve are enhanced F-waves (Roth et al., 1990; Ishikawa et al., 1994). Last, while the calculations deal in differences of only a millisecond or two, the conduction times might be more consistent with transmission all the way to the brainstem and back, rather than just to the site of demyelination (Moller and Jannetta, 1984; Moller, 1987).

## Focal Myoclonus Due to Root, Plexus, or Peripheral Nerve Lesions

Myoclonic jerking of the paraspinal muscles due to a malignant tumor involving the fifth thoracic root, without long tract signs of spinal cord involvement, has been described (Sotaniemi, 1985). Similar focal myoclonus of the legs has also occurred with lumbosacral radiculopathy and after lumbar laminectomy for lumbar stenosis and root lesions (Jankovic and Pardo, 1986). Rhythmic myoclonus of the quadriceps muscle has been reported due to a Schwann-cell sarcoma of the femoral nerve (Said and Bathien, 1977).

Focal myoclonus of the right arm due to a brachial plexus lesion has been described following radiotherapy for carcinoma of the breast followed by abduction trauma of the right shoulder (Banks et al., 1985). The latter case exhibited rhythmic muscle jerks at a rate of about five per second in the distribution of the axillary and radial nerves but not in other muscles innervated by the lateral and medial cords of the brachial plexus. Electromyographic analysis of this case indicated that the myoclonus arose from a generator located in a segment of the posterior cord of the brachial plexus, between the departure of the axillary nerve and distal to the emergence of the suprascapular nerve. Another patient developed myoclonus of one arm after an electrical injury to the left brachial plexus (Jankovic and Pardo, 1986). Myoclonus of an arm has even occurred after a thoracic sympathectomy (Jankovic and Pardo, 1986).

The clinical characteristics of myoclonus due to spinal cord, root, plexus, or peripheral nerve diseases are the following:

1. It is focal, being confined to the muscles that are innervated by the affected spinal cord segments or peripheral lower motor neurons.
2. It is usually spontaneous and rhythmic, and it often persists in sleep.

These observations suggest that it is the result of repetitive, spontaneous discharge of groups of anterior horn cells.

Swanson and colleagues (1962) suggested two mechanisms that might be responsible for spinal segmental myoclonus: (1) enhanced neuronal excitability due to direct cellular excitation by inflammation or tumor or (2) enhanced neuronal excitability due to removal of inhibition. The former seems unlikely, for spinal segmental myoclonus can occur without evidence of damage to anterior horn cells. Loss of inhibition of anterior horn cell pools seems more probable.

Posterior rhizotomy or hemicordectomy leads to abnormal spontaneous discharge of some spinal neurons in the deafferented segments, which tend to fire in bursts at high frequency (Loeser and Ward, 1967). However, these bursting spinal neurons are found in the dorsal horns, not in the ventral horns. Nevertheless, such spontaneous bursting of spinal interneurons following deafferentation might drive anterior horn cells to produce focal myoclonus.

Alternatively, loss of inhibitory spinal interneurons might liberate anterior horn cells to fire spontaneously in a rhythmic burst fashion. In the case described by Davis and colleagues (1981), spinal myoclonus occurred following ischemic damage to the cord, which at autopsy was found to have caused extensive loss of small and medium-sized interneurons, with relative preservation of large anterior horn cells. The loss of inhibitory spinal interneurons could well release anterior horn cells to discharge spontaneously, but what then determines their tendency to fire repetitively and rhythmically is less clear (Kiehn, 1991; Kiehn and Eken, 1997). Loss of spinal interneurons also is the pathologic change that is held to be responsible for alpha spinal rigidity.

## Muscle Spasms Associated with Reflex Sympathetic Dystrophy

In 1984, five patients were described who developed abnormal involuntary movements of a limb after injury (Marsden et al., 1984). All developed RSD (now often called complex regional pain syndrome, or CRPS) (Stanton-Hicks et al., 1995) with Sudeck atrophy and then abnormal muscle spasms or jerks of the affected limb, lasting years. Two patients exhibited myoclonic jerks of the injured leg; one had both jerks and more prolonged muscle spasms of the injured foot; the remaining two patients developed more complex dystonic spasms of the injured arm. All had severe persistent causalgic pain in the damaged limb as well as the vasomotor, sudomotor, and trophic changes that are typical of RSD. Jankovic and

Van der Linden (1988), Robberecht and colleagues (1988), and Schwartzman and Kerrigan (1990) also have drawn attention to a variety of involuntary movements associated with causalgia (CRPS II) and RSD (CRPS I). These include fixed abnormal dystonic postures due to sustained muscle spasms and tremor. Schwartzman and Kerrigan (1990) collected 43 patients with "dystonia," spasms, or tremor from 200 cases of RSD.

Bhatia and colleagues (1993) reviewed 18 patients with causalgia and dystonia, triggered by injury (usually trivial) in 15 patients and occurring spontaneously in 3 patients (Box 24-6). Most were young women. All had the typical burning causalgic pain with hyperpathia and allodynia, along with the vasomotor, sudomotor, and trophic changes in skin, subcutaneous tissue, and bone that are typical of RSD (Box 24-7). All these patients developed deforming and often grotesque dystonic postures in the affected limb (the arm in 6 patients, the leg in 12 patients), coincident with or after the causalgia. The dystonic spasms typically were sustained, producing a fixed dystonic posture, in contrast to the mobile spasms that are characteristic of primary torsion dystonia. Both the dystonia and the causalgia spread to affect other limbs in seven patients. All investigations were normal, and all modes of conventional treatment failed to relieve either the pain or the dystonia, but two patients recovered spontaneously. Therefore, there appears to be a relationship between causalgia, RSD, and a variety of involuntary movements, all precipitated by peripheral injury.

The classic clinical features of causalgia have been documented extensively (Schott, 1986b; Schwartzman and McLellan, 1987; Schwartzman, 1993). The mechanisms that are responsible for causalgia and RSD have been the subject of much speculation and appear to be relevant to the pathophysiology of the associated dyskinesias. At first sight, it would seem likely that some persisting peripheral abnormality must be responsible, but close analysis indicates that this is an inadequate explanation (Schwartzman and McLellan, 1987; Schott, 1995). Most authors now also invoke altered central

**Box 24-6** The causalgia-dystonia syndrome

18 cases, aged 12 to 51 years, 16 women and 2 men
  15 followed peripheral injury (often minor);
  3 spontaneous
None had a family history of this disorder
All had reflex sympathetic dystrophy (RSD) (see
  Box 24-7)
Painful fixed dystonia presented at or following onset of
  RSD, initially in the injured limb
Lower limb in 12; upper limb in 6
Contractures developed
Dystonia spread in 10 cases to other limbs, as did
  causalgia in 7 cases.
Brain and spinal cord imaging normal
No response to treatment
Two spontaneous recoveries (4 and 9 years after onset)

Reprinted with permission from Bhatia KP, Bhatt MH, Marsden CD: The causalgia-dystonia syndrome. Brain 1993;116: 843–851.

**Box 24-7** Reflex sympathetic dystrophy

Causalgia (spontaneous burning pain)
Allodynia (hyperpathia or pain on gentle touch)
Trophic changes (edema, cyanosis, hair loss, brittle
  nails, shiny thin skin)
Sudeck atrophy
Spread of pain
Emotional consequences
Relief by sympathetic block (possibly placebo effect)
Soft tissue injury
Infection
Fractures, sprains, dislocations
Surgery
Immobilization
Myocardial infarction (1%)
Nerve damage (5%)

Reprinted with permission from Bhatia KP, Bhatt MH, Marsden CD: The causalgia-dystonia syndrome. Brain 1993;116: 843–851.

mechanisms, triggered by peripheral trauma, as the cause of RSD and causalgia.

Nathan (1947) proposed that the pain of RSD might arise from abnormal stimulation of somatic sensory axons in damaged nerves. Peripheral mechanisms (at sites of nerve damage, including neuromas) that have been invoked to explain causalgia and RSD include the following (Schott, 1986b; Schwartzman and McLellan, 1987; Schwartzman, 1993):

1. Activation of low-threshold mechanoreceptor afferents (pain and allodynia) by ephatic sympathetic efferent activity
2. Activation of nociceptor afferents by ephatic sympathetic efferent activity
3. Ectopic pacemaker discharges in damaged demyelinated axons, sensitive to circulating catecholamines or those released by sympathetic activity (Devor, 1983)

All these mechanisms might explain causalgic pain in the distribution of damaged peripheral nerves, but the trivial trauma that provokes causalgia and dystonia often does not appear to cause detectable nerve damage. In these cases, it is assumed that the local trauma initiates changes in sensory input that have central consequences.

Schott (1986b, 1995) points out that causalgia is unlikely to arise solely from the peripheral nerve itself, for peripheral nerve section, rhizotomy, cordotomy, and even sympathectomy are unlikely to relieve the pain. He also reviews the numerous reports of causalgia provoked by disease of the central nervous system, such as strokes, multiple sclerosis, and spinal cord trauma. The spread of pain (and dystonia) within the limb and to other limbs, sometimes bilaterally, points to a central process at the spinal or supraspinal level. Persistent pain in a phantom limb also argues for a central origin. Peripheral nerve injuries have been shown experimentally to alter the pattern of neuronal activity not only in the dorsal horn (Devor and Wall, 1981a, 1981b) but also in dorsal column nuclei and in ventral thalamus and sensory cortex (Florence and Kaas, 1995; Kaas, 2000).

So trauma or damage to peripheral nerves is thought to give rise to abnormal impulse transmission in peripheral sensory and sympathetic nerves, which in turn leads to reorganization of central processing of sensory (and motor) information to cause causalgia (and dystonia). There is a close analogy between the postulated mechanisms that are responsible for hemifacial spasm and those that cause RSD and causalgia. The idea is that peripheral and central mechanisms interact to produce the motor, sensory, and sympathetic phenomena.

It is important to note that the whole issue of RSD is muddled in controversy. Certainly, the notion of a primary sympathetic dysfunction seems unlikely. This area has been marked by anecdotal reports and poor science. The view opposing RSD has been eloquently stated by Ochoa (1995, 1999; Ochoa and Verdugo, 1995) and by Lang and Fahn (1990). Many patients with this syndrome have significant psychiatric disease, and many of the movement disorders appear to be psychogenic. Verdugo and Ochoa prospectively studied 58 patients with CRPS I or II and a movement disorder (Verdugo and Ochoa, 2000). The patients exhibited various combinations of dystonic spasms, coarse postural or action tremor, irregular jerks, and choreiform movements. No case of CRPS II but only cases of CRPS type I displayed abnormal movements. In addition to an absence of evidence of structural nerve, spinal cord, or intracranial damage, all CRPS I patients with abnormal movements typically exhibited pseudoneurologic (nonorganic) signs. In some cases, malingering was documented by secret surveillance.

Abnormalities in clinical neurophysiologic testing were found by one group (van de Beek et al., 2002), but another study reported that changes are not dissimilar to findings that are seen in normal individuals who are mimicking an abnormal posture (Koelman et al., 1999).

Treatment of this disorder is very difficult. A report shows that intrathecal baclofen can be efficacious (van Hilten et al., 2000).

## Jumpy Stumps

Not only did Weir Mitchell (1872) describe causalgia after gunshot wounds of peripheral nerves; he also recorded tremor, jerks, and spasms of the remaining stump following amputation, sometimes associated with severe phantom pain. The "painful, jumpy stump" has since been described by others (Russell, 1970; Steiner et al., 1974; Marion et al., 1989; Kulisevsky et al., 1992), and even a phantom dyskinesia induced by metoclopramide has been reported (Jankovic and  Glass, 1985) (Video 24-3).

Jerking of the amputation stump (jactitation), coinciding with lancinating neuralgic stump pains, frequently occurs in the postoperative period but settles over weeks or months (Russell, 1970). The patients referred to previously, however, experienced spasms and jerks of the stump for prolonged periods—for example, up to 40 years in one of the patients reported by Marion and colleagues (1989), who also reviewed many similar cases described in the earlier literature. Jerking of the stump frequently was preceded by severe pain in the stump, appearing weeks or months after the surgery. Upper or lower limb stumps could be affected. The stump jerks could be induced by voluntary movement or sometimes by cutaneous stimuli.

Steiner and colleagues (1974) considered involuntary stump movements to be a form of segmental myoclonus, caused by afferent impulses arising from the severed nerves. Marion and colleagues (1989) concluded that they were due to either "the result of functional changes in spinal (or cortical) circuitry leading to redirection of afferent information through different spinal neurons, or structural reorganization of local neuronal circuitry by axonal sprouting following nerve injury."

## Belly Dancer's Dyskinesia

Belly dancer's dyskinesia, or the moving umbilicus syndrome, is another bizarre condition that is sometimes related to abdominal trauma. Iliceto and colleagues (1990) described five patients with odd abnormal movements of the abdomen (Video 24-4). One had diaphragmatic flutter (repetitive contractions at the rate of about 1 per second are seen on diaphragmatic screening), but the remainder did not. The latter exhibited regular rhythmic contractions of the abdominal wall, which had a sinuous, writhing, flowing character, often moving the umbilicus from side to side or in a circular rotatory fashion. The intensity of the abnormal movement may vary with respiration. Three of these four patients dated the onset of their abdominal dyskinesia to trauma (cholecystectomy and anal fistula, cystoscopic removal of a renal calculus, and cystectomy), and two had severe pain.

## Dystonia Induced by Peripheral Injury

A few reports have suggested that peripheral nerve lesions apparently cause typical arm dystonia (Schott, 1985; Scherokman et al., 1986), and action dystonia of the legs associated with severe lumbar canal stenosis has been described (Al-Kawi, 1987). However, caution must be exercised in attributing dystonia to a peripheral nerve injury, for nerve entrapment may be secondary to dystonia. Thus, for example, some 7% of patients with writer's cramp subsequently develop carpal tunnel compression of the median nerve as a consequence of their dystonia (Sheehy et al., 1988), and secondary entrapment neuropathies are not uncommon in those with any form of dystonia.

More convincing is the association of trauma with the onset of dystonia (Video 24-5). Sheehy and Marsden (1980) described three trauma-induced cases out of a series of 60 patients with torticollis and calculated that 9% of 414 cases of this focal dystonia had suffered preceding injuries. These authors (Sheehy and Marsden, 1982) also noted that writer's cramp could be precipitated by local hand injury and subsequently identified five such cases among 91 patients (Sheehy et al., 1988). Schott (1985) described four patients with axial or arm dystonia after local trauma and later (Schott, 1986a) described a further ten patients with movement disorders that appeared to have been precipitated by peripheral trauma; six of these had developed dystonia, including writer's and pianist's cramps, cranial segmental dystonia, axial segmental dystonia, and focal foot dystonia. The interval from injury to development of dystonia ranged from 24 hours to 3 years. In some patients, oromandibular dystonia has appeared after dental treatment (Thompson et al., 1986; Koller et al., 1989). Brin and colleagues (1986) briefly reported 23 patients in whom trauma precipitated dystonia in the injured region after an interval of between 1 day and 8 weeks. Jankovic and Van der Linden (1988) described a number of patients with dystonia and tremor induced by peripheral trauma; of 28 patients, 13 had persistent dystonia (4 of a hand, 5 of a foot, 1 of an arm, 1 of a leg, and 2 of craniocervical musculature) developing within 1 day to 12 months after a relevant injury. In blepharospasm, a history of preceding local ocular disease has been recorded in about 12% of cases (Grandas et al., 1988).

Thus, there appears to be a significant association between local trauma and the onset of a variety of focal dystonias in a proportion of patients with this illness, perhaps some 5% to 10% overall. The matter remains controversial, however, and is often debated (Jankovic, 2001; Weiner, 2001).

Of course, the vast majority of people who are subjected to local injury do not develop dystonia, so trauma alone is unlikely to be the cause. It seems more probable that trauma triggers the appearance of dystonia in those who are predisposed to develop this illness. Indeed, on occasion, trauma may trigger a focal dystonia in patients who subsequently progress to develop generalized dystonia.

Primary torsion dystonia is usually genetic in origin, so the trauma might be a significant trigger to onset of the illness in those who carry the abnormal gene. Fletcher and colleagues (1991b) examined the relationship between trauma and dystonia in 104 patients with primary generalized, multifocal, or segmental torsion dystonia. Genetic analysis of this population had indicated that the illness was caused by an autosomal-dominant gene with reduced (40%) penetrance in about 85% of cases (Fletcher et al., 1990). Seventeen (16.4%) of these 104 cases reported that their dystonia had been precipitated (14 cases) or exacerbated (5 cases) by local trauma. The dystonia appeared in the injured part of the body within days or up to 12 months after the trauma. Subsequently, the dystonia spread to other body regions. Some patients experienced a new dystonia in a different body part after a subsequent injury to that distant structure. Eight of these 17 patients had affected relatives and so were genetically at risk of developing dystonia before the injury. Brin and colleagues (1986) and Jankovic and Van der Linden (1988) also noted familial cases among patients with trauma-induced dystonia (i.e., 9 of 23 patients and 3 of 13 patients, respectively). All this evidence is consistent with the hypothesis that peripheral injury might precipitate dystonia in people who carry the idiopathic torsion dystonia gene or genes, although trauma among those with idiopathic torsion dystonia is no more frequent than that in a matched control population (Fletcher et al., 1991a).

The dystonia associated with trauma in these cases was similar in all respects to that occurring spontaneously. Inherited primary dystonia is thought to be due to basal ganglia dysfunction. If this is also the case in those who develop dystonia after injury, then it would seem that trauma might trigger abnormalities of the brain as well as the spinal cord.

There are possible mechanisms whereby peripheral injury might alter basal ganglia function. A major projection of the spinothalamic tract is to the ventrobasal nucleus of the thalamus, which projects to the somatosensory cortex. This system probably subserves discriminative pain perception, while spinoreticular pathways may be involved in large-scale somatic and autonomic responses to pain. The main projection of the nocioceptive component of the spinoreticular tract is to the nucleus gigantocellularis, in which (in the rat) nearly all cells respond to noxious stimuli (Benjamin, 1970). Neurons in nucleus gigantocellularis project principally to the centrum medianum and parafascicular thalamic nuclei, which are a major source of projections to the striatum (Guilbaud, 1985). Thus, nociceptive stimuli can gain access to the basal ganglia.

There also is direct experimental evidence that peripheral injury can alter basal ganglia chemistry. De Ceballos and colleagues (1986) found that a thermal injury to one hind limb in the rat causes early (24 hours) bilateral reduction of leu-encephalin immunoreactivity in the globus pallidus and later (1 week) bilateral (but most marked contralaterally) reduction of both met-encephalin and leu-encephalin immunoreactivity in the globus pallidus and of met-encephalin immunoreactivity in the caudate and putamen. These late changes in basal ganglia encephalin content may reflect alterations in basal ganglia function that could conceivably be responsible for peripheral trauma precipitating dystonia in genetically susceptible individuals.

## PAINFUL LEGS AND MOVING TOES

There is another condition in which injury to peripheral nerves and roots may cause the combination of pain in the leg and abnormal involuntary movement of the toes (Box 24-8). Spillane and colleagues (1971) described six patients with severe pain in one or both feet accompanied by characteristic writhing movements of the toes and sometimes of the feet. Three of these patients had a history that suggested lumbosacral root damage. Subsequently, more patients were described with local peripheral nerve damage, L5 herpes zoster, S1 root compression, and cauda equina lesions (Nathan, 1978); generalized peripheral neuropathy (Montagna et al., 1983); and as minor trauma to the legs (Schott, 1981). This condition may be associated with the neuropathy of AIDS (Pitagoras de Mattos et al., 1999). A similar condition has been recorded in the upper limb, with a painful arm and moving fingers, one example being due to a brachial plexus lesion associated with a breast carcinoma and radiotherapy (Verhagen et al., 1985).

Dressler and colleagues (1994) reviewed a series of 18 patients with the syndrome of painful legs and moving toes (Table 24-1). One case followed a bullet injury to the spinal cord and cauda equina; four cases were due to spinal nerve root injury (one with herpes zoster, two with lumbar disc prolapses, and one with an L5 hemangioma); four cases were due

---

**Box 24-8** Painful legs and moving toes

Adults 30 to 80 years of age; males and females
Unilateral or bilateral
Pain in feet first, followed days or years later by movements
Deep ache, burning, throbbing, crushing, tearing
Hyperpathia and allodynia
Sinuous, writhing, athetoid toe movements
Complex 1- to 2-Hz movement patterns of central origin
Very difficult to treat; some success has been claimed with the following:
   Nerve blocks, guanethidine infusions, transcutaneous electrical nerve stimulation
   Anticonvulsants, antidepressants, adenosine

**Table 24-1** Clinical features of patients with painful legs and moving toes

| Feature | N = 29[*] | N = 18[†] |
|---|---|---|
| Average age of onset | 57.7 (30–80 years) | 60.3 (28–76 years) |
| Male/female | 11:18 | 3:15 |
| Bilateral/unilateral | 15:14 | 10:8 |
| Lesions identified | | |
| Cord | 0 | 0 |
| Cauda equina[‡] | 14 | 8 |
| Peripheral neuropathy | 7 | 3 |
| Peripheral trauma | 6 | 4 |
| Unknown | 2 | 3 |

[*]Twenty-nine cases from various sources (Spillane et al., 1971; Nathan, 1978; Barnett et al., 1981; Schott, 1981; Wulff, 1982; Montagna et al., 1983; Schoenen et al., 1984).
[†]Cases from Dressler and colleagues, 1994.
[‡]Includes disc compression, herpes zoster, sacral cyst, hemangioma, and trauma.

to peripheral leg trauma; three cases were associated with an axonal peripheral neuropathy; and in six cases, no definite cause could be identified (although lumbosacral radiculopathies were suspected in at least four of these patients). Three other patients with identical toe movements but no pain also were described.

The age of onset usually is in middle or late life. Pain usually was the first symptom, preceding the movements by days to years. The pain has been described as a deep dull ache, burning, throbbing, crushing, searing, surging, or bursting. Sometimes there are associated sensations of pins and needles in the affected limb. The pain is very severe, leading patients to put their feet into ice boxes, wrap them with flannels, or other major measures. The onset may be unilateral, with subsequent spread to the opposite limb, or bilateral. In many patients, the pain and the movements appeared to be linked, with increasing pain associated with worsening movements. The pain typically is diffuse, not limited to a peripheral nerve or segmented dermatomal pattern. The characteristics of the pain and the common coexistence of hyperpathia and allodynia suggest causalgia (Schott, 1986b).

The moving toes symptom refers to sinuous, athetoid-like dystonic movements of the toes and, rarely, of the feet. The patient might complain that the toes are working inside the shoe, rubbing to cause blisters. The toe movements consist of complex sequences of flexion, extension, abduction, and adduction in various combinations at frequencies of 1 to 2 Hz (Video 24-6). The electromyographic characteristics of such muscle contractions cannot be explained by a peripheral nerve mechanism alone but point to an origin in the central nervous system.

The mechanism that has been proposed to explain this condition again is that of peripheral injury to nerves, plexus, or roots, causing an alteration in spinal and/or supraspinal sensory (the pain) and motor (the movements) machinery. However, the nature of the movements (slow, writhing, and sustained—i.e., dystonic) is quite different from the types of movements that are seen in hemifacial spasm (myoclonic jerks) or, indeed, in spinal myoclonus. Whether the movements in this condition arise in the spinal cord, as was suggested by Nathan (1978) and Schott (1981, 1986a), or supraspinally is unknown.

It is the pain that causes the major disability, and unfortunately, this is very difficult to treat. A few patients have responded to sympathetic blockade, but in the majority, this is ineffective. A course of guanethidine blocks into the affected limb is worth trying. Transcutaneous electrical nerve stimulation applied to the leg or foot might help the pain. Carbamazepine, diphenylhydantoin, amitriptyline, and phenothiazines occasionally help. There is one report of adenosine being useful (Guieu et al., 1994). One patient responded to gabapentin 600 mg three times per day (Villarejo et al., 2004). Epidural block may be helpful (Okuda et al., 1998), as may epidural spinal cord stimulation (Takahashi et al., 2002).

The syndrome can very rarely involve the upper extremity, in which case it is referred to as *painful arm and moving fingers* (Supiot et al., 2002) (Video 24-7).

## Acknowledgments

This chapter is the work of the U.S. government and is not copyrighted. This chapter has been extensively modified and updated from an original by C. D. Marsden.

## References

Adler CH, Hauser RA, Sethi K, et al: Ropinirole for restless legs syndrome: A placebo-controlled crossover trial. Neurology 2004;62:1405–1407.

Albanese A, Filippini G: Gabapentin improved sensory and motor symptoms in the restless legs syndrome. ACP J Club 2003;139:17.

Al-Kawi MZ: Focal dystonia in spinal stenosis. Arch Neurol 1987;44:692–693.

Allen R: Dopamine and iron in the pathophysiology of restless legs syndrome (RLS). Sleep Med 2004;5:385–391.

Allen RP, Picchietti D, Hening WA, et al: Restless legs syndrome: Diagnostic criteria, special considerations, and epidemiology: A report from the restless legs syndrome diagnosis and epidemiology workshop at the National Institutes of Health. Sleep Med 2003;4:101–119.

Allen RP, Walters AS, Montplaisir J, et al: Restless Legs Syndrome Prevalence and Impact: REST General Population Study. Arch Intern Med 2005;165:1286–1292.

Banks G, Neilsen VK, Short MP, Kowal CD: Brachial plexus myoclonus. J Neurol Neurosurg Psychiatry 1985;48:582–584.

Bara-Jimenez W, Aksu M, Graham B, et al: Periodic limb movements in sleep: State-dependent excitability of the spinal flexor reflex. Neurology 2000;54:1609–1616.

Barnett RE, Singh N, Fahn S: The syndrome of painful legs and moving toes. Neurology 1981;31:79.

Bassetti CL, Mauerhofer D, Gugger M, et al: Restless legs syndrome: A clinical study of 55 patients. Eur Neurol 2001;45:67–74.

Becker PM, Jamieson AO, Brown WD: Dopaminergic agents in restless legs syndrome and periodic limb movements of sleep: Response and complications of extended treatment in 49 cases. Sleep 1993;16:713–716.

Benjamin RM: Single neurons in the rat medulla responsive to nociceptive stimulation. Brain Res 1970;24:525–529.

Bhatia KP, Bhatt MH, Marsden CD: The causalgia-dystonia syndrome. Brain 1993;116:843–851.

Bjorvatn B, Leissner L, Ulfberg J, et al: Prevalence, severity and risk factors of restless legs syndrome in the general adult population in two Scandinavian countries. Sleep Med 2005;6: 307–312.

Bogan RK, Fry JM, Schmidt MH, et al: Ropinirole in the treatment of patients with restless legs syndrome: A US-based randomized, double-blind, placebo-controlled clinical trial. Mayo Clin Proc 2006;81:17–27.

Bonati MT, Ferini-Strambi L, Aridon P, et al: Autosomal dominant restless legs syndrome maps on chromosome 14q. Brain 2003; 126:1485–1492.

Brin MF, Fahn S, Bressman SB, Burke RE: Dystonia precipitated by peripheral trauma. Neurology 1986;36(suppl 1):119.

Cardoso F, Jankovic J: Peripherally induced tremor and parkinsonism. Arch Neurol 1995;52:263–270.

Chesson AL Jr, Wise M, Davila D, et al: Practice parameters for the treatment of restless legs syndrome and periodic limb movement disorder: An American Academy of Sleep Medicine Report: Standards of Practice Committee of the American Academy of Sleep Medicine. Sleep 1999;22:961–968.

Colosimo C, Bologna M, Lamberti S, et al: A comparative study of primary and secondary hemifacial spasm. Arch Neurol 2006;63: 441–444.

Comella CL: Restless legs syndrome: Treatment with dopaminergic agents. Neurology 2002;58:S87–S92.

Connor JR, Boyer PJ, Menzies SL, et al: Neuropathological examination suggests impaired brain iron acquisition in restless legs syndrome. Neurology 2003;61:304–309.

Davis BJ, Rajput A, Rajput ML, et al: A randomized, double-blind placebo-controlled trial of iron in restless legs syndrome. Eur Neurol 2000;43:70–75.

Davis SM, Murray NM, Diengdoh JV, et al: Stimulus-sensitive spinal myoclonus. J Neurol Neurosurg Psychiatry 1981;44:884–888.

de Ceballos ML, Baker M, Rose S, et al: Do enkephalins in basal ganglia mediate a physiological motor rest mechanism? Mov Disord 1986;1:223–233.

de Mello MT, Poyares DL, Tufik S: Treatment of periodic leg movements with a dopaminergic agonist in subjects with total spinal cord lesions. Spinal Cord 1999;37:634–637.

Defazio G, Abbruzzese G, Girlanda P, et al: Botulinum toxin A treatment for primary hemifacial spasm: A 10-year multicenter study. Arch Neurol 2002;59:418–420.

Desautels A, Turecki G, Montplaisir J, et al: Restless legs syndrome: Confirmation of linkage to chromosome 12q, genetic heterogeneity, and evidence of complexity. Arch Neurol 2005;62:591–596.

Devor M: Nerve pathophysiology and mechanisms of pain in causalgia. J Auton Nerv Syst 1983;7:371–384.

Devor M, Wall PD: Effect of peripheral nerve injury on receptive fields of cells in the cat spinal cord. J Comp Neurol 1981a;199:277–291.

Devor M, Wall PD: Plasticity in the spinal cord sensory map following peripheral nerve injury in rats. J Neurosci 1981b;1:679–684.

Dressler D, Thompson PD, Gledhill RF, Marsden CD: The syndrome of painful legs and moving toes. Mov Disord 1994;9:13–21.

Earley CJ, Allen RP, Beard JL, Connor JR: Insight into the pathophysiology of restless legs syndrome. J Neurosci Res 2000a;62:623–628.

Earley CJ, Connor JR, Beard JL, et al: Abnormalities in CSF concentrations of ferritin and transferrin in restless legs syndrome. Neurology 2000b;54:1698–1700.

Earley CJ, Connor JR, Beard JL, et al: Ferritin levels in the cerebrospinal fluid and restless legs syndrome: Effects of different clinical phenotypes. Sleep 2005;28:1069–1075.

Earley CJ, Heckler D, Allen RP: The treatment of restless legs syndrome with intravenous iron dextran. Sleep Med 2004;5:231–235.

Earley CJ, Heckler D, Allen RP: Repeated IV doses of iron provides effective supplemental treatment of restless legs syndrome. Sleep Med 2005;6:301–305.

Earley CJ, Yaffee JB, Allen RP: Randomized, double-blind, placebo-controlled trial of pergolide in restless legs syndrome. Neurology 1998;51:1599–1602.

Eisensehr 1, Wetter TC, Linke R, et al: Normal IPT and IBZM SPECT in drug-naive and levodopa-treated idiopathic restless legs syndrome. Neurology 2001;57:1307–1309.

Ekbom KA: Restless legs syndrome. Neurology 1960;1960:868–873.

Fletcher NA, Harding AE, Marsden CD: A genetic study of idiopathic torsion dystonia in the United Kingdom. Brain 1990;113:379–395.

Fletcher NA, Harding AE, Marsden CD: A case-control study of idiopathic torsion dystonia. Mov Disord 1991a;6:304–309.

Fletcher NA, Harding AE, Marsden CD: The relationship between trauma and idiopathic torsion dystonia. J Neurol Neurosurg Psychiatry 1991b;54:713–717.

Florence SL, Kaas JH: Large-scale reorganization at multiple levels of the somatosensory pathway follows therapeutic amputation of the hand in monkeys. J Neurosci 1995;15:8083–8095.

Garcia-Borreguero D, Larrosa O, de la Llave Y, et al: Treatment of restless legs syndrome with gabapentin: A double-blind, cross-over study. Neurology 2002;59:1573–1579.

Geller BD, Hallett M, Ravits J: Botulinum toxin therapy in hemifacial spasm: Clinical and electrophysiologic studies. Muscle Nerve 1989;12:716–722.

Grandas F, Elston J, Quinn N, Marsden CD: Blepharospasm: A review of 264 patients. J Neurol Neurosurg Psychiatry 1988; 51:767–772.

Guieu R, Sampieri F, Pouget J, et al: Adenosine in painful legs and moving toes syndrome. Clin Neuropharmacol 1994;17:460–469.

Guilbaud G: Thalamic nociceptive systems. Philos Trans R Soc Lond B Biol Sci 1985;308:339–345.

Guilleminault C, Flagg W: Effect of baclofen on sleep-related periodic leg movements. Ann Neurol 1984;15:234–239.

Hening W: The clinical neurophysiology of the restless legs syndrome and periodic limb movements. Part I: Diagnosis, assessment, and characterization. Clin Neurophysiol 2004;115:1965–1974.

Hening W, Allen R, Earley C, et al: The treatment of restless legs syndrome and periodic limb movement disorder: An American Academy of Sleep Medicine Review. Sleep 1999;22:970–999.

Hening W, Walters AS, Allen RP, et al: Impact, diagnosis and treatment of restless legs syndrome (RLS) in a primary care population: The REST (RLS epidemiology, symptoms, and treatment) primary care study. Sleep Med 2004;5:237–246.

Hening WA, Walters A, Kavey N, et al: Dyskinesias while awake and periodic movements in sleep in restless legs syndrome: Treatment with opioids. Neurology 1986;36:1363–1366.

Hening WA, Walters AS, Wagner M, et al: Circadian rhythm of motor restlessness and sensory symptoms in the idiopathic restless legs syndrome. Sleep 1999;22:901–912.

Iliceto G, Thompson PD, Day BL, et al: Diaphragmatic flutter, the moving umbilicus syndrome, and "belly dancer's" dyskinesia. Mov Disord 1990;5:15–22.

Ishikawa M, Ohira T, Namiki J, et al: [Neurophysiological study of hemifacial spasm: F wave of the facial muscles]. No To Shinkei 1994;46:360–365.

Jankovic J: Post-traumatic movement disorders: Central and peripheral mechanisms. Neurology 1994;44:2006–2014.

Jankovic J: Can peripheral trauma induce dystonia and other movement disorders? Yes! Mov Disord 2001;16:7–12.

Jankovic J, Glass JP: Metoclopramide-induced phantom dyskinesia. Neurology 1985;35:432–435.

Jankovic J, Pardo R: Segmental myoclonus: Clinical and pharmacological study. Arch Neurol 1986;43:1025–1031.

Jankovic J, Van der Linden C: Dystonia and tremor induced by peripheral trauma: Predisposing factors. J Neurol Neurosurg Psychiatry 1988;51:1512–1519.

Jost WH, Kohl A: Botulinum toxin: Evidence-based medicine criteria in blepharospasm and hemifacial spasm. J Neurol 2001;248 (suppl 1):21–24.

Kaas JH: The reorganization of somatosensory and motor cortex after peripheral nerve or spinal cord injury in primates. Prog Brain Res 2000;128:173–179.

Kaplan PW, Allen RP, Buchholz DW, Walters JK: A double-blind, placebo-controlled study of the treatment of periodic limb movements in sleep using carbidopa/levodopa and propoxyphene. Sleep 1993;16:717–723.

Kedia S, Moro E, Tagliati M, et al: Emergence of restless legs syndrome during subthalamic stimulation for Parkinson disease. Neurology 2004;63:2410–2412.

Kiehn O: Plateau potentials and active integration in the "final common pathway" for motor behaviour. Trends Neurosci 1991;14:68–73.

Kiehn O, Eken T: Prolonged firing in motor units: Evidence of plateau potentials in human motoneurons? J Neurophysiol 1997;78:3061–3068.

Koelman JH, Hilgevoord AA, Bour LJ, et al: Soleus H-reflex tests in causalgia-dystonia compared with dystonia and mimicked dystonic posture. Neurology 1999;53:2196–2198.

Koller WC, Wong GF, Lang A: Posttraumatic movement disorders: A review. Mov Disord 1989;4:20–36.

Kotagal S, Silber MH: Childhood-onset restless legs syndrome. Ann Neurol 2004;56:803–807.

Krishnan PR, Bhatia M, Behari M: Restless legs syndrome in Parkinson's disease: A case-controlled study. Mov Disord 2003;18:181–185.

Kulisevsky J, Marti-Fabregas J, Grau JM: Spasms of amputation stumps. J Neurol Neurosurg Psychiatry 1992;55:626–627.

Lang A, Fahn S: Movement disorder of RSD. Neurology 1990;40:1476–1477.

Levchenko A, Montplaisir JY, Dube MP, et al: The 14q restless legs syndrome locus in the French Canadian population. Ann Neurol 2004;55:887–891.

Liebetanz KM, Winkelmann J, Trenkwalder C, et al: RLS3: Fine-mapping of an autosomal dominant locus in a family with intrafamilial heterogeneity. Neurology 2006;67:320–321.

Littner MR, Kushida C, Anderson WM, et al: Practice parameters for the dopaminergic treatment of restless legs syndrome and periodic limb movement disorder. Sleep 2004;27:557–559.

Loeser D, Ward AA: Some effects of deafferentation on neurons of the cat spinal cord. Arch Neurol 1967;17:629–636.

Lugaresi E, Cirignotta F, Coccagna G, Montagna P: Nocturnal myoclonus and restless legs syndrome. Adv Neurol 1986;43:295–307.

Marion MH, Gledhill RF, Thompson PD: Spasms of amputation stumps: A report of 2 cases. Mov Disord 1989;4:354–358.

Marsden CD, Obeso JA, Traub MM, et al: Muscle spasms associated with Sudeck's atrophy after injury. Br Med J (Clin Res Ed) 1984;288:173–176.

Michaud M, Soucy JP, Chabli A, et al: SPECT imaging of striatal pre- and postsynaptic dopaminergic status in restless legs syndrome with periodic leg movements in sleep. J Neurol 2002;249:164–170.

Mitchell SW: Injuries of nerves and their consequences. New York, JB Lippincott, 1872.

Moller AR: Hemifacial spasm: Ephaptic transmission or hyperexcitability of the facial motor nucleus? Exp Neurol 1987;98:110–119.

Moller AR, Jannetta PJ: On the origin of synkinesis in hemifacial spasm: Results of intracranial recordings. J Neurosurg 1984;61:569–576.

Montagna P, Cirignotta F, Sacquegna T, et al: "Painful legs and moving toes" associated with polyneuropathy. J Neurol Neurosurg Psychiatry 1983;46:399–403.

Montplaisir J, Nicolas A, Denesle R, Gomez-Mancilla B: Restless legs syndrome improved by pramipexole: A double-blind randomized trial. Neurology 1999;52:938–943.

Nathan PW: On the pathogenesis of causalgia in peripheral nerve injuries. Brain 1947;70:145–170.

Nathan PW: Painful legs and moving toes: Evidence on the site of the lesion. J Neurol Neurosurg Psychiatry 1978;41:934–939.

Nielsen VK: Pathophysiology of hemifacial spasm: I. Ephaptic transmission and ectopic excitation. Neurology 1984a;34:418–426.

Nielsen VK: Pathophysiology of hemifacial spasm: II. Lateral spread of the supraorbital nerve reflex. Neurology 1984b;34:427–431.

Nielsen VK, Jannetta PJ: Pathophysiology of hemifacial spasm: III. Effects of facial nerve decompression. Neurology 1984;34:891–897.

Ochoa JL: Reflex? Sympathetic? Dystrophy? Triple questioned again. Mayo Clin Proc 1995;70:1124–1126.

Ochoa JL: Truths, errors, and lies around "reflex sympathetic dystrophy" and "complex regional pain syndrome." J Neurol 1999;246:875–879.

Ochoa JL, Verdugo RJ: Reflex sympathetic dystrophy: A common clinical avenue for somatoform expression. Neurol Clin 1995;13:351–363.

Okuda Y, Suzuki K, Kitajima T, et al: Lumbar epidural block for "painful legs and moving toes" syndrome: A report of three cases. Pain 1998;78:145–147.

Okun MS, Fernandez HH, Foote KD: Deep brain stimulation of the GPi treats restless legs syndrome associated with dystonia. Mov Disord 2005;20:500–501.

Ondo W: Ropinirole for restless legs syndrome. Mov Disord 1999;14:138–140.

Ondo W, Jankovic J: Restless legs syndrome: Clinicoetiologic correlates. Neurology 1996;47:1435–1441.

Ondo WG, Vuong KD, Jankovic J: Exploring the relationship between Parkinson disease and restless legs syndrome. Arch Neurol 2002;59:421–424.

Phillips B, Young T, Finn L, et al: Epidemiology of restless legs symptoms in adults. Arch Intern Med 2000;160:2137–2141.

Pieta J, Millar T, Zacharias J, et al: Effect of pergolide on restless legs and leg movements in sleep in uremic patients. Sleep 1998;21:617–622.

Pitagoras de Mattos J, Oliveira M, Andre C: Painful legs and moving toes associated with neuropathy in HIV-infected patients. Mov Disord 1999;14:1053–1054.

Pollmacher T, Schulz H: Periodic leg movements (PLM): Their relationship to sleep stages. Sleep 1993;16:572–577.

Poungvarin N, Devahastin V, Viriyavejakul A: Treatment of various movement disorders with botulinum A toxin injection: An experience of 900 patients. J Med Assoc Thai 1995;78:281–288.

Prinz PN: Sleep and sleep disorders in older adults. J Clin Neurophysiol 1995;12:139–146.

Robberecht W, Van Hees J, Adriaensen H, Carton H: Painful muscle spasms complicating algodystrophy: Central or peripheral disease? J Neurol Neurosurg Psychiatry 1988;51:563–567.

Roth G, Magistris MR, Pinelli P, Rilliet B: Cryptogenic hemifacial spasm: A neurophysiological study. Electromyogr Clin Neurophysiol 1990;30:361–370.

Rothdach AJ, Trenkwalder C, Haberstock J, et al: Prevalence and risk factors of RLS in an elderly population: The MEMO study: Memory and Morbidity in Augsburg Elderly. Neurology 2000;54:1064–1068.

Russell WR: Neurological sequelae of amputation. Br J Hosp Med 1970;6:607–609.

Rye DB, DeLong MR: Amelioration of sensory limb discomfort of restless legs syndrome by pallidotomy. Ann Neurol 1999;46:800–801.

Said G, Bathien N: [Rhythmic quadriceps myoclonia related to sarcomatous involvement of the crural nerve]. Rev Neurol (Paris) 1977;133:191–198.

Samii M, Gunther T, Iaconetta G, et al: Microvascular decompression to treat hemifacial spasm: Long-term results for a consecutive series of 143 patients. Neurosurgery 2002;50:712–718; discussion 718–719.

Sanders DB: Ephaptic transmission in hemifacial spasm: A single-fiber EMG study. Muscle Nerve 1989;12:690–694.

Schattschneider J, Bode A, Wasner G, et al: Idiopathic restless legs syndrome: Abnormalities in central somatosensory processing. J Neurol 2004;251:977–982.

Scherokman B, Husain F, Cuetter A, et al: Peripheral dystonia. Arch Neurol 1986;43:830–832.

Schoenen J, Gonce M, Delwaide PJ: Painful legs and moving toes: A syndrome with different physiopathologic mechanisms. Neurology 1984;34:1108–1112.

Schott GD: "Painful legs and moving toes": The role of trauma. J Neurol Neurosurg Psychiatry 1981;44:344–346.

Schott GD: The relationship of peripheral trauma and pain to dystonia. J Neurol Neurosurg Psychiatry 1985;48:698–701.

Schott GD: Induction of involuntary movements by peripheral trauma: An analogy with causalgia. Lancet 1986a;2:712–716.

Schott GD: Mechanisms of causalgia and related clinical conditions: The role of the central and of the sympathetic nervous systems. Brain 1986b;109:717–738.

Schott GD: An unsympathetic view of pain. Lancet 1995;345:634–636.

Schwartzman RJ: Reflex sympathetic dystrophy. Curr Opin Neurol Neurosurg 1993;6:531–536.

Schwartzman RJ, Kerrigan J: The movement disorder of reflex sympathetic dystrophy. Neurology 1990;40:57–61.

Schwartzman RJ, McLellan TL: Reflex sympathetic dystrophy: A review. Arch Neurol 1987;44:555–561.

Sheehy MP, Marsden CD: Trauma and pain in spasmodic torticollis. Lancet 1980;1:777–778.

Sheehy MP, Marsden CD: Writers' cramp: A focal dystonia. Brain 1982;105:461–480.

Sheehy MP, Rothwell JC, Marsden CD: Writer's cramp. Adv Neurol 1988;50:457–472.

Silber MH, Ehrenberg BL, Allen RP, et al: An algorithm for the management of restless legs syndrome. Mayo Clin Proc 2004;79:916–922.

Sotaniemi KA: Paraspinal myoclonus due to spinal root lesion. J Neurol Neurosurg Psychiatry 1985;48:722–723.

Spillane JD, Nathan PW, Kelly RE, Marsden CD: Painful legs and moving toes. Brain 1971;94:541–556.

Stanton-Hicks M, Janig W, Hassenbusch S, et al: Reflex sympathetic dystrophy: Changing concepts and taxonomy. Pain 1995;63:127–133.

Steiner JC, DeJesus PV, Mancall EL: Painful jumping amputation stumps: Pathophysiology of a "sore circuit." Trans Am Neurol Assoc 1974;99:253–255.

Stiasny K, Wetter TC, Winkelmann J, et al: Long-term effects of pergolide in the treatment of restless legs syndrome. Neurology 2001;56:1399–1402.

Supiot F, Gazagnes MD, Blecic SA, et al: Painful arm and moving fingers: Clinical features of four new cases. Mov Disord 2002;17:616–618.

Swanson PD, Luttrell CN, Magladery JW: Myoclonus: A report of 67 cases and review of the literature. Medicine (Baltimore) 1962;41:339–356.

Takahashi H, Saitoh C, Iwata O, et al: Epidural spinal cord stimulation for the treatment of painful legs and moving toes syndrome. Pain 2002;96:343–345.

Tan EK, Chan LL: Clinico-radiologic correlation in unilateral and bilateral hemifacial spasm. J Neurol Sci 2004;222:59–64.

Tan EK, Fook-Chong S, Lum SY, Lim E: Botulinum toxin improves quality of life in hemifacial spasm: Validation of a questionnaire (HFS-30). J Neurol Sci 2004;219:151–155.

Tan EK, Lum SY, Wong MC: Restless legs syndrome in Parkinson's disease. J Neurol Sci 2002;196:33–36.

Tan EK, Ondo W: Restless legs syndrome: Clinical features and treatment. Am J Med Sci 2000;319:397–403.

Telstad W, Sorensen O, Larsen S, et al: Treatment of the restless legs syndrome with carbamazepine: A double blind study. Br Med J (Clin Res Ed) 1984;288:444–446.

Thompson PD, Obeso JA, Delgado G, et al: Focal dystonia of the jaw and the differential diagnosis of unilateral jaw and masticatory spasm. J Neurol Neurosurg Psychiatry 1986;49:651–656.

Trenkwalder C, Collado Seidel V, Kazenwadel J, et al: One-year treatment with standard and sustained-release levodopa: Appropriate long-term treatment of restless legs syndrome? Mov Disord 2003;18:1184–1189.

Trenkwalder C, Hening WA, Walters AS, et al: Circadian rhythm of periodic limb movements and sensory symptoms of restless legs syndrome. Mov Disord 1999;14:102–110.

Trenkwalder C, Paulus W: Why do restless legs occur at rest? Pathophysiology of neuronal structures in RLS. Neurophysiology of RLS (pt 2). Clin Neurophysiol 2004;115:1975–1988.

Trenkwalder C, Walters AS, Hening W: Periodic limb movements and restless legs syndrome. Neurol Clin 1996;14:629–650.

van de Beek WJ, Vein A, Hilgevoord AA, et al: Neurophysiologic aspects of patients with generalized or multifocal tonic dystonia of reflex sympathetic dystrophy. J Clin Neurophysiol 2002;19: 77–83.

van Hilten BJ, van de Beek WJ, Hoff JI, et al: Intrathecal baclofen for the treatment of dystonia in patients with reflex sympathetic dystrophy. N Engl J Med 2000;343:625–630.

Verdugo RJ, Ochoa JL: Abnormal movements in complex regional pain syndrome: Assessment of their nature. Muscle Nerve 2000; 23:198–205.

Verhagen WI, Horstink MW, Notermans SL: Painful arm and moving fingers [letter]. J Neurol Neurosurg Psychiatry 1985;48:384–385.

Vetrugno R, Provini F, Plazzi G, et al: Propriospinal myoclonus: A motor phenomenon found in restless legs syndrome different from periodic limb movements during sleep. Mov Disord 2005;20:1323–1329.

Villarejo A, Porta-Etessam J, Camacho A, et al: Gabapentin for painful legs and moving toes syndrome. Eur Neurol 2004;51:180–181.

von Spiczak S, Whone AL, Hammers A, et al: The role of opioids in restless legs syndrome: An [11C]diprenorphine PET study. Brain 2005;128:906–917.

Wagner ML, Walters AS, Coleman RG, et al: Randomized, double-blind, placebo-controlled study of clonidine in restless legs syndrome. Sleep 1996;19:52–58.

Walters AS: Toward a better definition of the restless legs syndrome: The International Restless Legs Syndrome Study Group. Mov Disord 1995;10:634–642.

Walters AS, Hening WA, Kavey N, et al: A double-blind randomized crossover trial of bromocriptine and placebo in restless legs syndrome. Ann Neurol 1988;24:455–458.

Walters AS, Hickey K, Maltzman J, et al: A questionnaire study of 138 patients with restless legs syndrome: The "Night-Walkers" survey. Neurology 1996;46:92–95.

Walters AS, Wagner ML, Hening WA, et al: Successful treatment of the idiopathic restless legs syndrome in a randomized double-blind trial of oxycodone versus placebo. Sleep 1993;16:327–332.

Weiner WJ: Can peripheral trauma induce dystonia? No! Mov Disord 2001;16:13–22.

Wetter TC, Pollmacher T: Restless legs and periodic leg movements in sleep syndromes. J Neurol 1997;244:S37–S45.

Wetter TC, Stiasny K, Winkelmann J, et al: A randomized controlled study of pergolide in patients with restless legs syndrome. Neurology 1999;52:944–950.

Winkelmann J, Ferini-Strambi L: Genetics of restless legs syndrome. Sleep Med Rev 2006;10(3):179–183

Winkelmann J, Wetter TC, Collado-Seidel V, et al: Clinical characteristics and frequency of the hereditary restless legs syndrome in a population of 300 patients. Sleep 2000;23:597–602.

Wulff CH: Painful legs and moving toes: A report of 3 cases with neurophysiological studies. Acta Neurol Scand 1982;66:283–287.

# Chapter 25

# Wilson Disease

Wilson disease is an inborn error of copper metabolism that manifests as hepatic cirrhosis and basal ganglia damage (Wilson, 1912). Wilson disease is one of the few movement disorders that is at the present time curable, provided it is diagnosed and treated early. It presents in so many guises that any patient with a movement disorder under the age of 50 years should be considered to possibly have Wilson disease. It is sufficiently rare that the diagnosis is often missed. In a recent review of 307 patients, the average delay to diagnosis was 2 years, and misdiagnoses included schizophrenia, juvenile polyarthritis, rheumatic chorea, nephrotic syndrome, metachromatic leukodystrophy, congenital myopathies, subacute sclerosing panencephalitis, and neurodegenerative disease (Prashanth et al., 2004).

Wilson disease is inherited as an autosomal-recessive trait. The gene that is responsible lies on chromosome 13q14.3 (whereas that for ceruloplasmin is located on chromosome 8 [Wang et al., 1988]). The Wilson disease gene encodes for a copper-transporting P-type ATPase (ATP7B) (Petrukhin et al., 1993; Tanzi et al., 1993). At least 35 mutations of the gene have been detected, and more are being found often (Thomas et al., 1995; Shah et al., 1997; Curtis et al., 1999). The enzyme binds copper in its large N-terminal domain and aids in transport across the membrane (Sarkar, 2000; Ala et al., 2007). These mutations lead to failure to excrete copper from the liver into bile, causing systemic copper poisoning (Cuthbert, 1998; Loudianos and Gitlin, 2000). Intestinal absorption of copper is normal in Wilson disease (normal adults absorb about 1 to 5 mg of copper daily). Accordingly, reduced biliary excretion (by as much as 40%) causes a substantial positive net copper balance. As a result, there is increased circulating free copper and excessive urinary excretion of copper, but this is insufficient to prevent copper accumulation (the normal human body contains 80 mg of copper). Initially, the liver accumulates copper, causing progressive liver damage. Copper then overflows into brain and other sites (the eye, kidney, bones, and blood tissues being particularly vulnerable to copper toxicity).

In most cases, Wilson disease can be diagnosed by measurement of the serum concentration of the copper protein ceruloplasmin. Ceruloplasmin (molecular weight: 132,000 D), an alpha-2 globulin glycoprotein, contains six atoms of copper per molecule. Ceruloplasmin contains 0.3% copper in a fixed ratio of metal to protein (330 mg of ceruloplasmin carries 1000 µg copper/L). In Wilson disease, there may be defective incorporation of copper into ceruloplasmin. However, the defect in ceruloplasmin is not the primary abnormality in Wilson disease; some patients have normal levels, and the gene for the disease lies at a different site from that responsible for ceruloplasmin synthesis. Ceruloplasmin may often be low in the serum in Wilson disease because of the liver's reduced ability to secrete it into the blood as well as reduced ability to excrete it in the bile.

Drugs that remove copper from the body and/or prevent its absorption can reverse the manifestations of Wilson disease and prevent its appearance in asymptomatic affected siblings. More is said about this later.

The prevalence of heterozygous carriers, who have inherited only one abnormal gene, is around 1 in 100 to 200 of the population (Reilly et al., 1993). Heterozygotes do not develop Wilson disease but may exhibit mild abnormalities of copper metabolism. The prevalence of Wilson disease is estimated to be about 17 per million of the population.

The initial manifestations of the illness (Box 25-1) are neurologic in about 40% of patients (usually after the age of 12 years) (Brewer, 2000a). The remainder present with symptoms of liver disease (about 40%) (usually at an earlier age) or a psychiatric illness (about 15%). The psychiatric picture might show a change in personality or mood. Psychosis is rare. What determines these individual variations in clinical presentation is not clear. One factor has been determined: Patients with ApoE epsilon 3/3 genotype have a delayed onset of symptoms compared to all other ApoE genotypes (Schiefermeier et al., 2000). Symptoms usually appear between the ages of 11 and 25 years but can occur as early as 4 years and as late as 50 plus years (Starosta-Rubinstein et al., 1987; Stremmel et al., 1991; Walshe and Yealland, 1992).

The pathologic abnormalities in the brain are primarily in the basal ganglia, with cavitary necrosis of the putamen and caudate, associated with neuronal loss, axonal degeneration, and astrocytosis (Fig. 25-1). In addition, there is cortical atrophy. The liver develops a nodular cirrhosis.

Patients with neurologic abnormalities usually present in the second or third decade with (1) an akinetic-rigid syndrome resembling parkinsonism, (2) a generalized dystonic syndrome (pure chorea is uncommon), or (3) postural and intention tremor with ataxia, titubation, and dysarthria (pseudosclerosis) (Table 25-1 and Video 25-1). The tremor may be mild but is classically a slow, high-amplitude proximal tremor with the appearance of wing-beating when the arms are elevated with elbows flexed and the hands placed near the nose. Dysarthria and clumsiness of the hands are common presenting features. The speech abnormality may include rapid speech, hypophonia, and slurring. It is most unusual for the illness to present with a gait disorder. No two patients with Wilson disease are ever quite the same. The facile grinning face with open mouth and drooling saliva is characteristic. Early pseudobulbar features are common. Eye movements can be disordered with slow saccades (Kirkham and Kamin, 1974) and occasionally ophthalmoplegia (Gadoth and Liel, 1980). Vision and sensation are not affected, and paralysis does not occur, although pyramidal signs may be evident. Sphincter control is spared. Seizures are infrequent (Smith and Mattson, 1967). Cognitive changes are common, even to the extent of a frank dementia. Changes in school or work performance are

Box 25-1 Presentation of Wilson disease

**Liver Disease (40%)**
95% present under the age of 20 years (usually 7 to 15 years)
Acute hepatitis
Fulminant hepatitis
Chronic active hepatitis
Cirrhosis

**Neurologic Presentation (40%)**
30% present over the age of 20 years
Isolated tremor, dysarthria, drooling, clumsiness or gait disturbance (rarely, seizures)
A parkinsonian syndrome
A generalized dystonic syndrome
A pseudosclerotic syndrome (postural and intention tremor)

**Psychiatric Presentation (15%)**
Conduct disorder
Cognitive impairment
Dementia
Psychosis

**Others (5%)**
Ocular: Kayser-Fleischer ring, sunflower cataract
Renal: Aminoaciduria, renal tubular acidosis, calculi
Skeletal: Osteomalacia and rickets (blue nails)
Hematologic: Hemolytic anemia

Table 25-1 Number (percentage) of Wilson's disease patients with different initial symptoms and signs

| Number of Patients | Juveniles (65) | Adults (71) |
|---|---|---|
| **Symptoms** | | |
| Personality change | 21 (32) | 23 (32) |
| Speech defect | 63 (41) | 42 (30) |
| Drooling | 31 (20) | 22 (16) |
| Dysphagia | 14 (9) | 7 (5) |
| Hand tremor | 48 (31) | 55 (39) |
| Hand clumsy | 32 (21) | 20 (14) |
| Abnormal gait | 34 (22) | 18 (13) |
| Fall at work or school | 40 (26) | |
| **Signs** | | |
| Personality disorder | 14 (21) | 13 (18) |
| Dysarthria | 34 (52) | 19 (27) |
| Gait abnormal | 8 (12) | 5 (7) |
| Eye movement abnormal | 4 (6) | 4 (6) |
| Drooling | 18 (28) | 11 (15) |
| Parkinsonian facies | 15 (23) | 5 (7) |
| Open mouth | 10 (15) | 0 (0) |
| Bradykinesia | 6 (9) | 3 (4) |
| Tongue abnormal | 11 (17) | 9 (13) |
| UL tremor | 17 (26) | 23 (32) |
| UL dystonia | 14 (21) | 13 (18) |
| UL spontaneous movements | 8 (12) | 0 (0) |
| LL tremor | 2 (3) | 6 (8) |
| LL dystonia | 12 (18) | 0 (0) |
| LL spontaneous movements | 1 (1) | 1 (1) |
| Liver disease | 19 (29) | 8 (11) |

UL, upper limb; LL, lower limb.

Data from Walshe JM, Yealland M: Wilson's disease: The problem of delayed diagnosis. J Neurol Neurosurg Psychiatry 1992;55:692–696.

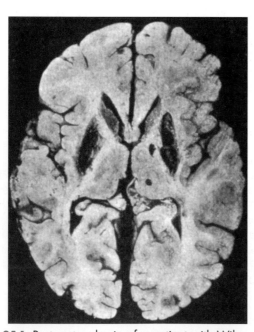

Figure 25-1 Postmortem brain of a patient with Wilson disease showing the cavitary necrosis of the basal ganglia. (From Wilson SAK: Progressive lenticular degeneration: A familial nervous disease associated with cirrhosis of the liver. Brain 1912;34:295–507, with permission.)

often the initial indication of the illness. Impulsiveness or antisocial behavior and other indications of personality change are common (Dening and Berrios, 1989; Dening, 1991; Akil and Brewer, 1995).

Many patients with neurologic complaints give a history of prior or concurrent liver disease. This may consist of a previous episode of acute hepatitis, chronic active hepatitis, portal hypertension, or asymptomatic hepatosplenomegaly (Scheinberg and Sternlieb, 1984). An unexplained hemolytic anemia, renal disease with hematuria, amino-aciduria, renal tubular defects, and calculi (Wiebers et al., 1979) or skeletal disease with osteoporosis/osteomalacia (Carpenter et al., 1983) are other clues.

Untreated, the condition progresses inexorably to death within a few years either from the complications of the liver disease or from severe neurologic involvement.

The diagnosis (Box 25-2) is established by discovery of a reduced serum ceruloplasmin. However, 5% of those with Wilson disease have a normal serum ceruloplasmin. The concentration of this copper-protein may be low in heterozygotes, severe protein loss, and severe liver disease of other cause and may be increased by pregnancy and estrogens. Serum total

**Box 25-2** The diagnosis of Wilson disease

1. Low serum ceruloplasmin (<20 mg/dL)
   False negatives in 5% of WD patients, pregnancy and the pill
   False positives in heterozygotes, severe protein loss, severe liver disease, Menkes disease
2. Kayser-Fleischer ring
   False negatives in Wilson disease with liver manifestations, local eye disease
   False positives in primary biliary cirrhosis
3. Raised 24-hour urinary copper excretion (>100 μg)
   False positives in cholestasis (Drugs)
4. Raised liver copper concentration (>250 μg/g dry weight)
   False positives in biliary cirrhosis, cholestasis (Histology is essential.)
5. Genetic linkage studies to chromosome 13

copper is low in many patients, and urinary copper excretion is nearly always raised. However, anything that causes cholestasis (particularly drugs) may raise the serum copper level and increase urinary copper excretion. When an expert examines the cornea with a slit lamp, virtually all patients with neurologic Wilson disease show Kayser-Fleischer rings in Descemet membrane (Fig. 25-2) (Wiebers et al., 1977). However, rare patients with neurologic Wilson disease but no Kayser-Fleischer ring have been described (Ross et al., 1985; Demirkiran et al., 1996). Occasionally, a Kayser-Fleischer ring is seen in only one eye (Madden et al., 1985). The yellow and brown copper deposits are seen at the limbus of the cornea, usually first visible and most dense at the upper and lower poles of the eye. Kayser-Fleischer rings are not present in all patients with the liver manifestations of Wilson disease, and other liver disease can produce Kayser-Fleischer rings

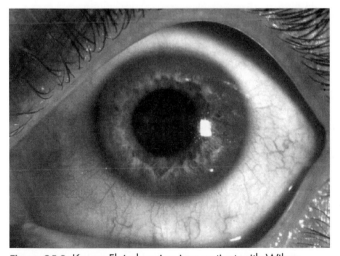

**Figure 25-2** Kayser-Fleischer ring in a patient with Wilson disease. The ring is composed of brown pigment at the outer circumference of the iris, which in a black-and-white photo appears as darkening. (See Color Plate 16 for the color version of this figure.) (From Scheinberg H, Sternlieb I: Wilson Disease. Philadelphia, Saunders, 1984, with permission.)

(Fleming et al., 1977). Computed tomography (Harik and Post, 1981; Williams and Walshe, 1981) or magnetic resonance imaging (MRI) (Starosta-Rubinstein et al., 1987; Alanen et al., 1999; Giagheddu et al., 2001) of the brain usually reveals changes in the basal ganglia, which are reversible with treatment. The caudate and putamen show increased T2 signal, and there may be similar changes in the substantia nigra pars compacta, periaqueductal gray matter, pontine tegmentum, and thalamus (Fig. 25-3A) (Saatci et al., 1997). Particularly striking are the putaminal lesions with a pattern of symmetric, bilateral, concentric-laminar T2 hyperintensity. Hyperintensity of the mesencephalon with sparing of the red nuclei and lateral aspect of the substantia nigra gives rise to the "face of the giant panda sign" (Fig. 25-3B) (Giagheddu et al., 2001). A "double panda sign" has also been described (Jacobs et al., 2003; Liebeskind et al., 2003). Diffusion-weighted MRI might be useful also (Favrole et al., 2006). Positron emission tomography using [18]F-fluorodopa shows reduced uptake in the striatum, indicating loss of the dopaminergic nigrostriatal pathway (Snow et al., 1991). Transcranial brain parenchyma sonography detects lenticular nucleus hyperechogenicity, likely to be caused by copper accumulation, in neurologically symptomatic and asymptomatic Wilson disease patients (Walter et al., 2005). Magnetic resonance spectroscopy is also abnormal (Lucato et al., 2005).

Following the above diagnostic tests, if there is any lingering doubt about the diagnosis of Wilson disease in a patient under the age of 50 who presents with neurologic problems, the first test would be a 24-hour urine copper excretion test. In Wilson disease, excretion is typically more than 100 μg/24 hours, and excretion less than 50 μg/24 hours would exclude the diagnosis (Brewer and Yuzbasiyan-Gurkan, 1992; Brewer, 2000a). The definitive investigation is a liver biopsy with histologic assessment of tissue and measurement of copper concentration. MRI is typically abnormal; in a series of eight patients with neurologic manifestations, seven were abnormal (Giagheddu et al., 2001). Genetic linkage studies to chromosome 13 can be valuable if other family members are available and the gene can be closely searched for a mutation (Farrer et al., 1991; Caca et al., 2001). However, since there are so many possible mutations, such testing is not commercially available. The method of single-stranded conformation polymorphism analysis is being tested to determine whether it can be useful in this situation; in 26 patients, an abnormality in the gene was found in 92% (Butler et al., 2001).

All siblings, who have a one in four chance of developing the illness, and cousins of known patients, should be screened for Wilson disease (Walshe, 1988). Clinical signs, the presence of a Kayser-Fleischer ring, and abnormalities of serum and urine copper metabolism indicate the need for prophylactic treatment (Scheinberg and Sternlieb, 1984). If there is doubt, a liver biopsy may be undertaken, although molecular genetic techniques might prove diagnostic.

## TREATMENT OF WILSON DISEASE

The treatments for Wilson disease have been reviewed (Walshe, 1999; Brewer, 2000b, 2006). The gold standard of treatment (Box 25-3) has been D-penicillamine (Shimizu et al., 1999; Walshe, 1999), slowly building up to around 1 g per day, along with pyridoxine 25 mg per day. D-Penicillamine

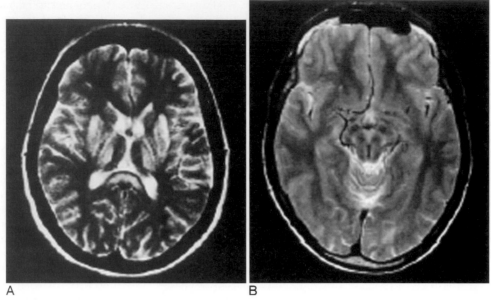

A          B

**Figure 25-3** MRI scans in Wilson disease showing a T2-weighted image of hyperintensity of the basal ganglia (**A**) and a T2-weighted image of the "face of the giant panda sign" due to hyperintensity of the mesencephalon sparing the red nuclei and the lateral part of the substantia nigra (**B**). (Modified with permission from Giagheddu M, Tamburini G, Piga M, et al: Comparison of MRI, EEG, EPs and ECD-SPECT in Wilson's disease. Acta Neurol Scand 2001;103:71–81.)

should be introduced gradually because about 20% of patients may develop early side effects. The commonest are fever, a rash, and lymphadenopathy. Gradual reintroduction of D-penicillamine in low dosage under steroid cover might overcome these problems. More serious is the development of bone marrow depression. Unfortunately, 20% to 40% of those

**Box 25-3** Treatment of Wilson disease

1. D-Penicillamine
   Low and slow: 1 g per day (0.5 to 2.0) before food
   Pyridoxine 25 mg per day
   Avoid copper-rich foods
   Monitor blood count and liver function tests, serum and urinary copper, Kayser-Fleischer ring
   Early side effects: Allergy (20%): Fever, rash, glands; marrow depression; neurologic deterioration (20% to 40%)
   Late problems: Nephrotoxicity (proteinuria, nephrotic syndrome); systemic lupus erythematosus; thrombocytopenia; Goodpasture syndrome; dermatopathy; myasthenia
2. Trientine
   1 to 2 g per day (250 to 500 mg four times a day)
   Iron deficiency
3. Zinc (sulfate or acetate)
   50 to 200 mg three times a day
   Gastrointestinal side effects
4. Tetrathiomolybdate
5. Liver transplant

with neurologic disability will exhibit deterioration in the initial months of penicillamine treatment (Brewer, 1999), believed to be caused by an overly rapid release of copper into plasma that then gets into brain. The neurologic deterioration can be severe; in one case, the patient developed marked dystonia (status dystonicus) and died (Svetel et al., 2001). With penicillamine treatment, clinical improvement usually occurs within about 3 months, but it may take 6 months to a year before noticeable change takes place.

Reducing copper intake obviously is wise (Shimizu et al., 1999), but strict diets are rarely followed. Copper-rich foods include liver, nuts, chocolate, coffee, and shellfish.

Successful decoppering can be monitored by an initial increase in urinary copper excretion, which subsequently falls, a reduction in the concentration of free copper in serum, and the fading of Kayser-Fleischer rings.

Late reactions to penicillamine treatment are usually seen after a year or so of therapy. The most common reaction is penicillamine dermatopathy, due to damage of collagen and elastin causing weakness of subcutaneous tissue so that slight trauma may cause bleeding, leaving brown papules with excessive wrinkling and thinning of the skin. A minority may develop proteinuria, which can progress to a frank nephrotic syndrome. Other problems include the emergence of a form of systemic lupus erythematosus, thrombocytopenia, Goodpasture syndrome, and myasthenia gravis.

An alternative to D-penicillamine is trientine (triethylene tetramine dihydrochloride) (Brewer, 1999; Shimizu et al., 1999), another chelator. Trientine undoubtedly is a valuable alternative for patients who are intolerant of D-penicillamine, but it has advantages in that the initial worsening might not occur (Brewer, 1999). Trientine is relatively safe (it can cause a sideroblastic anemia and can reactivate penicillamine-induced lupus) but is expensive and poorly absorbed.

Zinc and tetrathiomolybdate, which prevent the absorption of copper, are other alternatives. Zinc is an excellent agent for chronic use for mild cases and prevention (Hoogenraad, 2006) but might not be rapid enough for initiating therapy in someone with severe illness (Brewer, 1999, 2000a). Zinc is also the treatment of choice during pregnancy. Zinc can also be given safely in the pediatric age group (Brewer et al., 2001). Long-term follow-up of neurologically asymptomatic children who were treated for 10 years shows that zinc is well tolerated; liver disease improves, neurologic disorders do not develop, and growth is normal (Marcellini et al., 2005).

Tetrathiomolybdate is not easily available except experimentally (Brewer, 1999, 2005). An open-label study of 55 de novo patients reported treatment with doses of 120 to 410 mg per day for 8 weeks with follow-up for 3 years (Brewer et al., 2003). Only two patients (4%) showed initial neurologic deterioration, and overall neurologic improvement was excellent. Five patients had bone marrow suppression, and three had aminotransferase elevations, and the authors thought that this might have been precipitated by a too rapid dose escalation.

In desperate cases, injection of dimercaprol (British Anti-Lewisite) still might be life-saving (Shale et al., 1988; Scheinberg and Sternlieb, 1995). But because injections are painful, this cannot be used chronically (Walshe, 1999).

The role of these alternative agents in the treatment of Wilson disease is debated, and a nice formal debate was published in *Movement Disorders* (Brewer, 1999; LeWitt, 1999; Walshe, 1999). Brewer (1999) takes the strong view that D-penicillamine should not be used. He and others favor zinc, a combination of zinc and trientine, or tetrathiomolybdate on the grounds that such an approach reduces the chances of initial neurologic deterioration and causes fewer side effects than does D-penicillamine (Czlonkowska et al., 1996; Brewer, 1999, 2000a, 2005; Schilsky, 2001).

Liver transplantation has also been employed and cures Wilson disease (Schilsky et al., 1994; Shimizu et al., 1999; Podgaetz and Chan, 2003). The neurologic manifestations can be reversed in about 80% of cases, and liver transplantation can be undertaken for the neurologic disorder even with stable liver disease (Stracciari et al., 2000; Geissler et al., 2003). A series of 21 patients had a mean follow-up of 5.2 years and an actuarial follow-up of 10 years (Schumacher et al., 2001). All patients did well with the neurologic functioning, improving over 1 to 1.5 years. In a series of 24 patients with a mean follow-up period of 92 months, quality of life improved to the same level as in controls in the general population (Sutcliffe et al., 2003).

Symptomatic treatment with antiparkinsonian and antidystonic drugs such as levodopa, dopamine agonists, and anticholinergics may be of benefit.

## HEREDITARY DEFICIENCY OF CERULOPLASMIN

A rare condition, hereditary deficiency of ceruloplasmin, can cause a movement disorder. In this autosomal-recessive disorder due to gene defects in the ceruloplasmin gene (Yazaki et al., 1998), homozygotes develop iron overload (Miyajima et al., 1987; Harris et al., 1995). The disorder is estimated to occur in 0.5 person per million in Japan (Miyajima et al.,

1999). Ceruloplasmin oxidizes ferrous iron to ferric iron (so some call ceruloplasmin ferroxidase), which is stored in ferritin and hemosiderin. Ferric iron can be transported out of cells. The absence of ceruloplasmin leads to a low serum iron level with normal total iron binding capacity and sometimes to anemia. The serum ferritin level and liver and brain iron concentrations are increased. Brain MRI shows increased iron deposition in the striatum, substantia nigra, red nuclei, and dentate nuclei. T2 hypointensities can be marked, including the cerebral cortex (Grisoli et al., 2005). Clinical presentation has been with insulin-dependent diabetes, retinal degeneration, subcortical dementia, and a movement disorder that typically is a facial dyskinesia (blepharospasm and oral dystonia) and torticollis, rigidity, and sometimes ataxia (Miyajima et al., 1987; Kawanami et al., 1996). One patient has presented with parkinsonism (Kohno et al., 2000). Treatment is by iron chelation with desferrioxamine (Miyajima et al., 1997). One patient was successfully treated with repeated infusions of fresh frozen plasma (containing ceruloplasmin) (Yonekawa et al., 1999).

## Acknowledgments

This chapter is the work of the U.S. government and is not copyrighted. This chapter has been extensively modified and updated from an original written by C. D. Marsden.

## References

Akil M, Brewer GJ: Psychiatric and behavioral abnormalities in Wilson's disease. Adv Neurol 1995;65:171–178.

Ala A, Walker AP, Ashkan K, et al: Wilson's disease. Lancet 2007; 369(9559):397–408.

Alanen A, Komu M, Penttinen M, Leino R: Magnetic resonance imaging and proton MR spectroscopy in Wilson's disease. Br J Radiol 1999;72:749–756.

Brewer GJ: Penicillamine should not be used as initial therapy in Wilson's disease. Mov Disord 1999;14:551–554.

Brewer GJ: Recognition, diagnosis, and management of Wilson's disease. Proc Soc Exp Biol Med 2000a;223:39–46.

Brewer GJ: Wilson's Disease. Curr Treat Options Neurol 2000b;2: 193–204.

Brewer GJ: Neurologically presenting Wilson's disease: Epidemiology, pathophysiology and treatment. CNS Drugs 2005;19:185–192.

Brewer GJ: Novel therapeutic approaches to the treatment of Wilson's disease. Expert Opin Pharmacother 2006;7:317–324.

Brewer GJ, Dick RD, Johnson VD, et al: Treatment of Wilson's disease with zinc XVI: Treatment during the pediatric years. J Lab Clin Med 2001;137:191–198.

Brewer GJ, Hedera P, Kluin KJ, et al: Treatment of Wilson disease with ammonium tetrathiomolybdate: III. Initial therapy in a total of 55 neurologically affected patients and follow-up with zinc therapy. Arch Neurol 2003;60:379–385.

Brewer GJ, Yuzbasiyan-Gurkan V: Wilson disease. Medicine (Baltimore) 1992;71:139–164.

Butler P, McIntyre N, Mistry PK: Molecular diagnosis of Wilson disease. Mol Genet Metab 2001;72:223–230.

Caca K, Ferenci P, Kuhn HJ, et al: High prevalence of the H1069Q mutation in East German patients with Wilson disease: Rapid detection of mutations by limited sequencing and phenotype-genotype analysis. J Hepatol 2001;35:575–581.

Carpenter TO, Carnes DL Jr, Anast CS: Hypoparathyroidism in Wilson's disease. N Engl J Med 1983;309:873–877.

Curtis D, Durkie M, Balac P, et al: A study of Wilson disease mutations in Britain. Hum Mutat 1999;14:304–311.

Cuthbert JA: Wilson's disease: Update of a systemic disorder with protean manifestations. Gastroenterol Clin North Am 1998;27:655–681, vi–vii.

Czlonkowska A, Gajda J, Rodo M: Effects of long-term treatment in Wilson's disease with D-penicillamine and zinc sulphate. J Neurol 1996;243:269–273.

Demirkiran M, Jankovic J, Lewis RA, Cox DW: Neurologic presentation of Wilson disease without Kayser-Fleischer rings. Neurology 1996;46:1040–1043.

Dening TR: The neuropsychiatry of Wilson's disease: A review. Int J Psychiatry Med 1991;21:135–148.

Dening TR, Berrios GE: Wilson's disease: Psychiatric symptoms in 195 cases. Arch Gen Psychiatry 1989;46:1126–1134.

Farrer LA, Bowcock AM, Hebert JM, et al: Predictive testing for Wilson's disease using tightly linked and flanking DNA markers. Neurology 1991;41:992–999.

Favrole P, Chabriat H, Guichard JP, et al: Clinical correlates of cerebral water diffusion in Wilson disease. Neurology 2006;66:384–389.

Fleming CR, Dickson ER, Wahner HW, et al: Pigmented corneal rings in non-Wilsonian liver disease. Ann Intern Med 1977;86:285–288.

Gadoth N, Liel Y: Transient external ophthalmoplegia in Wilson's disease. Metab Pediatr Ophthalmol 1980;4:71–72.

Geissler I, Heinemann K, Rohm S, et al: Liver transplantation for hepatic and neurological Wilson's disease. Transplant Proc 2003;35:1445–1446.

Giagheddu M, Tamburini G, Piga M, et al: Comparison of MRI, EEG, EPs and ECD-SPECT in Wilson's disease. Acta Neurol Scand 2001;103:71–81.

Grisoli M, Piperno A, Chiapparini L, et al: MR imaging of cerebral cortical involvement in aceruloplasminemia. AJNR Am J Neuroradiol 2005;26:657–661.

Harik SI, Post MJ: Computed tomography in Wilson disease. Neurology 1981;31:107–110.

Harris ZL, Takahashi Y, Miyajima H, et al: Aceruloplasminemia: Molecular characterization of this disorder of iron metabolism. Proc Natl Acad Sci U S A 1995;92:2539–2543.

Hoogenraad TU: Paradigm shift in treatment of Wilson's disease: Zinc therapy now treatment of choice. Brain Dev 2006;28:141–146.

Jacobs DA, Markowitz CE, Liebeskind DS, Galetta SL: The "double panda sign" in Wilson's disease. Neurology 2003;61:969.

Kawanami T, Kato T, Daimon M, et al: Hereditary caeruloplasmin deficiency: Clinicopathological study of a patient. J Neurol Neurosurg Psychiatry 1996;61:506–509.

Kirkham TH, Kamin DF: Slow saccadic eye movements in Wilson's disease. J Neurol Neurosurg Psychiatry 1974;37:191–194.

Kohno S, Miyajima H, Takahashi Y, Inoue Y: Aceruloplasminemia with a novel mutation associated with parkinsonism. Neurogenetics 2000;2:237–238.

LeWitt PA: Penicillamine as a controversial treatment for Wilson's disease. Mov Disord 1999;14:555–556.

Liebeskind DS, Wong S, Hamilton RH: Faces of the giant panda and her cub: MRI correlates of Wilson's disease. J Neurol Neurosurg Psychiatry 2003;74:682.

Loudianos G, Gitlin JD: Wilson's disease. Semin Liver Dis 2000;20:353–364.

Lucato LT, Otaduy MC, Barbosa ER, et al: Proton MR spectroscopy in Wilson disease: Analysis of 36 cases. AJNR Am J Neuroradiol 2005;26:1066–1071.

Madden JW, Ironside JW, Triger DR, Bradshaw JP: An unusual case of Wilson's disease. Q J Med 1985;55:63–73.

Marcellini M, Di Ciommo V, Callea F, et al: Treatment of Wilson's disease with zinc from the time of diagnosis in pediatric patients: A single-hospital, 10-year follow-up study. J Lab Clin Med 2005;145:139–143.

Miyajima H, Kohno S, Takahashi Y, et al: Estimation of the gene frequency of aceruloplasminemia in Japan. Neurology 1999;53:617–619.

Miyajima H, Nishimura Y, Mizoguchi K, et al: Familial apoceruloplasmin deficiency associated with blepharospasm and retinal degeneration. Neurology 1987;37:761–767.

Miyajima H, Takahashi Y, Kamata T, et al: Use of desferrioxamine in the treatment of aceruloplasminemia. Ann Neurol 1997;41:404–407.

Petrukhin K, Fischer SG, Pirastu M, et al: Mapping, cloning and genetic characterization of the region containing the Wilson disease gene. Nat Genet 1993;5:338–343.

Podgaetz E, Chan C: Liver transplantation for Wilson's disease: Our experience with review of the literature. Ann Hepatol 2003;2:131–134.

Prashanth LK, Taly AB, Sinha S, et al: Wilson's disease: Diagnostic errors and clinical implications. J Neurol Neurosurg Psychiatry 2004;75:907–909.

Reilly M, Daly L, Hutchinson M: An epidemiological study of Wilson's disease in the Republic of Ireland. J Neurol Neurosurg Psychiatry 1993;56:298–300.

Ross ME, Jacobson IM, Dienstag JL, Martin JB: Late-onset Wilson's disease with neurological involvement in the absence of Kayser-Fleischer rings. Ann Neurol 1985;17:411–413.

Saatci I, Topcu M, Baltaoglu FF, et al: Cranial MR findings in Wilson's disease. Acta Radiol 1997;38:250–258.

Sarkar B: Copper transport and its defect in Wilson disease: Characterization of the copper-binding domain of Wilson disease ATPase. J Inorg Biochem 2000;79:187–191.

Scheinberg IH, Sternlieb I: Wilson's disease. Philadelphia, WB Saunders, 1984.

Scheinberg IH, Sternlieb I: Treatment of the neurologic manifestations of Wilson's disease. Arch Neurol 1995;52:339–340.

Schiefermeier M, Kollegger H, Madl C, et al: The impact of apolipoprotein E genotypes on age at onset of symptoms and phenotypic expression in Wilson's disease. Brain 2000;123(3):585–590.

Schilsky ML: Treatment of Wilson's disease: What are the relative roles of penicillamine, trientine, and zinc supplementation? Curr Gastroenterol Rep 2001;3:54–59.

Schilsky ML, Scheinberg IH, Sternlieb I: Liver transplantation for Wilson's disease: Indications and outcome. Hepatology 1994;19:583–587.

Schumacher G, Platz KP, Mueller AR, et al: Liver transplantation in neurologic Wilson's disease. Transplant Proc 2001;33:1518–1519.

Shah AB, Chernov I, Zhang HT, et al: Identification and analysis of mutations in the Wilson disease gene (ATP7B): Population frequencies, genotype-phenotype correlation, and functional analyses. Am J Hum Genet 1997;61:317–328.

Shale H, Fahn S, Sternlieb I, Scheinberg IH: Follow-up of "What Is It?" Case 1, 1987. Mov Disord 1988;3:370.

Shimizu N, Yamaguchi Y, Aoki T: Treatment and management of Wilson's disease. Pediatr Int 1999;41:419–422.

Smith CK, Mattson RH: Seizures in Wilson's disease. Neurology 1967;17:1121–1123.

Snow BJ, Bhatt M, Martin WR, et al: The nigrostriatal dopaminergic pathway in Wilson's disease studied with positron emission tomography. J Neurol Neurosurg Psychiatry 1991;54:12–17.

Starosta-Rubinstein S, Young AB, Kluin K, et al: Clinical assessment of 31 patients with Wilson's disease: Correlations with structural changes on magnetic resonance imaging. Arch Neurol 1987;44:365–370.

Stracciari A, Tempestini A, Borghi A, Guarino M: Effect of liver transplantation on neurological manifestations in Wilson disease. Arch Neurol 2000;57:384–386.

Stremmel W, Meyerrose KW, Niederau C, et al: Wilson disease: Clinical presentation, treatment, and survival. Ann Intern Med 1991;115:720–726.

Sutcliffe RP, Maguire DD, Muiesan P, et al: Liver transplantation for Wilson's disease: Long-term results and quality-of-life assessment. Transplantation 2003;75:1003–1006.

Svetel M, Sternic N, Pejovic S, Kostic VS: Penicillamine-induced lethal status dystonicus in a patient with Wilson's disease. Mov Disord 2001;16:568–569.

Tanzi RE, Petrukhin K, Chernov I, et al: The Wilson disease gene is a copper transporting ATPase with homology to the Menkes disease gene. Nat Genet 1993;5:344–350.

Thomas GR, Roberts EA, Walshe JM, Cox DW: Haplotypes and mutations in Wilson disease. Am J Hum Genet 1995;56:1315–1319.

Walshe JM: Diagnosis and treatment of presymptomatic Wilson's disease. Lancet 1988;2(8608):435–437.

Walshe JM: Penicillamine: The treatment of first choice for patients with Wilson's disease. Mov Disord 1999;14:545–550.

Walshe JM, Yealland M: Wilson's disease: The problem of delayed diagnosis. J Neurol Neurosurg Psychiatry 1992;55:692–696.

Walter U, Krolikowski K, Tarnacka B, et al: Sonographic detection of basal ganglia lesions in asymptomatic and symptomatic Wilson disease. Neurology 2005;64:1726–1732.

Wang H, Koschinsky M, Hamerton JL: Localization of the processed gene for human ceruloplasmin to chromosome region 8q21.13–q23.1 by in situ hybridization. Cytogenet Cell Genet 1988;47:230–231.

Wiebers DO, Hollenhorst RW, Goldstein NP: The ophthalmologic manifestations of Wilson's disease. Mayo Clin Proc 1977;52:409–416.

Wiebers DO, Wilson DM, McLeod RA, Goldstein NP: Renal stones in Wilson's disease. Am J Med 1979;67:249–254.

Williams FJ, Walshe JM: Wilson's disease: An analysis of the cranial computerized tomographic appearances found in 60 patients and the changes in response to treatment with chelating agents. Brain 1981;104:735–752.

Wilson SAK: Progressive lenticular degeneration: A familial nervous disease associated with cirrhosis of the liver. Brain 1912;34;295–507.

Yazaki M, Yoshida K, Nakamura A, et al: A novel splicing mutation in the ceruloplasmin gene responsible for hereditary ceruloplasmin deficiency with hemosiderosis. J Neurol Sci 1998;156:30–34.

Yonekawa M, Okabe T, Asamoto Y, Ohta M: A case of hereditary ceruloplasmin deficiency with iron deposition in the brain associated with chorea, dementia, diabetes mellitus and retinal pigmentation: Administration of fresh-frozen human plasma. Eur Neurol 1999;42:157–162.

# Chapter 26

# Psychogenic Movement Disorders
## Phenomenology, Diagnosis, and Treatment

## FUNDAMENTALS

An entire international symposium on psychogenic movement disorders was held in late 2004, and the subsequent publication of its proceedings is now available (Hallett et al., 2006). That volume covers all aspects of psychogenic movement disorders, beyond the scope of this chapter, and scholars in the field are encouraged to read it. Psychogenic movement disorders are caused by psychological factors rather than by an organic etiology. Other terms, such as *functional, nonorganic,* and *medically unexplained symptoms,* have been used. Although the term *functional* might be more convenient to convey to patients and their families—because of old stigmas attached to psychological disorders—the term *psychogenic* best describes the condition related to its etiology. This is much the same way that neurologists have labeled such disorders as postencephalitic parkinsonism, vascular parkinsonism, posttraumatic parkinsonism, and drug-induced parkinsonism. Why not label parkinsonism due to psychogenic etiology as psychogenic parkinsonism? It places the emphasis on etiology, thereby guiding the physician toward appropriate treatment. The term *functional* has been used in the past to denote organic diseases in which a specific cause was not determined and has been applied to organic illnesses such as chorea, epilepsy, and neuralgias (for a historical review, see Fahn, 2006a). Although today, for most clinicians, *functional* is synonymous with *psychogenic,* it might not be uniformly defined this way, so *psychogenic* is less ambiguous.

## Frequency

Movement disorder specialists are seeing increasing numbers of patients with movement disorders whose problems are secondary to psychogenic factors. As one might expect, bradykinetic disorders are less likely than hyperkinetic ones to have a psychogenic etiology unless one were to consider the phenomenon of deliberate slowness to be a bradykinetic disorder. Although deliberate slowness is common in psychogenic disorders, it is not usually the dominant feature, but when it is pure and without accompanying abnormal movements, it is considered in the category of psychogenic parkinsonism. Fixed postures, so-called psychogenic dystonia, account for a sizable proportion of psychogenic movement disorders, so a separate section of this chapter is devoted to the psychogenic dystonias.

Psychogenic findings in neurology have been estimated to occur in 1% to 9% of all neurologic diagnoses (Marsden, 1986; Lempert et al., 1990). Neurologists usually and appropriately recognize patients with psychogenic movement disorders, but the patients often do not accept this diagnosis and seek other opinions, going from physician to physician, seeking a diagnosis that is more to their liking. Therefore, a strategy is necessary for the best way to inform the patients of the diagnosis. This issue is discussed in this chapter. Another common situation is that many physicians do not offer the time-consuming care that is necessary to restore such patients to normality, preferring instead merely to diagnose the condition and have the referring physician deal with the healing.

Like other subspecialties in neurology, psychogenic movement disorders are not uncommon. In one large movement disorder clinic, these patients account for 10% of all nonparkinsonian new patient visits (Portera-Cailliau et al., 2006). Typically, patients are diagnosed by the predominant movement feature (e.g. psychogenic tremor, psychogenic dystonia, psychogenic myoclonus). When evaluated this way, tremor is the most common psychogenic phenomenology, followed by dystonia.

## Importance of an Accurate Diagnosis

The diagnosis of a psychogenic movement disorder is a two-stage process (Lang, 2006). The first stage is to make a positive diagnosis that the movements are psychogenic and not due to an organic illness. The second stage is to identify a psychiatric disorder that could explain the etiology of the abnormal movements and prepare the way for deciding the best course for therapy of the individual patient. The decision between abnormal movements due to a psychogenic cause and those due to an organic cause can be extremely difficult. It is unsatisfactory to pronounce as psychogenic strange movements that have never before been seen, since not even senior movement disorder specialists can profess to have seen the whole gamut of organic abnormal movements. An organic cause of the movements must be excluded (Fahn, 1994; Williams et al., 2005). But even then, neurologists have long advised, making a diagnosis of a psychogenic disorder depends not simply on failing to find an organic cause but on finding positive criteria (for a historical review, see Fahn 2006a).

An accurate diagnosis of psychogenic movement disorder, as opposed to diagnosing an organic movement disorder, is often one of the most difficult tasks in the movement disorder specialty. It is extremely important to be correct in the diagnosis because only then can the appropriate therapy be initiated. The results of an incorrect diagnosis are detrimental. If a patient has a psychogenic disorder that is misdiagnosed, the patient will be given inappropriate and potentially harmful medication and is also denied the proper treatment to overcome the disabling symptoms. By postponing the appropriate psychiatric treatment, the cycle of disability is perpetuated. Untreated patients with psychogenic movement disorders are at risk for becoming career invalids with chronic disability.

If the obverse occurs—that is, if a patient is given a diagnosis of a psychogenic movement disorder when, in fact, he or she suffers from an organic one—again the wrong treatment is given. In this situation, time-consuming and expensive psychotherapy, psychiatric medications, and possibly electroconvulsive therapy might be initiated instead of more appropriate pharmacotherapeutic agents that could provide relief. Moreover, a diagnosis of a psychogenic disorder can create emotional trauma for the patient and his or her family (Cooper, 1976). It is important to point out that no matter how much experience a clinician has had, encountering a new type of movement disorder for the first time does not automatically make this a psychogenic movement disorder. For example, task-specific jaw tremor (Miles et al., 1997) is rare, and even when it is encountered for the first time, a wise clinician should consider it to be organic (Video 26-1) and not psychogenic (Video 26-2).

Neurologic symptoms and signs are a common result of hysteria, and neurologists have long been fascinated by the brain's ability to be able to produce such clinical expressions on the basis of psychological disturbances. Many great neurologists, such as Charcot and Freud, intensively studied hysterical conversion reactions, using hypnosis as a tool in their investigations and treatment (Goetz, 1987). In their training, neurologists-to-be are taught to differentiate the clinical findings of psychogenic etiology from those of organic disorders (Gowers, 1893; Oppenheim, 1911a; DeJong, 1958a). However, textbooks in the past often considered some dyskinesias that are recognized today as organic, such as tics, writer's cramp, and other occupational cramps, and some other forms of dystonia, to be examples of hysteria (DeJong, 1958b).

Although there is a modest neurologic literature on psychogenic phenomenology, the literature dealing specifically with psychogenic movement disorders is rather sparse. For example, tremor as the result of a conversion reaction has been long recognized, at least since the days of Gowers (1893), but scientific reports on psychogenic tremor or other movement disorders are rarely described in the literature. Campbell (1979) pointed out that the amplitude of psychogenic tremor is more pronounced when attention is paid to it and that it lessens and may even disappear when the patient's attention is diverted to another subject or other part of the body. Distraction is a useful part of the examination, and lessening of severity by distraction can be very helpful diagnostically in trying to establish a diagnosis of psychogenic tremor. But in our experience, distraction does not always succeed in making the tremor disappear, so this maneuver is often not successful. Therefore, additional findings on examination are often necessary and can be just as helpful in considering the diagnosis of a psychogenic movement disorder; these are discussed in this chapter.

Although in the great majority of patients with a psychogenic movement disorder, all their clinical features result only from a psychogenic problem, some may have the psychogenic movement disorder on top of an organic movement disorder, as seen in Patient 5 in the series of psychogenic dystonias reported by Fahn and Williams (1988) and the cases of Ranawaya and colleagues (1990). Perhaps 10% to 15% of patients with a psychogenic movement disorder have an underlying organic movement disorder as well. This overlap is seen in patients with psychogenic seizures (pseudoseizures); 10% to 37% of patients have organic seizures as well (Krumholz and Niedermeyer, 1983; Lesser et al., 1983). Nevertheless, a useful rule of thumb is that if one part of the examination reveals nonorganicity, it is likely that other "abnormalities" on the examination might also be nonorganic. The term *organic* is used to mean "not due to a psychogenic etiology."

Perhaps the movement disorders with the highest prevalence rate of a psychogenic origin are the nonfamilial, "idiopathic," paroxysmal nonkinesigenic dyskinesias, as surveyed by Bressman and colleagues (1988). They found that of 18 patients with paroxysmal nonkinesigenic dystonias and with no known symptomatic etiology or positive family history for a paroxysmal dyskinesia, the dystonias were due to psychogenic causes in 11 patients. This represents 61% of such cases. The age at onset in these patients ranged from 11 to 49 years; 8 of the 11 patients were female. Thus, unless accompanied by a clear-cut family history, these paroxysmal dystonias are particularly commonly psychogenic, and their diagnosis is extremely difficult to make for reasons that are explained later in the chapter (Fahn and Williams, 1988).

Kotagal and colleagues (2002) conducted a study of paroxysmal events in children. Over a 6-year period, 883 patients were monitored in their pediatric epilepsy monitoring unit; 134 patients (15.2%) were documented to have paroxysmal nonepileptic events. Children in the preschool group (age 2 months to 5 years) (n = 26) were eventually diagnosed with stereotypies, hypnic jerks, parasomnias, and Sandifer syndrome. The school-age group (age 5 to 12 years) (n = 61) had diagnoses of psychogenic seizures, inattention or daydreaming, stereotypies, hypnic jerks, and paroxysmal dyskinesias. The adolescent group (age 12 to 18 years) (n = 48) had a diagnosis of psychogenic seizures in 40 patients (83%). The authors concluded that in patients with paroxysmal nonepileptic events, conversion disorder was seen in children older than 5 years of age, and its frequency increased with age, becoming the most common type of paroxysmal nonepileptic events among adolescents. In adolescents, conversion disorder was more common in females, whereas males predominated in the school-age group. Concomitant epilepsy with nonepileptic events occurred in all three age groups to a varying extent.

## Mass Hysteria

Today, neurologists encounter individual patients with psychogenic movement disorders. But historically, mass hysteria was common, probably more so than it is today. Mass hysteria still occurs, such as "shell shock" in wartime and mass hysteria during environmental events such as mass inoculations (Kharabsheh et al., 2001; Khiem et al., 2003). Symptoms can also be generated from mass concerns about medications and breast implants, in part owing to widespread publicity, although legal liability issues may also drive the development of symptoms. Mass hysteria resembling seizures occurred recently in 10 high school girls following the development of organic absence seizures in another student (Roach and Langley, 2004).

It is interesting to note that the term *chorea*, meaning "dancing" in Latin, comes from the dancing mania (a mass hysteria) that was seen in the Middle Ages and from which the term *St. Vitus' dance* was coined; this term subsequently was applied by Sydenham to describe the condition now referred to as *Sydenham chorea* (Hayden, 1981).

For further information, see the 2001 monograph by Halligan and colleagues, which is devoted to the topic of hysteria.

## Physiologic Basis for Psychogenic Neurologic Dysfunctions

It is intellectually intriguing that the brain can create neurologic deficits, such as paralysis, sensory loss, blindness, seizures, and movement disorders. This mysterious ability fascinated pioneers working on hysteria, such as Charcot and Freud. The ensuing 100-plus years offered little enlightenment, until recently, when newer technologies have begun to shed some light on the mechanism. Vuilleumier and colleagues (2001) utilized single photon emission computed tomography to measure regional cerebral blood flow with and without bilateral vibration in seven patients with unilateral psychogenic sensory loss and then again in the four fully recovered subjects after recovery. These studies revealed a consistent decrease of regional cerebral blood flow in the thalamus and basal ganglia contralateral to the deficit, which reverted to normal when the patients recovered. These results suggest that hysterical conversion deficits might entail a functional disorder in striatothalamocortical circuits controlling sensorimotor function and voluntary motor behavior. The same subcortical premotor circuits are involved in unilateral motor neglect after organic neurologic damage.

In an analogous situation, a patient who was diagnosed with psychogenic reduced visual acuity underwent a single photon emission computed tomography scan that revealed reduced regional cerebral blood flow in the bilateral visual association areas but not in the primary visual areas (Okuyama et al., 2002). The authors concluded that psychogenic visual disturbance is associated with functional suppression of the visual association area. A listing of functional imaging studies carried out on hysteria has been collated by Fink and colleagues (2006). These studies indicate that alterations in regional brain activity may accompany the expression of conversion symptoms.

The results in functional imaging studies are complemented by motor physiology studies. When cortical and spinal inhibition was evaluated in psychogenic and organic dystonia, both groups had similar results for reduced inhibition (Espay et al., 2006). Again, this suggests that the central nervous system accommodates its physiology to follow the motor pattern

## DEGREE OF CERTAINTY OF THE DIAGNOSIS OF A PSYCHOGENIC MOVEMENT DISORDER

Fahn and Williams (1988) categorized patients into four levels of certainty as to the likelihood of their having a psychogenic movement disorder. These four degrees of certainty are (1) documented psychogenic disorder, (2) clinically established psychogenic disorder, (3) probable psychogenic disorder, and (4) possible psychogenic movement disorder. Subsequent authors have used this classification (Koller et al., 1989; Ranawaya et al., 1990; Lang, 1995). The classification of Fahn and Williams is incorporated here, but with the criteria expanded somewhat, taking into account additional observations since the original publication.

## Documented Psychogenic Movement Disorder

Mere suspicion that the signs and symptoms are psychogenic is insufficient for the diagnosis of documented psychogenic disorder. For the disorder to be documented as being psychogenic, the symptoms must be completely relieved by psychotherapy, by the clinician's use of psychological suggestion, including physiotherapy, or by administration of placebos (again with suggestion being a part of the approach), or the patient must be witnessed as being free of symptoms when left alone and (as far as the patient knows) unobserved. This last feature would be a major factor in proving psychogenicity in those who are malingering or have a factitious disorder, since such patients would not likely obtain relief of symptoms by manipulation of the examiner. Insurance companies are increasingly using videotaped surveillance to protect themselves against fraud. There is now a published report of a patient with a clinical diagnosis of reflex sympathetic dystrophy who sued for financial compensation despite features of psychogenicity and was videotaped while under surveillance by a private investigator and shown to be completely free of the abnormal movements, allowing the case to be settled for a reduced amount (Kurlan et al., 1997). If the signs and symptoms disappear and do not return, that is fairly good evidence that the underlying psychiatric problem has been relieved. But it is not uncommon for the psychogenic movement disorder to return if the patient does not obtain complete relief of the psychiatric factors that led to the neurologic dysfunction.

A critical issue for using the relief of signs as a criterion for the definition is that most organic movement disorders rarely remit spontaneously and completely except for tics, tardive dyskinesia, infectious disorders (e.g., Sydenham chorea) and drug-induced reactions, and, rarely, essential myoclonus (Fahn and Sjaastad, 1991). Other organic disorders, such as Parkinson disease, Huntington disease, and essential tremor, are persistent and even progressive. Idiopathic torsion dystonia, except for torticollis (Jayne et al., 1984; Friedman and Fahn, 1986; Jahanshahi et al., 1990), rarely totally remits. On occasion, patients with other types of dystonia will show improvement, but this improvement is typically incomplete and temporary (Marsden and Harrison, 1974), although gradual, prolonged, incomplete improvement has been encountered in at least one patient (Eldridge et al., 1984).

The degree of remission that is seen in cases with documented psychogenic movement disorders is usually the dramatic, sudden improvement that occurs within a few days with supportive suggestion or placebo treatment. In a few patients with more chronic symptoms, improvement can be more gradual, occurring over weeks to months of "physiotherapy" used as a means of allowing the patient to relinquish the symptoms in a face-saving manner. Physiotherapy also can have physical benefits for patients who had developed weakness, spasms, or contractures based on chronic disuse and/or abnormal postures for extended periods, even though these were on a psychogenic basis.

## Clinically Established Psychogenic Movement Disorder

When the movement disorder is inconsistent over time (the features are different when the patient is observed at subsequent examinations) or is incongruent with a classic movement disorder, one becomes suspicious that the movements are psychogenic. If either inconsistency or incongruity is present and, in addition, the patient manifests any of the following, one can feel comfortable in believing that the disorder is psychogenic, and this has been referred to as clinically established psychogenic movement disorder. These additional manifestations are the following:

1. Other neurologic signs are present that are definitely psychogenic (e.g., false weakness, false sensory findings, and self-inflicted injuries).
2. Multiple somatizations are present.
3. An obvious psychiatric disturbance is present.
4. The movement disorder disappears with distraction.
5. Excessive (appearing deliberate) slowness of movement is present.

It should be noted that item 4 by itself is insufficient for a diagnosis of a documented or clinically established psychogenic disorder. This is because some organic movement disorders can be temporarily and voluntarily suppressed (Koller and Biary, 1989). Similarly, akathitic movements and paradoxical dystonia (Fahn, 1989) tend to disappear with active voluntary movement.

## Probable Psychogenic Movement Disorder

This definition contains four categories of patients:

1. Patients in whom the movements are inconsistent or are incongruent with any classic movement disorder, and there are no other features to provide further support for such a diagnosis of psychogenicity
2. Patients in whom the movements are consistent and congruent with an organic disorder, and the movements can be made to disappear with distraction when ordinarily distraction would not be expected to eliminate the movements if they were organic
3. Patients in whom the movements are consistent and congruent with an organic disorder, but other neurologic signs are present that are definitely psychogenic (e.g., false weakness, false sensory findings, or self-inflicted injuries)
4. Patients in whom the movements are consistent and congruent with an organic disorder, but multiple somatizations are present

The last two subdivisions contain psychiatric manifestations that make the clinician highly suspicious that the movements might also be psychogenic, but by themselves they are insufficient to give a higher degree of certainty to the diagnosis of a psychogenic movement disorder.

## Possible Psychogenic Dystonia

One can be suspicious that the movements are psychogenic if an obvious emotional disturbance is present, but this is not as compelling as the psychiatric features listed previously. For the category of a possible psychogenic disorder, the movements would be consistent and congruent with an organic movement disorder.

## Summary on the Degree of Certainty of the Diagnosis of a Psychogenic Paroxysmal Movement Disorder

Paroxysmal movement disorders present a special and difficult problem. Their natural history characteristically shows prolonged periods of cessation of the abnormal movements,

so their disappearance with placebo or by suggestion cannot by itself establish the diagnosis of a psychogenic disorder, since the remission could have been coincidental. However, if the paroxysms are frequent and the attacks are prolonged, then repeated trials with placebo can be informative. If such trials consistently produce remissions, then one can be convinced that the diagnosis is a documented psychogenic disorder.

The criteria for clinically established, probable, and possible psychogenic movement disorders would be the same for paroxysmal movement disorders and continual movement disorders. It is likely when both a paroxysmal movement disorder and a continual movement disorder are present in the same patient that the etiology is psychogenic.

## DEFINITIONS OF PSYCHIATRIC TERMINOLOGY

Definitions from DSM-IV are used regarding psychogenic movement disorders. Patients with psychogenic movement disorder can be subdivided into three categories: the somatoform disorders, the factitious disorders, and malingering.

## Somatoform Disorder

A somatoform disorder is one in which the physical symptoms are linked to psychological factors yet the symptom production is *not under voluntary control* (i.e., *not consciously produced*). The two main types of somatoform disorders that produce psychogenic neurologic problems are *conversion disorder* and *somatization disorder*; the latter is also known as hysteria or as Briquet syndrome. Other somatoform subsets are hypochondriasis, somatoform pain disorder, and body dysmorphic disorder.

In *conversion disorder*, psychological factors may be judged to play a primary etiologic role in a variety of ways. This may be suggested by a temporal relationship between the onset or worsening of the symptoms and the presence of an environmental stimulus that activates a psychological conflict or need. Alternatively, the symptom may be noted to free the patient from a noxious activity or encounter. Finally, the symptom may be noted to enable the patient to get support from the environment that otherwise might not be forthcoming.

A *somatization disorder* involves recurrent and multiple complaints of several years' duration for which medical care has been sought but that are apparently not due to any physical disorder. The dynamics are presumably the same as those of conversion disorder, and the symptoms may emerge from chronic, recurrent, untreated conversion disorder. There are four separate categories of symptoms that need to be present at some time for the diagnosis of a somatization disorder according to the DSM-IV-TR. They are (1) four sites or functions of pain, (2) two gastrointestinal symptoms, (3) one symptom related to sex or reproduction, and (4) at least one of 13 neurologic complaints, namely, problems with coordination, paralysis or weakness, feeling of an object in the throat, aphonia, urinary retention, hallucinations, anesthesia, diplopia, blindness, deafness, seizures, amnesia, and loss of consciousness. It should be noted that various movement disorders, such as tremor and sustained contractions, are not on this list of 13, and this should be included as one of the neurologic complaints. Other requirements are age at onset under 30 years and severe enough symptomatology that the patient has taken medications, consulted a physician, or altered his or her lifestyle because of it.

## Factitious Disorder

A factitious disorder is one in which the physical symptoms are *intentionally produced* (hence are under voluntary control) owing to psychological need. This group includes Munchausen syndrome. Factitious disorders are due to a mental disorder. They are generally associated with severe, dependent, masochistic, or antisocial personality disorders.

## Malingering

Malingering refers to *voluntarily produced* physical symptoms in pursuit of a goal such as financial compensation, avoidance of school or work, evasion of criminal prosecution, or acquisition of drugs. Malingering is not considered to be a mental disorder.

When a physician is faced with a patient who has a psychogenic movement disorder, it is often not possible to distinguish with certainty among somatoform, factitious, and malingering disorders. A patient's volitional intent is often impossible to determine with certainty.

## Depression

It is worth making some comment about depression. In our experience, many patients with a psychogenic movement disorder also have concurrent depression. Treatment of this depression is essential and is part of the overall strategy in outlining a treatment program for the patient. Often, lifting of the depression is necessary for the patient to obtain relief of the motor symptoms.

## CLUES SUGGESTING THE PRESENCE OF A PSYCHOGENIC MOVEMENT DISORDER

Often, there are clues from the history and neurologic examination that lead the clinician to suspect a diagnosis of psychogenic dystonia. Fahn and Williams (1988), Koller and colleagues (1989), and Factor and colleagues (1995) have enunciated many of these clues. Boxes 26-1 and 26-2 list these clues, as well as some additional ones.

 Abrupt onset of the movement disorder is quite common. The presence of more than one type of dyskinesia (item 5 in Box 26-1) is another important clue, often confounding clinicians (Video 26-3). Most of the time, patients with an organic movement disorder present with only a single type. A note of caution is warranted, however. Certain organic disorders progress to involve more than one type of abnormal movement. For example, Huntington disease can have chorea, bradykinesia, dystonia, and myoclonus (Penney et al., 1990). Neuroacanthocytosis often is manifested by both chorea and tics (Hardie et al., 1991). Some patients with childhood-onset tics may later develop torsion dystonia (Shale et al., 1986; Stone and Jankovic, 1991). Often, patients with idiopathic torsion dystonia will have dystonic tremor or rapid movements that resemble myoclonus or chorea (Fahn et al., 1987).

---

**Box 26-1** Clues relating to the movements that suggest a psychogenic movement disorder

1. Abrupt onset
2. Inconsistent movements (changing characteristics over time; pattern, body distribution, rapidly varying severity)
3. Incongruous movements and postures (movements that do not fit with recognized patterns or with normal physiologic patterns)
4. Presence of certain types of abnormal movements that are fairly common among individuals with psychogenic movement disorders, such as rhythmic shaking, bizarre gait, deliberate slowness carrying out requested voluntary movement, bursts of verbal gibberish, or excessive startle (bizarre movements in response to sudden, unexpected noise or threatening movement)
5. Presence of additional types of abnormal movements not known to be part of the primary or principal movement pattern that the patient manifests
6. Manifesting exhaustion, excessive fatigue
7. Delayed, often excessive, startle response to a stimulus
8. Spontaneous remissions
9. Decrease or disappearance of movements with distraction
10. Disappearance of tremors when handling treasured objects
11. Entrainment of the tremor to the rate of the requested rapid successive movement the patient is asked to perform
12. Response to placebo, suggestion, or psychotherapy
13. Manifestation of a paroxysmal disorder
14. Dystonia beginning as a fixed posture
15. Twisting facial movements that move the mouth to one side or the other (*Note:* Organic dystonia of the facial muscles usually does not move the mouth sidewise.)

---

Patients with tardive dyskinesia may have a combination of rhythmic oral-buccal-lingual movements plus dystonia and akathitic movements (Fahn, 1984). Box 1-12 in Chapter 1 lists the diseases that are composed of multiple types of movement disorders.

---

**Box 26-2** Clues relating to other medical observations that suggest a psychogenic movement disorder

1. False (give-way) weakness
2. False sensory complaints
3. Multiple somatizations or undiagnosed conditions
4. Self-inflicted injuries
5. Obvious psychiatric disturbances
6. Employed in the health profession or in health insurance claims
7. Presence of secondary gain, including continuing care by a devoted spouse
8. Litigation or compensation pending

The most common type of movements, whether isolated or in the presence of other types of movements, in patients with psychogenic movement disorders is shaking movements (item 4 in Box 26-1) that can resemble organic tremors or peculiar, atypical tremors (Video 26-4). This was the most common type of abnormal movement in the spectrum of psychogenic movement disorders reported by Lang (2006) and by Jankovic and Thomas (2006). Another note of caution about unusual tremors is that Wilson disease can also present with unusual tremors (Shale et al., 1987, 1988). Utterances of gibberish (Videos 26-5 and 26-6) can be another useful sign.

Item 4 in Box 26-1 also lists bizarre gaits as a feature of psychogenicity. After tremors and dystonia, bizarre gait disorders are the next most common type of unusual movement disorder encountered in patients with mixed features of movements. The psychogenic gait can show posturing (see Video 26-6), excessive slowness, and hesitation. There could be pseudo-ataxia or careful walking (like walking on ice). The latter resembles the fear-of-falling syndrome, which is discussed in more detail later. There can be sudden buckling of a leg, as if there is weakness (Vecht et al., 1991), but the failure to produce this dipping movement each time the patient steps on the leg would be evidence of inconsistency. Accompanying this bizarre gait would be a variability of impairment and excessive swaying when tested for the Romberg sign, without actually falling.

Another aspect of item 4 is excessive startle that could mimic hyperekplexia, excessive startle syndrome, jumping Frenchman syndrome (Video 26-7), or even reflex myoclonus (Andermann and Andermann, 1986). Thompson and colleagues (1992) determined the physiologic parameters that are typically seen in patients with psychogenic startles. There is a variable latency to the onset of the jerk; the latencies are greater than those seen in reflex myoclonus of cortical or brainstem origin; the latencies are longer than the fastest voluntary reaction time; there are variable patterns of muscle recruitment within each jerk; and there is significant habituation with repeated stimulation. This last point is probably not specific to psychogenic startle, since organic startles may also show habituation. Noise stimuli can induce other abnormal movements besides startle. Walters and Hening (1992) reported a case with psychogenic tremor following sudden, loud noise; the patient had a posttraumatic stress disorder.

Item 11 in Box 26-1 points out that in a patient with psychogenic tremor, when the patient is asked to carry out rapid successive movements, such as tapping the index finger on the thumb, the rate of the tremor becomes the same as the rapid successive movements (i.e., the tremor has become entrained). In contrast, an organic tremor is the dominant rate; it will gradually force the voluntary movements to be the same rate as the tremor.

Idiopathic torsion dystonia usually begins with action dystonia (Fahn et al., 1987), but psychogenic dystonia often begins with a fixed posture. Fixed postures are sustained postures that resist passive movement, and the presence of such fixed postures is highly likely to be due to a psychogenic dystonia (Fahn and Williams, 1988; Lang and Fahn, 1990; Schrag et al., 2004; Schrag, 2006). The posture can manifest so much rigidity that it is extremely difficult to move the limb about a joint (Video 26-8). Often, the psychogenic dystonia resembles reflex sympathetic dystrophy because there is accompanying pain and tenderness (Lang and Fahn, 1990; Schwartzman and Kerrigan, 1990; Bhatia et al., 1993; Schrag et al., 2004; Schrag, 2006). To make matters confusing, in many cases, psychogenic dystonia of a limb follows a minor trauma to that limb, similar to the pattern of reflex sympathetic dystrophy. On the other hand, organic dystonia of a body part can be preceded by an injury to that body part (Schott, 1985, 1986; Scherokman et al, 1986; Gordon et al., 1990; Goldman and Ahlskog, 1993), so it can be difficult to distinguish between organic and psychogenic dystonia. Fixed painful postural torticollis following trauma is not uncommon, and determining whether it is organic or psychogenic is difficult, but recent analysis indicates that many of these cases appear to be psychogenic in etiology (Sa et al., 2003).

Although a fixed dystonic posture, in which the joint cannot be passively extended or flexed, is often psychogenic, it might also be due to a contracture (which, of course, might also be the result of a psychogenic dystonia as well as an organic dystonia). The evaluation of such fixed postures in which the affected joint cannot be passively altered requires the aid of anesthesia to determine whether contractures are present (Fahn, 2006b). This technique not only aids in the diagnosis but also guides the clinician and patient in what to expect during therapy (Video 26-9).

In addition to the clues in the history and examination related to the movements themselves, which are presented in Box 26-1, clues in the nonmovment history and examination are often helpful to the clinician in the consideration of a psychogenic disorder (see Box 26-2).

The frequency with which patients with psychogenic movement disorders are employed in some capacity in the health professions is impressive (item 6 in Box 26-2). Many are nurses; another large group is employed in the health insurance industry, processing medical claims.

Another point that is worth commenting on is that many of the affected individuals have a devoted spouse who responds readily to their pressing needs (item 7 in Box 26-2). Some spouses carry a pager so that the patient can easily call them while they are at work. Others pamper the patient, who might even be wheelchair-bound, especially if the patient has psychogenic dystonia. Such devotion could be a secondary gain from having the movement disorder.

## DIAGNOSTIC APPROACH AND CLINICAL FEATURES

Psychogenic movement disorders are usually identified on the basis of (1) unusual motor phenomenology and other clues as listed in Box 26-1, (2) a discrepancy between the patient's disability and objective signs of motor deficit, and (3) the presence of psychiatric abnormalities. First, the neurologist bases the suspected diagnosis on identifying the different types of abnormal movements that are present in a given patient. The type of movement disorder is assigned on the basis of the phenomenology, which can consist of more than one type (item 5, Box 26-1). The neurologist must exclude possible organic causes for the abnormal movements so that both the neurologist and the patient feel comfortable that the diagnosis of a psychogenic movement disorder has been made with confidence. Then the consulting psychiatrist attempts to establish a psychiatric diagnosis. Finally, a suggested strategy for treatment is presented to the patient. In fact, explaining to the patient that the condition has the potential for a more favorable outcome with proper treatment than would an organic movement disorder may help the patient more readily accept the diagnosis of a psychogenic etiology.

**Table 26-1** Predominant movement feature in psychogenic movement disorders

| Predominant Movement Feature | n | Percent |
|---|---|---|
| Tremor | 467 | 37.5 |
| Dystonia | 365 | 29.3 |
| Myoclonus | 146 | 11.7 |
| Gait disorder | 114 | 9.2 |
| Parkinsonism | 60 | 4.8 |
| Tics | 29 | 2.3 |
| Other | 64 | 5.1 |
| Total | 1245 | 100 |

This is a tabulation of psychogenic movement disorders seen at eight centers; most centers report their patients by a single primary motor feature, but some report multiple features if more than one is present.

Data from Lang AE: General overview of psychogenic movement disorders: Epidemiology, diagnosis, and prognosis. In Hallett M, Fahn S, Jankovic J, et al: Psychogenic Movement Disorders—Neurology and Neuropsychiatry. Philadelphia, Lippincott Williams & Wilkins, 2006, pp 35–41.

The types of psychogenic movements seen in a review of the publications from eight movement disorder centers are presented in Table 26-1. Tremor was found to be the most common psychogenic phenomenology, followed by dystonia. Tics were the least common. Williams and colleagues (1995) reviewed the records of 131 patients with psychogenic movement disorders and listed their motor phenomenologies (Table 26-2). In their experience, dystonia, tremor, gait disturbances, paroxysmal dyskinesias, and myoclonus were the major motor types that were encountered. The difference from other centers that found tremor to be more common than dystonia may be that the Columbia group labeled movements on a hierarchical scale, whereby if any dystonia was present, regardless whether other movements like tremor were also present, the condition was coded as a dystonic one. Williams and colleagues found that 79% of patients had multiple types of abnormal movements and that only 21% had a single definable type (Table 26-3).

**Table 26-2** Principal motor phenomenology in 131 patients with psychogenic movement disorders

| Type of Movement | n | Percent of Organic Cases |
|---|---|---|
| Dystonia | 82 | 2.5 |
| Tremor | 21 | |
| Gait disorder | 14 | |
| Myoclonus | 11 | |
| Blepharospasm/facial movements | 4 | |
| Parkinsonism | 3 | <0.1 |
| Tics | 2 | |
| Stiff person | 1 | |
| Paroxysmal and undifferentiated movements | 14 | |

Total = 152, because more than one type was equally prominent.

Data from Williams DT, Ford B, Fahn S: Phenomenology and psychopathology related to psychogenic movement disorders. Adv Neurol 1995;65:231–257.

**Table 26-3** Phenomenology of psychogenic movements

| Clinical Feature | Percent of Patients |
|---|---|
| Single type | 21 |
| Multiple types | 79 |
| Continuous movements | 45 |
| Intermittent/paroxysmal | 55 |
| Fifteen patients with hand tremor (dominant hand) | 93 |
| Abrupt onset (usually inciting event) | 60 |
| Spread from initial site | 43 |

Data from Williams DT, Ford B, Fahn S: Phenomenology and psychopathology related to psychogenic movement disorders. Adv Neurol 1995;65:231–257.

Moreover, again in contrast with the vast majority of organic movement disorders, in 55% of the patients the movements were either intermittent or paroxysmal, while only 45% of the patients had only continuous movements. They also reported that the onset was abrupt in 60% of patients, usually with a specific inciting event. In 43% of patients, the movements spread beyond the initial site of involvement.

Factor and colleagues (1995) reviewed their 28 cases of psychogenic movement disorders. These represented 3.3% of all 842 consecutive movement disorder patients seen over a 6-year period. Tremor was most common (50%), followed by dystonia, myoclonus, and parkinsonism. Clinical clues included distractibility (86%) and abrupt onset (54%). Distractibility was more important in tremor and least important in dystonia. Other diagnostic clues included entrainment of tremor to the frequency of repetitive movements of another limb, fatigue of tremor, stimulus sensitivity, and a previous history of psychogenic illness.

The demographic pattern of the 131 patients reported by Williams and colleagues (1995) is presented in Box 26-3. Of the 131 patients, 87% were females; the mean age at onset was

**Box 26-3** Demographics of patients with psychogenic movement disorders

**Age at Onset**
Range: 4 to 73 years
Mean: 36.9 years

**Gender**
Male:female ratio = 22:109
Males = 13%
Females = 87%

**Presence of Some Organic Component**
13%

**Onset to Correct Diagnosis**
Mean: 4.9 years
Trimodal
    <6 months: 25%
    2 years: 40%
    23 years: 15%

Data from Williams DT, Ford B, Fahn S: Phenomenology and psychopathology related to psychogenic movement disorders. Adv Neurol 1995;65:231–257.

**Table 26-4** Clinical features in patients with psychogenic movement disorders

| Clinical Feature | Percent of Patients |
|---|---|
| Previously erroneously diagnosed as organic (3 with multiple sclerosis despite negative laboratory tests) | 75 |
| False weakness | 37 |
| False sensory exam | 8.7 |
| Pain and tenderness | 17.4 |
| Startle | 29 |
| Psychogenic seizures | 11.6 |
| Disabled | 65 |
| Head trauma | 25 |
| Peripheral trauma | 12.5 |

Data from Williams DT, Ford B, Fahn S: Phenomenology and psychopathology related to psychogenic movement disorders. Adv Neurol 1995;65:231–257.

37 years, with a range of 4 to 73 years. An organic component of a movement disorder was present in 13%. The mean duration before a correct diagnosis was made was 5 years.

An organic diagnosis was made originally in 75% of the patients with a psychogenic movement disorder (Table 26-4), including three patients who carried a diagnosis of multiple sclerosis despite the lack of any positive laboratory data detected by the treating neurologist. A number of neurologic findings presented as clues to psychogenicity. The most common was the presence of give-way weakness (37%). Next most common was a startle reaction that was nonphysiologic (29%). Pain and false sensory findings on examination were also encountered (see Table 26-4). Surprisingly, psychogenic seizures were concurrently present in 12% of the patients. The psychogenic movement disorder was disabling in 65% of the patients. A preceding history and inciting event of head trauma and peripheral trauma occurred in 25% and 12.5% of patients, respectively.

Williams and colleagues (1995) found that the most common psychiatric diagnosis was a somatoform disorder, particularly a conversion disorder (Table 26-5). Briquet syndrome (somatization disorder) was diagnosed in 12.5%, and there were even fewer patients with a factitious disorder (8%) or malingering (4%). An accompanying depression or anxiety was found in 71% and 17% of patients, respectively.

## PSYCHOGENIC DYSTONIA

It is, in some ways, ironic that torsion dystonia can sometimes be due to psychogenic causation. From its earliest beginnings, idiopathic torsion dystonia appeared to have been mistaken as a manifestation of a psychiatric disturbance (Schwalbe, 1908). Soon after Schwalbe's description in 1908 (see English translation by Truong and Fahn, 1988), however, Oppenheim (1911b) and Flatau and Sterling (1911) set matters right by emphasizing the organic nature of this disorder. Although some early publications on dystonia mentioned the "functional" nature of the symptoms (Destarac, 1901) or used the label *neurosis* (Ziehen, 1911), these terms were employed in those days in a manner different from that of today. *Functional* referred to a physiologic activation of the abnormal movements with voluntary motor activity, which would otherwise disappear when the patient was quiet at rest. *Neurosis* was a term that was used to indicate a neurologic, rather than a psychiatric, disorder but one without a structural lesion. Today, it is common for the term *functional* to be equivalent to *psychogenic* and for *neurosis* not to be used at all in neurology but to refer to certain psychiatric disorders.

Thus, for many decades, the organic nature of torsion dystonia was emphasized. Yet, possibly beginning in the 1950s, many patients with various forms of focal, segmental, and generalized dystonia began to be misdiagnosed as having a conversion disorder. Among 44 patients with idiopathic dystonia reviewed by Eldridge and colleagues (1969), 23 patients (52%) had previously been referred for psychiatric treatment (without benefit). Marsden and Harrison (1974) had a similar experience; 43% of their 42 patients were previously diagnosed as suffering from hysteria. Cooper and his colleagues (1976) reviewed their series of 226 patients and found that 56 patients (25%) had a diagnosis of psychogenic etiology at some time during their illness. Lesser and Fahn (1978) reviewed the records of 84 patients with idiopathic dystonia seen at Presbyterian Hospital in New York from 1969 to 1974 and found that 37 patients (44%) had previously been given a diagnosis that their movement abnormalities were due to an emotional disorder. These 37 patients consisted of 11 with generalized dystonia, 14 with segmental dystonia, and 19 with focal dystonia (14 with torticollis, 2 with oromandibular dystonia, and 3 with blepharospasm).

Although some authors (Meares, 1971; Tibbets, 1971) suggested that an underlying psychiatric illness might exist in patients with torticollis, others (Zeman and Dyken, 1968; Cockburn, 1971; Riklan et al., 1976) found no differences between dystonic patients and controls in regard to previous psychiatric history and current life adjustment or on psychiatric testing. Similarly, some authors (Crisp and Moldofsky, 1965; Bindman and Tibbets, 1977) considered hand dystonia (writer's cramp, occupational cramp) to be psychogenic. But Sheehy and Marsden (1982) studied 34 patients with writer's or other occupational cramps affecting the hand or arm. All patients underwent assessment by a psychiatric interview technique; these patients compared favorably with a control group,

**Table 26-5** Psychiatric aspects of psychogenic movement disorders

| Psychiatric Feature | Percent of disorder |
|---|---|
| Conversion disorder | 75 |
| Somatization disorder | 12.5 |
| Factitious disorder | 8.3 |
| Malingering | 4.2 |
| Accompanying | |
| Depression | 71 |
| Anxiety | 17 |
| Hypnotizable | |
| Highly | 36 |
| Mild-moderately | 41 |

Data from Williams DT, Ford B, Fahn S: Phenomenology and psychopathology related to psychogenic movement disorders. Adv Neurol 1995;65:231–257.

and the investigators concluded that their disorder was not psychiatric in origin. Another recent study involved psychiatric assessment in 20 subjects with focal hand dystonia, and it also concluded that none had any serious psychopathology (Grafman et al., 1991). Furthermore, patients with writer's cramp do not have increased anxiety (Harrington et al., 1988).

At the time of the first international symposium on dystonia, held in 1975, Fahn and Eldridge (1976) noted that no case of proven psychological dystonia had been reported. With the realization that patients with dystonia were being misdiagnosed as having a psychiatric disorder, knowledgeable neurologists became sensitive to this problem and, since then, seemed to avoid a diagnosis of hysterical dystonia. However, at the annual meeting of the American Academy of Neurology in 1983, Fahn and colleagues (1983) described ten patients as having documented psychogenic dystonia, five of them identified after the abstract to the meeting was submitted. Batshaw and colleagues (1985) had followed a patient who had been misdiagnosed as having an organic dystonia and who had had a stereotactic thalamotomy based on that diagnosis; these authors eventually recognized that their patient had psychogenic dystonia and reported her as a case of Munchausen syndrome. Fahn and Williams (1988) have described 22 cases of documented or clinically established psychogenic dystonia, including a case of a young girl who underwent a stereotaxic thalamotomy. Lang (1995) reported on 18 patients with documented or clinically established psychogenic dystonia, 14 of whom had a known precipitant. Involvement of the legs occurred in 12 patients, despite onset in adulthood. Ten of Lang's patients had paroxysmal worsening of dystonia or other abnormal movements. Pain was a prominent feature in 14 of 16 patients with this complaint.

Psychogenic dystonia is difficult to diagnose, since there are no laboratory tests to establish the diagnosis of organic idiopathic dystonia. A number of cortical and spinal reflex abnormalities have been reported in organic dystonia, all showing lack of inhibition or spread of cortical field (see Chapter 13). These abnormalities could be a useful way to differentiate psychogenic dystonia from organic dystonia; however, when these tests were applied to both groups to compare the differences, the results were similar in both groups—both showed a reduced inhibition (Espay et al., 2006). This supports the growing PET scan findings in psychogenic neurologic disorders that the central nervous system accommodates its physiology to follow the motor pattern.

Without laboratory analysis, diagnosis depends on clinical skill to differentiate organic and psychogenic dystonia. The clues listed in Boxes 26-1 and 26-2 should help to alert the clinician to the possibility of a psychogenic etiology. Clues that often point to an organic diagnosis, such as a sensory trick (gets antagonistic) that mitigates dystonia, can be very helpful but also occasionally misleading (Munhoz and Lang, 2004).

In a survey of 22 patients reported by Fahn (1994) on documented and clinically established cases of psychogenic dystonia, he found that 6 patients had paroxysmal dystonia and 16 had continual dystonia. Females outnumbered males by a ratio of 20:2. The youngest age at onset was 8 years, and the oldest was 58 years. Those with paroxysmal dystonia were, as a general rule, older than patients with continual dystonia.

# PSYCHOGENIC NONDYSTONIC MOVEMENT DISORDERS

## Psychogenic Tremor

As mentioned earlier, rhythmic movements, often appearing as shaking, are the most common abnormal movement in patients with psychogenic movement disorders. But what resembles organic tremor is also a common presentation. The tremor tends to be present equally with the affected limb at rest, with posture holding, and with action (Video 26-10). This fact helps  differentiate the condition from organic tremors, which typically dominate just one of these characteristic features. Also, psychogenic tremor tends to vary in pattern (for example, being vertical in the hands when the arm is at rest and being horizontal in the hands when the arm is held against gravity in front of the body) (Jankovic et al., 2006b). If distraction of the patient results in disappearance of the tremor, it is a helpful, but not a conclusive, sign that the tremor is psychogenic (Campbell, 1979). Many patients with organic tremor are able to temporally suppress tremor, even parkinsonian tremor. Furthermore, distractibility is often difficult to observe, and many patients are too aware to distract easily. Entrainment of the tremor to a new frequency may sometimes be seen when the patient is asked to touch his or her thumb to various fingers in a dictated pattern. Of 12 patients with psychogenic tremor compared with 33 with organic essential tremor studied by Kenney and colleagues (2007), psychogenic tremor was significantly more likely to start suddenly and to be associated with spontaneous remissions than was essential tremor. Family history of tremor was significantly more common in the essential tremor group; distraction with alternate finger tapping significantly decreased psychogenic tremor, but entrainment did not differentiate the two groups.

Koller and colleagues (1989) diagnosed 24 patients with psychogenic tremors. They described the tremors as complex; usually, they were present at rest, with posture, and with action. The onset was abrupt, and in all but one, the tremors lessened or were abolished with distraction. Fahn (1994) described that psychogenic tremors are sometimes paroxysmal and not always continuous. Deuschl and colleagues (1998) reviewed 25 cases of psychogenic tremor. Sudden onset and rare remissions were common. The "coactivation sign" and absent finger tremor were the most consistent criteria to separate them from organic tremors. Whereas most organic tremors show decreasing amplitudes when the extremity is loaded with additional weights, most psychogenic tremors show an increase of tremor amplitude (i.e., coactivation sign). Overall, psychogenic tremor in their series had a poor outcome. Kim and colleagues (1999) reviewed their series of 70 cases of psychogenic tremor. They emphasized the abrupt onset (73%), often with the maximal disability at onset (46%), and then took static (46%) or fluctuating (17%) courses. Tremor usually started in one limb and spread rapidly to a generalized or mixed distribution. Other features were spontaneous resolution and recurrence, as well as easy distractibility together with entrainment and response to suggestion. In addition to tremor in the limbs, psychogenic palatal tremor has been reported (Pirio Richardson et al., 2006).

Another electrophysiologic approach to aid in distinguishing between psychogenic and organic tremors is with accelerometry. Tremor is measured in one hand while the other hand either rests or taps to an auditory stimulus at 3 and

4 or 5 Hz. Psychogenic tremors showed larger tremor frequency changes and higher intraindividual variability during tapping (Zeuner et al., 2003). Motor control physiology can be useful to distinguish psychogenic from organic tremor (Deuschl et al., 2006).

About half of the psychogenic tremors are coherent between the two arms, suggesting to the authors that coherent tremors might be voluntary, while noncoherent tremors are involuntary (Raethjen et al., 2004). Voluntary tapping of the contralateral limb usually results in either dissipating the tremor or shifting the tremor frequency to that of the metronome (O'Suilleabhain et al., 1998).

## Psychogenic Gait

Morris and colleagues (2006) described key features of the psychogenic gait. These include exaggerated effort, fatigue with groans and sighs, extreme slowness, appearance of pain with grimaces, knee buckling, unusual postures, and astasia-abasia. Keane (1989) described 60 cases with psychogenic gait abnormality out of 228 patients with psychogenic neurologic problems. Among these abnormal gaits were 24 patients with "ataxia" (the most common gait abnormality), 9 patients with trembling, 2 patients with "dystonia," 2 patients with truncal "myoclonus," and 1 patient with camptocormia (markedly stooped posture). Among the myriad of associated psychogenic signs were 8 patients with tremor. A knee giving way, with recovery, was seen in 5 patients, and is a feature of a case that presented as an unknown, unusual movement disorder (Vecht et al., 1991). In a video review of psychogenic gaits, Hayes and colleagues (1999) emphasized certain features of the gait: exaggerated effort, extreme slowness, variability throughout the day, unusual or uneconomic postures, collapses, convulsive tremors, and distractibility. On the other hand, it is possible to misdiagnose as psychogenic an abnormal gait that is organic. Such happened to a patient with a gait disorder and episodic weakness that were thought to be psychogenic who was subsequently diagnosed with status cataplecticus due to narcolepsy (Simon et al., 2004).

## Fear of Falling

According to Keane (1989), Spiller (1933) referred to the syndrome of fear of falling as *staso-basophobia*. Fear of falling is a syndrome in which the patient can walk perfectly well if he or she is holding onto someone but is unable to walk without leaning against furniture or walls if alone. Sometimes, this could be purely due to a psychiatric problem, such as agoraphobia. Most of the patients we have seen with this problem developed the condition after they had fallen, usually from organic causes (such as loss of postural reflexes or ataxia), and were left with a marked fear of falling when walking without holding on. One of our patients with essential action myoclonus developed this disorder after suffering several falls and continued to have fear of falling even after successful treatment of the myoclonus with clonazepam. The freezing phenomenon (or motor blocks) that is seen in parkinsonism and the gait in action myoclonus patients are the other major conditions in which the gait also normalizes when the patient holds onto someone. The fear-of-falling syndrome is usually separated from the list of psychogenic movement disorders. But because, for many of these patients, the fear of falling is beyond what can be considered rational, there is a psychogenic

component. Women are more affected than men, and often the mistaken diagnosis is Parkinson disease (Kurlan, 2005).

## Psychogenic Myoclonus

Psychogenic myoclonus should be relatively easy to distinguish from organic myoclonus where access to a motor control physiology laboratory is available (Brown, 2006). The short duration of a myoclonic jerk (usually less than 100 msec) is almost impossible to duplicate voluntarily. The EMG pattern of voluntary jerks exhibits a triphasic pattern of activity between antagonistic muscles, whereas cortical myoclonus consists of short-duration 25 to 50 msec bursts of cocontracting antagonistic muscles (Thompson, 2006). Furthermore, the latency of reflex myoclonus is physiologically short (40 to 100 msec), whereas abnormal reactive voluntary jerks are much longer (Thompson, 2006).

Monday and Jankovic (1993) reported 18 patients with psychogenic myoclonus (although no electromyographic observations were reported to indicate that myoclonus was the actual type of abnormal movement), stating that this is the most common form of psychogenic movement disorder encountered in their clinic. The myoclonus was segmental in 10 patients, generalized in 7 patients, and focal in 1 patient. Psychogenic myoclonus accounted for 8.5% of the 212 patients with myoclonus in their clinic. Inconsistency with continuously changing pattern anatomically and temporally was common. The movements often increased with stress, anxiety, and exposure to noise or light. A Bereitschaftspotential preceding muscle jerks was found in five of six patients with a diagnosis of psychogenic myoclonic (Terada et al., 1995). The authors suggest that this is a positive sign for the diagnosis of psychogenic myoclonus, but because of the one patient who did not have a Bereitschaftspotential, its absence cannot be used to exclude the diagnosis.

Rhythmic palatal myoclonus has also been reported to be of a psychogenic etiology in rare cases (Williams, 2004; Pirio Richardson et al., 2006).

## Psychogenic Tics

Psychogenic movements can sometimes resemble tics, but this is one of the least common manifestations of a psychogenic movement disorder (Lang, 2006). It is more complicated when organic tics are also present. Dooley and colleagues (1994) described two children with Tourette syndrome who also had pseudo-tics, in whom the psychogenic movements resolved when the stressful issues in their lives were addressed.

## Psychogenic Parkinsonism

Psychogenic parkinsonism is relatively uncommon (see Table 26-2). Lang and colleagues (1995) reported 14 patients with this disorder. Eleven patients had tremor at rest, but the tremor did not disappear with movement of the limb, and the frequency and rhythmicity varied. Rigidity was present in six patients but without cogwheeling. All 14 patients had slowness of movement (bradykinesia) without the typical decrementing feature of organic bradykinesia (Video 26-11). One patient had evidence of some organic parkinsonism as well but required a fluorodopa positron emission tomography scan to be certain. Another study also reported the combination of organic and psychogenic parkinsonism and found that the dopaminergic SPECT imaging can help in distinguishing this disorder from pure psychogenic parkinsonism (Benaderette et al., 2006).

## APPROACHES TO THE PATIENT WHO IS SUSPECTED OF HAVING A PSYCHOGENIC MOVEMENT DISORDER

The following treatment plan has been developed over the years of attempting to manage patients with psychogenic disorders.

Ideally, the patient should be admitted to the hospital, specifically to the neurology unit where the treating neurologist is in control of the treating regimen. Informing the patient of the diagnosis on the initial visit in an outpatient setting often leads to disbelief and distrust by the patient. If this happens, the patient usually never returns and will continue to have symptoms and probably see a number of other physicians, looking for an organic diagnosis. The success rate of outpatient treatment is uncertain, but in this age of managed health care, the difficulty in obtaining permission to admit the patient to a hospital will force many patients to be treated in an outpatient setting.

Because of the difficulty in admitting the patient to the hospital, a new strategy has evolved over the past few years that appears to be a reasonable substitute for hospitalization. All necessary and reasonable tests should be performed to ensure that an organic basis for the symptoms has not been overlooked. This includes a sleep study with video recording if the family insists that the movements are present during sleep. The purpose of the sleep study is to observe objectively the movements and with electroencephalographic monitoring to determine whether the patient is asleep. It is possible that conversion reactions occur during sleep.

When the diagnosis seems certain during an outpatient evaluation, the next step is to inform the patient of the diagnosis. This is usually difficult for the physician and must be done in a tactful manner that will convince the patient and the family and avoid denial. It is helpful to ask the patient and family whether they have any thoughts about the possible cause of the symptoms. If there is mention that the condition might have resulted from "nerves" or stress, this provides an excellent opportunity for the physician to state that he or she has come to a similar conclusion. If there is no mention of stress, the physician will have to take another approach to inform the patient of the diagnosis. In this situation, one approach is to inform the patient (1) that he or she has a movement disorder (and specifically name the disorder—e.g., dystonia or tremor) and (2) that this disorder "can be attributed to many different etiologies." Then the clinician can proceed to explain that, in the patient's situation, all the evidence rules out a structural defect in the brain and that the variety of symptoms indicates that they are caused by brain physiology expressing pent-up emotions by producing the abnormal movements. The clinician can then explain that the mind controls the body by producing physiologic changes in the brain to allow these symptoms to emerge. It is important to point out that, because the symptoms are not due to a structural lesion, the probability for reversal of the abnormal physiology is great. This presents a positive view of the disorder, which can be strengthened by explaining that if the condition were

due to a structural change in the brain, the chance for full recovery would be small.

At this point, the physician can explain the treatment approach, pointing out that it is essential for the neurologist to work with a psychiatrist who can determine what the stress factors are that have allowed the brain physiology to be altered. If the psychiatrist determines that there is an underlying depression or anxiety, he or she will have the opportunity to treat those conditions with medications. It is important to explain to the patient that (1) the psychiatrist may want to utilize medications to alter the brain transmitters to hasten a normalization of brain physiology and (2) in addition to working with a psychiatrist, it will be essential for treatment to include physiotherapy to teach the muscles (essentially retrain the muscles) to move normally again.

Once the diagnosis and the therapeutic strategy have been explained, the physician must determine whether the patient sincerely wishes to seek improvement through an intensive treatment program that entails outpatient psychotherapy and outpatient physiotherapy. The responsibility for improvement should be placed with the patient by explaining that the patient must resolve to work on the treatment regimen if improvement is to be achieved. The patient should be told that unless improvement is evident at each follow-up visit, continuation of the program will be of no use.

Ideally, the psychiatric consultant should be experienced in and should have had success working with patients with a psychogenic movement disorder. It will be the psychiatrist who obtains clues about the possible psychodynamics underlying the symptoms, who determines whether the patient has insights that will be important for estimating the prognosis, who utilizes hypnosis or conducts an amobarbital interview in order to obtain more psychodynamic information, who discusses possible pharmacotherapeutic approaches, and who establishes the rapport with the patient that will be necessary for psychotherapy. A psychiatrist who has an interest in treating psychogenic movement disorders is critical to successful therapy.

*The psychiatrist cannot make the diagnosis of a psychogenic movement disorder. This diagnosis can be made only by the neurologist.*

The severity of the underlying psychiatric illness should not be underestimated by the neurologist. These patients are prone to committing suicide.

The presence of joint contractures does not exclude the diagnosis of a psychogenic movement disorder. This feature would require examination under deep anesthesia to determine whether there is an actual contracture (Fahn, 2006b). Knowing this information allows one to calculate the maximum amount of motor improvement that can be expected. Arrangements are made with an anesthesiologist to carry out the evaluation.

There is controversy about using placebos in the diagnosis or treatment of patients with psychogenic movement disorders (Jankovic et al., 2006a). Although the use of placebos can be an easy approach to making the correct diagnosis, it often angers patients, who feel that they have been "tricked." If the approach is used to help make the diagnosis, disclosure after the fact—explaining the rationale and the physician's desire to be certain about the diagnosis so that proper treatment can be initiated—is necessary. Patients will lose trust in the treating physician if they discover on their own that placebos have been used. Placebos can be used to exacerbate the abnormal movements as well as to relieve them (Levy and Jankovic, 1983). Using placebos to treat the symptoms can also lead to a loss of trust; this approach is no substitute for important psychotherapy to determine the root cause of, and consequently a cure for, the problem. If placebos are used to treat the condition, and the patient improves, it can then be difficult to explain the procedure to the patient. Patients can suffer serious clinical reversal when they learn what has taken place. If placebos are used to treat the symptoms, it is, therefore, important to inform the patient as soon as possible in order to ensure that the patients maintain confidence that you are working with them to achieve a speedy recovery. Many patients would lose faith in their doctor if they learned from another source that they had been treated with a placebo. For a variety of reasons, then, it is better to avoid the use of placebos and strive to obtain successful results by other means (Ford et al., 1995). Nonetheless, if it is determined that the risks outweigh the benefits, judicious use of a placebo can aid in making the correct diagnosis (Tan, 2004) to determine proper treatment.

If the patient is admitted to the hospital before receiving the diagnosis of a psychogenic movement disorder, he or she should not be allowed to leave the hospital without being informed of the diagnosis. The diagnosis should be discussed with the patient in the presence of the psychiatric consultant if necessary. It is usually incorrect to anticipate that the referring physician is in a better position to discuss the diagnosis and manage treatment. When outpatient treatment is the only available choice, the patient needs to be informed of the diagnosis before being referred to the psychiatrist. As noted previously, psychiatrists cannot make the diagnosis of a psychogenic movement disorder; their role is to establish the psychodynamics and to provide psychiatric treatment.

It is important to be consistently positive and absolute with the patient once the diagnosis is certain. If any uncertainty is conveyed, the patient will continue to doubt the diagnosis and fail to respond to therapy. Positive reinforcement should be given to assure the patient that the symptoms will progressively improve with time as the muscles "are being retrained to move more appropriately." However, if there is uncertainty about the diagnosis, another opinion should be sought.

As was mentioned previously, treatment should be initiated in the hospital if at all possible. But if hospitalization is not feasible, treatment may be given in the outpatient setting. Any combination of psychotherapy, positive reinforcement, physiotherapy, relaxation techniques, and *desensitization therapy* may be used. Desensitization therapy is a mechanism of treatment for patients who are stimulus-sensitive, such as those who have excessive startle, shakes, or myoclonus after exposure to a sensory stimulus. Introducing the stimulus in a mild, subclinical form that fails to induce the abnormal response is the starting point. Then the intensity of the stimulus should be increased over time until the patient is desensitized. Patients who are depressed will usually benefit from psychotherapy or antidepressant medication. For long-term care, often the patient has a need to belong to a group and will join the local chapter of the lay organization that deals with this disorder.

Factitious disorders and malingering are usually not benefited. Symptoms will disappear only when the patient is ready to give them up.

Somatoform disorders can usually be treated. In some patients, the symptom may return despite the patient's being aware that it is due to an emotional problem.

## RESULTS OF TREATMENT

Psychotherapy is the major treatment approach that is best suited for permanent benefit. Somatoform disorders have the best results from treatment. Factitious disorders and malingering yield poor results, and the patient improves only when he or she is ready to relinquish the symptoms. Williams and colleagues (1995) utilized psychotherapy in all patients, along with the following supplemental approaches: family sessions, 58%; hypnosis, 42%; physical therapy, 42%; and placebo therapy, 13% (Table 26-6). Psychotropic medication (antidepressants) was utilized in 71%. Two patients with treatment-resistant major depression received electroconvulsive therapy; one responded completely, and the other responded only partially. One fourth of the patients required more extensive psychiatric hospitalization because of suicidal ideation or because there was a poor response in reversing the psychodynamic pathology while on the neurology service.

Treatment by Williams and colleagues (1995) resulted in a permanent, meaningful benefit in 52% of patients, with complete relief, considerable relief, and moderate relief in 25%, 21%, and 8% of patients, respectively (Table 26-7). Some relapse occurred in over 20% of patients, and no improvement was seen in 12%. Of those who had been previously employed, 25% were able to resume full-time work, and 10% were able to work part time, with 15% functioning at home (see Table 26-7).

In the series of 28 cases of psychogenic movement disorders reported by Factor and colleagues (1995), 35% resolved, and this subgroup had a shorter duration of disease than did those who did not resolve. Of 56 patients with any type of psychogenic neurologic disorder other than pseudoseizures, Couprie and colleagues (1995) found that the long-term outcome was good in 96% of those who improved during a hospital stay and in only 30% of others and that rapid improvement was related to recent onset of symptoms. In a longitudinal study of 228 patients evaluated in the Baylor College of Medicine Movement Disorders Clinic, after a mean duration of follow-up of 3.4 ± 2.8 years, improvement of symptoms was noted in 56.6% patients, 22.1% worsened, and 21.3% remained the same at the time of follow-up. Positive social life perceptions, strong suggestion of effective treatment

**Table 26-6** Treatment of psychogenic movement disorders

| Patient Acceptance | Percent of Patients |
| --- | --- |
| Accepted diagnosis and treatment | 70 |
| Refused diagnosis and treatment | 30 |

**Psychiatrically Treated Patients**

| Type of Psychiatric Treatment | Percent of Patients |
| --- | --- |
| Family sessions | 58 |
| Hypnosis | 88 |
| Physiotherapy | 42 |
| Placebo | 13 |
| Antidepressants | 71 |
| Electroconvulsive therapy | 8 |

Data from Williams DT, Ford B, Fahn S: Phenomenology and psychopathology related to psychogenic movement disorders. Adv Neurol 1995;65:231–257.

Table 26-7 Results of treatment of psychogenic movement disorders

| Results of Treatment | Percent of Patients |
|---|---|
| Permanent, complete relief | 25 |
| Permanent, considerable relief | 21 |
| Permanent, moderate relief | 8 |
| Relapse | 4 |
| Partial relapse | 17 |
| No improvement | 12 |
| **Previously Employed** | |
| Now working full time | 25 |
| Now working part time | 10 |
| Functioning at home | 15 |
| Now disabled | 30 |

Data from Williams DT, Ford B, Fahn S: Phenomenology and psychopathology related to psychogenic movement disorders. Adv Neurol 1995;65:231–257.

by the physician, elimination of stressors, and treatment with antidepressant medications contributed to a favorable outcome. Using a "blinded" review of videos, psychiatric rating scales, and a psychogenic movement disorder scale, Hinson and colleagues (2006) demonstrated the efficacy of psychotherapy and medications in the treatment of patients with psychogenic movement disorders.

## OTHER MOVEMENT DISORDERS CAUSED BY PSYCHIATRIC CONDITIONS BUT NOT REGARDED AS PSYCHOGENIC MOVEMENT DISORDERS

A number of movement disorders are due to diseases that are classified as mental or psychiatric disturbances, in which the abnormal hypokinesia or hyperkinesia is not listed as a psychogenic movement disorder. Table 26-8 lists these, as well as the common underlying causes.

Table 26-8 shows that basically none of the aforementioned psychiatric conditions is a somatoform disorder, a factitious disorder, or a malingering state. Thus, the psychogenic movement disorders can be distinguished from the conditions listed in Table 26-8 on the basis of the underlying psychiatric state. It should be noted that even if a somatoform disorder, a factitious disorder, or a malingering state is only suspected and not officially diagnosed, the diagnosis of a psychogenic movement disorder can still be

Table 26-8 Movement disorders that are symptoms of psychiatric conditions and not classified as psychogenic movement disorders

| Psychiatric Condition | Movement Disorder |
|---|---|
| Schizophrenia, depression | Catatonia |
| Depression | Psychomotor slowness |
| Obsessive-compulsive disorder | Obsessional slowness, stereotypies |
| Agoraphobia, anxiety | Fear of falling |
| Schizophrenia, autism | Stereotypies |

made. Also, even if a psychiatric consultant cannot detect one of these disorders, a neurologist may still make the diagnosis on the grounds listed in Boxes 26-1 and 26-2.

## References

Andermann F, Andermann E: Excessive startle syndromes: Startle disease, jumping, and startle epilepsy. Adv Neurol 1986;43:321–338.

Batshaw ML, Wachtel RC, Deckel AW, et al: Munchausen's syndrome simulating torsion dystonia. N Eng J Med 1985;312:1437–1439.

Benaderette S, Fregonara PZ, Apartis E, et al: Psychogenic parkinsonism: A combination of clinical, electrophysiological, and [(123)I]-FP-CIT SPECT scan explorations improves diagnostic accuracy. Mov Disord 2006;21(3):310–317.

Bhatia KP, Bhatt MH, Marsden CD: The causalgia-dystonia syndrome. Brain 1993;116:843–851.

Bindman E, Tibbets RW: Writer's cramp, a rational approach to treatment? Br J Psychiatry 1977;131:143–148.

Bressman SB, Fahn S, Burke RE: Paroxysmal non-kinesigenic dystonia. Adv Neurol 1988;50:403–413.

Brown P: Clinical neurophysiology of myoclonus. In Hallett M, Fahn S, Jankovic J, et al (eds): Psychogenic Movement Disorders—Neurology and Neuropsychiatry, Philadelphia, Lippincott Williams & Wilkins, 2006, pp 262–264.

Campbell J: The shortest paper. Neurology 1979;29:1633.

Cockburn JJ: Spasmodic torticollis: A psychogenic condition? J Psychosom Res 1971;15:471–477.

Cooper IS: The Victim Is Always the Same. New York, Norton, 1976.

Cooper IS, Cullinan T, Riklan M: The natural history of dystonia. Adv Neurol 1976;14:157–169.

Couprie W, Wijdicks EFM, Rooijmans HGM, van Gijn J: Outcome in conversion disorder: A follow up study. J Neurol Neurosurg Psychiatry 1995;58:750–752.

Crisp AH, Moldofsky HA: A psychosomatic study of writer's cramp. Br J Psychiatry 1965;111:841–858.

DeJong RN: The Neurologic Examination: Incorporating the Fundamentals of Neuroanatomy and Neurophysiology, 2nd ed. New York, Hoeber-Harper, 1958a, pp 931–956.

DeJong RN: The Neurologic Examination: Incorporating the Fundamentals of Neuroanatomy and Neurophysiology, 2nd ed. New York, Hoeber-Harper, 1958b, pp 521–523.

Destarac: Torticolis spasmodique et spasmes fonctionnels. Rev Neurol 1901;9:591–597.

Deuschl G, Koster B, Lucking CH, Scheidt C: Diagnostic and pathophysiological aspects of psychogenic tremors. Mov Disord 1998; 13:294–302.

Deuschl G, Raethjen J, Kopper F, Govindan RB: The diagnosis and physiology of psychogenic tremor. In Hallett M, Fahn S, Jankovic J, et al (eds): Psychogenic Movement Disorders—Neurology and Neuropsychiatry, Philadelphia, Lippincott Williams & Wilkins, 2006, pp 265–273.

Dooley JM, Stokes A, Gordon KE: Pseudo-tics in Tourette syndrome. J Child Neurol 1994;9:50–51.

Eldridge R, Ince SE, Chernow B, et al: Dystonia in 61-year-old identical twins: Observations over 45 years. Ann Neurol 1984;16:356–358.

Eldridge R, Riklan M, Cooper IS: The limited role of psychotherapy in torsion dystonia: Experience with 44 cases. JAMA 1969;210:705–708.

Espay AJ, Morgante F, Purzner J, et al: Cortical and spinal abnormalities in psychogenic dystonia. Ann Neurol 2006;59(5):825–834.

Factor SA, Podskalny GD, Molho ES: Psychogenic movement disorders: Frequency, clinical profile, and characteristics. J Neurol Neurosurg Psychiatry 1995;59:406–412.

Fahn S: The tardive dyskinesias. In Matthews WB, Glaser GH (eds): Recent Advances in Clinical Neurology, vol 4. Edinburgh, Churchill Livingstone, 1984, pp 229–260.

Fahn S: Clinical variants of idiopathic torsion dystonia. J Neurol Neurosurg Psychiatry 1989;special suppl:96–100.

Fahn S: Psychogenic movement disorders. In Marsden CD, Fahn S (eds): Movement Disorders 3. Oxford, Butterworth-Heinemann, 1994, pp 359–372.

Fahn S: The history of psychogenic movement disorders. In Hallett M, Fahn S, Jankovic J, et al (eds): Psychogenic Movement Disorders—Neurology and Neuropsychiatry, Philadelphia, Lippincott Williams & Wilkins, 2006a, pp 24–31.

Fahn S: The role of anesthesia in the diagnosis and treatment of psychogenic movement disorders. In Hallett M, Fahn S, Jankovic J, et al (eds): Psychogenic Movement Disorders—Neurology and Neuropsychiatry, Philadelphia, Lippincott Williams & Wilkins, 2006b, pp 256–261.

Fahn S, Eldridge R: Definition of dystonia and classification of the dystonic states. Adv Neurol 1976;14:1–5.

Fahn S, Marsden CD, Calne DB: Classification and investigation of dystonia. In Marsden CD, Fahn S (eds): Movement Disorders 2. London, Butterworths, 1987, pp 332–358.

Fahn S, Sjaastad O: Hereditary essential myoclonus in a large Norwegian family. Mov Disord 1991;6:237–247.

Fahn S, Williams D: Psychogenic dystonia. Adv Neurol 1988;50:431–455.

Fahn S, Williams D, Reches A, et al: Hysterical dystonia, a rare disorder: Report of five documented cases. Neurology 1983;33(suppl 2):161.

Fink GR, Halligan PW, Marshall JC: Neuroimaging of hysteria. In Hallett M, Fahn S, Jankovic J, et al (eds): Psychogenic Movement Disorders—Neurology and Neuropsychiatry, Philadelphia, Lippincott Williams & Wilkins, 2006, pp 230–237.

Flatau E, Sterling W: Progressiver Torsionspasms bie Kindern. Z Gesamte Neurol Psychiatr 1911;7:586–612.

Ford B, Williams DT, Fahn S: Treatment of psychogenic movement disorders. In Kurlan R (ed): Treatment of Movement Disorders. Philadelphia, JB Lippincott, 1995, pp 475–485.

Friedman A, Fahn S: Spontaneous remissions in spasmodic torticollis. Neurology 1986;36:398–400.

Goetz CG: Charcot, the Clinician: The Tuesday Lessons. Excerpts from Nine Case Presentations on General Neurology Delivered at the Salpetriere Hospital in 1887–88 by Jean-Martin Charcot, translated with Commentary. New York, Raven Press, 1987, pp 102–122.

Goldman S, Ahlskog JE: Posttraumatic cervical dystonia. Mayo Clin Proc 1993;68:443–448.

Gordon MF, Brin MF, Giladi N, et al: Dystonia precipitated by peripheral trauma. Mov Disord 1990;5(suppl 1):67.

Gowers WR: A Manual of Diseases of the Nervous System, vol II, 2nd ed. Philadelphia, Blakiston, 1893, pp 984–1030.

Grafman J, Cohen LG, Hallett M: Is focal hand dystonia associated with psychopathology? Mov Disord 1991;6:29–35.

Hallett M, Fahn S, Jankovic J, et al (eds): Psychogenic Movement Disorders—Neurology and Neuropsychiatry, Lippincott Williams & Wilkins, Philadelphia, 2006.

Halligan PW, Bass C, Marsja JC (eds): Contemporary Approaches to the Study of Hysteria. Oxford, UK, Oxford University Press, 2001.

Hardie RJ, Pullon HWH, Harding AE, et al: Neuroacanthocytosis: A clinical, haematological and pathological study of 19 cases. Brain 1991;114:13–49.

Harrington RC, Wieck A, Marks IM, Marsden CD: Writer's cramp: Not associated with anxiety. Mov Disord 1988;3:195–200.

Hayden MR: Huntington's Chorea. Berlin, Springer-Verlag, 1981.

Hayes MW, Graham S, Heldorf P, et al: A video review of the diagnosis of psychogenic gait: Appendix and commentary. Mov Disord 1999;14:914–921.

Hinson VK, Weinstein S, Bernard B, et al: Single-blind clinical trial of psychotherapy for treatment of psychogenic movement disorders. Parkinsonism Relat Disord 2006;12(3):177–180.

Jahanshahi M, Marion M-H, Marsden CD: Natural history of adult-onset idiopathic torticollis. Arch Neurol 1990;47:548–552.

Jankovic J, Cloninger CR, Fahn S, et al: Therapeutic approaches to psychogenic movement disorders. In Hallett M, Fahn S, Jankovic J, et al (eds): Psychogenic Movement Disorders—Neurology and Neuropsychiatry, Philadelphia, Lippincott Williams & Wilkins, 2006a, pp 323–328.

Jankovic J, Vuong KD, Thomas M: Psychogenic tremor: Long-term outcome. CNS Spectr 2006b;11:501–508.

Jayne D, Lees AJ, Stern GM: Remission in spasmodic torticollis. J Neurol Neurosurg Psychiatry 1984;47:1236–1237.

Keane JR: Hysterical gait disorders: 60 cases. Neurology 1989;39:586–589.

Kenney C, Mejia N, Jankovic J: Clinical features that distinguish psychogenic and essential tremor. Mov Disord 2007 (in press).

Kharabsheh S, Al-Otoum H, Clements J, et al: Mass psychogenic illness following tetanus-diphtheria toxoid vaccination in Jordan. Bull World Health Organ 2001;79:764–770.

Khiem HB, Huan LD, Phuong NTM, et al: Mass psychogenic illness following oral cholera immunization in Ca Mau City, Vietnam. Vaccine 2003;21(31):4527–4531.

Kim YJ, Pakiam ASI, Lang AE: Historical and clinical features of psychogenic tremor: A review of 70 cases. Can J Neurol Sci 1999;26:190–195.

Koller W, Lang A, Vetere-Overfield B, et al: Psychogenic tremors. Neurology 1989;39:1094–1099.

Koller WC, Biary NM: Volitional control of involuntary movements. Mov Disord 1989;4:153–156.

Kotagal P, Costa M, Wyllie E, Wolgamuth B: Paroxysmal nonepileptic events in children and adolescents. Pediatrics 2002;110(4):e46.

Krumholz A, Niedermeyer E: Psychogenic seizures: A clinical study with follow-up data. Neurology 1983;33:498–502.

Kurlan R: "Fear of falling" gait: A potentially reversible psychogenic gait disorder. Cogn Behav Neurol 2005;18(3):171–172.

Kurlan R, Brin MF, Fahn S: Movement disorder in reflex sympathetic dystrophy: A case proven to be psychogenic by surveillance video monitoring. Mov Disord 1997;12:243–245.

Lang AE: Psychogenic dystonia: A review of 18 cases. Can J Neurol Sci 1995;22:136–143.

Lang AE: General overview of psychogenic movement disorders: Epidemiology, diagnosis, and prognosis. In Hallett M, Fahn S, Jankovic J, et al (eds): Psychogenic Movement Disorders—Neurology and Neuropsychiatry, Philadelphia, Lippincott Williams & Wilkins, 2006, pp 35–41.

Lang A, Fahn S: Movement disorder of RSD. Neurology 1990;40:1476–1477.

Lang AE, Koller WG, Fahn S: Psychogenic parkinsonism. Arch Neurol 1995;52:802–810.

Lempert T, Dietrich M, Huppert D, Brandt T: Psychogenic disorders in neurology: Frequency and clinical spectrum. Acta Neurol Scand 1990;82:335–340.

Lesser RP, Fahn S: Dystonia: A disorder often misdiagnosed as a conversion reaction. Am J Psychiatry 1978;153:349–452.

Lesser RP, Lueders H, Dinner DS: Evidence for epilepsy is rare in patients with psychogenic seizures. Neurology 1983;33:502–504.

Levy R, Jankovic J: Placebo-induced conversion reaction: A neurobehavioral and EEG study of hysterical aphasia, seizure and coma. J Abnorm Psychol 1983;92:243–249.

Marsden CD: Hysteria: A neurologist's view. Psychol Med 1986;16:277–288.

Marsden CD, Harrison MJG: Idiopathic torsion dystonia. Brain 1974;97:793–810.

Meares R: Features which distinguish groups of spasmodic torticollis. J Psychosom Res 1971;15:1–11.

Miles TS, Findley LJ, Rothwell JC: Electrophysiological observations on an unusual, task specific jaw tremor. J Neurol Neurosurg Psychiatry 1997;63:251–254.

Monday K, Jankovic J: Psychogenic myoclonus. Neurology 1993;43:349–352.

Morris JC, de Moore GM, Herberstein M: Psychogenic gait: An example of deceptive signaling. In Hallett M, Fahn S, Jankovic J, et al (eds): Psychogenic Movement Disorders—Neurology and Neuropsychiatry, Philadelphia, Lippincott Williams & Wilkins, 2006, pp 69–75.

Munhoz RP, Lang AE: Gestes antagonistes in psychogenic dystonia. Mov Disord 2004;19(3):331–332.

Okuyama N, Kawakatsu S, Wada T, et al: Occipital hypoperfusion in a patient with psychogenic visual disturbance. Psychiat Res 2002;114(3):163–168.

Oppenheim H: Textbook of Nervous Diseases for Physicians and Students, 5th ed., translated by Bruce H. Edinburgh, Otto Schulzle, 1911a, pp 1053–1111.

Oppenheim H: Uber eine eigenartige Krampfkrankheit des kindlichen und jugendlichen Alters (Dysbasia lordotica progressiva, Dystonia musculorum deformans). Neurol Centrabl 1911b; 30:1090–1107.

O'Suilleabhain PE, Matsumoto JY: Time-frequency analysis of tremors. Brain 1998;121:2127–2134.

Penney JB, Young AB, Shoulson I, et al: Huntington's disease in Venezuela: 7 years of follow-up on symptomatic and asymptomatic individuals. Mov Disord 1990;5:93–99.

Pirio Richardson S, Mari Z, Matsuhashi M, Hallett M: Psychogenic palatal tremor. Mov Disord 2006;21(2):274–276.

Portera-Cailliau C, Victor D, Frucht SJ, Fahn S: Movement disorders fellowship training program at University Medical Center in 2001–2002. Mov Disord 2006;21(4):479–485.

Raethjen J, Kopper F, Govindan RB, et al: Two different pathogenetic mechanisms in psychogenic tremor. Neurology 2004;63(5):812–815.

Ranawaya R, Riley D, Lang A: Psychogenic dyskinesias in patients with organic movement disorders. Mov Disord 1990;5:127–133.

Riklan M, Cullinan T, Cooper IS: Psychological studies in dystonia musculorum deformans. Adv Neurol 1976;14:189–200.

Roach ES, Langley RL: Episodic neurological dysfunction due to mass hysteria. Arch Neurol 2004;61(8):1269–1272.

Sa DS, MailisGagnon A, Nicholson K, Lang AE: Posttraumatic painful torticollis. Mov Disord 2003;18(12):1482–1491.

Scherokman B, Husain F, Cuetter A, et al: Peripheral dystonia. Arch Neurol 1986;43:830–832.

Schott GD: The relation of peripheral trauma and pain to dystonia. J Neurol Neurosurg Psychiatry 1985;48:698–701.

Schott GD: Mechanisms of causalgia and related clinical conditions: The role of the central nervous and of the sympathetic nervous systems. Brain 1986;109:717–738.

Schrag A: Psychogenic dystonia and reflex sympathetic dystrophy. In Hallett M, Fahn S, Jankovic J, et al (eds): Psychogenic Movement Disorders—Neurology and Neuropsychiatry, Philadelphia, Lippincott Williams & Wilkins, 2006, pp 53–61.

Schrag A, Trimble M, Quinn N, Bhatia K: The syndrome of fixed dystonia: An evaluation of 103 patients. Brain 2004;127:2360–2372.

Schwalbe W: Eine eigentumliche tonische Krampfform mit hysterischen Symptomen. Inaug Diss, Berlin, G. Schade, 1908.

Schwartzman RJ, Kerrigan J: The movement disorder of reflex sympathetic dystrophy. Neurology 1990;40:57–61.

Shale HM, Fahn S, Koller WC, Lang AE: What is it? Case 1—1987: Unusual tremors, bradykinesia, and cerebral lucencies. Mov Disord 1987;2:321–338.

Shale HM, Fahn S, Sternlieb I, Scheinberg IH: Follow-up of "What is it?" Case 1—1987. Mov Disord 1988;3:370.

Shale HM, Truong DD, Fahn S: Tics in patients with other movement disorders. Neurology 1986;36(suppl 1):118.

Sheehy MP, Marsden CD: Writer's cramp: A focal dystonia. Brain 1982;105:461–480.

Simon DK, Nishino S, Scammell TE: Mistaken diagnosis of psychogenic gait disorder in a man with status cataplecticus ("limp man syndrome"). Mov Disord 2004;19(7):838–840.

Spiller WG: Akinesia agera. Arch Neurol Psychiatry 1933;30:842–884.

Stone LA, Jankovic J: The coexistence of tics and dystonia. Arch Neurol 1991;48:862–865.

Tan EK: Psychogenic tics: Diagnostic value of the placebo test. J Child Neurol 2004;19(12):976–977.

Terada K, Ikeda A, Van Ness PC, et al: Presence of Bereitschaftspotential preceding psychogenic myoclonus: Clinical application of jerk-locked back averaging. J Neurol Neurosurg Psychiatry 1995;58:745–747.

Thompson PD: The phenomenology of startle, latah, and related conditions. In Hallett M, Fahn S, Jankovic J, et al (eds): Psychogenic Movement Disorders—Neurology and Neuropsychiatry, Philadelphia, Lippincott Williams & Wilkins, 2006, pp 48–52.

Thompson PD, Colebatch JG, Brown P, et al: Voluntary stimulus-sensitive jerks and jumps mimicking myoclonus or pathological startle syndromes. Mov Disord 1992;7:257–262.

Tibbets RW: Spasmodic torticollis. J Psychosom Res 1971;15:461–469.

Truong DD, Fahn S: An early description of dystonia: Translation of Schwalbe's thesis and information on his life. Adv Neurol 1988;50:651–664.

Vecht CJ, Meerwaldt JD, Lees AJ, et al: Unusual movement disorder, case 1, 1991: Unusual tremor, myoclonus and a limping gait. Mov Disord 1991;6:371–375.

Vuilleumier P, Chicherio C, Assal F, et al: Functional neuroanatomical correlates of hysterical sensorimotor loss. Brain 2001;124:1077–1090.

Walters AS, Hening WA: Noise-induced psychogenic tremor associated with post-traumatic stress disorder. Mov Disord 1992;7:333–338.

Williams DR: Psychogenic palatal tremor. Mov Disord 2004;19(3):333–335.

Williams DT, Ford B, Fahn S: Phenomenology and psychopathology related to psychogenic movement disorders. Adv Neurol 1995;65:231–257.

Williams DT, Ford B, Fahn S: Treatment issues in psychogenic-neuropsychiatric movement disorders. Adv Neurol 2005;96:350–363.

Zeman W, Dyken P: Dystonia musculorum deformans. In Handbook of Clinical Neurology, vol 6. Amsterdam, North-Holland, 1968, pp 517–543.

Zeuner KE, Shoge RO, Goldstein SR, et al: Accelerometry to distinguish psychogenic from essential or parkinsonian tremor. Neurology 2003;61(4):548–550.

Ziehen T: Ein fall von tonischer Torsionsneurose. Neurol Centrabl 1911;30:109–110.

# Appendix

# Video Legends

## CHAPTER 1

Video 1-1 **Akinesia/bradykinesia/hypokinesia.** A man with Parkinson disease (PD) seen in the morning prior to his first dose of levodopa, his last dose having been 12 hours earlier. He had lost facial expression, with lips parted, slow tongue movements, and very slow movements of his limbs, left worse than right. He was able to rise from a chair but walked very slowly.

Video 1-2 **Unilateral PD.** A man with signs and symptoms of PD on the right side of the body, including decreased shrug of the shoulder, rest tremor of the right hand that reemerges when the arm sustains a posture against gravity, flexed posture of the metacarpal-phalangeal joints and extension of the interphalangeal joints, decreased rapid successive movements with finger tapping, and decreased finger mobility. Handwriting becomes progressively smaller with continued writing. There is decreased armswing on walking.

Video 1-3 **Postural and action tremor in a patient with PD.** This man with PD has a tremor of his hands when he holds the arms up against gravity (postural tremor) and when he moves the arms (action tremor).

Video 1-4 **Jaw tremor as well as hand tremor in a patient with PD.** This man with PD has a pronounced tremor of his jaw. His right hand shows the typical abnormal hand posture and a rest tremor.

Video 1-5 **Masked face and drooling of saliva.** This young girl has juvenile parkinsonism due to Wilson disease. After initiation of penicillamine therapy, she became febrile and had a worsening of bradykinesia. She manifests an expressionless face with drooling of saliva (sialorrhea) due to lack of spontaneous swallowing. The second scene of this girl shows her before penicillamine therapy, with risus sardonicus (dystonic facial grin).

Video 1-6 **Myerson sign.** Tapping the glabella produces up to three blinks in normal subjects, which are then suppressed. But in patients with PD, blinking tends to persist, as shown here. This is a positive Myerson sign.

Video 1-7 **Apraxia of eyelid opening.** Opening the eyelids may be delayed in some patients with atypical parkinsonism, especially in progressive supranuclear palsy. Although a misnomer, because it is not an apraxia, it has been considered as a dystonia, as freezing, and as levator inhibition.

Video 1-8 **Square wave jerks.** With the patient looking straight ahead, the eyes are usually quiet. When quick, small-amplitude jerks appear, these are called square wave jerks. This patient has progressive supranuclear palsy.

Video 1-9 **Impaired ocular movements.** This patient has progressive supranuclear palsy. She has neck extension, facial dystonia with deep nasolabial folds, square wave jerks, impaired vertical gaze, and normal doll's eye movements.

Video 1-10 **Decreased shoulder shrug, decrementing rapid successive movements, and decreased armswing due to bradykinesia.** This man has left-sided greater than right-sided PD. There is decreased amplitude in raising the left shoulder and in executing hand and feet movements of the left limbs. In performing rapid successive movements, there is lack of smoothness with decrementing of these movements in the left upper and lower limbs. On walking, the amplitude of armswing is reduced, more so on the left.

Video 1-11 **Decreased rapid successive movements in juvenile Huntington disease.** A young man with juvenile-onset akinetic-rigid syndrome due to juvenile Huntington disease has bradykinesia, including masked facies and decreased rapid successive movements.

Video 1-12 **Overcoming akinesia.** This man has PD and has trouble initiating or maintaining movement. By chasing a bouncing ball, he can move quickly. By bouncing the ball on the floor and going after it, he is able to arise from the chair more quickly. By purposefully reaching for a handkerchief, he can initiate the movement of an arm that otherwise would be akinetic.

Video 1-13 **Shoulder rigidity manifested by decreased armswing with passive movement of the shoulders.** This is the same man as in Video 1-10. He has predominantly left-sided PD. When his shoulders are passively moved, the involved arm moves with decreased amplitude owing to rigidity.

Video 1-14 **Flexed posture.** This woman with PD has pronounced flexed posture of the limbs, neck, and trunk.

Video 1-15 **Normal pull test.** The pull test is performed to assess postural reflexes. This man (the same person as in Videos 1-10 and 1-13) with mild PD has a normal pull test. He recovered with one step.

Video 1-16 **Examples of abnormal (positive) pull tests. A,** This man failed to recover his balance in two steps or fewer. **B,** This woman's pull test showed more severe impairment; it took a less forceful pull to make her lose her balance. **C,** This women's pull test showed even greater abnormality; she failed even to step backward (retropulsion).

**Video 1-17 Festinating gait.** When walking, this man with PD is leaning forward too much, so his center of gravity is in front of his feet. The result is that he runs (festinates) to prevent falling. He stops by reaching a wall to support himself.

**Video 1-18 Freezing when turning and when starting to walk.** When walking, this man with PD has freezing of gait even when other signs of PD have responded to levodopa therapy. In these scenes, the patient is walking in the straight corridor without freezing of gait, but freezing occurs when he turns and sometimes when he starts to walk again.

**Video 1-19 Apraxia.** This patient has corticobasal ganglionic degeneration with apraxia of the left arm. The left arm does not know how to grab the pen from the right hand.

**Video 1-20 Cortical myoclonus.** This patient has corticobasal ganglionic degeneration involving the right arm. The fingers show spontaneous irregular tremor, often a manifestation of cortical myoclonus and not a true tremor. The examiner brings out cortical reflex myoclonus by applying a sudden stimulus to one of the fingers.

**Video 1-21 Alien limb.** This patient has corticobasal ganglionic degeneration. Without realizing it, the patient's left leg spontaneously elevates in the air. He was unaware of this until it was pointed out to him.

**Video 1-22 Blocking tics.** This patient has Tourette syndrome with both dystonic (e.g., grinding his teeth) and clonic (e.g., repetitive jerks of his right arm) tics. The patient also demonstrates the type of palilalia that is seen in Tourette syndrome, namely, a repetition of phrases. When a tic appears, his speech is interrupted (blocked). When the tic ceases, he resumes talking as if there had been no interruptions.

**Video 1-23 Catatonia.** This 16-year-old youth was found standing silently, without moving, in the family's kitchen. Because of the differential diagnosis of an acute form of parkinsonism, he was seen by the movement disorder group. The patient is virtually motionless yet has spontaneous, normal scratching movements. He does not move on command but moves easily when guided. There is no rigidity or tremor. Catatonia needs to be differentiated from parkinsonian akinesia.

**Video 1-24 Psychomotor slowness.** This youth was considered to have parkinsonism because of the expressionless facies, soft voice, and decreased armswing. But there was no rigidity, decrementing of rapid successive movements, tremor, loss of postural reflexes, or flexed posture. A fluorodopa PET scan was obtained that showed normal uptake in the striatum. Treatment with antidepressants resulted in loss of the expressionless facies and a return of normal motor speed.

**Video 1-25 Freezing when trying to arise from a chair.** This man with young-onset PD eventually developed freezing of gait and freezing when trying to initiate other movements. He found that clapping his hands will break the freeze that occurs when he tries to arise from a chair.

**Video 1-26 Freezing when trying to go through a doorway.** The same man with young-onset PD (see Video 1-25) would freeze when trying to walk through a doorway. He learned that dropping to the ground breaks the freeze.

**Video 1-27 Stepping over an inverted cane to overcome freezing of gait.** This man has a genetic disorder, lubag, which is X-linked dystonia-parkinsonism (DYT-3). Dystonia was the initial symptom, involving his back muscles. When parkinsonism later developed, this became the predominant problem, eliminating much of the dystonia. With the parkinsonism, he developed severe freezing of gait that interfered with his ability to walk. He built an inverted cane that he could step over, thereby avoiding freezing.

**Video 1-28 Freezing of speech (severe palilalia).** This man has PD. He eventually developed a problem with his speech, in which the first syllable would be repeated many times before the word could be said. This is a severe form of palilalia and resembles stuttering. In reading aloud, the palilalia is not present.

**Video 1-29 Primary freezing gait syndrome.** This man has no clear-cut signs of PD, only freezing of gait. Eventually, he developed impairment of postural reflexes and then other features of parkinsonism. Primary freezing gait syndrome often turns out to be progressive supranuclear palsy at autopsy. It has also been called pure akinesia and gait initiation syndrome.

**Video 1-30 Unilateral rigidity in corticobasal ganglionic degeneration.** This woman has extreme rigidity of the right arm with fixed curling of the fingers. The arm is useless. The symptom began insidiously and slowly worsened. Notice the typical slowly articulated speech with delays between words; this is common in corticobasal ganglionic degeneration and progressive supranuclear palsy.

**Video 1-31 Subacute rigidity, rash, fever, and myoclonus.** This 27-year-old man rapidly developed marked stiffness of muscles associated with a rash and fever. Examination revealed sensitivity to tapping the muscles or moving the joints with reflex myoclonus. Previously known as spinal neuronitis, this condition is now called progressive encephalomyelitis with rigidity and is a severe form of the stiff-person syndrome. This patient improved rapidly with corticosteroid therapy.

**Video 1-32 Stiff-person syndrome.** This man developed marked stiffness of muscles of his trunk, neck, and proximal limb muscles. It was difficult to move the joints surrounded by these muscles. The distal parts of the extremities were relatively spared.

**Video 1-33 Stiff-baby syndrome.** This neonate goes into muscle spasms when the body is touched. Breathing can stop owing to prolonged muscle firing, so continuous stimulation should be avoided. Although named stiff-baby syndrome, this disorder is due to hereditary hyperekplexia, a startle disorder. Even in utero, the fetus had spasms of the muscles.

**Video 1-34 Abdominal dyskinesias.** Continual movements of the abdominal muscles have been called belly dancer's dyskinesias. The patient seen in this video had back trauma and then developed these abdominal movements. To differentiate this from psychogenic movements, poly-EMG was carried out that revealed a spread rostrally and caudally from a spinal segment, firing at a physiologic rate. This led to a diagnosis of spinal myoclonus in this patient.

**Video 1-35   Akathitic movements.** This man has truncal rocking. He crosses and uncrosses his legs, and touches his cap repeatedly, with an urge to jump up out of a chair. He had been exposed to dopamine receptor blocking agents and now had tardive akathisia without other signs of tardive dyskinesia.

**Video 1-36   Akathitic movements associated with tardive dyskinesia and moaning.** This woman had been treated with antipsychotic medication and developed tardive dyskinesia (observe the mouthing movements). In addition, she is restless. She describes this symptom as being unable to sit still and having an urge to run. With this tardive dyskinesia, she has moaning, another way to express her discomfort.

**Video 1-37   Cerebellar ataxia and asynergia.** This man has a family history of cerebellar ataxia. It developed in this patient in adulthood and slowly progressed. There is a decomposition of limb movement (asynergia or limb ataxia), missing the target (dysmetria), titubation on standing, and a wide-based gait. He usually walks with two Canadian crutches to maintain his balance.

**Video 1-38   Athetoid cerebral palsy.** This child developed choreoathetosis due to perinatal difficulty. His limbs, trunk, and neck are continuously moving in a flowing fashion but slower than is seen with chorea.

**Video 1-39   Hemiballism.** This woman suffered a stroke involving the left subthalamic nucleus. The initial weakness was followed by the continual flailing movements of the right limbs. These hemiballistic movements are large-amplitude choreic movements and are present at rest. With active voluntary movement of the affected limbs, the movements can be partially suppressed.

**Video 1-40   Huntington disease.** This man has Huntington disease with its characteristic choreic movements. The movements are brief with an appearance of flowing from one body part to another. Note particularly the chorea in the forehead and relatively sparse movements in the lower face; the opposite would be typical in tardive dyskinesia, which also has a more rhythmic quality compared to the random nature of the chorea that is seen in Huntington disease. The patient has other features of the disease, such as his disheveled features and irregular gait.

**Video 1-41   Sydenham disease.** This girl has Sydenham disease, with flowing abnormal movements that are not identical to the chorea seen in Huntington disease. In Sydenham disease, the movements have a restless appearance rather than being discreet individual jerks.

**Video 1-42   Blepharospasm.** Owing to orbicularis contractions, the eyelids are showing excessive movements, from increased blinking to more sustained closing. Some contractions of the lower face (also innervated by cranial nerve VII)

can be seen, especially around the mouth, though less frequently and severely.

**Video 1-43   Cranial segmental dystonia (Meige syndrome).** When more than one cranial nerve's muscles are affected by dystonia, this becomes cranial segmental dystonia, often referred to as *Meige syndrome*. This man has blepharospasm, lower face dystonia, platysma contractions (also CN VII), and jaw-closing contractions (CN V).

**Video 1-44   Spasmodic dysphonia (dystonic adductor dysphonia).** This schoolteacher's voice is tight and strangulated, causing interruptions of her talking. This is due to excessive contractions of the adductor muscles of the larynx. After these muscles are injected with botulinum toxin to weaken them, the dysphonia is much improved and, in this case, eliminated. The speed of her talking became normal again.

**Video 1-45   Jerky torticollis (cervical dystonia).** This woman's head is twisted with the chin turned to the right shoulder, tilted with the left ear pulled to the left shoulder, and with jerky movements, particularly as she tries to overcome the pulling of the muscles.

**Video 1-46   Writer's cramp (arm and hand dystonia).** When writing, this woman's fingers, hand, forearm, and arm muscles contract excessively, producing tightness of the muscles that can be detected by palpation. This is an action dystonia; the dystonia appears with the specific action of writing, although a mild amount of flexion of the right metacarpal-phalangeal joints appears when she tries to hold the arms and hands out straight.

**Video 1-47   Truncal dystonia.** This boy developed marked kyphoscoliosis, with some lordosis, also with involvement of the hips (tortipelvis). The dystonia is worse with walking, and some leg involvement is now seen as well (therefore technically a crural segmental dystonia). When it is treated with a combination of antimuscarinic medication and baclofen, there is a marked reduction of the dystonia.

**Video 1-48   Segmental axial-brachial dystonia.** This boy developed marked flexion of his neck (antecollis), kyphoscoliosis, with also involvement of his arms and vocal cords. The legs are spared, so this is not generalized dystonia.

**Video 1-49   Segmental crural dystonia, worsening to become generalized dystonia.** This boy's dystonia involves both legs (left worse than right) and less involvement of his trunk. He is able to hop for a short distance on his right leg. One and a half years later (without any treatment), the dystonia is worse in both legs and the trunk and has spread to involve his arms. He is no longer able to sit or stand.

**Video 1-50   Oculogyric crises.** This girl has episodic attacks of oculogyric crises. The eyes turn up and stay in this fixed position for many minutes, with some ability to temporarily overcome the fixed upgaze.

**Video 1-51   Feeding dystonia.** Whenever this young man puts food in his mouth in an effort to eat, he involuntarily protrudes his tongue, which pushes the food out of his mouth, resulting in food being spilled and often biting his tongue. Notice that a piece of his tongue is missing, having been bitten off in the past. To get food to the back of his throat, he needs to tilt his head back to have the food reach his throat by gravity.

**Video 1-52  Paradoxical dystonia.** This woman is an example of paradoxical dystonia. In this situation, the dystonia appears at rest and is relieved by active movement. This woman has cervical dystonia that appears when she is not active and is sitting or lying. With movement, either walking or using her hands in activity, the dystonia disappears.

**Video 1-53.  Hemifacial spasm.** This man has tonic spasms of the left side of his face.

**Video 1-54  Hyperekplexia (excessive startle).** This 17-year-old youth required resuscitation at birth and had a seizure with cyanosis. He had poor suck, irritability, opisthotonic posturing when he was picked up, extremely exaggerated startle, and delayed developmental motor milestones. He had poor motor coordination and frequently fell. Since the age of 14, in response to a sudden stimulus, his trunk would flex, his arms would abduct, his muscles would stiffen, and he would fall forward or backward. There was progressive gait stiffness, and he became confined to a wheelchair because of frequent falls since the age of 16. This excessive reaction to sudden stimuli is known as hyperekplexia.

**Video 1-55  Periodic movements in sleep.** Periodic movements in sleep, previously called *nocturnal myoclonus*, are slow flexion contractions of the lower extremities that occur approximately every 20 seconds. They can be recorded by observing the patient during sleep. Sometimes, they are a cause of fractured sleeping. They are usually a component of restless legs syndrome. (From Walters AS, Hening WA, Chokroverty S: Review and videotape recognition of idiopathic restless legs syndrome. Mov Disord 1991;6:105–110. With permission from the Movement Disorder Society.)

**Video 1-56  Hypnogenic paroxysmal dyskinesia.** This youth is asleep. He is having bilateral ballistic movements. These occur during his sleep. The side of his bed is padded to prevent his injuring himself. His parents hear him move about and make noises; they awaken him to stop these movements. A seizure workup failed to reveal any epileptic discharges. Anticonvulsants were not helpful.

**Video 1-57  Jumpy stump.** This woman developed abnormal involuntary movements in her amputated limb.

**Video 1-58  Moving toes, painful leg.** This woman had a pressure injury to her sciatic nerve and eventually developed constant pain in that leg, along with these persistent movements of the toes of the ipsilateral foot. The movements themselves are not painful. They do not cease during sleep.

**Video 1-59  Moving fingers, painful hand.** This young woman had an injury to her right arm and eventually developed pain in that hand, along with the persistent movements of the fingers in that hand. The fingers involved change depending on the posture of that hand.

**Video 1-60  Asterixis (negative myoclonus).** This man had a hepatic encephalopathy that led to the development of "liver flap," that is, asterixis, which is a negative myoclonus. There are brief pauses while he is trying to maintain a sustained contraction, and these silent periods inhibit the voluntary sustained extension of the fingers.

**Video 1-61  Action and intention myoclonus.** This woman had developed myoclonic jerks when she moved a limb or held the limb up against gravity. When she aims for a target, so-called intention myoclonus appears, making it difficult to reach the target. There were no myoclonic jerks when the limbs were at rest. In contrast to action or intention tremor, with which this could be confused, myoclonus is lightning-like in speed, and the jerks are square-wave-like rather than sinusoidal-like tremor.

**Video 1-62  Palatal myoclonus.** This woman noticed that pressing on her nose in a certain way could trigger palatal myoclonus. This type of brainstem segmental myoclonus is rhythmic, at a rate of approximately 2 Hz. This is an example of primary palatal myoclonus.

**Video 1-63  Palatal myoclonus.** This man also has primary palatal myoclonus, associated with clicking in his ears. One can detect the rhythmic myoclonus by looking at his throat, either through his open mouth or by viewing the throat externally. The rhythmic movements spread beyond the palate and involve other muscles of deglutition and the esophagus, as can be seen in the fluoroscopic swallowing study using contrast medium.

**Video 1-64  Ocular myoclonus.** This man suffered a brainstem stroke involving the dentato-olivary pathway that caused secondary palatal myoclonus and ocular myoclonus. Both are rhythmic and synchronous with each other. The eyes move up and down vertically at a rate of approximately 2 Hz.

**Video 1-65  Opsoclonus (dancing eyes) and minipolymyoclonus.** This woman developed minipolymyoclonus and opsoclonus following a febrile illness. The lightning-like movements of the eyes are irregular and random, which are features of ordinary myoclonus in other parts of the body. Besides opsoclonus, she has associated minipolymyoclonus that look like very rapid, low-amplitude, irregular tremor.

**Video 1-66  Spinal segmental myoclonus.** This man has an irritable focus in the spinal cord from an infection that is inducing rhythmic myoclonus emanating from that focus. The synchronous contractions involving paraspinal and abdominal muscles can be localized to the involved muscle groups with electrophysiologic studies. The brief duration of the contractions can also be measured to confirm that the movements are of the brief duration of myoclonus.

**Video 1-67  Bouncing gait.** This man developed a seizure and then progressive ataxia and myoclonus in childhood (progressive myoclonic ataxia of Ramsay Hunt). His myoclonus consisted of both action myoclonus (as depicted in the finger to nose test) and negative myoclonus (affecting thigh muscles) when he stands or walks. The latter results in a bouncing quality when he attempts to walk.

**Video 1-68  Myokymia.** This man had a pontine glioma treated with radiation therapy. He now has myokymia of the left facial muscles. Because of left lower motor neuron facial weakness, there are contractures of those muscles. Because of myokymia producing continuous rippling movements, he has received injections of botulinum toxin into those muscles. As the effect of the last injection has worn off, the myokymia has returned. The rippling movements are most prominent in his chin, and some can be seen on the lateral edge of the left eye and on his left cheek.

**Video 1-69  Ocular myorhythmia.** The ocular movements seen in this man with Whipple disease is ocular myorhythmia, which manifests as pendular vergence oscillations. These are continuous, slow, regular (rhythmic) movements converging the eyes symmetrically. When the eyes diverge at the end of the movement, they never go beyond the midline.

**Video 1-70  Faciomasticatory myorhythmia.** This man with Whipple disease has rhythmic myoclonus of the facial, pharyngeal, and masticatory muscles. It is also called faciomasticatory myorhythmia. The ocular muscles can also be involved. It needs to be distinguished from hemifacial spasm, but that condition is unilateral and limited to muscles innervated by CN VII and is not continuous or rhythmic.

**Video 1-71  Paroxysmal kinesigenic dyskinesia.** This teenage girl can trigger brief choreic-ballistic movements by executing a sudden movement. In this attack, the legs are predominantly affected, but the arms and trunk show dystonic posturing. Note that there is a brief latency period between the triggering movement and the onset of the involuntary dyskinesias.

**Video 1-72  Paroxysmal nonkinesigenic dyskinesia.** This toddler has a variety of dystonic postures that can last hours and then clear. She manifests nuchal and truncal postures, and when these appear, they cause discomfort. There is no positive family history.

**Video 1-73  Tardive dyskinesia (TD).** The repetitive, fairly rhythmic nature of the truncal rocking movements and the complex movements around the mouth are highly characteristic of classic TD. The repetitive patterns separate these movements from the choreic movements of Huntington disease, which are random events and have the appearance of flowing from one part of the body to another. The repetitive nature of TD can qualify this for the stereotypic family of hyperkinesias.

**Video 1-74  Stereotypic hand movements in Rett syndrome.** This little girl has the mental retardation disorder of Rett syndrome. At this young age, the bringing together of the hands into the midline, with a hand-wringing maneuver, is typical of the stereotypies that are seen in this disorder at this age. As children with Rett grow older, the types of abnormal movements vary.

**Video 1-75  Stereotypy.** This infant has repeated movements with the left arm, of the same type, over and over again. This stereotypy suggests that this could be an early sign of autism, because stereotypies are very common in that disorder.

**Video 1-76  Abnormal movements in Kluver-Bucy syndrome.** This young woman developed encephalitis at the age of 18 and was in a coma for over 2 weeks. On awakening, she had an altered behavior consistent with the Kluver-Bucy syndrome and had abnormal involuntary movements of the right hand and arm. The fingers and hand are choreic, but there are also stereotypic repetitive movements of that arm.

**Video 1-77  Abnormal movements in a boy with normal intelligence.** This boy has choreic-like movements when sitting alone, but the movements disappear when he is asked a question or when he is asked to stand up and is spoken to. It is as if he were daydreaming with his thoughts elsewhere when he is not engaged, with the choreic-like movements as part of being involved with his thoughts.

**Video 1-78  Ocular tics.** This youth has intermittent single, brief ocular deviations. He has motor tics elsewhere as well.

**Video 1-79  Tics in Tourette syndrome.** This girl has both motor and phonic tics. The former are bursts of complex coordinated movements of her arms and other parts of her body. The phonic tics are simple sounds, but she also has verbalizations, including coprolalia, which prevents her from attending school.

**Video 1-80  Describing the urge to move and produce tics in Tourette syndrome.** This man has both motor and phonic tics. He suppresses them briefly when asked to do so and describes how an inner tension builds up that is very uncomfortable and leads him to release the tics, with a resultant lessening of the tension.

**Video 1-81  Dystonic tics.** This man's motor tics are bursts of brief sustained contractions of the neck and face. He has some control over them in that he can suppress them for a while. He has an urge that leads to tightness of neck and face muscles and also leads him to bring an arm up. His tics strongly resemble cranial-cervical segmental dystonia except that the dystonia is not continually present but occurs after an urge to make the movement.

**Video 1-82  Tremor at rest.** This man has Parkinson disease with its typical rest tremor, the right hand being affected worse than the left. This type of tremor almost always manifests itself when the patient is walking. Decreased armswing (more pronounced on the right) and dragging the right leg is also seen when he walks. When he is sitting, the tremor at rest in his right hand disappears as he raises that arm, and then the tremor reemerges after a latency period. The rest tremor of the left foot is also visible when the patient is sitting.

**Video 1-83  Postural and action tremor.** This man has essential tremor, with its typical tremor that is seen when the limb is held up against gravity and is accentuated when the limb is put into motion, such as with writing and pouring water. There is asymmetry, the tremor of the left arm being worse than the right.

**Video 1-84  Intention tremor.** This woman has multiple sclerosis with ataxia and intention tremor. In intention tremor, the tremor increases as the involved limb is approaching a target. In contrast to intention myoclonus, intention tremor is rhythmic, oscillatory, and sinusoidal rather than consisting of square-angled jerks. Intention tremor is the result of a lesion in the dentatorubrothalamic pathway.

**Video 1-85  Orthostatic tremor.** This woman has increasing discomfort in her legs and thighs on prolonged standing. This is due to 16-Hz tremor in the muscles of the lower extremities, which is present only on standing and disappears with sitting or walking. This condition is known as orthostatic tremor.

**Video 1-86  Dystonic tremor.** This man has Oppenheim dystonia due to mutation in the gene for TorsinA. The tremor in his right arm becomes manifest when he holds the arm up against gravity. In this way, it resembles postural tremor. The right arm tremor appears when the arm assumes postures that are in contrast to the direction that the dystonia tries to force it. When the patient places the arm in the position the dystonia wishes to place it in, the tremor is gone. This is the null point and should be sought in all cases of dystonic tremor, whether in the arm, the neck, or another body part.

**Video 1-87  Midbrain tremor.** This woman suffered a stroke that affected the region of the left midbrain to the left subthalamic nucleus. After she recovered from weakness,

tremor of the right arm developed. The tremor is quite pronounced at rest and is more proximal than the typical parkinsonian rest tremor, which is usually in the distal part of the limb. Holding the arm against gravity exacerbates the tremor amplitude. The passive spread of the tremor contractions make it appear that there is tremor of the left arm also, but we demonstrate that this is the result of the passive spread and not a true tremor of that arm. There is some suppression of right arm tremor when the arm is in the winged position, but the tremor increases when the arm is extended to reach a target.

**Video 1-88  Unusual tremor due to Wilson disease.** This man had a febrile illness, after which he noticed tremors of his hands and fingers. The tremors are present at rest and continue with posture holding and with action. He also has mild cerebellar dysarthria. Detection of Kayser-Fleischer rings led to the correct diagnosis of Wilson disease.

**Video 1-89  Worsening of Wilson disease tremor after initiating penicillamine treatment and improvement with BAL treatment.** This same patient as in the previous video (see Video 1-88) was begun with penicillamine therapy, but this led to a marked worsening of the tremor. Next, he was started on injections of British Anti-Lewisite (BAL), which resulted in remission of the symptoms.

## CHAPTER 4

**Video 4-1  Reemergent tremor.** This patient with Parkinson disease has tremor at rest in the right hand, which reemerges a few seconds after the arms assume horizontal position.

**Video 4-2  Camptocormia.** This patient with Parkinson disease has severe truncal flexion (camptocormia) when sitting and walking.

**Video 4-3  Camptocormia.** This patient with Parkinson disease has severe truncal flexion (camptocormia), which he is able to overcome by the "climbing-on-the-wall" maneuver and by lying down in the supine position.

**Video 4-4  Camptocormia.** This patient with Parkinson disease has marked dystonic camptocormia associated with

"involuntary pulling" of her trunk forward and contraction of the abdominal muscles. She received marked improvement after injection of botulinum toxin into the rectus abdominus muscles.

**Video 4-5  Freezing.** This patient with Parkinson disease has marked freezing, particularly on gait initiation and when turning. He also manifests marked retropulsion.

**Video 4-6  Freezing.** This patient with Parkinson disease and shuffling gait has marked freezing that he can overcome by means of visual cues when using an inverted L-shaped cane.

## CHAPTER 7

**Video 7-1  Deep brain stimulation (DBS) for essential tremor (ET).** This patient with long-standing severe ET is unable to write or hold a glass of water without spilling, but after the left ventral intermediate (VIM) DBS is turned on, her right hand tremor essentially resolves, and she is able to perform the various tasks without any difficulties.

**Video 7-2  DBS for ET.** This patient with essential tremor, an artist, had not been able to paint for many years before she underwent left thalamotomy, which markedly improved her right hand tremor, and she was able to paint again. The procedure was complicated by abnormal gait, however, and the tremor in

the right hand gradually recurred, although its amplitude was still lower than that of the left hand tremor. Both right and left hand tremor and her gait improved after bilateral VIM DBS.

**Video 7-3  DBS for multiple sclerosis (MS)–related tremor.** This young man with MS and large-amplitude, slow, postural, wing-beating and kinetic, cerebellar-outflow tremor, also known as myorhythmia, predominantly involving the right hand and arm, has a marked improvement with left VIM DBS.

**Video 7-4  DBS for PD.** This patient with advanced Parkinson disease, manifested by severe bradykinesia, difficulty rising from a chair, and a shuffling gait, has a marked improvement in these parkinsonian features when bilateral subthalamic nucleus (STN) DBS is turned on. The before and after video segments were taken during true "off" state when the patient has been without dopaminergic drugs for at least 12 hours. When levodopa is added to the effects of DBS, his motor symptoms are nearly completely controlled.

Video 7-5 **DBS for PD.** This patient with Parkinson disease enjoys nearly complete control of his Parkinson symptoms, but when the bilateral STN DBS is turned off, marked rest and postural arm and leg tremor and bradykinesia emerge; these symptoms instantly improve when the DBS is again turned on.

Video 7-6 **DBS-induced hemiballism.** This patient with Parkinson disease underwent right STN DBS; however, when the voltage was increased, he began to develop left hemiballism. When the DBS was turned off, the hemiballism improved.

## CHAPTER 10

Video 10-1 **Progressive supranuclear palsy (PSP).** This patient with PSP demonstrates typical dysarthria, deep facial folds, procerus sign, supranuclear ophthalmoparesis, and typical broad-based gait with extension of the knees and pivoting, rather than turning en bloc. Note that the head turning lags behind the body turning, probably because of perseveration of gaze.

Video 10-2 **PSP.** This patient with PSP shows prominent procerus sign and typical vertical ophthalmoparesis that can be easily overcome with oculocephalic maneuver.

Video 10-3 **PSP.** This patient with early stages of PSP still has well-preserved vertical gaze and horizontal saccades, but there is marked impairment of vertical saccades, particularly downward saccades, as demonstrated by optokinetic nystagmus. Note that when the tape moves in the upward direction, the corrective downward saccades are absent, but upward saccades are present when the tape moves in a downward direction.

Video 10-4 **PSP.** This patient with PSP demonstrates marked hypokinetic dysarthria associated with a hypernasal deep voice. He also has typical vertical ophthalmoparesis.

Video 10-5 **PSP.** This patient with PSP shows exaggeration of expression or "emotional incontinence" as part of her pseudobulbar affect. She also has typical hypokinetic dysarthria.

Video 10-6 **PSP.** This patient with PSP shows marked supranuclear vertical ophthalmoplegia with some limitation of lateral gaze. She also exhibits "the applause sign" as part of her preseverative automatic behavior.

Video 10-7 **PSP.** This patient with PSP and associated marked blepharospasm and apraxia of eyelid opening had a marked improvement in both conditions following botulinum toxin injections.

Video 10-8 **Multiple system atrophy (MSA).** This patient with MSA has scoliosis to the right, a slow and shuffling gait, and the "Pisa syndrome" manifested by leaning to the right when sitting. When her arms are held in a horizontal position, there is moderate myoclonus. She also has marked reddish discoloration of both hands, the so-called cold hand sign.

Video 10-9 **MSA.** This patient with MSA has a history of pronounced orthostatic hypotension, urinary incontinence, advanced bradykinesia, dysarthria, sleep apnea, and bluish discoloration of feet, the so-called cold feet sign. She has a subclavian line to maintain hydration, tracheostomy, and PEG, and she requires intermittent catheterization. Eating sweets or even anticipation of eating sweets, particularly chocolate, induced massive drooling and a marked drop in blood pressure.

Video 10-10 **Corticobasal degeneration (CBD).** This patient with CBD manifests marked, asymmetric apraxia.

Video 10-11 **CBD.** This patient with CBD is describing the alien hand syndrome. She also has marked asymmetric apraxia and characteristic "cortical" myoclonus.

Video 10-12 **Lytico-Bodig.** This woman, who has lived most of her life in Guam, has developed a slow and shuffling gait, hypokinetic dysarthria, facial and hand fasciculations, and distal atrophy. She also has some features of PSP, as is suggested by the absence of downward saccades when the optokinetic tape moves upward.

## CHAPTER 11

Video 11-1 **Hemiplegic gait secondary to a stroke.** This patient has a left hemiparesis. He walks with a stiff left leg. The leg circumducts to avoid hitting the ground in swing, and the landing of the foot is flat. (Courtesy of Mark Hallett, MD, NIH.)

Video 11-2 **Paraplegic gait secondary to hereditary spastic paraplegia.** This patient has hereditary spastic paraplegia. There is scissoring of the legs with bilateral circumduction of the legs in swing phase. (Courtesy of Mary Kay Floeter, MD, NIH.)

Video 11-3 **Two examples of gait in stiff-person syndrome. A,** The first patient with stiff-person syndrome is clearly very stiff in all joints and can barely walk, needing some support to aid her balance. She was filmed while having a gait study, and there are markers on her joints. **B,** The second patient is also very stiff, but his balance is better. (**A,** Courtesy of Marinos Dalakas, MD, NIH. **B,** Courtesy of Joseph Jankovic, MD.)

**Video 11-4** **Ataxic gait in a patient with degenerative ataxia.** This patient has a degenerative ataxia and walks with poor balance, a wide base, and irregular steps. There is also an occasional lurch. (Courtesy of Mark Hallett, MD, NIH.)

**Video 11-5** **Two examples of gait in patients with dystonia. A,** This first patient has neuroacanthocytosis. There is obvious dystonic posturing of the legs during walking. As is common in dystonia, she walks much better backward. **B,** The second patient is a young boy with an intermittent abnormal movement of the legs when walking, including occasional toe walking. A walking abnormality is often the opening symptom of childhood dystonia. (**A,** Courtesy of Adrian Danek, MD, NIH. **B,** Courtesy of Leon Dure, MD.)

**Video 11-6** **Gait in a patient with Huntington disease.** This patient with Huntington disease presented with a gait abnormality, called the dancing gait. Since this patient was a longtime dancer, the movement disorder was not recognized at first. (Courtesy of Mark Hallett, MD, NIH.)

**Video 11-7** **Myoclonic gait.** This patient has posthypoxic myoclonus. He has considerable negative and positive myoclonus while trying to walk; this is called the bouncy gait. The backpack carries physiologic recording equipment. (Courtesy of Mark Hallett, MD, NIH.)

**Video 11-8** **Three examples of frontal gait. A,** The first patient has a frontal gait disorder that is characterized by slowness and freezing while walking. She has particular difficulty with turns. **B,** The second patient also has a frontal gait disorder, but the freezing has a different character, with the legs rapidly moving in place. This is called the slipping clutch gait. **C,** The third patient has normal pressure hydrocephalus as the cause of his frontal gait disorder. Balance is poor, turning is difficult, and stepping is slow. **D,** The next segment shows this same patient after shunting. His walking has clearly improved considerably, and his turning is faster. (**A,** Courtesy of Mark Hallett, MD, NIH. **B–D,** Courtesy of William Weiner, MD.)

**Video 11-9** **Two examples of psychogenic gait. A,** The first patient has a classic psychogenic gait. Stepping is very irregular, and the knee buckling is a very frequent manifestation. Despite the claim of poor balance, her balance is clearly very good. She occasionally falls but never hurts herself. **B,** The second patient has a psychogenic tremor as well as a psychogenic gait. It appears that he is periodically pushed backward as he walks. (**A,** Courtesy of Mark Hallett, MD, NIH. **B,** Courtesy of Mark Hallett, MD, NIH.)

## CHAPTER 12

**Video 12-1** **Stiff-person syndrome.** This patient with stiff-person syndrome clearly demonstrates truncal rigidity. There is a marked lumbar lordosis, characteristic of most patients, and this does not reverse when the person bends over. (Courtesy of C. D. Marsden.)

**Video 12-2** **Progressive encephalomyelitis with rigidity.** This woman has progressive encephalomyelitis with rigidity. Note the severe stiffness and limited voluntary movement affecting the whole body. (Courtesy of C. D. Marsden.)

## CHAPTER 13

**Video 13-1** **Blepharospasm.** This man has increased blinking with intermittent closing of the eyelids. Blepharospasm is a focal dystonia of the upper face.

**Video 13-2** **Cervical dystonia.** This man has a tilt of his head with turning of his chin to the right. Cervical dystonia is a focal dystonia of the neck musculature and is commonly known as torticollis. He demonstrates a sensory trick in that when he raises his arms or touches his chin, there is a reduction of the torticollis.

**Video 13-3** **Dystonia of leg, with active voluntary movement.** This girl developed twisting of her left foot due to Oppenheim dystonia. It is present when the leg is carrying out activities. There is no dystonia when the foot is at rest. The twisting of the foot is present when she is walking forward, but it is not present when she walks backward or runs.

**Video 13-4** **Writer's cramp.** This young woman's dystonia started in one arm and manifests itself with the specific action of writing. Over time, it began to be present with other motor activities of the arm and when she holds her arm up against gravity. There is some suppression of the writer's cramp when she places the other hand on top of the involved one.

**Video 13-5** **Musician's cramp.** This young woman is a professional musician. Her instrument is the French horn. After years of practice and playing, the lips began to separate when playing certain notes. This dystonia involves the muscles that are engaged in playing the instrument. This focal dystonia is called *embouchure dystonia* to reflect the involvement of the muscles around the mouth.

**Video 13-6** **Action focal dystonia of the jaw when chewing.** This woman developed abnormal movements when she would bite and chew her food. The muscles of the jaw, lips, and tongue are involved. The dystonia is not present when her mouth is at rest.

**Video 13-7** **Truncal dystonia relieved by dancing or running.** This man's truncal dystonia appears to be a tardive dystonia that is due to exposure to neuroleptic medications. The dystonia is present when he is standing and is relieved when he is dancing or running.

**Video 13-8** **Truncal dystonia relieved temporarily by placing a hand on the back of her head.** This woman has Oppenheim dystonia with a dromedary gait (flexed trunk at the hips and extension of the upper trunk and head). This abnormal posture that occurs as she walks is partially relieved when she places a hand on the back of her head.

**Video 13-9** **Retrocollis dystonia relieved by touching the back of the head.** This patient has retrocollis due to tardive dystonia. He has learned that when he places a hand on the back of his head, the backward pulling of his head is suppressed. He and his family had a brace made that allows the back of his head to be cradled by a plastic cap, which allows him to keep his head from being pulled backward.

**Video 13-10** **Postural tremor of the arms associated with dystonia of the arms.** This man has bibrachial dystonia. It began in one arm and eventually spread to the other but nowhere else. This is a segmental dystonia. When the arms are involved with dystonia, it is not uncommon to see tremor in the arm with posture holding.

**Video 13-11** **Generalized torsion dystonia.** This woman is the sister of the previous patient (see Video 13-10). Both have Oppenheim dystonia, and both were the same age at onset (7 years). But this woman's dystonia began in one leg, while her brother's began in one arm. His did not progress beyond segmental bibrachial dystonia, while hers became generalized. She had multiple stereotactic thalamotomies that affected her speech.

**Video 13-12** **Generalized dystonia.** This man has Oppenheim dystonia that spread to become generalized, involving all limbs and trunk. He is still able to walk.

**Video 13-13** **Generalized dystonia.** This youth has Oppenheim dystonia that started in one leg. It gradually began to involve the other leg, trunk, and one arm.

**Video 13-14** **Generalized dystonia that evolved into a fixed posture.** This woman has Oppenheim dystonia that ultimately involved all parts of her body and led to a fixed kyphoscoliosis and postures of her limbs.

**Video 13-15** **Generalized dystonia with inability to walk or crawl.** This man has Oppenheim dystonia, and he eventually underwent thalamotomies for generalized dystonia. By sitting on flexed legs, he is able to keep his back straight. He can barely crawl, which is interfered with by extension of his back and neck.

**Video 13-16** **Aromatic amino acid decarboxylase deficiency.** These twins were diagnosed by Hyland and his colleagues (1992) with this autosomal-recessive disorder. A deficiency of this enzyme leads to a reduction in the production of dopamine, norepinephrine, epinephrine, and serotonin. (Hyland K, Surtees RAH, Rodeck C, Clayton PT: Aromatic L-amino acid decarboxylase deficiency: Clinical features, diagnosis, and treatment of a new inborn error of neutrotransmitter amine synthesis. Neurology 1992;42:1980–1988.)

**Video 13-17** **Onset of Oppenheim dystonia involving a leg.** When walking, this boy developed an abnormal lifting of the right leg when he carried that leg forward in his stride.

**Video 13-18** **Worsening of dystonia over time.** This is the same boy that was seen in the previous video segment (see Video 13-17), but now he is 2.5 years older. The dystonia has spread and now involves twisting of his trunk when he walks, along with increased torsion of his right leg. He is essentially unable to walk and needs to use the electric "pony" seen in the lower left corner of the video.

**Video 13-19** **A patient with dopa-responsive dystonia (DRD) in the morning.** This boy has DRD with diurnal fluctuations. In this scene, he is depicted at 9:45 A.M. His dystonia is minimal. Rapid successive movements and walking are performed well, but the pull test is abnormal.

**Video 13-20** **Same patient with DRD, now at night.** This is the same boy on the same day as the previous video segment (see Video 13-19). Now it is 8:00 P.M., and he has generalized dystonia, with marked involvement in his legs. He has difficulty walking and maintaining his balance. He has marked postural instability and cannot stand unassisted.

**Video 13-21** **A patient after treatment with levodopa.** This is the same boy as in Videos 13-19 and 13-20 but now on treatment with levodopa. He is essentially normal, including his response to the pull test.

**Video 13-22** **DRD manifesting in infancy.** This boy has never walked. He was considered to have cerebral palsy. The movements are very bradykinetic, his posture is flexed (trunk and limbs), and his postural reflexes are greatly impaired.

**Video 13-23** **Same patient after treatment with levodopa.** This is the same boy as in the previous video segment (see Video 13-22). He was treated with levodopa, and he began to walk immediately. His older sister, who was mildly affected with DRD, decided to be treated as well when she saw the dramatic improvement in her brother.

**Video 13-24** **Mother of a patient with DRD who presents with parkinsonism.** This woman was in good health until adulthood, when she developed features of Parkinson disease. Because she was the mother of a child with DRD, she was suspected of having adult-onset DRD. An FDOPA PET scan revealed normal FDOPA uptake. Treatment with levodopa at 300 mg per day was not effective, but 400 mg per day was very effective.

**Video 13-25** **Untreated DRD with onset in childhood, now an adult.** This 41-year-old woman was walking on her toes as a child. She was not diagnosed with DRD until recently being evaluated by a movement disorder specialty center. Although she had not received treatment for over 30 years, she responded well when placed on levodopa.

**Video 13-26** **Myoclonus-dystonia in a boy.** This boy has a combination of myoclonic jerks and torsion dystonia in his arms.

**Video 13-27** **Myoclonus-dystonia in the father of the previous boy.** This man is the father of the boy seen in the previous video segment (see Video 13-26). The father also has a combination of myoclonus and dystonia in his arms. The dystonia is more pronounced than the myoclonus.

**Video 13-28 Lubag causing severe oromandibular dystonia.** This Filipino man has lubag (X-linked dystonia-parkinsonism) (DYT3) with marked involvement of his jaw. He has jaw-opening dystonia, and he has to make his mouth close by placing a cloth in it as a sensory trick to enable him to bite down on the cloth.

**Video 13-29 Lubag with parkinsonism and lingual dystonia.** This Filipino man has lubag with lingual dystonia and parkinsonism.

## CHAPTER 14

**Video 14-1 Botulinum toxin (BTX) in cranial dystonia.** This patient with long-standing cranial dystonia improved markedly with BTX injections into the orbicularis oculi and jaw muscles when initially treated; the response has been sustained, and she has benefited without adverse effects for about 3 to 4 months after each injection during the next 15 years and beyond. This patient illustrates the persistent long-term benefits of BTX treatment. (From Mejia NI, Vuong KD, Jankovic J: Long-term botulinum toxin efficacy, safety and immunogenicity. Mov Disord 2005;20:592–597.)

**Video 14-2 BTX in cervical dystonia.** This young man had marked cervical dystonia manifested by retrocollis and torticollis to the left side, dystonic tremor, and marked hypertrophy of the right sternocleidomastoid muscle. He showed marked improvement with BTX injections into the right sternocleidomastoid muscle and both splenius capitus muscles.

**Video 14-3 BTX in anterocollis.** This patient with Parkinson disease and dystonic anterocollis improved markedly with BTX injections into the anterior scaleneus muscles. In addition to marked improvement in the patient's head posture and his range of neck movement, his drooling improved, possibly as a result of diffusion of BTX into the salivary glands.

**Video 14-4 Bilateral pallidotomy for generalized dystonia.** This 14-year-old girl with DYT1 dystonia had a disabling generalized dystonia manifested by a dromedary gait and camptocormia because of truncal dystonia; marked hand dystonia, which prevented her from writing; and severe jaw-opening dystonia with anarthria, which could be partially corrected when her mother forced her jaw closed. She had marked improvement in her dystonia following bilateral pallidotomy, with improvement in posture, gait, and speech. As a result of the surgery, she has been able to write again.

**Video 14-5 Bilateral DBS for generalized dystonia.** The previous patient (see Video 14-4) has continued to benefit from bilateral pallidotomy, but because of some progression of upper thoracic and cervical dystonia, she underwent bilateral GPi DBS, which again improved her axial dystonia. When the DBS is turned off, her dystonia recurs.

**Video 14-6 Bilateral pallidotomy for generalized dystonia.** This patient with DYT1 generalized dystonia manifested by right more than left dystonic tremor and dystonic camptocormia has a 14-year-old daughter who also suffers from progressive generalized dystonia involving the left more than the right side. The daughter's dystonia markedly improved following bilateral pallidotomy.

## CHAPTER 15

**Video 15-1 Huntington disease (HD).** This young patient with HD manifests jerk-like movements that randomly involve different body parts, the classic characteristics of chorea. In addition, she has a typical, irregular, dance-like gait.

**Video 15-2 HD.** This patient with moderately advanced HD has marked chorea and typical halting, slurred speech as well as an irregular dance-like gait with postural instability requiring assistance when walking.

**Video 15-3 HD.** This patient with HD demonstrated typical chorea. Eight years later, she is in an end stage of the disease, markedly demented, and dysarthric, and she has contracture of the right hand.

**Video 15-4 HD.** This patient with HD and moderate dementia demonstrates marked chorea, dysarthria, gait abnormality, and bilateral arm dystonia.

**Video 15-5 HD.** This patient with HD has marked chorea and inability to maintain tongue protrusion. She requires assistance with walking because of marked postural instability and chorea, which interferes with her gait and balance.

**Video 15-6 HD.** This patient with HD has mild chorea but a marked inability to maintain tongue protrusion. She also demonstrated "hung-up" and "pendular" reflexes.

**Video 15-7 HD.** This patient with HD has moderate generalized chorea, which he attempts to camouflage by voluntary or semivoluntary movements, such as touching his face and adjusting his glasses. This phenomenon is referred to as parakinesia.

**Video 15-8 HD.** This 14-year-old girl with HD demonstrates bradykinesia, myoclonus, dystonia in her feet, "hung-up" reflexes, and marked ataxia. She has occasional generalized seizures. These features are typical for juvenile HD.

**Video 15-9 HD.** This patient with a familial movement disorder presented with a 6-month history of facial and cervical tics and loud grunting vocalizations, initially diagnosed as adult-onset Tourette syndrome. His family history, however, suggested HD, which was confirmed by a DNA test.

**Video 15-10 HD.** This patient from Mexico, who has a strong family history of HD, demonstrates marked euphoria.

**Video 15-11 HD.** This patient, initially diagnosed with mental retardation, has juvenile HD, manifested chiefly by marked ataxia.

**Video 15-12 HD.** This patient with juvenile HD has marked blepharospasm and apraxia of eyelid opening as well as bradykinesia. Three years later, he has much more severe bradykinesia, postural instability, and spontaneous as well as stimulus-sensitive myoclonus. He also has childhood-onset generalized seizures.

**Video 15-13 HD.** This patient with HD and chorea markedly improved with tetrabenazine, at a dose of 50 mg per day.

## CHAPTER 16

**Video 16-1 Dentatorubral-pallidoluysian atrophy (DRPLA).** This patient has DRPLA documented by CAG expansion. Her mother and younger brother died of the same disease, and another brother was in a nursing home with the misdiagnosis of Huntington disease.

**Video 16-2 Neuroacanthocytosis.** This patient with documented neuroacanthocytosis demonstrates dysarthria, slow chorea, stereotypies (such as finger snapping), and peculiar posture and gait, reminiscent of "rubber man" syndrome.

**Video 16-3 Sydenham disease.** This 8-year-old girl with a history of abnormal movements, rheumatic fever, and heart disease at age 5 presents with a 1-month history of involuntary movements, which represent recurrence of Sydenham disease. In addition to chorea, she has pendular reflexes typically associated with chorea.

**Video 16-4 Sydenham disease.** This 13-year-old boy developed left hemichorea after a streptococcal throat infection documented by positive cultures and an ASO titer of 600. The Sydenham disease completely resolved in 6 months.

**Video 16-5 Levodopa-induced dyskinesia.** This young patient has Parkinson disease and severe generalized choreic levodopa-induced dyskinesia.

**Video 16-6 Post-pump chorea.** At 4 years of age, this boy with congenital transposition of great vessels developed involuntary movements on the fourth day after cardiac surgery that involved an intra-aortic balloon pump. The chorea markedly improved with tetrabenazine.

**Video 16-7 Post-pump chorea.** This patient demonstrates generalized chorea that occurred immediately after cardiovascular surgery to repair congenital heart disease that involved a pump.

**Video 16-8 Hepatic chorea.** This patient has severe generalized chorea associated with underlying liver disease.

**Video 16-9 Ballism.** This patient has left hemiballism due to stroke in the left hemisphere involving the subthalamic nucleus.

**Video 16-10 Ballism.** This patient has long-standing diabetes mellitus and right hemiballism associated with infarction of the left subthalamic nucleus. The involuntary movement markedly improved with tetrabenazine.

**Video 16-11 Cerebral palsy.** This patient has cerebral palsy and generalized chorea, athetosis, and dystonia associated with severe dysarthria but well-preserved cognitive functioning.

## CHAPTER 17

**Video 17-1 Facial tics.** This series of patients demonstrates a variety of facial tics, including blinking, oculogyric deviations, facial grimacing, and other facial and jaw involuntary movements.

**Video 17-2 Cervical tics.** This series of patients demonstrates a variety of tics involving chiefly the neck, including the so-called whiplash tics. If left untreated, such tics can result in secondary degenerative spine changes and even compression of the cervical roots and spinal cord.

**Video 17-3 Shoulder tics.** This series of patients demonstrates tics of shoulders that resemble focal dystonia, hence the term *dystonic tics*.

**Video 17-4 Limb tics.** This series of patients demonstrates simple or complex tics involving chiefly the arms and legs.

**Video 17-5 Truncal-abdominal tics.** This series of patients demonstrates tics involving the trunk and abdominal muscles. Some of the bending tics resemble intermittent, repetitive camptocormia.

**Video 17-6 Complex tics.** This series of patients demonstrates more complex and stereotypic tics.

**Video 17-7 Simple phonic tics.** This series of patients demonstrates simple vocalizations without linguistic meaning.

**Video 17-8 Complex phonic tics.** This series of patients shouts linguistically meaningful utterances, including coprolalia.

**Video 17-9 Shoulder tics.** This patient demonstrates a simple phonic tic and a typical shoulder tic that is clonic at times and other times is a more sustained, so-called dystonic tic, as demonstrated by the EMG recording.

**Video 17-10 Tonic (isometric) tics.** In addition to phonic tics, this pregnant woman experiences abdominal isometric contractions that have precipitated early labor.

**Video 17-11** **Blocking tics.** This patient demonstrates classic blocking tic, during which he suddenly becomes motionless. Most blocking tics are associated with isometric muscle contractions and may be viewed as variants of tonic tics.

**Video 17-12** **Complex motor tics.** This patient demonstrates complex motor behavior that consists of repetitive somersaults and other repetitive complex movements.

**Video 17-13** **Complex motor tics.** This patient demonstrates complex running and stereotypic behavior as part of his Tourette syndrome (TS).

**Video 17-14** **Peripherally induced tics.** This 43-year-old man suffered a left shoulder dislocation during a motorcycle accident 21 years ago. Within 2 weeks after the injury, he noticed the gradual onset of involuntary jerking movements of his left shoulder, which was markedly exacerbated after a second left shoulder injury 2 years later. The involuntary movements are phenomenologically identical to the dystonic tics that are typically associated with TS but without the involvement of any other body part and without phonic tics or the typical TS comorbidities, such as attention deficit disorder or obsessive-compulsive disorder.

**Video 17-15** **Coprolalia.** This patient with extremely severe coprolalia was the first reported case of the use of botulinum toxin, injected into the vocal cords, in the treatment of this disabling disorder. The premonitory sensation in the throat essentially completely resolved after botulinum toxin injections. The effects lasted about 3 to 4 months, and the patient was undergoing injections three or four times per year for several years.

**Video 17-16** **Self-injurious behavior.** This patient has severe self-injurious tics, a compulsion to avulse her cornea, as a result of which she has already become blind in the left eye. These actions are preceded by an intense urge, which she can partially control by squeezing a ball.

**Video 17-17** **Self-injurious behavior.** This patient with TS has a severe compulsion to eviscerate himself and to expose his intestines, which is accompanied by a sexual climax. This is an example of a life-threatening self-injurious behavior.

**Video 17-18** **Tics and tardive dystonia.** This patient with long-standing TS developed tardive dystonia as a result of the use of haloperidol for his tics.

**Video 17-19** **Treatment with botulinum toxin.** This patient with cervical, shoulder, and arm tics has had marked improvement not only in her motor tics but also in the premonitory urge.

## CHAPTER 18

**Video 18-1** **Subacute sclerosing panencephalitis (SSPE).** This patient has SSPE, proven by brain biopsy, and complex stereotypies.

**Video 18-2** **Animal stereotypies.** These zoo elephants and flamingos show repetitive, stereotypic behaviors.

**Video 18-3** **Williams syndrome.** This patient with Williams syndrome shows head and upper body stereotypy.

**Video 18-4** **Self-gratifying behavior.** This patient demonstrates stereotypic movements of her legs as part of self-gratifying or masturbatory behavior.

**Video 18-5** **Lesch-Nyhan syndrome.** This patient has Lesch-Nyhan syndrome and engages in self-injurious behavior.

**Video 18-6** **Lesch-Nyhan syndrome.** This patient has Lesch-Nyhan syndrome and engages in self-injurious behavior.

**Video 18-7** **Rett syndrome.** This patient with Rett syndrome shows typical hand and body stereotypies and an ataxic, toe-walking gait.

**Video 18-8** **Rett syndrome.** This patient with Rett syndrome shows typical hand stereotypies.

**Video 18-9** **Tardive akathisia.** This patient has stereotypies as part of tardive akathisia. Both the motor and sensory components improved with tetrabenazine.

## CHAPTER 19

**Video 19-1** **Reemergent tremor.** This patient has marked left arm rest tremor, which transiently resolves when arms are outstretched and in a wing-beating position and reemerges after a short latency. This reemergent tremor, typically seen in patients with Parkinson disease, resolved after treatment with levodopa.

**Video 19-2** **Task-specific tremor.** This patient, a draftsman, has primary handwriting tremor, manifested only while the patient is writing.

**Video 19-3** **Task-specific tremor.** This patient has a task-specific tremor that is present only while the patient is playing golf and attempting to putt.

**Video 19-4** **Cerebellar outflow tremor.** This patient has cerebellar outflow tremor of the left arm and right third nerve palsy as a result of a brainstem injury following a motorcycle accident.

**Video 19-5** **Orthostatic tremor.** This patient has no tremor when sitting or walking but is unable to stand for more than a few seconds because of sensations of uncomfortable "vibrations" and "cramps" in the legs on standing due to a high-frequency, about 14 Hz, tremor in the legs, demonstrated by EMG recording from the gastrocnemius muscle.

**Video 19-6  Dystonic tremor.** This patient has cervical and bilateral, right more than left, arm dystonia and associated dystonic irregular tremor.

**Video 19-7  Dystonic tremor.** This patient has cervical dystonia manifested by torticollis to the left and lateral head oscillation due to dystonic tremor. His tremor disappears when he allows his head to turn to the right to the position of the so-called null point.

**Video 19-8  Psychogenic tremor.** This young woman has had a sudden onset of severe tremor in the hands that is intermittent and changes frequency, amplitude, and direction. Also, the tremor is markedly distractible and exhibits entrainment, features that are characteristic of psychogenic tremor. Psychogenic etiology is also suggested by the exacerbation of the tremor by stress, manifested as a bizarre, "parkinsonian" gait. The patient expressed fear that she might be developing Parkinson disease.

**Video 19-9  Hereditary chin tremor.** This is a 74-year-old man with familial, childhood-onset chin tremor and a 3-year history of progressive hand tremor, gait difficulty, and other parkinsonian features. It is not clear whether the hereditary chin tremor predisposed him to the later development of Parkinson disease.

## CHAPTER 20

**Video 20-1  Withdrawal emergent syndrome.** This boy had been exposed to antipsychotic medication. When the medication was stopped abruptly, he developed restless movements that resembled those of Sydenham disease (see Video 1-41).

**Video 20-2  Withdrawal emergent syndrome.** This boy was treated with haloperidol to control Sydenham disease. When the medication was discontinued, the chorea returned. This happened each time haloperidol was stopped. He had been diagnosed as having persistent Sydenham disease. Because withdrawal emergent syndrome could be the correct diagnosis, the patient was treated with tetrabenazine for several months, simultaneously controlling the choreic movements and allowing the brain a respite from haloperidol. When tetrabenazine was then withdrawn, the abnormal movements were found to have disappeared, supporting the diagnosis that this was a case of withdrawal emergent syndrome and not persistent Sydenham disease.

**Video 20-3  Oral-buccal-lingual dyskinesia.** This woman had been exposed to antipsychotic drugs and developed abnormal, complex movements around the mouth that are of a rhythmic type, typical of classic tardive dyskinesia.

**Video 20-4  Oral-buccal-lingual dyskinesia with tongue popping.** This woman was given antipsychotic medications and subsequently developed pronounced movements of her mouth and tongue. The tongue would pop out of her mouth intermittently. When the tongue is at rest in her mouth, it is not quiet but is continuously moving (athetosis of the tongue). The tongue is able to remain protruded without darting back into the mouth, as would be typical in chorea. This lack of motor impersistence, so common in chorea (a form of negative chorea), is not present in classic tardive dyskinesia.

**Video 20-5  Rhythmic rocking movements of the trunk and marching in place.** This woman complained of abnormal movements of her trunk. These were rhythmic; therefore, a suspicion of tardive dyskinesia was entertained, supported clinically by the presence of mouth movements. But the patient denied knowingly having taken antipsychotic medications. A review of her pharmacist's records did reveal that she had been given such medications, which provides the basis for developing tardive dyskinesia. On standing, the patient's movements became those of marching in place, again rhythmically. When treated with reserpine, her truncal rocking movements were markedly reduced, but the slowness of her walking indicates the presence of some reserpine-induced parkinsonism.

**Video 20-6  Segmental jaw, neck, and arm dystonia, along with classic oral-buccal-lingual dyskinesia.** This woman has dystonia affecting her jaw (jaw-opening, affecting her speech), neck (chin being turned to her left), and twisting of the left arm. This is associated with classic oral-buccal-lingual dyskinesia.

**Video 20-7  Retrocollis as the feature of tardive dystonia.** This man developed extension of the neck as a feature of tardive dystonia. When tardive dystonia affects the neck muscles, retrocollis is a common result. Retrocollis more often is the result of tardive dystonia than of primary dystonia.

**Video 20-8  Retrocollis, opisthotonus, internal rotation of the arms, extension of the elbows, and flexion of the wrists.** This man has a form of tardive dystonia that is fairly specific for tardive dystonia. It consists of extension of the axial muscles (neck and trunk), with internal rotation of the arms, which are extended at the elbows and flexed at the wrists. This patient was also shown in Video 13-9 with a sensory trick.

**Video 20-9  A combination of dystonia with myoclonic or ballistic movements.** This woman has the opisthotonic movements with extension of the elbows and flexion of the wrists that are so typical of tardive dystonia. But these movements, though sustained for short periods, are brought about by very rapid movements that result in these postures.

**Video 20-10  Moaning as a manifestation of tardive akathisia.** This woman was given haloperidol to treat blepharospasm, resulting in the development of tardive dyskinesia (oral-buccal-lingual type) and persistent akathisia that leads her to moan loudly. She can suppress the moaning for brief periods when asked to do so while counting. Although treatment with tetrabenazine was effective in suppressing the akathisia and moaning, it produced unpleasant parkinsonism, with bradykinesia and lack of motivation. Electroconvulsive therapy was effective in controlling the akathisia but not the oral-buccal-lingual dyskinesias.

**Video 20-11  A combination of tardive dyskinesia and tardive akathisia.** This woman has tardive dyskinesia (oral-buccal-lingual dyskinesias and rhythmic truncal rocking and rhythmic foot movements). But her major difficulty is tardive akathisia, expressed by her as the feeling of restlessness and nervousness. Caressing her scalp is a typical feature of an akathitic movement, as is the squirming of her trunk. Treatment with tetrabenazine suppressed both the tardive dyskinesia and the tardive akathisia but induced parkinsonism in their place. To provide relief from the drug-induced parkin-

sonism, carbidopa/levodopa was added. This video segment demonstrates the degree of improvement that was accomplished by the combination of tetrabenazine and levodopa.

**Video 20-12  A combination of tardive dyskinesia, tardive dystonia, and tardive akathisia.** This woman was exposed to antipsychotic medications for anxiety and developed the combination of three different tardive phenomena. She has oral-buccal-lingual dyskinesia, but this is relatively minor and does not bother her. She has dystonic tightness of muscles around the mouth, including the jaw, and dystonia of the arms (internal rotation, elbow extension, and wrist flexion). The most distressing symptom is the akathisia. She feels unable to sit still, having the need to move about, and if kept from moving, she feels that she is going to explode inside.

## CHAPTER 21

**Video 21-1  Examples of different types of myoclonus. A,** This patient presented with just some focal twitching of the left hand; present at rest, it was increased with movement. Subsequently, dementia developed, and a brain biopsy proved Alzheimer disease. **B,** The second segment from this same patient taken 2 years later shows worsening of the myoclonus and difficulty in moving the arm. **C,** The next patient has a multifocal myoclonus from an unknown encephalopathy. She has myoclonus at rest, but it is brought out with kinetic movement. She also has sensory evoked myoclonus that is triggered by quick stretches to the finger flexors. (**A–C,** Courtesy of Mark Hallett, MD, NIH.)

**Video 21-2  Examples of negative myoclonus. A,** This patient has Lafora body disease and demonstrates negative myoclonus, also called asterixis. **B,** The second patient has negative myoclonus triggered by sensory stimuli. (**A,** Courtesy of Hiroshi Shibasaki, MD. **B,** Courtesy of Mark Hallett, MD, NIH.)

**Video 21-3  Spinal myoclonus.** The spinal myoclonus in this patient is of unknown etiology. Note the rhythmic jerking of the right shoulder area that is continuous, day and night. (Courtesy of Hiroshi Shibasaki, MD.)

**Video 21-4  Different types of palatal myoclonus (palatal tremor). A,** This first example is of symptomatic palatal myoclonus due to contractions of the levator palatini muscle. Note that the back edge of the palate moves but the roof does not. **B,** This second example is from another patient with symptomatic palatal myoclonus. In these patients, there is virtually always involvement of the seventh cranial nerve, here seen with a twitch at the corner of the mouth. **C,** The third patient has essential palatal myoclonus due to contractions of the tensor veli palatini muscle. Note the involvement of the roof of the palate. (**A** and **C,** From Deuschl G, Toro C, Hallett M: Symptomatic and essential palatal tremor: 2. Differences of palatal movements. Mov Disord 1994;9:676—678; used with permission. **B,** Courtesy of Mark Hallett, MD, NIH.)

**Video 21-5  Cortical tremor.** This patient has a rhythmic myoclonus on action that has an appearance similar to essen-

tial tremor. That it is cortical myoclonus is proven by physiologic recordings. (Courtesy of Mark Hallett, MD, NIH.)

**Video 21-6  Examples of propriospinal myoclonus. A,** Propriospinal myoclonus is characterized by occasional flexions of the trunk. They can be spontaneous or induced by sensory stimuli. **B,** In the second patient, the myoclonus is induced by tapping on the knee. (**A** and **B,** From Brown P, Thompson PD, Rothwell JC, et al: Paroxysmal axial spasms of spinal origin. Mov Disord 1991;6:43—48; used with permission.)

**Video 21-7  Hereditary hyperekplexia.** This young girl is from a large family with hereditary hyperekplexia. Taps to the nose produce head retraction. Noises, such as a clap, induce a whole-body startle that does not habituate. She was well treated with clonazepam and only partially withdrew from medication for this taping. (Courtesy of Mark Hallett, MD, NIH.)

**Video 21-8  Latah.** This is a sequence of four patients with Latah from a long videotape produced by Indiana University. In the first two segments, there are four people, of whom only one has Latah. (From a videotape entitled "Latah," Producer, director, ethnographer: Ronald C. Simons. Distributor: Instructional Support Services, Indiana University, Bloomington, IN 47405; used with permission.)

**Video 21-9  Posthypoxic myoclonus.** These two patients are some of the originals from the series by Lance and Adams. Note the large-amplitude positive and negative action myoclonus. (From Lance JW, Adams RD: Negative myoclonus in posthypoxic patients: Historical note. Mov Disord 2001;16:162—163; used with permission.)

**Video 21-10  Negative myoclonus and bouncy gait from posthypoxic myoclonus.** This patient with posthypoxic myoclonus has positive and negative myoclonus with arm movements. When the patient is standing and trying to walk, it is primarily the negative myoclonus that produces the bouncy gait. (Courtesy of Stanley Fahn, MD.)

**Video 21-11  SSPE.** This young boy has subacute sclerosing panencephalitis. He has whole-body jerks at long intervals.

The jerk has a long duration but rapid onset. (Courtesy of C. D. Marsden.)

**Video 21-12 Opsoclonus-myoclonus syndrome. A** and **B,** These two patients have the opsoclonus-myoclonus syndrome. Note the chaotic, but conjugate, movement of the eyes. (**A,** Courtesy of Stanley Fahn, MD. **B,** Courtesy of Mark Hallett, MD, NIH.)

**Video 21-13 Dystonic myoclonus.** This patient has a focal hand dystonia, a writer's cramp. In addition to the dystonic posturing, there are many myoclonic jerks. (Courtesy of Hiroshi Shibasaki, MD.)

**Video 21-14 Psychogenic myoclonus.** This patient has psychogenic myoclonus. Note that the movements are not really fully simple in nature. (Courtesy of Mark Hallett, MD, NIH.)

## CHAPTER 23

**Video 23-1 Paroxysmal torticollis in infancy.** This infant has a head tilt to his right shoulder. These episodes of torticollis in infants can last during sleep and for many months before they disappear.

**Video 23-2 Paroxysmal dystonia in infancy.** This infant has very brief jaw-opening episodes that last seconds. These are associated with tongue protrusions and some elevation of the arms. These eventually disappeared.

**Video 23-3 Primary paroxysmal kinesigenic dyskinesia.** This young man has had brief bursts of tightness of his muscles following sudden movement. They last a few seconds, and he can induce them by jumping up suddenly from a sitting position. There is a brief latency before development of the movements, which are accompanied by a tingling sensation.

**Video 23-4 Secondary paroxysmal kinesigenic dyskinesia.** This woman had a thalamic stroke. After recovering from it, she developed contralateral attacks of sustained postures following sudden movement.

**Video 23-5 Primary paroxysmal nonkinesigenic dyskinesia (PNKD).** This video segment shows the evolution of an attack of PNKD in a young boy, lasting up to 1 hour. The severity builds up gradually and then gradually subsides. There is some irritability or discomfort associated with the attack.

**Video 23-6 Secondary paroxysmal nonkinesigenic dyskinesia.** This man developed episodes of sustained jaw opening and tongue protrusions after recovering from

encephalitis. To break the attacks, the patient learned to induce a gag reflex.

**Video 23-7 Psychogenic PNKD.** This patient has complex ballistic and dystonic postures when he is startled. The postures could last for days. The stimuli that induce the reaction can be noise, light, or other sensory inputs. When an infusion of ACTH aborted the attacks and restored him to normal, he would receive these infusions after an attack. When he agreed to undergo a single-blind trial of ACTH or saline, he was found to respond favorably to each. His appearance after the saline infusion during the trial is shown.

**Video 23-8 Paroxysmal exertional dyskinesia.** This boy would develop sustained muscle contractions and postures after prolonged exercise. These attacks would last about one-half hour. In this office examination, hyperventilation was able to bring on one of these attacks. There is erythema due to blood vessel dilatation. The skin blanches when it is touched. The attacks cause much discomfort.

**Video 23-9 A burst of stereotypic arm and hand wiggling.** This boy has normal development and behavior, but when excited, he would have repetitive movements of his arms and hands. This pattern of abnormal movements are those of stereotypies.

**Video 23-10 Paroxysmal self-stimulatory behavior.** This infant girl would periodically apply her suprapubic region to the firm edge of furniture, such as the edge of a sofa. Her legs would often stiffen or assume a posture. The episodes last about a minute; she can be distracted from this activity.

## CHAPTER 24

**Video 24-1 Periodic limb movements.** This shows three examples of periodic limb movements. The first patient has movements while awake when lying down. While the patient is restless, there are some involuntary movements also present. The second patient has the classic periodic limb movements of sleep with a "triple flexion" of the leg occurring about every 20 seconds. The third patient illustrates that periodic movements when asleep can also affect the arms. (From Walters AS, Henning WA, Chokroverty S: Review of videotape recognition of idiopathic restless legs syndrome. Mov Disord 1991;6:105–110; used with permission.)

**Video 24-2 Hemifacial spasm.** This patient has hemifacial spasm. There are frequent twitching movements of the left

side of the face that are made worse by speaking. (Courtesy of Joseph Jankovic, MD.)

**Video 24-3 Jumpy stumps.** Here are two examples of jumpy stumps. In the first case, the movements are spontaneous. In the second case, the movements are action induced. The line on the thigh is drawn to indicate the middle of the thigh. (From Marion MH, Gledhill RF, Thompson PD: Spasms of amputation stumps: A report of 2 cases. Mov Disord 1989; 4:354–358; used with permission.)

**Video 24-4 Belly dancer's dyskinesia.** There are two patients illustrated here with involuntary movement of the abdomen. In the first patient, there is a rotatory movement of the umbilicus. In the second patient, the movement is a bit more irregular in its path. (From Iliceo G, Thompson PD, Day BL, et al: Diaphragmatic flutter, the moving umbilicus syndrome, and "belly dancer's" dyskinesia. Mov Disord 1990; 5:15–22; used with permission.)

Video 24-5 **Peripheral dystonia.** This patient developed dystonic posturing of the hand following trauma. The dystonia can be fixed for long periods. (Courtesy of Joseph Jankovic, MD.)

Video 24-6 **Painful feet and moving toes.** This is a patient with the painful feet and moving toes syndrome affecting his left foot. Typically, the pain is more of a problem to the patient than is the involuntary movement. In this case, the movements are somewhat regular, but they can be irregular. (Courtesy of Joseph Jankovic, MD.)

Video 24-7 **Painful arm and moving fingers.** While much less common than painful feet and moving toes, a similar syndrome can affect the arm, called painful arm and moving fingers. (Courtesy of Mark Hallett, MD, NIH.)

## CHAPTER 25

Video 25-1 **Examples of Wilson disease.** Here are four examples of patients with Wilson disease. **A,** The first has a parkinsonian presentation. The first thing that is apparent is his smile, the risus sardonicus. He has drooling, and all of his movements are very slow. **B,** The second patient has a dystonic presentation. He has generalized dystonia with some fixed postures, likely due to contractures. All his movements are very stiff. **C,** The third patient has the pseudosclerotic form, with prominent ataxia, looking like multiple sclerosis. Her speech is slow and dysarthric. **D,** The fourth patient has a very slow, irregular tremor. This type of tremor is not uncommon in Wilson disease. (**A,** Courtesy of Shyamal Das, MD. **B,** Courtesy of C. D. Marsden. **C** and **D,** Courtesy of Joseph Jankovic, MD.)

## CHAPTER 26

Video 26-1 **Task-specific jaw tremor.** This woman noticed that she has jaw tremor whenever she brings a glass of liquid to her mouth to drink. The video segment shows that the same event occurs even with an empty glass and pretending to drink. This is an organic task-specific jaw tremor.

Video 26-2 **Head shaking.** This woman has episodes of head shaking, during which time she becomes exhausted and fatigued. Her husband helps to stop these episodes.

Video 26-3 **Shaking movements and abnormal postures.** This woman had an abrupt onset of shaking movements and abnormal postures in different parts of her body. She denied any emotional problems. This combination of movements does not fit with a known organic movement disorder. She was admitted to the hospital from the emergency room, and after 3 days of psychotherapy, the movement disorder cleared.

Video 26-4 **Paroxysmal tremor.** This man developed tremor, was suspected to have Parkinson disease, and was referred for a second opinion. When he was examined as an outpatient, no tremor or other sign of parkinsonism was present, but he gave the history that the tremor comes and goes. He was admitted to the hospital to have a longer period of observation. The tremor developed as the physicians were making rounds.

Video 26-5 **Delayed startle, utterances of gibberish.** This woman complained of speaking gibberish at times. The examination detected a delayed reaction of complex movements to unexpected noise. The video segment also reveals some of the gibberish she had complained about.

Video 26-6 **Bent gait, episodes of shaking, startle reaction with gibberish.** This woman developed gibberish when startled and then a bent posture when she walked. Paroxysmal shaking movements were also present.

Video 26-7 **Jumping Frenchman syndrome.** This video segment depicts five individuals in Quebec who had jumping Frenchman syndrome. The video was made by Dr. Saint-Hilaire, who is examining the people. He gave permission for use and publication of the video.

Video 26-8 **Dystonic postures that persist in sleep.** This nurse developed twisting of one foot after tripping in a sidewalk pothole. The foot and ankle resisted passive movement, but the toes were supple. Psychotherapy was unsuccessful. A year later, the other foot developed a similar problem. Admission to the hospital revealed that the feet were postured during sleep, and the floor nurses were unable to move them. An EMG failed to reveal electrical activity, suggesting that the postures were now in a state of contracture. During an amobarbital test, the patient fell into a deep sleep; the feet relaxed and the abnormal postures disappeared. When the patient was later informed that there were no contractions and her feet were easily moveable in deep sleep, she quickly became normal and also euphoric with her sudden improvement.

Video 26-9 **Dystonia with fixed contractures.** This woman was referred for fixed postures of the legs and right hand. The clue that these were not organic was the inability to passively move her right thumb, but when she placed the pen in the hand, the right thumb extended slightly to allow the pen to be held. The patient underwent examination during deep anesthesia, and some of the abnormal posture was now seen to be complicated by contractures. When the patient was informed about these observations under anesthesia, she lost all the abnormal fixed postures that were not contractured.

Video 26-10 **Tremors of the hands.** This man developed tremor of his hands after his garage door struck him on the head as it was coming down to be closed. Because the tremors persisted in all positions (at rest, with posture, and with action) and because of the abnormal speech pattern, psychogenic tremor was suspected. After psychotherapy, the patient's speech and tremors improved.

Video 26-11 **Deliberate slowness, psychogenic parkinsonism.** This woman complained of marked slowness that was diagnosed elsewhere as Parkinson disease. Examination showed what appeared to be deliberate slowness. For example, when asked to perform the finger-to-nose maneuver, she did so very slowly. But when she was observed scratching her nose spontaneously, she performed this movement with normal speed. The repetitive successive movements were slow without the typical decrementing. Following psychotherapy, her chronic condition became normal.

# Index

*Note: Page numbers followed by b refer to boxes; page numbers followed by f refer to figures; page numbers followed by t refer to tables.*